Mosby's®
ONCOLOGY
NURSING ADVISOR

A Comprehensive Guide to Clinical Practice

3RD
EDITION

Susan Maloney-Newton, MS, APRN, AOCN, AOCNS
Senior Director
The Medical Affairs Company (TMAC);
President
Oncology Nursing Advisors, LLC
Dayton, Ohio

Margaret Hickey, MSN, MS, RN
President
MMH Communications, LLC
Pensacola Beach, Florida

Jeannine M. Brant, PhD, APRN, AOCN, FAAN
Executive Director
Clinical Science & Innovation
City of Hope Comprehensive Cancer Center
Duarte, California

ELSEVIER

Elsevier
3251 Riverport Lane
St. Louis, Missouri 63043

MOSBY'S® ONCOLOGY NURSING ADVISOR: A COMPREHENSIVE
GUIDE TO CLINICAL PRACTICE, THIRD EDITION

ISBN: 978-0-323-93446-6

Notice

Practitioners and researchers must always rely on their own experience and knowledge in evaluating
and using any information, methods, compounds or experiments described herein. Because of rapid
advances in the medical sciences, in particular, independent verification of diagnoses and drug dosages
should be made. To the fullest extent of the law, no responsibility is assumed by Elsevier, authors, editors,
or contributors for any injury and/or damage to persons or property as a matter of products liability,
negligence or otherwise, or from any use or operation of any methods, products, instructions, or ideas
contained in the material herein.

Previous editions copyrighted 2017 and 2009.

Executive Content Strategist: Lee Henderson
Senior Content Development Manager: Lisa Newton
Senior Content Development Specialist: Laura Selkirk
Publishing Services Manager: Deepthi Unni
Project Manager: Sheik Mohideen K
Design Direction: Patrick Ferguson

Printed in India

Last digit is the print number: 9   8   7   6   5   4   3   2   1

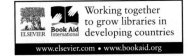

Acknowledgments

I am blessed to have the support of my loving partner, Steve; my three sons, Alex, Casey, and Jackson; and my adorable grandson, Kamden. They bring joy and laughter to my life and I am forever grateful. My Mom is my biggest fan and has taught me about cancer through the eyes of a caregiver. In my work, I am able to meet oncology nurse colleagues from across the US and globally, and I dedicate this resource to helping them improve the lives of patients with cancer.

Susan (Susie)

This book is dedicated to patients and families who live with a cancer diagnosis and the nurses who care for them. Special thanks and recognition are due to the expert oncology nurses who contributed chapters. Without their willingness to share their knowledge and experience, this book would not be possible. My sincere appreciation to my coeditors, Susie and Jeannine, for their partnership and support. Lastly, special thanks to my husband, Kenny, for his never-ending support and love.

Margaret (Margie)

Writing always takes a village. My heartfelt thanks go out to the nurses who contributed many hours of work to this book and for the dedication that went into each chapter. I hope and pray that it will be used to provide quality cancer care to patients and their families around the globe. I give special thanks to my family members who are always there for me—my husband, Rich; my daughter, Danielle, and her husband, Thomas and their four beautiful children (my grandkids!); my daughter, Annette, who is now an oncology nurse and contributed to this book, and her husband, Riley; my son, Zach; and his wife, Sara. You are the light of my life!

Jeannine

Authors

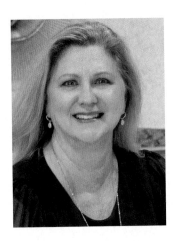

Susie Maloney-Newton, MS, APRN, AOCN, AOCNS, has worked as an Oncology Advanced Practice Nurse for 30 years. She is currently Senior Director at TMAC/The Medical Affairs Company, leading teams of clinicians throughout the country. She is also President of the consulting business Oncology Nursing Advisors, LLC. Susie is an international speaker, having taught across the US and in 10 countries. She has published six oncology nursing books and numerous articles and serves on the editorial board for two journals.

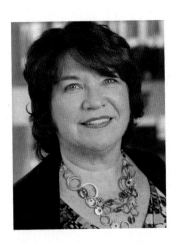

Margie Hickey, MSN, MS, RN, has more than 40 years of oncology nursing experience and has worked in all oncology settings caring for inpatients and outpatients undergoing cancer surgery, radiation therapy, and medical treatments, including chemotherapy, biotherapy, and immunotherapy. Currently self-employed, Margie provides communication and strategy support to patient organizations as well as medical communication and educational consulting services. Margie is currently Editor-in-Chief of *ORL—Head and Neck Nursing Journal*, the official peer-reviewed journal of the Society of Otorhinolaryngology and Head-Neck Nurses. Additionally, she has been an editor of six oncology nursing books and has authored more than 25 other publications.

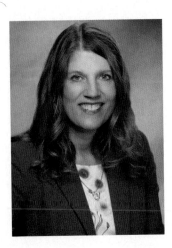

Jeannine M. Brant, PhD, APRN, AOCN, FAAN, has been an oncology nurse for almost 40 years and has worked as a staff nurse, infusion center nurse, clinical nurse specialist in inpatient and ambulatory settings, and a nurse scientist. She is an internationally recognized speaker, author, and researcher and has presented in Europe, China, and the Middle East. She is currently Executive Director of Clinical Science & Innovation at City of Hope in Duarte, California. She has more than 175 contributions to the literature and is an editor of the Oncology Nursing Society *Core Curriculum for Oncology Nursing*.

Contributors

Tahani Al Dweikat, EMHCA, BSN, RN, OCN, CCRP
Oncology Clinical Research Nurse
Nursing Research
City of Hope
Duarte, California

Paula Anastasia, MN, RN, AOCN
Advanced Practice Nurse
Gyn-Oncology
University of California—Los Angeles
Los Angeles, California;
Patient and Nurse Oncology Education Consultant
Palm Desert, California

Nimian Bauder, MSN, APRN, AGCNS-BC, NPD-BC, EBP-C
Clinical Nurse Specialist
Surgical Oncology/Medical Telemetry
City of Hope
Duarte, California

Laura Benson, MS, RN, ANP
President
Consulting
Conversations in Care, LLC
New Rochelle, New York

Carol Stein Blecher, MS, RN, APNC, AOCN, CBCN
Nurse Navigator
Nursing
Alliance Cancer Specialists
Bensalem, Pennsylvania;
Instructor, ADN Program
Bucks County Community College
Newtown, Pennsylvania;
Women's Health Screener
Trinitas Comprehensive Cancer Center
Trinitas Regional Medical Center
Elizabeth, New Jersey

Linda Buck, MSN, NP-C, AOCNP
Nurse Practitioner
Medical Oncology
City of Hope
Newport Beach, California

Darcy Burbage, DNP, RN, AOCN, CBCN
Oncology Clinical Nurse Specialist
Consultant
Newark, Delaware

Joshua Carter, BS, BSN, OCN, CBCN
Nurse Navigator
Breast Oncology
Stanford Healthcare
Palo Alto, California

Jesee Jay Castro, MSN, RN, CCRN-K
Director, Nursing
Intensive Care Unit, Evaluation Treatment Center, Rapid
    Response, Nurse Triage, and Dialysis
City of Hope
Duarte, California

Becky Collins, MS, RN, CHPN, CCM, CENP
Director of Programs and Pathways
Clinical Operations
Alternate Solutions Health Network
Kettering, Ohio

Francisco Conde II, PhD, APRN-Rx, AOCNP, FAAN
Oncology Nurse Practitioner
Hematology-Oncology
Straub Medical Center
Honolulu, Hawaii

Diane Cope, PhD, APRN, BC, AOCNP
Oncology Nurse Practitioner
Medical Oncology
Florida Cancer Specialists and Research Institute
Fort Myers, Florida

Grace Cullen, DNP, FNP-BC, AOCNP, ACHPN, PMGT-BC
Nurse Practitioner
Medicine
Detroit VA Medical Center
Detroit, Michigan

Kristin M. Ferguson, DNP, RN, OCN
Administrator
Stem Cell Transplant and Cellular Immunotherapy Program
MedStar Georgetown University Hospital
Washington, District of Columbia

Danielle M. Fournier, DNP, APRN, AGPCNP-BC, AOCNP
Advanced Practice Registered Nurse
Department of Cardiovascular and Thoracic Surgery
The University of Texas MD Anderson Cancer Center
Houston, Texas

Michele R. Gardom, DNP, RN, CENP
Outcomes and Impact Manager
Administration
Nurses on Boards Coalition
Pittsburgh, Pennsylvania

Rupa Ghosh-Berkebile, DNP, APRN-CNP, AOCNP
Nurse Practitioner
James Cancer Diagnostic Center
The Ohio State University, Wexner Medical Center—James
    Cancer Hospital and Solove Research Institute
Columbus, Ohio

Savanna Gilson, MSN, RN, OCN
Clinical Educator
Medical Surgical Oncology
PIH Health Whittier Hospital
Whittier, California

Terri Gross, RN, BS
Director of Quality and Informatics
Hospice of Dayton
Dayton, Ohio

Emily Groves, MSN, RN, CDCES, PHN
Nurse Manager
Nursing Administration
City of Hope
Duarte, California

Kristen Hurley, DNP, RN, CNP
Principal Medical Science Liaison
Medical Affairs
Kite, a Gilead Company
Sioux Falls, South Dakota

Annette Brant Isozaki, RN, MSN
Staff Nurse
Bone Marrow Transplant, CAR T Cell Therapy, and
    Investigational Therapy Unit
City of Hope
Duarte, California

Deborah Lynn Kirk, DNP, FNP-BC, NP-C, AOCN, FAANP
Associate Dean, Nursing
Associate Professor
Nurse Practitioner
School of Nursing and Midwifery
Edith Cowan University
Bunbury, Western Australia
Australia

Lisa Kottschade, MSN, APRN, CNP
Nurse Practitioner, Medical Oncology
Associate Professor of Oncology
Mayo Clinic
Rochester, Minnesota

Elizabeth Maggio, MSN, PhD, RN, OCN, NCTTP
Consultant
Oncology and Public Health Policy
Lexington, Kentucky

Suzanne M. Mahon, DNS, RN, AOCN, AGN-BC, FAAN
Professor, Internal Medicine
Division of Hematology/Oncology;
Professor, Adult Nursing
School of Nursing
Saint Louis University
St. Louis, Missouri

Kristen Maloney, PhD, RN, AOCNS
Clinical Director
Oncology Nursing
Hospital of the University of Pennsylvania
Philadelphia, Pennsylvania

Susie Maloney-Newton, MS, APRN, AOCN, AOCNS
Senior Director
The Medical Affairs Company (TMAC);
President
Oncology Nursing Advisors, LLC
Dayton, Ohio

Mary E. Murphy, AD, BSN, MS
Chief Nursing and Care Officer
Hospice of Dayton
Dayton, Ohio

Colleen O'Leary, DNP, AOCNS, EBP-CH
Associate Director, Evidence Based Practice
Professional Practice
The Ohio State University Comprehensive Cancer
    Center—Arthur James Cancer Hospital and Richard
    Solove Research Institute
Columbus, Ohio

Lisa S. Parks, MS, APRN-CNP, ANP-BC
Nurse Practitioner, Hepato-Biliary Surgery
Division of Surgical Oncology
The Ohio State University Wexner Medical
    Center—James Cancer Hospital and Solove
    Research Institute
Columbus, Ohio

Martha Polovich, PhD, RN, AOCN - Emeritus
Adjunct Associate Professor
Medicine/Occupational and Environmental Medicine
University of Maryland School of Medicine
Baltimore, Maryland

Julie Ponto, PhD, APRN, CNS, AGCNS-BC, AOCNS
Professor, Adult-Gerontology Clinical Nurse Specialist
  Program Coordinator
Department of Graduate Nursing
Winona State University—Rochester
Rochester, Minnesota

Holly M. Reames, MSN, RN
Medical Science Liaison
Medical Affairs
CTI Biopharma
Humble, Texas

Jill Reese, MS, APRN, AGCNS-BC, OCN
Advanced Practice Nurse, Clinical Nurse Specialist Board
  Certified
Foster J. Boyd Cancer Center
Clinton Memorial Hospital
Wilmington, Ohio

Jeanene (Gigi) G. Robison, MSN, RN, AOCN
Oncology Clinical Nurse Specialist
The Christ Hospital
Cincinnati, Ohio

Nezar Ahmed Salim, MSN
Nurse Educator
Oncology
George Washington University Hospital
Washington, District of Columbia

Emily Sanders, MSN, RN, CORLN
Head & Neck Oncology Program Manager
Oncology Administration
AdventHealth Cancer Institute
Orlando, Florida

Marlon Garzo Saría, PhD, RN, AOCNS, NEA-BC, NPD-BC,
FAAN
Director and Nurse Scientist
Nursing Professional Practice
Providence Saint John's Health Center
Santa Monica, California;
Deputy Chief Nurse
United States Air Force
March Air Reserve Base
California

Leah A. Scaramuzzo, MSN, RN, MEDSURG-BC, AOCN
Nursing Director, Oncology Clinical Development
Nursing Administration
Logan Health
Kalispell, Montana

Melissa Shackelford, MSN, RN, MPPM
Associate Director
Medical Affairs
Novocure Inc.
New York, New York

Terry Wikle Shapiro, MSN, RN, CRNP
Nurse Practitioner
Pediatric Stem Cell Transplant
Penn State Children's Hospital;
Clinical Instructor
Department of Pediatrics
Penn State College of Medicine
Hershey, Pennsylvania

Lisa Kennedy Sheldon, PhD, APRN-BC, AOCNP, CGNC,
FAAN
Global Nurse Consultant
Dogcove Consulting Group, LLC
Portsmouth, New Hampshire;
Oncology Nurse Practitioner
The Cancer Center
St. Joseph Hospital
Nashua, New Hampshire

Mary Steinbach, DNP, APRN, FNP-C
Lead Advance Practice Provider
Hematology/Bone Marrow Transplant
Huntsman Cancer Institute, University of Utah
Salt Lake City, Utah

Elizabeth Anderson Strand, MSN, APRN, BC
Nurse Practitioner
Medical Oncology
Lombardi Cancer Center, Medstar Georgetown Hospital
Washington, District of Columbia

Carrie Tompkins Stricker, PhD
Associate Professor
College of Nursing
Thomas Jefferson University
Philadelphia, Pennsylvania;
Executive Director
Canopy Cancer Collective
Scotts Valley, Pennsylvania

Wendy H. Vogel, MSN, FNP, AOCNP, FAPO
Executive Director, Oncology
Advanced Practitioner Society for Hematology and
  Oncology
Oncology Nurse Practitioner
Kingsport, Tennessee

Anna Weber, DNP, NP-C
Nurse Practitioner
Palliative Care
Billings Clinic
Billings, Montana

Jennifer S. Webster, MN, MPH, RN, AOCNS, NPD-BC
Oncology Clinical Specialist
Georgia Cancer Specialists
Northside Hospital Cancer Institute
Atlanta, Georgia

Laura S. Wood, MSN, RN, OCN
Oncology Nurse Specialist
Laura Wood Consulting, LLC
Medina, Ohio

Tyler Workman, MSN, AG-CNS, APRN-Rx
Clinical Educator
Clinical Trials Office
University of Hawaii Cancer Center
Honolulu, Hawaii

Laura J. Zitella, MS, RN, ACNP-BC, AOCN
Nurse Practitioner
Hematology, Blood and Marrow Transplant, and Cellular
    Therapy Program;
Associate Clinical Professor
Department of Physiological Nursing
University of California—San Francisco
San Francisco, California

Reviewers

Nimian Bauder, MSN, APRN, AGCNS-BC, NPD-BC, EBP-C
Clinical Nurse Specialist
Surgical Oncology/Medical Telemetry
City of Hope
Duarte, California

Joyce Jackowski, MS, FNP-BC
Nurse Practitioner
Venice, Florida

Preface

Welcome to the third edition of *Mosby's® Oncology Nursing Advisor*. This book is designed for the busy nurse who needs easy-to-access clinical information on a full range of oncology topics.

Mosby's® Oncology Nursing Advisor provides nurses access to almost any oncology topic in a streamlined, concise format. The third edition provides updated, evidence-based information on sections such as major cancers, principles of cancer management, and symptom management. New additions to the third edition include integrated information in consideration of diversity, equity, and inclusion; a chapter focused on social determinants of health; a survivorship chapter; and a chapter on cytokine release syndrome.

Working on this book has provided a venue to allow us to contribute to the oncology nursing body of knowledge. It has also enabled us to work with some of the brightest and best oncology nurses across the nation. We would like to thank the contributing authors, whose expertise and willingness to share their knowledge made this book possible. The contributing authors are truly content experts in their topic areas, and they showed great patience and persistence through the entire writing and editing process. While we—Susie, Margie, and Jeannine—are oncology advanced practice nurses with varied clinical backgrounds, it is the expertise and diverse experiences of the many contributing authors that make this book a solid resource for nurses.

Susie Maloney-Newton, MS, APRN, AOCN, AOCNS

Margie Hickey, MSN, MS, RN

Jeannine M. Brant, PhD, APRN, AOCN, FAAN

Contents

SECTION THREE: PRINCIPLES OF CANCER MANAGEMENT

SECTION FIVE: ONCOLOGIC EMERGENCIES

Cancer Epidemiology
Implications for Prevention, Early Detection, and Treatment

Suzanne M. Mahon

Introduction

Cancer continues to be a significant public health problem in the United States and throughout the world. The American Cancer Society (ACS) annually estimates the number of new cancer cases and deaths expected in the United States in the current year and provides evidence-based recommendations for prevention and early detection (ACS, 2021a). The *Cancer Facts & Figures* documents, which are updated regularly, provide an epidemiologic report of cancer in the United States that offers insight into trends in cancer and its care (Smith et al., 2017). Another major source of data is the Surveillance, Epidemiology, and End Results (SEER) program (https://seer.cancer.gov/). An understanding of its epidemiology is important to achieve the long-term public health goal of decreasing the morbidity and mortality associated with a diagnosis of cancer.

Epidemiology is the study of how disease is distributed in a population, factors that influence its distribution, and trends over time. Although it often receives little attention in formal educational programs, an understanding of epidemiology is essential to comprehend cancer biology, identify its risk factors, and develop prevention and treatment strategies. Epidemiologic studies encompass the basis of disease and the impacts of treatment, screening, and preventive measures on the natural history of the disease (see the box below).

Focus of Epidemiologic Studies

- Determine the extent of disease in a community, region, or defined area.
- Identify potential etiologic sources and risk factors for a disease.
- Study the natural history of the disease.
- Study the prognosis of the disease with and without treatment or intervention.
- Evaluate existing and new prevention and treatment measures and methods of health care delivery.
- Examine the cost-effectiveness of various prevention and treatment strategies.
- Provide the basis for public health policy and regulatory decisions about health care spending and environmental issues.

Data from Celentano, D. D., & Szklo, M. (2019). *Gordis epidemiology* (6th ed.). Philadelphia, PA: Elsevier.

Epidemiologists think that illness, disease, and poor health are not always random events. Some people have risk factors that are associated with an increased propensity for developing a disease. Risk assessment is a critical component of epidemiology. Concepts and commonly used epidemiologic terms are shown in the box below.

Terms Used in Cancer Epidemiology

Absolute risk: The occurrence of the cancer in the general population (i.e., incidence or mortality rate).

Asymptomatic: The person being screened and the examiner are unaware of signs or symptoms of cancer in the individual before the screening test is initiated.

Attributable risk: The number of cases of cancer that could be prevented with the manipulation of known risk factors.

Cancer prevention strategy:

Primary cancer prevention: Measures to avoid carcinogen exposure, to improve health practices, and, in some cases, to provide chemoprevention agents. Primary prevention may also include the use of chemoprevention or prophylactic surgery to prevent or significantly reduce the development of a malignancy.

Secondary cancer prevention: Identification of persons at risk for malignancy and implementation of appropriate screening recommendations. Terms often used interchangeably in secondary cancer prevention are *early detection* and *cancer screening*.

Tertiary cancer prevention: Efforts that are aimed at persons with a history of malignancy, including monitoring for and preventing recurrence and screening for second primary cancers. In many cases, those who have had a diagnosis of cancer and who carry a pathogenic variant in a cancer susceptibility gene are at significantly higher risk for a second malignancy.

Cancer screening test: A method or strategy used to detect a specific cancer. It may be a single modality, but often it is a combination of tests. Laboratory tests of blood or body fluids, imaging tests, physical examination, and invasive procedures are sometimes used for screening tests.

Cost-effectiveness: A financial indicator that is achieved if the costs of the screening program are less than the costs in the unscreened group.

Diagnostic tests: Tests used in those with symptoms of cancer or abnormal screening test results to determine their cause.

Effectiveness: A measure derived by comparing the outcomes to determine whether the benefits outweigh the risks and harms and the actual costs of the benefits.

False negative: A test result indicating that the tested person does not have a particular characteristic when he or she actually does have it (e.g., a negative mammogram result for a woman with early breast cancer).

False positive: A test result indicating that the tested person has a particular characteristic when he or she actually does not have it (e.g., a very suspicious mammogram result for a woman who does not have breast cancer).

Incidence: The number of cancers that develop in a population during a defined period, such as 1 year.

Mortality rate: The number of persons who die of a particular cancer during a defined period, such as 1 year.

Terms Used in Cancer Epidemiology—cont'd

Outcomes: Health and economic results that occur related to screening. Outcomes may include the benefits, harms, and costs of screening or genetic testing and its incurred diagnostic evaluations. They may be short or long term in nature.

Prevalence: The number of cancers that exist in a defined population at a given point in time.

Relative risk: A statistical estimate that compares the likelihood of development of a cancer in a person who has a specific risk factor with the likelihood in a person who does not have the specific risk factor.

Sensitivity: Ability of a screening test to detect individuals with the characteristic or symptom. It is calculated by dividing the total number of true positives by the total number of individuals in the population.

Specificity: Ability of a screening test to correctly identify patients without the characteristic or symptom. It is calculated by dividing the total number of true negatives by the total number of individuals in the population.

Target population: Number of people in a defined group who are capable of developing the disease and are therefore appropriate candidates for screening. *Population* may refer to the general population or to a specific group of people defined by geographic, physical, or social characteristics. For example, nurses who provide cancer genetics counseling need to assess whether a person is of Ashkenazi Jewish background. This special population of Jewish people is at higher risk for three specific pathogenic variants associated with hereditary breast cancer (National Comprehensive Cancer Network, 2022b).

True negative: Test result indicating that the tested person does not have a particular characteristic when the person indeed does not have it (e.g., a negative mammogram result for a woman in whom cancer does not develop during the next 12–24 months).

True positive: Test result indicating that the tested person has a particular characteristic that the person indeed does have (e.g., a suspicious mammogram for a woman in whom a subsequent biopsy demonstrates a breast malignancy).

Validity: Degree to which a test measures what it is supposed to measure.

Data from Celentano, D. D., & Szklo, M. (2019). *Gordis epidemiology* (6th ed.). Philadelphia, PA: Elsevier; Mahon, S. M. (2021a). *Understanding genomic and hereditary cancer risk: A handbook for oncology nurses.* Pittsburgh, PA: Oncology Nursing Society.

Types of Epidemiology

Two types of epidemiology are often applied in cancer: descriptive epidemiology and analytic epidemiology.

Descriptive Epidemiology

Descriptive epidemiology provides information about the occurrence of disease in a population or its subgroups and trends in the frequency of disease over time. The information includes incidence and mortality rates and survival data. Sources of data include death certificates, cancer registries, surveys, and population censuses (Celentano & Szklo, 2019). Descriptive measures are useful for identifying populations and subgroups at high and low risk for a disease and for monitoring time trends. They can be especially helpful in understanding the natural history of rare tumors providing leads for analytic studies designed to investigate factors responsible. There are several common descriptive terms used in epidemiology that oncology nurses frequently encounter.

Incidence

Incidence refers to the number of new cases of disease that occur during a specified period of time in a defined population at risk for the disease. Incidence rates also provide information about the risk of a disease or condition one has by virtue of being a member of a specified population. The ACS publishes projected incidence rates annually for common cancers in its annual *Cancer Facts & Figures* publication (ACS, 2021a). The table below provides examples of the incidence of the most commonly diagnosed cancers in the United States. The ACS estimated that about 1,898,160 new cases of cancer would occur in the United States in 2021 (ACS, 2021a).

Mortality Rates

The table below shows the projected number of deaths from cancer in the United States in 2021. The *mortality rate* is the number of persons who die of a particular cancer during a specified period. The ACS (2021a) estimated that approximately 608,570 Americans would die of cancer during 2021. This translates to about 1670 deaths per day.

Many epidemiologists consider the incidence and mortality rates together when making public health decisions. For example, breast cancer affects one in eight women (i.e., 281,550 new cases) and results in 43,600 deaths annually (ACS, 2021a).

Estimated Incidence and Mortality Statistics for Selected Cancers, United States, 2021

New Cases Men	Deaths Men	New Cases Women	Deaths Women
Prostate: 248,530	Lung: 69,410	Breast: 281,550	Lung: 62,470
Lung: 119,100	Prostate: 34,130	Lung: 116,660	Breast: 43,600
Colorectal: 79,520	Colorectal: 28,520	Colorectal: 69,980	Colorectal: 24,460
Bladder: 64,280	Pancreas: 25,270	Uterus: 66,570	Pancreas: 22,950
Melanoma: 62,260	Liver: 20,300	Melanoma 43,850	Ovary: 13,770
Kidney: 48,780	Leukemia: 13,900	Non-Hodgkin lymphoma: 35,903	Uterine: 12,940
Non-Hodgkin lymphoma: 45,630	Esophagus: 12,410	Thyroid: 32,130	Liver: 9930
Oral cavity: 38,800	Bladder: 12,260	Pancreas: 28,480	Leukemia: 9760
Leukemia: 35,530	Non-Hodgkin lymphoma: 12,170	Kidney: 27,300	Non-Hodgkin lymphoma: 8550
Pancreas: 31,950	Brain and central nervous system: 10,500	Leukemia: 25,560	Brain and nervous system: 8100
All sites: 970,250	All sites: 319,420	All sites: 927,910	All sites: 289,150

Data from American Cancer Society. (2021a). *Cancer facts & figures 2021.* Atlanta, GA: American Cancer Society.

It accounts for 30% of new cases of cancer among women and 15% of deaths annually (ACS, 2021a). In comparison, pancreatic cancer affects 28,480 women and results in 22,950 deaths annually (ACS, 2021a). It accounts for 3% of new cases of cancer among women but 8% of deaths annually. Examination of these figures suggests either that pancreatic cancer is diagnosed at a later stage on average than breast cancer or that treatment is less effective, or both.

Age-Specific Rates

Age-specific rates provide valuable insight and information about how disease risks vary among groups and populations (see the figure below). This often is extremely helpful when conveying information about risk to an individual. It also helps when considering recommendations for initiating screening. For example, the median age for developing breast cancer is 63 years of age. Approximately 90% of breast cancer cases are diagnosed after the age of 45, and this is a consideration in screening recommendations. For example, mammography is often recommended to begin at age 40 because most cases occur at this age or older (ACS, 2021a).

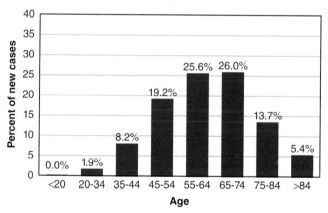

Percentage of New Cases of Breast Cancer Over Selected Age Intervals. The percentage of new cases of breast cancer by age group demonstrates how the risk for breast cancer changes over time. (From SEER Stat Fact Sheets. [2018]. Female breast cancer. Available at https://seer.cancer.gov/statfacts/html/breast.html [accessed December 20, 2021].)

Prevalence

The *prevalence* of a disease or condition is the proportion of individuals in a specific population who have the disease or condition at a specific point or during a defined period of time. Prevalence includes both newly diagnosed and existing (i.e., previously diagnosed or current) cases of a particular disease. Cancer prevalence data provide information on the impact that cancer has on a population and can help inform the scope of cancer health services needed for a specific community or population. For example, more than 3.8 million US women with a history of breast cancer were alive on January 1, 2019 (ACS, 2019a). Breast cancer survivors often have an increased risk for osteoporosis due to chemotherapy, endocrine therapy, and premature menopause. Knowing that a large number of breast cancer survivors are at risk is useful for

developing recommendations for screening and management to prevent long-term complications that may stem from osteoporosis (Whitton-Smith et al., 2021).

Case-Fatality Rates

Cancer case-fatality rates are often an important indicator of the effectiveness of a particular cancer detection or treatment method and the impact of the cancer in a defined population. Cancer case-fatality rates provide information about the likelihood of dying from cancer among those diagnosed with the disease (Celentano & Szklo, 2019). *Case-fatality rates* are different from mortality rates. The mortality rate represents an entire population at risk for cancer-related deaths and includes both those who do and those who do not have cancer. Cancer case-fatality rates include only those who have the disease. The cancer case-fatality rate is higher among men than women (189.5 per 100,000 men and 135.7 per 100,000 women). When comparing groups based on race/ethnicity and sex, cancer case-fatality rate is highest in African American men (227.3 per 100,000) and lowest in Asian/Pacific Islander women (85.6 per 100,000) (ACS, 2021a).

Risk Factor

A *risk factor* is a trait or characteristic that is associated with a statistically significant increased likelihood of developing a disease (Celentano & Szklo, 2019). However, having a risk factor does not mean that a person will develop a disease or malignancy, nor does the absence of a risk factor mean that a person will not develop a disease or malignancy. Risk factors are becoming increasingly important because screening guidelines are often based on an individualized cancer risk assessment.

Absolute Risk

Absolute risk is a measure of the occurrence of cancer, in terms of incidence (i.e., new cases) or mortality rate (i.e., deaths), in the general population over a specific time period. Absolute risk is helpful when a patient needs to understand what the chances are for all persons in a population of having a particular disease. Absolute risk can be expressed as the number of cases for a specified denominator (e.g., 131 cases of breast cancer per 100,000 women annually) or as a cumulative risk up to a specified age (e.g., one in eight women will develop breast cancer if they live to age 85 years) (ACS, 2019a). Another way to express absolute risk is to discuss the average risk of having breast cancer at a certain age. For example, the absolute risk of breast cancer increases with age: 12 out of 10,000 women ages 40 to 44 versus 23 out of 10,000 women ages 50 to 54 will be diagnosed with breast cancer in the next year. Risk estimates are much different for a 54-year-old woman than for an 85-year-old woman because approximately 70% of the cases of breast cancer occur after the age of 55 years (see the figure in the left column).

Certain assumptions are made to reach an absolute risk value for a particular cancer. For example, the one-in-eight risk of breast cancer describes the average risk among White

American women, and its calculation takes into consideration other causes of death over the life span. This figure overestimates breast cancer risk for some women with no risk factors and underestimates the risk for women with several risk factors.

The statistic means that the average woman's breast cancer risk is just 1.2% up to age 40 years, 3.7% from age 40 to 60 years, 3.5% from age 60 to 69 years, and 3.9% from age 70 years on. The 12.3%, or one-in-eight, risk is obtained by adding the risk in each age category (1.2% + 3.7% + 3.5% + 3.9% = 12.3%). When a woman who has an average risk reaches age 40 years without a diagnosis of breast cancer, she has passed through 1.2% of her risk, so her lifetime risk is 12.3% 1.2% = 11.1%. When she reaches age 70 years without a diagnosis of breast cancer, her risk is 12.3% − 1.2% − 3.7% − 3.5% = 3.9%. Time must always be considered for the absolute risk figure to be meaningful. The 12.3% figure represents the lifetime risk of developing breast cancer (ACS, 2019a). Absolute risk is useful to help a patient understand how common a particular cancer is in the general population.

Relative Risk

The term *relative risk* refers to a comparison of the incidence or mortality rate among those with a particular risk factor compared to those without the risk factor. By using relative risk factors, individuals can determine their risk factors and better understand their personal chances of developing a specific cancer compared to someone without the risk factors.

If the risk for a person who has no known risk factors for a disease is 1.0%, the risk for those with known risk factors can be evaluated in relation to this figure. This can be illustrated by considering several relative risk factors for breast cancer. A woman who has her first menstrual period before age 12 years has a 1.3% relative risk for development of breast cancer compared to a woman who has her first menstrual period after age 15 years (ACS, 2019a). For a woman with a known *BRCA2* pathogenic variant, the relative risk is

estimated to be 8% compared with a woman who has no relatives with premenopausal breast cancer. This means she is eight times more likely to develop breast cancer than the woman without risk factors (National Comprehensive Cancer Network [NCCN], 2022a). The table in the left column below shows some of the relative risk calculations for developing breast cancer.

Attributable Risk

Attributable risk is the amount of disease within the population that could be prevented by alteration of a particular risk factor. Attributable risk has important implications for public health policy. More attention is being directed to assessment and management of attributable risk because it is a valuable means of primary cancer prevention.

A risk factor may be associated with a very large relative risk but be restricted to a few individuals; therefore, changing it would benefit only a small group. Conversely, some risk factors that can be altered may decrease the morbidity and mortality rates associated with malignancy in a large number of people. Smoking is a perfect example. The ACS estimates that about 30% of all cancer deaths in the United States and as much as 40% in parts of the South and Appalachia are still caused by smoking (ACS, 2021b). Altering this risk factor could significantly alter the morbidity and mortality associated with cancer in the future.

Odds Ratio

The odds ratio is a measure of association that provides information similar to that found in relative risk calculations. *Odds ratios* are an estimate or measure of the chance of having a specific exposure (usually to an environmental agent) among those who have the disease compared to the chance among those who do not have the disease. It is most used in cohort studies to address whether an association exists between the exposure and the disease (Celentano & Szklo, 2019).

Analytic Epidemiology

Descriptive epidemiology helps to identify variations and trends in the distribution of cancer in a population. When analyzed, descriptive epidemiologic data provide information to formulate hypotheses about the health of a population. *Analytic epidemiology* provides strategies to test these hypotheses to find the reasons or determinants that are associated with variations identified in descriptive epidemiology (Celentano & Szklo, 2019). Analytic epidemiology strives to determine whether an association exists between a particular exposure or carcinogen and disease status.

Analytic epidemiologic studies can be observational or interventional in nature. Observational studies include cohort, case-control, and cross-sectional studies. Cohort studies follow a group of people over time. They can be retrospective or prospective in design. A case-control study is a retrospective study in which exposures and risk factors for persons with a disease are compared to those for persons who do not have the disease. In interventional studies, participants receive or do not receive a specific exposure (e.g., drug, treatment, lifestyle change), and changes in disease status are compared. Interventional studies are often referred to as clinical trials, and they may be randomized (randomly assigns participants into an experimental group or a control group) or blinded

Relative Risk of Developing Breast Cancer

Risk Factors	Associated Relative Risk[*]
BRCA1 and *BRCA2* or other inherited gene pathogenic variants	5–30
Two first-degree relatives diagnosed with breast cancer	3–7.1
Mother diagnosed before age 60	2–4
Mother diagnosed after age 60	1.5–2
High breast density	3–5
Atypical hyperplasia	4–5
Nulliparity	1.3–3
First pregnancy after age 30	1–3
First period before age 12	1.2–2.0
Last menstrual period after age 55	1.3
Drinking 2–4 drinks/day	1.2–1.4

[*]Adding relative risk scores does not give a total risk score.
Data from American Cancer Society. (2019a). *Breast cancer facts & figures 2019-2020*. Atlanta, GA: American Cancer Society; NCCN. (2021a). Breast cancer risk reduction version 1.2021. Available at https://www.nccn.org/login?ReturnURL=https://www.nccn.org/professionals/physician_gls/pdf/breast_risk.pdf (accessed December 20, 2021).

(single blinded, when the researchers but not the subjects know who is receiving the active medication or treatment; or double blinded, when neither the researchers nor the subjects know who is receiving the active medication or treatment).

Risk Assessment

A cancer risk assessment may include review of a person's medical history, history of exposures to carcinogens in daily living, and detailed family history. After the information is gathered, it must be interpreted into understandable terms for the patient. This often is accomplished by calculating absolute risk, relative risk, attributable risk, or specific risk values for various cancers.

Family History

A *family history* should focus on first- and second-degree relatives and should include at least three generations. It includes an assessment of both paternal and maternal sides of the family because many autosomal dominant syndromes can be passed through the father or the mother (Mahon, 2021a). This lineage is typically displayed in a pedigree (see the figure below).

First-degree relatives include parents, siblings, and children. Because first-degree relatives share 50% of their genes, these are the relatives most likely to inherit similar genetic information. Information about second-degree relatives can also be helpful. Second-degree relatives include grandparents, aunts, and uncles.

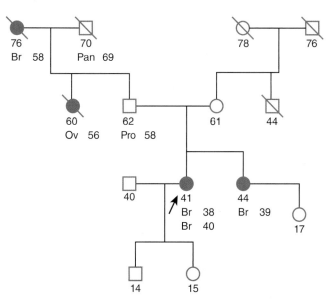

Pedigree. In a typical pedigree constructed to evaluate hereditary risk factors, the *squares* represent males and *circles* represent females. The *arrow* represents the proband or spokesperson for the family. *Slashes* represent deceased persons. *Solid circles* and *squares* represent persons with cancer. The age and anatomic site of diagnosis are recorded.

Second-degree relatives have 25% of their genes in common. Older second-degree relatives can provide important information about genetic risk because an early-onset cancer would likely have manifested in the older person if a hereditary trait exists in the family. The pedigree should also include nieces and nephews because younger family members can provide information about childhood cancers that also has implications for the genetic risk assessment.

Third-degree relatives (i.e., cousins, great-aunts, great-uncles, and great-grandparents) can be included in the family history, although reports about these relatives are not always accurate. Third-degree relatives share 12.5% of the same genes.

Ethnicity should be recorded. Some ethnicities are associated with an increased risk of malignancies. For example, persons of Ashkenazi Jewish ancestry have an increased risk for developing breast cancer (NCCN, 2022b).

After all information is documented, it should be stored in a standard pedigree format (see the figure in the left column). The pedigree can be helpful in families with multiple cases of malignancy to help teach concepts of genetics, clarify relationships, provide a quick reference, and calculate the risk of having a cancer-causing pathogenic variant. The availability of software to generate these pedigrees has made updating the information simple (Mahon, 2021a).

The family history provides an organized way to document data such as whether a relative is alive or dead, age at death if applicable, significant medical diagnoses, and diagnosis of cancer. Space can be provided to describe in detail the specific type of cancer, age at diagnosis, and other characteristics (e.g., whether a breast cancer was premenopausal or bilateral). Specific information may influence recommendations for screening. Obtaining a detailed family history is useful for cancer risk assessment and is the first step in identifying families with a possible hereditary predisposition to malignancy and other illnesses. Health care providers should ask patients about specific relatives and their health individually rather than asking a general question such as, "Have any of your relatives been diagnosed with cancer?"

After gathering the family history, it is important to recheck whether any of the patient's relatives have been diagnosed with any type of cancer. Patients often forget to provide these details and reiterating the question can prompt recall of valuable information. Those who have multiple family members diagnosed with cancer, especially at a younger age, should be referred to a health care provider with expertise in genetics. Genetics professionals assess genetic risk, provide counseling before and after genetic testing, and follow up to ensure that all at-risk family members are informed about their potential increased risk of developing cancer. Patients and family members can be offered the option of undergoing genetic testing to better clarify their risk.

Genetic testing for hereditary cancer syndromes is an important component of cancer risk assessment. In persons with a documented hereditary cancer syndrome, the risk of cancer can be substantially increased. For example, a woman with a known pathogenic variant in the *BRCA1* gene has an estimated 85% lifetime chance of developing breast cancer and an estimated 50% lifetime risk of developing ovarian cancer (NCCN, 2022b). She may want to consider primary prevention measures to better manage her risk, such as risk reducing mastectomies or bilateral salpingo-oophorectomy. Identification of persons with a suspected or known hereditary risk factor often results in substantial change in cancer prevention and early detection recommendations.

Medical History and Lifestyle Factors

Assessment of medical history and personal lifestyle factors that may increase the risk of cancer should be documented.

The inventory can include information such as menstrual history, hormonal exposures, and exposure to carcinogens such as ultraviolet light or tobacco. Many risk factors are not within an individual's control (e.g., age at menarche) and are not amenable to primary prevention efforts. Some lifestyle factors are within the control of the individual and can be affected by providing education about primary prevention efforts.

After all risk data are collected, the clinician must assimilate the risk factors and provide information to the patient about their effect on each of the major cancers. For example, early menarche, nulliparity, and late menopause are risk factors for breast and endometrial cancer (ACS, 2021a). Communication of risk should include a discussion about the presence of these risk factors and the risk of developing both cancers. Risk can be communicated to patients in several different formats. Often it is best to explain the implications of a patient's medical history and lifestyle in terms of absolute risk, relative risk, and attributable risk.

For some cancers, it is possible to combine risk factors in well-tested models to calculate the risk of developing cancer at a specific age or over a lifetime. This is often done for breast cancer, colon cancer, and malignant melanoma. These tools combine risk factors to provide an estimate of the risk of developing a particular malignancy (National Cancer Institute, n.d.). These calculations can be utilized to compare a patient's risk for developing malignancy based on their risk factors with risk of developing the malignancy in the general population. For patients with increased risk, modifications to general screening guidelines are often recommended. The breast cancer risk assessment tool is available at https://bcrisktool.cancer.gov/calculator.html. Risk assessment tools are also available for colorectal cancer (https://ccrisktool.cancer.gov/) and for melanoma (https://mrisktool.cancer.gov/).

Oncology nurses can use these models to help individuals put their risk in perspective. The clinician is responsible for using the model that most accurately reflects the person's risk factors and for helping the individual to understand the strengths and limitations of the model in calculating risk and quickly stratifying risk to determine whether screening measures need to be modified.

Levels of Cancer Prevention

There are three levels of cancer prevention. *Primary prevention* refers to evading disease by methods such as immunization against childhood and other diseases, avoiding tobacco products, or reducing exposure to ultraviolet rays. Primary prevention measures can reduce the risk of cancer but do not guarantee that a person will not develop a malignancy. Primary prevention measures include adopting a healthier lifestyle, using chemoprevention (e.g., tamoxifen to prevent breast cancer), and undergoing prophylactic surgery if there is a genetic susceptibility to cancer (e.g., bilateral mastectomies in a woman without a diagnosis of breast cancer who has a known pathogenic variant in the *BRCA1* or *BRCA2* gene).

More attention is being directed toward primary prevention by reducing attributable risk. In addition to eliminating tobacco use to reduce smoking-related deaths, efforts are being targeted at human papillomavirus (HPV) vaccination, reduction of exposure to ultraviolet light, improved nutrition, and increased physical activity (ACS, 2021b). At least 42% of newly diagnosed cancers in the United States (estimate 797,000 cases in 2021) are potentially avoidable, including the 19% of cancers caused by smoking and at least 18% caused by a combination of excess body weight, alcohol consumption, poor nutrition, and physical inactivity (ACS, 2021b).

Secondary prevention refers to the early detection and treatment of subclinical, asymptomatic, or early disease in persons without signs or symptoms of cancer. Forms of secondary cancer prevention include the use of a Papanicolaou test (Pap smear) to detect cervical cancer, a mammogram to detect a nonpalpable breast cancer, and colonoscopy to remove polyps and detect early colon cancers. Cancer screening is aimed at asymptomatic persons with the goal of finding disease when it is most easily and effectively treated in its early stages.

Screening tests seek to decrease the morbidity and mortality associated with cancer. After a positive screening test result, further diagnostic testing is required to determine whether a malignancy exists. This is the traditional definition of cancer screening. Some also consider screening for genetic or molecular markers that put the individual at high risk for cancer as a specialized form of cancer screening (NCCN, 2022a).

Tertiary prevention refers to management of an illness such as cancer to prevent progression, recurrence, or other complications. In cancer care, examples of tertiary prevention include monitoring for early signs of recurrence by measuring levels of tumor markers or detecting second primary malignancies early in long-term survivors. An estimated 16.9 million persons are alive with a diagnosis of cancer (ACS, 2021a). Because of this ever-growing population, there has been a push to develop cancer survivor care plans that include a component of tertiary prevention (Mahon, 2021b).

Accuracy of Screening Tests

In addition to communicating about cancer risks with patients, nurses must explain the accuracy of screening tests. It is not enough to recommend a screening test. Patients need to understand what the possibilities are regarding a truly positive or truly negative test result.

Individuals often inquire about recommendations for a specific cancer screening test, such as a mammogram or a Pap smear. Specific recommendations often vary among organizations such as the ACS, the U. S. Preventive Services Task Force (USPSTF), the NCCN, and the National Cancer Institute (NCI) (ACS, 2021a; National Cancer Institute, n.d.; NCCN, 2021a, 2021b, 2021c; NCCN, 2022a, 2022b, 2022c; USPSTF, 2021). These recommendations are readily available for comparison at https://www.ahrq.gov/gam/index.html.

The specific criteria used by these organizations to make recommendations vary, which is why the recommendations are not universal and are very confusing for the general public. However, there is consensus for some requirements and characteristics included in acceptable screening tests. When screening recommendations are presented, it is important to include the rationale, strengths, and limitations of the test and to present this information in light of the individual's risk of developing cancer (see the box below).

Considerations for Cancer Screening Tests

- The disease should be an important health problem. There is little doubt that cancer is a significant health problem, but some types of cancers are more significant health problems than other types. For example, the estimated incidence of breast cancer is 2,815,500 new cases annually, and that of lung cancer is 235,760 new cases, making both cancers highly significant (ACS, 2021a). The mortality rate associated with these cancers is also high, with an estimated 43,600 deaths annually from lung cancer.
- The disease should have a preclinical stage before symptoms become obvious. In breast cancer, mammography can detect the cancer before it is palpable. Although lung cancer has a high incidence, only 15% of lung cancers are diagnosed at a localized stage, for which the 5-year survival rate is 59% (ACS, 2021a).
- The disease should be treatable, and there should be a recognized treatment for lesions identified after screening. Breast cancer is clearly a disease that responds to surgery, chemotherapy, and radiation therapy, especially when it is detected early (ACS, 2021a). More importantly, when breast cancer is detected early, it can often be treated with less radical surgery, such as lumpectomy. The same is not true of lung cancer.
- The test must be clinically relevant. The test must be able to detect a condition for which intervention at a preclinical stage can improve outcome.
- The test must be accurate. The sensitivity and specificity must be acceptable.
- The test must be cost-effective.
- The test must be acceptable to individuals being screened. Highly invasive, painful, or risky procedures usually are unacceptable. The test must be widely available and easily accessible. Most women are willing to tolerate the discomfort and risks associated with mammography.

The accuracy of screening tests is described by several terms. A true-positive (TP) test result is a normal test result for cancer in an individual who has the disease. A true-negative (TN) test result is a normal or negative screening result for cancer in an individual who is subsequently found not to have the disease within a defined period after the last test. A false-negative (FN) test result is a normal test result for cancer in an individual who, in fact, has the cancer. A false-positive (FP) test result is an abnormal test result for cancer screening in an individual who does not have the disease.

Sensitivity

An understanding of true and false test results is necessary to calculate information about sensitivity and specificity. The *sensitivity* of a screening test is its ability to detect those individuals who have cancer. It is calculated by taking the number of TP results and dividing it by the total number of cancer cases (i.e., TP and FN cases). For example, a screening test given to 1000 persons resulting in 85 TPs and 15 FNs has a sensitivity of 0.85. This is calculated as 85/(85 + 15) = 0.85. Most people are unwilling to accept a test with a high FN rate because many cancers will be missed.

Specificity

The *specificity* of a test is its ability to identify those individuals who do not have cancer. It is calculated by dividing the TN by

the sum of the total number of individuals in the population who do not have cancer (i.e., TN and FP cases). For example, if a test is given to 1000 persons and there are 775 TNs and 225 FPs, the specificity is 0.78, which is calculated as 775/(775 + 225) = 0.78. A high FP test rate can result in unnecessary follow-up testing and anxiety in persons who have a positive screening result.

Positive and Negative Predictive Values

The *positive predictive value* is the measure of the validity of a positive test. It is the proportion of positive tests that are TP cases. The predictive value of a test depends on the disease prevalence. As the prevalence of a cancer increases in the population, the positive predictive value of the screening tests increases, although its sensitivity and specificity remain unchanged.

The *negative predictive value* is the measure of the validity of a negative test. This refers to the proportion of negative tests that are TNs.

Bias

Bias affects screening tests. *Selection bias* occurs during clinical trials that evaluate the effectiveness of screening tests. Ideally, those screened should be similar to those not screened to determine the effectiveness of the tests. This problem is minimized with randomization. *Lead-time bias* refers to the bias that arises by adding the time gained as a result of early diagnosis to survival time. *Length bias* occurs because of the preferential diagnosis of more indolent cases of cancer through screening. This may be especially true with the identification of in situ cancers that never become a health threat (e.g., identification of early prostate cancers that may never progress enough to cause morbidity or mortality). There is a lack of consensus regarding the utility of prostate cancer screening (ACS, 2021a). Because of length bias, persons may have indolent cancers that are diagnosed early but could have taken years to progress, resulting in the appearance of longer survival times. *Overdiagnosis bias* occurs with excess screening. FP rates and overzealous screeners may inflate the detection and diagnosis of early-stage cancers.

Outcomes

Outcomes of cancer screening are considered in epidemiologic studies. If there are no differences in outcome, particularly with respect to morbidity and mortality rates, it is often inappropriate to offer a screening maneuver. Similarly, some agencies consider cost-benefit analyses to determine purely on a financial basis whether years of life are saved, and costs of treatment are reduced with early detection of cancer through a screening test. Quality of life is another significant outcome that should be considered in these analyses.

Selection of a Screening Test

Understanding these principles is necessary to help patients comprehend the strengths and limitations of the test they are using to screen for a particular cancer. The perfect screening test does not exist. For example, the overall sensitivity of screening mammography is 87% (NCCN, 2021b). Other considerations drive screening recommendations. The cancer being screened for should have a high prevalence and incidence, significant mortality and morbidity rates and cost, and availability of an effective treatment if detected early.

Many individuals still choose to undergo a screening examination despite a lower sensitivity and specificity in the hope that it will be effective for them. Screening for ovarian cancer is an excellent example. Highly specific and sensitive screening tests are unavailable for the early detection of ovarian cancer. Many women, however, still want an annual pelvic examination to assess for ovarian masses. The test is relatively inexpensive to perform and is usually well tolerated. Some clinicians are better at detecting ovarian masses than others, but many ovarian cancers cannot be detected by this examination, even when it is performed by a skilled clinician. As long as a woman realizes the test may fail to detect ovarian cancer and is willing to accept this limitation, the pelvic examination may be considered to be effective by some.

Some steps can be taken by health care providers to improve the accuracy of screening tests. The establishment of certification and federal guidelines in the areas of radiology and laboratory services is an example. Guidelines are in place for mammography centers and laboratories providing cancer screening services to ensure that a minimum acceptable standard is met so that the screen is as accurate as possible.

The person conducting the examination or interpreting the laboratory or radiologic test result also affects the effectiveness of a cancer screening test. For example, some health care professionals are better at performing clinical examinations than others and are more likely to detect a subtle physical change. Monitoring the quality of clinical examinations is important. Monitoring and improving the quality of physical examinations in the clinical setting are far more challenging but important to improve the sensitivity and specificity of the examination.

Screening quality may be improved by developing standardized instructions for patient preparation. This may improve patient compliance and help obtain the best possible screening data. Examples include avoiding the use of deodorant before mammography, having a thorough colon evacuation prior to colonoscopy, and instructing a patient to avoid douching for 24 hours before a Pap smear.

Cancer Screening Recommendations

A screening protocol or recommendation defines how cancer screening tests should be used. A protocol usually describes the target population being served, the screening recommendation to be applied, and the interval at which the test should be applied. Screening protocols can vary among organizations and practitioners. The table below illustrates a comparison of ACS, NCCN, and USPSTF recommendations for early detection of cancer in asymptomatic individuals.

Comparison of Screening Guidelines for the Early Detection of Cancer in Asymptomatic People

Target Organ	American Cancer Society	United States Preventive Task Force	National Comprehensive Cancer Network
Breast	• Women should have the opportunity to begin annual mammography screening between the ages of 40 and 44. • Women should undergo regular screening mammography, starting at age 45. • Women ages 45–54 should be screened annually. • Women aged 55 and older can transition to biennial screening or have the opportunity to continue annual screening. Continue screening as long as overall health is good and life expectancy is 10+ years.	• Recommends biennial screening mammography for women aged 50–74 years.	• For ages 20–39, breast awareness and CBE every 1–3 years. • For ages 40+, annual clinical breast exam, breast awareness, and annual mammography.
Cervix	• For women ages 21–29, screening should be done every 3 years with conventional or liquid-based Pap tests. • For women ages 30–65, screening should be done every 5 years with both the HPV test and the Pap test (preferred) or every 3 years with the Pap test alone (acceptable). • Women ages 65+ who have had ≥3 consecutive negative Pap tests or ≥2 consecutive negative HPV and Pap tests within the past 10 years, with the most recent test occurring within the past 5 years, and women who have had a total hysterectomy should stop cervical cancer screening.	• Women ages 21–65 years should be screened with cytology (Pap smear) every 3 years. • Women ages 30–65 years can be screened with cytology every 3 years or co-tested (cytology + HPV testing) every 5 years. • Women 65+ years should not be screened.	• Same as American Cancer Society (ACS) recommendations.

Comparison of Screening Guidelines for the Early Detection of Cancer in Asymptomatic People—cont'd

Target Organ	American Cancer Society	United States Preventive Task Force	National Comprehensive Cancer Network
Colon	• FOBT with at least 50% test sensitivity for cancer, or FIT with at least 50% test sensitivity for cancer annually *or* • Stool DNA test every 3 years starting at age 50 years *or* • Flexible sigmoidoscopy every 5 years, starting at age 50 years performed alone or combined with FOBT or FIT annually *or* • Double-contrast barium enema every 5 years starting at age 50 years *or* • Colonoscopy every 10 years starting at age 50 years *or* • CT colonography every 5 years starting at age 50 years.	• Adults aged 45–49 can consider colon screening. • Adults aged 50–75 years can be screened with high-sensitivity FOBT annually, flexible sigmoidoscopy every 5 years, or colonoscopy every 10 years.	• Colonoscopy every 10 years *or* • Annual FOBT or FIT *or* • Flexible sigmoidoscopy with or without FOBT *or* • FIT every 5 years.
Lung	• Current or former smokers ages 55–74 and in good health with at least a 30 pack-year history who currently smoke or who have quit in the past 15 years can consider LDCT. • This is not a substitute for smoking cessation.	• Asymptomatic adults ages 55–80 who have a 20 pack-year smoking history and currently smoke or have quit smoking within the past 15 years should screen annually with LDCT. • Discontinue screening when the patient has not smoked for 15 years.	• Age 55–74 and >30 pack-year history with smoking cessation of <15 years, or age 50+ years with a >20 pack-year history and one other risk factor other than secondhand smoke. • Annual LDCT every 2 years until the patient can no longer tolerate definitive treatment.
Prostate	• Men ages 50+ can consider DRE and PSA if they have at least a 10-year life expectancy and have been fully informed of the risks and benefits.	• Recommend against PSA screening for prostate cancer in men aged 70 and older. • For men aged 55–69 years, the decision to undergo periodic PSA-based screening for prostate cancer should be an individual one.	• For ages 50+, DRE and PSA every 1–2 years.

BSE, Breast self-examination; *CBE*, clinical breast examination; *CT*, computed tomography; *DRE*, digital rectal examination; *FIT*, fecal immunochemical test; *FOBT*, fecal occult blood test; *HPV*, human papillomavirus; *LDCT*, low-dose helical computed tomography; *MRI*, magnetic resonance imaging; *Pap*, Papanicolaou smear; *PSA*, prostate-specific antigen test.

Data from American Cancer Society. (2021a). *Cancer facts & figures 2021*. Atlanta, GA: American Cancer Society; United States Preventive Services Task Force. (2021). A and B recommendations. Available at https://www.uspreventiveservicestaskforce.org/uspstf/recommendation-topics/uspstf-and-b-recommendations (accessed December 12, 2021); National Comprehensive Cancer Network. (2021b). Breast cancer screening and diagnosis version 1.2021. Available at https://www.nccn.org/guidelines/guidelines-detail?category=2&id=1421 (accessed December 20, 2021); National Comprehensive Cancer Network. (2021c). Colorectal cancer screening version 2.2021. Available at https://www.nccn.org/guidelines/guidelines-detail?category=2&id=1429 (accessed December 20, 2021); National Comprehensive Cancer Network. (2021d). Prostate cancer early detection version 2.21. https://www.nccn.org/guidelines/guidelines-detail?category=2&id=1460 (accessed December 20, 2021); National Comprehensive Cancer Network. (2022c). Lung cancer screening version 1.2022. Available at https://www.nccn.org/guidelines/guidelines-detail?category=2&id=1441 (accessed January 11, 2016).

Screening guidelines change over time. The ACS has been publishing guidelines for early cancer detection for more than 20 years (ACS, 2021a). Although the specific recommendations have changed over the years, the focus of the guidelines has changed very little. They mandate that health care providers use the guidelines to select the best screening tests for an individual of average risk and modifications be made in some cases (e.g., for an individual who has a particularly high risk for a specific malignancy). For example, a woman with a known hereditary predisposition gene for hereditary nonpolyposis colorectal cancer (HNPCC) should begin having an annual colonoscopy at 25 years of age instead of following the population recommendation of a colonoscopy every 7 to 10 years beginning at 45 years of age (NCCN, 2022a). Her risk for development of colorectal cancer approaches 85% over a lifetime, and in individuals with this genetic pathogenic variant for colon cancer it develops in as little as 12 to 18 months after the development of a polyp. Polyps increase the risk of colorectal cancer in patients with HNPCC by at least 25% by age 50 years and up to 82% by age 70 years. Aggressive screening is imperative to decrease the morbidity and mortality rates associated with the disease. Similarly, the ACS and NCCN recommend breast MRI in addition to mammography for any woman whose estimated lifetime risk of breast cancer is greater than 20% (ACS, 2021a; NCCN, 2022b).

Clinicians must remember that screening protocols are guidelines and that the recommendations vary across agencies (see the table above). Screening recommendations are not practice standards to be used with every individual. The goal of the ACS and NCCN standards is the detection of malignancy. The USPSTF uses very strict criteria for evidence of effectiveness. Cost-effectiveness of the screening recommendations is an important consideration for this group. When providing information on cancer screening recommendations, nurses need to inform the individual why a certain recommendation is being selected.

Means to Express Cancer Prognosis and Outcomes

Patient survival is a primary means of assessing the effectiveness of screening tests and treatment. Because patients usually have had cancer for different lengths of time, survival rates are often expressed separately by stage. The figure below shows an example of relative survival rates by stage at diagnosis for breast cancer.

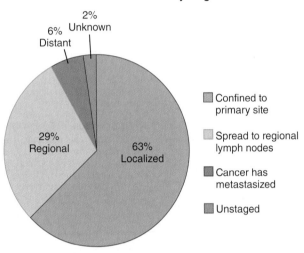

Percent of Cases by Stage

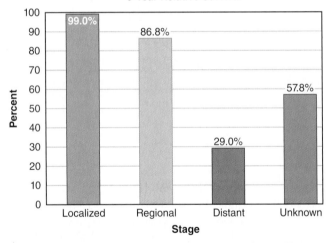

5-Year Relative Survival

Five-Year Relative Survival for Breast Cancer by Stage. Five-year survival rates for persons with breast cancer by stage at diagnosis. (From SEER Stat Fact Sheets. Female breast cancer. https://seer.cancer.gov/statfacts/html/breast.html [accessed December 21, 2021].)

The difference between living 6 months and living 10 years after diagnosis is important to patients and health care providers. Length of survival is often a function of disease stage at diagnosis, clinical characteristics of the disease, comorbidities, and treatments used to manage the disease.

The *observed survival rate*, which is also known as the *overall survival rate*, is a measure of the proportion of patients who survive all causes of death after a cancer diagnosis for a defined period of study. The cause- or disease-specific survival rate is a measure of the proportion of persons who do not die of the specific disease under study, such as cancer, during a defined period.

The *relative survival rate* is a ratio of the observed survival rate and the expected survival rate for a patient cohort. It is the observed survival rate for individuals with a specific cancer relative to the survival rate that is expected for people of similar age, race, and sex in the general population during the same period of observation (see the figure in the left column).

The 5-year survival rate represents the proportion of patients who did not experience a defined event (usually death) during the first 5 years after diagnosis. Selection of the 5-year mark is arbitrary (ACS, 2021a). Because a significant number of persons historically die during the first 5 years after diagnosis, health care providers use this period as an indicator of successful treatment and management of the disease.

Ethnic Differences

Knowledge of the overall trends in cancer incidence and mortality rates, particularly among individuals in certain age groups and racial or ethnic groups, can help oncology nurses identify populations at risk. These groups may require specialized prevention or early detection programs. If they live in identifiable communities, efforts can be made to provide more targeted prevention and early detection intervention strategies that are culturally acceptable.

Data on the differences in stage at diagnosis, prognosis, incidence, and mortality rates are readily available from the SEER program and from the ACS. The figure below illustrates

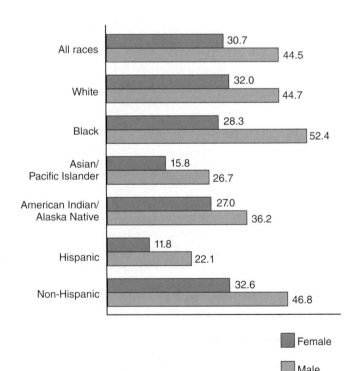

Number of New Cases of Lung Cancer per 100,000 Persons by Race or Ethnicity and Sex. The graph shows the distribution of lung cancer cases by race and ethnicity for men and women. (From SEER Stat Fact Sheets. Lung and bronchus https://seer.cancer.gov/statfacts/html/lungb.html [accessed December 21, 2021].)

differences in mortality rates and incidence among several ethnic groups. This information can be particularly helpful when screening programs that target populations at risk are developed.

Epidemiology Resources

Each year, the ACS publishes *Cancer Facts and Figures*. It is an invaluable resource that nurses can use to quickly gather estimated incidence data about cancer cases. The information is presented in several different formats, including the estimated projected number of new cases of specific cancers (i.e., incidence) and estimated mortality rates. The incidence rates are also given by state. Oncology nurses can obtain this publication free of charge from the local unit of the ACS or online at www.cancer.org and may find it helpful to better understand the incidence of specific cancers in the geographic areas of the country in which they practice. The publication also offers detailed information about primary and secondary cancer prevention of major tumors and projected survival data by stage.

Similar resources are available for specific cancers such as breast or colon cancer, for which detailed information is provided (ACS, 2019a, 2020). Other resources detail cancer risks for specific racial or ethnic groups (ACS, 2018a, 2019b). Resources are also available for prevention statistics and global cancer statistics (ACS, 2018b, 2021b).

Another source of commonly cited data is the SEER program. Data have been collected by the SEER program for incidence, mortality rates, and survival rates from 1973 through 2018. Data from the SEER geographic areas are used to represent an estimated 26% of the U.S. population. Approximately 250,000 new cases are added yearly. This information can be obtained easily at the NCI's web site https://seer.cancer.gov/.

Conclusion

Knowledge and integration of epidemiologic concepts are essential in oncology nursing practice. The concepts have implications for risk assessment, prevention recommendations, screening strategies, and monitoring of therapeutic effectiveness.

Epidemiologic data are presented in numerous formats. Nurses can use this information when educating patients, devising screening or prevention programs, conducting clinical research, and monitoring the effectiveness of therapy.

References

American Cancer Society. (2018a). *Cancer facts & figures 2018-2020 for Hispanics/Latinos*. Atlanta, GA: American Cancer Society.

American Cancer Society. (2018b). *Global cancer facts & figures* (4th ed.). Atlanta, GA: American Cancer Society.

American Cancer Society. (2019a). *Breast cancer facts & figures 2019-2020*. Atlanta, GA: American Cancer Society.

American Cancer Society. (2019b). *Cancer facts & figures for African Americans—2019-2021*. Atlanta, GA: American Cancer Society.

American Cancer Society. (2020). *Colorectal cancer facts & figures 2020-2022*. Atlanta, GA: American Cancer Society.

American Cancer Society. (2021a). *Cancer facts & figures 2021*. Atlanta, GA: American Cancer Society.

American Cancer Society. (2021b). *Cancer prevention and early detection facts & figures 2021-2022*. Atlanta, GA: American Cancer Society.

Celentano, D. D., & Szklo, M. (2019). *Gordis epidemiology* (6th ed.). Philadelphia, PA: Elsevier.

Mahon, S. M. (2021a). *Understanding genomic and hereditary cancer risk: A handbook for oncology nurses*. Pittsburgh, PA: Oncology Nursing Society.

Mahon, S. M. (2021b). Survivorship care: More than checking a box. *Clinical Journal of Oncology Nursing, 25*(6), 3–4. https://doi.org/10.1188/21.CJON.S2.3-4.

National Cancer Institute. (n.d.). The breast cancer risk assessment tool. Available at https://bcrisktool.cancer.gov/ (accessed December 20, 2021).

National Comprehensive Cancer Network. (2021a). Breast cancer risk reduction version 1.2021. Available at https://www.nccn.org/login?ReturnURL=https://www.nccn.org/professionals/physician_gls/pdf/breast_risk.pdf (accessed December 21, 2021).

National Comprehensive Cancer Network. (2021b). Breast cancer screening and diagnosis version 1.2021. Available at https://www.nccn.org/guidelines/guidelines-detail?category=2&id=142 1 (accessed December 20, 2021).

National Comprehensive Cancer Network. (2021c). Colorectal cancer screening version 2.2021. Available at https://www.nccn.org/guidelines/guidelines-detail?category=2&id=1429 (accessed December 20, 2021).

National Comprehensive Cancer Network. (2021d). Prostate cancer early detection version 2.21. Available at https://www.nccn.org/guidelines/guidelines-detail?category=2&id=1460 (accessed December 20, 2021).

National Comprehensive Cancer Network. (2022a). NCCN Clinical Practice Guidelines in Oncology (NCCN Guidelines®): Genetic/familial high-risk assessment: Colorectal [v.1.2022]. Available at https://www.nccn.org/professionals/physician_gls/pdf/genetics_colon.pdf (accessed December 20, 2021).

National Comprehensive Cancer Network. (2022b). Genetic/familial high-risk assessment: Breast, ovarian, and pancreatic version 1.2022. Available at https://www.nccn.org/guidelines/guidelines-detail?category=2&id=1503 (accessed December 20, 2021).

National Comprehensive Cancer Network. (2022c). Lung cancer screening version 1.2022. Available at https://www.nccn.org/guidelines/guidelines-detail?category=2&id=1441 (accessed December 20, 2021).

Smith, R. A., Andrews, K. S., Brooks, D., Fedewa, S. A., Manassaram-Baptiste, D., Saslow, D., … Wender, R. C. (2017). Cancer screening in the United States, 2017: A review of current American Cancer Society guidelines and current issues in cancer screening. *CA: A Cancer Journal for Clinicians, 67*(2), 100–121. https://doi.org/10.3322/caac.21392.

United States Preventive Services Task Force. (2021). A and B recommendations. Available at https://www.uspreventiveservicestaskforce.org/uspstf/recommendation-topics/uspstf-and-b-recommendations (accessed December 12, 2021).

Whitton-Smith, A., Schmidt, R., Howlett, K., Hatfield, R., & Mahon, S. M. (2021). Breast cancer: Survivorship care case study, care plan, and commentaries. *Clinical Journal of Oncology Nursing, 25*(6), 34–42. https://doi.org/10.1188/21.CJON.S2.34-42.

Cancer Pathophysiology

Grace Cullen

Introduction

Cancer is a state of cellular deviation from the normal rules of growth and reproduction marked by uncontrolled cellular division, tissue invasion, and inappropriate use of bodily resources that can lead to death. It is a genetic disease that is comprised of a complex series of processes and pathways involving multiple factors. It is one of the leading causes of death in the world and has been one of the largest utilizers of health care resources.

Cell Cycle

Genetic information is typically retained, repaired, and passed to daughter cells during the cell cycle process. However, mistakes that can be made by the cycle or its regulating system can result in uncontrollable cellular growth leading to cancer. Somatic cells are commonly associated with this cell cycle which involves two main phases: interphase and mitosis. Subdivisions during interphase are important to cell division

The Cell Cycle. (From Herlihy, B. [2022]. *The human body in health and illness* [7th ed.]. Elsevier.)

and maintenance of genetic material. These subdivisions include G1, S, and G2. Cells may also go into a fourth phase, G0, where they die and no longer divide (Mercadante & Kasi, 2021) (see the figure in the left column below).

Cell-to-cell adhesion and cell-to-extracellular matrix interactions are important in maintaining balance in healthy tissues. Proteins that mediate these activities are collectively referred to as cell adhesion molecules (CAMs) that consist of four major groups: cadherins, integrins, selections, and immunoglobulins. They physically anchor cells and integrate signals between the extracellular microenvironment and cells. These include biochemical cues as adhesion proteins can be ligand-activated receptors as well as initiate mechanotransduction triggered by physical environment changes. Mutations and changes in the expression of these adhesion proteins, particularly cadherins and integrins, are largely associated with diseases, including cancer (Janiszewska et al., 2020).

Stem cells are nonspecialized cells that can exist in the embryo and the adult cell in the human body. They can self-renew and differentiate into any cell of the organism. There are several steps to their specialization, and their developmental potency is reduced with each step. Therefore, a unipotent stem cell cannot differentiate into as many cell types as a pluripotent stem cell. Stem cell specialization is influenced by internal factors such as signals controlled by genes in the deoxyribonucleic acid (DNA), and external factors, such as physical contact between cells or chemical secretions from surrounding tissue. Stem cells can also act as the body's internal repair mechanism, with the formation of new stem cells being unrestricted for as long as an organism is alive. Formation of new stem cells is influenced by their location. For instance, they can constantly divide in the bone marrow, but in organs such as the pancreas, they only divide under special physiologic conditions (Zakrzewski et al., 2019).

Totipotent stem cells have the highest differentiation potential and can divide and differentiate into cells of the entire organism. They can form both embryonic and extra-embryonic structures. An example is a zygote which is formed after a sperm fertilizes an egg. These cells can develop into any of the three germ layers (endoderm, mesoderm, and ectoderm) which make up the cellular blueprint for tissues and organs during embryonic development, or form a placenta (Zakrzewski et al., 2019; Ferretti & Hadjantonakis, 2019).

After about 4 days, the blastocysts inner cell mass becomes pluripotent stem cells. These cells form the germ layers but not extra-embryonic structures, like the placenta. Examples of pluripotent stem cells are embryonic stem cells, which originate from the inner cell mass of preimplantation embryos, and induced pluripotent stem cells, which originate from the epiblast layer of implanted embryos. Induced pluripotent stem cells are artificially generated from somatic cells and function just like pluripotent cells. They show promising utility in regenerative medicine. Pluripotent cells function in a sequence that ends in cells with less potency, such as the multipotent, oligopotent, and unipotent stem cells (Zakrzewski et al., 2019).

Although multipotent stem cells have less ability at differentiation than pluripotent cells, they specialize in distinct cells of specific lineages. An example is a hematopoietic stem cell which develops into different types of blood cells. After they differentiate, hematopoietic stem cells become oligopotent, which restricts their ability to differentiate within cells of their lineage but can still differentiate into several cell types. For instance, a myeloid stem cell can divide into white but not red blood cells (Zakrzewski et al., 2019).

Unipotent stem cells have the lowest ability for differentiation among stem cells but can divide repeatedly which makes their role in future use for regenerative medicine promising. They can only form on cell type, an example of which are dermatocytes (Zakrzewski et al., 2019).

Nonembryonic or somatic stem cells (also called "adult" stem cells) are found in a tissue or organ and can differentiate to yield the specialized cell types of that tissue or organ. They serve as an internal repair system that generates replacement cells for those that are lost through normal wear and tear, injury, or disease. They are generally associated with specific anatomic locations and may not divide for long periods of time until they are activated by a normal need for more cells for maintenance and repair of tissues (National Institutes of Health, 2016).

Among the types of somatic stem cells are mesenchymal stem cells which can be found in many tissues. In the bone marrow, they can differentiate into the bone, cartilage, and fat cells. They act pluripotently and can specialize in any of the germ layers. Neural cells produce nerve cells and their supporting cells, the oligodendrocytes and astrocytes. Hematopoietic stem cells form the different blood cells (red, white, and platelets). Skin stem cells can form keratinocytes that create a protective layer for the skin (Zakrzewski et al., 2019) (see the figure below).

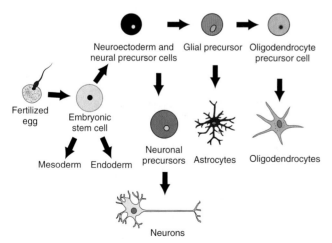

Stem Cells and Neural Precursor Cells. (From Winn, R. H. [2023]. *Youmans & Winn neurological surgery* [8th ed.]. Elsevier.)

Terminally differentiated somatic cells can be reprogrammed to become pluripotent again by downregulating genes that promote genome stability, such as *P53*. They can propagate indefinitely and differentiate into any kind of cell and be an unlimited resource for replacing lost or diseased tissue. Induced pluripotent stem cells can bypass the need for embryos in stem cell therapy. They can be autologous, or made from the patient's own cells, and not lead to the risk of immune rejection. Because of this, they have a promising use in restorative medicine. Among the conditions that may benefit from stem cell therapy that is being evaluated at this time are macular degeneration, osteoarthritis, neurodegenerative diseases, diabetes, fertility diseases, and cardiovascular accidents (Zakrzewski et al., 2019).

Use of stem cell therapy is not without its challenges, including ethical concerns, risk of immunologic rejection of the stem cells by the patient's body, the possibility of complications that may be associated with obtaining stem cells, such as pain or the risk of morbidity in both the patient and the donor, and the chances of oncogene (OCG) expression when cells are reprogrammed (Zakrzewski et al., 2019).

Deoxyribonucleic Acid

DNA is the material through which genetic information is stored and transmitted. Two aspects of DNA's structure were identified by Watson and Crick in the 1950s. This includes the pairing of the nucleotide bases in a complementary fashion (e.g., adenine with thymine, and cytosine with guanine) and its double-helical nature (Watson & Crick, 1953). Insight into DNA's structure, such as the equivalent ratios of purines and pyrimidines found in the molecule, provided a framework for the understanding of the mechanism of DNA replication. The remarkable structure of DNA, from the nucleotide up to the chromosome, plays a crucial role in biologic function (Ghannam et al., 2021).

When the DNA structure is changed or mutated, proteins encoded by the mutated DNA undergo alteration that can adversely impact the survival of the cell or organism. This mutation can take many forms, such as big or small insertions or deletion of base pairs, or insertions and inversions of whole DNA segments between or within chromosomes. As a consequence, the proteins that are encoded by genes with mutations may have changes in their amino acid sequence that can alter their function and subsequently lead to adverse impacts in the cell (Ghannam et al., 2021).

Damage to the cellular DNA can result from intrinsic factors such as naturally occurring reactive oxygen species, reactive nitrogen and carbonyl species, lipid peroxidation products, and the chemical lability of DNA. Extrinsic factors that can result in DNA damage include exposure to ultraviolet (UV) light, ionizing radiation, chemicals in the air, food, and water, and cancer chemotherapeutics. Cells can sustain greater than 100,000 spontaneous DNA lesions daily. Most DNA lesions are single-strand damage that includes damage to the base and single-strand breaks. Double-strand DNA breaks are not common. Double-strand breaks can be due to stress from replication, creation of single-strand gaps or breaks during repair of single-strand lesions, and exposure to ionizing radiation. Clustered or complex lesions are rare and can result from exposure to ionizing radiation or certain chemicals, like bleomycin. Clustered lesions are more challenging to repair with the DNA repair mechanisms than dispersed lesions and are more mutagenic (Nickoloff et al., 2020).

Exogenous or induced damage is from external factors influencing the cell. Common causes are radiation such as UV light exposure (UVA and UVB) and ionizing radiation, thermal disruptions, toxins and drugs that cause base-pair mismatches, and intercalation that inhibits replication. UV damage can cause the cross-linking of adjacent cytosine and thymine bases, leading to the formation of harmful dimers. Certain toxins and drugs can also cause chemical associations leading to single- or double-strand breakage in the composition of DNA. Thermal disruption of DNA by exposure to high temperatures can lead to higher rates of depurination as well as single-strand breaks. Environmental toxins, such as cigarette smoke, contain carcinogens like benzo[a]pyrene that can be oxidized by cellular enzymes and lead to DNA damage (Lewis & Dimri, 2021).

The damage to DNA requires correction for cells to continue to appropriately function. Without regular repair, the integrity of the genome will be compromised. The cell can take different actions to repair DNA. Most of these errors are corrected by DNA polymerase during replication with its proofreading mechanism that allows for it to read the most recently placed base before adding the next. If the base does not pair correctly with the base on the template strand, then the exonuclease mechanism of DNA cuts the phosphodiester bond holding that section of the strand and releases the nucleotide. This process is not perfect and can be flawed, and incorrect bases are commonly left in the newly synthesized DNA strand. Mismatch repair proteins correct this by locating incorrectly matched nucleotides and removing them before placing the correct nucleotides in place (Lewis & Dimri, 2021).

Damage to the DNA is different from DNA mutations in that the single- and double-strand breakages in a damaged DNA are repairable. DNA repair can occur through the actions of enzymes in the cell because they have a repair template present either in the complementary strand of a damaged DNA molecule or a homologous chromosome that can be copied and used to create the correct base pairs and orders in the double helix. In DNA mutations, there is a permanent alteration to the base-pair sequence of the DNA that is irreparable by enzymes because there is no template available for the correct base-pair sequence to be integrated into the strand. Mutations can influence how genes are expressed, while damage can cause either a halt in gene function or damage to the cell. DNA damage can also lead to mutations, but while mutations can lead to harmful byproducts, they do not cause direct damage to the mutated gene or DNA molecule (Lewis & Dimri, 2021).

Unrepaired damage to DNA molecules can often lead to carcinogenesis, the development of cancer cells that can easily spread and replicate through mitosis. DNA repair mechanisms can be impaired by carcinogens in the body. Studies are underway targeting DNA repair pathways that have undergone mutagenetic changes to fight the tumor and induce malignant cell death (Lewis & Dimri, 2021).

Cell Surface and Membrane Changes

Some of the acquired characteristics of cancer cells involve surface and membrane changes. The cells that make up a multicellular organism interact with each other and with the extracellular matrix (ECM). The structure of the ECM differs by tissue type, and it is essential for the growth and survival of normal cells. For example, ECM components interact and combine with growth factors, controlling their availability to the cells. Without these interactions with the ECM, normal cells will undergo apoptosis. Malignant neoplastic cells can survive and reproduce without the usual interactions with the ECM. Cancer cells produce plasminogen activator, which helps to break down plasminogen to plasmin. Plasmin can cause the release of growth factors in cancer cells, leading to proliferation of these mutant cells or gain of function (Pickup et al., 2014).

Matrix Metalloproteinases

Matrix metalloproteinases (MMPs) are a family of proteases (enzymes that degrade proteins) that regulate the microenvironment of cells by controlling growth factors and their receptors. They are active in cell adhesion and apoptosis, and they can degrade the protein components of the ECM and basement membranes. Some MMPs generate specific signals that promote tumor development and the growth of new blood vessels (angiogenesis) to support tumor growth. Increased expression of MMPs correlates with a poor prognosis and more a invasive disease (Kessenbrock et al., 2015).

Carcinogens

Carcinogens are environmental agents that can increase the chance of mutational events and cause tumors. Agents are considered *carcinogenic* if they can contribute to the development of cancers and *oncogenic* if they can cause tumors. Carcinogens typically work on the DNA where genes are encoded, making them mutagenic as well. The process of carcinogenesis is believed to involve multiple steps and more than a single carcinogen. Neoplastic activity does not need the continued presence of a carcinogen once it has been established. This is the reason why causative agents are not typically found in the resulting tumors (although mutational clues may be present), except for some carcinogenic viruses whose genetic material can remain in the tumors and some insoluble substances like asbestos, which does not go away from the tissues (Arends, 2019).

Identification of Carcinogens

Tumor formation is felt to require both environmental and inherited factors, but about 70% to 85% are associated with environmental factors. Much of what is known about carcinogens comes from indirect evidence because it typically takes a long time from exposure to the development of clinical signs and symptoms, sometimes as much as two to three decades.

Among the evidence used are epidemiologic studies, assessment of occupational risks, direct accidental exposure, laboratory animal testing, transforming effects on cell cultures, mutagenicity testing in bacteria, genome sequencing, and mutational signature analysis (Arends, 2019).

Epidemiologic Evidence

Certain types of cancer are more common in certain countries, regions, or communities, and this is determined by studying tumor incidence using diagnostic records, cancer registries, or physical inspection. Findings of a high tumor incidence in a population should prompt comparisons of lifestyle, diet, and occupational risks with a population that has a lower tumor incidence. Factors such as population movement of migrants should be considered, particularly when trying to distinguish between racial or hereditary factors and environmental factors (Arends, 2019).

For instance, hepatocellular carcinoma (HCC), the most common type of liver cancer, has the highest incidence in Africa and Asia. While hepatitis B virus (HBV) and hepatitis C virus (HCV) have been identified as the most crucial risk factors in the development of HCC, other factors such as excessive alcohol use have also been found to contribute to the development of HCC. Calculation of the personal attributable fraction (PAF) estimates how individual risk factors can contribute to the burden of HCC. The global HBV PAF is 56%, while the HBV PAF for Eastern Asia is about 69% and only approximately 7% for North America. This can be due in part to more active HBV vaccination programs in North America. On the other hand, the global PAF for alcohol-related HCC is about 26% and even higher at 39% in Eastern Europe, while it is only 13% in South Asia (McGlynn et al., 2021).

Occupational and Behavioral Risks

Some cancers can be more common in people with certain lifestyle choices and occupations. For instance, there is a linear dose-response relationship found between the number of cigarettes smoked daily and the risk of developing lung cancer. The risk of cervical cancer is increased with multiple sexual partners due to higher risk of sexually transmitted infections like human papillomavirus (HPV) (Huang et al., 2020). High-risk genotypes of HPV (HPV 16 and 18) are associated with cervical cancer and its precursor, cervical intra-epithelial neoplasia (CIN). This has led to the use of HPV immunization in reducing the incidence of cervical cancer (Arends, 2019).

Examples of occupational carcinogens are many including exposure to asbestos. Inhalation of asbestos fibers has been associated with asbestosis, pleural plaques, malignant mesothelioma, and lung carcinoma. Mesothelioma most frequently occurs in the pleura but can also be found in the peritoneum. Other manufacturing-related risks include exposure to beta-naphthylamine used in the manufacturing of rubber and has been associated with bladder carcinoma (Arends, 2019). Exposure to benzene has been associated with leukemia and nasopharyngeal cancer. Exposure to formaldehyde and sulfuric acid has been linked to laryngeal cancer and kidney cancer, respectively (Li et al., 2021).

Oncogenic Viruses

Many human tumors are associated with viruses and tend to be more common in younger people and those who are immunosuppressed. Oncogenic RNA viral genome is reverse transcribed into DNA by reverse transcriptase prior to integration. An oncogenic DNA viral genome is then directly integrated into the host cell DNA. Examples are Epstein-Barr virus (EBV), which has been associated with Burkitt lymphoma and nasopharyngeal cancer; HBV and HCV, which have been associated with HCC; and HPV in cervical and oral cancer (Arends, 2019).

Radiant Energy

Exposure to ionizing radiation has been associated with an increased risk of different cancers, including leukemia and others. A nuclear reactor explosion in Ukraine in the 1980s led to the release of large quantities of radioactive material into the atmosphere, including radioactive iodine. Iodine is a substance concentrated by the thyroid gland when thyroid hormone is synthesized. Four years after the nuclear incident, there was a dramatic increase in the incidence of thyroid carcinoma among children living in the area. Nowadays, nonradioactive iodine is given to people immediately after accidental exposure to radioactive iodine to compete for uptake by the thyroid gland (Arends, 2019).

UV light has been associated with skin cancer, including malignant melanoma, basal cell carcinoma, and squamous cell carcinoma (Losquadro, 2017). Although radiant UV light is a carcinogen, the risk of developing skin cancer is decreased among people with naturally pigmented skin due to the protective effect of melanin against UV light. Patients with xeroderma pigmentosum, a rare congenital deficiency of one family of the nucleotide excision repair enzymes, are at a higher risk of developing skin cancer due to a genetic inability of skin cells to repair DNA damage from UV light exposure (Arends, 2019).

Hormones

Exogenous estrogens have been known to promote mammary and endometrial carcinomas. Androgenic and anabolic steroids have been associated with hepatocellular tumors. Estrogenic steroids can make otherwise asymptomatic, preexisting lesions such as adenomas and focal nodular hyperplasia abnormally vascular, causing them to be present clinically (Arends, 2019).

Bacteria, Parasites, and Miscellaneous Carcinogens

Helicobacter pylori (*H. pylori*) is largely associated with gastritis and peptic ulcers and is also associated with the development of gastric mucosa-associated lymphoid tissue lymphomas and gastric adenocarcinoma. Although the molecular mechanisms in which *H. pylori* can influence cellular pathways remain unknown, there is some evidence to suggest that bacteria can suppress *p53* and DNA damage repair activities leading to carcinogenesis (Zella & Gallo, 2021).

Opisthorchis viverrini and *Clonorchis sinensis* cause an inflammatory reaction and epithelial hyperplasia in the bile ducts and are implicated with cholangiocarcinoma particularly in the Far East, where they are more common. *Schistosoma haematobium* has been associated with bladder cancer and is commonly found in Egypt (Arends, 2019).

Host Factors in Carcinogenesis

Aging. The incidence of cancer increases with age, with a median age of 66 years at the time of a cancer diagnosis. In the United States, the incidence of cancer in people 65 years of age and older is almost nine times that of people younger than 65 years of age. Worldwide, approximately 80% of cancers are diagnosed in people 50 years of age or older (Krasnick et al., 2022). The major reason for this is the accumulation of mutations over time. The more division a cell goes through over time, it will allow for more mistakes to occur. Cancer treatment is also less well studied in the elderly, and they are typically underrepresented in clinical trials (Krasnick et al., 2022).

Obesity and Physical Activity

Epidemiologic studies have shown that obesity is a risk factor for different sites of cancer. Immune, metabolic, endocrine, and inflammatory properties of excess adipose tissue appear to contribute to the increased incidence of malignancy among overweight or obese individuals. For instance, greater amounts of adipose tissue can lead to increased levels of free fatty acids in the circulation. Liver, muscle, and other tissues subsequently increase their use of fats for energy production, leading to a lesser need for uptake and metabolism of glucose and resulting in hyperglycemia. This functional insulin resistance leads to an increase in pancreatic insulin secretion. Studies have shown that chronic hyperinsulinemia increases the risk for colon and endometrial cancer and probably other tumors such as the pancreas and kidney (Krasnick et al., 2022).

Obesity can also cause an increase in the adipocyte-derived stem cell and adipose tissue deposition in the tumor microenvironment that can lead to ECM deposition, alteration in immune profiles, as well as increased supply of growth factors, nutrients, and cytokines that promote tumor growth. Adipocyte-derived stem cells can also promote fibrosis and become associated with fibroblasts, which have been associated with a more aggressive cancer biology. Increased adiposity in the omentum for patients who are obese has also been associated with a proinflammatory state that can promote cancer at different sites through immune cell activation and inflammatory signaling pathways. Obesity is associated with increased estrogen levels, and circulating levels of estrogen are associated with cancers of the breast (in postmenopausal women) as well as the endometrium (Krasnick et al., 2022).

Physical activity has also been shown to improve the regulation of the cell cycle and DNA repair pathways in patients undergoing surveillance for prostate cancer. Decreased physical activity has also been associated with an increased incidence of many types of cancer, including esophageal adenocarcinoma, colorectal adenocarcinoma, gallbladder, and liver cancer (Krasnick et al., 2022).

Race

The exact mechanism of how race plays a role in the development of cancer is complicated by the fact that racial difference coincides with difference in place of residence, diet, and cultural influences. For instance, oral cancer is common in India and South Asia, not because of their race but because of the practice of using smokeless tobacco. Tobacco comes from the leaves of two plant species, *Nicotiana tabacum and Nicotiana rustica*. Although the most important and addictive ingredient of tobacco is nicotine, the more severe health impact of smokeless tobacco comes from other chemicals, such as tobacco-specific nitrosamines (TSNAs). Higher arsenic levels have also been found in the blood of patients who chew tobacco (Muthukrishnan & Warnakulasuriya, 2018).

A study conducted among all Black populations in the United States, including US-born African Americans, African and Afro-Caribbean immigrants, showed heterogeneity by place of birth in US cancer mortality profiles. US-born African Americans had the highest mortality rates for common and infection-related cancers, while Afro-Caribbean immigrants had intermediate rates and African immigrants had the lowest rates. Prostate cancer was more common among West Africans, and liver cancer was higher among East Africans (Pinheiro et al., 2020).

Constitutional Factors

Inherited Predisposition

Some risks are inherited such as women inheriting mutant *BRCA1* (chromosome 17) or *BRCA2* (chromosome 13) genes being at greater risk for developing breast cancer. Familial *adenomatous polyposis coli* (*APC*) is an autosomal-dominant, inherited predisposition to develop several adenomatous polyps of the large bowel due to mutant *APC* gene (chromosome 5), with a risk of colon and rectum adenocarcinoma arising from these polyps up to 100% of the time if not resected. A malignant tumor of the eye in children, retinoblastoma, can be due to an abnormality of the *RB1* gene (chromosome 13) and is often bilateral. Autosomal recessive inheritance of one of the mutated *FANC* genes has been associated with Fanconi anemia which can give rise to leukemia and congenital defects (Arends, 2019).

Sex

Certain cancers can be more common in one gender over the other, such as breast cancer, which is more common in women than men, likely due to a higher mammary epithelial volume and promoting effects of estrogens in females (Arends, 2019). Cases of renal cell carcinoma among men account for two-thirds of global cases and deaths. This may be due in part to modifiable risk factors such as smoking, hypertension, and obesity among men (Padala et al., 2020).

Premalignant Lesions and Conditions

Premalignant lesions are local abnormalities that increase the risk of a malignant tumor developing at that site, such as adenomatous polyps of the colon and rectum and epithelial dysplasia in different sites, including the skin and cervix. These lesions are partially neoplastic cells which have yet to achieve a full malignant neoplastic state. Screening can detect these premalignant lesions, allowing for earlier diagnosis, treatment, and improved outcomes (Arends, 2019).

Premalignant conditions are also associated with a higher risk of malignant tumors, such as chronic ulcerative colitis, which increases the risk for colorectal cancer and can be predicted by the finding of premalignant lesions or dysplasia in biopsies. Conditions such as hepatic cirrhosis from different causes can increase the risk of HCC. Congenital abnormalities, such as undescended testis, pose an increased risk for neoplasm than a normally located testis.

Transplacental Carcinogenesis

Transplacental carcinogenesis is the administration of a carcinogen to a pregnant woman, but the carcinogenic effect is exhibited by the child on reaching young adulthood. An example is the use of diethylstilbestrol, a synthetic estrogenic compound, among pregnant women from the 1940s to the 1970s to prevent miscarriages. These babies were successfully delivered to full term but went on to develop vaginal clear cell adenocarcinoma in their early adult years (Arends, 2019).

Cellular and Molecular Events in Carcinogenesis

Oncogenes and Tumor-Suppressor Genes

Tumor suppressor genes (TSGs) are largely disrupted by copy number deletions and loss--function (nonsense and frameshift) mutations, while OCGs are mainly activated by focal amplifications and missense mutations. TSGs are often biallelically inactivated (*two-hit theory*), while OCGs are frequently activated by dominant-acting heterozygous single events. In TSGs, loss-of-function mutations are distributed throughout their length, whereas in OCGs, missense mutations affect specific hotspots, which include few highly recurrent (major) positions (such as *KRAS* G12, G13, and Q61) and a much larger number of rare (minor) positions. Minor hotspot mutations are functionally weak and rare as individuals but account for a significant portion of the accumulated mutations. However, little is known as to why such minor mutations are frequently observed in cancer despite their weak function (Saito et al., 2021).

Advances in cancer genomics have enabled the identification and characterization of many cancer genes and the associated mutations driving each patient's tumor. Defective TSGs and hyperactive OCGs are associated with cell proliferation and apoptosis through genetic variations like somatic mutations and deletions during the development of cancer. They usually perform their cellular functions jointly. TSGs have the highest mutation frequency in most tumor types with OCG only being second. Even though they have different mutation patterns, they have similar and stronger protein-protein characteristics relative to the essential and control proteins in the whole human interactome. They have also been found to have the most direct interactions with cancer drug targets. OCG mutations are usually dominant, so one mutant copy is usually enough to start switching a cellular activity. Although TSG mutations have been found to be recessive following the two-hit hypothesis of needing both copies of TSGs to mutate to cause loss of function, there has been increasing evidence that even partial inactivation of TSGs can lead to tumorigenesis (Zhu et al., 2015).

The development of cancer is driven by the accumulation of somatic mutations and other genetic alterations that impair cell-division checkpoints, resulting in abnormal cell proliferation and eventually tumorigenesis (drivers). Identification of cancer genes provides insights into the processes involved in tumorigenesis as well as possible therapy targets. Like any other gene in the genome, cancer genes are expected to accumulate passenger mutations that do not contribute to or even hinder cancer progression. Thus, although cancer genes often harbor driver mutations, only a small number of them are actual drivers (Iranzo et al., 2018).

One question that comes up about cancer-driver mutations is their specificity in different cancer types. Some tumors show recurrent mutation patterns, such as the oncogenic fusion *BCR-ABL* in chronic myeloid leukemia or the inactivation of specific tumor suppressors, for example, *RB1* in retinoblastoma. Other tumors appear to be the product of interchangeable mutations in a pool of genes involved in key signaling pathways, such as the receptor tyrosine kinase *RAS/RAF* pathway in lung adenocarcinoma. Between these two, intermediate degrees of specificity are observed in many cancer types. Also, even though numerous studies on cancer mutations have resulted in extensive lists of genes that are mutated in various cancers, a quantitative understanding of the extent to which the current tumor classification reflects the existence of specific sets of driver mutations is scarce. An increase in driver mutations is noted with advancing age, largely between 60 and 70 years (Iranzo et al., 2018).

Growth Factor Receptors

Besides cell cycle regulation involving OCGs and TSGs, interaction with tumor- or stroma-derived growth factors is essential for growth inhibition. For instance, breast cancer cell proliferation by co-culture with fibroblasts is inhibited by $1,25(OH)_2 D_3$. Transforming growth factor-β (TGFβ) is involved in cell cycle and apoptosis and works by interfering the series of events that lead to inhibiting the ability of cells to enter the S phase. It has been shown to suppress c-myc, cyclin A and E, and CDK 2 and 4 expression. It has also been associated with the inhibition of p110. Vitamin D_3 compounds induce dephosphorylation of the retinoblastoma gene product, and vitamin D_3 growth inhibition of MCF-7 breast cancer cells is inhibited by TGFβ neutralizing antibody (van Driel et al., 2018).

Signal Transducers: Kinases and Transcription Factors

Kinases are enzymes that catalyze many significant processes, such as signal transduction, transcription, and metabolism. Mutations in signal transducers such as kinases and other proteins can result in uncontrolled cellular proliferation. Nuclear transcription factors are proteins that bind to specific DNA sequences and regulate the expression of genes that are associated with cellular growth, proliferation, metabolism, differentiation, and apoptosis. Overexpression of the transcription factor *MYC* is a common mutation typically associated with cancer and leads to uncontrolled growth and a loss of apoptosis (Yu et al., 2014).

Physiologic Changes in Tumorigenesis

Sustained Proliferation Signaling

Cells in normal tissues typically receive signals for growth from themselves (autocrine), by neighboring cells (paracrine), or through systemic (endocrine) factors. The growth of tumor depends on the response of tumor cells to paracrine, endocrine, and autocrine factors. These include angiogenesis factors, growth factors, chemokines, cytokines, hormones, enzymes, and cytolytic factors that can promote or reduce tumor growth. An example of hormone signaling impacting cancer growth is evident in breast cancer, wherein an overexpression of the nuclear estrogen receptor leads to estrogen-dependent tumor cell proliferation. Taking away the supply of estrogen from the tumor or blocking the receptor leads to decreased tumor cell proliferation and induces cell death (Krasnick et al., 2022).

To maintain proliferation, growth signaling pathways, including extracellular growth signals, transmembrane transducers of those signals, or intracellular signaling pathways that translate those signals into action, are altered. Growth factors are also overexpressed in cancer and enable cancer cells to grow with low levels of growth factors that do not normally trigger proliferation (Krasnick et al., 2022).

Many OCGs mimic normal growth signaling and induce mitogenic signals without stimulation from upstream regulators. For example, *KRAS* (*Kirsten rat sarcoma viral* OCG homologue), seen in a variety of cancers, has activating mutations leading to receptor-independent signaling (Krasnick et al., 2022; Huang et al., 2021). This *KRAS* signaling cascade leads to different protumor activities such as sustained proliferation, immune evasion, resistance to apoptosis, cell migration, and metastasis. *BRAF* (v-raf murine sarcoma viral OCG homolog B1) is another mutated OCG whose activating mutations lead to constitutive activation, upregulation of MEK and ERK signaling, and increased transcription of protumor survival and proliferation factors and pathways (Krasnick et al., 2022; Eachkoti et al., 2018).

These mutations have been associated with cancers such as melanoma, colorectal, and thyroid cancer. Finally, negative feedback mechanisms can be disrupted, thereby enhancing proliferative signaling by failing to regulate normal signaling pathways (Krasnick et al., 2022).

Evading Growth Suppressors

Cell division is a tightly regulated process that involves both stimulatory and inhibitory signals. Tumor cells acquire stimulatory growth signals and overcome growth-inhibitory signals. Many antiproliferative signals involve the retinoblastoma protein (pRb). This protein can block cell division by binding E2F transcription factors that control the expression of genes essential for progression from G_1 into the S phase of the cell cycle. Disruption of the pRb pathway can liberate E2Fs and lead to cell proliferation by rendering cells insensitive to antigrowth factors that normally operate along this pathway (Krasnick et al., 2022).

Cancer cells can also turn off the expression of integrins and other CAMs that send antigrowth signals. Tumor cells can avoid terminal differentiation through overexpression of the OCG c-*myc* which encodes a transcription factor that regulates expression of cyclins and cyclin-dependent kinases. In colon cancer carcinogenesis, mutations of *APC*, a negative regulator of β-catenin, can lead to processes that block the terminal differentiation of enterocytes in colonic crypts (Krasnick et al., 2022).

Avoiding Immune Destruction

Cancer cells can avoid immune system detection and attack, a mechanism that is influenced by the expression of cell surface proteins. Protein kinases such as ATM and ATR are DNA damage sensors that are required to upregulate cell surface ligands. In the setting of cancer, this mechanism is altered, leading to disruption of cancer immune surveillance and increase in cancer cell resistance to phagocytosis (Huang & Zhou, 2021).

The immune-oncology cycle also works by improving the activity of T lymphocytes and is triggered by tumor antigens carried by antigen-presenting cells (APCs). APCs can capture, process, and present exogenous antigen to T cells. Dendritic cells (DCs), macrophages, and B cells are considered the three major types of APCs. In solid tumor, antigen uptake and presentation are largely performed by DC and macrophages, but only DCs can migrate to the lymph nodes and initiate T cell activation and antitumor activity, as well as regulate T cell response within tumors during therapy (Gardner et al., 2020).

Resisting Cell Death

Most cells die due to activation of programmed cell death that exist for this purpose. The term *apoptosis* refers to the process of cells dying from physiologic suicide rather than from catastrophic events such as freezing or burning which is typically a result of necrosis. Apoptopic and mitotic activities are both present in rapidly growing tumors, but a more active mitotic process can lead to an enlarging tumor. On their own, mutations that prevent a cell from killing itself are not enough to cause a normal cell to become fully malignant, but they can promote neoplasia. Activation of the tumor suppressor *p53* can transcriptionally activate apoptosis. Overexpression of the apoptosis inhibitor BCL-2 or defects in *p53* can lead to further genetic damage that can enhance neoplastic transformation. Loss of function mutations to *p53* not only prevent apoptosis but also impair its ability to activate the DNA repair pathways, leading to cell cycle arrest (Strasser & Vaux, 2020).

When a cell that is not able to kill itself undergoes another mutation that promotes cell proliferation such as a chromosome translocation that causes overexpression of c-MYC, the combined effect will lead to the rapid growth of a malignant clone. Genetic instability increases the diversity among growing malignant cells. Chemotherapy or radiation therapy selects malignant cells that have a higher threshold for activating their intrinsic cell death mechanism and facilitates resistance to treatment (Strasser & Vaux, 2020).

Defects in tumor necrosis factor (TNF) receptor or death receptors, such as FAS, are seen in humans with autoimmune lympho-proliferative syndrome and increase their predisposition to B-cell malignancies (Strasser & Vaux, 2020).

Enabling Replicative Immortality

Studies of primary cultured fibroblasts showed that cells with longer telomeres had longer replication potentials, leading to longevity. Exogenous expression of the telomerase holoenzyme TERT can bypass the cellular growth mechanism and immortalize primary cells. The upregulation of telomerase has been linked to familial cancer risk. Overexpression of OCGs, such as *Myc* or *KRAS*, was compared in short- and long-telomere mice and showed that long-telomere mice developed more aggressive tumors and had decreased survival (McNally et al., 2019).

Inducing Angiogenesis

Malignant cells depend on the circulatory system for survival, and tumor progression is frequently accompanied by ingrowth of blood vessels. Tumor vascularization can occur through the existing vasculature or creation of new blood vessels through several cellular and molecular mechanisms. Large numbers of pro- and antiangiogenic factors regulate vascular homeostasis and when they are in balance, the vasculature is dormant and endothelial cells do not proliferate. Blood vessel formation is triggered by domination of the pro-angiogenic signaling, a term referred to as the "angiogenic switch" in tumors. This process sparks a rapid growth of malignant cells along with new blood vessel formation. An example of which is an expression of the simian virus 40 large T (SV40T) OCG in pancreatic insulinoma. In this model, tumors start as non-angiogenic clusters of dysplastic cells, some of which develop into small angiogenic tumor islets that can evolve into large, vascularized tumors and spread to other organs such as the lung. Additional genetic alterations of tumor cells can also activate the angiogenic switch and lead to increased growth and hypoxia or expression of pro-angiogenic factors, or tumor-related inflammation and recruitment of immune cells (Lugano et al., 2020).

The aorta, arteries, capillaries, and veins make up the vascular system that is responsible for transporting blood throughout the body. The capillary networks have narrow walls and help in gas exchange between the tissues and blood. Capillary venules facilitate transmigration of immune cells into tissues. The capillary wall consists of an endothelial cell layer supported by pericytes and surrounded by a basement membrane. Angiogenesis typically starts from the capillaries and plays a vital role in tumor growth, existence, and spread (Lugano et al., 2020).

There are several cellular processes that can lead to blood vessel formation in tumors. New capillaries can form from parental vessels through multiple steps, a mechanism known as sprouting angiogenesis. It starts from selection of a tip cell, where a cell from a parent vessel becomes the leading migratory cell and blocks neighboring cells from adopting the tip cell fate through a lateral inhibition process. The tip cell then travels through the chemotactic path and is followed by trailing stalk cells. The luminal space of the sprout then connects with the parent vessel, and the developing sprout then connects with other vessels—a process referred to as anastomosis. Endothelial cells are normally dormant but can engage in sprouting angiogenesis by the pro-angiogenic vascular endothelial growth factor (VEGF). The tip and stalk cell selection are regulated by an interaction between VEGF and Dll4/Notch pathways (Lugano et al., 2020).

Intussusceptive angiogenesis is where transluminal tissue pillars grow from existing blood vessels and fuse to redesign the vascular plexus. This was first detected in the remodeling of lung capillaries but has also been seen in melanoma, colorectal carcinoma, glioma, and mammary tumors. The mechanism of intussusceptive angiogenesis is not well understood but can be triggered by growth factors such as VEGF, PDGF (platelet-derived growth factor), and erythropoietin. Intussusceptive angiogenesis is believed to increase the complexity and number of microvascular structures within a tumor that leads to its growth (Lugano et al., 2020; Yeola et al., 2021).

Vasculogenesis is the process of blood vessel formation in the embryo resulting from differentiation and association of endothelial progenitor cells (EPCs). Mediation by hematopoietic cells from the bone marrow or recruitment of EPCs results in formation of new vessels that support tumor growth. EPCs are largely unipotent adult stem cells that can proliferate, self-renew, repair endothelial tissue, and engage in neovascularization. Vasculogenesis in tumors results from an interaction between tumor cells and EPCs in the bone marrow. VEGF from the tumor mobilizes VEGFR2+EPCs from the bone marrow. Factors released by tumors, such as chemokines C-C motif ligand (CCL) 2 and CCL 5, attract EPCs to the tumor and trigger neovascularization (Lugano et al., 2020).

The process whereby rapidly growing tumor cells form vessel-like structures is known as vascular mimicry. They are formed without endothelial cells and provide an alternate source of blood supply and nutrients to tumors. These endothelial-like tumor cells secrete collagens IV and VI that aid in stabilization and formation of tubular structures. Vascular mimicry is triggered by different mechanisms. In melanoma, mitochondrial reactive oxygen species can activate Met proto-OCG when subjected to hypoxia, resulting in vascular mimicry. Vascular mimicry has also been noted after antiangiogenic therapy and is thought to be the tumor's attempt at neovascularization following hypoxia. Vascular mimicry has been associated with poor prognosis among patients with cancer, but additional studies of this mechanism have been limited due to the challenges of differentiating it from normal endothelial cell lining (Lugano et al., 2020).

Normal physiologic blood vessel formation is a tightly controlled process that ends when the need for new blood vessels is met. Tumor angiogenesis, on the other hand, is poorly regulated because of the constant activity of pro-angiogenic factors in the tumor microenvironment. The vascular tree is orderly divided into arteries, arterioles, capillaries, venules, and veins. In the presence of pro-angiogenic tumor signaling, this orderly division can be disrupted, vessels may fail to mature and prune, the vessel diameter can vary, and blood flow can be impaired, resulting in hypoxia. Endothelial junctions can be disrupted in tumor vessels, leading to increased permeability. Vessels can be more fragile, increasing the likelihood of bleeding (Lugano et al., 2020).

Activating Invasion and Spread

The adhesion theory of invasion indicates that endothelial cells lining the blood vessels in certain organs permit extravasation by expressing adhesion molecules that bind tumor cells. Another theory is that chemokines secreted by the target organ can enter the circulation and attract tumor cells that express receptors for the chemokines. Studies have also shown that primary tumors create microenvironments in distant organs that promote the growth of tumor cells before they arrive. This process is achieved by a series of events that include increasing vascular permeability in microvessels of organs and attracting bone marrow-derived cell subsets that contribute to local tissue remodeling and recruitment of cancer cells (Krasnick et al., 2022).

The epithelial-to-mesenchymal transition (EMT) is a cell-biologic program influenced by transcription factors where epithelial cells turn into more mesenchymal cell states. This process is dependent on extracellular signals and intracellular gene circuitry. This system is not only involved in cancer progression but also in wound healing, tissue fibrosis, embryonic morphogenesis, and can give rise to cancer stem cells. EMT is used by cancer cells to downregulate the expression of cellular adhesion molecules, allowing the cancer cells to invade surrounding tissue, the bloodstream, and metastasize. Once at the site of distant metastasis, cells in EMT can extravasate and undergo mesenchymal-epithelial transition, allowing them to assume their original epithelial phenotype for clonal expansion and metastasis. Invasion and metastasis are also influenced by extracellular proteases that regulate extracapsular membrane turnover. Tumor progression involves an increased expression of proteases, decreased expression of protease inhibitors, and conversion of inactive forms of proteases into active enzymes. Matrix metalloproteases are overexpressed in a variety of cancers (Krasnick et al., 2022).

Deregulating Cellular Energetics and Metabolomics

Altered metabolism of cancer cells allows them to have the energy required for growth. They can limit their energy metabolism to glycolysis even in the presence of oxygen (aerobic glycolysis). Because glycolysis has a lower energy yield compared with aerobic metabolism through mitochondrial oxidative phosphorylation, cancer cells significantly increase the rate of glycolysis to meet the rapid metabolism of a dividing tumor. For instance, upregulating the expression of glucose transporters such as GLUT1 leads to an increased rate of glycolysis by tumor cells. This principle has been helpful in cancer diagnosis or staging by visualizing uptake of glucose by positron emission tomography (PET) with F-fluorodeoxyglucose (Krasnick et al., 2022).

Genomic Instability and Mutation

Under normal circumstances, the genome is maintained by caretaker genes. Alterations in this process can lead to the loss of ability to detect DNA damage, loss of ability to directly repair damaged DNA, and failure to inactivate or stop mutagenic molecules before DNA damage happens. Caretaker genes such as *TP53*, a TSG that is key in detecting and resolving mutations, can mutate and result in an increased risk of developing certain cancers (Krasnick et al., 2022).

Tumor-Promoting Inflammation

Pro-tumorigenic inflammation contributes to cancer formation by blocking antitumor immunity, making the tumor microenvironment conducive to tumor formation and by releasing signals that directly promote tumors on the epithelial and cancer cells. Tumors can cause upregulation of inflammatory mediators and recruit other immune cells that have tumor-promoting properties such as macrophages, monocytes, neutrophils, or innate lymphoid cells. Inflammation and tissue repair immune responses have been associated with tumor incidence, growth, and proliferation. Macrophages clear apoptotic cells, release chemotactic molecules to recruit other cell types as needed, regulate immune responses and barrier, and support the stem cell (Greten & Grivennikov, 2019).

There are interdependent mechanisms involved in inflammatory tissue response. Macrophages and DCs in tissues can locally proliferate in cases of mild insult to the tissue. Strong insult to the tissue can result in recruitment of immune cells from the bone marrow, including monocytes, neutrophils, and monocyte-derived cells, as well as from the secondary lymphoid tissues such as lymphoid cells. Recruited or locally intensified inflammatory cells can then activate, differentiate, and polarize based on their microenvironment. In tumors, this process of recruitment and growth can persist due to OCG-driven stress, apoptosis, and microbial signals (Greten & Grivennikov, 2019).

Some cancers follow chronic inflammation, infection, or autoimmunity at the same tissue or organ. Examples of which are inflammatory bowel diseases (IBDs), chronic hepatitis, Helicobacter-induced gastritis, or schistosoma-induced bladder inflammation that increase the risk of colorectal cancer, hepatic cancer, gastric cancer, or bladder cancer, respectively. Other examples are inhalation of particles, tobacco smoke, and asbestos that can lead to lung and airway inflammation and increase the risk of lung cancer and mesothelioma. Low-grade inflammation from chronic conditions, such as obesity, hyperglycemia, and hyperlipidemia, can also increase the risk of cancers, such as liver, pancreatic, colon, and breast, among others (Greten & Grivennikov, 2019).

Clinical Effects of Tumors

Tumors can cause structural and functional changes to the body that can lead to symptoms and even death. Understanding of how tumors can cause these changes is crucial to appropriate symptom and disease management.

Local

Local effects of tumors often include compression and displacement of nearby tissues. Malignant tumors can also cause destruction as they invade normal structures. Sometimes, even benign tumors can threaten the function of vital structures, such as functionally inactive adenomas of the pituitary gland that can impair the function of the nearby pituitary tissue, leading to hypopituitarism. Malignant invasion and destruction of blood vessels can lead to fatal consequences.

Metabolic

Tumor Type-Specific

Well-differentiated endocrine tumors frequently retain the functionality of their parent cells; clinical effects are common because of the total number of functioning cells exceeding that in the normal organ. Examples include thyrotoxicosis from a thyroid adenoma, Cushing syndrome from an adrenocortical adenoma, and hyperparathyroidism from a parathyroid adenoma. Paraneoplastic syndromes are unexpected or inappropriate metabolic effects of a tumor such as secretion of adrenocorticotropic hormone (ACTH) or antidiuretic hormone (ADH) by small cell carcinoma of the lung.

Nonspecific

Weight loss is common in cancer and is likely multifactorial. Cachexia, a catabolic clinical state among patients with cancer, is marked by severe weight loss and debility and is believed to be due to tumor-driven humoral factors interfering with protein metabolism and leading to muscle loss (sarcopenia). It can occur earlier in the course of the disease, such as in the case of lung cancer. Weight loss can also be a result of nutritional challenges posed by certain malignancies, such as the dysphagia associated with an obstructing esophageal mass. Cancer has also been associated with a higher rate of glycolysis. Venous thrombosis is commonly associated with mucus-producing adenocarcinomas such as those of the pancreas. Deposition of immune complexes from a tumor antigen can cause glomerular injury. Neuropathies and myopathies have also been associated with malignant neoplasms (Arends, 2019).

Pathophysiology of Metastasis

Metastasis is the process wherein the malignant tumors spread from their original site (primary tumor) to form other tumors (secondary tumors) at distant sites. The secondary tumors tend to exceed the total mass of the primary tumor. Metastasis can sometimes be detected due to accompanying symptoms of bone pain from skeletal metastases or lymphadenopathy from lymph node metastases. Metastasis is a process that occurs in a series of steps, and only a certain portion of neoplastic cells in a malignant tumor can have all the properties needed to complete this process. Metastatic tumors in humans are often histologically less well differentiated than the primary tumor, supporting the theory that there is a clonal evaluation of the metastatic phenotype.

The steps involved in the metastatic sequence include detachment of tumor cells from their neighbors, invasion of surrounding connective tissue to reach the blood and lymphatic vessels, intravasation into the lumen of vessels, evasion of host defense mechanisms (such as T lymphocytes in the blood and tissues), adherence to a remote endothelium, extravasation from the vessel lumen into the surrounding tissue, and growth and survival of the tumor in its new environment. Once able to grow and form a nodule larger than a few millimeters in diameter, the process of angiogenesis begins (Arends, 2019).

A study conducted among patients with renal cell carcinoma showed that subclones originate from the interior of the tumor instead of the margin, with the center of the tumor exhibiting more proliferation, necrosis, and somatic copy number alteration (SCNA). This shows that heightened central tumor necrosis increases SCNA acquisition, resulting in subclones that can withstand harsh microenvironmental conditions and be better suited to initiate secondary metastatic sites. Tumor necrosis is associated with chronic hypoxia and has been linked to poor survival outcomes among patients with cancer. Hypoxia in the tumor microenvironment is known to promote metastasis by inducing genome doubling in cancer cell lines and increasing rates of allelic loss and shortening telomeres (Zhao et al., 2021).

After evaluating macroscopic images of the tumor, the pattern of cancer growth among these patients was also found not to be simply linear (from the interior tumor to the exterior margins), but evolutionary, in which subclones have been found to originate from both the central tumor regions as well as its margin. Genetic and spatial distance analysis revealed that tumor subclones are more genetically similar to subclones nearby than those that are farther away (Zhao et al., 2021).

Distant metastases account for 90% of deaths from cancer. For metastasis to take place, primary tumor cells must separate from the primary tumor, enter the vasculature (intravasation), travel to distant sites, and inhabit destination organ sites. This process is not random. Tumor cells can only grow in environments where their growth is supported. For instance, malignant melanoma typically metastasizes to the brain, and ocular malignant melanoma usually metastasizes to the liver (Krasnick et al., 2022).

Routes of Metastasis

Metastasis can happen through the blood stream (hematogenous) from perfusion of organs by blood that has been drained from the tumor. It can also occur in regional lymph nodes through the lymphatic system. It can also occur in pleural, pericardial, or peritoneal cavities (transcoelomic) in the form of a neoplastic effusion. Implantation can also occur by accidentally spilling tumor cells during invasive procedures like surgery. Carcinomas tend to spread via the lymphatic system, and sarcomas tend to have a hematogenous spread.

Hematogenous Metastasis

The liver, lung, bone, and brain are the most common sites of metastasis. Primary cancers of the lung, breast, kidney, thyroid, and prostate tend to metastasize to the bone. Metastases tend to be in multiple areas, whereas primary tumors are usually solitary. Solid tumors also rarely metastasize to the spleen or skeletal muscles, despite their rich blood supply.

Lymphatic Metastasis

Tumor cells can also travel through the lymphatic channel, settle, and grow in the periphery of a lymph node, gradually replacing it. Metastatic lymph nodes are typically firmer and larger than a normal node and can be tangled together by tumor tissue and the connective tissue's response to it. These can lead to edema in the area and interrupt lymphatic flow and drainage. It should be noted that lymph nodes can also enlarge outside the setting of cancer.

Transcoelomic Metastasis

Transcoelomic metastasis occurs in the pleural, peritoneal, and pericardial activities and is accompanied by effusion of fluid into the cavity involved. The fluid is high in protein (exudative) and contains neoplastic cells. This is typically diagnosed by cytologic examination of the fluid that is aspirated from the cavity. The tumor cells can also develop into nodules on the mesothelial surface of the cavity. Ascites or peritoneal effusions are commonly associated with abdominal tumor as well as primary tumor in the ovaries. Breast and lung carcinomas are commonly associated with breast pericardial and pleural effusions (Arends, 2019).

Prognostic Indices

Information on tumor characteristics, such as tumor type, cellular differentiation or grade, and stage, is used to evaluate the extent of malignant disease, identify appropriate and effective treatments, and aid in prognostication. Tiny deposits of a malignant tumor can escape detection even with the use of sophisticated tests and lie clinically dormant in the body for years after treatment. This makes it challenging to refer to a cancer patient as being cured, and prognosis is typically discussed in terms of survival or being disease-free in years.

Tumor Type

The tumor type is usually determined by the appearance of the cell and its relationship to the surrounding structure that can help identify a precursor from a direct origin. For instance, a primary breast adenocarcinoma will typically appear as a gland-forming neoplasm and signify ductal carcinoma in situ if neoplastic cells are noted within the breast ducts near the tumor. Squamous cell carcinoma is usually associated with keratin production and may be in continuity with adjacent squamous epithelium that may appear as carcinoma in situ or dysplasia or intraepithelial neoplasia.

Some tumor types may be further classified based on their different behaviors such as Hodgkin and non-Hodgkin lymphoma. These two types of lymphoma are further classified histologically, as well. Molecular pathologic or immunohistochemical analysis is used for tumor typing when no obvious differentiated features are found on routine light microscopy (Arends, 2019).

Tumor Grade

The grade of a tumor is measured by the appearance of its cells under the microscope, also referred to as cellular differentiation. The higher the grade, the less differentiated or more abnormal the cells appear. Tumors with a higher grade also grow and spread faster. Grades are usually assigned a number that typically ranges from 1 to 4 (American Cancer Society [ACS], 2022).

Tumor Stage or Extent of Spread

The extent to which the cancer spreads, or tumor stage, is assessed using histopathologic tumor evaluation, and clinical and radiologic assessment. The TNM staging system is frequently used, where "T" refers to the primary tumor and is suffixed by a number corresponding to the tumor size or anatomic extent. This number depends on the organ carrying the tumor. "N" refers to the lymph node status and is suffixed by a number indicating the number of nodes or group of nodes that contain metastases. The anatomic extent of distant metastasis corresponds to "M" (Arends, 2019). For instance, a T1 lung cancer consists of a tumor that is less than 3 cm in its greatest dimension, N0 stands for no regional node involvement, and M0 indicates no distant metastases (Grant & Griffin, 2019). TNM status is typically used to arrive at a stage score. For example, a stage 1 tumor is typically confined to the organ of origin, whereas a stage 4 tumor has widely disseminated. Molecular evaluation is also a helpful tool to aid in prognostication (Arends, 2019).

Clinical Pathologic Staging

Tumor size, number of sites, and degree of metastasis are determined by pathologic examination of tissue obtained at surgery. Pathologic examination provides the clinician with information about the cellular characteristics of the tumor.

Conclusion

Cancer development is a highly complex process that involves multiple factors. Although some causes of cancer may be unavoidable, there are many contributing factors that can potentially be avoided to mitigate the risk of developing this potentially fatal disease. Avoiding risk factors and participating in screening activities are helpful in minimizing the likelihood of developing cancer. Over time, the more that is learned about how cancer develops, the more it can aid in further enhancement of diagnostics, therapeutics, and improve overall outcomes.

References

American Cancer Society (ACS). (2022). Cancer staging. Available at https://www.cancer.org/treatment/understanding-your-diagnosis/staging.html.

Arends, M. J. (2019). Neoplasia and carcinogenesis. In S. S. Cross (Ed.), *Underwood's pathology: A clinical approach* (7th ed., pp. 177–217). Elsevier.

Eachkoti, R., Farooq, S., Syeed, S. I., Wani, H. A., Majid, S., & Pampori, M. R. (2018). Prevalence and prognostic relevance of BrafV600E mutation in colorectal carcinomas from Kashmir (North India) valley. *Mutagenesis*, *33*(3), 225–230,

Ferretti, E., & Hadjantonakis, A. K. (2019). Mesoderm specification and diversification: From single cells to emergent tissues. *Current Opinion in Cell Biology*, *61*, 110–116.

Gardner, A., Pulido, A. M., & Ruffell, B. (2020). Dendritic cells and their role in immunotherapy. *Frontiers in Immunology*. https://doi.org/10.3389/fimmu.2020.00924 (accessed April 17, 2022).

Ghannam, J. Y., Wang, J., & Jan, A. (2021). Biochemistry, DNA structure. In *StatPearls*. StatPearls Publishing. 2022. Available at https://www.ncbi.nlm.nih.gov/books/NBK538241/.

Grant, L. A., & Griffin, N. (2019). TNM staging of common cancer. In L. A. Grant, & N. Griffin (Eds.), *Grainger & Allison's diagnostic radiology essentials* (2nd ed., pp. 970–985). Elsevier.

Greten, F. R., & Grivennikov, S. I. (2019). Inflammation and cancer: Triggers, mechanisms, and consequences. *Immunity, 51*(1), 27–41.

Huang, L., & Zhou, P. K. (2021, July 9). DNA damage repair: Historical perspectives, mechanistic pathways and clinical translation for targeted cancer therapy. *Signal Transductions and Targeted Therapy, 6*, 254. https://doi.org/10.1038/s41392-021-00648-7.

Huang, L., Guo, Z., Wang, F., & Fu, L. (2021). KRAS mutation: From undruggable to druggable in cancer. *Signal Transduction and Targeted Therapy, 6*, 386. Available at https://www.nature.com/articles/s41392-021-00780-4 (accessed April 16, 2022).

Huang, Y., Wu, X., Lin, Y., Li, W., Liu, J., & Song, B. (2020). Multiple sexual partners and vaginal microecological disorder are associated with HPV infection and cervical carcinoma development. *Oncology Letters, 20*(2), 1915–1921.

Iranzo, J., Martincorena, I., & Koonin, E. V. (2018). Cancer-mutation network and the number and specificity of driver mutations. *Proceedings of the National Academy of Sciences of the United States of America, 115*(26), E6010–E6019.

Janiszewska, M., Primi, M. C., & Izard, T. (2020). Cell adhesion in cancer: Beyond the migration of single cells. *Journal of Biological Chemistry, 295*(8), 2495–2505.

Kessenbrock, K., Wang, C. Y., & Werb, Z. (2015). Matrix metalloproteinases in stem cell regulation and cancer. *Matrix Biology, 44-46*, 184–190.

Krasnick, B. A., Goedegebuure, S. P., & Fields, R. (2022). Tumor biology and tumor markers. In C. M. Townsend, R. D. Beauchamp, B. M. Evers, & K. L. Mattox (Eds.), *Sabiston: Textbook of surgery: The biological basis of modern surgical practice* (21st ed., pp. 656–686). Elsevier.

Lewis, T., & Dimri, M. (2021). Biochemistry, DNA repair. *StatPearls.* Available at https://www.ncbi.nlm.nih.gov/books/NBK560563/ (accessed November 20, 2021).

Li, N., Zhai, Z., Zheng, Y., Lin, S., Deng, Y., Xiang, G., … Yang, S. (2021). Association of 13 occupational carcinogens in patients with cancer, individually and collectively, 1990-2017. *JAMA Network Open, 4*(2), e2037530.

Losquadro, W. D. (2017). Anatomy of the skin and the pathogenesis of nonmelanoma skin cancer. *Facial Plastic Surgery Clinics of North America, 25*(3), 283–289.

Lugano, R., Ramachandran, M., & Dimberg, A. (2020). Tumor angiogenesis: Causes, consequences, challenges and opportunities. *Cellular and Molecular Life Sciences: CMLS, 77*(9), 1745–1770.

McGlynn, K. A., Petrick, J. L., & El-Serag, H. B. (2021). Epidemiology of hepatocellular carcinoma. *Hepatology (Baltimore, Md.), 73*(Suppl 1), 4–13.

McNally, E. J., Luncsford, P. J., & Armanois, M. (2019). Long telomeres and cancer risk: The price of cellular immortality. *The Journal of Clinical Investigation, 129*(9), 3474–3481.

Mercadante, A., & Kasi, A. (2021). Genetics, cancer cell cycle phases. In *StatPearls.* Available at https://www.ncbi.nlm.nih.gov/books/NBK563158/. (accessed November 20, 2021).

Muthukrishnan, A., & Warnakulasuriya, S. (2018). Oral health consequences of smokeless tobacco use. *The Indian Journal of Medical Research, 148*(1), 35–40.

National Institutes of Health (NIH). (2016). *Stem cell basics.* Available at https://stemcells.nih.gov/info/basics/stc-basics/. (accessed November 30, 2021).

Nickoloff, J. A., Sharma, N., & Taylor, L. (2020). Clustered DNA double-strand breaks: Biological effects and relevance to cancer radiotherapy. *Genes, 11*(1), 99.

Padala, S. A., Barsouk, A., Thandra, K. C., Saginala, K., Mohammed, A., Vakiti, A., … Barsouk, A. (2020). Epidemiology of renal cell carcinoma. *World Journal of Oncology, 11*(3), 79–87.

Pickup, M. W., Mouw, J. K., & Weaver, V. M. (2014). The extracellular matrix modulates the hallmarks of cancer. *EMBO Reports, 15*(12), 1243–1253.

Pinheiro, P. S., Medina, H., Callahan, K. E., Kwon, D., Ragin, C., Sherman, R., … Jemal, A. (2020). Cancer mortality among US blacks: Variability between African Americans, Afro-Caribbeans, and Africans. *Cancer Epidemiology, 66*, 101709.

Saito, Y., Koya, J., & Kataoka, K. (2021). Multiple mutations within individual oncogenes. *Cancer Science, 112*(2), 483–489.

Strasser, A., & Vaux, D. L. (2020). Cell death in the origin and treatment of cancer. *Molecular Cell, 78*(6), 1045–1054.

Van Driel, M., van Leeuwen, J. P. T. M., Muñoz, A., & Feldman, D. (2018). Overview of vitamin D actions in cancer. In D. Feldman (Ed.), *Vitamin D volume 2: Health, disease and therapeutics* (4th ed., pp. 711–742). Elsevier.

Watson, J. D., & Crick, F. H. (1974). Molecular structure of nucleic acids: A structure for deoxyribose nucleic acid. Published in Nature, number 4356 April 25, 1953. *Nature, 248*(5451), 765.

Yeola, A., Subramanian, S., Oliver, R. A., Lucas, C. A., Thomas, J. A. I., Yan, F., … Pimanda, J. E. (2021). Induction of muscle-regenerative multipotent stem cells from human adipocytes by PDGF-AB and 5-azacytidine. *Science. Advances, 7*(3). eabd1929.

Yu, H., Lee, H., Herrmann, A., Buettner, R., & Jove, R. (2014). Revisiting STAT3 signalling in cancer: New and unexpected biological functions. *Nature Reviews Cancer, 14*, 736–746.

Zakrzewski, W., Dobrzyński, M., Szymonowicz, M., & Rybak, Z. (2019). Stem cells: Past, present, and future. *Stem Cell Research & Therapy, 10*(68), 1–16.

Zella, D., & Gallo, R. C. (2021). Viruses and bacteria associated with cancer: An overview. *Viruses, 13*(6), 1039.

Zhao, Y., Fu, X., Lopez, J. I., Rowan, A., Au, L., Fendler, A., … Litchfield, K. (2021). Selection of metastasis competent subclones in the tumour interior. *Nature Ecology & Evolution, 5*(7), 1033–1045.

Zhu, K., Liu, Q., Zhou, Y., Tao, C., Zhao, Z., Sun, J., & Xu, H. (2015). Oncogenes and tumor suppressor genes: Comparative genomics and network perspectives. *BMC Genomics, 16*(Suppl 8), 2–9.

Cancer Genetics/Genomics

Suzanne M. Mahon

Precision Medicine

Genetic (study of a gene) and genomic (the study of all a person's genes) science are the backbone of precision medicine. Precision medicine is an emerging approach for disease treatment and prevention that considers individual variability in genes, environment, and lifestyle. This approach enables the selection of treatment and prevention strategies more accurately in an individual patient. It contrasts with a one-size-fits-all approach, in which disease treatment and prevention strategies are developed for the average person, with less consideration for the differences between individuals. Understanding genomic science is critical to the practice of precision medicine and the effective treatment of malignancy.

Molecular Genetics

Genes, the smallest functional units of inherited information in living organisms, are the controlling factors for cellular development and function. Genes are made up of deoxyribonucleic acid (DNA) and provide the instructions for making proteins by using different combinations of amino acids, and they regulate when and where a protein is produced (i.e., regulatory sequence). The process of making proteins is called protein synthesis.

Proteins are large, complex molecules that perform essential roles in cellular maintenance, growth, and function. Various types of proteins catalyze biochemical reactions (i.e., enzymes such as transferases), provide structure in the cytoskeleton and muscles (e.g., actin, tubulin), participate in immune responses (e.g., antibodies), act as messengers (e.g., hormones), and store or transport ligands (e.g., hemoglobin).

In humans, genes vary in size from a few hundred DNA bases to more than 2 million bases. The Human Genome Project, which determined the sequence of the human genome and identified the genes that it contains, estimated that humans have between 20,000 and 25,000 genes (Gates et al., 2021). Every person has two copies of each gene, one inherited from each parent. Most genes are the same in all people, but a small number of genes (<1% of the total) are slightly different between people. Alleles are forms of the same gene with small differences in their sequence of DNA bases. These small differences contribute to each person's unique physical features.

Protein Synthesis

DNA is a large, self-replicating molecule located primarily in the nucleus and a smaller amount in the mitochondria of each cell. The condensed, coiled forms (i.e., chromosomes) contain smaller units (i.e., genes) that provide codes (i.e., instructions) for the construction of every protein in the body. Commonly used genetic terms are shown in the box below.

Terms Used in Genetics

Allele: One of several forms of a gene at a particular location on a chromosome.

Amino acid: Basic building block of all proteins. The genetic code encodes the 20 standard amino acids used by cells to build proteins and can produce nonstandard amino acids that are substituted for standard forms.

Aneuploidy: The gain or loss of chromosomes from the normal 46.

Anticipation: The signs and symptoms of some genetic conditions tend to become more severe and appear at an earlier age as the disorder is passed from one generation to the next.

Autosomal dominant: Mendelian inheritance pattern in which an affected individual possesses one copy of a mutant allele and one normal copy, with a 50% chance that the allele and associated disorder or disease will be passed to offspring.

Autosomal recessive: A trait or disorder that appears only in people who have received two copies of a mutant or altered gene (i.e., one from each parent).

Autosome: Chromosome that is not a sex chromosome. Humans have 22 pairs of autosomal chromosomes.

Base pairs: A nucleotide is composed of a molecule containing phosphoric acid, sugar, and a base. The bases are designated by the letters A, T, G, and C, representing adenine, thymine, guanine, and cytosine, respectively.

Biallelic: Both alleles of a gene are affected.

Chromosome: Threadlike structure of nucleic acids and proteins in the nucleus of the cell that contains genes. Humans have 23 pairs of chromosomes; 22 pairs are autosomes, and 1 pair is a set of sex chromosomes.

Codon: A group of three nucleotides that form a unit of genetic code in a deoxyribonucleic acid (DNA) or ribonucleic acid (RNA) molecule.

Deletion: Type of chromosomal abnormality in which a piece of DNA is removed or omitted from a gene, which disrupts the normal structure and function of the gene.

DNA sequencing: Determination of the exact order of the base pairs (i.e., adenine, guanine, cytosine, and thymine) in a segment of DNA.

Duplication: Type of chromosomal abnormality in which a piece of DNA is abnormally copied one or more times.

Exon: Region of a gene that contains part of the code for producing a protein. Each exon codes for a specific portion of the complete protein.

Fluorescence in situ hybridization (FISH): Laboratory process that involves painting chromosomes or sections of chromosomes with fluorescent molecules. It is a useful technique for identifying chromosomal abnormalities and gene mapping.

Frameshift: Type of chromosomal abnormality in which there is an addition or loss of DNA bases that changes a gene's reading frame that codes for one amino acid.

Terms Used in Genetics—cont'd

Gene: Functional and physical unit of heredity that is passed from parent to offspring and contains information necessary for making a specific protein.

Genome: Entire set of genetic instructions found in a cell. In humans, the genome consists of 23 pairs of chromosomes, found in the nucleus, as well as a small chromosome found in the cells' mitochondria. Each set of 23 chromosomes contains approximately 3.1 billion bases of DNA sequence.

Genotype: Genetic identity that may or may not be physically manifested in outward characteristics.

Germline: Inherited material that comes from the egg or sperm and is passed to offspring.

Heterozygous: Possessing two different forms of a particular gene; one is inherited from each parent.

Homozygous: Possessing two identical forms of a particular gene; one is inherited from each parent.

Insertion: Type of chromosomal abnormality in which an extra piece of DNA is inserted into a gene, resulting in the disruption of the normal structure and function of that gene.

Intron: Segment of DNA or RNA that does not code for proteins and interrupts the sequence of genes.

Karyotype: Visual presentation of the chromosomal complement of an individual, including all chromosomes and abnormalities.

Microsatellite: A repetitive, short sequence of DNA that is used as a genetic marker to track inheritance patterns in families.

Missense: Type of chromosomal abnormality in which one amino acid is substituted for another.

Monosomy: Form of aneuploidy in which there is only one copy of a particular chromosome instead of two.

Next-generation sequencing (NGS): Laboratory technique in which many strands of DNA are sequenced at the same time, generating far more data per instrument run than the Sanger method.

Nonsense: Point mutation in a sequence of DNA that results in a stop codon that prematurely ends the process of building a protein.

Oncogene: Pathogenic variant of a gene that leads to transformation of normal cells into cancer cells.

Penetrance: Penetrance refers to the likelihood that a clinical condition will occur when a particular genotype is present. For adult-onset diseases, penetrance is usually described by the individual carrier's age, sex, and organ site.

Pharmacogenomics: The study of the relationship between genetic variations and how our body responds to medications.

Phenotype: Set of observable characteristics or traits of an organism resulting from the interaction of its genotype with the environment.

Polymerase chain reaction (PCR): Laboratory technique that is a fast, relatively inexpensive means for making an unlimited number of copies of any piece of DNA.

Polymorphism: A variant with a frequency in the general population of greater than 1%.

Precision medicine: A form of medicine that uses information about a person's own genes or proteins to prevent, diagnose, or treat disease. In cancer, precision medicine oncology uses specific information about a person's tumor to help make a diagnosis, plan treatment, find out how well treatment is working, or make a prognosis. Also called personalized medicine, precision medicine, or precision health.

Proband: Person who serves as the starting point for the genetic study of a family. Risks are calculated based on an individual's relation to the proband.

Promoter: DNA sequence that defines where transcription of a gene begins. Transcription is initiated in the promoter part of the gene by binding enzymes and proteins called transcription factors.

Sanger sequencing: Original sequencing technology that helped scientists to determine the human genetic code. Now automated, it is still used to sequence short pieces of DNA.

Single-nucleotide polymorphisms (SNPs): Each SNP (pronounced *snip*) represents a variation in a single nucleotide. SNPs normally occur about once in every 300 nucleotides in an individual's DNA. These variations usually are found in the DNA between genes functioning as biologic markers, helping scientists locate genes associated with disease. There are about 10 million SNPs in the human genome.

Somatic cells: All cells in the body except the reproductive cells.

Translocation: Breaking and removal of a large segment of DNA from one chromosome, followed by the segment's attachment to a different chromosome. This can alter gene expression.

Trisomy: The most common form of aneuploidy, it is the presence of an extra chromosome in each cell.

Tumor suppressor gene: A protective gene that usually limits the growth of tumor cells. If mutated, it may not be able to keep a cancer from growing (e.g., *BRCA* genes).

Variable expression: Many genetic disorders have a wide variety of signs and symptoms, but not all individuals with the same disorder express them to the same degree.

Variant: An alteration in the most common DNA nucleotide sequence. The term variant can be used to describe an alteration that may be benign, pathogenic, or of unknown significance. The term variant is the preferred term used in place of the term mutation.

Data from NCI Dictionary of Cancer Terms, by the National Cancer Institute (NCI). Available at https://www.cancer.gov/publications/dictionaries/cancer-terms. Copyright by NCI, n.d.; NCI Dictionary of Genetic Terms, by the National Cancer Institute (NCI). Available at https://www.cancer.gov/publications/dictionaries/genetics-dictionary. Copyright by NCI, n.d.; NHGRI Talking Glossary Dictionary of Terms, by the National Human Genome Research Institute, (NHGRI). Available at https://www.genome.gov//genetics-glossary/c#glossary. Copyright by NHGRI, n.d.; PDQ Cancer Genetics Overview by the National Cancer Institute (NCI). Available at https://www.cancer.gov/about-cancer/causes-prevention/genetics/overview-pdq#_146. Copyright by NCI, n.d.

The double-helix form of DNA is a pair of molecules consisting of polymers (i.e., long chains) of interlocking nucleotides, called chromatin. Nucleotides are the basic structural units of nucleic acids such as DNA and ribonucleic acid (RNA). The chemical building blocks consist of a phosphate, a five-carbon sugar, and a base (i.e., adenine [A], guanine [G], thymine [T], or cytosine [C]). Arrangement of the bases can be likened to a genetic alphabet that is used to create the language of intercellular and intracellular communication (see figure on the next page).

Protein synthesis is the process by which genes serve as codes to produce amino acids and proteins. This activity occurs in the ribosomes, which are ribonucleoprotein complexes found in the cytoplasm of the cell. Proteins are formed by peptide bonds between individual amino acids in a linear strand. To accomplish protein synthesis, a particular DNA sequence (i.e., gene) for a specific protein is transcribed into a piece of RNA. RNA consists of a sugar-phosphate backbone with a nucleotide attached. Although RNA is similar to DNA, it uses the nucleotide base U instead of T and has a hydroxyl group attached to its ribose sugar.

Protein synthesis consists of two phases: transcription and translation. The overall process arranges amino acids into proteins through the action of several types of RNA and various

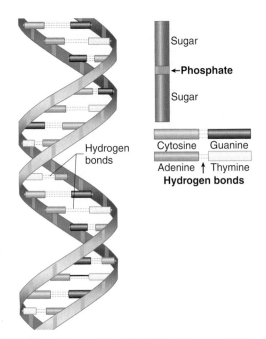

Sugar

←**Phosphate**

Sugar

Cytosine   Guanine

Adenine ↑ Thymine

Hydrogen bonds

Hydrogen bonds

Model of Deoxyribonucleic Acid (DNA). A base pair is two chemical bases bonded to one another, forming a rung of the DNA ladder. The DNA molecule consists of two strands that wind around each other like a twisted ladder. Each strand has a backbone made of alternating sugar (i.e., deoxyribose) and phosphate groups. Attached to each sugar is one of four bases: adenine (A), cytosine (C), guanine (G), or thymine (T). Adenine forms a base pair with thymine, and cytosine forms a base pair with guanine. The two strands are held together by hydrogen bonds between the bases. (Modified from Patton, K. T., Bell, F., Thompson T., & Williamson, P. [2022]. *Anatomy & physiology* [11th ed.]. St. Louis: Elsevier.)

enzymes. Initially, the cells receive a message to produce a specific protein. Transcription begins when the enzyme RNA polymerase attaches to a segment of the DNA (i.e., gene) and creates a transcription bubble, which separates ("unzips") the two strands of the DNA helix, as also occurs during cell division. RNA polymerase moves along the strand of exposed gene and transcribes the subunits of DNA by adding matching RNA nucleotides to the complementary nucleotides of the DNA strand. The new strand is called messenger RNA (mRNA). The previously exposed segment of DNA closes and remains in the nucleus of the cell. Before the transcribed mRNA moves from the nucleus into the cytoplasm, nuclear enzymes remove introns (i.e., noncoding sections) and splice together exons (i.e., sequences that code for proteins). This process is repeated as long as the signal to make the desired protein remains viable.

In the translation phase, the information contained in the mRNA is converted into a sequence of amino acids in proteins. The copies of mRNA enter the cytoplasm through channels (i.e., pores) in the nucleus, bind to ribosomal RNA (rRNA) found in the cytoplasm, and are decoded. The mRNA is encoded with information about the particular arrangement of amino acids that makes up the final protein. During translation, a molecule of transfer RNA (tRNA) matches the strand of mRNA and carries the correct amino acids to the ribosome. Three nucleotide bases (i.e., codons) are read at a time, and each codon represents a specific

amino acid. As each codon is decoded, the corresponding amino acid is activated. The amino acids are brought into the proper sequence as the entire message is read, and the newly formed polypeptide chain then folds into its final three-dimensional shape based on chemical bonds formed between amino acids. The total number of amino acids in a specific protein and the exact code that links them together determine the nature and activity of the protein. Different sequences of amino acids change the shape of the proteins and therefore their function (see figure on the next page).

Gene Variants

A gene variant is a permanent change in the DNA sequence that makes up a gene. This type of genetic change used to be known as a gene mutation, but because changes in DNA do not always cause disease, it is thought that gene variant is a more accurate term (Friend et al., 2021). Variants can affect one or more DNA building blocks (nucleotides) in a gene. Gene variants can be inherited from a parent or occur during a person's lifetime.

Inherited variants are passed from parent to child and are present throughout a person's life in virtually every cell in the body (McClary, 2020). These variants are also called germline variants because they are present in the parent's egg or sperm cells, which are also called germ cells. When an egg and a sperm cell unite, the resulting fertilized egg cell contains DNA from both parents. Any variants that are present in that DNA will be present in the cells of the child that grows from the fertilized egg.

Noninherited variants occur at some time during a person's life and are present only in certain cells, not in every cell in the body. Because noninherited variants typically occur in somatic cells (cells other than sperm and egg cells), they are often referred to as somatic variants. These variants cannot be passed to the next generation. Most malignancies are not inherited and are due to changes that are acquired over time resulting in somatic pathogenic variants that can occur as cells divide. These variants can also arise from exposure to carcinogenic substances that damage DNA, such as certain chemicals in tobacco smoke, and radiation including ultraviolet rays from the sun. Genetic changes that occur after conception are called somatic (or acquired) changes.

There are many kinds of DNA changes. Some changes affect just one unit of DNA, called a nucleotide. One nucleotide may be replaced by another, or it may be missing entirely. Other changes involve larger stretches of DNA and may include rearrangements, deletions, or duplications of long stretches of DNA (see figure on the next page). In general, malignant cells have more genetic changes than normal cells. But each person's malignancy has a unique combination of genetic alterations. Some of these changes may be the result of cancer, rather than the cause. As the cancer continues to grow, additional changes will occur. Even within the same tumor, cancer cells may have different genetic changes.

Germline and Somatic Variants

Many different pathogenic variants occur in malignant cells. Malignancies may develop resulting from the conversion of

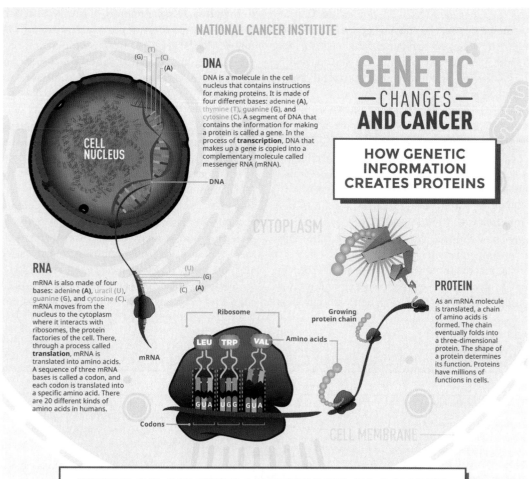

NATIONAL CANCER INSTITUTE

GENETIC
—CHANGES—
AND CANCER

HOW GENETIC INFORMATION CREATES PROTEINS

DNA

DNA is a molecule in the cell nucleus that contains instructions for making proteins. It is made of four different bases: adenine (A), thymine (T), guanine (G), and cytosine (C). A segment of DNA that contains the information for making a protein is called a gene. In the process of **transcription**, DNA that makes up a gene is copied into a complementary molecule called messenger RNA (mRNA).

CELL NUCLEUS

CYTOPLASM

DNA

RNA

mRNA is also made of four bases: adenine (A), uracil (U), guanine (G), and cytosine (C). mRNA moves from the nucleus to the cytoplasm where it interacts with ribosomes, the protein factories of the cell. There, through a process called **translation**, mRNA is translated into amino acids. A sequence of three mRNA bases is called a codon, and each codon is translated into a specific amino acid. There are 20 different kinds of amino acids in humans.

mRNA

Ribosome

LEU TRP VAL

Amino acids

GUA UGG GUA

Codons

Growing protein chain

PROTEIN

As an mRNA molecule is translated, a chain of amino acids is formed. The chain eventually folds into a three-dimensional protein. The shape of a protein determines its function. Proteins have millions of functions in cells.

CELL MEMBRANE

TYPES OF GENETIC MUTATIONS IN CANCER

DNA alterations can affect the structure, function, and amount of the corresponding proteins. All of these effects can change a cell's behavior from normal to cancerous. For example, a genetic alteration can intensify or eliminate the protein's function, which could make cells divide uncontrollably. Many different kinds of genetic mutations are found in cancer cells, including missense, nonsense, and frameshift mutations and chromosome rearrangements.

MISSENSE MUTATION

Original	C T A	T G G	G T A	DNA
	LEU (leucine)	TRP (tryptophan)	VAL (valine)	Amino Acids
Mutation	C T A	T G T	G T A	DNA
	LEU (leucine)	CYS (cysteine)	VAL (valine)	Amino Acids

A missense mutation is a change of a single DNA base that results in a change in the amino acid sequence. Sometimes a single amino acid change can greatly alter the protein's function.

NONSENSE MUTATION

Original	C T A	T G G	G T A	DNA
	LEU (leucine)	TRP (tryptophan)	VAL (valine)	Amino Acids
Mutation	C T A	T G A	G T A	DNA
	LEU (leucine)	● (stop)		Amino Acids

A nonsense mutation is a change of a single DNA base that creates a "stop" codon, which terminates translation. The result is a shortened protein that may not function or that may have an abnormal function.

FRAMESHIFT MUTATION

Original	C T A	T G G	G T A	DNA
	LEU (leucine)	TRP (tryptophan)	VAL (valine)	Amino Acids
Mutation	C T A	A T G	G G T	DNA
	LEU (leucine)	MET (methionine)	GLY (glycine)	Amino Acids

A frameshift mutation results from the addition or removal of DNA bases that shifts the DNA sequence and the corresponding amino acid sequence. The result is a protein whose sequence, structure, and function are very different from those of the original protein.

CHROMOSOME REARRANGEMENTS

DNA is wound tightly into structures called chromosomes. Chromosome rearrangements can occur when a piece of a chromosome breaks and is lost entirely (deletion), moves to a different chromosomal location (translocation), flips directions (inversion), or is repeated (duplication). These rearrangements can alter several genes at once. For example, they can generate fusion genes, in which parts of two separate genes are joined together. Proteins made from fusion genes sometimes cause cancer.

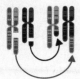

cancer.gov/genetics

Genetic Changes and Cancer. (From National Cancer Institute [NCI]. How genetic changes lead to cancer. Updated October 12, 2017. Available at https://www.cancer.gov/about-cancer/causes-prevention/genetics/genetic-changes-infographic.)

protooncogenes to oncogenes (NCI Dictionary of Cancer Terms, n.d.). Protooncogenes (i.e., normal genes before they are altered by genetic changes) regulate normal cell growth, whereas oncogenes (i.e., altered genes) are associated with abnormal cell growth, leading to increased cellular proliferation and uncontrolled growth.

Some tumors arise because of the inactivation of both alleles of tumor suppressor genes, which play an important role in slowing or stopping abnormal cell growth. Tumor suppressor genes include caretaker genes, which maintain integrity of the genetic material, and gatekeeper genes, which regulate proliferation and cell life (McClary, 2020).

Mismatch repair (MMR) genes repair mistakes that occur during DNA replication (Schmitt, 2020). When MMR genes are damaged, genetic stability is altered, and tumor cells replicate. Some variants interfere with apoptosis.

Somatic variants can spontaneously arise in any cell in the body except germ cells (i.e., eggs and sperm) at any time during the patient's life. This type of genetic alteration is limited to the descendants of the original cell that developed the variant, and it is not present in other cells in the patient's body (McClary, 2020). Because the alteration is not in the germ cells, the variant cannot be passed from parent to child. Somatic variants are responsible for most malignancies. Sporadic cancers occur from multiple somatic alterations in a cell. Acquired somatic variants develop in DNA during a person's lifetime.

The other type of variant is referred to as a germline variant, which occurs in the patient's germ cells and can be passed to future generations. A patient who inherits a germline pathogenic variant has that altered variant in all the cells of his or her body because the variant was present at conception. Germline variants are associated with hereditary cancer predisposition syndromes and account for approximately 10% of all malignancies (McClary, 2020). Common germline variants associated with the risk of developing cancer are shown in the table below.

Some genetic changes are described as new (de novo) variants; these variants are recognized in a child but not in either

Germline Variants Associated With Increased Cancer Risk

Gene/Syndrome	Associated Cancers and Risk
APC (familial adenomatous polyposis)	Colorectal (up to 93%), duodenal or periampullary (4%–12%), gastric, thyroid, pancreatic, brain, liver, desmoid tumors, gastrointestinal polyps (100s–1000s)
ATM	Breast (25%–50%), colon, pancreatic, ovarian, prostate (ataxia telangiectasia with two pathogenic variants)
BARD1	Breast, ovarian
BMPR1A	Colon (60%), gastric (20%), small bowel, pancreatic and multiple gastrointestinal polyps
BRCA1/2	Breast—female (90%), ovarian (60%), pancreatic (17%), prostate (35%), melanoma, breast—male, endometrial
BRIP1	Breast, ovarian, prostate
CDH1	Gastric (50%–85%), breast (30%–50%), colon
CDK4	Melanoma, pancreatic, breast, nonmelanoma skin
CDKN2A	Melanoma, pancreatic
CHEK2	Breast (lobular)—female (30%–50%), prostate, colon, breast—male, ovarian, thyroid
EPCAM/MLH1/MSH2/MSH6/PMS2 (Lynch syndrome)	Colon (60%–75%), endometrial (40%–70%), ovarian, gastric, pancreatic, female breast, biliary tract, urothelium, small bowel, brain, sebaceous neoplasms
HOXB13	Prostate
MEN1 (multiple endocrine neoplasia type 1)	Parathyroid (85%), pancreatic (40%), adrenal (15%–35%), pituitary (30%–80%)
MUTYH (MUTYH-associated polyposis—recessive syndrome)	Biallelic (two pathogenic copies)—Colon (50%–80%), small bowel (5%) Monoallelic (one pathogenic copy)—Colon
NF1 (neurofibromatosis type 1)	Neurofibromas (100%), breast
NF2 (neurofibromatosis type 2)	Vestibular schwannomas
PALB2	Breast—female (60%), pancreatic, colon, ovarian, pancreas, male breast
PTEN (Cowden syndrome)	Breast—female (50%), thyroid (35%), endometrial (10%), colon, gastric, melanoma, kidney, prostate, gastrointestinal polyps
RAD51C/RAD51D	Breast, ovarian, prostate
RB1 (retinoblastoma)	Retinoblastoma, osteosarcoma, melanoma, pineoblastoma
RET (multiple endocrine neoplasia type 2)	Medullary thyroid (100%), pheochromocytoma (40%–50%), parathyroid (30%)
SDHA, SDHB, SDHC, SDHD/SDHF (paraganglioma-pheochromocytoma [PGL-PCC] syndrome)	Paraganglioma (48%–84%), pheochromocytoma
STK11 (Peutz-Jeghers syndrome)	Breast—female (55%), colon (40%), pancreatic (40%), gastric (20%), small bowel (13%), endometrial
TP53 (Li Fraumeni syndrome)	Breast—female (85%), sarcoma, brain, hematologic malignancies, adrenocortical malignancies. Overall risk for malignancy in females is 95% and 88% in males
VHL (von Hippel–Lindau syndrome)	Renal (70%), pancreatic (17%) neuroendocrine tumors, hemangioblastoma, pheochromocytoma

Data from LaDuca, H., Polley, E. C., Yussuf, A., Hoang, L., Gutierrez, S., Hart, S. N., … Dolinsky, J. S. (2020). A clinical guide to hereditary cancer panel testing: Evaluation of gene-specific cancer associations and sensitivity of genetic testing criteria in a cohort of 165,000 high-risk patients. *Genetics in Medicine*, 22(2), 407–415; Shane-Carson, K., & Jeter, J. M. (2019). Hereditary risk for cancer. In D. S. Alberts & L. M. Hess (Eds.), *Fundamentals of cancer prevention* (4th ed.). Cham: Springer International Publishing.

parent (NCI Dictionary of Genetics Terms, n.d.). In some cases, the variant occurs in a parent's egg or sperm cell but is not present in any of their other cells. In other cases, the variant occurs in the fertilized egg shortly after the egg and sperm cells unite. (It is often impossible to tell exactly when a de novo variant happened.) As the fertilized egg divides, each resulting cell in the growing embryo will have the variant. De novo variants are one explanation for genetic disorders in which an affected child has a variant in every cell in the body, but the parents do not, and there is no family history of the disorder.

Variants acquired during development can lead to a situation called mosaicism, in which a set of cells in the body has a different genetic makeup than others. In mosaicism, the genetic change is not present in a parent's egg or sperm cells, or in the fertilized egg, but happens later, anytime from embryonic development through adulthood. As cells grow and divide, cells that arise from the cell with the altered gene will have the variant, while other cells will not. When a proportion of somatic cells have a gene variant and others do not, it is called somatic mosaicism. Depending on the variant and how many cells are affected, somatic mosaicism may or may not cause health problems. When a proportion of egg or sperm cells have a variant and others do not, it is called germline mosaicism. In this situation, an unaffected parent can pass a genetic condition to their offspring.

Biomarker Testing

Precision medicine is based on biomarker testing. Biomarker testing for a patient with a diagnosis of cancer can provide information that might identify individuals with hereditary risk, facilitate cancer diagnosis, provide prognostic information, and facilitate selection of treatments that are most likely to be effective by identifying oncogenic driver variants with actionable targets. This leads to the identification of patient-specific treatment options and management when certain biomarkers are present.

A biomarker is a molecule that can be measured in blood, other bodily fluids, or tissues. A biomarker can be an indicator of normal or abnormal biologic processes. Biomarkers have been used for decades in cancer care including the detection of estrogen and progesterone in breast cancer samples to guide treatment or prostate-specific antigen (PSA) which can be utilized to monitor the effectiveness of prostate cancer treatment.

There are a host of biomarkers associated with specific cancer types, disease diagnosis or prognosis, and treatment decisions and monitoring. Some biomarkers are not tumor-specific (tumor-agnostic). Some common biomarkers include:

- BRAF in melanoma, colon, or lung cancers
- KRAS and EGRF in colorectal and lung cancers
- HER2+ amplification in breast cancer
- ALK+ in non–small cell lung cancer and lymphoma
- Germline BRCA pathogenic variants in breast, ovarian, prostate, or pancreatic cancers
- Microsatellite instability-high (MSI-H) and MMR deficiencies in colorectal and other cancers

- NTRK in non–small cell lung cancer, thyroid, colon, pancreatic, breast, or other cancers
- Diagnosis, treatment selection, recurrence, and relapse detection are now biomarker driven in many cancers.

Classification Germline and Somatic Variants

Biomarkers can be classified as somatic (i.e., indicative of the acquired cellular and genomic alterations that drive cancer pathogenesis) or germline (i.e., indicative that the genomic alteration is present from birth and in every cell of the body) (Li et al., 2017). US Food and Drug Administration (FDA) created the BEST (Biomarkers, EndpointS, and other Tools) resource (FDA-NIH Biomarker Working Group, 2016) as a classification system to facilitate consistent use of terms. The box below describes these classifications.

Variant Classifications

Germline Variant Classification

- *Pathogenic Variant:* Directly contributes to the development of disease. Additional evidence is not expected to alter the classification of this variant. (Note: Not all pathogenic variants are fully penetrant.)
- *Likely Pathogenic Variant:* Very likely to contribute to the development of disease, but scientific evidence is currently insufficient to prove this conclusively.
- *Variant of Uncertain Significance:* There is not enough information at this time to support a more definitive classification of this variant.
- *Likely Benign Variant:* Not expected to have a major effect on disease, but the scientific evidence is currently insufficient to prove this conclusively.
- *Benign Variant:* Does not cause disease. Additional evidence is not expected to alter classification of this variant.

Somatic Variant Classification (Based on Actionability)

Tier I: Variants of Strong Clinical Significance

- *Level A Evidence:* FDA-approved therapy. Included in professional guidelines.
- *Level B Evidence:* Well-powered studies with consensus from experts in the field.

Tier II: Variants of Potential Clinical Significance

- *Level C Evidence:* With FDA-approved therapies for different tumor types or investigational therapies. Multiple published small studies with some consensus.
- *Level D Evidence:* Preclinical trials or a few case reports without consensus.

Tier III: Variants of Unknown Significance

- Not observed at a significant allele frequency in the general or specific subpopulation databases, or pan-cancer or tumor-specific variant databases. No convincing published evidence of cancer association.

Tier IV: Variants of Known Insignificance (i.e., Likely Benign or Benign)

- Observed at significant allele frequency in the general or specific subpopulation databases. No existing published evidence of cancer association.

Data from Li, M. M., Datto, M., Duncavage, E. J., Kulkarni, S., Lindeman, N. I., Roy, S., ... Nikiforova, M. N. (2017). Standards and guidelines for the interpretation and reporting of sequence variants in cancer: A joint consensus recommendation of the Association for Molecular Pathology, American Society of Clinical Oncology, and College of American Pathologists. *The Journal of Molecular Diagnostics, 19*(1), 4–23; FDA-NIH Biomarker Working Group. (2016). BEST (Biomarkers, EndpointS, and other Tools) Resource [Internet]. Food and Drug Administration (US), co-published by National Institutes of Health (US), Bethesda, MD. Available at https://www.ncbi.nlm.nih.gov/books/NBK326791/.

Biomarkers as part of precision medicine have many implications for care including:

- *Prognostic:* Identifies the likelihood of a clinical event, disease recurrence, or progression in patients who have the disease or medical condition
- *Predictive:* Identifies individuals who are more likely than those without the biomarker to experience a favorable or unfavorable effect from exposure to a medical product or an environmental agent
- *Pharmacodynamic/Response:* Shows whether an individual developed a biologic response to a medical product or an environmental agent
- *Safety:* Measured before or after an exposure to a medical product or an environmental agent to indicate the likelihood, presence, or extent of toxicity

Management of Germline Pathogenic Variants Associated With Hereditary Cancer Syndromes

Identification of a pathogenic variant in a family helps risk management and treatment planning for individuals with cancer and at-risk, unaffected family members. Genetic testing is not used in routine screening of a population because of the expense of testing and the complex counseling needs of families (Colas et al., 2019). It is best used to help selected individuals from high-risk families to make good decisions about cancer screening and prevention strategies. Key indicators of hereditary cancer syndromes are shown in the table on this page.

Genetic testing is best carried out by one of several types of credentialed genetics professionals. Geneticists are physicians with board certification in genetics from the American Board of Medical Genetics. Licensed genetics counselors are health care professionals with specialized graduate degrees in the areas of medical genetics and counseling who have been certified by the American Board of Genetic Counseling. Credentialed genetic nurses have specialized education and training in genetics and are credentialed by the American Nurses Credentialing Commission (ANCC) by portfolio and have the Advanced Genetics Nursing–Board Certified (AGN-BC) credential or by portfolio from Nurse Portfolio Credentialing Commission as an Advanced Clinical Genomics Nurse (ACGN) credentials. These professionals provide genetic risk assessment services, pedigree construction, and before and after genetic test counseling and coordinate follow-up for other at-risk family members.

Selection of the appropriate genetic test depends on risk factor assessment. This includes an assessment of the risk of developing the cancer and, in many cases, calculations of the risk of carrying a pathogenic variant as well as considering standardized guidelines from organizations such as the National Comprehensive Cancer Network. Genetic risk assessment begins with the construction of a pedigree as shown in the figure on the next page. The pedigree is an excellent means to educate a family about autosomal dominant transmission, and if a pathogenic variant is detected in the family, the pedigree provides a useful tool to identify other family members at risk who should be offered genetic testing. It should be updated as the family history changes.

Key Indicators of Hereditary Risk of Developing Cancer

Indicator	Examples
Cancer occurring at a younger age than expected in the general population	Breast cancer before age 50 Colon cancer before age 50 Endometrial cancer before age 50
More than one primary cancer	Breast and ovarian cancer Colon and endometrial cancer Synchronous colon cancer
Evidence of autosomal dominant inheritance pattern	Two or more generations affected Both men and women affected
Bilateral cancer in a paired organ	Breast cancer Ovarian cancer Thyroid cancer
Rare cancers	Ovarian Pancreatic Medullary thyroid cancer Paraganglioma Pheochromocytoma Male breast cancer Retinoblastoma
Any pattern of cancer associated with a known cancer syndrome	Hereditary breast and ovarian cancer Lynch syndrome Li-Fraumeni syndrome von Hippel–Lindau syndrome Multiple endocrine neoplasia types 1 and 2
Cancers occurring more frequently in a family than expected in the absence of known environmental and lifestyle risk factors	Cluster of the same cancers, especially in close relatives Breast cancer Colon cancer Pancreatic cancer Kidney cancer Melanoma
Presence of nonmalignant changes associated with a hereditary risk	More than 20 adenomatous polyps in a lifetime Hamartomas Dysplastic nevi
Presence of indicators on pathology report	Triple negative breast cancer Prostate cancer Gleason score 7 or higher Microsatellite instability on a colon or endometrial cancer specimen

Data from LaDuca, H., Polley, E. C., Yussuf, A., Hoang, L., Gutierrez, S., Hart, S. N., … Dolinsky, J. S. (2020). A clinical guide to hereditary cancer panel testing: Evaluation of gene-specific cancer associations and sensitivity of genetic testing criteria in a cohort of 165,000 high-risk patients. *Genetics in Medicine, 22*(2), 407–415; Shane-Carson, K., & Jeter, J. M. (2019). Hereditary risk for cancer. In D. S. Alberts & L. M. Hess (Eds.), *Fundamentals of cancer prevention* (4th ed.). Cham: Springer International Publishing.

Ethnicity should be assessed and recorded because some groups (e.g., those of Ashkenazi Jewish ancestry) may be at increased risk for certain hereditary cancer syndromes. This is known as the *founder effect,* which is the accumulation of random genetic changes in an isolated population as a result of its proliferation from only a few parent colonizers (McClary, 2020).

After the pedigree is constructed, risks for developing cancers are calculated based on the family history, personal history, and likelihood of having a pathogenic variant. If the family history suggests a germline pathogenic variant or the family meets designated criteria from a professional agency

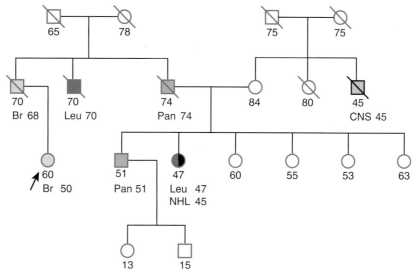

Components of a Pedigree. *Squares* represent males, and *circles* represent females. A *slash* represents a deceased person. *Solid circles* and *squares* represent diagnoses of cancer. The family member's current age or age at death is shown, as well as the age at a cancer diagnosis. The *arrow* represents the proband, or spokesperson, for the family. Three generations showing maternal and paternal sides are included. If information is known about ethnicity, it can be included. Ideally, all cancer diagnoses are verified by pathology reports or death certificates. *Br*, Breast cancer; *CNS*, central nervous system malignancy; *Leu*, leukemia; *NHL*, non-Hodgkin lymphoma; *Pan*, pancreatic cancer.

or Medicare criteria, the family can be offered the option of genetic testing (LaDuca et al., 2020). Typical elements of genetic counseling before germline genetic testing are described in the box below.

Counseling includes an extensive discussion about what recommendations will likely be made based on each genetic testing outcome and about the implications of testing for germline pathogenic variants for the patient and the entire family. If a pathogenic variant is identified, the immediate family members should inform other relatives that they may be at increased risk. This is an extensive process; a typical pretest counseling session takes approximately 75 to 90 minutes.

Recommendations for cancer prevention and early detection are based on the test results. The results may or may not be informative, and several outcomes of testing are possible (see the table on the next page). Recommendations may include increased surveillance, chemoprevention options, lifestyle strategies to decrease risk, and in some cases, prophylactic surgery. In cases of indeterminate results, participation in clinical trials may be an option. If a pathogenic variant is detected, other family members should be offered testing which is referred to as cascade testing (Srinivasan et al., 2020). In some cases, other family members may benefit from modified recommendations for cancer prevention and early detection.

Typical Elements of Pretest Genetic Counseling

- Explore patient concerns, motivations, and expectations regarding the genetic testing process.
- Clarify misconceptions about the process or concepts.
- Construct a pedigree.
- Document lifestyle and medical history risk factors.
- Perform a targeted physical examination for features associated with hereditary syndromes.
- Discuss factors that limit interpretation and assessment, such as adoption, estrangement from the family, or a small family structure.
- Present basic risk information about developing cancers.
- Present basic information about suspected syndromes.
- Present calculations for the risk of having a pathogenic variant or discuss clinical criteria that suggest hereditary risk.
- Discuss principles of genetics such as autosomal transmission, penetrance, founder effect, and the difference between germline and somatic pathogenic variants.
- Identify and discuss who are the best individuals to test in the family. It is best to begin testing a person who is affected with the disease or cancer because there is a much higher probability of identifying the pathogenic variant.
- Discuss alternatives to testing, including not testing.
- Discuss specimen collection, which is usually done with a buccal (saliva) specimen or a blood specimen.

- Discuss potential test outcomes of testing, which can include
  - *True Positive:* The person carries the pathogenic variant.
  - *True Negative:* The person does not carry a pathogenic variant known to be in the family.
  - *Noninformative Negative:* The person was the first one tested in a family and tested negative for pathogenic variants. This means the person does not carry a known pathogenic variant but could have another pathogenic variant for which testing has not been completed.
  - *Variant of Unknown Significance:* The person has a change in genetic material, but it is not clear whether it is associated with a particular disease or malignancy.
- Discuss possible management strategies for each outcome.
- Discuss testing costs, insurance coverage, and preauthorization.
- Discuss possible discrimination issues, especially for life, disability, and long-term care insurance.
- Discuss the potential benefits, risks, and limitations of genetic testing.
- Assess psychosocial support, including resources from the family, community, and religious affiliation.
- Offer opportunities to ask questions for clarification.

Potential Outcomes of Genetic Testing

Result	Implications for Individuals	Implications for Family Members
Positive result (pathogenic or likely pathogenic variant)	Individuals have increased risk of developing cancer. Encourage patients to adopt a healthier lifestyle. Consider risk-reducing surgery or using chemoprevention agents. Enables individuals to make decisions about more intensive early detection measures.	First-degree relatives have a 50% chance of having the pathogenic variant. Single-site testing would clarify if the family member has the pathogenic variant and associated increased risk. Single-site testing has a lower cost. Positive results do not inform about what type of cancer will develop or when, but informs only that the risk is higher. Cancer screening should start earlier and occur more often than usually recommended. Instruct patients on symptoms to report.
True negative (no pathogenic variant detected in an individual of a family with a known pathogenic variant)	In most cases, these individuals will not need screening greater than that recommended for the general population. Encourage patients to adopt a healthier lifestyle. Individuals do not need to consider risk-reducing surgery or chemoprevention.	Offspring from this individual are not at risk for carrying the known pathogenic variant. No further testing is necessary. Unless offspring have risk from the other parent, their risk for developing cancer is like that of the general population. Provides psychological relief regarding risk for developing cancer and that offspring will not inherit the pathogenic variant.
Negative result (no pathogenic variant identified in family)	The cancer may be the result of a different pathogenic variant from the one tested, or the cancer seen in the family occurs because of nonhereditary reasons. Results are difficult to interpret and must be considered in conjunction with personal risk factors and family history.	Testing is not typically available to other unaffected members in the family because they will also likely test negative especially if they do not have a diagnosis of cancer. Individuals are managed based on their personal and family history as their risk could still be increased. Individuals may consider participating in research studies or high-risk registries.
Genetic variant of unknown significance (VUS)	Test identifies a change in the genetic material; it is not clear if it is a harmless or harmful change. Results do not provide meaningful information. The test result is not actionable.	Meaningful testing will not be available to other family members. Results may create uncertainty and anxiety about the usefulness of cancer-risk reduction strategies. Individuals are managed based on their personal family history as their risk could still be increased. Individuals may consider participation in a research study or hereditary cancer registry.

Data from Colas, C., Golmard, L., de Pauw, A., Caputo, S. M., & Stoppa-Lyonnet, D. (2019). Decoding hereditary breast cancer benefits and questions from multigene panel testing. *Breast*, *45*, 29–35; LaDuca, H., Polley, E. C., Yussuf, A., Hoang, L., Gutierrez, S., Hart, S. N., … Dolinsky, J. S. (2020). A clinical guide to hereditary cancer panel testing: Evaluation of gene-specific cancer associations and sensitivity of genetic testing criteria in a cohort of 165,000 high-risk patients. *Genetics in Medicine*, *22*(2), 407–415.

Somatic Variants in Cancer Treatment

Diagnosis. Somatic genetic testing is sometimes done on tumor specimens to clarify the diagnosis. For example, identification of the *BRAF* V600E variant in a thyroid tumor specimen is diagnostic for papillary thyroid carcinoma (Araque et al., 2020). The presence of a somatic *BRAF* variant in a colorectal tumor showing high-microsatellite instability suggests the tumor is sporadic and not a case of hereditary nonpolyposis colorectal cancer (HNPCC), which is sometimes referred to as Lynch syndrome (Schmitt, 2020).

Prognosis. Somatic variant profiles can help clarify the prognosis for some malignancies. Patients who have activating variants in *KRAS* who have adenocarcinomas of the lung, colon, and pancreas often have a poor prognosis (Luo, 2021; Meng et al., 2021; Xie et al., 2021). Women diagnosed with breast cancer that is estrogen receptor negative, progesterone receptor negative, and nonamplified *HER2* (i.e., triple-negative breast cancer) may have a more aggressive form of breast cancer that can sometimes be more difficult to treat (Howard & Olopade, 2021).

Risk of Recurrence. Understanding what the risk of recurrence is for a cancer and the potential benefits of systemic therapy can help patients make treatment decisions. Systemic therapy can have toxic short-term and long-term effects. Genetic evaluation of breast, prostate, and colon malignant tumors can estimate the chance of recurrence and the potential benefit of systemic therapy (PDQ Cancer Genetics Overview, n.d.). For example, the Oncotype DX test for stage I or II breast cancers that are estrogen receptor positive, progesterone receptor positive, and nonamplified *HER2* examines 21 genes in a tumor to determine a *recurrence score*. The recurrence score corresponds to the likelihood of breast cancer recurrence within 10 years of the initial diagnosis, and it is reported as low, intermediate, or high risk (Syed, 2020). This can also help inform whether a patient is likely to benefit from systemic therapy.

Treatment. Biomarker tests can enable the selection of a cancer treatment based on the genomic signature of the malignancy. Some cancer treatments, including targeted therapies and immunotherapies, may only work for individuals whose cancers have certain biomarkers. Testing the tumor or performing a liquid biopsy can provide information about the genomic changes driving the growth of the malignancy. Increasing numbers of somatic variants have been identified that indicate whether a tumor will be susceptible or resistant to anticancer therapy. For example, activating variants in kinase genes (e.g., *EGFR*, *KIT*, and *BRAF*) or translocations that lead to overexpression of kinases (e.g., *ALK*) often result in susceptibility of the tumor cells to small-molecule inhibitors that are selective for the affected kinase. Tyrosine kinase inhibitors (TKIs) are a class of medications that block the enzyme tyrosine kinase. TKIs are a form of targeted therapy that lessens the risk of damage to healthy cells and increases the likelihood of treatment success. Similarly individuals with a malignancy that has certain genetic changes in the *EGFR* gene can get treatments that target those changes, called EGFR inhibitors. In this case, biomarker testing can find out whether someone's cancer has an *EGFR* gene change that can be treated with an EGFR inhibitor.

Pharmacogenomics

There is a growing body of knowledge about how some alleles in germline DNA contribute to therapeutic responses. Pharmacogenomics is the study of how gene variants affect a person's response to drugs. This relatively new field combines pharmacology and genomics to develop effective, safe medications and doses that can be tailored to a person's genetic makeup. Response to drug therapy varies from person to person. It can be difficult to predict who will benefit from a medication, who will not respond at all, and who will experience negative side effects (i.e., adverse drug reactions). For example, a dihydropyrimidine dehydrogenase deficiency can limit dosages and sometimes lead to life-threatening toxicity in persons receiving 5-fluorouracil (Miteva-Marcheva et al., 2020). Identification of patients who carry these variants can guide treatment selection to avoid unnecessary toxicity.

Conclusion

Knowledge of genetics is revolutionizing cancer care. Understanding these concepts is essential in oncology nursing practice. Nurses need to be able to identify patients and families with possible germline pathogenic variants and refer them to genetics professionals for evaluation. Patients should understand the difference between germline and somatic variants.

More tests are being developed to analyze tumor specimens for somatic changes to provide information for diagnosis, prognosis, and effective treatment selection. Pharmacogenomics is an emerging field that offers a way to select the best treatment with the least toxicity.

References

Araque, K. A., Gubbi, S., & Klubo-Gwiezdzinska, J. (2020). Updates on the management of thyroid cancer. *Hormone and Metabolic Research, 52*(8), 562–577.

Colas, C., Golmard, L., de Pauw, A., Caputo, S. M., & Stoppa-Lyonnet, D. (2019). "Decoding hereditary breast cancer" benefits and questions from multigene panel testing. *Breast, 45*, 29–35.

FDA-NIH Biomarker Working Group. (2016). BEST (Biomarkers, EndpointS, and other Tools) Resource [Internet]. Silver Spring (MD): Food and Drug Administration (US), co-published by National Institutes of Health (US), Bethesda, MD. Available at https://www.ncbi.nlm.nih.gov/books/NBK326791/.

Friend, P., Dickman, E., & Calzone, K. (2021). Using a genomics taxonomy: Facilitating patient care safety and quality in the era of precision oncology. *Clinical Journal of Oncology Nursing, 25*(2), 205–209.

Gates, A. J., Gysi, D. M., Kellis, M., et al. (2021). A wealth of discovery built on the Human Genome Project—By the numbers. *Nature, 590*, 212–215.

Howard, F. M., & Olopade, O. I. (2021). Epidemiology of triple-negative breast cancer: A review. *The Cancer Journal, 27*(1), 8–16.

LaDuca, H., Polley, E. C., Yussuf, A., Hoang, L., Gutierrez, S., Hart, S. N., … Dolinsky, J. S. (2020). A clinical guide to hereditary cancer panel testing: Evaluation of gene-specific cancer associations and sensitivity of genetic testing criteria in a cohort of 165,000 high-risk patients. *Genetics in Medicine, 22*(2), 407–415.

Li, M. M., Datto, M., Duncavage, E. J., Kulkarni, S., Lindeman, N. I., Roy, S., … Nikiforova, M. N. (2017). Standards and guidelines for the interpretation and reporting of sequence variants in cancer: A joint consensus recommendation of the Association for Molecular Pathology, American Society of Clinical Oncology, and College of American Pathologists. *The Journal of Molecular Diagnostics, 19*(1), 4–23.

Luo, J. (2021). KRAS mutation in pancreatic cancer. *Seminars in Oncology, 48*(1), 10–18.

McClary, L. M. (2020). *Essentials of medical genetics for nursing and health professionals*. Sudbury, MA: Jones & Bartlett Learning.

Meng, M., Zhong, K., Jiang, T., Liu, Z., Kwan, H. Y., & Su, T. (2021). The current understanding on the impact of KRAS on colorectal cancer. *Biomedicine & Pharmacotherapy, 140*, 111717.

Miteva-Marcheva, N., Ivanov, H. Y., Dimitrov, D. K., & Stoyanova, V. K. (2020). Application of pharmacogenetics in oncology. *Biomarker Research, 8*, 32.

NCI Dictionary of Cancer Terms. (n.d.). Available at https://www.cancer.gov/publications/dictionaries/cancer-terms.

NCI Dictionary of Genetic Terms. (n.d.). Available at https://www.cancer.gov/publications/dictionaries/genetics-dictionary.

PDQ Cancer Genetics Overview. (n.d.). Available at https://www.cancer.gov/about-cancer/causes-prevention/genetics/overview-pdq#_146.

Schmitt, M. L. (2020). Molecular biomarkers: A review of multiple applications in clinical care of colorectal cancer. *Clinical Journal of Oncology Nursing, 24*(6), 635–643.

Srinivasan, S., Won, N. Y., Dotson, W. D., Wright, S. T., & Roberts, M. C. (2020). Barriers and facilitators for cascade testing in genetic conditions: A systematic review. *European Journal of Human Genetics, 28*(12), 1631–1644.

Syed, Y. Y. (2020). Oncotype DX breast recurrence score®: A review of its use in early-stage breast cancer. *Molecular Diagnosis & Therapy, 24*(5), 621–632.

Xie, M., Xu, X., & Fan, Y. (2021). KRAS-mutant non-small cell lung cancer: An emerging promisingly treatable subgroup. *Frontiers in Oncology, 11*, 672612.

Breast Cancer

Linda Buck

Invasive Breast Cancer

Definition

Invasive breast cancer, also referred to as infiltrating breast cancer, has spread beyond the basement membrane of the duct or lobule of the breast and into the surrounding tissue. Invasive breast cancer is considered a systemic disease because of its ability to spread to distant sites through the vascular or lymphatic systems. The breast includes the following anatomic areas (see the figure below):

- Nipple
- Areola
- Duct and ductal
- Lactiferous sinus and lactiferous duct
- Lobules
- Alveolus
- Adipose tissue
- Suspensory ligaments of Cooper
- Pectoralis major and minor muscles
- Associated lymph nodes

Incidence

(American Cancer Society, 2022c)

- In the United States, breast cancer is the most common cancer and the second leading cause of cancer deaths among women.
- An estimated 287,850 new cases of invasive breast cancer were diagnosed in the United States in 2022. This represents 31% of all new cases of cancer in women.
- The incidence is highest among White women, followed by Black women.
- The incidence increases up to the seventh decade. The median age of development is 62.
- Male breast cancer accounts for fewer than 1% of all breast cancers. An estimated 2710 new diagnoses and 530 deaths occurred in the United States in 2022.

Etiology and Risk Factors

Breast cancer is a heterogeneous disease with no single cause. Several factors are commonly associated with an increased risk of breast cancer (Łukasiewicz et al., 2021):

- Sex: More than 99% of cases occur in women
- Age: Risk increases with age, which is the strongest risk factor

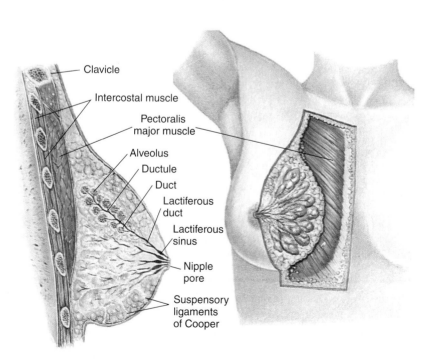

Anatomy of the Breast. (From Perry, S. E., Lowdermilk, D. L., & Cashion, K. [2023]. *Maternal child nursing care* [7th ed.]. St. Louis: Elsevier.)

Labels: Clavicle, Intercostal muscle, Pectoralis major muscle, Alveolus, Ductule, Duct, Lactiferous duct, Lactiferous sinus, Nipple pore, Suspensory ligaments of Cooper

- Race: Highest risk in White, non-Hispanic women; highest mortality in Black women
- Personal history of breast cancer: Three- to fourfold increased risk of a second primary breast cancer
- Family history of breast cancer is associated with a greater risk if:
  - One first-degree relative is affected, which doubles the risk.
  - Two first-degree relatives are affected, which increases the risk threefold.
  - The relative has bilateral breast cancer.
  - The relative with breast cancer is male.
  - The relative's breast cancer was diagnosed before menopause.
- Inherited genetic mutations account for up to 10% of all breast cancers (Łukasiewicz et al., 2021):
  - *BRCA1* (17q21): Lifetime risk of developing breast cancer in some families is as high as 80%; average risk is 55% to 65%.
  - *BRCA2* (13q14): Lifetime breast cancer risk is approximately 45%.
  - Other rare genetic mutations may increase risk but far less than *BRCA* mutations (see the table below).
- History of receiving ionizing radiation to the chest (e.g., patient with a history of Hodgkin lymphoma treated with mantle irradiation).
- Hormonal factors:
  - Menarche before age 12 or menopause after age 55
- First term pregnancy after age 30
- Nulliparity
- Use of oral contraceptives before age 20 years, with use lasting 6 years or more
- Hormone replacement therapy with estrogen plus progestin for more than 5 years
- Use of diethylstilbestrol (DES) to prevent miscarriage from 1940 to 1971
- Overweight and obese women have a higher incidence of breast cancer.
  - Postmenopausal overweight (body mass index [BMI] >25–30) women are at 1.5 times higher risk for breast cancer than women with a BMI less than 25.
  - Postmenopausal obese (BMI >30) women are at two times higher risk for breast cancer than women with a BMI less than 25.
- Proliferative breast disease, atypical hyperplasia, or previous in situ disease
- Dense breast tissue on mammography
- Smoking and drinking 10 g (i.e., one drink) of alcohol per day increase the breast cancer risk by 10% for each drink.
- Risks specific to men include radiation exposure, gene mutations, family history of breast cancer, obesity, testicular disorders, and Klinefelter syndrome (i.e., extra copy of the X chromosome in boys).

Inherited Genetic Mutations That Increase Breast Cancer Risk

Gene	Normal Function	Mutation
ATM	Helps to repair damaged DNA	One mutated copy has been linked to a high rate of breast cancer in some families.
TP53	Encodes the TP53 (p53) protein, which acts as a tumor suppressor and stops growth of abnormal cells	Inherited mutations cause Li-Fraumeni syndrome, which carries an increased risk of cancer, including breast cancer.
CHEK2	Encodes the checkpoint kinase 2 (CHK2) protein, which act as a tumor suppressor	Mutations can lead to Li-Fraumeni syndrome. With or without the syndrome, CHEK2 mutations can lead to a twofold increase in breast cancer risk.
PTEN	Encodes a tumor suppressor enzyme found in most tissues, which helps to regulate cellular growth	Inherited mutation can cause Cowden syndrome, a rare disorder that increases the risk of benign and malignant breast tumors and growths in the gastrointestinal tract, thyroid, uterus, and ovaries.
CDH1	Encodes a protein called epithelial cadherin (E-cadherin), which is found in the membrane that surrounds epithelial cells and helps neighboring cells stick to one another (i.e., cell adhesion) to form organized tissues	Inherited mutations cause hereditary diffuse gastric cancer and, in women, an increased risk of invasive lobular breast cancer.
STK11	Encodes a tumor suppressor protein called serine/threonine kinase 11	Defects can lead to Peutz-Jeghers syndrome, which causes pigmented spots on the lips and in the mouth, gastrointestinal and urinary polyps, and an increased risk of cancer, including breast cancer.
PALB2	Encodes a protein that works with the BRCA2 protein to repair damaged DNA and stop tumor growth	Mutations can lead to an increased risk of breast cancer.
XRCC2	Involved in DNA repair	Associated with Fanconi anemia, premature ovarian failure, spermatogenic failure

Data from Łukasiewicz, S., Czeczelewski, M., Forma, A., Baj, J., Sitarz, R., & Stanisławek, A. (2021). Breast cancer—epidemiology, risk factors, classification, prognostic markers, and current treatment strategies—an updated review. *Cancers, 13*(17), 4287.

Signs and Symptoms

Breast cancer in its early stages is usually asymptomatic. Later signs and symptoms include the following (Harbeck et al., 2019):

- A firm, painless, possibly immobile lump
- Pain is uncommon in early stages of disease
- Changes in the size or shape of the breast
- Swelling on all or part of the breast
- May have peau d'orange (orange peel appearance) with inflammatory breast cancer
- Spontaneous, unilateral nipple discharge that is clear, black, pink, or bloody
- Presence of enlarged, firm, nontender lymph nodes
- Skin changes such as dimpling, edema, erythema, ulceration, or thickening
- Nipple changes such as inversion, scaling, ulceration, pain, thickening, or color changes
- Symptoms of metastases to distant sites include shortness of breath, cough, loss of appetite, abnormal liver function test results, headaches, and back pain

Diagnostic Workup

A diagnostic mammogram is used for the detection of breast lesions. The diagnostic workup is completed to stage the breast cancer and develop an appropriate treatment plan (Esserman & Joe, 2022).

- Clinical breast examination includes bilateral breasts, axillae, and supraclavicular and infraclavicular areas.
- Workup may include ultrasonography, mammography with spot compression and magnification views, or magnetic resonance imaging (MRI).
- Digital breast mammography using tomosynthesis can help localize lesions, especially in noncalcified lesions.
- Biopsy is done for a pathologic diagnosis. Core needle biopsy is the preferred initial approach. Other options include using fine needle aspiration (FNA) for a palpable lesion. Stereotactic core-needle biopsy with imaging guidance or surgical incisional or excisional biopsy is used for nonpalpable lesions. Biopsy techniques are reviewed in the table below.
- Imaging studies to assess the extent of disease may include a chest radiograph, bone scan, computed tomography (CT) of the chest and abdomen, and MRI of the brain.
- Laboratory tests include a complete blood count and chemistry panel.

Breast Biopsy Techniques

Type of Biopsy	Analysis Method	Rationale for Use
Core needle biopsy (preferred method)	Histology	Allows more thorough evaluation of the tumor
Fine-needle aspiration	Cytology	Must be used for a palpable lesion, can be a stereotactic fine-needle aspiration
Open	Histology	Recommended for lesions that are difficult to obtain via a core or fine-needle aspiration

Histopathology

- Breast cancer is a heterogeneous disease with many histologic subtypes. The more common subtypes of invasive breast cancer include the following (American Cancer Society, 2022c):
  - Invasive ductal carcinoma: 70% to 80% of all breast cancers
  - Invasive lobular carcinoma: 10% to 15% of all breast cancers
  - Medullary carcinomas: 5% to 7% of malignant breast tumors
  - Less common subtypes include the following:
    - Paget disease occurring in the nipple with intraductal or invasive ductal carcinoma
    - Tubular, mucinous, and papillary carcinomas
    - Angiosarcoma and phyllodes tumors of the breast (rare)
  - Inflammatory breast cancer is not a subtype but a special manifestation that typically manifests with dramatic and diffuse skin edema, erythema, hyperemia, and induration of the underlying tissue.
- Identification of prognostic factors is essential for determining the appropriate treatment of an individual woman's breast cancer (Łukasiewicz et al., 2021):
  - Axillary lymph node status: Prognosis worsens with increased involvement.
  - Tumor size: Increased risk of recurrence with increasing size.
  - Hormone receptor status: Tumors without estrogen receptors (ER−) and progesterone receptors (PR−) are associated with a poorer prognosis.
  - Deoxyribonucleic acid (DNA) ploidy: Aneuploid tumors with an abnormal amount of DNA and an unorganized dividing pattern have a poorer prognosis.
  - High S-phase fraction or higher division rate predicts a poorer outcome.
  - Histopathologic grading: Considers the nuclear pattern, morphologic features, and mitotic activity; the higher the grade, the worse the prognosis.
  - Molecular subtypes that are being investigated and targeted for future therapies:
    - Luminal A type: 40% of all breast cancers; typically, they are slower growing and have a hormone profile of ER+/PR+ and HER2−.
    - Luminal B type: 10% to 20% of all breast cancers are ER+/PR+ and have a high proliferation rate.
    - Ki-67 and PR are useful for luminal subtyping.
    - Basal-like (triple-negative breast cancer—TNBC): 10% to 20% of breast cancers; are ER−/PR−/HER2− evaluation of cytokeratin 5/6 and epidermal growth factor receptor is used to identify basal-like breast cancer among the TNBC.
    - HER2 enriched: 10% of all breast cancers; are ER−/PR−/HER2+ and tend to be more aggressive.
- Molecular and biologic factors that may be associated with a poor prognosis include the following:
  - TNBC: ER−/PR−/HER2−
  - Loss of functioning of tumor suppression genes such as TP53 and NME/NM23

- Overexpression of oncogenes such as HER2 and epidermal growth factor receptor
- Roles of proteases such as cathepsin D and urokinase plasminogen activator in tumor cell invasion and metastasis

Clinical Staging

- Clinical staging is based on the size of the primary tumor (T), the presence of palpable lymph nodes with cancer in the axilla (N), and distant metastases (M). The size, nodes, and location of the cancer determine the overall disease stage (I–IV).
- Pathologic staging can be more accurate and is recommended by the American Joint Committee on Cancer Staging (AJCC) and can be found in the AJCC manual (American Cancer Society, 2022b).

Treatment

There are a variety of therapies for breast cancer patients. Treatment is determined by the size of the tumor, the stage of the disease, menopausal and hormone receptor status, and the histology of the cancer, including tumor markers. Treatment goals depend on whether the breast cancer is localized, metastatic, or recurrent (National Comprehensive Cancer Network, 2022).

Surgery

- Surgical resection of the tumor with breast-conserving surgery includes a lumpectomy or partial mastectomy with a sentinel node biopsy.
- Evidence has shown that breast-conserving surgery with postoperative irradiation is as effective as a total mastectomy with lymph node dissection for early-stage breast cancer.
- Bilateral mastectomies with immediate reconstruction may be used in younger women with *BRCA*-associated early breast cancer in one breast.
- A summary of surgical procedures can be found in the table below.

Radiation Therapy

- Radiation therapy (RT) is the treatment of choice to achieve local control of cancer.
- To reduce the risk of recurrence and eradicate any remaining microscopic cancer cells, RT is given after surgery or chemotherapy.
- Accelerated partial breast irradiation (APBI) may be used. APBI delivers a higher concentrated dose of radiation to the tumor bed over a shorter period than other methods.
- APBI can be delivered intraoperatively with one treatment or postoperatively with an inserted balloon over 5 days. Clinical trials are being conducted in the United States before this can be recommended as the standard of care.
- In the setting of metastatic disease, irradiation is used to treat solitary bone metastasis and for emergency treatment of spinal cord compression.

Systemic Therapy

(National Comprehensive Cancer Network, 2022)

- The goal of systemic treatment is to destroy or control cancer cells throughout the body.
- Systemic treatment includes chemotherapy, hormonal therapy, biologic, and targeted therapy, which may be given in neoadjuvant, adjuvant, and metastatic settings.
- Treatments are chosen based on factors such as age, health, size of tumor, nodal involvement, hormone receptor status, *HER2* status, and other factors.
- Oncotype Dx can be used for predictive and prognostic evaluation in early-stage breast cancer and to determine the risk/benefit ratio of chemotherapy.
- Breast cancer index (BCI) is used to determine the benefit of extended hormone therapy beyond 5 years.
- Hormonal therapies provide a response rate of 50% to 70% for women with ER+ and PR+ tumors.
- Hormonal therapies include tamoxifen, anastrozole, exemestane, fulvestrant, and letrozole.
- Some agents have been approved to enhance the efficacy of hormonal therapies after disease progression.

Breast Cancer Surgical Procedures

Treatment	Procedure
Breast-Conserving Surgeries (BCS)	
• Lumpectomy	Excision of tumor with small margin of normal tissue around it to remove cancer or abnormal tissue from the breast
• Partial mastectomy (e.g., partial/segmental mastectomy, lumpectomy, wide local excision, or quadrantectomy)	Excision of tumor with a wider margin of surrounding tissue but not the full breast itself
• Lymph node sampling (sentinel lymph node biopsy—SNLB or axillary lymph node dissection—ALND)	Can be done with any surgery / For sentinel node biopsy—dye is injected and identified at the sentinel nodes; if positive nodes are removed
Mastectomies	
• Nipple-areolar sparing mastectomy	Removal of the breast tissue sparing uninvolved nipple-areolar complex
• Skin sparing	Removes above plus limited overlying skin, at-risk biopsy scar
• Total (simple) mastectomy	Removes all breast tissue, including skin, gland, nipple-areolar complex
• Modified radical mastectomy	Removes breast plus axillary node dissection
• Radical mastectomy	Removes above plus underlying pectoral muscles

Data from Kaidar-Person, O., Offersen, B. V., Boersma, L. J., de Ruysscher, D., Tramm, T., Kühn, T., . . . Poortmans, P. (2021). A multidisciplinary view of mastectomy and breast reconstruction: Understanding the challenges. *The Breast, 56*, 42–52.

- Everolimus, a mammalian target of rapamycin (mTOR) inhibitor, plus exemestane is indicated for postmenopausal women with HER−/ER+/PR+ advanced breast cancer after progression on letrozole or anastrozole.
- Palbociclib, a CDK 4-6 inhibitor, plus letrozole is indicated for postmenopausal women with HER2−/ER+ advanced disease. The drug targets CDK4 and CDK6, which are involved in promoting the growth of cancer cells.
- Targeted therapies are used for the treatment of invasive breast cancer.
  - Early-stage disease: CDK 4-6 inhibitor abemaciclib is used in the adjuvant setting for patients at high risk of recurrence; PARP inhibitor Olaparib is used in the adjuvant setting for patients with a germline *BRCA* mutation who are at high risk for recurrence.
  - Triple-negative disease: Pembrolizumab is used in high-risk diseases.
  - Metastatic disease: PARP inhibitors (olaparib, talazoparib, rucaparib), mTOR inhibitor (everolimus), CDK 4-6 inhibitors (palbociclib, ribociclib, abemaciclib), PIK3CA inhibitor (alpelisib), and HER-2 inhibitor (neratinib, lapatinib).
- Chemotherapy may be given to reduce the size of a tumor before surgery (i.e., neoadjuvant chemotherapy), to eliminate occult tumor cells after primary surgery (i.e., adjuvant), or for palliation in the setting of metastatic cancer.
  - Agents commonly combined and used in the adjuvant and neoadjuvant settings are doxorubicin, epirubicin, paclitaxel, docetaxel, cyclophosphamide, carboplatin, fluorouracil, and methotrexate.
  - For metastatic disease, the same agents may be used as single agents. Other frequently used agents are capecitabine, gemcitabine, and vinorelbine.

Prognosis

The prognosis for breast cancer depends on many factors, including stage of disease, histologic diagnosis and grade of the cancer, hormone receptor status, HER2 protein overexpression status, menopausal status, and the overall health of the individual.

- The 5- and 10-year survival rate continues to improve (90% and 84%, respectively; 10% lower in Black women).
- Survival is lower for Black women than for White women at every stage of disease.
- Five-year relative survival has improved in White women from 76% (1975-1977) to 92% (2009-2015) and in Black women from 62% to 83% over the same time; while the gap has narrowed, a substantial gap continues to exist, especially for late-stage disease (American Cancer Society, 2022a).
- Among the many known prognostic factors, stage of disease is one of the best indicators of prognosis. Five-year survival rates for stage at diagnosis for individuals with breast cancer who receive appropriate treatment are as follows:
  - 99% for localized disease
  - 86% for regional disease
  - 27% for patients diagnosed with metastatic disease

Prevention and Surveillance

- Breast cancer screening includes clinical examinations, self-evaluations, and mammograms:
  - Screening mammograms are obtained between the ages of 40 and 44 years.
  - Women ages 45 to 54 should get mammograms every year.
  - Women 55 and older can switch to a mammogram every other year, or they can choose to continue yearly mammograms. Screening should continue as long as a woman is in good health and is expected to live at least 10 more years.
  - Women at high risk should begin screening mammography earlier.
  - Little evidence exists regarding the efficacy of breast self-examination (BSE); women should be familiar with how their breasts normally look and feel and should report any changes to a health care provider right away.
- Several trials have been conducted to evaluate breast cancer prevention:
  - The Exemestane for Breast Cancer Prevention in Postmenopausal Women trial showed early positive results of a 65% decrease in developing invasive cancer versus placebo.
  - The Breast Cancer Prevention Trial (BCPT or National Surgical Adjuvant Breast and Bowel Project 1 [NSABP-1]) showed a 49% risk reduction in breast cancer for women with a known high risk of breast cancer who took 20 mg of tamoxifen daily compared with those taking a placebo.
  - The Study of Tamoxifen and Raloxifene (STAR) trial (i.e., NSABP-P2) was a randomized trial comparing two drugs for reducing the incidence of breast cancer among high-risk, postmenopausal women. The initial results of STAR showed that raloxifene and tamoxifen were equally effective in reducing invasive breast cancer risk, but after an average of 81 months (i.e., 5 years of medication and 21 months of follow-up), raloxifene had reduced the risk by about 38% and tamoxifen had reduced the risk by about 50%.
  - The Multiple Outcomes of Raloxifene Evaluation (MORE) trial examined the effects of raloxifene versus placebo on the risk of osteoporosis and showed a reduced risk of osteoporosis and fractures. In a secondary end point of the trial, raloxifene also produced a 65% reduction in the risk of invasive breast cancer.
  - Prophylactic mastectomy accompanied by immediate reconstruction or oophorectomy may be appropriate for some women at high risk for breast cancer due to their genetic profiles.

References

American Cancer Society. (2022a). *Breast cancer facts and figures 2019-2020.* Available at https://www.cancer.org/content/dam/cancer-org/research/cancer-facts-and-statistics/breast-cancer-facts-and-figures/breast-cancer-facts-and-figures-2019-2020.pdf.

American Cancer Society. (2022b). *Breast cancer stages*. Available at https://www.cancer.org/cancer/breast-cancer/understanding-a-breast-cancer-diagnosis/stages-of-breast-cancer.html.

American Cancer Society. (2022c). *Cancer facts & figures 2022*. Available at https://www.cancer.org/content/dam/cancer-org/research/cancer-facts-and-statistics/annual-cancer-facts-and-figures/2022/2022-cancer-facts-and-figures.pdf.

Esserman, L. J., & Joe, B. N. (2022). Diagnostic evaluation of suspected breast cancer. Available at https://www.uptodate.com/contents/diagnostic-evaluation-of-suspected-breast-cancer?search=breast%20cancer&source=search_result&selectedTitle=4~150&usage_type=default&display_rank=4.

Harbeck, N., Penault-Llorca, F., Cortes, J., Gnant, M., Houssami, N., Poortmans, P., … Cardoso, F. (2019). Breast cancer. *Nature Reviews Disease Primers, 5*(1), 67.

Kaidar-Person, O., Offersen, B. V., Boersma, L. J., de Ruysscher, D., Tramm, T., Kühn, T., . . . Poortmans, P. (2021). A multidisciplinary view of mastectomy and breast reconstruction: Understanding the challenges. *The Breast, 56*, 42-52. https://doi.org/10.1016/j.breast.2021.02.004.

Łukasiewicz, S., Czeczelewski, M., Forma, A., Baj, J., Sitarz, R., & Stanisławek, A. (2021). Breast cancer-epidemiology, risk factors, classification, prognostic markers, and current treatment strategies—An updated review. *Cancers, 13*(17), 4287. https://doi.org/10.3390/cancers13174287.

National Comprehensive Cancer Network. (2022). Breast cancer, v.3. Available at https://www.nccn.org/professionals/physician_gls/pdf/breast.pdf.

Noninvasive Breast Cancer

Definition

Noninvasive breast cancers, also referred to as in situ carcinomas, are precancerous lesions confined to the duct or lobule in the breast. The two types of in situ carcinomas are ductal carcinoma in situ (DCIS) and lobular carcinoma in situ (LCIS) (American Cancer Society, 2022b; Badve & Gökmen-Polar, 2019; National Comprehensive Cancer Network, 2022).

- DCIS is a precancerous condition in which abnormal cells are found in the lining of a breast duct. DCIS may become invasive cancer and spread to other tissues.
- In LCIS, the abnormal cells are found only in the lobules of the breast. LCIS is 7 to 12 times more likely to progress to invasive breast cancer in the same or the opposite breast.

Incidence

- DCIS accounts for about 20% to 25% of all new breast cancer cases and about 5% of male breast cancers. Over 60,000 women are diagnosed each year with DCIS in the United States (American Cancer Society, 2022a).
- Treatment is controversial as 20% to 53% of women with untreated DCIS are ultimately diagnosed with invasive breast cancer (American Cancer Society, 2022a; Miller et al., 2022).
- The incidence of LCIS is difficult to estimate because it is usually an incidental finding and is therefore likely to be underdiagnosed (American Cancer Society, 2022b).

Etiology and Risk Factors

- The cause of noninvasive breast cancers is thought to be the same as for invasive breast cancer. The increased risk of death with DCIS is ipsilateral recurrence of invasive breast cancer.

Signs and Symptoms

(Badve & Gökmen-Polar, 2019; Thomas, 2018)

- Most women with noninvasive breast cancer do not have palpable lesions or symptoms.
- Rarely, a woman with DCIS is seen for a lump, nipple discharge, or Paget disease of the breast.
- LCIS is asymptomatic and is usually found by chance in tissue obtained during a breast biopsy or other surgical procedure.
- LCIS, although uncommon, occurs predominantly in premenopausal patients at an average age of about 45 years.

Diagnostic Workup

(Salvatorelli et al., 2020; Thomas, 2018; van Seijen et al., 2019)

- DCIS is typically diagnosed from routine mammograms.
- The mammogram shows an unusual cluster of calcifications.
- A needle-localization or needle-core biopsy may be required.
- Although not standard of care, some centers conduct sentinel node biopsies in cases of high-grade DCIS because there are reports of positive nodes in some cases.
- LCIS is usually diagnosed coincidently from tissue taken during a biopsy or breast surgery.

Histopathology

- DCIS is a precancerous condition in which abnormal cells are found in the lining of a breast duct.
- DCIS may become invasive cancer and spread to other tissues, although it is not known how to predict which lesions will become invasive.
- DCIS is further divided into noncomedo and comedo carcinomas and into low-, intermediate-, or high-grade lesions (Salvatorelli et al., 2020).
- LCIS is a precancerous condition in which abnormal cells are found in the lobules of the breast. It seldom progresses to an invasive cancer but having LCIS in one breast increases the risk for breast cancer in both breasts (Thomas, 2018).

Clinical Staging

- Applying AJCC staging classification system for breast cancer, a noninvasive cancer is stage 0.

Treatment

- Challenges exist in treatment as it is difficult to discern harmless lesions from potentially invasive ones (van Seijen et al., 2019).
- Treatment for DCIS depends on the extent and grade of disease, the classification, the patient's health, and the medical history.
- Breast-conserving surgery is the standard treatment for DCIS and is intended to completely remove all cancer cells with 2 mm free margins being recommended.
- Adjuvant treatments, such as RT and hormonal therapy, may be given to reduce the risk of DCIS recurring (Salvatorelli et al., 2020; van Seijen et al., 2019).
- Women with LCIS may be given the option of a lumpectomy or mastectomy.
- Many clinicians advocate local excision with close follow up that includes mammography twice a year and a clinical examination every 3 to 4 months.
- Women with LCIS may be given hormone therapy to reduce the risk of recurrence in the affected and bilateral breast (Thomas, 2018).

Prognosis

- The prognosis for women with noninvasive breast cancer is almost 100% survival at 5 years after diagnosis.
- Women with DCIS or LCIS carry an 8- to 10-fold risk for invasive breast cancer.
- DCIS classified as noncomedo, low-grade carcinoma carries a better prognosis than a high-grade, comedo carcinoma.
- LCIS is associated with a small but increased risk of invasive breast cancer (Badve & Gökmen-Polar, 2019).

Prevention and Surveillance

Information about the prevention of noninvasive breast cancers has not been specifically reported. It is thought to be the same as that for invasive breast cancer (Thomas, 2018).

References

American Cancer Society. (2022a). *Cancer facts & figures 2022*. Available at https://www.cancer.org/content/dam/cancer-org/research/cancer-facts-and-statistics/annual-cancer-facts-and-figures/2022/2022-cancer-facts-and-figures.pdf.

American Cancer Society. (2022b). *Lobular carcinoma in situ (LCIS)*. Available at https://www.cancer.org/cancer/breast-cancer/non-cancerous-breast-conditions/lobular-carcinoma-in-situ.html.

Badve, S. S., & Gökmen-Polar, Y. (2019). Ductal carcinoma in situ of breast: Update 2019. *Pathology, 51*(6), 563–569.

Miller, K. D., Nogueira, L., Devasia, T., Mariotto, A. B., Yabroff, K. R., Jemal, A., … Siegel, R. L. (2022). Cancer treatment and survivorship statistics, 2022. *CA: A Cancer Journal for Clinicians, 72*(5), 409–436. https://doi.org/10.3322/caac.21731.

National Comprehensive Cancer Network. (2022). Breast cancer, v.3. Available at https://www.nccn.org/professionals/physician_gls/pdf/breast.pdf.

Salvatorelli, L., Puzzo, L., Vecchio, G. M., Caltabiano, R., Virzì, V., & Magro, G. (2020). Ductal carcinoma in situ of the breast: An update with emphasis on radiological and morphological features as predictive prognostic factors. *Cancers, 12*(3), 609. https://www.mdpi.com/2072-6694/12/3/609.

Thomas, P. S. (2018). Diagnosis and management of high-risk breast lesions. *Journal of the National Comprehensive Cancer Network, 16*(11), 1391–1396. https://doi.org/10.6004/jnccn.2018.7099.

van Seijen, M., Lips, E. H., Thompson, A. M., Nik-Zainal, S., Futreal, A., Hwang, E. S., … PRECISION Team. (2019). Ductal carcinoma in situ: To treat or not to treat, that is the question. *British Journal of Cancer, 121*(4), 285–292. https://doi.org/10.1038/s41416-019-0478-6.

Central Nervous System Cancers

Marlon Garzo Saria

Definition

Central nervous system (CNS) malignancies are a histologically complex group of cancers that include brain and other CNS tumors with over 100 types as listed in the World Health Organization classification of central nervous system tumors (WHO CNS5) (Ostrom, Francis, et al., 2021). This chapter provides an overview of these diseases and addresses specific CNS malignancies in detail.

Incidence

(Ostrom, Cioffi, et al., 2021)
- The Central Brain Tumor Registry of the United States (CBTRUS) estimates that 25,690 cases of primary malignant CNS tumors and 62,500 cases of nonmalignant tumors will be diagnosed in 2021 (see the figure below).
  - Glioblastoma multiforme (GBM) is the most common malignant CNS tumor, accounting for 49.1% of malignant tumors.
  - The most prevalent nonmalignant tumor is meningioma, accounting for 54.5% of nonmalignant tumors.
- Incidence rates by age and gender at birth vary significantly based on tumor type.
  - The median age for GBM is 65, meningioma is 66, but the incidence of GBMs is greater among males, and the incidence of meningioma is higher in females. The median age for oligodendrogliomas is 43.

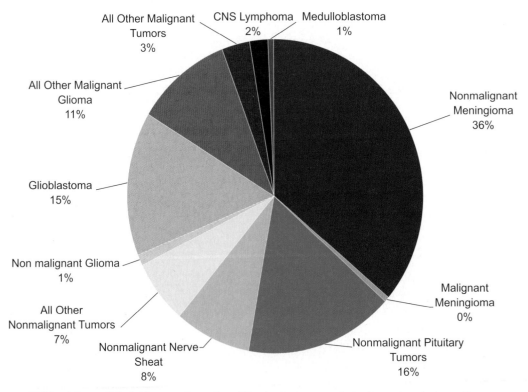

Epidemiology of Brain Tumors. Every slice of the pie chart represents the frequency of a type of tumor. *CNS,* Central nervous system. (From Campanella, R., Guarnaccia, L., Caroli, M., Zarino, B., Carrabba, G., La Verde, N., . . . Marfia, G. [2020]. Personalized and translational approach for malignant brain tumors in the era of precision medicine: The strategic contribution of an experienced neurosurgery laboratory in a modern neurosurgery and neuro-oncology department. *Journal of the Neurological Sciences, 417,* 117083.)

Etiology and Risk Factors

The only consistent risk factor for brain and other CNS tumors identified in adults is exposure to high doses of ionizing radiation.

- Radiofrequency field-emitting cellphones were classified as a possible carcinogen by the International Agency for Research on Cancer (IARC) in 2011, but most epidemiologic studies since the publication of the IARC report have found no significant associations.
- Extremely low frequency magnetic fields (ELFs) and power lines have also been studied; none have been consistently associated with the risk of brain and other CNS tumors.
- There are a number of Mendelian cancer syndromes that have been associated with increased risk of brain and CNS tumors: neurofibromatosis types 1 and 2, tuberous sclerosis, von Hippel–Lindau syndrome, Li-Fraumeni syndrome, and Turcot syndrome.
- Infections have been epidemiologically evaluated in glioma: polyomavirus family, including BK, JC, and SV40; herpesvirus including varicella zoster virus, Epstein-Barr virus, herpes simplex 1 and 2; cytomegalovirus; and *Toxoplasma gondii*.
- Diet, vitamins, alcohol use, tobacco use, and environmental exposures have been studied, but little information has been produced about the causes of CNS tumors, especially gliomas.

Signs and Symptoms

- Signs and symptoms are related to increased mass in the cranial vault and increased intracranial pressure.
- Symptoms include headache, nausea, vomiting, altered level of consciousness, cognitive impairment, dizziness, and seizures.
- Later sections of this chapter outline the specific signs and symptoms by tumor type.
- Focal signs and symptoms related to tumor location include seizures, weakness, sensory changes, visual changes, behavioral and personality changes, and endocrine abnormalities (see the figure below).

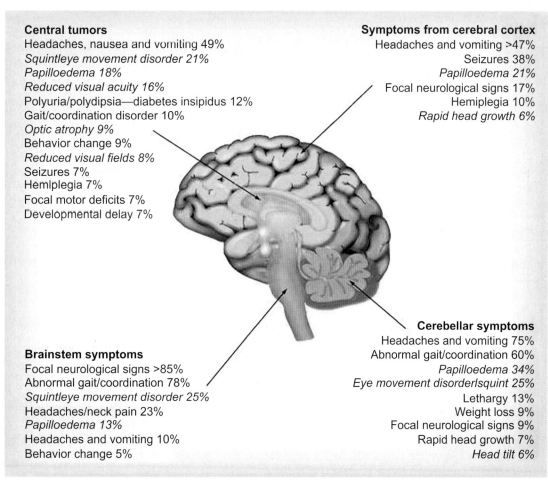

Central tumors
Headaches, nausea and vomiting 49%
Squint/eye movement disorder 21%
Papilloedema 18%
Reduced visual acuity 16%
Polyuria/polydipsia—diabetes insipidus 12%
Gait/coordination disorder 10%
Optic atrophy 9%
Behavior change 9%
Reduced visual fields 8%
Seizures 7%
Hemiplegia 7%
Focal motor deficits 7%
Developmental delay 7%

Symptoms from cerebral cortex
Headaches and vomiting >47%
Seizures 38%
Papilloedema 21%
Focal neurological signs 17%
Hemiplegia 10%
Rapid head growth 6%

Brainstem symptoms
Focal neurological signs >85%
Abnormal gait/coordination 78%
Squint/eye movement disorder 25%
Headaches/neck pain 23%
Papilloedema 13%
Headaches and vomiting 10%
Behavior change 5%

Cerebellar symptoms
Headaches and vomiting 75%
Abnormal gait/coordination 60%
Papilloedema 34%
Eye movement disorder/squint 25%
Lethargy 13%
Weight loss 9%
Focal neurological signs 9%
Rapid head growth 7%
Head tilt 6%

Brain Function and Symptoms Associated With Lesion Location. (From Walker, D., Hamilton, W., Walter, F. M., & Watts, C. [2013]. Strategies to accelerate diagnosis of primary brain tumors at the primary-secondary care interface in children and adults. *CNS Oncology, 2*[5], 447–462. https://doi.org/10.2217/cns.13.36. Copyright by Future Medicine Ltd.)

Diagnostic Workup

- Neurologic examination
- Magnetic resonance imaging (MRI) of the brain or spine
- Biopsy or craniotomy for a tissue diagnosis (American Cancer Society, 2020)
  - Tumors may look so characteristically obvious on an MRI scan that a biopsy is not needed
  - Tumor may be in a part of the brain that would make it hard to biopsy (e.g., brainstem).
  - In rare cases, a positron emission tomography (PET) scan or magnetic resonance spectroscopy (MRS) may give enough information so that a biopsy is not needed.
- Optional or additional radiologic studies
  - MRS
  - PET

Histopathology

- Classification of CNS tumors was historically based on histologic features only; however, advances in the understanding of molecular features led to the incorporation of molecular alterations into the diagnostic criteria (Gritsch et al., 2022) (see the figure below).
  - Molecular classification is highly relevant since patients with CNS tumors are now considered for inclusion in clinical trials of targeted drugs based on genetic profile of the underlying tumor.
- Incorporation of relevant diagnostic markers, including histopathologic and molecular information, should be considered standard practice for tumor classification (National Comprehensive Cancer Network, 2022).

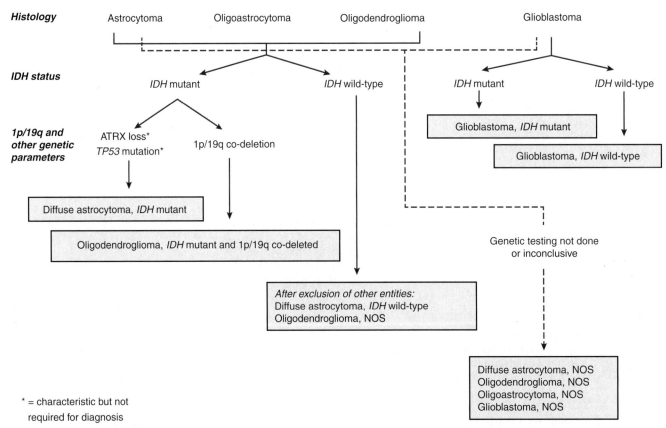

Simplified Algorithm to Classify the Diffuse Gliomas as a Function of Histologic and Genetic Features. Of note, the diagnostic flow does not necessarily proceed from histology to molecular genetic features because molecular signatures may outweigh histologic characteristics in achieving an integrated diagnosis. *IDH,* Isocitrate dehydrogenase; *NOS,* not otherwise specified. (Redrawn from Louis, D. N., Perry, A., Reifenberger, G., von Deimling, A., Figarella-Branger, D., Cavenee, W. K., . . . Ellison, D. W. [2016]. The 2016 World Health Organization classification of tumors of the central nervous system: A summary. *Acta Neuropathologica. 131*[6], 803–820.)

- For decades, CNS tumor grading has been distinct from the grading of other, non-CNS cancers. WHO CNS5 brought CNS tumor grading closer to how grading is done for non-CNS neoplasms but has retained some key aspects of traditional CNS tumor grading.
  - Two specific aspects of CNS tumor grading have changed for WHO CNS5: Arabic numerals are employed (rather than Roman numerals) and neoplasms are graded within types rather than across different tumor types (Louis et al., 2021).
- WHO CNS5 featured several changes in the classification, diagnostic criteria, nomenclature, and grading of diffuse gliomas. Adult-type diffuse gliomas are genetically defined and include astrocytoma, isocitrate dehydrogenase (IDH)-mutant, oligodendroglioma, IDH-mutant and 1p/19q codeleted, and glioblastoma, IDH-wildtype (Santosh & Rao, 2022).

Clinical Staging

- Because of the very low incidence of metastases, most CNS tumors do not require staging.
- If indicated, CNS staging involves imaging of the spine and obtaining cerebrospinal fluid (CSF) to identify evidence of metastasis.

Treatment

- Treatment, which varies based on tumor type, includes surgery, radiation, and chemotherapy.
- Molecular markers are used by neuropathologists to facilitate characterization of gliomas and/or by neuro-oncologists to guide treatment decisions.
- Treatment options being studied in clinical trials include immunotherapy and targeted agents.
- Clinical trials are evaluating the efficacy of using the tumor characteristics of proliferation, angiogenesis, and invasion to select treatments.
- Concomitant medications used for brain tumors often include steroids, especially dexamethasone, for control of cerebral edema or symptom management and anticonvulsants for patients in the acute postoperative period and those who have seizures.

Prognosis

- Prognosis depends on the tumor type and grade.
- Age, functional status, and neurocognitive status at diagnosis are strong prognostic indicators.
- The 5-year relative survival rate following diagnosis of a malignant brain and other CNS tumor was 66.9% (Ostrom, Francis, et al., 2021).

Prevention and Surveillance

- There are no known preventive measures to reduce the incidence of primary CNS tumors.
- Surveillance for CNS malignancies is discussed under the individual tumor types.

References

American Cancer Society. (2020). *Brain and spinal cord tumors in adults.* Available at https://www.cancer.org/cancer/brain-spinal-cord-tumors-adults.html.

Gritsch, S., Batchelor, T. T., & Gonzalez Castro, L. N. (2022). Diagnostic, therapeutic, and prognostic implications of the 2021 World Health Organization classification of tumors of the central nervous system. *Cancer, 128*(1), 47–58.

Louis, D. N., Perry, A., Wesseling, P., Brat, D. J., Cree, I. A., Figarella-Branger, D., … Ellison, D. W. (2021). The 2021 WHO classification of tumors of the central nervous system: A summary. *Neuro-Oncology, 23*(8), 1231–1251.

National Comprehensive Cancer Network. (2022). *NCCN clinical practice guidelines in oncology (NCCN guidelines)—Central nervous system cancers version 1.2022.* Available at https://www.nccn.org/professionals/physician_gls/pdf/cns.pdf.

Ostrom, Q. T., Cioffi, G., Waite, K., Kruchko, C., & Barnholtz-Sloan, J. S. (2021). CBTRUS statistical report: Primary brain and other central nervous system tumors diagnosed in the United States in 2014-2018. *Neuro-Oncology, 23*(12 Suppl 2), iii1–iii105.

Ostrom, Q. T., Francis, S. S., & Barnholtz-Sloan, J. S. (2021). Epidemiology of brain and other CNS tumors. *Current Neurology and Neuroscience Reports, 21*(12), 68.

Santosh, V., & Rao, S. (2022). A review of adult-type diffuse gliomas in the WHO CNS5 classification with special reference to astrocytoma, IDH-mutant and oligodendroglioma, IDH-mutant and 1p/19q codeleted. *Indian Journal of Pathology & Microbiology, 65*(Supplement), S14–S23.

Walker, D., Hamilton, W., Walter, F. M., & Watts, C. (2013). Strategies to accelerate diagnosis of primary brain tumors at the primary-secondary care interface in children and adults. *CNS Oncology, 2*(5), 447–462.

Astrocytoma, Isocitrate Dehydrogenase-Mutant

Definition

Diffuse astrocytomas represent the most common group of infiltrative primary brain tumors in adults (Recht et al., 2022). Astrocytoma, IDH-mutant is a diffusely infiltrating astrocytic glioma that harbors IDH1 or IDH2 mutations. In the new WHO CNS5 classification, astrocytoma, IDH-mutant is genetically defined and classified as adult-type diffuse gliomas with oligodendroglioma, IDH-mutant and 1p/19q codeleted, and glioblastoma, IDH-wildtype (Santosh & Rao, 2022).

Incidence

- WHO-CNS5 grading criteria had not yet been incorporated into registry reporting. Brain tumor molecular data are available for the first time in 2022 from the US cancer registries and CBTRUS for diagnosis year 2018 in the United States (Iorgulescu et al., 2022).
- The three WHO CNS5 subtypes (i.e., grades) are astrocytoma, IDH-mutant CNS WHO grade 2; astrocytoma, IDH-mutant CNS WHO grade 3; and astrocytoma, IDH-mutant CNS WHO grade 4 (Santosh & Rao, 2022).

Etiology and Risk Factors

(Kapoor & Gupta, 2021)

- There is no known cause for astrocytomas, but the following are considered risk factors:
  - Exposure to ionizing radiation; children who receive prophylactic radiation for acute lymphocytic leukemia (ALL) may have 22 times more chance of developing CNS malignancy within about 5 to 10 years.

- Genetic disorders, including Turcot syndrome, p53 mutations (Li-Fraumeni), and NF1 syndrome.

Signs and Symptoms

(Kapoor & Gupta, 2021)

- Symptoms are classified into two categories: general and focal.
  - General symptoms include early morning headache, nausea, vomiting, cognitive difficulties, personality changes, and gait disorders.
  - Localizing symptoms include seizures, aphasia, or visual field defects.

Diagnostic Workup

(Kapoor & Gupta, 2021)

- Full neurologic examination
- MRI of the brain or spine; gadolinium contrast-enhanced MR imaging recommended
- Biopsy or craniotomy for a tissue diagnosis

Histopathology

(Santosh & Rao, 2022)

- Astrocytoma, IDH-mutant tumors are diffusely infiltrating
- Mutations in IDH1 and 2 genes are the important driver mutations in the initiation and progression of most adult diffuse gliomas.
- Astrocytoma, IDH-mutant, CNS WHO grade 2 tumors are well-differentiated, mild to moderately cellular astroglial tumors, composed of fibrillary, protoplasmic, and gemistocytic astrocytes in varying proportions.
- Astrocytoma, IDH-mutant, CNS WHO grade 3 tumors are more cellular, show anaplastic features including multinucleated tumor cells, nuclear atypia, and significant mitosis. The defining feature of these tumors is an absence of microvascular proliferation and necrosis.
- Astrocytoma, IDH-mutant, CNS WHO grade 4 show necrosis and/or microvascular proliferation along with the histologic features of grade 3 tumors. Several times, they have focal oligodendroglioma-like areas.

Clinical Staging

- There is no standard staging system for brain tumors since they rarely spread to other parts of the body.

Treatment

- A multidisciplinary review of treatment planning as soon as pathology is available is highly recommended.
- Maximal safe resection is the preferred initial approach for patients with suspected diffuse gliomas of all grades, even for tumors discovered incidentally (National Comprehensive Cancer Consortium [NCCN], 2022a; Recht et al., 2022).
- Surgery alone is not curative in patients with diffuse gliomas, even for grade 2 tumors, and additional therapy (i.e., radiation and chemotherapy) is ultimately required in nearly all patients.
- WHO grade 2, low risk, Karnofsky Performance Status (KPS) ≥60 (NCCN, 2022a)
  - Clinical trial
  - Observe

- WHO grade 2, high risk, KPS ≥60 (NCCN, 2022a)
  - Clinical trial
  - Radiation therapy (RT) with adjuvant PCV (procarbazine/lomustine/vincristine)
  - RT with adjuvant temozolamide
  - RT with concurrent and adjuvant temozolamide
  - Observe
- WHO grade 3 or 4, KPS ≥60 (NCCN, 2022a)
  - Clinical trial
  - RT with adjuvant temozolamide
  - RT with concurrent and adjuvant temozolamide
- Any grade, KPS ≤60 (NCCN, 2022a)
  - RT
  - Temozolamide
  - Palliative or best supportive care

Prognosis

- IDH-mutant astrocytomas in adults are treatable but incurable tumors, and the vast majority are life-limiting (Recht et al., 2022).
- Favorable for low-grade tumors; survival times approaching 7 to 8 years after surgery (Kapoor & Gupta, 2021).
- Radiotherapy of partially resected tumors increases postoperative survival rates; survival rates after post-surgery radiation are nearly double that of only surgical intervention.

Prevention and Surveillance

- There are no known preventative measures to reduce the incidence of primary CNS tumors.
- Active surveillance after surgery alone typically involves an MRI with contrast every 3 to 4 months.
- After patients have completed the prescribed therapy, they should be monitored according to the NCCN Survivorship Care for Cancer-Related Late and Long-Term Effects (NCCN, 2022b).

References

Iorgulescu, J. B., Sun, C., Neff, C., Cioffi, G., Gutierrez, C., Kruchko, C., … Barnholtz-Sloan, J. S. (2022). Molecular biomarker-defined brain tumors: Epidemiology, validity, and completeness in the United States. *Neuro-Oncology*, 24(11), 1989–2000.

Kapoor, M., & Gupta, V. (2021). Astrocytoma. *StatPearls [Internet]*. https://www.ncbi.nlm.nih.gov/books/NBK559042/.

National Comprehensive Cancer Network (NCCN). (2022a). NCCN clinical practice guidelines in oncology (NCCN guidelines)—Central nervous system cancers, version 1.2022. Available at https://www.nccn.org/professionals/physician_gls/pdf/cns.pdf.

National Comprehensive Cancer Network (NCCN). (2022b). NCCN clinical practice guidelines in oncology (NCCN guidelines)—Survivorship, version 1.2022. Available at https://www.nccn.org/professionals/physician_gls/pdf/survivorship.pdf.

Recht, L., van den Bent, M., & Shih, H. A. (2022). Treatment and prognosis of IDH-mutant astrocytomas in adults. In *UpToDate*. Available at https://www.uptodate.com/contents/treatment-and-prognosis-of-idh-mutant-astrocytomas-in-adults?search=astrocytoma&source=search_result&selectedTitle=2~75&usage_type=default&display_rank=2.

Santosh, V., & Rao, S. (2022). A review of adult-type diffuse gliomas in the WHO CNS5 classification with special reference to astrocytoma, IDH-mutant and oligodendroglioma, IDH-mutant and 1p/19q codeleted. *Indian Journal of Pathology & Microbiology*, 65(Supplement), S14–S23.

Glioblastoma, IDH-Wildtype

Definition

Glioblastoma is the most common malignant primary brain tumor in adults. The 2021 revision of the WHO CNS5 classified glioblastoma into two separate diagnoses based primarily on IDH mutation status: glioblastoma, IDH-wildtype, CNS WHO grade 4, and astrocytoma, IDH-mutant, CNS WHO grade 4.

Incidence

(Melhem et al., 2022)

- Glioblastoma accounts for 14.5% of all primary CNS tumors and 48.6% of all malignant primary CNS tumors, with an annual age-adjusted incidence rate of 3.23 per 100,000 population
  - Incidence exponentially increases beyond 40 years of age, with a mean age of diagnosis at 65, and peaking between 75 and 84 years.
  - GBM is 1.59 times more common in males and 1.99 times more common in Caucasians compared to African American patients.

Etiology and Risk Factors

(Melhem et al., 2022)

- Ionizing radiation in medium-to-high doses, particularly in children, was consistently found to be a risk factor.
- Mendelian inherited syndromes (e.g., Lynch syndrome, neurofibromatosis, tuberous sclerosis) are identified in less than 4% of adult and pediatric cases.

Signs and Symptoms

(Dietrich, 2022)

- Clinical presentation often includes subacute neurologic signs and symptoms that progress over days to weeks and vary according to the location of the tumor within the brain.
- Most common presenting symptoms include headache (50%–60%), seizures (20%–50%), and focal neurologic symptoms such as memory loss, motor weakness, visual symptoms, language deficits, and cognitive and personality changes (10%–40%).

Diagnostic Workup

- MRI with gadolinium remains the gold standard diagnostic modality for GBM evaluation (Melhem et al., 2022).
- Advanced imaging techniques can assist with differential diagnosis:
  - Diffusion-weighted imaging (DWI)—calculate apparent diffusion coefficient (ADC) values, which assess tumor cellularity through measuring water diffusivity; GBM has a significantly lower ADC value as compared to gliomas of lower grades.
  - Perfusion-weighted imaging (PWI)—reflects the state of the tumor vascular bed.
  - Dynamic susceptibility contrast MRI measures cerebral blood volume (CBV), a surrogate marker of total tumor vascularity; differentiates GBM from lower-grade gliomas; compared to IDH-mutant tumors, IDH-wildtype tumors are associated with significantly higher relative CBV values.
  - Dynamic contrast-enhanced MRI measures the permeability surface area which reflects the leakiness of vasculature; differentiate GBM from lower-grade gliomas.
  - MRS can be useful in detecting metabolic alterations within GBM.
  - PET—clinical applicability includes the delineation of tumor extent, especially in normal-appearing tissue where it can aid in radiotherapy and surgical planning; amino acid PET may be used in assessing treatment response.

Histopathology

(Dietrich, 2022)

- Glioma classification has relied on histopathology, with the hallmarks of GBM being an astroglial tumor with features of microvascular proliferation and/or necrosis.
- WHO CNS5 classified diffuse astrocytic gliomas based on molecular lineage; a mutation in IDH 1 or 2 (IDH1/2) has become a defining branch point in adult-type diffuse glioma diagnosis.
- The distinction between IDH-mutant and wildtype gliomas has also become clearer, with the omission of "secondary" or IDH-mutant GBM in favor of the term diffuse IDH-mutant astrocytoma, WHO grade 4.
- Other mutations that have distinct prognostic and therapeutic implications include BRAF V600E mutations, FGFR alterations, or MYB or MYBL1 rearrangements.
- MGMT promoter methylation status is the most predictive and prognostic molecular biomarker; roughly 40% of IDH-wildtype glioblastomas will be methylated.

Clinical Staging

- Glioblastoma is not categorized by stages.

Treatment

Newly Diagnosed Glioblastoma Multiforme

- Well-known standard of care for newly diagnosed GBM is maximal safe surgical resection followed by concurrent chemoradiation with TMZ, and adjuvant TMZ (Melhem et al., 2022).
- Tumor-treating fields (TTF) are wearable scalp transducers that deliver local low-intensity, intermediate-frequency (200 kHz) alternating electrical fields that have an antimitotic effect, and work synergistically with concurrent chemotherapies (Melhem et al., 2022).
- The addition of bevacizumab conferred a statistically significant advantage of 3 months in progression-free survival but no improvement in overall survival (Melhem et al., 2022).
- Patients with unfavorable prognostic markers such as advanced age or poor performance status have a worse prognosis and are vulnerable to treatment toxicities (Melhem et al., 2022).
- There is no universally accepted salvage therapy for recurrent GBM; consider individualized consideration of

re-operation, re-irradiation, and systemic therapy options (Melhem et al., 2022).

Prognosis

- MGMT methylation predicts response to standard of care therapy with temozolamide; 50% increase in median overall survival (Batchelor, 2022).

Prevention and Surveillance

(Abdalla et al., 2020)

- Currently, there is no standard of care for the management of the inevitable tumor recurrence that leads to almost no improvement in the survival rates of patients with glioblastoma over time.

References

Abdalla, G., Hammam, A., Anjari, M., D'Arco, D. F., & Bisdas, D. S. (2020). Glioma surveillance imaging: Current strategies, shortcomings, challenges and outlook. *BJR Open, 2*(1), 20200009.

Batchelor, T. (2022). Initial treatment and prognosis of IDH-wildtype glioblastoma in adults. In *UpToDate*. Available at https://www.uptodate.com/contents/initial-treatment-and-prognosis-of-idh-wildtype-glioblastoma-in adults?sectionName=MGMT%20methylation%20status&search=glioblastoma&topicRef=15246&anchor=H1781604552&source=see_link#H1781604552.

Dietrich, J. (2022). Clinical presentation, diagnosis, and initial surgical management of high-grade gliomas. In *UpToDate*. Available at https://www.uptodate.com/contents/clinical-presentation-diagnosis-and-initial-surgical-management-of-high-grade-gliomas?search=glioblastoma&topicRef=5207&source=see_link.

Melhem, J. M., Detsky, J., Lim-Fat, M. J., & Perry, J. R. (2022). Updates in IDH-wildtype glioblastoma. *Neurotherapeutics: The Journal of the American Society for Experimental NeuroTherapeutics, 19*(6), 1705–1723.

Medulloblastoma

Definition

WHO CNS5 revised the classification of medulloblastomas to reflect clinical and biologic heterogeneity (Louis et al., 2021). Occurring primarily in the cerebellum, medulloblastomas are the most common malignant brain tumor of childhood.

Incidence

(Fangusaro & Pomeroy, 2022a)

- Medulloblastoma is rare with approximately 500 children diagnosed annually in the United States.
- Accounts for approximately 10% of all CNS primary tumors in children less than 19 years of age.
  - Peak incidence is between 5 and 9 years
  - Seventy percent of patients are diagnosed before the age of 20

Etiology and Risk Factors

- Five to 6% of medulloblastomas, with significant variation by molecular subtype, occur in association with a cancer predisposition syndrome such as nevoid basal cell carcinoma syndrome (NBCCS), caused by germline mutations in the patched-1 (PTCH1) gene; Li-Fraumeni syndrome, caused by mutations in the tumor protein p53 (TP53) gene; or familial adenomatous polyposis (FAP), caused by inactivating mutations in the adenomatous polyposis coli (APC) gene (Fangusaro & Pomeroy, 2022a).

Signs and Symptoms

- Clinical presentation includes signs and symptoms of increased intracranial pressure and cerebellar dysfunction evolving over a period of weeks to a few months.
- Nocturnal or morning headaches, nausea, vomiting, and altered mental status.
- Dizziness and double vision from cerebellar, brainstem, or cranial nerve involvement.
- Prolonged elevation of intracranial pressure can lead to papilledema and complete or partial loss of vision.

Diagnostic Workup

- MRI typically demonstrates a midline or paramedian cerebellar mass that enhances after contrast administration, and approximately one-third of patients will have evidence of tumor dissemination through the subarachnoid space either by imaging or CSF examination.
- Medulloblastomas may be missed on computed tomography (CT) scan.
- Cytopathologic examination of the CSF may reveal neoplastic cells.
- A diagnosis of medulloblastoma requires histopathologic confirmation at the time of surgical resection.

Histopathology

(Louis et al., 2021)

- Previous histopathologic classifications of medulloblastoma have now been combined by the WHO CNS5 into one section that describes them as morphologic patterns of an inclusive tumor type, medulloblastoma, histologically defined.

Clinical Staging

- There is no standard staging system for childhood medulloblastoma.

Treatment

(Fangusaro & Pomeroy, 2022b)

- Age, extent of disease, histopathologic subtype, and molecular subtype are used to stratify patients with medulloblastoma into risk groups and determine appropriate therapy.
- Optimal initial treatment of patients with medulloblastoma includes both general measures to alleviate increased intracranial pressure and specific therapy directed against the tumor.
  - CSF shunt to relieve hydrocephalus is usually deferred until after a surgical resection.
- Maximal safe resection is a key component of the treatment of all patients with medulloblastoma.
- RT is an integral component of the initial management of patients with medulloblastoma.
- Chemotherapy has an important role in the multimodality management of children with medulloblastoma:
  - Used after surgery to delay or avoid irradiating the developing brain and spinal cord in young children.
  - Adjuvant chemotherapy is used following surgery and RT to decrease the incidence of recurrence and minimize craniospinal radiation exposure in average-risk children.
  - Used with RT to treat high-risk diseases.

Prognosis

(Fangusaro & Pomeroy, 2022a, 2022b)

- The modified Chang criteria, which are based upon the size of the primary tumor and the extent of nervous system and extraneural spread, are useful in estimating the prognosis, which is progressively worse in the presence of more advanced disease.
- The presence of lung or liver metastases, the presence of CNS disease, and a shorter interval between original diagnosis and the development of these metastases are considered negative prognostic indicators.
- With modern multimodality therapy, approximately 75% of all children diagnosed with medulloblastoma will survive into adulthood.

Prevention and Surveillance

- Following completion of therapy and restaging, patients are seen at periodic intervals to monitor for treatment complications and disease recurrence.
- Every 3 months for the first 1 to 2 years, then every 6 to 12 months for the next 5 to 10 years, then every 1 to 2 years, or as clinically indicated (Fangusaro & Pomeroy, 2022b).

References

Fangusaro, J., & Pomeroy, S. (2022a). Clinical presentation, diagnosis, and risk stratification of medulloblastoma. In *UpToDate*. Available at https://www.uptodate.com/contents/clinical-presentation-diagnosis-and-risk-stratification-of-medulloblastoma?search=medulloblastoma&source=search_result&selectedTitle=2~69&usage_type=default&display_rank=2.

Fangusaro, J., & Pomeroy, S. (2022b). Treatment and prognosis of medulloblastoma. In *UpToDate*. Available at https://www.uptodate.com/contents/treatment-and-prognosis-of-medulloblastoma?sectionName=Surgery&search=medulloblastoma&topicRef=5219&anchor=H3177285&source=see_link#H3177285.

Louis, D. N., Perry, A., Wesseling, P., Brat, D. J., Cree, I. A., Figarella-Branger, D., … Ellison, D. W. (2021). The 2021 WHO classification of tumors of the central nervous system: A summary. *Neuro-Oncology, 23*(8), 1231–1251.

Meningioma

Definition

Meningioma is considered a single type in WHO CNS5, with its broad morphologic spectrum reflected in 15 subtypes (Louis et al., 2021).

Incidence

(Park, 2022)

- Most frequent primary CNS tumors; they account for approximately one-third of all primary brain and spinal tumors.
- Incidence of meningioma increases progressively with age, with a median age at diagnosis of 65 years; it is more common in women, with a female-to-male ratio of approximately two or three to one.
- Rare in children except in those with hereditary syndromes such as neurofibromatosis type 2 (NF2) or previous RT.
- WHO grade 1, 80% to 85%; WHO grade 2, 15% to 18%; WHO grade 3, 1% to 3%.

Etiology and Risk Factors

(Park, 2022)

- Exposure to ionizing radiation is the most important acquired risk factor for meningioma; latency period for patients who received prior RT is more than 20 years in many cases.
- Genetic predisposition, including NF2, schwannomatosis, and multiple endocrine neoplasia type 1 (MEN1).
- Hormonal factors, low-dose estrogen and progestin exposure, high-dose cyproterone.
- Other risk factors including a history of breast cancer, obesity, head trauma, and cell phones.

Signs and Symptoms

(Park, 2022)

- Symptoms correspond to the location of the mass and is associated with the duration of time over which the tumor develops. Meningiomas are frequently extremely slow growing and are often asymptomatic.
- Presenting symptoms include seizures (30%), focal findings, that is, visual changes, loss of hearing or smell, mental status changes, extremity weakness, and obstructive hydrocephalus.

Diagnostic Workup

(Park, 2022)

- MRI: Extra-axial, dural-based mass that is isointense or hypointense to gray matter on T1 and isointense or hyperintense on proton density and T2-weighted images.
- CT scan: Well-defined extra-axial mass that displaces the normal brain.
- ^{18}F-Fluorodeoxyglucose (FDG) PET scanning is of limited diagnostic value.
- A definitive diagnosis of meningioma requires histologic confirmation.

Histopathology

(Louis et al., 2021)

- Criteria defining atypical or anaplastic (i.e., grades 2 and 3) meningioma should be applied regardless of the underlying subtype.
- Chordoid and clear cell meningioma are noted to have a higher likelihood of recurrence than the average CNS WHO grade 1 meningioma and have hence been assigned to CNS WHO grade 2.
- Molecular biomarkers are also associated with classification and grading of meningiomas, including SMARCE1 (clear cell subtype), BAP1 (rhabdoid and papillary subtypes), and KLF4/TRAF7 (secretory subtype) mutations, telomerase reverse transcriptase (TERT) promoter mutation and/or homozygous deletion of CDKN2A/B (CNS WHO grade 3), H3K27me3 loss of nuclear expression (potentially worse prognosis), and methylome profiling (prognostic subtyping).
- WHO CNS5 classification:
  - WHO grade 1: Benign meningiomas
  - WHO grade 2: Meningiomas include specific morphologic subtypes (clear cell and chordoid meningiomas), tumors with increased mitotic activity (4–19 mitoses per 10 high-powered fields) or brain invasion, and tumors with three or more of the following features: increased

cellularity, small cells with a high nuclear-to-cytoplasmic ratio, prominent nucleoli, uninterrupted patternless or sheet-like growth, and foci of spontaneous or geographic necrosis.
- WHO grade 3: Malignant meningiomas have ≥20 mitoses per 10 high-powered fields; malignant characteristics resembling carcinoma, sarcoma, or melanoma; or a high-risk molecular feature (TERT promotor mutation or homozygous cyclin-dependent kinase inhibitor 2A/B [CDKN2A/B] deletion).

Clinical Staging

- There is no formal staging system for meningiomas.

Treatment

- Management requires a balance between definitive treatment of the tumor and avoidance of neurologic damage from the treatment.
- Known or presumed benign (WHO grade 1) meningioma: Initial management may consist of observation, surgery, surgery plus RT, or RT alone (Park & Shih, 2022).
- WHO grades 2 and 3: Complete surgical resection is preferred when a meningioma is in an accessible location, since complete resection of the tumor and its dural attachment can be curative, and the extent of resection is consistently identified as an independent prognostic factor for both progression-free and overall survival (Shih & Park, 2022).
  - Adjuvant RT is a standard component of initial therapy in patients with subtotally resected atypical meningiomas to improve local control (Shih & Park, 2022).
  - Adjuvant RT is a standard component of initial management for all malignant meningiomas, regardless of the extent of resection, to improve local control and overall survival (Shih & Park, 2022).

Recurrent Meningiomas

(Wen, 2022)
- Inhibition of progesterone and androgen receptors has not been demonstrated to alter the natural history of recurrent meningiomas.
- A variety of chemotherapy agents, including hydroxyurea, temozolomide, and combinations such as cyclophosphamide, doxorubicin, and vincristine have not shown evidence of significant activity.
- The use of somatostatin analogues has not shown clear benefit.
- Molecularly targeted agents (e.g., platelet-derived growth factor inhibitors, epidermal growth factor receptor tyrosine kinase inhibitors, vascular endothelial growth factor inhibitors, and mechanistic target of rapamycin [mTOR] inhibitors) have not demonstrated clinically useful efficacy but are still under investigation.
- There is growing interest in the use of immunotherapy.
- Whenever possible, consider enrollment in clinical trials. For patients who are ineligible for trials, options are limited to hydroxyurea, octreotide, or possibly a VEGF inhibitor.

Prognosis

- WHO grade 1: Results of treatment vary depending on the location of the meningioma as well as the therapeutic approach; optimal therapy needs to be individualized based upon the anatomic location of the tumor and patient-specific considerations (Park & Shih, 2022).
- WHO grades 2 and 3: Atypical and malignant meningiomas are associated with an increased risk of local recurrence and decreased overall survival compared with grade 1 meningiomas (Shih & Park, 2022).

Prevention and Surveillance

- Brain MRI with contrast is the best modality to monitor for evidence of recurrence or for progression of residual disease.
- WHO grade 1 (Park & Shih, 2022)
  - For asymptomatic or minimally symptomatic patients managed with active surveillance, repeat the imaging procedure in 3 to 6 months, annually for 3 to 5 years, and every 2 to 3 years thereafter if there is no evidence of progression.
  - For patients whose initial management consisted of surgery and/or RT, imaging should be repeated in the postoperative period, annually for 3 to 5 years, and then every 2 to 3 years, so that any evidence of recurrent or progressive disease can be detected while the disease burden is relatively limited.
- WHO grades 2 and 3 (Shih & Park, 2022)
  - Cranial imaging (preferably MRI) is used following initial treatment to monitor for evidence of recurrence or progression of residual disease.
    - Atypical meningioma, obtain an MRI at 3, 6, and 12 months postoperatively, then every 6 to 12 months for 5 years, then every 1 to 3 years.
    - Malignant meningioma, obtain MRIs every 3 to 6 months for 3 to 5 years after initial therapy, then every 6 to 12 months.

References

Louis, D. N., Perry, A., Wesseling, P., Brat, D. J., Cree, I. A., Figarella-Branger, D., & Ellison, D. W. (2021). The 2021 WHO classification of tumors of the central nervous system: A summary. *Neuro-Oncology, 23*(8), 1231–1251.

Park, J. K. (2022). Epidemiology, pathology, clinical features, and diagnosis of meningioma. In *UpToDate*. Available at https://www.uptodate.com/contents/epidemiology-pathology-clinical-features-and-diagnosis-of-meningioma?search=meningioma&source=search_result&selectedTitle=1~116&usage_type=default&display_rank=1.

Park, J. K., & Shih, H. A. (2022). Management of known or presumed benign (WHO grade 1) meningioma. In *UpToDate*. Available at https://www.uptodate.com/contents/management-of-known-or-presumed-benign-who-grade-1-meningioma?search=meningioma&topicRef=5220&source=see_link.

Shih, H. A., & Park, J. K. (2022). Management of atypical and malignant (WHO grade 2 and 3) meningioma. In *UpToDate*. Available at https://www.uptodate.com/contents/management-of-atypical-and-malignant-who-grade-2-and-3-meningioma?search=meningioma&topicRef=5220&source=see_link.

Wen, P. Y. (2022). Systemic treatment of recurrent meningioma. In *UpToDate*. Available at https://www.uptodate.com/contents/systemic-treatment-of-recurrent-meningioma?search=meningioma&topicRef=5220&source=see_link.

Metastases to the Brain and Spinal Cord Parenchyma

Definition

Metastatic tumors are tumors that spread to the brain or spinal cord from a primary neoplasm located in other organs of the body. The WHO CNS5 section on metastatic tumors is divided into those that preferentially affect the brain and spinal cord parenchyma versus those that favor the meninges. Given progress in the treatment of specific systemic cancers, attention has been paid to those immunohistochemical and molecular diagnostic markers that are helpful for diagnosis and/or for guiding therapies of these tumors (Louis et al., 2021).

Incidence

(Loeffler, 2022a)

- Brain metastases are the most common intracranial tumors in adults, accounting for significantly more than one-half of brain tumors.
- Incidence may be increasing, due to both improved detection of small metastases by MRI and better control of extracerebral disease resulting from improved systemic therapy.

Etiology and Risk Factors

- Most common primary tumors responsible for brain metastases are carcinomas, which include lung, breast, kidney, and colorectal cancers, as well as melanoma.
- Most common mechanism of metastasis to the brain is by hematogenous spread.

Signs and Symptoms

- Clinical features vary widely among patients with brain metastases. Brain metastases should be suspected in any cancer patient who develops neurologic symptoms or behavioral abnormalities.
- Presenting symptoms include headaches, focal neurologic dysfunction, cognitive dysfunction, seizures, and stroke.

Diagnostic Workup

(Loeffler, 2022a)

- Imaging studies provide useful information, but a brain biopsy is necessary in some cases for a definitive diagnosis.
- Contrast-enhanced MRI is the preferred imaging study for the diagnosis of brain metastases.

Histopathology

- Refer to primary tumor; ancillary immunohistochemical analysis is the most effective tool for characterizing a metastatic neoplasm of unknown origin.

Clinical Staging

- Staging evaluation will be based on the primary tumor.

Treatment

(Loeffler, 2022b)

- Treatment of patients with brain metastases is similar to the approach used in those with primary brain tumors.

- Key components include the control of peritumoral edema and increased intracranial pressure with corticosteroids, the treatment of seizures, and the management of venous thromboembolic disease.
- Single brain metastasis—surgical resection or stereotactic radiosurgery (SRS) rather than whole brain radiation therapy (WBRT) alone.
- Two to four small brain metastases (<3 cm)—SRS alone rather than SRS plus adjunctive WBRT or WBRT alone.
- Five to 10 small brain metastases—SRS alone
- Greater than 10 brain metastases—WBRT remains the mainstay of treatment for many good performance status patients who are not eligible for SRS or surgery due to a high a number of tumors or multiple bulky tumors and who do not have good systemic therapy options.
- Patients with poor performance status or a relatively short life expectancy—individualized treatment based on symptoms, patient preferences, intracranial disease burden, and the availability of additional systemic therapies.

Prognosis

(Loeffler, 2022b)

- Based on most recent data, median survival exceeds 6 months for all major cancer types and ranges from approximately 8 to 16 months, depending on the primary tumor.

Prevention and Surveillance

(Loeffler, 2022b)

- Brain metastases should be followed with brain MRI or contrast-enhanced CT if MRI is not possible to detect early evidence of recurrence or new lesions, particularly when adjunctive WBRT has been omitted.

References

Loeffler, J. S. (2022a). Epidemiology, clinical manifestations, and diagnosis of brain metastases. In *UpToDate*. Available at https://www.uptodate.com/contents/epidemiology-clinical-manifestations-and-diagnosis-of-brain-metastases?topicRef=5212&source=see_link.

Loeffler, J. S. (2022b). Overview of the treatment of brain metastases. In *UpToDate*. Available at https://www.uptodate.com/contents/overview-of-the-treatment-of-brain-metastases.

Louis, D. N., Perry, A., Wesseling, P., Brat, D. J., Cree, I. A., Figarella-Branger, D., … Ellison, D. W. (2021). The 2021 WHO classification of tumors of the central nervous system: A summary. *Neuro-Oncology, 23*(8), 1231–1251.

Oligodendroglioma, IDH-Mutant and 1p/19q Codeleted

Definition

Oligodendroglioma, IDH-mutant and 1p/19q codeleted, classified as CNS WHO grade 2 or 3, is defined as a "diffusely infiltrating glioma with IDH1 or IDH2 mutation and codeletion of chromosome arms 1p and 19q" (Santosh & Rao, 2022).

Incidence

- Oligodendrogliomas comprise approximately 5% of all neuroepithelial tumors of the CNS, accounting for about 1000 diagnoses in the United States every year.
- They commonly present in adults between 25 and 45 years old (van den Bent, 2022a).

Etiology and Risk Factors

There is no known cause for brain tumors, but the following are considered risk factors:

- Therapeutic ionizing radiation to the head
- Genetic disorders, including neurofibromatosis types 1 and 2, tuberous sclerosis, von Hippel–Lindau syndrome, and Li-Fraumeni syndrome.

Signs and Symptoms

(van den Bent, 2022a)

- Oligodendrogliomas are slow-growing, infiltrative tumors that may be asymptomatic for many years.
- For those who present with symptoms, seizures are the most common.
- As the disease progress, symptoms vary based on tumor location, size, and rate of tumor growth.

Diagnostic Workup

- Neurologic examination
- MRI of the brain and spine with contrast
- Biopsy or craniotomy for a tissue diagnosis
- Molecular characterization

Histopathology

(Santosh & Rao, 2022; van den Bent, 2022a)

- Oligodendrogliomas contain both an IDH1 or IDH2 mutation and whole-arm codeletion of chromosomes 1p and 19q.
- The WHO grading system distinguishes two histopathologic grades of oligodendroglioma: grade 2 (low grade) and grade 3 (anaplastic) oligodendroglioma.
  - Grade 2 tumors do not have features of anaplasia.
  - Grade 3 tumors are characterized by the presence of anaplastic features (high cell density, mitosis, nuclear atypia, microvascular proliferation, and necrosis) and are associated with a modestly worse prognosis compared with grade 2 tumors.

Treatment

(NCCN, 2022)

- Appropriate treatment depends on the grade of the tumor, extent of resection, and age of the patient.
- Maximal resection is the preferred approach, but depending upon the location and extent of the tumor, only a partial resection or even just a biopsy may be safely feasible.
- Surgery is not curative in patients with oligodendrogliomas, and additional therapy (i.e., RT and chemotherapy) is ultimately required in all patients.
- WHO grade 2, low risk, KPS ≥60
  - Consider clinical trial
  - Observe
- WHO grade 2, high risk, KPS ≥60
  - Consider clinical trial
  - RT with adjuvant PCV (procarbazine/lomustine/vincristine) systemic therapy
  - RT with adjuvant temozolamide
  - Observe
- WHO grade 3, KPS ≥60
  - Consider clinical trial
  - RT with neoadjuvant or adjuvant PCV (procarbazine/lomustine/vincristine) systemic therapy
  - RT with concurrent and adjuvant temozolamide
  - RT with adjuvant temozolamide
- Any grade, KPS ≤60
  - RT with concurrent and adjuvant temozolamide
  - Temozolamide
  - Palliative or best supportive care

Prognosis

- Prognosis depends on the grade of the oligodendroglioma. Compared with other diffuse gliomas, oligodendrogliomas are highly chemosensitive (van den Bent, 2022b).
- Oligodendrogliomas with noncanonical IDH1 and IDH2 mutations may have improved outcomes compared with IDH1 R132H-mutant tumors.
- In oligodendrogliomas with 1p/19q codeletion, the presence of polysomy of chromosomes 1 and 19 may identify a subset of patients with a poorer prognosis.
- The presence of CDKN2A/B deletion has been associated with shorter progression-free and overall survival.
- Despite the prolonged clinical course seen with oligodendroglial tumors, almost all are life-limiting due to tumor relapse, eventual acceleration of tumor growth, and resistance to existing therapies.

Prevention and Surveillance

- There are no known preventive measures to reduce the incidence of primary CNS tumors.
- After oligodendroglioma patients have completed the prescribed therapy, they are monitored according to the NCCN guidelines, which are based on the management of the most aggressive portion of the tumor (NCCN, 2022).
  - WHO grade 2: Brain MRI every 3 to 6 months for 5 years, then every 6 months.
  - WHO grade 3: Brain MRI 2 to 8 weeks after radiation, then every 2 to 4 months for 3 years, then every 3 to 6 months.
  - Any grade, KPS ≤60: Brain MRI 2 to 8 weeks after radiation, then every 2 to 4 months for 3 years, then every 3 to 6 months.

References

National Comprehensive Cancer Network (NCCN). (2022). NCCN clinical practice guidelines in oncology (NCCN guidelines)—Central nervous system cancers, version 1.2022. Available at https://www.nccn.org/professionals/physician_gls/pdf/cns.pdf.

Santosh, V., & Rao, S. (2022). A review of adult-type diffuse gliomas in the WHO CNS5 classification with special reference to astrocytoma, IDH-mutant and oligodendroglioma, IDH-mutant and 1p/19q codeleted. *Indian Journal of Pathology & Microbiology*, 65(Supplement), S14–S23.

van den Bent, M. (2022a). Clinical features, diagnosis, and pathology of IDH-mutant, 1p/19q-codeleted oligodendrogliomas. In *UpToDate*. Available at https://www.uptodate.com/contents/clinical-features-diagnosis-and-pathology-of-idh-mutant-1p-19q-codeleted-oligodendrogliomas?search=oligodendroglioma%20idh%20mutant%20incidence&source=search_result&selectedTitle=1~150&usage_type=default&display_rank=1.

van den Bent, M. (2022b). Treatment and prognosis of IDH-mutant, 1p/19q-codeleted oligodendrogliomas in adults. In *UpToDate*. Available at https://www.uptodate.com/contents/treatment-and-prognosis-of-idh-mutant-1p-19q-codeleted-oligodendrogliomas-in-adults?search=Oligodendroglioma,%20IDH-mutant%20and%201p%2F19q%20codeleted&source=search_result&selectedTitle=2~150&usage_type=default&display_rank=2.

Gastrointestinal System Cancers

Lisa S. Parks

Anal Cancer

Definition

The anus is the most distal portion of the large intestine and connects the large intestine and the rectum. The anal canal is 3.5 to 4 cm in total length and is divided into two sections: the anatomic canal and the surgical canal. The anatomic canal is 2 cm from the dentate or pectineal line and extends distally to the anal verge. The surgical canal is defined as the region from the dentate line, extending 2 cm proximal to the anorectal ring. The superior extent of the surgical canal can be palpated on digital rectal examination (DRE) as a tight muscular junction. The dentate line is the defining structure between the anatomic and surgical canals and is important because it distinguishes the lymphatic drainage of tumors and transition in mucosa (Young et al., 2020). Eighty-five percent of all anal cell cancers are squamous cell (Symer & Yeo, 2018). From the anal verge distally toward the perineum is defined as skin tissue and can give rise to melanoma and lymphoma (Lu et al., 2020). Squamous cell anal cancer accounts for 80% of all anal cancers (Young et al., 2020).

Incidence

- The incidence of anal cancer is rare and accounts for 0.5% of all cancer diagnoses and 3% of all gastrointestinal (GI) malignancies (Symer & Yeo, 2018; Young et al., 2020).
- This number has doubled over the past 25 years due to persistent infection with human papilloma virus (HPV). Ninety-one percent of anal cancers are attributed to HPV. This may be due to certain subpopulations, such as individuals with human immunodeficiency virus (HIV), men and women with a history of receptive anal intercourse, and women with a history of vulvar, vaginal, or cervical dysplasia or cancer (Siegel et al., 2021).
- Women are approximately 1.6 times more likely to develop anal cancer than men. In the United States, women and patients of lower socioeconomic status present with more advanced stages, shortening survival compared to patients from higher socioeconomic status or men (Siegel et al., 2021).
- Anal intraepithelial neoplasia (AIN) is a precursor lesion to anal cancer and includes two categories. AIN I is a low-grade squamous cell intraepithelial neoplasia, and AIN II is a high-grade squamous cell intraepithelial neoplasia (Symer & Yeo, 2018).

Etiology and Risk Factors

- Infection with HPV-16 and HPV-18 is strongly linked to anal cancer.
- Two HPV viral proteins, E6 and E7, are closely linked to oncogenesis in squamous epithelia. By preventing apoptosis and causing cell cycle arrest, these proteins contribute to the progression to cancer (Symer & Yeo, 2018).
- Persons with a history of multiple sex partners and a history of smoking are at higher risk (Lu et al., 2020).
- Other risk factors not previously discussed include immunosuppression after solid organ transplantation, autoimmune disorders, and hematologic malignancies (Symer & Yeo, 2018).
- History of chronic inflammation such as Crohn disease, anal fistulas, and chronic fissures.

Signs and Symptoms

- Anal cancer is often asymptomatic.
- Forty-five percent of patients with anal cancer present with rectal bleeding (National Comprehensive Cancer Network [NCCN], 2022).
- Thirty percent of patients have rectal pain or the sensation of a rectal mass (NCCN, 2022).
- Nonspecific symptoms include perirectal itching, nonhealing perirectal wounds/ulcers, rectal incontinence and urge, and rectal tenesmus.
- Enlarged inguinal lymph nodes.

Diagnostic Work-up

Early identification of anal cancer leads to a better prognosis. Diagnosis of anal cancer includes

- *History and physical examination* focusing on the inguinal lymph nodes—for women, including a gynecologic examination.
- *HIV testing* if the patient's HIV status is unknown.
- *Digital rectal examination*
- *Endoscopy*
  - *Anoscopy* using an anoscope inserted into the anal canal to visualize the anus and lower rectum.
  - *Rigid proctosigmoidoscopy* visualizes the anal cancer and distal sigmoid colon after a bowel preparation with a laxative or enema.
- *Biopsy* is performed for histologic confirmation
  - *Excisional biopsy*: The entire mass should be removed with a 0.5 cm margin for a mass up to 2 cm in diameter with the sphincter if adjacent organs have not been infiltrated.

- *Tissue biopsy* may be performed but not an excisional biopsy if the mass is large and infiltrating. Performing an excisional biopsy may delay chemoradiation therapy.
- *Fine-needle aspiration (FNA)* with a sample of the surrounding lymph nodes in the groin or anal area can be performed to detect cancer spread.
- *Ultrasound* to assess for infiltration into surrounding structures.
- *Computed tomography (CT) of the chest, abdomen, and pelvis* to assess metastatic disease.
- *Magnetic resonance imaging (MRI)* for more detailed imaging of the anal canal.
- *Positron emission tomography (PET)* is a nuclear imaging test that uses a radioactive tracer. PET assesses the increased metabolic activity of highly metabolic cancer cells to locate sites of metastatic disease.

Histopathology

The cell types from the surgical canal are glandular and transitional and can lead to development of adenocarcinoma. Keratinized or nonkeratinized squamous cells can lead to squamous cell carcinoma (SCC).

- Glandular tissue, which consists of irregular crypts and smooth muscle fibers in the lamina propria, is found in the proximal anus.
- The transitional cells of the anus are located between uninterrupted squamous epithelia mid anus. Transitional epithelia contain features of both small basal cells and squamous epithelium. This epithelium has the appearance of glistening wrinkled tissue and produces very small amounts of mucin.
- The transitional tissue has anal glands in the submucosa and endocrine cells with occasional melanocytes. This tissue expresses cytokeratin 7 positive (CK7+) and cytokeratin 20 negative (CK20−).
- The distal aspect of the anus consists of the dentate line to the squamous mucocutaneous junction. It is composed of nonkeratinizing squamous epithelium without appendages or glands. The lower region contains melanocytes, keratin, hair, and apocrine glands.

Clinical Staging

Anal cancer is staged according to the tumor, node, and metastasis (TNM) system developed by the American Joint Committee on Cancer (AJCC) (Dahl et al., 2020). Tumor staging describes the size of the primary tumor in centimeters. Nodal staging describes the extent of tumor spread to nearby or local lymph nodes. Metastasis staging notes spread of the cancer to other distant sites.

- T1 disease shows invasion through the mucosa and submucosa with no extension into the muscularis propria
- T2 disease shows invasion into the muscularis propria
- T3 disease shows invasion through the muscularis propria into the perirectal tissues
- T4 disease shows the tumor involves the visceral peritoneum or anterior peritoneal reflection (Nougaret et al., 2019)

The nodal presence of lymph nodes is used in the TNM staging:
- N0—no lymph nodes present
- N1a—metastasis in one regional lymph node
- N1b—metastasis in two to three regional lymph nodes
- N1c—there are no positive regional lymph nodes, but there are tumor deposits in the subserosa, mesentery, or nonperitonealized pericolic or perirectal/mesorectal tissues
- N2a—metastasis in four to six regional lymph nodes
- N2b—metastasis in seven or more regional lymph nodes (Nougaret et al., 2019)

Treatment

Treatment goals for anal cancer include preservation and function of the anal sphincter.

- Stage I anal cancer is excised locally with a safety margin of 1.0 cm as treatment.
- In stage 2 (T2,3N0) anal cancer, chemoradiation is the gold standard. Mitomycin/5-fluorouracil (5-FU) or mitomycin/capecitabine is administered concurrently with radiation.
- In stage 3c or stage 4 (T3 to T4N0) or any T with positive nodes, NCCN recommends 5-FU/mitomycin + radiation; capecitabine/mitomycin + radiation; 5-FU/cisplatin + radiation (NCCN, 2023; Rose, 2018).
- Metastatic anal cancer: Palliative radiation can be administered with chemotherapy for local control of a symptomatic bulky tumor primary. The NCCN recommends chemotherapy, 5-FU or capecitabine, and radiation to the primary site for local control and a number of systemic regimens. These include carboplatin + paclitaxel as the preferred regimen with other regimens including 5-FU + cisplatin, FOLFCIS (5-FU, leucovorin, and cisplatin), mFOLFOX6 (5-FU, oxaliplatin, and leucovorin), modified DCF (docetaxel, cisplatin, and 5-FU). Checkpoint inhibitors, nivoloumab and pembrolizumab, are preferred secondary therapies if not previously administered.
- Surgery is reserved for residual or recurrent anal cancer. An abdominoperineal resection (APR) is the standard procedure performed. If complete resection is not possible, palliative options should be discussed, including diverting ostomy for obstruction.

Prognosis

Four factors have been identified as prognostic factors for anal cancer.

- Older age is associated with a poor survival rate.
- Higher tumor stage with lymph node involvement results in poor survival and higher relapse rates.
- Large tumor size and narrow margins of the resected tumor are predictive for cancer recurrence.
- Patients with a lower tumor burden and involved lymph nodes have a better prognosis than those with node negative disease but a high tumor burden.

Prevention

Prevention of infection with HPV is an important intervention for prevention of anal cancer. A quadrivalent HPV vaccine has been available since 2006. In 2014, a nonvalent vaccine was approved. In the United States, only 50% of eligible adolescents aged 13 to 17 years have received one or more doses (Symer & Yeo, 2018). Other recommendations include

- Smoking or tobacco cessation
- Use of condoms during intercourse, although HPV is transmitted by skin-to-skin contact and still can be transmitted with wearing of a condom
- Avoidance of multiple sexual partners
- Avoidance of anal intercourse
- Screening for HIV (Siegel et al., 2021; Symer & Yeo, 2018).

Surveillance

- Following primary treatment
  - Patients are reevaluated using DRE between 8 and 12 weeks after completion of chemoradiation. Patients are classified as having a complete remission, persistent disease, or progressive disease. Patients with persistent disease without progression can be reevaluated in 4 weeks.
  - Patients who have not shown a complete clinical response after 6 months and have not progressed following completion of chemoradiation may be followed at 3-month intervals.
  - Patients with complete remission should be evaluated every 3 to 6 months for 5 years with DRE, anoscopy, and inguinal node palpation.
  - Annual chest, abdominal, and pelvic CT with contrast is recommended for 3 years for patients with stage 2b, stage 3 b and c, stage 4 (T3 or T4), or node positive cancers.
- Following treatment of recurrence
  - Following APR, patients should be reevaluated every 3 to 6 months for 5 years, including inguinal node palpation. Annual chest, abdomen, and pelvic CT for 3 years.
  - After treatment of inguinal node recurrence, patients should have a DRE with inguinal node palpation every 3 to 6 months for 5 years. Anoscopy should be performed every 6 to 12 months, and annual chest, abdominal, and pelvic CT with contrast imaging is recommended for 3 years.

References

Dahl, O., Myklebust, M. P., Dale, J. E., Leon, O., Serup-Hansen, E., Jakobsen, A., … Johnsson, A. (2020). Evaluation of the stage classification of anal cancer by the TNM 8th version versus the TNM 7th version. *Acta Oncologica*, 59(9), 1016–1023.

Lu, Y., Wang, X., Li, P., Zhang, T., Zhou, J., Ren, Y., … Zou, H. (2020). Clinical characteristics and prognosis of anal squamous cell carcinoma: A retrospective audit of 144 patients from 11 cancer hospitals in southern China. *BioMed Central (BMC) Cancer*, 20(1), 679.

National Comprehensive Cancer Network (NCCN). (2023). Anal carcinoma (version 1.2023). https://www.nccn.org/professionals/physician_gls/pdf/anal.pdf.

Nougaret, S., Jhaveri, K., Kassam, Z., Lall, C., & Kim, D. H. (2019). Rectal cancer MR staging: Pearls and pitfalls at baseline examination. *Abdominal Radiology*, 44(11), 3536–3548.

Rose, P. (2018). Concurrent chemotherapy and radiation therapy for anal cancer: Retrospective chart audit of treatment-related toxicities. *Cancer Nurses Society of Australia*, 19(2), 3–8.

Siegel, R., Werner, R. N., Koswig, S., Gaskins, M., Rödel, C., Aigner, F., & German Anal Cancer Guideline Group. (2021). Clinical practice guideline: Anal cancer—Diagnosis, treatment and follow-up. *Deutsches Arzteblatt International*, 118(13), 217–224. https://doi.org/10.3238/arztebl.m2021.0027.

Symer, M., & Yeo, H. (2018). Recent advances in the management of anal cancer. *F1000Research*, 7, 1572.

Young, A. N., Jacob, E., Willauer, P., Smucker, L., Monzon, R., & Oceguera, L. (2020). Anal cancer. *Surgical Clinics of North America*, 100(3), 629–634.

Cholangiocarcinoma

Definition

Cholangiocarcinomas are rare tumors arising from the epithelium of the bile ducts and can involve any part of the biliary tree. They are classified based on their anatomic location, clinical presentation, and molecular features. The three locations of cholangiocarcinoma include intrahepatic cholangiocarcinoma (IHCC), extrahepatic cholangiocarcinoma (EHCC), which includes perihilar, and distal cholangiocarcinoma.

- IHCCs arise above the second-order bile ducts and are proximal to the common bile duct.
- Perihilar cholangiocarcinomas are located between the second-degree bile ducts and the cystic duct, where it inserts into the common bile duct.
- Distal cholangiocarcinoma is located between the cystic duct and the ampulla of Vater.

Sixty percent of cholangiocarcinomas are perihilar, 30% arise in mid or distal common bile duct, and 6% to 10% are intrahepatic (Khan & Dageforde, 2019).

Incidence

Cholangiocarcinoma is the second most common hepatic malignancy after hepatocellular carcinoma (HCC). It comprises 3% of GI malignancies and accounts for 10% to 25% of all hepatobiliary malignancies. Cholangiocarcinoma affects men more than women and rarely occurs before the age of 40. It most typically presents itself in the seventh decade of life (Khan & Dageforde, 2019).

Etiology and Risk Factors

Cholangiocarcinomas are aggressive tumors and usually present at an advanced disease stage. Etiology is unknown. Khan and Dageforde (2019) cite risk factors which include

- Primary sclerosing cholangitis (PSC)—Due to ongoing inflammation and bile stasis
- Choledochal cysts—Patients with these cysts have a 10- to 50-fold increased risk secondary to reflux of pancreatic enzymes, bile stasis, and increased concentration of intraductal bile acids in dilated ducts, leading to malignant transformation.
- Viral hepatitis and cirrhosis—Patients with hepatitis B and C and cirrhosis have a 10-fold increase in risk.
- Hepatolithiasis—Prolonged irritation of stones, bile stasis, and cholangitis lead to a 10% increased risk.
- Parasitic infections—Hepatobiliary flukes in Southeast Asia can increase risk.
- Inflammatory bowel disease (ulcerative colitis and Crohn's), choledocholithiasis, diabetes, obesity, heavy alcohol use, smoking.

Signs and Symptoms

- IHCC diagnosis is often incidental. Patients usually present with symptoms of fullness and rarely have pain.
- Patients with EHCC present with symptoms of obstructive jaundice, tea-colored urine, clay-colored stools, cholangitis, pruritus. They may also have vague abdominal pain, weight loss, anorexia, abnormal liver functions, such as elevated alkaline phosphatase and serum bilirubin.

Diagnostic Work-up

Work-up for Intrahepatic Cholangiocarcinoma

- Triple-phase CT scan
  - On CT, IHCC is hypodense and has peripheral rim enhancement in the arterial phase and hypoattenuation on the venous and delayed phases.
- MRI/magnetic resonance cholangiopancreatography (MRCP)
  - On MRI, IHCC is hypointense on T1 and hyperintense on T2 weighted image
  - The most recent guidelines from the NCCN recommend the triple phase CT scan or MRCP (Benson et al., 2021)
- Tumor markers, such as CA 19-9, can be used, but they are not highly sensitive or specific. Patients with unresectable cholangiocarcinoma have significantly higher levels than resectable patients, meaning that these patients have a poorer prognosis. Only about 20% to 40% of IHCC patients are candidates for surgical resection (Zhao et al., 2021). Tumor markers, such as CA 19-9 and carcinoembryonic antigen (CEA), are used in surveillance in patients who have an elevated level on initial presentation.

Work-up for Extrahepatic Cholangiocarcinoma (Perihilar and Distal)

- Laboratory testing includes a complete blood count (CBC), a coagulation profile, and liver function tests. Serum alkaline phosphatase levels are often elevated, which suggests an obstructive jaundice pattern.
- Endoscopic retrograde cholangiopancreatography (ERCP) with brushings and biopsy
- Fluorescence in situ hybridization (FISH)
- Endoscopic ultrasound (EUS)

Histopathology

Cholangiocarcinoma arises from a malignant transformation of a cholangiocyte. There are two histopathologic subtypes of the disease: those with cylindrical, mucin-producing glands, and those with cuboidal, non-mucin-producing glands. Cholangiocarcinomas are commonly a mixture of these two types (Rhee et al., 2019).

Genetic Alterations

Different genetic alterations in each disease subtype lead to their distinct biologic behavior. These genetic alterations determine which molecularly targeted therapies may be utilized in the patient's treatment (Rahnemai-Azar et al., 2017; Rizvi et al., 2018).

Intrahepatic Cholangiocarcinoma

- *IDH1, IDH2, FGFR1, FGFR2, FGFR3, EPHA2, and BAPI*

Extrahepatic Cholangiocarcinoma

- *ARiD1B, ELF3, PBRM1, PRKACA, PRKACB*

Clinical Staging

- Vascular invasion, numbers of tumors, and extent of lymph node involvement determine the staging classification. The AJCC eighth edition defined the stages as distal (dCCA), perihilar (pCCA), and IHCC (iCCA; NCCN, 2022).
- In Tx the primary tumor cannot be assessed.
- In situ tumors (Tis) have been expanded to include high-grade biliary intraepithelial neoplasia (BiIIN-3).
- T1 in dCCA, the tumor invades the bile duct wall with a depth of less than 5 mm, and in pCCA, the tumor is confined to the bile duct with extension up to the muscle layer through fibrous tissue.
- T1a in iCCA includes a solitary tumor greater than 5 cm without vascular invasion.
- T1b is a solitary tumor greater than 5 cm without vascular invasion.
- T2 in pCCA, the tumor invades the bile duct wall and invades beyond the wall of the bile duct to surrounding adipose tissue and adjacent hepatic parenchyma.
- With iCCA, T2 is a solitary tumor with intrahepatic vascular invasion of multiple tumors, with or without vascular invasion.
- In pCCA, T2a defines a tumor beyond the wall of the bile duct to surrounding adipose tissue, while T2b tumor invades adjacent hepatic parenchyma.
- In dCCA, T3 is a tumor that invades the bile duct wall with a depth of 12 mm. In pCCA, T3 tumor invades unilateral branches of the portal vein (PV) or hepatic artery while in iCCA, tumor perforates the visceral peritoneum.
- T4 in dCCA is a tumor which involves the celiac axis, superior mesenteric artery (SMA), and/or common hepatic artery. In pCCA with T4, tumor invades the main PV, its branches bilaterally, the common hepatic artery and in iCCA, the tumor involves the local extrahepatic structures by direct invasion (Forner et al., 2019; Lee et al., 2020).
- NX means that the regional lymph nodes could not be assessed.
- N0 is defined as no regional lymph node metastasis.
- With N1, there is metastasis to one to three regional lymph nodes, and in N2, there is metastasis to four or more regional lymph nodes (Forner et al., 2019; Lee et al., 2020).

Treatment

- Surgical resection is the only chance for cure in cholangiocarcinoma, with a disease-free survival (DFS) of 12 to 36 months. Surgical resection includes a partial hepatectomy with a bile-duct resection, a regional lymphadenectomy, and a Roux-en-Y hepaticojejunostomy with perihilar cholangiocarcinoma.
- Patients with distal cholangiocarcinoma undergo a Whipple procedure for surgical resection. Predictors of short DFS include large tumor size, the presence of multiple liver lesions, and regional lymph node involvement.

- Cirrhosis is an independent factor associated with unfavorable survival.
- Liver transplantation can be used in patients with early IHCC.
- Locoregional therapies, such as transarterial chemoembolization (TACE) and transarterial radioembolization (TARE) with yttrium 90, are used in advanced IHCC and are associated with an overall survival of 12 to 15 months.
- First-line chemotherapy includes gemcitabine and cisplatin, with advanced cholangiocarcinoma not amenable to locoregional or surgical options. Median survival with this option is 11.7 months.
- For patients with resected cholangiocarcinoma, postoperative external beam radiation therapy (EBRT) with concurrent chemotherapy is used, especially in node-positive or margin-positive patients.
- Molecular targeted therapies are currently being studied for use in cholangiocarcinoma.

Prognosis

Five-year survival is 18%.

Prevention

There is no standard surveillance for cholangiocarcinoma. Patients with PSC should be screened annually.

References

Benson, B., D'Angelica, M., Abbott, D., Anaya, D., Anders, R., Are, C., ... Darlow, S. (2021). Hepatobiliary cancers, version 2.2021, NCCN clinical practice guidelines in oncology. *National Comprehensive Cancer Network, 19*(5), 541–565. https://doi.org/10.6004/jnccn.2021.0022.

Forner, A., Vidili, G., Rengo, M., Bujanda, L., Ponz-Sarvisé, M., & Lamarca, A. (2019). Clinical presentation, diagnosis and staging of cholangiocarcinoma. *Liver International: Official Journal of the International Association for the Study of the Liver, 39*(Suppl 1), 98–107. https://doi.org/10.1111/liv.14086.

Khan, A. S., & Dageforde, L. A. (2019). Cholangiocarcinoma. *Surgical Clinics of North America, 99*, 315–335.

Lee, J. W., Lee, J. H., Park, Y., Lee, W., Kwon, J., Song, K. B., ... Kim, S. C. (2020). Prognostic predictability of American joint committee on cancer 8th staging system for perihilar cholangiocarcinoma: Limited improvement compared with the 7th staging system. *Cancer Research Treatment, 52*(3), 886–895.

Rahnemai-Azar, A. A., Weisbrod, A., Dillhoff, M., Schmidt, C., & Pawlik, T. M. (2017). Intrahepatic cholangiocarcinoma: Molecular markers for diagnosis and prognosis. *Surgical Oncology, 26*, 125–137.

Rhee, H., Kim, M. J., Park, Y. N., & An, C. (2019). A proposal of imaging classification of intrahepatic mass-forming cholangiocarcinoma into ductal and parenchymal types: Clinicopathologic significance. *European Radiology, 29*, 3111–3121.

Rizvi, S., Khan, S. A., Hallemeier, C. L., Kelley, R. K., & Gores, G. J. (2018). Cholangiocarcinoma—evolving concepts and therapeutic strategies. *Natural Reviews of Clinical Oncology, 15*(2), 95–111.

Zhao, J., Chen, Y., Wang, J., Wang, J., Wang, Y., Chai, S., ... Zhang, W. (2021). Preoperative risk grade predicts the long-term prognosis of intrahepatic cholangiocarcinoma: A retrospective cohort analysis. *Biomedical Central Surgery, 21*(1), 113.

Colorectal Cancer

Definition

Colorectal cancer (CRC) arises as adenocarcinoma from glandular epithelial cells of the large intestine in the colon and rectum. The development of CRC may occur over several years due to dysregulation of several signaling pathways. Malignant cells arising in the large intestine are defined as CRC (Ahmad et al., 2021).

Incidence

- CRC is the third most common detected cancer and the second most common cause of cancer-related mortality globally in men and women (Zhou & Rifkin, 2021).
- The incidence and mortality of CRC in developed countries have decreased due to CRC screening with colonoscopy (Ahmad et al., 2021).
- In 2020, 11% of all colon cancer diagnoses and 15% of all rectal cancer diagnoses are estimated to occur in patients under the age of 50 with the median age of 44. Seventy-five percent of all CRCs occurring under the age of 50 occur between the ages of 40 and 49 (Patel et al., 2021).

Etiology and Risk Factors

- Epidemiologic research estimates that 50% of colon cancer risk is preventable by modifying risk factors. Modifiable risk factors of CRC include smoking, excess alcohol intake, obesity, lack of physical activity, and poor dietary habits. These dietary habits include eating processed and charred red meat, having a low fiber intake, eating a high fat diet, lack of fruits, vegetables, and dairy products, which provide calcium and vitamin D (Zhou & Rifkin, 2021).
- Twenty percent of colon cancer is associated with familial history and first-degree relatives of patients with colorectal adenomas or invasive CRC. These patients are at a higher risk for development of CRC.
- Inflammatory bowel disease, such as ulcerative colitis and Crohn disease, has an increased risk of developing colon cancer (NCCN, 2022).

Hereditary Colorectal Cancer

It is estimated that 20% to 30% of CRC is familial, with 5% to 10% related to a known genetic syndrome. Hereditary CRC is divided into nonpolyposis and polyposis syndromes.

- Hereditary nonpolyposis CRC (HNPCC) or Lynch syndrome is the most common hereditary CRC syndrome, but it only accounts for 2% to 3% of all CRC (Wells & Wise, 2017). Mean age of onset of CRC is age 45. These cancers are proximal to the splenic flexure and have a high degree of microsatellite instability (MSI) and poor differentiation.
- Familial adenomatous polyposis (FAP) accounts for 0.5% to 1% of all CRC. It is characterized by development of greater than 100 colorectal adenomatous polyps and follows an autosomal-dominant inheritance pattern (Wells & Wise, 2017).

Signs and Symptoms

- Abdominal pain and rectal bleeding are the most frequent complaints of patients presenting with CRC (Holtedahl et al., 2021).
- Patients with proximal or right colon cancer may have vague symptoms (Holtedahl et al., 2021).
- Other symptoms include abdominal bloating, constipation, diarrhea, fatigue, weight loss, and anorexia.

Diagnostic Work-up

- Comprehensive history, including family history and social history to screen for risk factors.

- Physical examination with examination of lymph nodes.
- CBC CEA.
- DRE
- Test for occult blood in stool.
- Colonoscopy with biopsy of any suspicious masses.
- Transrectal ultrasound to stage rectal masses.
- CT of the abdomen, pelvis, and chest. MRI may be considered if contrasted CT scan are contraindicated (Moe & Bohnenkamp, 2020).

Histopathology

The World Health Organization (WHO) defines different subtypes of CRC based on their histopathologic appearance.

- *Glandular:* If gland formation is observed without excessive mucus production. This type of cancer usually metastasizes to the liver.
- *Mucinous:* Mucus production occurs in more than 50% of tumors. These account for 10% of CRC and are found primarily in the right colon. High rates of *MSI, BRAF, KRAS, and PIK3CA* mutations are present. These cancers have low response rates to neoadjuvant chemoradiation therapy and high rates of incomplete surgical resection (Sagaert et al., 2018).
- *Medullary:* Poorly differentiated solid sheets or nests of malignant cells with pushing borders and prominent epithelial lymphocytic infiltration. These are rare tumors occurring in the right colon and are associated with MSI (60%) and BRAF (80%). It is associated with lack of nodal positivity or extramural invasion (Sagaert et al., 2018).
- *Signet ring:* Accounts for less than 1% of CRC. It is characterized by proliferation of signet rings with intracellular mucin pools that push the nucleus to the periphery. These cells appear in younger patients and are found in the right colon. MSI is present in 40% of cases. Signet ring tumors tend to metastasize at an early stage and to multiple sites, such as the liver, ovaries, and peritoneum (Sagaert et al., 2018).

Tumor Grading

CRC tumors can be graded as well, moderately, or poorly differentiated based on the percentage of gland formation.

- Well-differentiated tumors have glandular structures in 95% of the tumors.
- Moderately differentiated tumors have glandular structures in 50% to 95% of the tumors.
- Poorly differentiated tumors display a loss of glandular structures in at least 50% of the tumors (Sagaert et al., 2018).

Clinical Staging

TNM staging is widely used to stratify patients into prognostic groups.

- Tis—lamina propria involvement with no extension through the muscularis mucosa
- T1—tumor invades the submucosa but not through the muscularis propria
- T2—tumor invades the muscularis propria

- T3—tumor invades the muscularis propria into the pericolorectal tissues
- T4—tumor invades the visceral peritoneum, including gross perforation of the bowel through tumor and other organs or structures
- N1—metastasis in one to three regional lymph nodes
- N2—metastasis in four or more regional lymph nodes
- M0—no distant metastasis
- M1—distant metastases (Macedo et al., 2021)

Molecular Biomarkers

Molecular biomarkers are characteristics of tumors that serve as an indicator of normal biologic behavior, pathogenic processes, and response to pharmacologic treatment. The College of American Pathologists, American Society of Clinical Oncology (ASCO), and NCCN recommend that all newly diagnosed with CRC should undergo biomarker testing (Schmitt, 2020).

- MSI is a deficiency of the mismatch repair (MMR) pathway. During DNA synthesis, MMR proteins recognize errors between newly formed and original DNA strands and correct these errors. The MSI pathway accounts for 15% of sporadic CRC (Sagaert et al., 2018; Schmitt, 2020). These tumors are often in the proximal colon, poorly differentiated with a high number of tumor-infiltrating lymphocytes. They have a better prognosis due to the lack of lymph node and distant metastasis.
- MMR proteins are dependent on four genes: *MLH1, PMS2, MSH2,* and *MSH6.* Inactivation of one or more MMR genes allows for errors to accumulate in DNA sequencing or microsatellites. These uncorrected errors lead to MSI and neoplasia.
- *KRAS,* a proto-oncogene, acts as a regulator of the epidermal growth factor receptor (EGFR), regulating cell growth, proliferation, migration, and differentiation. Forty to 45% of CRC patients have *KRAS* mutations affecting codons 12 and 13.
- *BRAF* mutations occur in 10% of all CRC patients and are a down regulator of the EGFR pathway. The NCCN (2022) recommends *BRAF* analysis in *KRAS* wild-type tumors.
- Human epidermal growth factor receptor 2 (HER2) is a signaling protein. Overexpression of this protein leads to activation of oncogenic signaling pathways, promoting cellular proliferation, survival, and angiogenesis. About 3% of CRCs display overexpression of HER2.

Treatment

Surgery

A colectomy may be performed via an open or minimally invasive approach with a laparoscope or robot. According to NCCN (2022) guidelines, for locally advanced cancer or acute bowel obstruction or perforation, a minimally invasive approach should not be used. During the colectomy, a thorough exploration of the abdomen should be completed. Lymph nodes at the origin of vessels supplying the area of the colon where the mass exists should be removed for pathologic examination. A minimum of 12 lymph nodes should be examined (NCCN, 2022).

A colostomy may be performed to temporarily divert stool from a colonic anastomosis. These diverting ostomies are usually reversed in 6 to 12 weeks. In rectal cancer, the ostomy may be an end colostomy and is permanent after the rectum is removed.

Chemotherapy

Chemotherapy before surgery is termed neoadjuvant, while chemotherapy delivered after surgery is adjuvant. First-line systemic therapy is FOLFOX (folinic acid, leucovorin, 5-FU, and oxaliplatin). Monoclonal antibodies, such as bevacizumab, panitumumab, or cetuximab, may be added for those patients with wild-type KRAS exon 2 and vascular endothelial growth factor (VEGF) pathways (Ahmad et al., 2021; NCCN, 2022).

Immunotherapy

Pembrolizumab (anti-PD1) has shown favorable responses in MSI-high subtypes. However, in the treatment of microsatellite stable (MSS) type of CRCs, immunotherapy alone has not shown positive results (Jin et al., 2020).

Prognosis

- According to the American Cancer Society (ACS), the overall 5-year survival rate for CRC is 65% (Simard et al., 2019).
- Patients who present with localized or regional disease have a survival rate of 71% to 90% (Simard et al., 2019).
- Tumor deposits reported in 4.9% to 41.8% of patients are associated with a poor prognosis (Liu et al., 2019).
- According to the National Cancer Institute's Surveillance, Epidemiology, and End Results (SEER), there has been a 51% increase in young-onset CRC since 1994 (Simard et al., 2019).

Prevention and Surveillance

Prevention

The United States Preventative Service Task Force (USPSTF) currently recommends screening for CRC starting at age 50 and continuing until age 75 (The Lancet Gastroenterology Hepatology, 2021). The task force also recommends CRC screening should be offered selectively to adults aged 76 to 85 years with clinicians reviewing the patient's overall health and screening history (The Lancet Gastroenterology Hepatology, 2021). The ACS in 2018 recommended lowering the age of initial screening to 45 years of age. The USPSTF recommends use of high-sensitivity fecal occult blood testing, fecal immunochemical testing (FIT), and stool DNA testing plus FIT, colonoscopy, CT colonography, and flexible sigmoidoscopy for CRC screening.

Surveillance

The NCCN, ACS, and ASCO recommend surveillance during the first 5 years of treatment.

- All survivors, regardless of stage, should undergo colonoscopy 1 year following surgical resection, which should be repeated at 3 years and then every 5 years (Simard et al., 2019).

- Patients with stage II to IV disease should have a complete history and physical examination, CEA and proctoscopy, plus EUS.
- Patients with rectal cancer not treated with radiation should undergo MRI every 3 to 6 months for 2 years, then every 6 months for 2 years. CT of the chest, abdomen, and pelvis is recommended every 6 to 12 months for 3 to 5 years for stages II to III and every 3 to 6 months for stage IV disease (Simard et al., 2019).

References

Ahmad, R., Singh, J. K., Wunnava, A., Al-Obeed, O., Abdulla, M., & Srivastava, S. K. (2021). Emerging trends in colorectal cancer: Dysregulated signaling pathways (review). *International Journal of Molecular Medicine, 47*(3), 14.

Holtedahl, K., Borgquist, L., Donker, G. A., Buntinx, F., Weller, D., Campbell, C., … Parajuli, R. (2021). Symptoms and signs of colorectal cancer, with differences between proximal and distal colon cancer: A prospective cohort study of diagnostic accuracy in primary care. *Biomedical Central Family Practice, 22*(1), 148.

Jin, K., Ren, C., Liu, Y., Lan, H., & Wang, Z. (2020). An update on colorectal cancer microenvironment, epigenetic and immunotherapy. *International Immunopharmacology, 89*, 107041.

Liu, F., Zhao, J., Li, C., Wu, Y., Song, W., Guo, T., … Xu, Y. (2019). The unique prognostic characteristics of tumor deposits in colorectal cancer patients. *Annals of Translational Medicine, 7*(23), 1–9.

Macedo, F., Sequeira, H., Ladeira, K., Bonito, N., Viana, C., & Martins, S. (2021). Metastatic lymph node ratio as a better prognostic tool than the TNM system in colorectal cancer. *Future Oncology, 17*(12), 1519–1532.

Moe, L., & Bohnenkamp, S. (2020). Overview of colon cancer for the medical-surgical nurse. *MedSurg Nursing, 29*(1), 58–60.

National Comprehensive Cancer Network (NCCN). (2022). Colon cancer (version 1.2022). Available at https://www.nccn.org/professionals/physician_gls/pdf/coloncarcinoma.

Patel, S. G., Murphy, C. C., Lieu, C. H., & Hampel, H. (2021). Early age onset colorectal cancer. *Advances in Cancer Research, 151*, 1–37.

Sagaert, X., Vanstapel, A., & Verbeek, S. (2018). Tumor heterogeneity in colorectal cancer: What do we know so far? *Pathobiology, 85*(1-2), 72–84.

Schmitt, M. (2020). Molecular biomarkers. *Clinical Journal of Oncology Nursing, 24*(6), 635–643.

Simard, J., Kamath, S., & Kircher, S. (2019). Survivorship guidance for patients with colorectal cancer. *Current Treatment Options in Oncology, 20*(38), 1–15.

The Lancet Gastroenterology Hepatology. (2021). USPSTF recommends expansion of colorectal cancer screening. *The Lancet Gastroenterology Hepatology, 6*, 1

Wells, K., & Wise, P. (2017). Hereditary colorectal cancer syndromes. *Surgical Clinic of North America, 97*, 605–625.

Zhou, E., & Rifkin, S. (2021). Colorectal cancer and diet: Risk versus prevention, is diet an intervention? *Gastroenterology Clinics of North America, 50*, 101–111.

Esophageal Cancer

Definition

Esophageal cancer is described by its anatomic location, of which there are five. The *cervical esophagus* is defined from the oropharynx to the sternal notch (15–20 cm from the teeth incisors). The *upper esophagus* is located from the sternal notch to the lower border of the azygos vein (20–25 cm). The *middle esophagus* is from the azygos vein to the lower border of the inferior pulmonary veins (25–30 cm). The *lower esophagus* is from the inferior pulmonary veins to the stomach (30–40 cm), and the *gastroesophageal junction* (Shemmeri & Fabian, 2021).

The esophageal wall is composed of three layers: mucosa, submucosa, and muscularis propria. The muscularis propria is contiguous with the periesophageal connective tissue or adventitia. There is no serosa, which facilitates local tumor invasion into the pleura, pericardium, diaphragm, and peritoneum (Betancourt-Cuellar et al., 2021).

Incidence

- Esophageal cancer is the ninth most common malignancy and the seventh most common cause of cancer death (Waters & Reznik, 2022).
- Esophageal cancer is less common in the United States, and adenocarcinoma has surpassed SCC as the most common type of cancer in the United States (Ahmad et al., 2022).
- Squamous cell carcinoma of the esophagus (ESSC) remains the most common type of esophageal cancer in the Middle East, Central Asia, southern former Soviet countries, and China (Waters & Reznik, 2022).
- The two most common histologic types of esophageal cancer, ESSC and adenocarcinoma, account for 90% of all esophageal cancers worldwide (Waters & Reznik, 2022).

Etiology and Risk Factors

The geographic differences in types of esophageal cancer worldwide show that ethnicity, genetics, and lifestyle play a role in cancer development.

- Barrett esophagus—a metaplastic transformation from the normal squamous mucosa to a columnar lining is the only known precursor of esophageal cancer. Only 5% of esophageal cancer patients had known Barrett esophagus.
  Risk factors include:
- White race—has a twofold risk of developing esophageal adenocarcinoma than Hispanics, and a three- to fourfold risk when compared with Blacks (Huang & Yu, 2018)
- Male sex—a 38-fold increase in males over females (Huang & Yu, 2018)
- Gastroesophageal reflux disease (GERD)—10% of patients will develop esophageal cancer (Huang & Yu, 2018).
- Cigarette smoking—total packs per year correlated with increased risk
- Obesity
- Excessive alcohol consumption
- Diet high in red meat

Hereditary Syndromes

- Tylosis (focal nonepidermolytic palmoplantar keratoderma [PPK] or Howel-Evans syndrome) is a rare autosomal dominant syndrome caused by gene mutation in the *RHBDF2* gene. This syndrome is associated with a higher lifetime risk of developing SCC of the middle or distal esophagus (NCCN, 2023; Ajani et al., 2023).
- Familial Barrett esophagus (FBE) may be associated with one or more autosomally inherited dominant susceptibility alleles.
- Fanconi anemia (FA) is an autosomal recessive disorder. It is caused by mutations in 1 of 15 genes, with *FANCA, FANCC, FANCG, and FANCD2* being the most common.

Signs and Symptoms

Most early esophageal cancers are asymptomatic and found incidentally. Advanced tumors may present with dysphagia or bleeding.

Diagnostic Work-up

- Upper EUS with biopsy remains the gold standard for diagnosis. It assesses the depth of tumor invasion and locoregional lymph node involvement (Bhatt et al., 2020).
- PET scan identifies metastatic sites.
- PET/CT is recommended by the NCCN (2023), Ajani et al., (2023).

Histopathology

Esophageal cancer is classified as SCC or adenocarcinoma. SCC is more likely to localize at or above the tracheal bifurcation, has a propensity for early lymph node spread, and is associated with a poorer prognosis (NCCN, 2023; Ajani et al., 2023).

Molecular Biomarkers

The role of micro RNAs (miRNAs) and long noncoding RNAs (lncRNAs) plays an important role in the development and progression of esophageal cancer. Further research to understand the clinical applications of miRNAs and lncRNAs is needed to diagnose and treat esophageal cancer (see table below).

Important Noncoding RNAs in Human Esophageal Cancer

Noncoding RNAs	Functions
lncRNA MALAT1	Enhances cell proliferation, G_2/M cell cycle arrest, migration, and invasion
lncRNA PEG10	Increases cell proliferation and migration
lncRNA TP73-AS1	Decreases cell apoptosis and induces chemo-resistance
lncRNA CASC9	Increases cell migration and invasion
lncRNA H19	Promotes cell proliferation and invasion and induces epithelial to mesenchymal transition
miR-373	Enhances cell proliferation, G_1-phase cell proportion, migration, and invasion
miR-26b	Enhances cell proliferation, cell-cycle transition, and migration
miR-100	Inhibits cell proliferation, migration, invasion, and suppresses tumor growth
miR-98	Restores radiosensitivity
miR-124	Increases cell apoptosis after radiotherapy

lncRNA, Long noncoding RNAs.
From Hou, X., Wen, J., Ren, Z., & Zhang, G. (2017). Non-coding RNAs: New biomarkers and therapeutic targets for esophageal cancer. *Oncotarget, 8*(26), 43572.

Clinical Staging

- The eighth edition of the AJCC TNM staging is utilized for esophageal cancer.
  - Tis—high-grade dysplasia
  - T1a—tumor is confined to the submucosa
  - T1b—tumor is confined to the submucosal components
  - T2—tumor invades the muscularis propria
  - T3—tumor invades the adventitia
  - T4—tumor invades adjacent structures
  - T4a—tumor is potentially resectable invasion of the pleura, pericardium, or diaphragm
  - T4b—tumor is unresectable invasion of other adjacent structures, such as aorta, vertebral body, or trachea (Betancourt Cuellar et al., 2023).
- N0 to N3 describe the number of lymph node metastasis. Regional lymph nodes are defined as any periesophageal

lymph nodes from the upper esophageal sphincter to the celiac axis. Lymph nodes outside the above region are considered distant metastases.

- Supraclavicular lymph nodes are considered M1 disease (Betancourt Cuellar et al., 2023).

Treatment

Surgery

The type of esophageal resection is determined by the tumor location. The two most common surgical approaches are transthoracic and transhiatal esophagectomy. The NCCN (2023), Ajani et al., (2023) recommends that esophagectomy should always be performed at high-volume centers with experienced surgeons. Minimally invasive esophagectomy (MIE) includes laparoscopy and robotic-assisted techniques during some of the esophagectomy procedure. MIE may be associated with decreased postoperative mortality, shorter recovery times, and increased long-term survival (NCCN, 2023; Ajani et al., 2023).

Endoscopic Therapies

Therapies include endoscopic mucosal resection (EMR) or endoscopic submucosal dissection (ESD), which can be used in the treatment of early-stage esophageal and esophago gastric junction (EGJ) cancers. Radiofrequency ablation (RFA) alone or in combination with endoscopic resection is an effective treatment option to completely eradicate residual dysplasia.

Radiation

The NCCN (2023), Ajani et al., (2023) recommends that radiation therapy alone should be used only for palliation or for patients who are medically unable to receive chemotherapy. Proton beam therapy (PBT) is an emerging radiation therapy which limits exposure to adjacent organs while allowing high radiation doses.

Systemic Therapy

Systemic therapy is used in both the neoadjuvant and adjuvant setting and includes the use of chemotherapy and immunotherapy before and after surgery. Due to the poor prognosis of treatment with surgery alone, multiple approaches have become the standard of care for an increased survival benefit in local advanced esophageal cancer (Lee et al., 2022). This treatment can provide palliation as well as improved survival. Systemic therapy is selected based on the patient's performance status (PS), comorbidities, and the toxicity profile of the selected agents (NCCN, 2023; Ajani et al., 2023), since the risk of complications and a reduced quality of life can be a therapy outcome.

Neoadjuvant

Neoadjuvant chemoradiation is preferred for cancers of the esophageal-gastric-junction (EGJ) and neoadjuvant chemotherapy is used for distal esophagus and EGJ cancers (NCCN, 2023; Ajani et al., 2023). This North American standard of care for chemotherapy prior to surgery is a result of the CROSS (Chemoradiotherapy for Oesphageal Cancer followed by Surgery Study) trial (Lee et al., 2022) Neoadjuvant chemotherapy added to radiation includes paclitaxel and carboplatin, or 5-FU and oxaliplatin (NCCN, 2023; Ajani et al., 2023). Other options include 5-FU and cisplatin, irinotecan and cisplatin, paclitaxel and fluoropyrimidine, and 5-FU and capecitabine (NCCN, 2023; Ajani et al., 2023). Two drug regimens are preferred due of lower toxicity versus multiple agents. For three agent therapy, patients must have an excellent PS and be accessible for frequent monitoring of a wide range and degree of severity of side effects (NCCN, 2023; Ajani et al., 2023).

Neoadjuvant chemotherapy includes 5-FU, leucovorin, oxaliplatin, and docetaxel (FLOT) or fluoropyrimidine and oxaliplatin (NCCN, 2023; Ajani et al., 2023). NCCN recommendations for second- and third-line therapies can be found in the NCCN guidelines (NCCN, 2023; Ajani et al., 2023).

Adjuvant

The role of adjuvant therapy has limited guidelines or randomized evidence and is institution and patient dependent (Lee et al., 2022). Adjuvant therapy is considered for patients who received surgery and are found to have positive lymph nodes or resection margins. It is used in palliative treatment for disease control.

Immunotherapy

Since, 2017, immunotherapy has been used as a third line treatment combined with systemic treatment (Ge et al., 2022). In patients with HER2 overexpression, trastuzumab should be added to chemotherapy regimens (NCCN, 2023; Ajani et al., 2023). Postoperative treatment may include nivolumab after neoadjuvant chemoradiation and clear surgical margins. Nivolumab is a monoclonal PD-1 antibody approved by the FDA in May 2021 for resected esophageal cancer or EGJ tumors with residual disease (NCCN, 2023; Ajani et al., 2023) and is used in the adjuvant treatment setting. Pembrolizumab is a PD-1 antibody approved by the FDA in March 2021 and can be used first line in combination with chemotherapy. There are still no biomarkers that can estimate the clinical outcomes of immunotherapy.

The NCCN panel encourages participation in well-designed clinical trials investigating novel therapies to propel further advanced in esophageal cancer (NCCN, 2023; Ajani et al., 2023).

Prognosis

The prognosis of esophageal cancer globally is poor due to the advanced stage at time of discovery, severe malnutrition due to digestive obstruction, and lower socioeconomic status (Vendrely et al., 2018).

- The overall 5-year survival rate is 10%, and postesophagectomy 5-year survival rate is 15% to 40% (Huang & Yu, 2018).

Prevention and Surveillance

- There are currently no screening guidelines for ESCC and low-level evidence for screening EAC (Uhlenhopp et al., 2020).
- Prevention strategies include the elimination of very hot food/drink, alcohol, and tobacco. The addition of fruits and vegetables to the diet would assist in prevention but may be difficult in developing countries, where more than 80% of ESCC deaths occur (Uhlenhopp et al., 2020).
- The NCCN (2023), Ajani et al., (2023) states that surveillance strategies remain controversial. Ninety percent of recurrences occur within the first 2 years after local therapy completion.

- Follow-up should include a complete history and physical examination every 3 to 6 months for the first 2 years, every 6 to 12 months for years 3 to 5, and then annually. CBC, chemistry, upper endoscopy, and imaging studies should be performed as clinically indicated.
- Nutritional assessment and counseling are recommended.
- Routine surveillance is not recommended for more than 5 years (NCCN, 2023; Ajani et al., 2023).

References

Ahmad, M. U., Javadi, C., & Poultsides, G. A. (2022). Neoadjuvant treatment strategies for resectable proximal gastric, gastroesophageal junction and distal esophageal cancer. *Cancers, 14*(7), 1755.

Ajani, J., D'Amico, T., Bentrem, D., Cooke, D., Corver, C., Das, P., … Pluchino, L. (2023). Esophageal and esophagogastric junction cancers, version 2.2023. *Journal of the Comprehensive Cancer Network, 21*(4), 393–422. https://doi.org/10.6004/jccn.2023.0019.

Betancourt-Cuellar, S. L., Benveniste, M. F. K., Palacio, D. P., & Hofstetter, W. L. (2021). Esophageal cancer: Tumor-node-metastasis staging. *Radiologic Clinics of North America, 59*(2), 219–229.

Betancourt Cuellar, S. L., Benveniste, M. F., Truong, M., Nguyen, Q. N., Atiyah, A., Hofstetter, W. L., & Erasmus, J. J. (2023). Liver injury in patients with distal esophageal carcinoma after precision radiation therapy: Systematic review of FDG-PET/CT patterns. *American Journal of Clinical Oncology, 46*(1), 25–30. https://doi.org/10.1097/COC.0000000000000960.

Bhatt, A., Kamath, S., Murthy, S. C., & Raja, S. (2020). Multidisciplinary evaluation and management of early stage esophageal cancer. *Surgical Oncology Clinics of North America, 29*(4), 613–630.

Ge, F., Huo, Z., Cai, X., Hu, Q., Chen, W., Lin, G., … Liu, J. (2022). Evaluation of clinical and safety outcomes of neoadjuvant immunotherapy combined with chemotherapy for patients with resectable esophageal cancer: A systematic review and meta-analysis. *JAMA Network Open Oncology, 5*(11), e22397781-18. https://doi.org/10.1001/jamanetworkopen 2022.39778.

Huang, F. L., & Yu, S. J. (2018). Esophageal cancer: Risk factors, genetic association, and treatment. *Asian Journal of Surgery, 41*(3), 210–215.

Lee, Y., Samarasinghe, Y., Lee, M., Thiru, L., Shargall, Y., Finley, C., … Agzarian, J. (2022). Role of adjuvant therapy in esophageal cancer patients after neoadjuvant therapy and esophagectomy. *Annals of Surgery, 275*(1), 91–98. https://doi.org/10.1097/SLA.0000000000005227.

National Comprehensive Cancer Network (NCCN). (2023). Esophageal and esophagogastric junction cancers (version 2.2023). Available at https://www.nccn.org/professionals/physician_gls/pdf/esophageal.pdf.

Shemmeri, E., & Fabian, T. (2021). Staging of esophageal malignancy. *The Surgical Clinics of North America, 101*(3), 405–414.

Uhlenhopp, D. J., Then, E. O., Sunkara, T., & Gaduputi, V. (2020). Epidemiology of esophageal cancer: Update in global trends, etiology and risk factors. *Clinical Journal of Gastroenterology, 13*(6), 1010–1021. https://doi.org/10.1007/s12328-020-01237-x.

Vendrely, V., Launay, V., Najah, H., Smith, D., Collet, D., & Gronnier, C. (2018). Prognostic factors in esophageal cancer treated with curative intent. *Digestive and Liver Disease, 50*(10), 991–996.

Waters, J. K., & Reznik, S. I. (2022). Update on management of squamous cell esophageal cancer. *Current Oncology Reports, 24*(3), 375–385.

Gallbladder Cancer

Definition

Gallbladder cancer is a rare biliary tract malignancy in most western countries but is widespread in other regions of the world. It arises from the biliary epithelium.

Incidence

- Gallbladder cancer constitutes 1.7% of all cancer deaths worldwide. Gallbladder cancer has an unusual geographic distribution with substantial geographic variation.
- Chile, northern India, Poland, southern Pakistan, Japan, and Israel have the highest rates of gallbladder cancer.
- In the United States, the highest incidence is found in Native Americans and Hispanic populations in New Mexico.
- There is a three to six times higher incidence in females compared to males.
- Two-thirds of persons diagnosed with gallbladder cancer are over the age of 65, with the average age of 72 (Hickman & Conteras, 2019; Schmidt et al., 2019).

Etiology and Risk Factors

Environmental exposures and lifestyle behaviors have been linked to a higher risk of developing gallbladder cancer.

- Gallstones or cholelithiasis are one of the most strongly associated risk factors in 70% to 90% of cases. This is thought to be due to chronic epithelial irritation and mucosal damage. The size of the gallstone influences the risk of gallbladder cancer. Gallstones greater than 3 cm are associated with a 9.2 to 10.1 times greater risk of gallbladder cancer (Shukla et al., 2018).
- Porcelain gallbladder is associated with an extremely high risk of cancer development.
- PSC is associated with a 2% lifetime incidence of developing gallbladder cancer.
- Anomalous pancreaticobiliary ductal junction or biliopancreatic malfunction.
- *Salmonella typhi* or *Helicobacter bilis* carriers have a 12-fold risk of developing gallbladder cancer.
- Diabetes and obesity.
- Environmental factors: fungal aflatoxins, ochratoxin, arsenic.
- Mirizzi syndrome.
- Family history of gallstones—the clustering of gallbladder cancer within families is suggestive of genetic role.
- Tobacco consumption.
- Excessive intake of fried foods.
- Gallbladder polyps (Schmidt et al., 2019).

Signs and Symptoms

- Weight loss
- Jaundice

Diagnostic Work-up

- CT of the chest, abdomen, and pelvis
- The NCCN recommends PET/CT when findings on imaging studies are equivocal (NCCN, 2023)
- Liver function tests
- Serum levels of CEA, cancer antigen 19-9 (CA 19-9), and cancer antigen 125 (CA 125) can be elevated, but diagnostic sensitivity and specificity are low
- Staging laparoscopy

Incidental Finding at Surgery

- Frozen section of gallbladder if suspicious for cancer
- Intraoperative staging with resection of any suspicious lymph nodes and cystic duct node
- Further surgery should be delayed until full imaging and pathology work-up is complete
- Contrasted CT of chest, abdomen, and pelvis

Incidental Findings on Pathology

- Contrasted CT/MRI of chest, abdomen, and pelvis for T1b or greater stage
- Observation for T1a patients with R0 resection
- Staging laparoscopy for T1b or greater

Unresectable on Imaging or Staging Laparoscopy

- Biopsy if tissue is not available

Histopathology

- Eighty-five to 97% of these cancers are adenocarcinomas.
  - Adenocarcinomas can be papillary, tubular, mucinous, or signet ring.
- Other histologies include squamous cell, anaplastic, adenosquamous cell, neuroendocrine, and sarcoma carcinoma.
- Most gallbladder cancers, approximately 60% are found in the fundus, 30% in the body, and 10% in the neck.
- Molecular and genetic alterations have been noted in gallbladder cancer. These include
  - KRAS—affects codons 12, 13, and 61.
  - Mutation at codon 12 occurs in 8% to 80% of gallbladder cancer
  - TP53—mutations occur in 27% to 70% of gallbladder cancer (Sharma et al., 2017)
  - HER2

Clinical Staging

The TNM classification is used for gallbladder cancer staging.
- T1—tumor invades the lamina propria or muscular layer
- T2a—tumor invades the perimuscular connective tissue of the peritoneal side without involvement of the serosa (visceral peritoneum)
- T2b—tumor invades the perimuscular connective tissue on the hepatic side with no extension into the liver
- T3—tumor perforates the serosa (visceral peritoneum) and/or directly invades the liver and/or one other adjacent organ or structure
- T4—tumor invades the main PV or hepatic artery or invades two or more extrahepatic organs or structures
- N0—no regional lymph node metastasis
- N1—metastasis to one to three regional lymph nodes
- N2—metastasis to four or more regional lymph nodes
- M0—no distant metastasis
- M1—distant metastasis including peritoneum, liver, lungs, pleura, periaortic, pericaval, SMA, and celiac artery lymph nodes (Wang et al., 2020)

Treatment

Staging laparotomy is endorsed by both the NCCN guidelines and the 2014 American Hepato-Pancreato-Biliary Association (AHPBA) to identify nodal disease and peritoneal implants.

Surgical

Most gallbladder cancers are diagnosed on pathologic review. If cancer is diagnosed by frozen section during the initial surgery, the surgeon should inspect the peritoneal cavity for distant spread and biopsy any suspicious lymph nodes (Hickman & Contreras, 2019). Surgery is the only curative treatment (Javle et al., 2019). The table below summarizes the principles driving surgery for gallbladder cancer.

Surgical Principles in the Treatment of Gallbladder Cancer

Surgical Principle	Key Points
Staging Laparoscopy	Highest yield in T3 or greater or positive margins after cholecystectomy
Laparotomy	Metastases to celiac axis or aortocaval nodes
Hepatic Resection	Standard resection is segments IVB and V
Lymphadenectomy	All nodes in the porta hepatitis and at least six nodes for complete staging
Bile Duct Resection	Routine resection is not recommended but may be necessary for complete resection
Port-site Resection	Routine resection is not recommended because port-site disease is a marker for intra-abdominal spread
Extent of Resection	• T1 tumors—cholecystectomy • T1b and greater—radical cholecystectomy (hepatic resection + portal lymphadenectomy + cholecystectomy) • Surgical morbidity 50% and perioperative mortality 5%

Data from National Comprehensive Cancer Network (NCCN). (2023). Biliary tract cancers (version 1.2023). Available at https://www.nccn.org/professionals/physician_gls/pdf/btc.pdf; Hickman, L., & Contreras, C. (2019). Gallbladder cancer: Diagnosis, surgical management, and adjuvant therapies. *The Surgical Clinics of North America, 99*(2), 337–355.

Systemic Therapy

Chemotherapy is recommended in conjunction with surgery, neoadjuvant and adjuvant therapy. Additionally, chemotherapy or a clinical trial is the standard of care for patients with unresectable or metastatic gallbladder cancer.

- Gemcitabine or gemcitabine + cisplatin is commonly used as neoadjuvant chemotherapy for patients with resectable gallbladder cancer (Hickman & Contreras, 2019). The NCCN (2023) also states that gemcitabine/oxaliplatin, gemcitabine/capecitabine, capecitabine/oxaliplatin, and 5-FU/oxaliplatin may be used.
- Adjuvant chemotherapy is recommended by the NCCN following resection of gallbladder cancer; capecitabine or oxaliplatin + gemcitabine and nab-paclitaxel are utilized after surgical resection (Azizi et al., 2021; NCCN, 2023).
- NCCN recommends chemotherapy in unresectable or metastatic gallbladder cancer, gemcitabine and cisplatin are preferred first-line therapies, followed by subsequent treatment with the FOLFOX regimen (leucovorin calcium [folinic acid], fluorouracil, and oxaliplatin) (NCCN, 2023).
- Targeted therapeutic agents are used in gallbladder cancer. Erlotinib has been used alone and in combination with bevacizumab. The table below provides a listing of mutations in gallbladder cancer and the agents which target these mutations.

Targeted Genetic Variants in Gallbladder Cancer

Targetable Gene Variants	Potential Therapeutics
EGFR	Afatinib
	Erlotinib
	Cetuximab
HER2	Trastuzumab
	Lapatinib
	Pertuzumab
TP53	Bevacizumab
ERBB3	Seribantumab
	Pertuzumab
	Trastuzumab
PTEN, PIK3CA	Everolimus (mTOR inhibitor)
KRAS	Trametinib
	Selumetinib
ARID1A	Everolimus (mTOR inhibitor)
	Pembrolizumab (anti-PDL1) for tumors with microsatellite instability
CDKN2A/B Loss	Palbociclib

EGFR, Epidermal growth factor receptor; *HER2*, human epidermal growth factor receptor 2; *mTOR,* mammalian target of rapamycin.
Data from Jain, A., & Javle, M. (2016). Molecular profiling of biliary tract cancer: A target rich disease. *Journal of Gastrointestinal Oncology, 7*(5), 797–803; Sicklick, J. K., Fanta, P. T., Shimabukuro, K., & Kurzrock, R. (2016). Genomics of gallbladder cancer: The case for biomarker-driven clinical trial design. *Cancer Metastasis Reviews, 35*(2), 263–275; Hickman, L., & Contreras, C. (2019). Gallbladder cancer: Diagnosis, surgical management, and adjuvant therapies. *The Surgical Clinics of North America, 99*(2), 337–355.

Palliative Therapy

- Ensure adequate biliary drainage with external drainage catheters
- Nutritional support
- Endoscopic biliary stents (Hickman & Contreras, 2019)

Prognosis

- The prognosis for gallbladder cancer is poor.
- T1a and T1b have a 5-year survival of 86% and T2 with 56%; and T3 cancer of 19% and T4 is 14%.
- The 5 years survival ranges from 50% for stage 1 to 2% for stage 4b based on the National Cancer Database of the American College of Surgeons (Schmidt et al., 2019).

Prevention and Surveillance

- There is no standardized screening for gallbladder cancer.
- NCCN (2023) recommends imaging every 6 months for 2 years and then annually up to 5 years.

References

Azizi, A. A., Lamarca, A., McNamara, M. G., & Valle, J. W. (2021). Chemotherapy for advanced gallbladder cancer (GBC): A systematic review and meta-analysis. *Critical Reviews in Oncology/Hematology, 163*, 103328.

Hickman, L., & Contreras, C. (2019). Gallbladder cancer: Diagnosis, surgical management, and adjuvant therapies. *The Surgical Clinics of North America*, 99(2), 337–355.

Javle, M., Zhao, H., & Abou-Alfa, G. K. (2019). Systemic therapy for gallbladder cancer. *Chinese Clinical Oncology, 8*(4), 44.

National Comprehensive Cancer Network (NCCN). (2023). Biliary Tract Cancers (version 2.2023). Available at https://www.nccn.org/professionals/physician_gls/pdf/btc.pdf.

Schmidt, M. A., Marcano-Bonilla, L., & Roberts, L. R. (2019). Gallbladder cancer: Epidemiology and genetic risk associations. *Chinese Clinical Oncology, 8*(4), 1–14.

Sharma, A., Sharma, K. L., Gupta, A., Yadav, A., & Kumar, A. (2017). Gallbladder cancer epidemiology, pathogenesis and molecular genetics: Recent update. *World Journal of Gastroenterology, 23*(22), 3978–3998.

Shukla, S. K., Singh, G., Shahi, K. S., Bhuvan, & Pant, P. (2018). Staging, treatment, and future approaches of gallbladder carcinoma. *Journal of Gastrointestinal Cancer, 49*(1), 9–15.

Wang, J., Bo, X., Shi, X., Suo, T., Xin, Y., Nan, L., … Liu, H. (2020). Modified staging classification of gallbladder carcinoma on the basis of the 8th edition of the American Joint Commission on Cancer (AJCC) staging system. *European Journal of Surgical Oncology, 46*, 527–533.

Gastric Cancer

Definition

Gastric cancer is classified by anatomic locations, which include the cardia, fundus, body, antrum, or pylorus. Tumors can manifest as malignant ulcers or polypoid lesions, or they can spread throughout the submucosal layers producing a rigid, nondistendable stomach called linitis plastica.

Incidence

- Gastric cancer is the fifth leading cancer in the world and the third leading cause of cancer-related death (Carvalho et al., 2021).
- The incidence of gastric cancer varies widely across geographic regions, with the highest incidence observed in East Asia, some Eastern European countries, and South American countries, which account for 70% of gastric cancers (NCCN, 2023).
- During the past 5 decades, there has been a decline in gastric cancer (Petryszyn et al., 2020).
- The lowest incidence is in North America and Africa (NCCN, 2023).
- Most patients with gastric cancer (50%) are diagnosed in late stages (NCCN, 2023).

Etiology and Risk Factors

- The incidence of gastric cancer is two times higher in males than females (Smyth et al., 2020).
- Epstein-Barr virus-associated gastric cancer comprises 1.3% to 30.9% of all gastric cancers depending on geographic distribution, with a global average of 8.9% of all gastric cancers (Yang et al., 2020).
- *Helicobacter pylori (H. pylori)* is the major cause of noncardia gastric cancer. Chronic infection of the gastric mucosa leads to progression from atrophic gastritis and intestinal metaplasia to cancer (Smyth et al., 2020).
- A positive association between GERD and proximal (cardia) gastric cancer has been shown (Smyth et al., 2020).
- Other risk factors include age greater than 60 years old, low socioeconomic status, cigarette smoking, alcohol consumption, diet high in nitrates and smoked foods that are high in sodium and deficient in vitamins A and C, familial predisposition, previous gastric surgery, and pernicious anemia (Smyth et al., 2020).
- Most gastric cancers are sporadic, with 1% to 3% being hereditary. These hereditary syndromes include hereditary diffuse gastric cancer (HDGC), gastric adenocarcinoma and proximal polyposis of the stomach (GAPPS), and familial intestinal gastric cancer (FIGC).
  - Germline mutations and deletions within the E-cadherin gene (*CDH1*) are the main cause of HDGC, which affects 14% to 40% of families.
  - FIGC is characterized by an autosomal dominant inheritance pattern of intestinal gastric cancer (IGC) without

gastric polyposis and is defined according to gastric cancer incidence as agreed by the International Gastric Cancer Linkage Consortium.

- Diagnostic criteria analogous to the Amsterdam criteria for hereditary nonpolypoid colorectal cancer (HNPCC): at least three relatives should have IGC and one of them should be a first-degree relative of the other two. At least two successive generations should be one of the relative and should be diagnosed before the age of 50.
- Gastric cancer has been identified in the tumor spectrum of Lynch syndrome, Li-Fraumeni syndrome, Peutz-Jeghers syndrome, FAP, juvenile polyposis, and hereditary breast and ovarian cancer (Carvalho et al., 2021).

Signs and Symptoms

- Patients with gastric cancer are difficult to diagnose due to their unspecific symptoms. This leads to later stage of disease at diagnosis.
- The most common symptoms are indigestion, anorexia, early satiety, weight loss, and abdominal pain.
  - Dysphagia or regurgitation may occur in proximal gastric cancer or cancers of the gastroesophageal junction.
  - Anemia may be present in bleeding tumors (Cainap et al., 2019).

Diagnostic Work-up

- *HER2* gene and/or HER2 protein expression has been implicated in the development of gastric cancer. HER2 testing is recommended at the time of diagnosis.
- An upper endoscopy is the gold standard of diagnosis, with a thorough examination of the gastric mucosa and biopsy of suspicious lesions.
- EUS is necessary if early versus more advanced disease by gross endoscopic appearances.
- Laparoscopy allows for visualization of the peritoneal surface, biopsy of suspicious lesions, and evaluation for microscopic disease by cytology from peritoneal washings.
- CT of the chest, abdomen, and pelvis is performed for cancer staging.
- Positron emission tomography (PET) is used more often now in staging but has low sensitivity in making a diagnosis of gastric cancer. PET grossly underestimates the extent of disease, and negative uptake does not rule out presence of metastatic disease (Hoshi, 2020).

Histopathology

- Early- and advanced-stage gastric cancer are characterized by morphologic diversity, resulting in multiple classification systems.
- The WHO has many histologic subtypes of gastric cancer: tubular, parietal cell, papillary, micropapillary, mucoepidermoid, mucinous, poorly cohesive, signet ring, medullary with lymphoid stroma, hepatoid, and Paneth cell.
- The macroscopic appearance of early gastric cancers includes type 1 (protruded), type 2 (superficial), and type 3 (excavated). Type 2 lesions are divided into elevated, flat, or depressed.
- The Borrmann classification uses four types: polypoid without ulceration and broad base (type I), ulcerated with

elevated borders and sharp margins (type II), ulcerated with diffuse infiltration at the base (type III), and diffusely infiltrative thickening of the wall (type IV). The Borrmann type appears to be an independent prognostic factor (Smyth et al., 2020).

- With the Asian Cancer Research Group, gastric cancers are classified in four subgroups: MSI, MSS, epithelial mesenchymal transition (EMT), and TP53 mutations, negative or positive (Smyth et al., 2020).

Clinical Staging

The AJCC eighth edition of TNM is used for clinical staging

- It is recommended that greater than 15 lymph nodes are obtained at the time of surgery for more accurate staging
- Tumor (T) Category
  - T1 tumor invades the lamina propria, muscularis mucosae, or submucosa
    - T1a tumor invades the lamina propria or muscularis mucosae
    - T1b tumor invades the submucosa
  - T2 tumor invades the muscularis propria
  - T3 tumor invades the adventitia
  - T4 tumor invades the adjacent structures
    - T4a tumor invades the pleura, pericardium, azygos vein, diaphragm, or peritoneum
    - T4b tumor invades aorta, vertebral body, or trachea
- Nodal (N) Category
  - N0—no regional lymph nodes
  - N1—metastasis in one to two regional lymph nodes
  - N2—metastasis in three to six regional lymph nodes
  - N3—metastasis in greater than seven regional lymph nodes
- Metastasis (M) category
  - M1—distant metastasis (Hayes et al., 2017)

Treatment

- Surgery remains the only option for curing gastric cancer. Minimally invasive surgeries, such as laparoscopic and robotic gastrectomy, have become options after selection criteria by the surgeon (Smyth et al., 2020).
- Neoadjuvant chemotherapy increases the chance for a curative resection and eliminates early microscopic spread. Based on the Medical Research Council Adjuvant Gastric Infusional Chemotherapy trial (MAGIC), this has become the standard of treatment for patients with locally advanced gastric cancer (Smyth et al., 2020).
- The addition of radiotherapy does not result in better overall survival after gastrectomy (Smyth et al., 2020).
- Recurrence is common following surgical resection, even with negative margins in early-stage disease. Chemotherapy can provide improved survival and quality of life. Chemotherapy drugs that are active in gastric cancer, include 5-FU, capecitabine, S-1, trifluridine–tipiracil, platinums, taxanes, and irinotecan. First-line therapy with a platinum-fluoropyrimidine agent is preferred (Smyth et al., 2020).
- Targeted therapies, such as trastuzumab and ramucirumab, have shown promising results in clinical trials. Trastuzumab has been evaluated in patients with HER2-positive gastric

cancer and shown a significant improvement in overall survival. Ramucirumab is a vascular endothelial growth factor receptor 2 (VEGFR-2) antibody that has shown to improve survival for patients progressing on first-line therapy.

- Immune checkpoint inhibitors include nivolumab, which is a monoclonal antibody against PD-1 and is approved as a third-line treatment (Smyth et al., 2020).
- Cytoreductive surgery and heated intraperitoneal chemotherapy is currently an option being studied to address peritoneal disease (Johnston & Beckman, 2019).

Prognosis

- Five-year survival in gastric cancer is 31%.
- The presence of lymphovascular invasion is the strongest predictor of lymph node metastasis.
- Peritoneal spread of gastric cancer is a poor prognostic indicator.
- Other poor prognostic factors include submucosal invasion, poor differentiation, ulceration, and large tumor size.

Prevention and Surveillance

- Eradication through treatment of *H. pylori*
- Patients with familial risk and an E-cadherin gene variant (*CDH1*) may be offered a prophylactic gastrectomy. Other high-risk patients may undergo periodic esophagogastroduodenoscopy (EGD) surveillance with biopsies.
- Lifestyle changes including tobacco cessation, avoidance of alcohol and salted, smoked foods, and foods with nitrates.
- In Asian countries where gastric cancer is high, screening with EGD is performed.
- CA72-4 is the most correlated marker for gastric cancer with a sensitivity of 50% and an accuracy of 77%. This may be used as a screening test in high-risk patients.

References

Cainap, C., Vlad, C., Seicean, A., Balacescu, O., Seicean, R., Constantin, A. M., Balacescu, L., Crisan, O., Marta, M. M., & Cainap, S. (2019). Gastric cancer: adjuvant chemotherapy versus chemoradiation. A clinical point of view. *Journal of B.U.ON.: official journal of the Balkan Union of Oncology, 24*(6), 2209–2219.

Carvalho, J., Oliveira, P., Senz, J., São José, C., Hansford, S., Teles, S. P., … Oliveira, C. (2021). Redefinition of familial intestinal gastric cancer: Clinical and genetic perspectives. *Journal of Medical Genetics, 58*, 1–11.

Hayes, T., Smyth, E., Riddell, A., & Allum, W. (2017). Staging in esophageal and gastric cancer. *Hematology/Oncology Clinics of North America, 31*(3), 427–440.

Hoshi, H. (2020). Management of gastric adenocarcinoma for general surgeons. *Surgical Clinics of North America, 100*, 523–534.

Johnston, F. M., & Beckman, M. (2019). Updates on management of gastric cancer. *Current Oncology Reports, 21*(8), 67.

National Comprehensive Cancer Network. (2023). Gastric cancers (version 1.2023). Available at https://www.nccn.org/professionals/physician_gls/pdf/gastric.pdf.

Petryszyn, P., Chapelle, N., & Matysiak-Budnik, T. (2020). Gastric cancer: Where are we heading. *Digestive Diseases, 38*, 280–285.

Smyth, E. C., Nilsson, M., Grabsch, H. I., van Grieken, N. C., & Lordick, F. (2020). Gastric cancer. *The Lancet, 396*(10251), 635–648.

Yang, J., Liu, Z., Zeng, B., Hu, G., & Gan, R. (2020). Epstein-Barr virus-associated gastric cancer: A distinct subtype. *Cancer Letters, 495*, 191–199.

Gastrointestinal Stromal Tumor

Definition

Gastrointestinal stromal tumors (GISTs) are rare sarcomas of the soft tissue and account for 80% of all GI sarcomas (Arshad et al., 2021). They are the most common mesenchymal neoplasm of the GI tract and can occur anywhere along the GI tract. The most common site is the stomach (60%) followed by the small intestine (30%), colon (1–2%), and rectum (4%) (Mantese, 2019; Park et al., 2017). GISTs originate from interstitial cells of Cajal or a common precursor cell. These cells are present throughout the GI tract, where they function as pacemaker cells to coordinate peristalsis. It is not clear whether these tumors arise from mature cells or their precursors. GISTs develop through oncogenic gain or function mutations in *KIT* or platelet-derived growth factor (*PDGFR*) genes that lead to activation of the tyrosine kinase receptor (Mantese, 2019).

Incidence

Worldwide incidence of GIST is estimated to be 1 to 2 per 100,000 and they account for 0.1% to 3% of all GI malignancies. From 2001 to 2015, the incidence of GIST has increased, possibly due to incidental discovery of small GISTs during routine upper and capsule endoscopy (Mantese, 2019).

Etiology and Risk Factors

- GISTs can occur at any age but are most commonly diagnosed in people over the age of 60 years (Gheorghe et al., 2021; Mantese, 2019).
- Men and women are equally affected.
- Risk factors for development of GIST include inherited familial GIST syndrome and primary familial GIST syndrome.
  - Familial GIST is an autosomal dominant pattern.
- A smaller subset of GISTs arise from mutational inactivation of neurofibromatosis-1 protein (NF1).

Signs and Symptoms

- GISTs are usually asymptomatic until they reach a size of 6 cm.
- Large GISTs are often vascular and may present with abdominal pain and/or GI bleeding. Bleeding may occur in the lower bowel or abdominal cavity.
- Less common presentations include nausea, pleuritic chest pain, pelvic pain, small bowel obstruction, fatigue, anemia, and abdominal fullness.
- Familial GIST often presents with hyperpigmentation, urticarial, pigmentosa, and an increase in nevi.

Diagnostic Work-up

- CT scan is the diagnostic modality of choice. GISTs larger than 5 cm appear exophytic and hypervascular, and those less than 5 cm are usually endoluminal polypoid masses. CT scans also identify local invasion and metastasis (Mantese, 2019).

- On MRI, small GISTs appear as round tumors with strong arterial enhancement. Large GISTS appear as lobulated tumors with mild heterogeneous gradual enhancement with intratumoral cystic change.
- Diagnosis using immunohistochemistry directed to the expression of KIT protein (95%), a receptor tyrosine kinase protein, also known as stem-cell growth factor receptor, or CD117, that is expressed on interstitial cells of Cajal (Gheorghe et al., 2021).
- Some GISTs (70%) express CD34, a transmembrane phosphoglycoprotein (Gheorghe et al., 2021).

Histopathology

Macroscopically, GISTs are of white color, well defined, not encapsulated, and firm. In small tumors, the tumor's surface is consistent. Large tumors may have areas of hemorrhage and necrosis. These large tumors may ulcerate.

- There are three types of GISTs:
  - Spindle cell type (70%)
  - Epithelioid type (20%)
  - Mixed type (10%) (Gheorghe et al., 2021; Koo et al., 2016)
- The pathologic diagnosis of GIST is based on the histologic profile of the tumor. It is recommended to be obtained via surgical resection rather than preoperative biopsy.

Immunohistochemical Clarification of Gastrointestinal Stromal Tumors

- These markers contribute to the differentiation of GISTs from other subepithelial tumors in the GI tract
  - KIT (CD117)
  - DOG-1 and protein kinase C theta (PKC-theta) (Gheorghe et al., 2021)

Molecular Classification

- Seventy-five percent of GISTs have KIT mutations in exons 11 and 9
- Ten percent of cases have *PDGFRA* mutations
- Ten to 15% are *KIT/PDGFRA* wild type
  - Twenty to 40% have *SDH* mutations
  - Thirteen percent have *BRAF* or *NF1* mutations (Gheorghe et al., 2021)

Clinical Staging

The TNM staging for GIST from AJCC eighth Edition:
Tumor (T)
- T1—tumor greater than 5 cm in greatest dimension
- T2—tumor greater than 5 cm and less than 10 cm in greatest dimension
- T3—tumor greater than 10 cm and less than 15 cm in greatest dimension
- T4—tumor greater than 15 cm in greatest dimension
Nodal (N)
- N0—no regional lymph node metastasis or unknown lymph node status

- N1—regional lymph node metastasis
Metastasis (M)
- M0—no distant metastasis
- M1—distant metastasis (Cates, 2018)

Treatment
Surgery

Surgery is the first-line treatment for patients, with localized and resectable GISTs with a 60% cure rate. GISTs are fragile tumors, and caution must be used during surgery to preserve the capsule, preventing rupture and dissemination of tumor cells into the abdominal cavity (Mantese, 2019).

- Surgical resection is recommended with tumors greater than 2 cm or with irregular margins, ulceration, bleeding, necrosis.
- Endoscopic enucleation can be used for type I and possibly for type II GISTs (Gheorghe et al., 2021).
- Surveillance is recommended for tumors less than 2 cm (Koo et al., 2016).

Systemic Therapy

- The purpose of adjuvant therapy is to reduce or delay the growth of microscopic tumors after complete resection of a GIST. For tumors of high risk of recurrence, it has been used up to 3 years for therapy (Koo et al., 2016).
- Neoadjuvant treatment with imatinib, a KIT and PDGFR inhibitor, may be used to shrink tumors prior to surgery. There is no predetermined duration of imatinib in this setting, but it has been used up to 12 months prior to surgery.
  - It is also used for localized GISTs when complete resection is not possible, to preserve the rectum, esophagus, duodenum, or to avoid a total gastrectomy (Koo et al., 2016).
- Tumor resistance is either primary or secondary. Primary resistance is progression on imatinib within 6 months of therapy. Secondary resistance is progression beyond 6 months on imatinib therapy (Khoshnood, 2019; Koo et al., 2016). Sunitinib is a secondary line of therapy based on mutational status. Resistance to sunitinib develops quickly.
- Regorafenib is a third-line medication after treatment failure to imatinib and sunitinib. It is a multikinase inhibitor active against KIT and EGFR. Resistance to regorafenib also develops quickly.
- Fourth-line therapy utilizes ripretinib, which is a KIT and PDGFRA switch control kinase inhibitor that blocks initiating and resistance KIT mutations in exons 9, 11, 13, 14, 17, and 18.
- Immunotherapies are being investigated in clinical trials for their efficacy and safety in treating GIST (Arshad et al., 2021).
- Postoperative radiation with chemotherapy is useful when there is a single, progressing liver or intraabdominal lesion.
- Embolization and RFA can be used to treat liver metastasis.

Prognosis

- Large tumor size, high mitotic count, and histologic subtype (spindle cell) influence the 5-year DFS. These factors are also associated with a 6.2% recurrence after curative surgery.
- Overall, the GIST 5-year survival rate is 67.5% (Mantese, 2019).

Prevention and Surveillance

- No preventative strategies have been established for GIST related to risk factor modification.
- For patients diagnosed with GIST in the high or intermediate risk groups, postoperative surveillance for the first 3 years after surgery includes an abdominal and pelvic CT scan every 3 to 4 months.
- From 3 to 5 years after surgery, an abdominal and pelvic CT scan every 6 months.
- Annual assessment after 5 years.
- The role of PET surveillance for metastasis has not been established (Gheorghe et al., 2021).

References

Arshad, J., Costa, P. A., Barreto-Coelho, P., Valdes, B. N., & Trent, J. C. (2021). Immunotherapy strategies for gastrointestinal stromal tumor. *Cancers*, *13*(14), 3525.

Cates, J. M. M. (2018). The AJCC 8th edition staging system for soft tissue sarcoma of the extremities or trunk: A cohort study of the SEER database. *Journal of the National Comprehensive Cancer Network*, *16*(2), 144–152.

Gheorghe, G., Bacalbasa, N., Ceobanu, G., Ilie, M., Enache, V., Constantinescu, G., … Diaconu, C. C. (2021). Gastrointestinal stromal tumors—A mini review. *Journal of Personalized Medicine*, *11*(8), 694. https://doi.org/10.3390/jpm11080694.

Khoshnood, A. (2019). Gastrointestinal stromal tumor—a review of clinical studies. *Journal of Oncology Pharmacy Practice*, *25*(6), 1473–1485.

Koo, D. H., Ryu, M. H., Kim, K. M., Yang, H. K., Sawaki, A., Hirota, S., … Kang, Y. K. (2016). Asian consensus guidelines for the diagnosis and management of gastrointestinal stromal tumor. *Cancer Research Treatment*, *48*(4), 1155–1166.

Mantese, G. (2019). Gastrointestinal stromal tumor: Epidemiology, diagnosis, and treatment. *Gastroenterology*, *35*(6), 555–559.

Park, C. H., Kim, G. H., Lee, B. E., Song, G. A., Park, D. Y., Choi, K. U., … Jeon, T. Y. (2017). Two staging systems for gastrointestinal stromal tumors in the stomach: Which is better? *Biomedical Central Gastroenterology*, *17*(141), 1–8.

Hepatocellular Carcinoma

Definition

Hepatocellular carcinoma (HCC) is a primary tumor of the liver.

Incidence

- HCC is a leading cause of cancer worldwide. In men, it is the fifth leading cause of cancer death, and in women, it is the seventh leading cause of cancer death.
- In Asia, it is the most common cause of cancer deaths. High incidence regions include sub-Saharan Africa, East and Southeast Asia, with half of all hepatocellular cancers occurring in China (Fujiwara et al., 2018).
- Over the last 2 years, HCC cases in the United States have increased threefold and have dramatically increased in Europe as well (Mokdad et al., 2017).

Etiology and Risk Factors

- Eighty-five percent of patients diagnosed with HCC have cirrhosis of the liver (Fujiwara et al., 2018).
- Patients infected with hepatitis B virus (HBV) or with aflatoxin B1 exposure may develop HCC without underlying cirrhosis. Aflatoxin is a mycotoxin produced by certain molds found in peanuts, soybeans, and corn.
- Hepatitis C virus (HCV), nonalcoholic steatohepatitis, or fatty liver disease (NAFLD) can lead to cirrhosis and HCC.
- Risk factors include male gender, obesity, diabetes, alcohol abuse, tobacco abuse, hereditary hemochromatosis, porphyria cutanea tarda, alpha-I antitrypsin deficiency, Wilson disease, and stage IV primary biliary cirrhosis.

Signs and Symptoms

- Patients with HCC have symptoms related to chronic liver disease.
- Patients with cirrhosis and decompensation of the liver may exhibit hepatic encephalopathy, ascites, or jaundice.
- Patients with HCC without cirrhosis may have dull abdominal pain, weight loss, weakness, anorexia, and malaise.
- At the time of diagnosis, 15% of cases will have extrahepatic spread. The areas of spread include the lungs, intra-abdominal lymph nodes, bones, and adrenal glands.
- HCC is often diagnosed in later stages, and subsequently, only 10% to 15% of patients have curative options at the time of diagnosis (Wang & Wei, 2020).

Diagnostic Work-up

- Diagnosis of HCC is unique, and the histopathologic tissue analysis is not mandatory. An HCC diagnosis can be established with imaging if the tumor is greater than 2 cm (O'Brien, 2021).
- Percutaneous biopsy of the tumor may not be feasible due to location of the tumor, or comorbidities of liver disease such as clotting disorders or ascites.
- Abdominal CT or MRI is the standard imaging method used to identify HCC. HCC is perfused by the hepatic artery and not by the PV. Therefore, arterial hypervascularity and nonperipheral contrast in the arterial phase with washout of contrast in the portal venous phase are the classic patterns observed.
- A serum α-fetoprotein (AFP) level greater than 500 ng/mL is diagnostic of HCC (Wang & Wei, 2020).
- Liquid biopsy has not been used outside of clinical trials for management of HCC.

Histopathology

- Histologic subtypes are characterized by distinct morphology, specific immunohistochemical profile, and have specific clinical correlates (Vyas & Zhang, 2020) (see table below).

Key Histologic and Molecular Features of Specific Hepatocellular Carcinoma Subtypes

Subtype	Histologic Criteria	Molecular Alteration
Fibrolamellar	Band of lamellar fibrosis, large, eosinophilic with prominent nucleoli	PRKACA activation, most commonly due to DNAJ81-PRKACA fusion
Scirrhous	>50% tumor shows dense fibrosis. Pericellular fibrosis	*TSC1/2* Mutations, TGF-β signaling activation
Steatohepatic	>50% tumor shows steatohepatic features	IL-6/JAK/STAT activation
Macrotrabecular	Thickened trabecular involving >50% of the tumor	*TP53* mutations and FGF19 amplifications
Lymphocyte-rich	Lymphocytes > tumor cells	None
Neutrophil-rich	Neutrophilic infiltrate in the tumor	None
Chromophobe	Chromophobic to eosinophilic cytoplasm with nuclear atypia	Alternate lengthening of telomeres
Clear cell	>80% tumor with glycogen-rich clear cells	None
Cirrhotomimetic	Multiple tumor nodules in a cirrhotic liver	None
Fibronodular	Multiple distinct nodules in single tumor. Popcorn appearance	None

Data from Vyas M, Zhang, X. (2020). Hepatocellular carcinoma: Role of pathology in the era of precision medicine. *Clinics of Liver Disease, 24*(4), 591–610.
JAK, Janus-activated kinase.

Major Cancers   2

Clinical Staging

- There are multiple staging systems commonly used in HCC. The two most frequently used systems are:
  - The AJCC TNM system which characterizes tumor features and metastases. This has been validated by AHPBA for patients undergoing hepatic resection or liver transplantation.
  - The Barcelona Clinic Liver Cancer (BCLC) system which combines tumor characteristics with assessment of severity of liver disease and functional status of the patient. This scoring system is used in nonsurgical patients with advanced disease.

Treatment

Treatments for HCC are often used in combination or to bridge between various therapies.

Surgery

- Surgical resection is a potentially curative option for solitary HCC or unilobar disease without vascular invasion or metastases and without portal hypertension or impaired liver function. Resection is limited to tumors less than 5 cm (Forner et al., 2019).
- A cure is not always achieved with resection, which has a 5-year recurrence rate of 70%. Recurrence is often multifocal (Hartke et al., 2017).
- According to AJCC, stages IIIB or higher are considered incurable and surgically unresectable.
- No clear benefit has been seen with neoadjuvant or adjuvant chemotherapy in preventing HCC recurrence.

Liver Transplantation

- Liver transplantation is the treatment of choice for patients with early-stage HCC (<5 cm or up to three lesions <3 cm), impaired liver function, and/or portal hypertension (Parikh & Pillai, 2021).
- Liver transplantation will treat both HCC and cirrhosis.

- The 5-year overall survival rate is 75%, and the recurrence rate is less than 15% following a liver transplant for HCC (Hartke et al., 2017).
- Priority for the waiting list for a transplant is based on the Model for End Stage Liver Disease (MELD) score (a calculation of INR, creatinine, and bilirubin). It does not predict mortality of HCC.
- A MELD "exception" has been developed to assign points based on tumor burden.

Locoregional Therapies

- Local treatments with RFA are considered a standard of care for very early tumors not suited for surgery (BCLC 0 and A).
- TACE is standard therapy for patients with BCLC stage B HCC, who have compensated liver function with a large single nodule less than 5 cm or multifocal HCC without vascular invasion or extrahepatic spread.
- TARE is also used to treat patients with BCLC stage B HCC. The most common technique uses yttrium 90 microspheres.
- Intraoperative microwave ablation (MWA) is the treatment option for a small number of patients with single nodule, normal liver function, and no underlying cirrhosis
- Stereotactic body radiation (SBRT), which delivers large ablative doses of radiation, is used to treat BCLC stage B HCC.

Systemic Therapies

- Conventional chemotherapy has provided limited clinical benefit for patients with advanced/metastatic HCC.

Targeted Therapies

- Used to treat patients with advanced disease (stage 3B and 4) (presence of extrahepatic spread, macrovascular invasion) who are not candidates for locoregional therapies.
- Sorafenib and lenvatinib are multikinase inhibitors that exert anti-proliferative and anti-angiogenic effects, and these agents are recommended options by the NCCN, 2023.

- Second-line therapy includes regorafenib and cabozantinib, multikinase inhibitors, inhibit angiogenesis, cellular proliferation, and provide immunomodulary effects.

Immunotherapy

- The checkpoint inhibitors, nivolumab and pembrolizumab, are fully humanized IgG4 monoclonal antibodies targeting programmed death-1 (PD-1) approved for use in patients with HCC. They are recommended as subsequent lines of therapy for disease progression after chemotherapy. In patients who progress on one of these agents' efficacy can be enhanced by combining these agents with acceptable toxicity using ipilimumab and tremelimumab (Sangro et al., 2021; Wong et al., 2021).
- Oncologic virus vaccine clinical trials have been studied in advanced HCC and to date have shown no overall survival benefit. However, vaccines continue to be studied for therapy in patients with less advanced disease.

Prognosis

- Prognostic factors for HCC include tumor size, number, vascular invasion, extrahepatic spread, and severity of underlying liver disease as defined by bilirubin levels and portal hypertension.
- Overall, 5-year survival with HCC is less than 20%.

Prevention and Surveillance

- HBV and HAV vaccination is a primary prevention method.
- Treatment with antiviral therapies for treatment of HBV- and HCV-infected patients.
- NCCN (2023) guidelines recommend cross-sectional imaging of the chest, abdomen, and pelvis every 3 to 6 months for 2 years, then every 6 to 12 months after therapy. Surveillance may be required indefinitely for patients with an ongoing risk of developing a new HCC. Elevated AFP levels are associated with poor prognosis and should be measured every 6 to 12 months.

References

Forner, A., Da Fonseca, L. G., Díaz-González, Á., Sanduzzi-Zamparelli, M., Reig, M., & Bruix, J. (2019). Controversies in the management of hepatocellular carcinoma. *JHEP Reports: Innovation in Hepatology, 1*(1), 17–29.

Fujiwara, N., Friedman, S. L., Goossens, N., & Hoshida, Y. (2018). Risk factors and prevention of hepatocellular carcinoma in the era of precision medicine. *Journal of Hepatology, 68*(3), 526–549.

Hartke, J., Johnson, M., & Ghabril, M. (2017). The diagnosis and treatment of hepatocellular carcinoma. *Seminars in Diagnostic Pathology, 34*(2), 153–159.

Mokdad, A. A., Hester, C. A., Singal, A. G., & Yopp, A. C. (2017). Management of hepatocellular in the United States. *Chinese Clinical Oncology, 6*(2), 1–13.

National Comprehensive Cancer Network (NCCN). (2023). Hepatocellular carcinoma (version 1.2023). Available at https://www.nccn.org/professionals/physician_gls/pdf/hcc.pdf.

O'Brien, B. (2021). Developments in hepatocellular cancer treatment. *Journal of Advanced Practitioners in Oncology, 12*(3), 310–314.

Parikh, N. D., & Pillai, A. (2021). Recent advances in hepatocellular carcinoma treatment. *Clinical Gastroenterology and Hepatology, 19*, 2020–2024.

Sangro, B., Sarobe, P., Hervás-Stubbs, S., & Melero, I. (2021). Advances in immunotherapy for hepatocellular carcinoma. *Nature Review Gasetoentoerology and Hepatology, 18*(8), 525–543.

Vyas, M., & Zhang, X. (2020). Hepatocellular carcinoma: Role of pathology in the era of precision medicine. *Clinics of Liver Disease, 24*(4), 591–610.

Wang, W., & Wei, C. (2020). Advances in the early diagnosis of hepatocellular carcinoma. *Genes and Diseases, 7*, 308–319.

Wong, J. S. L., Kwok, G. G. W., Tang, V., Li, B. C. W., Leung, R., Chiu, J., … Yau, T. (2021). Ipilimumab and nivolumab/pembrolizumab in advanced hepatocellular carcinoma refractory to prior immune checkpoint inhibitors. *Journal for Immunotherapy of Cancer, 9*(2), e001945.

Pancreas Cancer

Definition

Pancreatic cancer ductal adenocarcinomas evolve from precursor lesions such as pancreatic intraepithelial neoplasms, intraductal papillary mucinous neoplasms, and mucinous cystic neoplasms. These ductal cancers account for more than 90% of pancreatic cancers. Neuroendocrine tumors (NETs) can also be found in the pancreas; however, these malignancies will be discussed in the chapter, Neuroendocrine Cancers.

Incidence

- Pancreatic ductal adenocarcinoma is currently the third leading cause of cancer deaths. There is a trend for higher incidence rates in developed countries compared to developing countries.
- Pancreatic adenocarcinoma is expected to become the second leading cause of cancer-related deaths in the United States by 2030.
- Approximately 60% to 70% of pancreatic cancers occur in the head of the pancreas and 15% each in the body and tail of the pancreas.
- At the time of diagnosis, most pancreatic cancers have already spread beyond the pancreas, with lymph node and distant metastases frequently present.

Etiology and Risk Factors

The large disparities in pancreatic cancer incidence between nations suggest that environmental factors play a significant role. Risk factors include

- Age: 70 to 80 years of age
- Gender: males
- In the United States, there is a 50% to 90% increased risk in the African American population
- Blood type: A or B
- Tobacco use
- Heavy alcohol consumption
- Type 2 diabetes mellitus
- Obesity
- History of chronic pancreatitis
- Ten percent of pancreatic cancer patients have a family history of the disease. Pancreatic cancer is familial if two or more first-degree relatives have been diagnosed. These patients have a 9 times greater risk which increases to 32 times greater risk if three or more first-degree relatives have been diagnosed. There are four main gene alterations, including
  - *KRAS*: 90% of all pancreatic cancers have this activating mutation

- Inactivating mutations *TP53, CDKN2A*, and *SMAD4* (50%–80%)
- *BRCA1, BRCA2, Palb2, ATM* genes
- Mutations in *STK11* (Peutz-Jeghers syndrome)

Signs and Symptoms

In the early stages of pancreatic cancer, signs and symptoms are often absent or vague. As the cancer progresses, patients may notice nausea and epigastric pain radiating to the back. Painless jaundice may develop with clay-colored stools and tea-colored urine. Unexplained weight loss may develop with floating fatty stools (steatorrhea). In 10% of patients, new onset of diabetes mellitus or pancreatic endocrine insufficiency can occur. In advanced disease, gastric outlet obstruction can occur (Goess & Friess, 2018; NCCN, 2022).

Diagnostic Work-up

- EUS has the highest sensitivity for identifying solid pancreatic lesions.
  This is combined with biopsy or FNA for tissue diagnosis.
- Pancreas protocol triple-phase CT imaging of the arterial, portal venous, and delayed phases detect pathology. The cancerous lesion is enhanced compared to surrounding structures.
- ERCP is performed if biliary obstruction is noted from the tumor with biliary stent placement during the procedure to relieve the biliary obstruction.
- MRI/MRCP. Pancreas protocol MRI with contrast can characterize CT-indeterminate liver lesions and when suspected pancreatic tumors are not visible on CT (NCCN, 2022).
- CA 19-9 is the most common serum tumor marker expressed in pancreatic cancer. It is not appropriate to use as a screening tool because of its low specificity and sensitivity. It can become elevated in inflammatory processes like chronic pancreatitis.

Histopathology

- The pancreas is composed of exocrine and endocrine glands.
- Exocrine glands release enzymes into the small intestine to aid in digestion and account for 95% of pancreatic cells.
- The endocrine function of the pancreas is carried out by the islets of Langerhans, which synthesize and release hormones into the bloodstream. These hormones regulate glucose, lipid, and protein metabolism.
- Ninety percent of pancreatic cancers are in the exocrine pancreas and manifest as infiltrating ductal adenocarcinoma.

Clinical Staging

Clinical staging is determined by tumor, regional lymph node involvement, and the presence or absence of metastasis (TNM) using the AJCC criteria (Kwon et al., 2018).

Tumor (T)
- T1—tumors have a tumor diameter of less than 2 cm
- T2—tumors have a diameter of greater than 2 cm but less than 4 cm
- T3—tumors have a diameter of greater than 4 cm

- T4—tumor involves the celiac axis or the SMA (unresectable)
Nodal Involvement (N)
- N0—no regional lymph node metastasis
- N1—metastasis in one to three regional lymph nodes
- N2—metastasis in greater than four regional lymph nodes
Metastasis (M)
- M0—no distant metastasis
- M1—distant metastasis

Treatment

Neoadjuvant Therapy

The rationale for neoadjuvant therapy is to eliminate micrometastases and shrink the primary tumor, which may downstage the tumor to be resectable. Various therapies include gemcitabine plus or minus nab-paclitaxel, FOLFIRINOX (folinic acid, fluorouracil, irinotecan, oxaliplatin), or chemoradiation. Chemoradiation often includes gemcitabine and cisplatin combined with 55 Gy of radiation.

Surgery

Surgical resection is the only treatment that offers a potential cure for pancreatic cancer.

- Ten to 20% of patients present with clear resectable tumors, and 30% to 40% of patients are described as borderline resectable (NCCN, 2022). A tumor is resectable when it does not involve major arteries and veins and has clear fat planes around the arteries.
- For those tumors involving the pancreatic head, the surgery involves a pancreaticoduodenectomy or Whipple procedure.
- For those tumors involving the body or tail of the pancreas, a near-total or distal pancreatectomy is usually performed.
- Surgery has historically been an open procedure but can be performed laparoscopically or robotically.
- Borderline resectable tumors show venous involvement with distortion or narrowing of the superior mesenteric vein (SMV) or PV. These tumors may require occlusion of the veins with suitable proximal and distal vessels allowing for a safe surgical resection and replacement of the occluded vessel with a graft of the blood vessel. Tumor encasement of the short segment of the hepatic artery without tumor extending into the celiac axis or tumor abutment of the SMA is also classified by the NCCN (2022) as borderline resectable.
- Pancreatic metastases are unresectable disease.

Adjuvant Therapy

After surgery adjuvant chemotherapy has emerged as the gold standard of care.
- Gemcitabine
- Gemcitabine/Capecitabine
- 5-FU/Leucovorin for periampullary tumors
- FOLFIRONOX

Palliative Therapy

A palliative care team is helpful to establish goals of care and assist with transition to hospice.
- Nab-paclitaxel + gemcitabine
- Gemcitabine

- Clinical trials are always an option.
- Biliary obstruction occurs in 65% to 75% of cancer patients. Placement of a biliary stent can alleviate this symptom.
- Gastric outlet obstruction occurs in 10% to 25% of pancreatic cancer patients. An intestinal stent or palliative gastrostomy tube may be placed.

Prognosis

The diagnosis of pancreatic cancer offers a dismal prognosis with a 5-year survival rate of 2% to 9%, ranking last among all cancer sites in terms of prognostic outcomes for patients (McGuigan et al., 2018).

Prevention and Surveillance

- The USPSTF in 2019 recommends against screening for pancreatic cancer in asymptomatic adults. The USPSTF found no evidence that screening for pancreatic cancer or treatment of screen-detected pancreatic cancer improves disease-specific morbidity or mortality.
- There are currently no accurate, validated biomarkers for early detection of pancreatic cancer.
- The International Cancer of the Pancreas Screening Consortium recommends that individuals meeting the definition of familial pancreatic cancer may be appropriate for screening. There is disagreement as to when screening should begin for this high-risk population, with just over half of the consensus voting that screening should begin at 50 years of age.
- NCCN (2022) recommends a complete history and physical examination for symptom assessment every 3 to 6 months for 2 years, then every 6 to 12 months. CA 19-9 testing and contrast-enhanced CT scans every 3 to 6 months for 2 years after surgical resection.

References

Goess, R., & Friess, H. (2018). A look at the progress of treating pancreatic cancer over the past 20 years. *Expert Review of Anticancer Therapy*, *18*(3), 295–304.

Kwon, W., He, J., Higuchi, R., Son, D., Lee, S. Y., Kim, J., … Jang, J. Y. (2018). Multinational validation of the American Joint Committee on Cancer 8th edition pancreatic cancer staging system in a pancreas head cancer cohort. *Journal of Hepato-Biliary-Pancreatic Sciences*, *25*(9), 418–427. https://doi.org/10.1002/jhbp.577.

McGuigan, A., Kelly, P., Turkington, R. C., Jones, C., Coleman, H. G., & McCain, R. S. (2018). Pancreatic cancer: A review of clinical diagnosis, epidemiology, treatment and outcomes. *World Journal of Gastroenterology*, *24*(43), 4846–4861.

National Comprehensive Cancer Network. (2022). Pancreatic cancers (version 1.2022). Available at https://www.nccn.org/professionals/physician_gls/pdf/pancreatic.pdf.

Genitourinary Cancers

Francisco Conde II and Tyler Workman

Bladder Cancer

Definition

Bladder cancer is the second most common urologic malignancy after prostate cancer and the fourth most common cancer in men. Most bladder cancers are transitional cell or urothelial carcinomas, and they are often discovered in the early stages of the disease. Bladder cancer can metastasize to the lymph nodes, bones, lung, liver, and peritoneum.

Incidence

(American Cancer Society [ACS], 2022)
- More than 81,800 Americans were diagnosed with bladder cancer in 2022, and more than 17,100 died of the disease.
- Incidence rates decreased by about 1% per year from 2009 to 2018.
- Incidence rates are high in the United States and in southern and western Europe.

Etiology and Risk Factors

(Lenis et al., 2020; Saginala et al., 2020; National Cancer Institute [NCI], 2022)
Risk factors include the following:
- Age: The median age at diagnosis is 73 years, and 9 of 10 people with bladder cancer are older than 55 years of age.
- Sex and race: The incidence is two times higher among White men than Black men, and it is four times higher among men than women.
- Cigarette smoking:
  - The risk is four times higher among smokers than nonsmokers.
  - Almost half (47%) of bladder cancer in men and women is attributed to cigarette smoking.
- Obesity: Obesity increases the risk of bladder cancer by 10%.
- Industrial chemical exposures: Workers in the rubber, dye, paint, leather, aluminum, petroleum, and printing industries are at increased risk for bladder cancer.
- Arsenic: High levels of arsenic in drinking water increase the risk of bladder cancer.
- Cyclophosphamide: Long-term exposure to the chemotherapy drug is associated with an increased risk of bladder cancer.
- Radiation: Pelvic exposure increases the risk of bladder cancer.
- Parasitic infection: Chronic bladder irritation and infections, particularly by *Schistosoma hematobium* (causes schistosomiasis), increases risk.
- Genetics: The risk of bladder cancer is increased for people with Cowden disease, Lynch syndrome, or mutations in the breast cancer (BRCA) 1 and 2, *CHEK2, ERCC3, FGFR3,* and retinoblastoma (*RB*) genes (Carlo et al., 2019).

Signs and Symptoms

- Patients with bladder cancer often have hematuria and other urinary symptoms:
  - Urinary frequency
  - Dysuria
  - Urgency
  - Altered stream
- Patients with advanced disease may have the following:
  - Palpable mass
  - Bone pain
  - Pelvic or rectal pain
  - Acute renal failure

Diagnostic Work-up

- Standard work-up:
  - History and physical examination
  - Cystoscopy with biopsy and urine cytology
- Additional work-up for patients with noninvasive bladder cancer:
  - Imaging of the upper tract collecting system
  - Computed tomography (CT) or magnetic resonance imaging (MRI) of the abdomen and pelvis before performing transurethral resection of a bladder tumor (TURBT)
- Additional work-up for patients with invasive bladder cancer:
  - Complete blood count (CBC) and chemistry profile
  - Imaging of the chest and upper tract collecting system
  - CT or MRI of the abdomen and pelvis
  - Bone scan if the alkaline phosphatase level is elevated or the patient has bone pain
  - Positive emission tomography (PET)/CT scan in whom metastatic disease is suspected.

Histopathology

(Al-Husseini et al., 2019)
- Approximately 95% of bladder cancers are transitional cell or urothelial carcinomas.
- Five percent of bladder cancers consist of squamous cell carcinoma, adenocarcinoma, and small cell carcinoma.
- Bladder cancer is typically divided into two groups: non-muscle invasive bladder cancer (NMIBC) or muscle-invasive bladder cancer (MIBC). Tumors are further classified according to histologic grade (low or high).

- NMIBC bladder cancers are superficial tumors (T1, Tis, or Ta) and are usually low grade. Approximately 75% patients have NMIBC bladder cancer.
- Muscle-invasive disease (T2 to T4) tends to be more aggressive and invades the muscularis propria.

Clinical Staging

The American Joint Committee on Cancer (AJCC) tumor-node-metastasis (TNM) system is used for staging bladder cancer. The AJCC TNM system for bladder cancer describes the extent of the primary tumor (T), whether the cancer has spread to nearby lymph nodes (N), and the absence or presence of distant metastasis (M) (Amin et al., 2017).

- Stage 0: The cancer is noninvasive papillary carcinoma or carcinoma in situ.
- Stage I: The cancer has invaded the lamina propria and has not spread to the lymph nodes or any distant site.
- Stage II: The cancer has invaded the muscularis propria and has not spread to the lymph nodes or any distant site.
- Stage III: The cancer has invaded the perivesical tissue or may have invaded the prostate, seminal vesicles, uterus, or vagina. The cancer may not have spread to the lymph nodes or may have spread to the lymph nodes in the true pelvis and common iliac lymph nodes. The cancer has not spread to any distant site.
- Stage IV: The cancer has invaded the pelvic wall or abdominal wall, has spread beyond the common iliac lymph nodes, and has spread to any distant site.

Risk Stratification for Nonmuscle Invasive Bladder Cancer
(Chang et al., 2016)

- Based on the American Urological Association (AUA) Risk Stratification
- Risk is classified as low risk, intermediate risk, and high risk.
- Low risk includes those with papillary urothelial neoplasm of low malignancy potential (PUNLMP) or those with low-grade urothelial carcinoma and solitary tumor measuring greater than 3 cm.
- Intermediate risk includes those with low-grade urothelial carcinoma, solitary tumor measuring greater than 3 cm, multifocal tumors, or recurrence within 1 year. It also includes those with high-grade urothelial carcinoma and solitary tumor measuring greater than 3 cm.
- High risk includes those with high-grade urothelial carcinoma with solitary tumor measuring greater than 3 cm, multifocal tumors, bacillus Calmette-Guérin (BCG) failure in high-grade patient, any variant histology, any lymphovascular invasion, or any prostatic urethral involvement.

Grading

For urothelial histologic types, the recommended grading system is based on low- and high-grade designations:

- LG: Low grade
- HG: High grade

For squamous cell carcinoma and adenocarcinoma, the following grading system is recommended:

- GX: Grade cannot be assessed
- G1: Well differentiated
- G2: Moderately differentiated
- G3: Poorly differentiated

Treatment

(National Comprehensive Cancer Network [NCCN], 2022)

Surgery

- TURBT is the standard treatment for nonmuscle invasive bladder cancers.
- For patients with muscle-invasive tumors, partial or radical cystectomy with pelvic lymph node dissection is performed.
  - In men, radical cystectomy involves removal of the bilateral pelvic lymph nodes, bladder, prostate gland, and seminal vesicles.
  - In women, radical cystectomy involves removal of the bilateral pelvic lymph nodes, uterus, fallopian tubes, ovaries, bladder, urethra, and segment of the interior vaginal wall.
- After surgical removal of the bladder, patients require an ileal conduit or a continent urinary diversion such as a Kock pouch or an Indiana pouch.

Radiation Therapy

- Radiation therapy may be used in the following:
  - If the patient prefers bladder preservation, radiation therapy is given concurrently with chemotherapy such as 5-fluorouracil (5-FU) and mitomycin or low dose gemcitabine.
  - Patients who are not surgical candidates.
  - As adjuvant therapy following cystectomy in selected patients, such as positive lymph nodes, positive margins.
  - To treat symptoms caused by metastatic bladder cancer.
- Patients must have an empty bladder for simulation and treatment.
- The radiation dose to the whole bladder ranges from 39.6 to 50.4 Gy plus an additional boost for a total between 60 and 66 Gy.

Intravesical Therapy

Intravesical therapy is used as prophylactic or adjuvant therapy to decrease recurrence, delay progression, and eradicate residual disease after transurethral resection. It is given immediately after surgery and as induction with or without maintenance therapy.

- Immediate postoperative intravesical chemotherapy is administered to reduce recurrence.
  - Single instillation of chemotherapy is administered within 24 hours of surgery (ideally within 6 hours).
  - Mitomycin and gemcitabine are drugs commonly used for intravesical chemotherapy.
- Induction or adjuvant intravesical chemotherapy or BCG
  - Commonly used agents are BCG, mitomycin, and gemcitabine.

- If there is a BCG shortage, BCG should be prioritized for induction of high-risk patients. Alternatives to BCG include mitomycin and gemcitabine.
- Initiated 3 to 4 weeks after TURBT with or without maintenance.
- Intravesical BCG or chemotherapy is given weekly for 6 weeks.
- Maintenance intravesical BCG
  - After a 6-week induction course of BCG, maintenance intravesical BCG is given at 3, 6, 12, 24, 30, and 36 months.

Systemic Therapies
Chemotherapy

- Systemic chemotherapy may be given in several settings:
  - Neoadjuvant chemotherapy to downstage a tumor before surgery
  - Adjuvant therapy after cystectomy for muscle-invasive lesions
  - For metastatic disease
  - Concurrently with radiation therapy as a radiosensitizer
- Commonly prescribed chemotherapy regimens for cisplatin eligible patients:
  - Dose-dense methotrexate, vinblastine, doxorubicin, and cisplatin (DDMVAC) followed by avelumab maintenance therapy
  - Gemcitabine and cisplatin followed by avelumab maintenance therapy
- Commonly prescribed chemotherapy regimens for cisplatin ineligible patients:
  - Gemcitabine and carboplatin followed by avelumab maintenance therapy
  - Gemcitabine
  - Gemcitabine and paclitaxel

Immune Checkpoint Inhibitors and Targeted Therapy

Immune checkpoint inhibitors and targeted therapies can be given to patients with metastatic disease who have relapsed after receiving first-line chemotherapy.

- Commonly prescribed checkpoint inhibitor agents are atezolizumab, avelumab, nivolumab, and pembrolizumab (Lopez-Beltran et al., 2021).
  - Avelumab is also approved as maintenance therapy for patients with locally advanced or metastatic bladder cancer that has not progressed with first-line cisplatin-containing chemotherapy.
  - Atezolizumab and pembrolizumab are also approved as a first-line treatment option for patients with locally advanced or metastatic bladder cancer who are not eligible for cisplatin-containing chemotherapy.
- Commonly prescribed targeted therapy agents are erdafitinib, enfortumab vedotin, and sacituzumab govitecan.

Prognosis

- For all stages combined, the 5-year relative survival rate is 77%.
- The 5-year survival rate is 70% for patients with localized disease at diagnosis.
- For patients with regional and distant disease, the 5-year survival rates are 38% and 6%, respectively.

Prevention and Surveillance

- There are no known prevention measures, but risk reduction is possible by smoking cessation, avoiding exposure to industrial chemicals and arsenic, maintaining good hydration, increasing physical activity, and eating a healthy diet that is rich in fruits and vegetables.
- There are no screening recommendations for people at average risk. Those at increased risk may be screened by cystoscopy or urine cytology.
- The National Comprehensive Cancer Network (NCCN) surveillance guidelines for NMIBC and muscle invasive bladder cancer are summarized in the tables National Comprehensive Cancer Network Surveillance Guidelines for Non-Muscle Invasive Bladder Cancer and National Comprehensive Cancer Network Surveillance Guidelines for Muscle Invasive Bladder Cancer, respectively.

National Comprehensive Cancer Network Surveillance Guidelines for Nonmuscle Invasive Bladder Cancer

AUA Risk Stratification	Test or Procedure	Frequency
Low Risk	Cystoscopy	At 3 and 12 months in year 1, then annually up to year 5. As clinically indicated after 5 years.
	Imaging of chest, abdomen, and pelvis	Baseline imaging, then as clinically indicated.
	Blood tests and urine tests	Not applicable
Intermediate Risk	Cystoscopy	At 3, 6, and 12 months in year 1, every 6 months in year 2, then annually up to year 5. As clinically indicated after 5 years.
	Imaging of chest, abdomen, and pelvis	Baseline imaging, then as clinically indicated.
	Urine cytology	At 3, 6, and 12 months in year 1, every 6 months in year 2, then annually up to year 5. As clinically indicated after 5 years.
	Blood tests	Not applicable

Continued

National Comprehensive Cancer Network Surveillance Guidelines for Nonmuscle Invasive Bladder Cancer—cont'd

AUA Risk Stratification	Test or Procedure	Frequency
High Risk	Cystoscopy	Every 3 months for years 1–2, then every 6 months for years 3–5, then annually for years 6–10. As clinically indicated after 10 years.
	Imaging of chest, abdomen, and pelvis	Baseline imaging and at 12 months in year 1, then every 1–2 years for years 2–10. As clinically indicated after 10 years.
	Urine cytology	Every 3 months in years 1–2, then every 6 months for years 3–5, then annually for years 6–10. As clinically indicated after 10 years.
	Blood tests	Not applicable

AUA, *American Urological Association.*
Data from National Comprehensive Cancer Network. NCCN Clinical Practice Guidelines in Oncology: Bladder cancer v1. 2022. Available at https://www.nccn.org/professionals/physician_gls/pdf/bladder.pdf.

National Comprehensive Cancer Network Surveillance Guidelines for Muscle Invasive Bladder Cancer

Test or Procedure	Frequency
Urine tests: Urine cytology	Every 6–12 months for 2 years, then as clinically indicated.
Blood tests: CBC, complete metabolic panel, liver function tests, creatinine, and electrolyte levels	Every 3–6 months for 2 years, then annually.
Imaging of chest, abdomen, and pelvis	Every 3–6 months for 2 years, then annually for 3 years.
For post-bladder preservation: cystoscopy	Every 3 months for 2 years, then every 6 months for years 3–4, then annually from years 5–10. As clinically indicated after 10 years.
For continent diversion	Monitor for vitamin B_{12} deficiency yearly.

CBC, Complete blood count.
Data from National Comprehensive Cancer Network. NCCN Clinical Practice Guidelines in Oncology: Bladder cancer v1. 2022. Available at https://www.nccn.org/professionals/physician_gls/pdf/bladder.pdf.

References

Al-Husseini, M. J., Kunbaz, A., Saad, A. M., Santos, J. V., Salahia, S., Iqbal, M., & Alahdab, F. (2019). Trends in the incidence and mortality of transitional cell carcinoma of the bladder for the last four decades in the USA: A SEER-based analysis. *BMC Cancer, 19*(1), 46.

American Cancer Society (ACS). (2022). *Cancer facts & figures, 2022.* Atlanta, GA: American Cancer Society.

Amin, M. B., Edge, S., Greene, F., Byrd, D. R., Brookland, R. K., Washington, M. K., ... Meyer, L. R. (Eds.). (2017). *AJCC cancer staging manual* (8th ed.). New York: Springer.

Carlo, M. I., Ravichandran, V., Srinavasan, P., Bandlamudi, C., Kemel, Y., Ceyhan-Birsoy, O., ... Rana, S. (2019). Cancer susceptibility mutations in patients with urothelial malignancies. *Journal of Clinical Oncology, 38*(5), 406–414.

Chang, S. S., Boorjian, S. A., Chou, R., Clark, P. E., Daneshmand, S., Konety, B. R., ... Skinner, E. C. (2016). Diagnosis and treatment of non-muscle invasive bladder cancer: AUA/SUO guideline. *Journal of Urology, 196*(4), 1021–1029.

Lenis, A. T., Lec, P. M., & Chamie, K. (2020). Bladder cancer: A review. *Journal of the American Medical Association, 324*(19), 1980–1991.

Lopez-Beltran, A., Cimadamore, A., Blanca, A., Massari, F., Vau, N., Scarpelli, M., ... Montironi, R. (2021). Immune checkpoint inhibitors for the treatment of bladder cancer. *Cancers, 13*(1), 131.

Saginala, K., Barsouk, A., Aluru, J. S., Rawla, P., Padala, S. A., & Barsouk, A. (2020). Epidemiology of bladder cancer. *Medical Sciences, 8*(1), 15.

National Cancer Institute. (2022). *Cancer stat facts: Bladder cancer.* Available at https://seer.cancer.gov/statfacts/html/urinb.html (accessed March 21, 2022).

National Comprehensive Cancer Network (NCCN). (2022). Bladder cancer (version 1.2022). Available at https://www.nccn.org/professionals/physician_gls/pdf/bladder.pdf.

Kidney Cancer

Definition

Kidney cancer is among the 10 most common cancers in both men and women in the United States. Eighty to 85% of kidney cancers arise from the renal cortex and are referred to as renal cell carcinomas (RCC). The subtypes of RCC include clear cell, papillary, chromophobe, oncocytic, collecting duct, and renal sarcomas. The second most common RCC type is transitional cell carcinomas (TCC) of the renal pelvis making up about 8% of all cases. Other types of kidney cancers include Wilms tumor (nephroblastoma) which is common in children and renal medullary cancer which is a rare form of RCC seen in sickle cell disease. Kidney cancer can metastasize to the brain, lung, lymph nodes, liver, adrenal gland, and bone (American Cancer Society [ACS], 2022; National Cancer Institute, 2022; Atkins et al., 2022).

Incidence

- Kidney cancer accounts for approximately 4% of all adult malignancies.
- About 79,000 new cases of kidney cancer and 14,000 deaths occur in the United States each year.
- Incidence rate has been increasing in the United States, while the size of RCC tumors has been decreasing in size. This is attributed to noninvasive abdominal imaging modalities finding.
- Overall lifetime risk of developing kidney cancer is 1 in 63 (1.6%).
- The incidence is high in North America and Europe, specifically the Czech Republic, and is low in Asian and South American countries.

Etiology and Risk Factors

(Atkins et al., 2022)
Risk factors include the following:
- Age: The average age at diagnosis is 64 years. Diagnosis is rare among people before 45 years of age.

- Sex: The incidence is higher among men (1 in 46) than women (1 in 80).
- Race: African Americans and American Indians/Alaska Natives have higher rates of kidney cancer.
- Cigarette smoking:
  - Compared to nonsmokers the risk for RCC increases about 50% in male and 20% in female smokers.
- Obesity: Accounts for over 30% of kidney cancers.
- Genetics: The risk of kidney cancer is increased for people with von Hippel–Lindau (VHL) disease, hereditary papillary RCC, Birt-Hogg-Dubé syndrome, and hereditary leiomyomatosis and renal cell cancer.
- Industrial chemical exposures: Workers exposed to cadmium, uranium, asbestos, and petroleum byproducts, specifically trichloroethylene, are at increased risk for kidney cancer.
- Hypertension is a risk factor.
- Hemodialysis and renal transplantation: An increased risk of kidney cancer is seen in people who are on long-term hemodialysis for end-stage renal disease, as well as after renal transplantation.

Signs and Symptoms

(Atkins, 2022b)

- More than 50% of kidney cancers are discovered as an incidental finding on radiographic imaging tests in asymptomatic individuals.
- Hematuria, flank pain, and palpable flank mass are the classic triad of symptoms. Other symptoms may include fever, loss of appetite, unintentional weight loss, anemia, bone pain, adenopathy, and varicocele.

Diagnostic Work-up

- History and physical examination
- CBC and comprehensive metabolic panel
- Urinalysis
- Abdominal or pelvic CT
- Abdominal MRI is used if inferior vena cava involvement is suspected.
- Chest imaging
- Bone scan if the alkaline phosphatase level is elevated or the patient has bone pain.
- Brain MRI if the patient has signs and symptoms that suggest brain metastasis.
- If urothelial carcinoma is suspected, urine cytology, ureteroscopy, and biopsy should be considered.
- Consider needle biopsy of small lesions to confirm a cancer diagnosis and guide treatment strategies.

Histopathology

(Atkins et al., 2022)

- Ninety percent of kidney cancers arise from the renal parenchyma and are referred to as RCC or renal adenocarcinomas. Major subtypes of RCC include:
  - Clear cell carcinoma: 75% to 80%
  - Papillary: 10% to 15%
  - Chromophobe: 5% to 10%
  - Oncocytic: 3% to 7%
  - Collecting duct: Very rare

- Translocation RCC: Very rare
- Unclassified: Up to 5%
- About 10% of kidney cancers occur in the renal pelvis and ureter.
  - Urothelial carcinomas, also known as TCC, account for more than 90% of upper urinary tract tumors.
  - Squamous cell carcinomas: 8%
  - Tend to be more invasive at diagnosis and have a poorer prognosis than urothelial carcinomas
  - Adenocarcinomas: Below 2%
- Renal sarcoma: Less than 1% of kidney cancers
  - Begins in the blood vessels or connective tissue of the kidneys
- Wilms' tumors: Almost always found in children and very rarely in adults

Clinical Staging

The AJCC TNM system is used for staging kidney cancer (Amin et al., 2017).

- Stage I: The cancer is limited to the kidney. The tumor measures less than 7 cm and has not spread to any lymph nodes or distant sites.
- Stage II: The cancer is still limited to the kidney, but the tumor measures greater than 7 cm. The cancer has not spread to any lymph nodes or distant sites.
- Stage III: The cancer has spread into the major veins or perinephric tissue, but not into the adrenal gland or Gerota fascia. Tumors with this spread are considered stage III no matter the size of the tumor or lymph node involvement. Also, any lymph node involvement is considered stage III also regardless of tumor size.
- Stage IV: The cancer has invaded past the Gerota fascia or has spread to any distant site.

Grading

- The Fuhrman grading system is used and has a scale of 1 (well differentiated) through 4 (undifferentiated).
- Grade 1 tumors are usually slow growing, less aggressive, and tend to have a good prognosis, whereas grade 4 tumors are the most aggressive and have a worse prognosis.

Risk Classification

- Treatment decisions can be influenced by a tumor's risk group. The two main models utilized to categorize risk factors are provided in the tables below and on the next page.

International Metastatic Renal Cell Carcinoma Database Consortium (IMDC) Criteria

Prognostic Factors	Risk Groups
• <1 year from time of diagnosis to systemic therapy	**Favorable-Risk Group** • No prognostic factors
• Performance status <80%	**Intermediate-Risk Group**
• Hemoglobin less than lower limit of normal	• One or two prognostic factors
• Calcium, neutrophils, or platelets greater than upper limit of normal	**Poor-Risk Group** • Three to six prognostic factors

Adapted from Grimm, M. O., Leucht, K., & Foller, S. (2021). Risk stratification and treatment algorithm of metastatic renal cell carcinoma. *Journal of Clinical Medicine, 10*(22), 5339.

Memorial Sloan Kettering Cancer Center (MSKCC) Prognostic Model

Prognostic Factors	Risk Groups
• Interval from diagnosis to treatment of <1 year • Performance status <80% • Lactate dehydrogenase >1.5 times the upper limit of normal. • Corrected serum calcium greater than the upper limit of normal • Hemoglobin less than the lower limit of normal	**Favorable-Risk Group** • No prognostic factors **Intermediate-Risk Group** • One or two prognostic factors **Poor-Risk Group** • Three or more prognostic factors

Data from Motzer, R. J. (2022). Memorial Sloan-Kettering Cancer Center (MSKCC/Motzer) score for metastatic renal cell carcinoma. Available at https://www.mdcalc.com/calc/2153/memorial-sloan-kettering-cancer-center-mskcc-motzer-score-metastatic-renal-cell-carcinoma-rcc.

Treatment

- Active surveillance: monitoring of tumors using abdominal imaging with delayed intervention when indicated.
  - Should be considered for elderly patients with limited life expectancy or those with significant comorbidities that places them at excessive risk for invasive interventions.

Surgery

- Radical nephrectomy is the mainstay of treatment for localized disease. This involves removal of the kidney, perirenal fat, regional lymph nodes, and ipsilateral adrenal gland.
  - Preferred surgery if the tumor extends into the inferior vena cava.
  - Techniques include open, laparoscopic, and robotic-assisted surgeries.
- Partial nephrectomy or nephron-sparing surgery
  - Preferred surgery for stage I disease.
  - Outcomes are comparable to radical nephrectomy.
  - Advantages over radical nephrectomy include preservation of renal function, reduction in overall mortality, and decreased frequency of cardiovascular events.
  - Contraindicated in patients with locally advanced disease or if the tumor is in an unfavorable location.
- Ablative therapy: include cryotherapy and radiofrequency ablation.
  - Option for patients with stage I disease who are not surgical candidates.
- Nephrectomy with surgical metastasectomy: used (1) in patients with RCC and a solitary site of metastasis in either the lung, bone, or brain or (2) in patients who were disease-free after nephrectomy and later developed a solitary recurrence.

Local Therapies

- Radiation therapy may be used for palliation, such as bone metastasis.

Systemic Therapies

(George & Jonasch, 2022)

- Both oral and intravenous therapies are used to prevent recurrence in high-risk disease in the adjuvant setting, along with patient who are unable to get surgery due to other comorbidities, unresectable or metastatic.
- Checkpoint inhibitors are a type of immunotherapy that work to block different checkpoint proteins and are utilized in both the adjuvant and unresectable metastatic setting.
  - Pembrolizumab, a PD-L1 inhibitor is used as adjuvant therapy for up to 1 year for patients with intermediate and high-risk clear cell carcinoma. May also be used in the metastatic setting.
  - Ipilumumab (a CTLA4 inhibitor) + nivolumab (a PD-L1 inhibitor) are used in relapsed or unresectable stage IV clear cell renal carcinoma who have excellent performance status and normal organ function (NCCN, 2022).
- Combination therapy
  - Immunotherapy plus targeted therapy, such as antiangiogenic therapy is used for patients with metastatic RCC.
  - Regimens include pembrolizumab with axitinib; pembrolizumab with lenvatinib, and cabozantinib.
  - Single agent antiangiogenic therapies may be used in individuals who want to avoid immunotherapy side effects or prefer convenience of oral therapy alone.
- Chemotherapy:
  - Not a standard treatment for kidney cancer. It may be used in patients who have failed immunotherapy and/or targeted therapy; however, it is rarely utilized due to only very limited activity in disease response and the growth of other immunotherapy and targeted therapy combinations.

Prognosis

- Prognostic factors include disease stage, tumor size, histologic type and grade, histologic tumor necrosis, number and location of metastatic sites, prior nephrectomy, performance status, substantial weight loss, elevated serum calcium and lactate dehydrogenase levels, low hemoglobin, and thrombocytosis.
- For all stages combined, the 5-year relative survival rate is 76% (ACS, 2022).
- The 5-year survival rate by stage at diagnosis (ACS, 2022):
  - Local: 93%
  - Regional: 71%
  - Distant: 14%

Prevention and Surveillance

- There are no recommendations for specific screening and prevention of kidney cancer. However, increasing levels of physical activity, maintaining a healthy weight, tobacco-free or smoking cessation, and diets high in fruits and vegetables may reduce the risk of kidney cancer. A family history of RCC, particularly in individuals less than 50 years old, may indicate a hereditary predisposition to the disease. Patients with a family history or hereditary RCC (i.e., VHL disease) should be closely monitored.
- The NCCN surveillance guidelines for kidney cancer are summarized in the table on the next page.

National Comprehensive Cancer Network Surveillance Guidelines for Kidney Cancer

Test or Procedure	Frequency
History and physical	Stage I—Annually Stage II–III—Every 3–6 months for 3 years, then annually
Blood tests: Complete metabolic panel and other tests as indicated	Stage I—Annually, as clinically indicated Stage II–III—Every 3–6 months for 3 years, then annually
Chest and abdominal imaging (CT or MRI) Note—Additional imaging may be considered for higher risk factors such as grade 4 disease or positive margins.	Stage I—Baseline, then annually for 3 years Stage II–III—Baseline, then every 3–6 months for at least 3 years, then annually up to 5 years

CT, Computed tomography; *MRI*, magnetic resonance imaging.
Data from the National Comprehensive Cancer Network. NCCN Clinical Practice Guidelines in Oncology: Kidney cancer v4.2022. Available at https://www.nccn.org/professionals/physician_gls/pdf/kidney.pdf.

References

American Cancer Society (ACS). (2022). *Cancer facts & figures, 2022*. Atlanta, GA: American Cancer Society.

Amin, M. B., Edge, S., Greene, F., Byrd, D. R., Brookland, R. K., Washington, M. K., … Meyer, L. R. (Eds.). (2017). *AJCC cancer staging manual* (8th ed.). New York: Springer.

Atkins, M. (2022a). *Overview of the treatment of renal cell carcinoma*. Available at https://www.uptodate.com/contents/overview-of-the-treatment-of-renal-cell-carcinoma?search=kidney%20cancer%20treatment&source=search_result&selectedTitle=1~150&usage_type=default&display_rank=1#H2582328022.

Atkins, M. (2022b). Clinical manifestations, evaluation, and staging of renal cell carcinoma. Available at https://www.uptodate.com/contents/clinical-manifestations-evaluation-and-staging-of-renal-cell-carcinoma?search=kidney%20cancer%20&source=search_result&selectedTitle=2~150&usage_type=default&display_rank=2#H1.

Atkins, M., Bakouny, Z., & Choueiri, T. (2022). Epidemiology, pathology, and pathogenesis of renal cell carcinoma. Available at https://www.uptodate.com/contents/epidemiology-pathology-and-pathogenesis-of-renal-cell-carcinoma.

George, D., & Jonasch, E. (2022). *Systemic therapy of advanced clear cell renal carcinoma*. Available at https://www.uptodate.com/contents/systemic-therapy-of-advanced-clear-cell-renal-carcinoma?sectionName=INITIAL%20TREATMENT%20OPTIONS&search=kidney%20cancer%20treatment&topicRef=15719&anchor=H1689558199&source=see_link#H2478406856.

Grimm, M. O., Leucht, K., & Foller, S. (2021). Risk stratification and treatment algorithm of metastatic renal cell carcinoma. *Journal of Clinical Medicine*, *10*(22), 5339.

Motzer, R. J. (2022). *Memorial Sloan-Kettering Cancer Center (MSKCC/Motzer) score for metastatic renal cell carcinoma*. Available at https://www.mdcalc.com/calc/2153/memorial-sloan-kettering-cancer-center-mskcc-motzer-score-metastatic-renal-cell-carcinoma-rcc.

National Cancer Institute. (2022). *Cancer stat facts: Kidney and renal pelvis cancer*. Available at https://seer.cancer.gov/statfacts/html/kidrp.html.

National Comprehensive Cancer Network (NCCN). (2022). Kidney cancer (version 4.2022). Available at https://www.nccn.org/professionals/physician_gls/pdf/kidney.pdf.

Penile Cancer

Definition

Carcinoma of the penis is an uncommon malignancy in the United States. Ninety-five percent of cancers of the penis are squamous cell carcinomas that may evolve from the prepuce, glans, or shaft of the penis. Metastasis occurs primarily in regional lymph nodes (i.e., femoral, inguinal, pelvic, and iliac), and it rarely spreads to distant sites such as the lungs, liver, bones, and brain.

Incidence

(America Cancer Society [ACS], 2022a)

- Carcinoma of the penis accounts for less than 1% of all malignancies in men.
- Approximately 2070 Americans were newly diagnosed with penile cancer, and 470 died of the disease in 2022.
- More common among men over 50 years old.
- More common in Africa, South America, and Asia. The incidence is low in North America and Europe.

Etiology and Risk Factors

(Douglawi & Masterson, 2019; Thomas et al., 2021)

- The exact cause of penile cancer is unknown.
- Risk factors include the following:
  - Risk increases with age with a median age at diagnosis of 68 years.
  - Not being circumcised
  - Men with phimosis have an increased risk of penile cancer between 25% and 60%.
  - Having multiple sex partners
  - A history of sexually transmitted diseases, including human immunodeficiency virus (HIV) and human papillomavirus (HPV).
    - Between 45% and 80% of penile cancer cases are related to HPV infection.
  - Tobacco smokers are 3 to 4.5 times more likely to develop penile cancer.
  - Lichen sclerosis
  - Chronic inflammation
  - Patients with psoriasis treated with psoralens plus ultraviolet A (UVA) light are at increased risk for penile cancer.
- Premalignant lesions associated with squamous cell carcinoma of the penis include the following:
  - Balanitis xerotica obliterans
  - Cutaneous horn
  - Giant condyloma
  - Bowenoid papulosis

Signs and Symptoms

(National Comprehensive Cancer Network [NCCN], 2022)

- Most often presents as a palpable, visible lesion on the penis.
- Lesions occur most commonly on the glans (34.5%), prepuce (13.2%), shaft (5.3%), and overlapping sites (4.5%). 42.5% were unspecified.
- There may be penile pain, bleeding, discharge, or a foul odor.
- Lesion may be nodular, ulcerative, or fungating.
- Patients with advanced disease may have palpable lymph nodes and constitutional symptoms such as weight loss.

Diagnostic Work-up

- The following tools are essential for the diagnosis and staging of penile cancer:
  - History and physical examination are important to assess risk factors and characteristics of the lesion, such

as diameter, number of lesions, location, morphology, and relationship to other structures (submucosal, corpora spongiosa, cavernosa, and/or urethra), and presence of palpable lymph nodes.
- A biopsy specimen is obtained from the penile lesion.
- HPV status is assessed.
- Imaging includes ultrasonography, CT, and MRI.

Histopathology

- Squamous cell carcinoma is the most common histologic form of penile cancer.
- Can be further subdivided into various subtypes: verrucous, papillary squamous, warty, basaloid, adenosquamous, sarcomatoid, and other rare subtypes.
- The verrucous subtype has low malignant potential.
- Adenosquamous and sarcomatoid variants have a worse prognosis.

Clinical Staging

The AJCC TNM system is used for staging penile cancer. The AJCC TNM system for penile cancer describes the extent of the primary tumor (T), whether the cancer has spread to nearby lymph nodes (N), and the absence or presence of distant metastasis (M) (Amin et al., 2017).
- Stage 0: The cancer is noninvasive localized squamous cell carcinoma or carcinoma in situ.
- Stage I: The cancer has invaded the lamina propria, is not high grade, and has not spread to the lymph nodes or any distant site.
- Stage II: The cancer is high grade and has invaded the blood vessels, lymph vessels, nerves, corpus spongiosum, or corpora cavernosum. It has not spread to the lymph nodes or any distant site.
- Stage III: The cancer has spread to the inguinal lymph nodes but has not spread to any distant site.
- Stage IV: The cancer has invaded the scrotum, prostate, or pubic bone. It has spread beyond the inguinal lymph nodes, and/or has spread to any distant site.

Grading

- Grading is based on the three-tiered World Health Organization/International Society of Urological Pathology grading system:
  - Grade 1: Well differentiated
  - Grade 2: Moderately differentiated
  - Grade 3: Poorly differentiated
- Any proportion of anaplastic cells is categorized as grade 3.
- Higher grade is an important predictor for metastatic nodal involvement.

Treatment

- Treatment depends on the disease stage at diagnosis.
- Penile preserving treatments
  - Topical therapy with topical 5-FU cream as first line therapy or imiquimod 5% as the second-line topical agent.
  - Laser therapy

- Glansectomy or removal of the glans penis may be considered for patients with distal tumors on the glans or prepuce.
- Wide local excision of penile tumors on the shaft.
- Mohs micrographic surgery
- Radiation therapy: Patients should be circumcised before starting radiation therapy to prevent radiation-related complications.
- Penectomy: Partial or total penectomy with or without inguinal lymph node dissection
- Chemotherapy: Used in patients with advanced or metastatic disease
  - Preferred first-line combination chemotherapy regimens include paclitaxel, ifosfamide, and cisplatin (TIP regimen) and cisplatin plus 5-FU.
  - Single-agent chemotherapy includes capecitabine, cisplatin, 5-FU, mitomycin C, docetaxel, paclitaxel, or cetuximab.

Prognosis

(ACS, 2022b)
- For all stages combined, the 5-year relative survival rate is 65%.
- The 5-year survival rate is 79% for patients with localized disease at diagnosis.
- For patients with regional and distant disease, the 5-year survival rates are 50% and 9%, respectively.

Prevention and Surveillance

- Although there is no proven way to prevent penile cancer, measures can be taken to decrease risk.
  - Avoidance of HPV and HIV exposure
  - Smoking cessation
  - Good personal hygiene, especially completely cleaning under the foreskin
  - Circumcision
- There are no screening recommendations, but penile cancers usually start in the skin and can be detected early.
  - The area underneath the foreskin should be kept clean and regularly examined.
  - Any reddened or scaly lesion or sore should be reported promptly to the medical team.
- Follow-up surveillance for all patients includes clinical examination of the penis and inguinal nodes.
  - Imaging is not routinely recommended for those with early disease, but it may be used after an abnormal finding or if a recurrence is suspected.
  - CT of the chest, abdomen, and pelvis is recommended for those with inguinal or pelvic lymph node metastases.

References

American Cancer Society (ACS). (2022a). *Cancer facts & figures, 2022.* Atlanta, GA: American Cancer Society.

American Cancer Society (ACS). (2022b). *Survival rates for penile cancer.* Available at https://www.cancer.org/cancer/penile-cancer/detection-diagnosis-staging/survival-rates.html.

Amin, M. B., Edge, S., Greene, F., Byrd, D. R., Brookland, R. K., Washington, M. K., ... Meyer, L. R. (Eds.). (2017). *AJCC cancer staging manual* (8th ed.). Springer.

Douglawi, A., & Masterson, T. A. (2019). Penile cancer epidemiology and risk factors: A contemporary review. *Current Opinion in Urology, 29*(2), 145–149.

National Comprehensive Cancer Network (NCCN). (2022). Penile cancer (version 2.2022). Available at https://www.nccn.org/professionals/physician_gls/pdf/penile.pdf.

Thomas, A., Necchi, A., Muneer, A., Tobias-Machado, M., Tran, A. T. H., Van Rompuy, A. S., … Albersen, M. (2021). Penile cancer. *Nature Reviews Disease Primers*, 7(1), 11.

Prostate Cancer

Definition

Prostate cancer is the most common cancer among men in the United States. The cancer affects the prostate, a lobular gland that serves as a secondary male sex organ. The prostate is located just below the bladder and in front of the rectum. The primary function of the prostate is to produce fluid that forms part of semen. The fluid is alkaline, which helps neutralize the acidity of the vaginal tract, thereby prolonging the lifespan of the sperm.

Among men with prostate cancer, approximately 60% are diagnosed at age 65-year-old or older (National Cancer Institute, 2022). And most men, approximately 84% are diagnosed limited to regional disease (Cancer.Net, 2022). Metastasis can occur through direct extension into the seminal vesicles, urethral mucosa, bladder wall, and external sphincter. The cancer may also spread through the regional lymph nodes. Prostate vasculature is often the method of spread when the cancer invades the pelvic bones, lumbar spine, liver, or lungs.

Incidence

(American Cancer Society [ACS], 2022a; National Cancer Institute, 2022)

- About 268,490 new cases of prostate cancer and 34,500 deaths occurred in the United States in 2022.
- Overall, 1 in 8 men in the United States are diagnosed with prostate cancer, and 1 in 41 dies of the disease.
- African American men have a highest incidence rate and at least double mortality rate compared with men of other racial groups.

Etiology and Risk Factors

(ACS, 2022b)
Several risk factors for prostate cancer have been identified.

- Age older than 50 years, with a median age at diagnosis of 67 years.
- Ethnicity: African American men are at higher risk than all other ethnic groups, and Asian men who live in Asia have the lowest risk (2%).
- Geography: It is more common in North America, northwestern Europe, Australia, and the Caribbean Islands.
- Family history:
  - The risk for prostate cancer is 2.1 to 2.4 times greater for men whose fathers had prostate cancer and 2.9 to 3.3 times higher for those whose brothers had the disease.
  - About 40% of early-onset prostate cancer and 5% to 10% of all prostate cancers are hereditary.
- Pathologic variants in genes:
  - *BRCA1* or *BRCA2* genetic variant
  - Lynch syndrome (also known as hereditary nonpolyposis colorectal cancer)
  - *HOXB13* genetic variant
  - *ATM* genetic variant
  - *PALB2* genetic variant
  - *CHEK2* genetic variant
- Diet: High intake of dairy products may increase the risk of prostate cancer.
- The degree to which factors such as obesity, recurring prostatitis, sexually transmitted infections, benign prostatic hypertrophy (BPH), prostatic intraepithelial neoplasia, vasectomy, and environmental exposures (e.g., herbicides such as Agent Orange) contribute to prostate cancer is inconclusive.

Signs and Symptoms

Because the signs and symptoms of prostate cancer can often be confused with normal signs of aging, BPH, or prostatitis an accurate diagnosis is imperative. The most common signs and symptoms of prostate cancer include the following:
- Weak or interrupted urinary stream
- Urinary frequency
- Nocturia
- Difficulty beginning urination
- Dysuria
- Hematuria
- Blood in semen
- Bone pain in the hips, spine, ribs, or other areas.
- Weakness or numbness in the legs or feet
- Shortness of breath
- Fatigue

Diagnostic Work-up

A physical examination is the primary measure for diagnosing prostate cancer because men often seek treatment for urinary symptoms. Diagnostic measures of prostate cancer include the following:
- Digital rectal examination (DRE)
- Prostate-specific antigen (PSA) blood test
- Transrectal ultrasound allows the provider to visualize the prostate, estimate prostate size, and detect tumors that cannot be felt by DRE.
- Prostate biopsy is required to diagnose prostate cancer. Ten to twelve tissue samples are taken from several places in the prostate.
- Bone scans, CT, MRI, and prostate-specific membrane antigen (PSMA) PET scans are used to evaluate metastatic disease.

Histopathology

More than 95% of prostate cancers are adenocarcinomas. The remaining 5% are squamous cell carcinomas, transitional cell tumors, and carcinosarcomas (rare).

Clinical Staging

- The AJCC TNM system for prostate cancer describes the extent of the primary tumor (T), whether the cancer has spread to nearby lymph nodes (N), and the absence or presence of distant metastasis (M).

- The AJCC anatomic prognostic groups incorporate the TNM system, PSA values, and histology Gleason grade group (Amin et al., 2017).
- The table below provides the definition of histologic grade group.

Definition of Histologic Grade Group

Grade Group	Gleason Score	Gleason Pattern
1	<6	<3 + 3
2	7	3 + 4
3	7	4 + 3
4	8	4 + 4, 3 + 5, 5 + 3
5	9 or 10	4 + 5, 5 + 4, 5 + 5

- Stage I: The cancer is confined within the prostate and has not spread to the lymph nodes or any distant site. PSA is less than 10 ng/mL, and grade group is 1.
- Stage II: The cancer is confined within the prostate and has not spread to the lymph nodes or any distant site. PSA is less than 20, and grade group is 1 to 4.
- Stage III: The cancer is confined within the prostate and has not spread to the lymph nodes or any distant site. PSA is greater than 20, and grade group is 1 to 4. This stage also includes tumors that have grown outside the prostate and might have invaded the seminal vesicles or other adjacent structures, such as the external sphincter, rectum, bladder, levator muscles, and/or pelvic wall regardless of any PSA value.
- Stage IV: The cancer has spread to the lymph nodes and/or has spread to any distant site regardless of any PSA value or grade group.

Grading

- The Gleason score is a measurement of the tumor's grade, which describes its aggressiveness.
  - The score is derived from the two most common malignant histologic patterns in the tumor, and each is assigned a grade. Scores range from 1 to 5, and the more differentiated that a cell is, the higher the grade. The two scores are added together, giving a final score between 2 and 10.
  - Higher Gleason scores are associated with more aggressive tumors.

Treatment

Treatment options include active surveillance, surgery, radiation therapy, hormonal therapy or androgen-deprivation therapy (ADT), chemotherapy, immunotherapy, and targeted therapy. The choice of treatment is determined by several factors: presence of symptoms, stage of disease, life expectancy, comorbidities, effect on quality of life, probability that the tumor can be cured by single-modality therapy, and patient's preference.

Observation

- Goal of observation is to maintain quality of life by avoiding side effects of unnecessary treatment.
- Applicable to elderly or frail patients who have other major health problems and are likely to die of other health issues before succumbing to the cancer.

- Involves monitoring the course of the cancer with a history and physical examination until symptoms develop. If symptoms develop, palliative treatment may be considered.

Active Surveillance

- Unlike observation, active surveillance may be indicated in younger patients with indolent or slow-growing cancer who wish to defer or avoid treatment and its potential side effects.
- It involves actively monitoring the disease with PSA, DRE, prostate biopsy, and imaging studies with the expectation to deliver curative therapy if the cancer progresses.
- In active surveillance, PSA is monitored every 6 months. DRE, prostate biopsy, and multiparametric MRI are performed annually unless clinically indicated.

Surgery

- If surgery is indicated, the most common option is a radical prostatectomy, in which the entire prostate is removed.

Radiation

- If radiation therapy is recommended, two types are used.
  - External beam radiation therapy targets the prostate and regional lymph nodes. It requires the implantation of gold seed markers in the prostate to accurately deliver radiation to the desired treatment areas.
  - Brachytherapy uses small radioactive implants that are placed directly in the prostate to deliver localized radiation therapy to the gland. Brachytherapy can be delivered by an implanted catheter at a high dose (which uses iridium-192 radioactive material) or a low dose (which uses iodine-125, cesium 131, or palladium-103 radioactive material).

Systemic Therapies

- Radiopharmaceuticals are drugs that contain radioactive elements. These include the following:
  - Lutetium Lu 177 vipivotide tetraxetan or ^{177}Lu-PSMA-617
  - Strontium-89
  - Samarium-153
  - Radium-223
- ADT can be achieved by surgery (i.e., orchiectomy) or by medical castration through the administration of pharmacologic agents.
  - The goal is to achieve a serum testosterone level below 0.5 ng/mL to decrease or inhibit prostate cancer cell proliferation.
  - The table below provides a list of commonly used pharmacologic agents for ADT.

Common Pharmacologic Agents for Androgen-Deprivation Therapy

Degarelix	LHRH antagonist	Subcut: 240 mg; maintenance 80 mg subcut
Relugolix	LHRH antagonist	PO: Loading dose 360 mg on the first day of treatment followed by 120 mg daily

Common Pharmacologic Agents for Androgen-Deprivation Therapy—cont'd

Generic Name	Drug Class	Dosage and Route
Goserelin acetate implant	LHRH agonist	Subcut: 3.6 mg every 28 days; 10.8 mg every 12 weeks
Histrelin	LHRH agonist	Implant: 50 mg implant every 12 months
Leuprolide acetate	LHRH agonist	IM or Subcut: 5 mg/day; 7.5 mg every month; 22.5 mg every 3 months; 30 mg every 4 months; 45 mg every 6 months
Triptorelin pamoate	LHRH agonist	IM: 3.75 mg every 4 weeks; 11.25 mg every 12 weeks; 22.5 mg every 24 weeks
Abiraterone	Nonsteroidal antiandrogen	PO: 1000 mg/day with prednisone 5 mg once daily
Enzalutamide	Nonsteroidal antiandrogen	PO: 160 mg daily
Bicalutamide	Nonsteroidal antiandrogen	PO: 50 mg daily
Darolutamide	Nonsteroidal antiandrogen	PO: 600 mg twice a day
Flutamide	Nonsteroidal antiandrogen	PO: 250 mg every 8 hr
Nilutamide	Nonsteroidal antiandrogen	PO: 300 mg daily for 30 days, followed by 150 mg once a day

IM, intramuscular injection; *PO*, by mouth; *subcut*, subcutaneous injection.
Adapted from Skidmore-Roth, L. (2022). *Mosby's 2022 nursing drug reference* (35th ed.). Elsevier.

- Chemotherapy is used in patients with high-volume, ADT-naïve, metastatic disease or in patient whose disease has become resistant to ADT.
  - Commonly used chemotherapy agents include docetaxel, cabazitaxel, mitoxantrone, and carboplatin.
- Immunotherapy may be used in patients with metastatic castrate-resistant prostate cancer who are asymptomatic or have mild symptoms.
  - Immunotherapy agents include sipuleucel-T and pembrolizumab.
- Targeted therapy is used in patients who has a homologous recombination repair (*HRR*) mutation or *BRCA* mutation (Sayegh et al., 2022; Sandhu et al., 2021).
  - Targeted therapy agents include olaparib and rucaparib.

Prognosis

There are about 3.2 million prostate cancer survivors in the United States. The prognosis for men with prostate cancer depends on disease stage.

- If the cancer is localized within the prostate and regional tissues, including seminal vesicles (stages I through III), the 5-year survival rate is greater than 99% (ACS, 2022a).
  - The survival rate drops to 31% for patients diagnosed with distant metastases (ACS, 2022a).
  - The survival rate drops for African American patients who are diagnosed at younger ages with more advanced diseases.

- Although the prognosis for survival is often good, most prostate cancer survivors have long-term effects of the disease.
  - If the patient underwent prostatectomy or medical castration with ADT, late effects could include urinary incontinence, sexual dysfunction, bowel issues, gynecomastia, and osteoporosis.
  - Psychological effects may include fear of recurrence and depression about sexual dysfunction. Worry about the loss of masculinity can lead to relationship issues with a partner.

Prevention and Surveillance

- There are no known medical measures to prevent prostate cancer. However, the risk may be reduced by maintaining a healthy weight, being physically active, eating foods with more fruits and vegetables, and limiting red meats and processed foods.

Screening Recommendations

- There are differences in recommendations regarding prostate cancer screening among various organizations, such as the American Cancer Society (ACS), AUA, United States Preventive Services Taskforce (USPSTF), and the NCCN. Since recommendations vary, the ACS's screening guidelines are presented.
- The ACS recommends that men make an informed decision with their health care provider about whether to be screened for prostate cancer.
- Based on the ACS recommendations, screening involves getting a PSA blood test and a DRE. For men who are at average risk and have a life expectancy of more than 10 years, PSA and DRE should be performed annually starting at the age of 50. For those at high risk (e.g., African Americans and men with a first-degree relative diagnosed with prostate before age 65), screening should begin at 45 years of age. Men with known or likely to carry *BRCA1* or *BRCA2* genetic mutations may begin screening at age 40 (ACS, 2022b).
- DRE
  - Palpation of the prostate can assess for tumors and detect BPH and prostatitis.
  - The sensitivity of DRE is 51%, and the specificity is 59% (Naji et al., 2018).
- PSA blood test
  - The test measures a protein released by epithelial cells in the prostate.
  - The measurement is not prostate cancer specific, and the PSA level can be elevated in cases of advanced age, BPH, or prostatitis.
  - The PSA blood test has a sensitivity of 67.5% to 80%, which suggests that 20% to 30% of prostate cancers are misdiagnosed if only this test is used (Brosman, 2020). Age-adjusted values are used to increase specificity.
  - Other methods to increase PSA sensitivity include measuring PSA velocity, PSA density, and free PSA levels.
  - Increasing PSA values often indicate the need for a prostate biopsy.

Surveillance

- Surveillance recommendations for stages I through III prostate cancer following initial definitive treatment include a PSA test every 6 to 12 months for 5 years and an annual DRE. The DRE may be omitted if the PSA value is undetectable.
- For patients with metastatic disease, a history, physical examination, and PSA test every 3 to 6 months are recommended. Imaging should be performed for new symptoms or a rising PSA value.

References

American Cancer Society (ACS). (2022a). *Cancer facts & figures, 2022.* Atlanta, GA: American Cancer Society.

American Cancer Society (ACS). (2022b). *Prostate cancer.* Available at https://www.cancer.org/cancer/prostate-cancer.%20html (accessed March 26, 2022).

Amin, M. B., Edge, S., Greene, F., Byrd, D. R., Brookland, R. K., Washington, M. K., ... Meyer, L. R. (Eds.). (2017). *AJCC cancer staging manual* (8th ed.). Springer.

Brosman, S. A. (2020). Prostate-specific antigen testing. In *Medscape.* Available at https://emedicine.medscape.com/article/457394-overview#a7.

Cancer.Net. (2022). *Prostate cancer statistics. Cancer.Net.* Available at https://www.cancer.net/cancer-types/prostate-cancer/statistics.

Naji, L., Randhawa, H., Sohani, Z., Dennis, B., Lautenbach, D., Kavanagh, O., ... Profetto, J. (2018). Digital rectal examination for prostate cancer screening in primary care: A systematic review and meta-analysis. *Annals of Family Medicine*, 16(2), 149–154.

National Cancer Institute. (2022). *Cancer stat facts: Prostate cancer.* Available at https://seer.cancer.gov/statfacts/html/prost.html (accessed March 26, 2022).

National Comprehensive Cancer Network (NCCN). (2022). Prostate cancer (version 3.2022). Available at https://www.nccn.org/professionals/physician_gls/pdf/prostate.pdf.

Sandhu, S., Moore, C. M., Chiong, E., Beltran, H., Bristow, R. G., & Williams, S. G. (2021). Prostate cancer. *Lancet*, 398(10305), 1075–1090.

Sayegh, N., Swami, U., & Agarwal, N. (2022). Recent advances in the management of metastatic prostate cancer. *Journal of Oncology Practice*, 18(1), 45–55.

Skidmore-Roth, L. (2022). *Evolve Resources for Mosby's 2022 nursing drug reference* (35th ed.). Saint Louis: Elsevier.

Testicular Cancer

Definition

Testicular cancer is an uncommon malignancy that forms in the tissues of one or both testes. It is the most common cancer in young men between the ages of 15 and 35 years.

Primary germ cell tumors (GCTs) constitute 95% of all testicular neoplasms. Testicular tumors are organized into the more common but slow-growing seminomas and the nonseminomas, which are rare but more aggressive than seminomas. The remaining 5% of neoplasms are stromal tumors, which develop in the stroma, the structural and hormone-producing tissue of organs. Although they account for only 5% of testicular malignancies, they make up 20% of childhood testicular tumors.

Testicular cancer metastasizes through the lymphatic system to the retroperitoneal lymph nodes. Distant metastasis sites include the lungs, liver, bones, and brain.

Incidence

- Testicular cancer accounts for 0.5% of all cancers in men each year and for 5% of all urologic tumors.
- About 9910 new cases of testicular cancer and 460 deaths are expected to occur in the United States in 2022 (National Cancer Institute [NCI], 2022a).
- In the United States, the chance for a man to develop testicular cancer is 0.4% (NCI, 2022a).
- Testicular malignancies have been on the rise in the United States over the past decade, increasing on average of 0.7% per year (NCI, 2022a).
- The incidence is four to five times higher among White males than African American males and more than three times higher than among Asian American males. White males of Scandinavian descent are at highest risk (NCI, 2022b).
- Neoplasms occur more often in the right testicle than in the left.
- Peak age of incidence is between 20 and 34 years of age (American Cancer Society [ACS], 2018).
- Between 70% and 75% of patients have stage I, 20% have stage II, and 10% have stage III disease at diagnosis. There is no stage IV based on the AJCC staging system.

Etiology and Risk Factors

The exact cause of testicular cancer is unknown, but several risk factors have been identified:

- Cryptorchidism
  - Higher risk for patients with abdominal cryptorchid testes than inguinal cryptorchid testes
  - Boys who had orchiopexy performed after age 13 were at higher risk (Pettersson et al., 2007).
  - The malignancy often occurs in the undescended testicle.
  - Researchers do not think cryptorchidism plays a direct role in testicular cancer. Instead, an unknown factor is thought to cause the malignancy and cryptorchidism.
- Two percent of men who develop a GCT in one testis eventually develop a GCT in the other testicle.
- Klinefelter syndrome
  - Genetic disorder manifested by testicular atrophy, gynecomastia, and absence of spermatogenesis.
  - Increases the risk of a mediastinal GCT.
- Testicular feminization syndrome increases the risk of a testicular GCT.
- HIV infection
- HPV infection
- Family history of testicular malignancies, particularly in a father or brother.

Signs and Symptoms

- The most common symptoms of testicular malignancy are a palpable mass in the scrotum found on testicular self-examination and a feeling of heaviness in the scrotum or lower abdomen.
- The tumor or mass in the testicle can cause pain.
- Other signs include swelling in the scrotum similar to epididymitis or orchitis, gynecomastia (i.e., breast growth and tenderness), and early signs of puberty in young boys.
- Advanced-disease symptoms can include lower back pain (indicating the disease has spread to lymph nodes), urinary obstruction, bone pain, shortness of breath, headaches, seizures, and weight loss.

Diagnostic Work-up

- Physical examination, including testicular palpation.
- Ultrasound of the testicles to help visualize inner structures and distinguish between cancer and benign conditions.
- Increased blood levels of tumor markers.
  - α-Fetoprotein (AFP), elevated only in cancers with a nonseminoma component.
  - β-Human chorionic gonadotropin (β-hCG).
  - Lactate dehydrogenase, which can indicate widespread disease.
- Transillumination of the scrotum to help establish the diagnosis.
- Surgical intervention with a radical inguinal orchiectomy to remove the testicle and spermatic cord for pathologic evaluation.
  - Surgery can lead to a definitive diagnosis, stage the cancer, and provide curative treatment if the cancerous cells are removed.
- CT scan to evaluate regional lymph nodes.
- Chest radiograph to evaluate possible metastasis.
- Bone scan.

Histopathology

- GCTs account for 95% of testicular malignancies.
- GCTs are classified as seminomas or nonseminomas.
  - Seminomas are considered only if the tumor is 100% within the sperm-producing cells (ACS, 2018).
  - Nonseminomas have four subtypes: embryonal carcinomas, yolk-sac tumors, teratomas, and choriocarcinomas. Most nonseminoma tumors consist of a mixture of subtypes, but this does not affect how the cancer is treated.
    - An embryonal carcinoma is identified in approximately 40% of all testicular neoplasms, and it increases levels of AFP (ACS, 2018).
    - Yolk sac tumors, which get their name from their resemblance to an embryonic yolk sac, are the most common form of cancer in children and infants.
    - Teratomas are further grouped as mature teratomas, immature teratomas, and those with elements of a somatic (non-germ cell) malignancy.
    - Choriocarcinoma is rare, but it is the most aggressive form of testicular cancer.
  - These cancers usually spread initially to the retroperitoneal lymph nodes.
  - Non–GCTs comprise the remaining 5% and include Leydig cell tumors and Sertoli cell tumors, which are often benign.

Clinical Staging

The two main staging systems for testicular cancer are the International Germ Cell Cancer Collaborative Group (IGCCCG) Risk Classification (see the table in the right column) and the AJCC TNM staging system (Amin et al., 2017). Based on the criteria developed by the IGCCCG, the prognosis can be good, intermediate, or poor. The prognosis helps to determine treatment options and has been incorporated into the AJCC anatomic prognostic groups.

International Germ Cell Cancer Consensus Group Risk Classification

Prognosis	Nonseminoma	Seminoma
Good	Testicular or retroperitoneal primary tumors No metastases to organs other than lungs and/or lymph nodes AFP <1000 ng/mL β-hCG <5000 mIU/ML LDH <3 × upper limit or normal	Any primary site No metastases to organs other than lungs and/or lymph nodes Normal serum AFP
Intermediate	Testicular or retroperitoneal primary tumors No metastases to organs other than lungs and/or lymph nodes AFP 1000–10,000 ng/mL Or β-hCG 5000–50,000 mIU/ML or LDH 3–10 × upper limit or normal	Any primary site Metastases to organs other than lungs and/or lymph nodes Normal serum AFP
Poor	Mediastinal primary site Metastases to organs other than lungs and/or lymph nodes AFP >10,000 ng/mL β-hCG >50,000 mIU/mL LDH >10 × upper limit or normal	No seminoma patients have a poor prognosis.

AFP, α-Fetoprotein; *β-hCG*, β-human chorionic gonadotropin; *LDH*, lactate dehydrogenase.

Data from Mead, G. M., & Stenning, S. P. (1997). The International Germ Cell Consensus Classification: A new prognostic factor-based staging classification for metastatic germ cell tumours. *Clinical Oncology (Royal College of Radiologists (Great Britain)*, 9(4), 207–209.

Treatment

Treatment depends on the tumor stage. A radical inguinal orchiectomy is often performed for diagnosis and treatment. Depending on the tumor type, staging, and degree of metastasis, further therapy may include additional surgery (e.g., regional lymph node dissection), radiation therapy, or chemotherapy.

- Seminomas are more responsive to radiation therapy, whereas nonseminomas are more sensitive to chemotherapy.
- Retroperitoneal radiation therapy cures almost 100% of patients with stage I seminoma; however, this approach may lead to overtreatment and a higher rate of recurrence.
- The NCCN guidelines prefer active surveillance for pT1 to pT3 (i.e., stages IA and IB) seminomas and for clinical stage IA nonseminomas (NCCN, 2022).
  - Chemotherapy is used for patients with bulkier or metastatic diseases.

- The AJCC staging system and the IGCCCG risk assessment help to determine which chemotherapy regimens to use.
- The most used regimens include three cycles of etoposide and cisplatin (EP) or four cycles of bleomycin, etoposide, and cisplatin (BEP).
- These combination therapies have cure rates of 70% to 80%, but their toxicity, especially with the BEP regimen, is substantial.
  - Pulmonary fibrosis is the most severe toxicity, often manifesting as pneumonitis. This is common in elderly patients and those receiving high doses of BEP (e.g., 300 to 400 units), but it is also possible in young adults receiving lower doses.
  - The risk of toxicity increases when supplemental oxygen is given for other issues.
  - Other adverse effects include hypotension, mental confusion, fever, chills, and wheezing.

Prognosis

- Testicular cancer has an overall 5-year survival and cure rate of 95%.
- Eighty percent of patients with metastatic disease have a 95% survival rate.
- The rate is lower for the aggressive choriocarcinoma subtype of nonseminoma tumors, dropping below 80%.
- Survivors of testicular cancer are at a risk for late recurrence (i.e., relapse more than 2 years after remission).

Prevention and Surveillance

- There are no known prevention measures.
- The USPSTF and the ACS do not recommend testicular cancer surveillance for adolescent or adult males.
- The ACS recommends a testicular examination as part of the physical examination and routine cancer-related checkup by the health care team.
- Men with risk factors may consider doing a monthly testicular self-examination.
- Men should promptly report a lump on the testicle to the health care team.
- Testicular self-examination instructions can be found in the box on this page.
- The surveillance of patients with testicular cancer varies based on clinical staging, treatment regimen, and tumor type. There are three main methods:
  - History and physical examinations
  - Abdominal and pelvic CT scans
  - Chest radiographs

- For seminomas, NCCN v2 (2022) recommends follow-up for with history and physical, abdominal or pelvic CT frequently in the first year, biannually in year 2 and 3 and annually thereafter.
- For nonseminomas, NCCN v2 (2022) recommends follow-up for with history and physical with tumor markers every 2 months for the first year, every 3 months in year 2, then biannually in years 3 and 4, then annually thereafter. It is also recommended to conduct imaging with abdominal and pelvic CT biannually in years 1 and 2, then annually thereafter. Chest imaging as clinically indicated.

Instructions for Testicular Self-Examination

- Self-examination should be done during or after a bath or shower, when the skin of the scrotum is relaxed.
- Check one testicle at a time, holding it between the thumbs and fingers of both hands and rolling it gently between the fingers.
- Look and palpate for lumps (i.e., hard, rounded, and smooth) or a change in the testicle's size, shape, or consistency.
- It is normal for testicles to vary slightly in size or for one to hang lower than the other. Each testicle has an epididymis that can feel like a small bump on the upper or middle outer side. It may be confused with an abnormal lump. Concerns should be reported to the health care team.
- A testicle can increase in size for reasons other than cancer. Hydroceles and varicoceles can sometimes cause swelling or lumps around the scrotum. Concerns should be discussed with the health care team.

Data from American Cancer Society. (2022). *Testicular cancer early detection, diagnosis, and staging*. Available at https://www.cancer.org/content/dam/CRC/PDF/Public/8845.00.pdf.

References

American Cancer Society (ACS). (2018). *Testicular cancer*. Available at https://www.cancer.org/cancer/testicular-cancer.html.

American Cancer Society (ACS). (2022). *Testicular cancer early detection, diagnosis, and staging*. Available at https://www.cancer.org/content/dam/CRC/PDF/Public/8845.00.pdf.

Amin, M. B., Edge, S., Greene, F., Byrd, D. R., Brookland, R. K., Washington, M. K., … Meyer, L. R. (Eds.). (2017). *AJCC cancer staging manual* (8th ed.). Springer.

Mead, G. M., & Stenning, S. P. (1997). The International Germ Cell Consensus Classification: A new prognostic factor-based staging classification for metastatic germ cell tumours. *Clinical Oncology (Royal College of Radiologists [Great Britain])*, 9(4), 207–209.

National Cancer Institute (NCI). (2022a). *Testicular cancer*. Available at https://www.cancer.gov/types/testicular.

National Cancer Institute (NCI). (2022b). *Testicular cancer treatment: Health professional*. Available at https://www.cancer.gov/types/testicular/hp/testicular-treatment-pdq.

National Comprehensive Cancer Network (NCCN). (2022). *Testicular cancer*. Available at https://www.nccn.org/professionals/physician_gls/pdf/testicular.pdf.

Pettersson, A., Richiardi, L., Nordenskjold, A., Kaijser, M., & Akre, O. (2007). Age at surgery for undescended testis and risk of testicular cancer. *New England Journal of Medicine, 356*, 1835–1841.

Gynecologic Cancers

Paula Anastasia

Cervical Cancer

Definition

The corpus cervix is the organ between the top of the vagina and the bottom of the uterus. Precancerous lesions usually begin as cervical intraepithelial neoplasia (CIN) or adenocarcinoma in situ, which can become invasive (American Cancer Society [ACS], 2022). Cervical cancer cells are most likely to arise at the transformation zone, where the glandular cells of the endocervix (opening of the cervix that leads to uterus) and the squamous cells of the exocervix (outer part of cervix) come together or merge (ACS, 2022).

The etiology is often due to human papillomavirus (HPV) infection, which accounts for more than 95% of cases (World Health Organization [WHO], 2022).

Most cervical cancers are slow growing and progress over 15 to 20 years, although for women who are immunocompromised, development may occur within 5 to 10 years (WHO, 2022). Carcinoma of the cervix has three main routes of spread:

- Direct extension to the uterus, vagina, parametria, bladder, or rectum
- Lymphatic spread
- Hematogenous spread to the lungs, liver, or bowel

Incidence

- According to the ACS (2022), about 14,100 new cases of cervical cancer and 4280 related deaths will occur in the United States in 2022.
- The average age at diagnosis is 50 years old.
- Minority and lower socioeconomic groups, including Latino, African Americans, native Americans, and Alaskan Natives, who do not have routine screening, have a higher incidence of cervical cancer.
- Globally, cervical cancer is the fourth most common cancer, and it is the fourth most common cancer-related death among women (WHO, 2022).
- Less developed countries have a greater incidence of cervical cancer.
- The incidence of cervical cancer is expected to continue to decline among women who receive the HPV vaccine (National Cancer Institute [NCI], 2022a).

Etiology and Risk Factors

- HPV infection is responsible for most cervical cancers. Other sexually transmitted contributing factors include herpes simplex virus 2 and chlamydia trachomatis. Although it is estimated that up to 80% of sexually active adults are exposed to the virus, most individuals clear the virus within 2 years.
  - More than 40 strains of *genital* HPV have been identified. Of those, 16, 18, 31, 33, 34, 35, 39, 45, 51, 52, 56, 58, 59, 66, 68, and 70 are high-risk HPV types. HPV 16 and 18 are responsible for more than half of cervical cancer cases (Centers for Disease Control and Prevention [CDC], 2021).
    - Globally, HPV 16 and 18 are attributed to 71% of cases, while HPV types 31, 33, 45, 52, and 58 account for 19% of cervical cancer cases (CDC, 2021).
- Many of the risk factors for cervical cancer are the same as those for sexually transmitted diseases (ACS, 2022).
  - Early age of sexual activity (<18 years).
  - Multiple sexual partners (>5).
  - Sexual partners who have had multiple partners.
  - Cigarette smoking.
  - Compromised immune system such as human immunodeficiency virus (HIV), organ transplant recipient, or autoimmune disorder.
  - Lower socioeconomic status due to potential lack of access to screening.
  - Long-term use of oral contraceptives (>5 years); risk decreases when oral contraceptives discontinued.
  - Diethylstilbestrol (DES) may increase risk for rare clear cell adenocarcinoma of cervix and vagina in the female offspring of women who took DES while pregnant.

Signs and Symptoms

(WHO, 2022)
- Presenting symptoms
  - New irregular or heavy bleeding
  - Bleeding after intercourse
  - Change in vaginal discharge to watery, mucous, purulent, or odorous fluid
- Late symptoms
  - Pain radiating to the flank or leg
  - Pelvic pressure and urinary changes such as hematuria
  - Vaginal hemorrhage and development of uremia

Diagnostic Work-up

(ACS, 2022)
- A pelvic examination should be performed for any woman with symptoms of cervical cancer.
- On speculum examination, the cervix may appear normal or have an obvious visible lesion.
- Cervical cytology or Papanicolaou testing (i.e., Pap smear) and HPV testing are used in combination for cervical cancer screening.

- Women with symptoms of cervical cancer or an abnormal Pap will undergo colposcopy of the cervix. A colposcope is a magnifying device for visualizing the cervix.
- If the cervix appears abnormal, biopsies of the cervix or endocervical canal are obtained.
- If the biopsies confirm a malignancy, a more comprehensive procedure such as a conization with or without a hysterectomy may be indicated.
- A bimanual pelvic and rectovaginal examination is required to assess the tumor size and vaginal or parametrial involvement.
- Imaging methods such as magnetic resonance imaging (MRI), computed tomography (CT), and positron emission tomography (PET) are used for staging.

Histopathology

- According to the National Comprehensive Cancer Network (NCCN, 2022), the most common histology is squamous cell carcinoma, which arise from the squamous epithelial cells, and represent more than 80% of cervical cancer. This includes both squamous cell carcinoma, HPV-associated, and HPV-independent.
- Adenocarcinomas, which originate from glandular cells, comprise close to 20% of tumors. There are subcategories of these glandular tumors including, adenocarcinoma, HPV-associated or HPV-independent, gastric type, endometrioid, and mucoepidermoid (Bhatla et al., 2021).
- These statistics are approximate calculations as there are rare histologies reported which include clear cell, germ cell tumors, adenosarcoma, primary sarcoma of the cervix, and a mix of squamous and adenocarcinoma cells called adenosquamous carcinoma (NCI, 2022a).

Clinical Staging

- Historically, cervical cancer was staged clinically because surgical staging was infrequent in developing countries where there is an increased incidence but fewer resources (Bhatla et al., 2018).
- Surgical staging for women with low-level disease and microinvasive disease may include fertility-sparing approaches or radical trachelectomy.
- Sentinel lymph node mapping remains controversial but may be useful in early-stage disease.
- The 2018 International Federation of Gynecology and Obstetrics (FIGO) staging system was revised to include the use of imaging and pathologic assessments. Several changes were made. A parallel tumor-node-metastasis (TNM) staging system is used by the American Joint Committee Commission on Cancer (AJCC).
- Microinvasive disease (stages IA1 and IA2 which are stromal invasion >3.0 mm but not >5.0 mm, with a horizontal spread ≤7.0 mm) is made on microscopic examination of cone biopsy specimen, obtained by loop electrosurgical excision procedures (LEEP) or cold knife conization, or on a trachelectomy or hysterectomy specimen (Bhatla et al., 2021).
- Stage I: cervical carcinoma confined to uterus. Tumor size has been stratified further into three subgroups: IB1 ≤2 cm, IB2 less than 2 to ≤4 cm, and IB3 greater than 4 cm.

- Stage II: Stage II cervical carcinoma invades beyond uterus but not to pelvic wall or to lower third of vagina. Stage IIA does not involve the parametrium, Stage IIA1 is lesion ≤4 cm/Stage IIA2 is lesion greater than 4 cm. Stage IIB has parametrial invasion.
- Stage IIIA: Tumor involves lower third of vagina, no extension to pelvic wall; however, IIIB extends to pelvic wall. Lymph node positivity, which correlates with poorer oncologic outcomes, assigns the case to stage IIIC—pelvic nodes IIIC1 and paraaortic nodes IIIC2. Micrometastases are included in stage IIIC.
- Stage IVA tumor invades mucosa of bladder or rectum or extends beyond true pelvis and Stage IIIB involves distant metastasis (Bhatla et al., 2019).

Treatment

Early-Stage Disease

- Early-stage cervical cancer includes all stage I and stage IIA disease.
- Primary treatment is surgery with a modified or radical hysterectomy; the need for adjuvant therapy depends on stage, grade, and carcinoma within the lymphatic and or blood vessels known as lymph-vascular space invasion (LSVI).
- Sentinel lymph node mapping may be considered for stage IB and IIA disease, usually in tumors that are 2 cm or less (NCCN, 2022).
- Fertility preservation approaches may be considered for select patients who have been counseled regarding disease risk and consultation with a reproductive endocrinology fertility specialist. After childbearing is complete, a hysterectomy may be recommended.
  - Conservative approaches to preserve fertility may include cold knife conization, LEEP, or trachelectomy.
    - A trachelectomy removes the cervix, parametrium, and upper 2 cm of the vagina. The uterus is left intact. A cerclage is placed to help maintain the pregnancy. Vaginal radical trachelectomy has been used in selected patients with lesions 2 cm or less (NCCN, 2022).
    - If a pregnancy goes to term, the baby is delivered by cesarean section.
- For women who no longer desire fertility, a hysterectomy is recommended. The choice of simple or modified radical hysterectomy with pelvic lymph node dissection depends on positive surgical margins and LVSI.
- No adjuvant therapy is indicated if lymph nodes, surgical margins, and parametria are negative.
- Adjuvant treatment for clinical IB3 or IIA2 tumors consists of external beam radiation and concurrent chemoradiation with a platinum-containing (cisplatin preferred) regimen

Advanced Stage Disease

- Advanced cervical cancer is defined as stage IIB to IVA disease, whereas IIB may be referred to locally advanced disease (Bhatla et al., 2021).
- Imaging studies such as PET and CT are recommended to confirm spread of disease.
- If needed, a needle biopsy or laparoscopic surgical staging of lymph nodes is performed.

- Recommended management of bulky tumors in select patients or advanced disease consists of pelvic external beam radiation therapy, and/or brachytherapy (e.g., internal intracavitary radiation therapy), concurrently with cisplatin chemotherapy in lieu of a hysterectomy.
- Controversy remains about whether a completion hysterectomy is required after external beam radiation therapy and concurrent chemotherapy. Studies show a decrease in the rate of pelvic recurrence but more morbidity and no overall survival benefit.

Recurrent or Metastatic Disease

- Patients with recurrent disease may be candidates for surgery, radiation therapy, or systemic therapy, depending on the extent of spread and prior treatment.
- Local recurrence after chemoradiation therapy may involve surgical intervention with an exenteration.
- Patients with distant metastasis at presentation or present with recurrent disease are usually given systemic therapy. Palliative radiation therapy may be indicated in situations such as bone metastasis or uncontrolled vaginal bleeding.

Radiation Therapy

- Adjuvant external beam radiation therapy is indicated for patients with stage IA to IIA disease who have tumor-negative lymph nodes after hysterectomy but have risk factors such as a large tumor ($\geq$4 cm) and LVSI. The radiation dose is approximately 45 cG.
- Vaginal cuff brachytherapy is recommended if there are positive vaginal margins.
- For patients with positive common iliac or paraaortic lymph nodes or bulky tumors, extended field radiation therapy up to the renal vessels is suggested, along with concurrent platinum-containing chemotherapy. Vaginal brachytherapy may also be recommended if positive vaginal margins exist.
- Brachytherapy (i.e., internal intracavitary radiation therapy) may be used for patients after hysterectomy and for patients with an intact cervix.
- Patient selection and radiation dose are determined by patient risk factors such as positive surgical margins.

Systemic Therapy

- The NCI issued an alert in 1999 recommending the use of concurrent chemotherapy (cisplatin-based) and radiation for patients with cervical cancer citing a survival advantage compared with radiation therapy alone (Nwachukwu et al., 2018).
- In five randomized phase III trials, four showed an overall survival advantage for concurrent cisplatin-based therapy and radiation, with the risk of death deceased by 30% to 50% in the combined approach.
- The NCI recommendation applied to women diagnosed with staged IB-IVA cervical cancer and women with stage IA and stage IIA who have metastatic disease in the pelvic lymph nodes, positive parametrial disease, or positive surgical margins.
- Chemoradiation therapy is usually given weekly while the patient is receiving daily radiation therapy.

- In addition to many platinum-based and non-platinum-based (cisplatin or carboplatin, and paclitaxel, with or without bevacizumab) chemotherapy agents approved for cervical cancer, Pembrolizumab in combination with chemotherapy for persistent, recurrent, or metastatic cervical cancer was approved in 2021 for patients whose tumors express PD-L1 (programmed death ligand). Pembrolizumab was also approved as a single agent in 2018 for patients with recurrent or metastatic cervical cancer with disease progression whose tumors express PD-L1. Other options include platinum combination with topotecan, topotecan combination with paclitaxel or taxane, fluorouracil, gemcitabine, pemetrexed, tisotumab vedotin, and larotrectinib or entrectinib for tumors that text positive for neurotropic tyrosine receptor kinase (NTRK) gene fusion.
- The FDA granted accelerated approval in 2021 for tisotumab vedotin-tftc, an antibody-drug conjugate directed to tissue factor, a protein highly prevalent in multiple solid tumors, including cervical cancer. This indication is for patients with recurrent or metastatic cervical cancer with disease progression on or after chemotherapy (Coleman et al., 2021).

Prognosis

(NCI, 2022b)

- The prognosis for patients with cervical cancers depends on the stage of disease, recurrence, and comorbid conditions.
- Women with HIV have more aggressive disease and a poorer prognosis.
- C-myc overexpression associated with squamous cell carcinoma have a poorer prognosis.
- Race and socioeconomic characteristics are relevant because of greater reference exposure to other risk factors and more advanced disease at diagnosis, which reduces likelihood of undergoing curative therapy.
- The 5-year relative survival rate is 66.5 % overall with survival for localized disease as high as 91.8%, and decreased survival for distant disease 17.6% (NCI, 2022b)

Prevention and Surveillance

Prevention

- Prevention includes healthy lifestyle choices, such as absence of smoking, limited sexual partners and/or condom use, vaccination against HPV, and screening Pap smears with co-testing HPV (ACS, 2022; NCCN, 2022; WHO, 2022).
- The HPV vaccine is FDA approved for both females and males aged 9 to 45.
  - 9-valent HPV (Gardasil9, 9vHPV) protects against 9 HPV types including types 16 and 18 that cause most HPV cancers. The other seven HPV types are 6, 11, 31, 33, 45, 52, and 58 (CDC, 2021; WHO, 2022).
- The American Cancer Society (2022) recommends administering HPV vaccine between ages 9 and 12 for best effectiveness, and it does not recommend HPV vaccination for people older than 26 years.

Screening

- Cervical cancer screening is less straightforward in the transgender community and currently the World

Profession Association of Transgender Health (WPATH) has no guidelines on cancer screening. Transmasculine patients who have their cervix should still follow ACS cervical cancer screening (Sterling & Garcia, 2020).

- U.S Preventive Services Task Force (2018) and The American College of Obstetricians and Gynecologists updated their guidelines in 2018 and 2021, respectively. They are similar to ACS guidelines but recommend cytology alone every 3 years for age 21 to 29. American Cancer Society (2022) Screening Guidelines for Cervical Cancer were updated in 2020 and recommend first cytology screening with HPV testing at age 25.
  - Women aged 25 to 65 may follow one of these guidelines:
    - Primary HPV testing every 5 years
    - HPV co-testing with a Pap test every 5 years
    - Pap test alone, every 3 years
  - After age 65, Pap testing may be discontinued if prior screening with HPV is negative, defined as two consecutive, negative primary HPV, or two negative co-tests, or three negative cytology in the previous 10 years, with the most recent negative test less than 5 years.
  - If one has had a hysterectomy (removal of uterus and cervix), screening (Pap smear, HPV) is no longer necessary, unless there is a history of CIN2 or more severe diagnosis, including cervical cancer. If the cervix is intact but the uterus has been removed, cervical cancer screening guidelines should continue (ACS, 2022).

Surveillance

(NCCN, 2022)

- Patients diagnosed with invasive cervical cancer should have a physical examination every 3 to 6 months by a gynecologic oncologist for 2 years and then yearly for the next 3 to 5 years.
- Cervical/vaginal cytology should be done at least annually.
- Imaging is usually indicated if patients have symptoms of recurrence (i.e., pelvic or back pain, vaginal discharge, persistent cough, or chest pain).
- Patient education includes lifestyle wellness choices, including maintaining a healthy weight, proper nutrition, smoking cessation, and safe sexual practices.
- Patients who have had brachytherapy may have cervical stenosis and may benefit from a vaginal dilator. Education should include sexual health, vaginal lubrication and moisturizers, and effects of hormonal changes.
- Ongoing surveillance and assessment of physical and psychosocial effects after cancer should include a multidisciplinary survivorship care plan.

References

American Cancer Society (ACS). (2022). *Cancer facts and figures 2022*. American Cancer Society.

Bhatla, N., Aoki, D., Sharma, N., & Sankaranarayanan, R. (2021). Cancer of the cervix uteri: 2021 update. *International Journal of Gynecology Obstetrics*, 155(1), 28–44.

Bhatla, N., Berek, J. S., Cuello Fredes, M., Denny, L. A., Grenman, S., Karunaratne, K., Kehoe, S. T, Konishi, I., Olawaiye, A. B., Prat, J., Sankaranarayanan, R., Brierley, J., Mutch, D., Querleu, D., Cibula, D., Quinn, M., … Natarajan, J. (2019). Revised FIGO staging for carcinoma of the cervix uteri. *International Journal of Gynaecology and Obstetrics: The Official Organ of the International Federation of Gynaecology and Obstetrics*, 145(1), 129–135.

Centers for Disease Control and Prevention. (2021). *Cancers associated with human papillomavirus, United States 2014–2018*. USCS Data Brief, no 26. US Department of Health and Human Services: Centers for Disease Control and Prevention.

Coleman, R. L., Lorusso, D., Gennigens, C., González-Martín, A., Randall, L., Cibula, D., Lund, B., Woelber, L., Pignata, S., Forget, F., Redondo, A., Vindeløv, S. D., Chen, M., Harris, J. R., Smith, M., Nicacio, L. V., Teng, M. S. L., Laenen, A., Rangwala, R., … Vergote, I. (2021). Efficacy and safety of tisotumab vedotin in previously treated recurrent or metastatic cervical cancer (innovaTV 204/GOG-3023/ENGOT-cx6): A multicentre, open-label, single-arm, phase 2 study. *Lancet Oncology*, 22(5), 609–619.

National Cancer Institute (NCI). (2022a). *Cervical cancer treatment-for health professionals (PDQ)*. https://www.cancer.gov/types/cervical/hp.

National Cancer Institute (NCI). (2022b). *SEER cancer stat facts: Cervical cancer, 2011–2017*. https://seer.cancer.gov/statfacts/html/cervix.html.

National Comprehensive Cancer Network (NCCN). (2022). *Clinical practice guidelines in oncology: Cervical cancer, version 1.2022*. https://www.nccn.org/professionals/physician_gls/pdf/cervical.pdf.

Nwachukwu, C. R., Mayadev, J., & Viswanathan, A. N. (2018). Concurrent chemoradiotherapy for stage IIIB cervical cancer-global impact through power. *JAMA Oncology*, 4(4), 514–515.

Sterling, J., & Garcia, M. M. (2020). Cancer screening in the transgender population: A review of current guidelines, best practices, and a proposed care model. *Translational Andrology and Urology*, 9(6), 2771–2785.

U.S. Preventive Services Task Force (USPSTF). (2018). Screening for cervical cancer. U.S Preventive Services Task Force Recommendation Statement. *Journal American Medical Association*, 320(7), 674–686. https://doi:10/100/jama.10897. and The American College of Obstetricians and Gynecologists updated their guidelines in 2021.

World Health Organization. (2022, February 22). *Cervical cancer*. https://www.who.int/news-room/fact-sheets/details/cervical-cancer.

Endometrial Cancer

Definition

Uterine carcinoma is often referred to as *endometrial cancer*. Endometrial cancer arises from the lining of the uterus and is most often confined to the body (corpus) of the uterus at the time of diagnosis. A small percentage of uterine carcinomas are sarcomas arising from endometrial glands and stroma or from the uterine muscle (e.g., leiomyosarcoma) (Siegel et al., 2022).

Incidence

(NCCN, 2022a)

- Endometrial carcinoma is the most common gynecologic malignancy, the fourth most common type of female cancer, and the sixth leading cause of female cancer–related death in the United States.
- According to the American Cancer Society, about 65,950 cases of endometrial cancer and 12,550 deaths will occur in the United States in 2022 (Siegel et al., 2022).
- Endometrial adenocarcinomas are the most common type (90%), with endometrial sarcomas accounting for 6% of all endometrial cancer cases in the United States.
- Endometrial cancer occurs most commonly in postmenopausal women, although 25% of cases occur before menopause, and 5% occur in patients younger than 40 years.
- The rates for new endometrial cancer statistics have not changed significantly over the past 10 years; however, mortality has increased 1% annually from 2015 to 2019.

- Researchers found that, from 2010 to 2017, deaths of women from all racial and ethnic groups from endometrial cancer increased 1.8% per year. Deaths from non-endometroid subtypes of uterine cancer, which are more aggressive, increased by 2.7% per year. Endometrioid cancer mortality rates were stable during this period. Black women had more than twice the rate of deaths from uterine cancer overall and of non-endometrioid subtypes compared with other racial and ethnic groups.

Etiology and Risk Factors

(ACS, 2022a)

- The incidence of endometrial cancer is higher in Western than Eastern countries.
- In the United States, more Black women than White women will be diagnosed, and have a higher incidence of dying from endometrial cancer (ACS, 2022b; Clarke et al., 2022; Siegel et al., 2022).
- Several factors increase the risk of endometrial carcinoma:
  - Unopposed estrogens
  - Obesity
    - Hypertension and type 2 diabetes may be a result of obesity and contribute to endometrial cancer risks
  - Nulliparity
  - Polycystic ovarian syndrome
  - Late onset menopause
  - Complex endometrial hyperplasia
  - Use of tamoxifen
- Lynch syndrome (e.g., hereditary nonpolyposis colorectal cancer) is caused by inherited pathogenic variant in one or more of the DNA mismatch repair genes *MLH1, MSH2, MSH6,* and *PMS2.*
  - According to the NCCN (2022b) patients with Lynch syndrome have up to 60% lifetime risk of endometrial cancer compared with the general population. For example, patients with PMS2 pathogenic variant have a 13% to 26% cumulative risk and patients with MSH6 have a 16% to 49% cumulative risk by age 80.
  - The syndrome also predisposes people to other cancers, including colon, ovarian, stomach, small intestine, and hepatobiliary cancers.
  - Genetic counseling and testing for Lynch syndrome should be considered for women with endometrial cancer who are diagnosed younger than age 50 or who have synchronous endometrial cancer and Lynch syndrome–associated cancers.
  - Relevant family history includes one or more first-degree relatives with Lynch syndrome–associated cancer and one member diagnosed before the age of 50 years.
  - Another identifier is endometrial or colorectal cancer diagnosed at any age in two or more first- or second-degree relatives with Lynch syndrome.

Signs and Symptoms

- The most common sign of endometrial cancer is abnormal vaginal bleeding.

- Vaginal bleeding in a postmenopausal woman or abnormal or prolonged menses in a premenopausal woman is usually what prompts a visit to the gynecologist and is the rationale why endometrial cancer is frequently diagnosed at an early stage.
- Signs and symptoms of advanced disease:
  - Pelvic pressure
  - Urinary changes
  - Leg swelling
  - Vaginal bleeding
  - Shortness of breath
  - Other symptoms indicating uterine enlargement or extrauterine tumor spread

Diagnostic Work-up

(NCCN, 2022a)

- Women with possible endometrial cancer should have a pelvic examination to evaluate the size and mobility of the uterus.
- Ultrasound may provide additional information such as thickness of the uterine lining or other causes of bleeding such as a uterine myoma.
- The standard procedure to diagnose endometrial carcinoma is endometrial sampling, although there is a 10% false-negative rate. Assessment often can be done in the office setting.
- Patients who are symptomatic and have a negative office biopsy require fractional dilation and curettage (D&C).
- A hysteroscopy may be helpful in identifying a polyp as the cause of bleeding.
- Imaging such as CT or MRI may assist in determining extrauterine spread.

Histopathology

(NCCN, 2022a; NCI, 2022)

- Endometrial carcinomas are divided into two categories.
  - Type 1 is associated with unopposed estrogen stimulation and may arise from complex, atypical hyperplasia.
  - Type 2 is not associated with unopposed estrogen and most likely develops from atrophic endometrium.
- Endometrioid carcinoma, composed of malignant glandular epithelial components, represents 75% to 80% of endometrial carcinomas, including subtypes such as ciliated, secretory, villoglandular, and adenocarcinoma with squamous differentiation.
- Uterine papillary serous and clear cell histologic types represent 10% and 4%, respectively, of endometrial carcinomas and have a worse prognosis than other types.

Clinical Staging

- Disease stage is often the single strongest predictor of outcome for women with endometrial adenocarcinoma.
- FIGO staging guidelines were updated in 2017 (see the table on the next page).
- Risk factors include older age, LVSI, size of tumor, and cervical and glandular involvement.
- Other unfavorable risk factors include high-grade tumors, myometrial invasion greater than 50%, and clear cell or serous histology.

International Federation of Gynecology and Obstetrics (FIGO) Classification of Endometrial Carcinoma

Stage	Definition
I	Tumor limited to uterus
IA	Tumor limited to endometrium or invades <50% of myometrium
IB	Tumor invades ≥50% myometrium
II	Tumor invades stromal connective tissue of cervix and is confined to uterus
III	Tumor involves serosa, vagina, and/or adnexa
IIIA	Tumor involves serosa and/or adnexa (direct extension or metastasis)
	Positive cytology does not change stage
IIIB	Tumor involves the vagina or parametrial
IIIC	Tumor metastases to pelvic and/or paraaortic lymph nodes
IIIC1	Positive pelvic nodes
IIIC	Positive paraaortic lymph nodes with or without positive pelvic lymph nodes
IV	Tumor invades bladder or bowel mucosa and/or distant metastases
IVA	Tumor invasion of bladder and or bowel mucosa
IVB	Distant metastasis

Adapted from Koskas, M., Amant, F., Mirza, M. R., & Creutzberg, C. L. (2021). Cancer of the corpus uteri: 2021 update. *International Journal of Gynecology Obstetrics, 155*(51), 45–60.

Treatment

(NCCN, 2022a)

- The standard treatment is a total hysterectomy and bilateral salpingo-oophorectomy unless the patient is a candidate for fertility-sparing options.
- The procedures can be performed minimally invasive through various approaches (laparoscopic, robotic, vaginal, or abdominal) and determined by patient factors and physician preferences.
- Pelvic and paraaortic lymph nodes are assessed for nodal metastasis and usually lymphadenectomy for high-risk patients. Sentinel lymph node mapping is done in select cases and in institutions with expertise in procedure.
- Biomarkers postoperative that may assist with treatment decisions include tumor testing for dMMR, MSI, Her2Neu, and programmed death ligand (PD-L1).
- Postoperative treatment is determined by stage, grade, tumor type, LVSI, and myometrial invasion.
- Adjuvant treatment with radiation therapy is determined by risk and site of recurrence, and methods may include external beam radiation therapy or brachytherapy, or both.
- Vaginal brachytherapy is often recommended for patients with tumors confined to the uterus, or in palliative situations.
- Patients with uterine confined disease, or advanced disease without extrauterine disease and not appropriate for surgery, may be treated with external beam radiation with or without brachytherapy. Hormonal therapy may also be recommended.
- Patients who have advanced disease unlikely to be optimally resected, such as nodal, bowel or bladder involvement are usually referred for external beam radiation, with or without brachytherapy and systemic therapy. The goal is to reduce tumor burden and reevaluate for surgical resection. If surgery is not an option, palliative approaches are considered.

- Standard of care systemic therapy is carboplatin and paclitaxel. The addition of bevacizumab may also be considered in metastatic settings. Other options include platinum-based combination with a taxane, or doxorubicin. Single agents may include a platinum, doxorubicin or liposomal doxorubicin, a taxane, topotecan, or temsirolimus.

Recurrent Disease

(ACS, 2022a; NCCN, 2022a)

- The treatment for recurrent endometrial cancer depends on the anatomic site and whether local or regional spread has occurred.
- Systemic therapy for recurrent disease may include platinum-based combination with a taxane, or doxorubicin. Single agents may include a platinum, doxorubicin or liposomal doxorubicin, a taxane, topotecan, or temsirolimus.
- For patients with serous histology and Her2neu positive disease, trastuzumab in addition to carboplatin and paclitaxel is preferred.
- Immunotherapy, such as pembrolizumab, nivolumab, avelumab, or dostarlimab, is an option for recurrent disease for patients whose tumors have mismatch repair deficient (dMMR) or microsatellite instability-high (MSI-H). The combination of pembrolizumab and lenvatinib, an oral kinase inhibitor, is FDA approved in the recurrent setting for patients whose tumor has intact MMR genes, or MSI stable (Makker et al., 2020).
- Hormonal therapies, such as progestin, tamoxifen, megestrol, or aromatase inhibitors are options for treating recurrent or metastatic disease. The oral combination of everolimus and letrozole is a treatment option for endometroid histology.

Prognosis

- Prognosis and survival for most women with early-stage disease is excellent with appropriate intervention.
- The overall 5-year survival rate for endometrial cancer is 84% in white women and 63% for Black women. Close to half (44%) of endometrial cancers in Black women are diagnosed at an advanced stage (or are unstaged), compared to 29% in White women (ACS, 2022b). Survival is lower for Black women for every stage of diagnosis.
- More than 70% of cases are diagnosed at an early stage, for which the 5-year relative survival rate is 94.9%. For those with regional spread to lymph nodes, the 5-year relative survival rate is 69.8% (NCI, 2022)
- Grade of tumor and depth of invasion are important prognostic considerations.

Prevention and Surveillance

(ACS, 2022a; NCCN, 2022a; NCCN, 2022b)

Prevention

- All women at menopause should be informed about the risks and symptoms of endometrial cancer.
- Women who have a history of breast cancer and are prescribed tamoxifen should be educated about their risk of endometrial cancer and should notify the physician if abnormal bleeding occurs.

- Patients who are on estrogen replacement therapy with an intact uterus should be counseled about using combination estrogen and progestin therapy.
- Women with Lynch syndrome should have an annual screening with an endometrial biopsy beginning at 30 to 35 years of age or 10 years before the age of the first family member diagnosed with endometrial cancer.
- Approximately 5% of women with endometrial cancer have a germline pathogenic variant for Lynch syndrome. Genetic counseling and testing should be considered for women younger than age 50, and/or family history of endometrial and/or colorectal cancer (NCCN, 2022b).

Surveillance
(NCCN, 2022a)

- Patients diagnosed with endometrial cancer should have physical examinations every 3 to 6 months by a gynecologic oncologist for 2 years and then yearly for the next 3 to 5 years. In patients with advanced, extrauterine disease, or serous histology, a serum CA125 blood test if initially elevated, may be helpful in monitoring clinical response (NCCN, 2022a).
- Pap smears are no longer performed unless an abnormality is visualized.
- Imaging is usually indicated if patients have symptoms of recurrence (e.g., pelvic or back pain, vaginal discharge, persistent cough, chest pain).
- Patient education includes healthy wellness choices, including increased cardiovascular activities, and maintaining more plant-based food choices to prevent obesity. Support groups and referral to a weight loss specialist may be of interest to patients.
- Women with endometrial cancer should be counseled about the risks and benefits of hormone replacement.
- Patients who have had brachytherapy may have cervical stenosis and may benefit from use of a vaginal dilator. Ongoing open discussion about sexual health is recommended.
- Coordination of care among health care providers and well woman surveillance, including breast and colon health, can improve survival outcomes and cost-effective practices.

References

American Cancer Society (ACS). (2022a). *Cancer facts and figures 2022.* American Cancer Society.

American Cancer Society (ACS). (2022b). *Cancer facts & figures for African American/Black People 2022–2024.* American Cancer Society.

Clarke, M. A., Devesa, S. S., Hammer, A., & Wentzensen, N. (2022). Racial and ethnic differences in hysterectomy-corrected uterine corpus cancer mortality by stage and histologic subtype. *JAMA Oncology, 8*(6), 895–903.

National Cancer Institute (NCI). (2022). *Endometrial cancer treatment-for health professionals (PDQ).* https://www.cancer.gov/types/uterine/hp.

National Comprehensive Cancer Network (NCCN). (2022a). *Clinical practice guidelines in oncology: Uterine neoplasms version 1.2022.* https://www.nccn.org/professionals/physician_gls/pdf/uterine.pdf.

National Comprehensive Cancer Network (NCCN). (2022b). *Clinical practice guidelines in oncology: Genetic/Familial High-Risk Assessment: Breast, Ovarian, and Pancreatic, version 2.2022.* https://www.nccn.org/professionals/physician_gls/pdf/genetics_bop.pdf.

Koskas, M., Amant, F., Mirza, M. R., & Creutzberg, C. L. (2021). Cancer of the corpus uteri: 2021 update. *International Journal of Gynecology Obstetrics, 15*(51), 45–60.

Makker, V., Taylor, M. H., Aghajanian, C., Oaknin, A., Mier, J., Cohn, A. L., Romeo, M., Bratos, R., Brose, M. S., DiSimone, C., Messing, M., Stepan, D. E., Dutcus, C. E., Wu, J., Schmidt, E. V., Orlowski, R., Sachdev, P., Shumaker, R., & Casado Herraez, A. (2020). Lenvatinib plus pembrolizumab in patients with advanced endometrial cancer. *Journal of Clinical Oncology, 38*(26). 2981–2892.

Siegel, R. L., Miller, K. D., Fuchs, H. E., & Jemal, A. (2022). Cancer statistics, 2022. *CA: A Cancer Journal for Clinicians, 72*(1), 7–33.

Ovarian Cancer

Definition

Ovarian cancer is the fifth leading cause of cancer-related death among women in the United States. Fallopian tube carcinoma (FTC) and primary peritoneal carcinoma (PPC) are separate but similar diseases, and they are usually included in statistical and treatment data when referring to epithelial ovarian cancer (EOC). It is now accepted that the origin of the majority of EOC and PPC may have started in the fallopian tube. Serous tubal intraepithelial carcinoma (STIC) is the genesis of most high-grade serous EOC or FTC (National Cancer Comprehensive Network [NCCN], 2022a).

Incidence

- According to the American Cancer Society (ACS, 2022) as many as 19,880 women will be diagnosed with ovarian cancer and 12,810 will die of their disease in the United States.
- Ovarian cancer is the most fatal of the gynecologic malignancies because it is typically diagnosed in an advanced stage due to lack of effective screening modalities (National Cancer Institute [NCI], 2022b).
- The majority of patients who undergo optimal surgical debulking and combination platinum-based therapy will achieve a remission, despite advanced stage at diagnosis.
- Although the rate of cure has not improved, survival times have increased as a result of better surgical and medical management and more effective systemic therapy.

Etiology and Risk Factors
(ACS, 2022)

- The most important risk factor for EOC is a family history of the disease, especially if two or more first-degree relatives have EOC.
- Epidemiologic studies have identified endocrine, environmental, and genetic factors as important in the development of ovarian cancer.
- Epidemiologically established risk factors include the following (ACS, 2022; NCI, 2022a):
  - Nulliparity
  - Family history
  - Deleterious germline mutation or pathogenic variant (e.g., *BRCA1, BRCA2, RAD51C, RAD51D, BRIP1, PALB2, ATM,* and Lynch syndrome)
  - Early menarche and late menopause
  - Endometriosis
  - Increasing age (average age at diagnosis of 63 years)
  - Obesity as a risk factor has shown inconsistent cause and effect
  - Smoking is associated with mucinous carcinoma of the ovary.

- Women who are nulligravida and have used fertility medications may have an increased risk of ovarian cancer.
- The use of hormone replacement therapy, especially with a combination of estrogen and progesterone, may increase a woman's risk.
- Hereditary ovarian cancer attributed to a pathogenic variant in the *BRCA1* and *BRCA2* genes accounts for up to 15% of ovarian cancer cases (NCCN, 2022b). These genes are normally involved in repair of mistakes in DNA that occur during cell division.
  - The cumulative lifetime risk of developing ovarian cancer in a woman with a germline *BRCA1* (gBRCA1) pathogenic variant is 48.3% and 20 % for carriers of a germline *BRCA2* (gBRCA2) pathogenic variant by age 70.
  - Other cancers associated with g*BRCA1* pathogenic variants include breast cancer in women, and prostate cancer in men.
  - *gBRCA2* pathogenic variant are associated with male and female breast cancer, melanoma, pancreatic cancer, and prostate cancer in men.
  - Ashkenazi Jewish ancestry have a higher likelihood of pathogenic variants in the *BRCA1* and BRCA2 gene than other groups.

Signs and Symptoms

Development of early-stage ovarian cancer rarely causes symptoms. Later-stage ovarian cancer manifests as nonspecific symptoms that may mimic benign conditions such as constipation or irritable bowel. Women usually do not recognize these as serious until disease has become advanced. Common symptoms of ovarian cancer include (Goff et al., 2007; NCCN, 2022a):

- Bloating or increased abdominal girth
- Urinary changes such as urgency or frequency
- Abdominal or pelvic discomfort
- Difficulty eating or early satiety

Any of these symptoms that are persistent for 2 or more weeks suggest a need for clinical assessment.

Diagnostic Work-up

- The diagnosis of ovarian cancer is often a series of steps beginning with a history and physical, and confirmation of a tissue biopsy or cytology (ACS, 2022; NCCN, 2022a). A bimanual pelvic examination is necessary, but although a pelvic examination may not be helpful in cases of early-stage disease or upper abdominal disease.
- Transvaginal ultrasound may show an abnormal pelvic mass or ascites, prompting further imaging with CT or MRI.
- The OVA1 blood test is used as a triage test for patients with an adnexal mass, and an elevated result should prompt practitioners to recognize that a referral to a gynecologic oncologist is warranted. It is not recommended as a screening test for ovarian cancer (NCCN, 2022a).
- The cancer antigen 125 (CA125) blood test biomarker is nonspecific. Levels may be elevated in nongynecologic cancers; therefore, the test should not be used as a screening modality. However, a confirmed diagnosis of EOC and an elevated CA125 test result may serve as a useful marker to evaluate treatment response (NCI, 2022a).
- Patients with advanced disease may have increased abdominal girth and ascites at presentation, suggesting a need for paracentesis and cytology to confirm the diagnosis.
- Symptoms such as shortness of breath consistent with a pleural effusion may also lead to diagnostic confirmation by thoracentesis and cytology.
- If a gynecologic malignancy is suspected, surgical intervention should be performed by a gynecologic oncologist, as opposed to a general surgeon (NCCN, 2022a).
- It is recommended that all women with a confirmed diagnosis of ovarian cancer, regardless of family history, have multi-gene testing to rule out a gBRCA1 or 2 (ASCO, 2020).

Histopathology

- EOC encompasses a group of diseases (e.g., FTC, primary peritoneal cancer) that have different molecular behaviors. Ovarian cancer is not a single disease. EOC, which arises from cells that line or cover the ovaries, represents 90% of ovarian cancers. Less common histopathologic types include low-malignant-potential or borderline tumors, germ cell tumors, adenocarcinomas, sarcomas, and sex cord–stromal tumors.
- EOC has four main subtypes including serous, endometrioid, clear cell, and mucinous carcinomas. Serous tumors are classified as high grade or low grade, with high grade being the most common (NCCN, 2022a).
- EOC histology consistent with high grade serous is more likely to be associated with carriers of a germline BRCA pathogenic variant than other histology (NCCN, 2022b).
- The cancers may arise from lesions that originated in the fimbriae of the fallopian tubes rather than the surface of the ovary. They are often referred to as *extrauterine adenocarcinomas of müllerian epithelial origin.*
- Clear cell and endometrioid EOCs are often associated with endometriosis and have different molecular profiles from serous carcinomas.
- Endometrioid cell types can be seen in patients with Lynch syndrome.
- Synchronous uterine carcinoma and EOC are seen in 15% to 20% of patients with endometrioid-type tumors.
- Mucinous subtypes may account for up to 15% of EOCs, but 80% of them are benign or borderline tumors.

Clinical Staging

- The FIGO system is used for staging EOC, FTC, and PPC, throughout the world. This was approved by the AJCC. The AJCC classification uses the TNM system for ovarian cancer, epithelial ovarian, fallopian tube, and primary peritoneal cancers are categorized as one disease, although the recommendations call for designating the primary site when possible.
- Aside from select group of patients diagnosed with stage I, grade 1 ovarian tumors, of which survival is over 90%, most patients will require surgical intervention and systemic treatment (NCCN, 2022a).

- Stage I disease will have tumor limited to one of both ovaries. Subcategories of stage I will be determined by ovarian rupture and positive cytology.
- Stage II disease involves one or both ovaries with or without pelvic implants.
- Stage III involves one or both ovaries or tubes or primary peritoneal cancer with microscopically confirmed peritoneal metastasis outside the pelvis or lymph nodes. Size and extent of peritoneal metastasis and retroperitoneal nodes will determine if stage III A-C.
- Stage IV includes distant spread, with or without peritoneal metastases, positive pleural washings, or distant spread to extra-abdominal organs and lymph nodes (AJCC, 2017).

Treatment

(NCCN, 2022a)

- Primary treatment for stage II through IV ovarian cancer involves surgical cytoreductive staging, including hysterectomy, bilateral salpingo-oophorectomy, possible omentectomy, and pelvic and paraaortic lymph node dissection.
- Overall survival is improved for women who have complete surgical debulking to no residual disease (R0) by a gynecologic oncologist. Histology and grade are helpful prognostic indicators.
- Women who present with large bulky disease, who may not achieve upfront optimal surgical success, are offered neoadjuvant systemic therapy followed by interval cytoreductive surgery and additional systemic therapy.
- In select situations, hyperthermic intraperitoneal chemotherapy (HIPEC) is considered at the time of interval debulking surgery, for patients with stage III disease after receiving neoadjuvant chemotherapy. Adjuvant chemotherapy is still warranted postoperatively.
- Chemotherapy with a taxane and platinum-based drug is the standard of care. The addition of bevacizumab may be used depending on patient factors such as ascites, pleural effusion, or large bulky disease.
- Among women with stage III ovarian cancer, an increased overall survival time of 16 months was demonstrated for those receiving intraperitoneal cisplatin and paclitaxel.
- For women with stage I or early disease, management may remove only one ovary. Adjuvant chemotherapy with three to six cycles of a taxane and platinum-based drug is indicated after surgery.
- For patients with stage I disease who desire fertility, referral to a reproductive, endocrinology and infertility specialty should be included in the treatment plan. It is possible for the unaffected ovary and/or uterus to remain intact, thus allowing for future assisted reproductive approaches.
- Patients with advanced ovarian, fallopian tube, or PPC who have undergone complete surgical staging and systemic chemotherapy should be recommended maintenance therapy.
- Maintenance therapy is becoming a standard of care option for stage III or IV cancer; however, it is not unreasonable for select patients with stage II disease to be considered for maintenance medication.
- It is recommended that patients who received bevacizumab in upfront setting with combination taxane and platinum continue bevacizumab as a maintenance therapy. Patients who receive bevacizumab upfront, and have a gBRCA1 or 2 pathogenic variant, may receive a maintenance parp inhibitor added concurrently with bevacizumab (Harter et al., 2022).
- Maintenance therapy with a parp inhibitor is indicated for patients in complete or partial remission following surgery and systemic therapy. The choice of parp inhibitor is determined by patient biomarkers including gBRCA1 or 2 pathogenic variant, and somatic tumor biomarkers.

Recurrent Disease

- More than 70% of patients with advanced ovarian cancer will have a recurrence (ACS, 2022; NCCN, 2022a). Long-term survival is achievable, especially in patients with platinum-sensitive disease.
- EOC that recurs more than 6 months after primary chemotherapy is referred to as platinum-sensitive disease, for which there are many treatment options. These women have a better prognosis than patients who have recurrent disease less than 6 months after primary systemic therapy.
- There are several options for platinum-sensitive disease (NCCN, 2022a; Tew et al., 2020).
  - Systemic platinum-based combination with any of the following:
    - Taxane-based therapy
    - Gemcitabine
    - Pegylated liposomal doxorubicin (PLD)
    - Bevacizumab added to one of the platinum-based combinations
- Other options for recurrent disease include a parp inhibitor such as niraparib, olaparib, or rucaparib.
- The patient's residual side effects from prior therapy, biomarker status such as germline, or somatic mutations may influence decision choices.
- Immunotherapy, such as pembrolizumab or dostarlimab, is an option for recurrent platinum-sensitive disease for patients whose tumors have mismatch repair deficient (dMMR) or microsatellite instability-high (MSI-H).
- Surgical intervention may be indicated if the patient recurs more than 6 months since prior therapy and has small, localized area of disease. Systemic therapy would be necessary postoperatively.
- When EOC, FTC, or PPC recurs less than 6 months after platinum-based chemotherapy, it is defined as platinum-resistant disease, whereas disease progression while currently receiving first-line therapy is defined as platinum refractory disease.
- For women with platinum-resistant or platinum-refractory disease, switching to a non-platinum therapy is recommended. The average response rate is less than 20%.
- There are several options for platinum-resistant disease including (NCCN, 2022a):
  - PLD with or without bevacizumab
  - Weekly paclitaxel, with or without bevacizumab

- Topotecan
- Docetaxel
- Gemcitabine
- Pemetrexed
- Oral etoposide
- Hormonal therapy
- Immunotherapy
- Parp inhibitor
- The choice of systemic therapy for patients with platinum-resistant or platinum-refractory disease is based on the side effect profile and the patient's toxicity experience from previous chemotherapy. The patient's performance status, renal and hepatic function, and patient's goals of care must also be considered.
- The role of radiation therapy for women with recurrent ovarian cancer is not commonly used; however, it may be recommended for an isolated tumor or for palliative symptom relief (NCI, 2022a).
- Clinical trials should be considered for patients with recurrent disease, regardless of the standard of care options.

Prognosis

(NCCN, 2022a)

- Survival outcomes are improved with complete surgical staging to R0 and is performed by a gynecologic oncologist in a high-volume facility (Bristow et al., 2014).
- Favorable prognostic factors of EOC:
  - Early stage
  - Younger age at diagnosis
  - Well-differentiated tumor
  - Serous histology
  - Optimally debulked tumor to no visible disease
- The 5-year survival rate for patients with EOC correlates with tumor stage. Five-year survival rates diminish greatly with advancing disease stage.
- According to the NCI (2022b), the 5-year survival rate for ovarian cancer increased from 33% to 48% among non-Hispanic White women but decreased from 44% to 41% in Black women between the years 1975 and 2016.
- Overall 5-year relative survival rates for women diagnosed with EOC is 49.7% (NCI, 2022b).
- Patients with early or local disease have a 5-year survival rate of 93.1%; however, only about 17% of ovarian cancers are diagnosed at a local stage (NCI, 2022b).
- Palliative care improves quality of life for patients with advanced disease.

Prevention and Surveillance

Prevention

There are no effective early detection methods to prevent ovarian cancer, but epidemiologically established factors that decrease the risk of EOC include the following (ACS, 2022; NCCN, 2022a):

- Younger age (<25 years) at first pregnancy and first birth.
- Breastfeeding.
- Use of oral contraceptives for 5 or more years.

- Women with a gBRCA1 or 2 deleterious mutation are recommended to undergo risk reducing surgery with a bilateral salpingo-oophorectomy.
- For premenopausal women who have not completed childbearing, a bilateral salpingectomy may be considered, and a completion bilateral oophorectomy when childbearing is completed.
- Referral to a reproductive endocrinologist (REI) specialist for egg harvesting and assisted reproductive technologies should be done before risk reducing surgery.

Surveillance

(NCCN, 2022a)

- Women who have completed primary therapy should be evaluated by their gynecologic oncologist or medical oncologist every 3 months for 2 years, every 3 to 6 months for 3 years, and annually after 5 years.
- CA125, if elevated at time of diagnosis is obtained, every 3 months. A complete blood count and chemistry panel are obtained as clinically indicated.
- Imaging with chest, abdomen, pelvic CT or combination PET/CT is recommended if suspected signs of recurrence.
- Pap smears are no longer indicated for ovarian cancer surveillance.
- Coordination of care among health care providers and well-woman surveillance can improve survival outcomes and cost-effective practices.
- Women who have a germline pathogenic variant should have their recommended screening surveillance (e.g., breast MRI, mammography) to prevent secondary hereditary malignancies (NCCN, 2022b).

References

American Cancer Society (ACS). (2022). *Cancer facts and figures 2022.* American Cancer Society.

American Joint Committee on Cancer. (2017). Ovary, fallopian tube, and primary peritoneal carcinoma. In M. B. Amin, S. B. Edge, F. L. Greene, et al. (Eds.), *AJCC Cancer Staging Manual* (8th ed., pp. 689–698). American College of Surgeons.

American Society of Clinical Oncology (ASCO). (2020). *ASCO guidelines for Germline and somatic tumor testing in epithelial ovarian cancer.* https://www.asco.org/sites/new-www.asco.org/files/content-files/practice-and-guidelines/documents/2020-Germline-Somatic-Testing-OvCa-Summary-Table.pdf.

Bristow, R. E., Chang, J., Ziogas, A., Randall, L. M., & Anton-Culver, H. (2014). High-volume ovarian cancer care: Survival impact and disparities in access for advanced-stage disease. *Gynecologic Oncology, 132*(2), 403–410.

Goff, B. A., Mandel, L., Drescher, C. W., Urban, N., Gough, S., Schurman, K. M., et al. (2007). Development of an ovarian cancer symptom index: Possibilities for earlier detection. *Cancer, 109*(2), 221–227.

Harter, P., Mouret-Reynier, M. A., Pignata, S., Cropet, C., González-Martín, A., Bogner, G., Fujiwara, K., Vergote, I., Colombo, N., Nøttrup, T. J., Floquet, A., El-Balat, A., Scambia, G., Alia, E. M. G., Fabbro, M., Schmalfeldt, B., Hardy-Bessard, A.-C., Runnebaum, I., Pujade-Lauraine, E., & Ray-Coquard, I. (2022). Efficacy of maintenance olaparib plus bevacizumab according to clinical risk in patients with newly diagnosed, advanced ovarian cancer in the phase III PAOLA-1/ENGOT-ov25 trial. *Gynecologic Oncology, 164*(2), 254–264.

National Cancer Institute (NCI). (2022a). *Ovarian epithelial, fallopian tube, and primary peritoneal cancer treatment—Health professional version.* https://www.cancer.gov/types/ovarian/hp.

National Cancer Institute (NCI). (2022b). *SEER cancer stat facts: Ovarian cancer, 2011–2017.* https://seer.cancer.gov/statfacts/html/ovary.html.

National Comprehensive Cancer Network (NCCN) (2022a). *NCCN clinical practice guidelines in oncology: Ovarian cancer, fallopian tube cancer, and primary peritoneal cancer, version 1.2022.* https://www.nccn.org/professionals/physician_gls/pdf/ovarian.pdf.

National Comprehensive Cancer Network (NCCN). (2022b). *NCCN clinical practice guidelines in oncology: Genetic/Familial High Risk Assessment: Breast, ovarian cancer, and pancreatic cancer, version 2.2022.* https://www.nccn.org/professionals/physician_gls/pdf/genetics_bop.pdf.

Tew, W. P., Lacchetti, C., Ellis, A., Maxian, K., Banerjee, S., Bookman, M., Jones, M. B., Lee, J.-M., Lheureux, S., Liu, J. F., Moore, K. N., Muller, C., Rodriguez, P., Walsh, C., Westin, S. N., & Kohn, E. C. (2020). PARP inhibitors in the management of ovarian cancer: ASCO guidelines. *Journal of Clinical Oncology, 38*(30), 3468–3493.

Vaginal Cancer

Definition

Primary vaginal cancer is rare. Metastatic disease to the vagina due to direct extension from the cervix or endometrium is more common. Due to the proximity of the vagina and the cervix, vaginal cancer that originates at the apex and involves the cervix may be classified as cervical cancer subsequently underestimating the reported number of vaginal cancers.

Incidence

(ACS, 2022)

- Vaginal cancer represents only 1% of all female genital tract malignancies.
- It is estimated in 2022 that there will be 8870 new cases of vaginal cancer and 1630 deaths in the United States due to vaginal cancer (ACS, 2022).
- Squamous cell carcinoma represents 85% of cases; other less common types include melanoma, sarcoma, and adenocarcinoma.
- The mean age at diagnosis is 60 years, although the disease can be present in women as young as 20 or 30 years of age.

Etiology and Risk Factors

(Adams et al., 2021; NCI, 2022)

- More than 70% of vaginal cancers are associated with HPV infection, and the risk factors are similar to those for cervical cancer (e.g., multiple sexual partners, cigarette smoking).
- Women who have a history of precancerous cells known as vaginal intraepithelial neoplasia (VAIN) are at a higher risk.
- Diethylstilbestrol (DES) may increase risk for rare clear cell adenocarcinoma of cervix and vagina in the female offspring of women who took DES while pregnant.
- The use of DES in pregnant women was commonly prescribed between 1940 and 1971 to prevent miscarriages. Women with a known exposure to DES should be screened for vaginal cancer.
- Women with a history of a gynecologic malignancy are at risk for a vaginal cancer metastasis, or secondary vaginal cancer. In rare cases, a primary vaginal cancer occurs without having spread from another site.

Signs and Symptoms

- Vaginal cancer is slow growing. Many women with vaginal cancer have no symptoms, but the cancer may manifest as a mass or lesion on a routine gynecologic examination or be confirmed on a Pap smear.
- Vaginal bleeding is the most common patient reported symptom.
- Postcoital spotting, irregular or postmenopausal bleeding, and dysuria are associated symptoms.
- Pelvic pain and enlarged inguinal nodes are late symptoms that are usually related to tumor extension beyond the vagina.

Diagnostic Work-up

- Patients with a suspected vaginal malignancy should undergo a thorough physical examination with speculum inspection.
- The posterior wall of the upper one-third of the vagina is the most common site of primary vaginal carcinoma.
- The lesion may appear as a mass or an ulcer.
- A biopsy is usually attainable in the clinic/office setting. When the vagina is stenosed, an examination and biopsy under anesthesia may be required.
- Other physical assessments include palpating the groin for enlarged lymph nodes.
- Imaging, such as CT scan, MRI, or PET scan, may be recommended to evaluate lymphadenopathy or other possible involvement.

Histopathology

- Most primary vaginal carcinomas are squamous cell neoplasms and occur in women after menopause.
- Adenocarcinomas (e.g., clear cell) can occur in women in their 20s.
- Melanoma is uncommon but occurs in women in the sixth decade of life.

Clinical Staging

- Primary malignancies of the vagina are staged clinically.
- A chest radiograph, bimanual and rectovaginal examination, cystoscopy, proctoscopy, and intravenous pyelogram are used by FIGO to determine the extent of disease.
- Stage I vaginal carcinoma is limited to the vaginal wall.
- Stage II involves the subvaginal tissue.
- Stage III involves the subvaginal tissue and extends to the pelvic wall.
- Stage IVA involves the pelvis and or mucosa of the bladder or rectum.
- Stage IVB spreads to distant organs (FIGO Committee on Gynecologic Oncology, 2014).

Treatment

(NCI, 2022)

- Specific treatment plans are based on the stage and extent of disease.
- Early-stage disease (stage I) treatment options:
  - Lesions less than 0.5 cm thick may be treated with wide local excision and upper vaginectomy. Vaginal brachytherapy or external beam radiation therapy may be recommended as adjuvant treatment after surgery.
  - External bream radiation therapy only.
  - Internal radiation or brachytherapy.

- For larger lesions, greater than 0.5 cm, radical vaginectomy and pelvic lymphadenectomy with or without vaginal reconstruction may be an option.
  - If lesion is in lower third of the vagina, a lymph node dissection may be performed.
  - Adjuvant radiation, consisting of external beam and/or brachytherapy, may be recommended post surgery.
- Advanced disease (Stage II-IVA) (NCI, 2022)
  - Radiation consisting of external beam therapy with or without brachytherapy.
  - Platinum chemotherapy may be given with radiation.
  - In select cases, a vaginectomy or pelvic exenteration may be recommended.

Recurrent Disease

- Although the prognosis is usually poor for a vaginal recurrence, surgery or radiation therapy may be an option, depending on the foci of disease.
- Pelvic exenteration with or without vaginal reconstruction may be indicated for selected patients.
- There are no standard of care chemotherapy regimens recommended for recurrent disease; however, platinum combinations and immunotherapy may be considered.
- Ongoing clinical trials are options to consider.

Prognosis

(ACS, 2022)

- Prognosis depends on the disease stage and symptoms at the time of diagnosis.
- The 5-year relative survival rate is 66% for localized disease and 54% for regional disease.
- For patients who have metastatic disease or disease that has metastasized from another malignancy, the prognosis is poor. The 5-year relative survival rate is 24%.
- Reports have indicated survival rates are similar to those for patients with cervical cancer.
- Women with DES-associated cancers have a good prognosis with treatment.
- Women with non-DES adenocarcinoma have a less favorable prognosis.

Prevention and Surveillance

Prevention

- Many women have no known risk factors, precluding prevention.
- Women who smoke should be educated about smoking cessation programs.
- Healthy sexual practices should be addressed. This includes addressing the risk of multiple sexual partners and recommendation for condoms to reduce the spread of HPV infection.
- Recommend HPV vaccination.
- Women who have had prior in utero DES exposure should have routine gynecologic examinations.

Surveillance

- Women with early-stage disease should be examined by a gynecologic oncologist every 6 months for 2 years and then annually.

- Patients with advanced disease should be examined by a gynecologic oncologist every 3 months.
- Imaging studies are not recommended for detecting recurrence unless patients are symptomatic.

References

American Cancer Society (ACS). (2022). *Cancer facts and figures, 2022.* American Cancer Society.

Adams, T. S., Rogers, L. J., & Cuello, M. A. (2021). Cancer of the vagina: 2021 update. *International Journal of Gynecology and Obstetrics, 155*(1), 19–27.

FIGO Committee on Gynecologic Oncology. (2014). Current FIGO staging for cancer of the vagina, fallopian tube, ovary, and gestational trophoblastic neoplasia. *International Journal of Gynaecology and Obstetrics, 125*(2), 97–98.

National Cancer Institute (NCI). (2022). *Vaginal cancer treatment—for health professionals (PDQ).* https://www.cancer.gov/types/vaginal/hp/vaginal-treatment-pdq.

Vulvar Cancer

Definition

The vulva is the external female genitalia, which includes the labia minora and majora, introitus, clitoris, vaginal vestibule, perineal body, and their supporting subcutaneous tissues. Primary malignant tumors of the vulva account for 4% of all gynecologic cancers (Siegel et al., 2022).

Incidence

- Most vulvar cancers occur in postmenopausal women, but reports show a trend toward younger age at diagnosis.
- According to the ACS (2022), 6330 women will be diagnosed with vulvar cancer and 1560 women will die of the disease in the United States.
- The rate of new cases of vulvar cancer has been rising by 0.5% and death rates by 0.7% each year for the past 10 years. It is more common in White women than in Black women.

Etiology and Risk Factors

(ACS, 2022)

- The incidence for vulvar cancer remains low, but the risk increases in the older population. The median age at diagnosis is 69.
- The peak incidence of invasive vulvar cancer occurs in the seventh decade of life.
- Cigarette smoking, infection with HPV types 16 and 18, and human immunodeficiency virus (HIV) infection are associated with the development of vulvar cancer.
- Preinvasive conditions such as vulvar intraepithelial neoplasia (VIN), squamous intraepithelial lesions (SIL), and lichen sclerosis can increase the risk of developing vulvar cancer.
- Younger women may have warty squamous cell carcinoma and are associated with persistent infection with HPV 16, 18, 31, or 33.

Signs and Symptoms

(ACS, 2022)

- Most women with vulvar cancer have pruritus and a pigmented lesion.
- Many women ignore or deny obvious symptoms and lesions for long periods and are diagnosed with advanced disease.

- The presentation in these cases usually is local pain, bleeding, and surface drainage from the tumor.
- The labia majora account for 50% of vulvar cancers, and the labia minora account for 15% to 20% of cases.
- Women who have squamous interepithelial lesions of the cervix, vagina, or anus should have inspection of the vulva as part of a colposcopy visit.

Diagnostic Work-up

- Initial evaluation includes the following:
  - Detailed physical examination with measurements of the primary tumor
  - Assessment for extension to adjacent mucosal or bony structures
  - Assessment for possible involvement of the inguinal lymph nodes
  - Suspicious vulvar lesions should be biopsied
- Presentation with small cancers and clinically negative groin nodes requires few diagnostic studies other than those for preoperative clearance.
- Additional radiographic studies such as CT or MRI of pelvis and groin may be helpful and should be considered for those with large primary tumors or suspected metastases.
- Because neoplasia of the female genital tract is often multifocal, evaluation of the vagina and cervix, including cervical cytologic screening, should always be performed in women with vulvar neoplasms.

Histopathology

(ACS, 2022; NCCN, 2022)

- The vulva is covered by keratinized squamous epithelium, and 85% of malignant vulvar tumors are squamous cell carcinomas.
- Melanoma is the second most common, accounting for 5% to 10% of cases.
- The remaining tumors are a diverse set of rare lesions that include basal cell carcinoma, adenocarcinomas, Paget disease of the vulva, and sarcomas arising from connective tissue.

Clinical Staging

(NCCN, 2022; Olawaiyem et al., 2021)

- FIGO uses a modified TNM and surgical staging scheme for vulvar carcinoma.
- The staging system incorporates the major identified prognostic factors of increasing primary tumor volume, lymph node metastasis, and distant spread.
- Stage I includes tumor confined to the vulva. Stage IA-IB is confined to vulva or perineum and is determined by stromal invasion.
- Stage II tumor of any size extends to the lower one-third of vagina, urethra, and anus, but nodes are negative.
- Stage III tumor of any size with extension to upper part of adjacent perineal structures, or with any nonfixed, nonulcerated lymph nodes. Stage IIIA-IIIB determines amount of lymph node involvement.
- Stage IVA-IVB tumor fixed to bone, or fixed, ulcerated lymph node metastases, or distant metastases.

Treatment

- Early vulvar cancers are managed with radical wide local excision of the tumor. This is as effective as a radical vulvectomy in preventing local recurrence, with the goal of reduced psychosexual morbidity.
- Limited resections are proposed for certain subsets with early or low-risk disease.
- All women who have stage IB or resectable stage II cancers should have an inguinofemoral lymphadenectomy.
- Most surgeons limit the initial procedure to radical vulvectomy and bilateral inguinal lymphadenectomy and do not proceed with pelvic node therapy unless metastasis is demonstrated in the inguinal node area.
- Sentinel node mapping is often done in early vulvar cancer in order to prevent full lymphadenectomy. The criteria include small less than 4 cm unifocal tumors confined to the vulva, stromal invasion greater than 1 mm, and no evidence of positive groin nodes on imaging (NCCN, 2022).
- Some gynecologic oncologists recommend pelvic lymph node irradiation for patients with positive inguinal nodes, but controversy still surrounds this approach.
- Combined radiation therapy and surgery, radiation therapy alone, or only local surgery have been used to treat this disease.
- No adequate prospective studies comparing therapies or their combinations are available for analysis.
- Systemic therapy has been used primarily as a salvage therapy for advanced disease. Options included neoadjuvant treatment with cisplatin and 5-fluorouracil or other combinations. Targeted therapies are being evaluated, such as epidermal growth factor receptor (EGRF) and inhibitors of angiogenesis. HPV-associated cancer are targets for E6 and E7 HPV oncogenes and possible immunotherapy (NCCN, 2022; Olawaiyem et al., 2021).

Recurrent Disease

(NCCN, 2022)

- Isolated or local recurrence is often treated with surgical re-excision and has a 5-year survival rate of up to 60%. If surgery is not an option, local radiation therapy may be an alternative.
- Women with inguinal and pelvic recurrences have a much worse prognosis and, depending on their performance status and comorbidities, they are treated with chemotherapy.
- No standard of care chemotherapy regimens are recommended for recurrent vulvar disease, and data are extrapolated from those for metastatic or recurrent cervical cancer.
- The most common chemotherapy regimen recommended is carboplatin and paclitaxel. The use of targeted therapy is being explored.
- Palliative care should be initiated at the time of diagnosis.

Prognosis

- Survival in cancer of the vulva is directly related to the extent of disease at the time of diagnosis and when treatment is started.
- The overall 5-year relative survival is 70.3% and 5-year survival for localized disease is 86.8%, followed by regional 48.4% and distant at 22.9% (NCI, 2022).

Prevention and Surveillance

Prevention
- Prevention of vulvar cancer is predicated on a healthy lifestyle of smoking cessation and safe sexual practices.
- Women should be counseled at a young age about the relationship between HPV infection and vulvar cancer and about incidence reduction resulting from HPV vaccination.
- HPV vaccine.

Surveillance
(NCCN, 2022)
- Follow-up and survival guidelines are extrapolated from cervical cancer guidelines because vulvar cancer is rare.
- Patients should have a physical examination and review of symptoms by their practitioner or gynecologic oncologist every 6 months for 2 years and then yearly thereafter.
- A Pap smear should be performed yearly, but no other blood tests or scans are indicated unless the patient has symptoms of recurrent disease.

References

American Cancer Society (ACS). (2022). *Cancer facts and figures 2022.* American Cancer Society.

Bhatla, N., Aoki, D., Sharma, D. N., & Sankaranarayanan, R. (2018). Cancer of the cervix uteri. *International Journal of Gynaecology and Obstetrics: The Official Organ of the International Federation of Gynaecology and Obstetrics, 143*(Suppl 2), 22–36.

National Cancer Institute (NCI). (2022). *SEER cancer stat review: Vulva cancer, 2011–2017.* https://seer.cancer.gov/statfacts/html/vulva.html.

National Comprehensive Cancer Network (NCCN). (2022). *Vulvar cancer (squamous cell carcinoma) Version1.2022.* https://www.nccn.org/professionals/physician_gls/pdf/vulvar.pdf.

Olawaiyem, A. B., Cotler, J., Cuello, M. A., Bhatla, N., Okamoto, A., Wilailak, S., Purandare, C. N., Lindeque, G., Berek, J. S., & Kehoe, S. (2021). FIGO staging for carcinoma of the vulva: 2021 revision. *International Journal of Gynecology and Obstetrics, 155*(1), 43–47.

Olawaiyem, A. B., Cuello, M. A., & Rogers, L. J. (2021). Cancer of the vulva: 2021 update. *International Journal of Gynecology and Obstetrics, 155*(1), 7–18.

Salani, R., Khanna, N., Frimer, M., Bristow, R. E., & Chen, L. M. (2017). An update on post-treatment surveillance and diagnosis of recurrence in women with gynecologic malignancies: Society of Gynecologic Oncology (SGO) recommendations. *Gynecologic Oncology, 146*(1), 3–10.

Siegel, R. L., Miller, K. D., Fuchs, H. E., & Jemal, A. (2022). Cancer statistics, 2022. *CA: A Cancer Journal for Clinicians, 72*(1), 7–33.

Head and Neck Cancers

Emily Sanders

Laryngeal Cancer

Definition

The larynx is an intricate neuromuscular organ located between the pharynx and trachea. It has three main functions. It prevents passage of food into the airway during swallowing, modulates air passing through the vocal cords to facilitate phonation, and regulates the flow of air into lungs during respiration. The larynx acts as a sphincter to prevent aspiration. The true and false cords, epiglottis, and aryepiglottic folds close, and the larynx moves slightly upward and forward to protect the trachea and prevent respiration during swallowing. A sound is created when the true vocal cords make contact with each other and air from the lungs passes between them. Phonation occurs when this sound is converted to recognizable speech by the contraction and relaxation of muscles in the oral cavity and tongue.

The larynx is divided into three anatomic regions (see the figure below) (Mu et al., 2021):

- The supraglottic larynx, which includes the epiglottis, false vocal cords, laryngeal ventricles, aryepiglottic folds, and arytenoids. Approximately 35% of laryngeal cancers occur in this region.

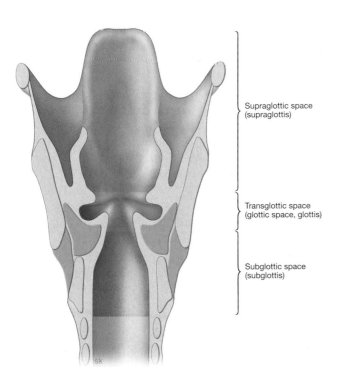

- The glottis includes the true vocal cords and the anterior and posterior commissures. Approximately 60% of laryngeal cancers occur in this region.
- The subglottic region begins about 1 cm below the true vocal cords and extends to the lower border of the cricoid cartilage or the first tracheal ring. Approximately 5% of laryngeal cancers occur in this region.

Incidence

- The American Cancer Society (ACS, 2022) reports the incidence of laryngeal cancer in the United States annually and the estimated 2022 statistics are as follows.
- In 2022, 12,470 new cases of laryngeal cancer are estimated to occur. Of those new cases, there will be 9820 men and 2650 women that will be diagnosed. Laryngeal cancer accounts for 0.7% of all new cancer cases.
- The estimated deaths attributed to laryngeal cancer in 2022 are 3820. Within that total, 3070 are men and 750 are women. Laryngeal cancer accounts for 0.6% of all cancer deaths.
- Men are five times more likely to develop laryngeal cancer than women, and race also plays a role, as Black men are more likely to develop laryngeal cancer than White men.
- Laryngeal cancer is most diagnosed in individuals over the age of 55 and the average age at diagnosis is 66 years old.
- As fewer people are smoking, the rate of newly diagnosed laryngeal cancer cases has been dropping by 2% to 3% annually. The death rate has also fallen 2% to 3% over the past 10 years.
- The lifetime risk of developing laryngeal cancer is about 1 in 190 for men and 1 in 830 for women, although a number of other factors can affect the risk of developing the disease.
- Surveillance, Epidemiology, and End Results Program (SEER) (National Cancer Institute, 2022b) data reports that there were an estimated 90,176 people living with laryngeal cancer in the United States in 2019.

Etiology and Risk Factors

- Cigarette smoking is the single most important risk factor for laryngeal cancer.
- Combined alcohol and tobacco use increases the risk of laryngeal cancer as alcohol and tobacco are thought to act synergistically. Although alcohol is not a carcinogen, it is thought to damage the mucosa and allow increased cellular permeability to known carcinogens.
- Studies have shown that exposure to asbestos and inorganic mists (such as fertilizer) are risk factors for the development of laryngeal cancer. Other suggested agents that may increase the risk are wood dust, diesel engine exhaust, coal products, cement, and paint fumes (Boffetta and Donato, 2020).

The Larynx. (S. Klebe in Paulsen/Waschke. Sobotta Atlas der Anatomie. 25. Edition 2022 © Elsevier GmbH.)

Signs and Symptoms

- Sore throat or throat irritation
- Dysphagia
- Odynophagia
- Referred otalgia
- Hoarseness or changes in voice
- Cervical lymphadenopathy
- Weight loss
- Aspiration
- Dyspnea
- Stridor
- Hemoptysis
- Nonmalignant conditions such as vocal cord polyps or cysts and sarcoidosis can mimic the symptoms associated with malignant lesions.

Diagnostic Workup

- Physical examination of the head and neck
- Thorough palpation of the neck for evidence of metastatic disease
- In-office mirror examination and direct flexible laryngoscopy of the upper aerodigestive tract
- Imaging studies, including computed tomography (CT) scan with contrast, magnetic resonance imaging (MRI), and positron emission tomography (PET) scan
- Rigid laryngoscopy under general anesthesia with possible biopsy of suspicious lesions
- Fine-needle aspiration (FNA) biopsy of any enlarged lymph nodes in the neck.

Histopathology

Most of the malignant lesions found in the larynx are squamous cell carcinomas (SCC) and are subtyped into keratinizing and nonkeratinizing. They are then graded from well differentiated to poorly differentiated.

Clinical Staging

Staging of laryngeal cancer is based on clinical and radiographic information obtained before treatment to estimate the extent of the disease and uses the American Joint Committee on Cancer (AJCC) guidelines based on the tumor-node-metastasis (TNM) classification system.

- Cancers that are classified as early stage (stage I or II) are confined to one or both vocal cords.
- Locally advanced disease is classified as stage III.
- Moderately advanced local disease that invades structures beyond the larynx or metastatic disease is classified as stage IV.

Treatment

- Early-stage lesions are treated with radiation therapy or surgery alone. Both approaches yield similar survival rates for early glottic and supraglottic lesions.
- Radiation therapy is confined to a small treatment area for small, superficial lesions of the glottis.
- Treatment of locally advanced or moderately local advanced disease often involves a multimodal approach. The choice of treatment is determined by determining prognosis, as well as the outcome and predicted functional results, as well as by the availability of a multidisciplinary team with experience in treating this type of malignancy. Consideration is given to the efficacy of treatment and quality of life issues, such as preservation of the ability to voice.
- If it is determined that clear margins would not be achieved in surgery, the disease is deemed unresectable.
- Treatment for patients with recurrent disease depends on the tumor location, size, and any prior treatment in the area.

Surgery

- Surgical excision must encompass the gross tumor and microscopic disease within 5 mm in order to be considered a clear, negative margin. Adequate margins are a good predictor of the risk for tumor recurrence.
- If positive regional nodes are identified, lymph node dissection is usually done.
- Early glottic lesions can be managed surgically with a cordectomy to remove the affected vocal cord. This should be attempted only if the lesion is superficial and does not extend to the anterior commissure or the arytenoid cartilage.
  - Transoral robotic surgery (TORS) is a minimally invasive procedure used to resect small, well-circumscribed lesions in the glottic and supraglottic area.
  - A carbon dioxide laser can be used transorally with ridged endoscopes to target small lesions in the supraglottic and glottic areas.
  - A wider-field supraglottic laryngectomy may be necessary and may include a tracheostomy in order to secure the airway.
- Locally advanced lesions are better managed with surgery followed by adjuvant radiation therapy or combined radiation and chemotherapy.
- Moderately locally advanced-stage cancers that involve the thyroid cartilage or other structures outside the larynx require a total laryngectomy.
  - Removal of the entire larynx may also involve partial or total removal of the thyroid gland, parathyroid glands, or other involved structures.
  - A permanent tracheostoma is created by suturing the trachea to the skin of the anterior neck. Postoperative adjuvant treatment is usually indicated.
- Postoperative rehabilitation, including voice aids for patients who have undergone total laryngectomy, is important to ensure the best quality of life.

Radiation Therapy

- Most early lesions can be successfully treated by radiation alone or surgery alone (Alfouzan, 2021).
- Radiation therapy is a reasonable choice to preserve the voice, leaving surgery for salvage if needed (Gamez, 2020).
- External beam radiation therapy is commonly used for treating the primary site and regional lymph nodes.
- Treatment may successfully treat the cancer but leave the patient with a nonfunctioning larynx.

- Intensity-modulated radiation therapy (IMRT) may be considered, as it lessens toxicity by limiting radiation exposure of the normal tissue surrounding the lesion.
- Acute side effects from radiation of the area may include fatigue, skin inflammation, lymphedema, xerostomia, odynophagia, as well as dysphagia, which could require feeding tube insertion during treatment.
- Late side effects from radiation can lead to dystonia, esophageal strictures, limited range of motion of the neck, carotid artery stenosis, and tracheostomy dependence. Hypothyroidism can occur if the thyroid gland was involved in the radiation field.
- Research suggests that there is a significant loss of local control when radiation therapy was not delivered according to the planned schedule and lengthening the radiation schedule should be avoided if possible (National Cancer Institute, 2022b).
- Patients should be counseled on smoking cessation prior to beginning radiation therapy, as lower response rates and shorter survival durations have been shown in those that continue to smoke during their course of radiation (National Cancer Institute, 2022b).

Systemic Therapies

Historically, surgery and radiation therapy have formed the foundation of therapy, with chemotherapy enhancing the effectiveness of radiation.

- Postoperative chemotherapy with radiation therapy is used for patients at high risk for recurrence, metastasis to the lymph nodes, or when surgical resection is inadequate and there is gross tumor remaining, or negative margins were not able to be achieved.
- Platinum-based chemotherapy with concurrent radiation therapy is the standard care for locally advanced nonresectable lesions.
- Neoadjuvant chemotherapy for locally advanced disease can be given before concurrent chemoradiation or for those patients with persistent disease following radiation.
- Molecularly targeted therapies are available for patients with head and neck cancers.
  - Epidermal growth factor receptor (EGFR) is expressed by most head and neck tumors, and drugs that target EGFR can be used to treat advanced laryngeal cancers.
- Immunotherapy drugs can be used to help the cells in a person's own immune system to seek and destroy cancer cells. These are typically used for patients with metastatic spread or those who have recurrent disease.
- Patients with distant disease are usually treated with palliative measures using concurrent chemoradiation.

Prognosis

- The prognosis for early-stage localized laryngeal cancers that have not spread to lymph nodes is very good, with a 5-year relative survival rate of 78.3% (National Cancer Institute, 2022a).
  - Based on data, the overall 5-year survival rate from 2012 to 2018 data is 61% (National Cancer Institute, 2022a).

- Adverse prognostic factors for laryngeal cancers include advanced stage of disease and metastases to lymph nodes.
  - Lymphatic invasion, which occurs in 26% of patients at the time of diagnosis, increases the risk of death and the 5-year survival rate falls to 46.2% (National Cancer Institute, 2022a).
  - Metastasis to bone and other distant areas increases the risk of death.
  - Distant metastases can occur even if the primary tumor is controlled.
- Other prognostic factors include sex, age, performance status, and pathologic features of the tumor, such as grade and depth of invasion.
- Comorbid conditions such as diabetes, hypertension, decreased pulmonary function, and malnutrition compromise successful treatment outcomes.
- Patients treated for laryngeal cancers are at the highest risk of recurrence in the first 2 to 3 years. Recurrences after 5 years are rare and usually represent new primary malignancies.

Prevention and Surveillance

The risk of developing laryngeal malignancies can be greatly reduced by avoiding certain risk factors.

- Use of tobacco in any form is the most significant cause of upper aerodigestive tract malignancies.
- Heavy alcohol abuse contributes to the increased risk, especially when used with tobacco.
- Exposure to known carcinogenic chemicals and wood dust must be eliminated by using proper ventilation and protective gear (Boffetta and Donato, 2020).
- Although it is a rare risk factor for cancers arising in the larynx, human papillomavirus (HPV) infection can be linked to some cases of laryngeal cancer.
  - The rate of HPV infection of the upper aerodigestive tract is increased among individuals who have oral sex and multiple sex partners (Irani, 2020).
  - Tobacco users are more prone to HPV infection because of a compromised immune system and because tobacco smoke injures respiratory cells.
  - Research is being conducted to show if HPV vaccination may decrease the risk of cancers in the upper aerodigestive tract.
- Poor nutrition and the vitamin deficiencies associated with alcohol abuse and malnutrition contribute to the risk of developing laryngeal malignancies.

References

American Cancer Society. (2022). *Key statistics for laryngeal and hypopharyngeal cancers.* Available at https://www.cancer.org/cancer/laryngeal-and-hypopharyngeal-cancer/about/key-statistics.html.

Boffetta, P., & Donato, F. (2020). Occupational risk factors of laryngeal cancer. In S. Anttila, & P. Boffetta (Eds.), *Occupational cancers* (pp. 193–204). Switzerland: Springer Nature.

Gamez, M. E., Blakaj, A., Zoller, W., Bonomi, M., & Blakaj, D. M. (2020). Emerging concepts and novel strategies in radiation therapy for laryngeal cancer management. *Cancers, 12*(6), 1651.

Irani, S. (2020). New insights into oral cancer-risk factors and prevention: A review of literature. *International Journal of Preventive Medicine, 11*, 202.

Mu, Z., Wang, X., & Huang, J. (2021). Applied anatomy and physiology of larynx. In Z. Mu, & J. Fang (Eds.), *Practical otorhinolaryngology—Head and neck surgery* (pp. 213–216). Singapore: Springer Nature.

National Cancer Institute. (2022a). *Cancer stat facts: Laryngeal cancer.* Available at https://seer.cancer.gov/statfacts/html/laryn.html.

National Cancer Institute. (2022b). *Laryngeal cancer treatment (adult) (PDQ)–health professional version.* Available at https://www.cancer.gov/types/head-and-neck/hp/adult/laryngeal-treatment-pdq#_1.

Oropharyngeal Cancers

Definition

The area that encompasses the oropharynx begins with the oral cavity (see the figure below). The oral cavity begins at the skin-vermilion junctions of the anterior lips to the junction of the hard and soft palates above and stretches to the line of circumvallate papillae below. The oral cavity includes:

- Lips
- Mobile anterior two-thirds of tongue
- Cheek or buccal mucosa
- Floor of the mouth
- Retromolar trigone
- Gingiva
- Hard palate

The pharynx is a muscular tube that connects the nasal cavity to the upper aerodigestive tract and is about 5 cm in length (see the figure on the next page). This structure begins at the skull base and ends below the cricoid cartilage near the level of C6. It contains three distinct areas, the nasopharynx, oropharynx, and hypopharynx, any of which can develop malignancies.

- The nasopharynx lies behind the nose and is located between the base of the skull and the soft palate and is a continuation of the nasal cavity. It humidifies and filters inspired air and directs the air to the larynx and then on to the lungs. The eustachian tube openings are found on the left and right lateral walls of the nasopharynx and lead into the middle ear.
- The oropharynx is the middle part of the pharynx, located between the soft palate and the superior border of the epiglottis to the level of the hyoid bone. It contains the base of the tongue, the lingual tonsils, and the palatine tonsils found in the oral cavity. The oropharynx is involved in the voluntary and involuntary phases of swallowing.
- The hypopharynx is the lower part of the pharynx, located between the upper part of the epiglottis and the upper border of the cricoid cartilage. It becomes part of the esophagus at the level of C6. It is located behind the larynx and communicates with it by the laryngeal inlet. The piriform sinuses are found on each side in this area.

Pharyngeal structures include mucosa, lymphoid tissue, and a longitudinal muscle layer that includes the stylopharyngeus muscle, palatopharyngeus muscle, and salpingopharyngeus muscle. These muscles elevate the larynx during swallowing. A circular muscle layer consists of the superior, middle, and inferior constrictor muscles. These muscles contract sequentially and propel a food bolus into the esophagus.

The pharyngeal plexus innervates the pharynx. It consists of branches of the glossopharyngeal nerve (CN IX), branches of the vagus nerve (CN X), and sympathetic fibers of the superior cervical ganglion.

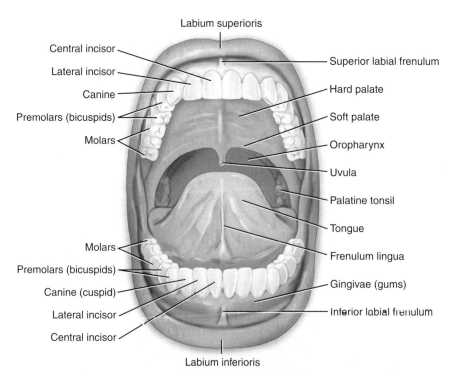

The Oral Cavity. (From Shiland, B. J. [2015]. *Medical assistant: Digestive system, nutrition, financial management and first aid* [2nd ed.]. St. Louis: Elsevier.)

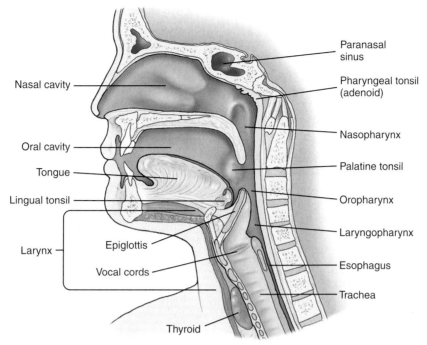

The Upper Respiratory System. (From Shiland, B. J. [2023]. *Mastering healthcare terminology* [7th ed.] Elsevier.)

Incidence

- Statistics for oral cancer are commonly combined with pharyngeal cancers. The ACS reports the incidence of oral cavity and pharynx cancers in the United States annually. In 2022, it is estimated that there will be 54,000 reported new cases of oral cavity and pharynx cancer. There will be 38,700 men and 15,300 women that are estimated to be diagnosed (ACS, 2022a). SEER data lists that oral cavity and pharynx cancers account for 2.8% of all new cancer cases (National Cancer Institute, 2022a).
- About 11,230 people are estimated to die from oral cavity and pharynx cancer in 2022 (National Cancer Institute, 2022a). Within that total, 7870 will be men and 3360 will be women (ACS, 2022a). Oral cavity and pharynx cancers account for 1.8% of all cancer deaths (National Cancer Institute, 2022a).
- Based on 2014 to 2018 data (ACS, 2022a), the annual age-adjusted incidence of oral cavity and pharyngeal cancer is 11.9 new cases per 100,000 men and women.
- Based on data from 2015 to 2019, the annual age-adjusted mortality rate is 2.5 deaths per 100,000 men and women (ACS, 2022a).
- Oral cavity and pharynx cancer are most frequently diagnosed among people between the ages of 55 and 64 and the median age at diagnosis is 64 (National Cancer Institute, 2022a).
- Men are twice as likely as women to be diagnosed with oral cavity and pharynx cancer and it is most common in white men.
- Nasopharyngeal cancer is quite rare. There is less than one case per 100,000 worldwide annually. However, in certain parts of the world, including parts of South Asia, the Middle East, and North Africa, it is more common. In some parts

of China, there may be as many as 21 cases per 100,000 people (National Cancer Institute, 2022c).
- From 2010 to 2019, oral cavity and oropharyngeal cancer rates are increasing by about 1% each year due to the relationship related to HPV infection (National Cancer Institute, 2022a).

Etiology and Risk Factors

- Oral cavity and pharyngeal carcinomas are more common in individuals who abuse alcohol and smoke. They are 30 times more likely to develop oral cavity and pharyngeal malignancies than people who do not drink or smoke.
  - Cigarette smoking is one of the strongest risk factors for head and neck cancers.
  - Use of oral tobacco products is linked to oral cavity cancers such as the buccal mucosa, the alveolar ridge, and the inner surfaces of the lips.
  - The carcinogens found in tobacco have a synergistic effect when combined with alcohol. While alcohol is not a carcinogen, it damages the mucosa and allows increased cellular permeability to tobacco carcinogens.
- Cigarette smoking is the single most important risk factor for head and neck cancer.
- More than three-fourths of head and neck cancers in the United States are related to tobacco and alcohol use. Alcohol and tobacco are thought to act synergistically. Alcohol is not a carcinogen, but it suppresses the immune system and damages the mucosa, increasing cellular permeability to known carcinogens such as tobacco.
- Nasopharyngeal cancer is rare. Risk factors are gender, race/ethnicity and where you live, diet, infection with the Epstein-Barr virus (EBV), family history, tobacco and alcohol use, and workplace exposures.

- Twice as many males than females are diagnosed with nasopharyngeal cancer.
- Nasopharyngeal cancer is most common in southern China, Singapore, Vietnam, Malaysia, the Philippines, Northwest Canada, and Greenland. In the United States, it is most common among Pacific Islanders and people of Asian ancestry.
- HPV infection (i.e., HPV16) has been linked to many oropharyngeal and some nasopharyngeal cancers, and many of those diagnosed with HPV-related oral cancers have never smoked and have no history of alcohol abuse. HPV cancers are often diagnosed in those younger than 50.
  - Compared with HPV-negative oropharyngeal cancers, HPV-related oropharyngeal cancers affect younger patients that have less comorbidities, a higher socioeconomic status, and a history of multiple sexual partners and orogenital sexual practice.
- Diets very high in salt-cured fish and meat or low in fruits and vegetables increase the risk of developing nasopharyngeal cancer.
- Sun exposure is a risk factor for cancer of the lip.

Signs and Symptoms

Oropharyngeal cancer signs and symptoms differ for the anatomic site of the tumor as follows:

Nasopharynx
(ACS, 2022d)
- Neck mass
- Unilateral otalgia, tinnitus, pain or feeling of fullness in the ear
- Recurrent serous otitis media
- Nasal obstruction or stuffiness
- Epistaxis
- Headaches
- Facial pain or numbness
- Trouble opening the mouth
- Blurred vision or diplopia
- Dyspnea or difficulty talking

Oral Cavity and Oropharynx
(ACS, 2022b)
- A sore on the lip or in the mouth that does not heal
- Pain in the mouth that does not go away
- A lump or thickening in the lips, mouth, or cheek
- A white or red patch on the gums, tongue, tonsil, or lining of the mouth (leukoplakia)
- Trouble moving the jaw or tongue
- Numbness of the tongue, lip, or other area of the mouth
- Swelling or pain in the jaw
- Dentures that start to fit poorly or become uncomfortable
- Loosening of the teeth or pain around the teeth
- Persistent sore throat or globus feeling
- Dysphagia
- Neck adenopathy
- Hemoptysis
- Unilateral otalgia
- Unexplained weight loss

Hypopharynx and Cervical Esophagus
(ACS, 2021; National Organization of Rare Diseases, 2019)
- Hoarseness
- Neck adenopathy
- Dyspnea or airway obstruction
- Persistent sore throat
- Dysphagia
- Otalgia
- Halitosis
- Choking
- Unexplained weight loss
- Indigestion/heartburn (cervical esophagus)
- Chest pain (cervical esophagus)

Diagnostic Workup

- Physical examination of the oral cavity and neck including thorough palpation of the neck, oral cavity, and tongue. Use of the mirror allows the examiner to view the base of the tongue and the supraglottic regions.
- Flexible fiberoptic endoscopy of the upper aerodigestive tract is used to look at areas that cannot easily be seen with mirrors.
- Imaging may be done with a CT with contrast. MRI may be indicated if the patient is allergic to contrast material or to determine the possibility of an intracranial extension. A PET scan is not commonly used in the diagnostic phase unless there is concern for disease metastasis.
- Biopsy is performed for suspicious lesions.
- FNA biopsy of any enlarged lymph nodes in the neck.

Histopathology

- Precancerous lesions of the oral cavity may include leukoplakia, erythroplakia, and mixed erythroleukoplakia.
- SCCs are the most common cell type arising in the pharynx. They are further categorized into the subtypes of keratinizing and nonkeratinizing. While not true for every SCC, most keratinizing SCCs are non-HPV-related and most nonkeratinizing SCCs are HPV-related.
- Verrucous carcinomas are rare and, when found, usually present in the buccal mucosa or in the gums. Verrucous carcinomas are slow growing.
- Mucosal melanomas may arise on the gingiva or hard palate. These are typically free of symptoms and may be found incidentally during a routine dental evaluation.
- Sarcomas may arise from the hard palate or mandible.
- Lymphomas may also start in the nasopharynx.

Clinical Staging

Staging of oropharyngeal cancers is based on clinical and radiographic information obtained before treatment to estimate the extent of the disease and uses the AJCC guidelines based on the TNM classification system.

Cancers That Are Not HPV Related
- Early stages (stage I or II) are confined to the primary site.
- Locally advanced disease that has a tumor greater than 4 cm or a tumor that extends past the diagnosed site is classified as stage III, as are tumors with a single metastatic lymph node.

- Moderately advanced local disease that invades surrounding structures or metastatic disease is classified as stage IV.

Cancers That Are HPV Related
(De Felice, 2019)
- HPV oropharyngeal cancers are categorized separately as their prognosis is more favorable. These cancers are often diagnosed when a patient presents with a painless neck mass and may have a microscopic primary tumor. Therefore, an adjustment was required for the staging system.

Treatment
Treatment often involves a multimodal approach. Depending on the site and extent of the primary tumor and the status of the lymph nodes, the treatment of lip and oral cavity cancer may be surgery alone, radiation therapy alone, the two modalities combined, or a combination of surgery, radiation, and chemotherapy.

Patients who have been diagnosed with oral cavity cancers should stop smoking and discontinue use of any oral tobacco products. Continued use during treatment will cause susceptibility to poor wound healing, high risk of infection, as well as enhanced side effects from radiation and chemotherapy.

The choice of treatment should be determined by the anticipated functional and cosmetic results and by the availability of the medical expertise required. Treatment plans for all disease stages should be discussed at a multidisciplinary tumor conference involving surgeons, radiation oncologists, medical oncologists, pathologists, and specialized nursing personnel.
- Early cancers (stages I and II) are highly curable with surgery or radiation therapy alone. The choice of treatment is determined by the stage of disease, anticipated functional and cosmetic results of surgery, comorbid conditions, and recommendations of a multidisciplinary team (National Cancer Institute, 2022b).
- Most patients with locally advanced or metastatic tumors (stage III or IV) require a multimodality approach that includes surgery, radiation, and chemotherapy (National Cancer Institute, 2022b).
- The risk of local recurrence or distant metastases is high and requires close monitoring. Treatment for patients with recurrent lesions depends on the location and size of the recurrent lesion as well as what their prior treatment was. Immunotherapy also has a role in managing recurrent disease.
- Patients with recurrent disease should be considered for clinical trials when available (National Cancer Institute, 2022b).

Surgery
- Lesions of the oral cavity usually are surgically resected. Resection encompasses gross tumor and a final pathologic margin of 5 mm for tumors with a surgeon-measured margin of 1 cm. Adequate margins are a good predictor of the risk for tumor recurrence.
- TORS or transoral laser microsurgery (TLM) are minimally invasive procedures used to resect small, well-circumscribed lesions at the base of the tongue or tonsillar regions.
- When the tumor is too large for a minimally invasive procedure, an open procedure is done to remove the tumor in its entirety and obtain clear margins. If an opening was left, then a prosthodontic appliance (palatal obturator) may be used to occlude the area.
- Large cancers when resected leave a large defect that may require surgical reconstruction with free tissue transfer, commonly referred to as a free flap. A soft tissue free flap may be harvested from the radial forearm, the anterior-lateral thigh, or the rectus abdominis muscle. If bone is required, such as in a mandibular cancer resection, the fibula bone, scapula, or osteocutaneous radial forearm may be used. The free tissue and/or bone are then transplanted to the defect area and venous and arterial anastomosis are done under a microscope to ensure that the transplanted tissue remains viable.
- If positive regional nodes are identified, cervical lymph node dissection (commonly referred to as a neck dissection) is done. Other factors that are considered to determine the need for neck dissection include the depth of invasion greater than 4 mm and tumor stage at the time of diagnosis.
- Surgical excision must encompass the gross tumor and microscopic disease.
- Postoperative speech and swallowing rehabilitation are important to ensure the best quality of life.
- Nasopharyngeal tumors are not commonly treated with surgery due to the geographic area in which it is located.

Radiation Therapy
Patients who smoke while on radiation therapy appear to have lower response rates and shorter survival durations than those who do not. Patients should be counseled to stop smoking before beginning radiation therapy.
- External beam radiation therapy or brachytherapy (which uses interstitial implants) may be used. Local implants can be successful in treating small, superficial cancers.
  - Acute side effects of external beam radiation may include oral mucositis, decreased oral intake leading to malnutrition and dehydration, as well as an increase in narcotic pain medications. Fournier (2020) lists long-term side effects including dysphagia, xerostomia, dental caries, osteoradionecrosis, trismus, cervical fibrosis and dystonia, lymphedema, and carotid artery stenosis.
- IMRT and intensity-modulated proton therapy (IMPT) are the latest technologic advancements in external beam radiation therapy. These techniques spare more of the surrounding normal tissue and minimize side effects (Moreno et al., 2019).
  - IMRT and IMPT both deliver precise radiation to the tumor while minimizing the dose to the surrounding tissue. Studies have shown that IMPT is superior in sparing of the head and neck organs, leading to decreased feeding tube dependency (Grant et al., 2020).
  - Side effects caused by traditional external beam radiation therapy are dramatically diminished with the use of IMRT or IMPT.

- Radiation therapy may be used in the postoperative setting if positive margins were identified in the final pathology and re-resection is not feasible, or if there is extranodal extension present.
- Radiation therapy alone is indicated to treat nasopharyngeal carcinoma. For advanced nasopharyngeal carcinomas, chemotherapy will be given together with radiation therapy.
- External beam radiation therapy or brachytherapy (which uses interstitial implants) may be used. Local implants can be successful in treating small, superficial cancers.
- For HPV-related oropharyngeal cancers, radiation dose escalation studies are currently under investigation with the intent to reduce radiation toxicities. There are also several studies under investigation to treat the ipsilateral neck without treating the primary site if margins were adequately resected, and there is no perineural invasion or extracapsular spread noted on pathology leading to a much more desirable and optimized quality of life (De Felice et al., 2019).
- Research suggests that there is a significant loss of local control when radiation therapy is not delivered according to the planned schedule. Lengthening the radiation schedule should be avoided whenever possible.

Chemotherapy

- Chemotherapy is not commonly used alone as the primary treatment modality for oropharyngeal cancers.
- Neoadjuvant or induction chemotherapy concurrent with radiation therapy (chemoradiation) may be used before surgery.
- Adjuvant chemoradiation therapy may be indicated postoperatively to eradicate any microscopic disease as well as decrease the risk of recurrence.
- For patients who have advanced disease for which surgery would be too debilitating and compromise functional and cosmetic outcomes, chemotherapy plus radiation therapy may produce a better outcome than radiation alone.
- Chemotherapy or immunotherapy with or without radiation can be used for metastatic or recurrent disease with the goal being to slow the growth of the cancer and provide symptom relief.
  - The preferred chemotherapy agents are high-dose cisplatin or carboplatin with 5-FU. If cisplatin cannot be used, then docetaxel and cetuximab can be considered.
  - Immunotherapy agents may include pembrolizumab or nivolumab.
- For locally advanced nasopharyngeal cancers, chemotherapy with concurrent radiation therapy is the treatment of choice. First-line agent is cisplatin, and if the patient is not tolerant, then carboplatin will be used as an alternative.

Prognosis

- Based on 2012 to 2018 SEER data, the overall 5-year survival rate for oral cavity and pharyngeal cancers combined is 68% (ACS, 2022a).
  - Recent evidence suggests that prognosis and survival rate for patients with HPV-positive tumors is better than HPV-negative tumors and additional research continues.
- Survival rates for pharyngeal cancers are dependent on tumor site and stage (ACS, 2022c):
  - When the tumor is localized and confined to the primary site, the 5-year survival rate is 86.3%. If it has spread to the regional lymph nodes, the 5-year survival rate drops to 69%.
- Prognostic factors include tumor size, depth of invasion, the presence of vascular invasion, margins of resection, tumor morphology, and lymph node metastases.
  - If lymph nodes are positive, prognostic factors include the number of positive nodes, the size of the largest node, laterality of nodes, and the presence of extracapsular extension.
  - The consequences of tumor extending beyond the limits of the primary site into adjacent tissues can be challenging to manage. Patients are prone to severe malnourishment, chronic pain, immobility, and depression.
- For nasopharyngeal cancer, data from the ACS (2022c) from 2011 to 2017 shows that the overall 5-year survival rate is 62%. A further breakdown of survival data is dependent on how the cancer was found at time of diagnosis:
  - Localized (contained to the nasopharynx): 81%
  - Regional (metastasis to nearby structures or lymph nodes): 73%
  - Distant (metastatic spread to a distant organ): 48%

Prevention and Surveillance

- Primary prevention of head and neck cancer requires cessation of alcohol and tobacco use.
  - Individuals who have had one cancer in a region are at an increased risk for other cancers with related risk factors, including other head and neck cancers, lung cancer, and esophageal cancer.
  - According to Andreasen et al. (2019), smoking can reduce the sensitivity of radiation and therefore increase toxicity and morbidity while decreasing a favorable long-term prognosis. Patients who continue to smoke are also at a greater risk for cancer recurrence.
  - Patients should be referred for counseling and support to address issues related to tobacco and alcohol use.
- Patients with oropharyngeal cancer should be followed closely during the first 2 years following completion of treatment to maintain close surveillance. Follow-up recommendations suggest that provider should have patients follow-up every 1 to 3 months for the first year, then every 2 to 6 months during year 2, and then lengthen the time between visits to 4 to 8 months during years 3 to 5. At year 5, patients may be examined annually (Joo et al., 2019). Patients are encouraged to see a provider at any time if they notice any concerning changes, as most recurrences are reported by the patient.
- While HPV vaccination has been shown to prevent 90% of oral HPV infections, there is not enough evidence to show a correlation that shows a reduced risk of oropharyngeal cancer in relation to HPV vaccination.

References

American Cancer Society. (2022a). *Cancer statistics center: Oral cavity and pharynx.* Available at https://cancerstatisticscenter.cancer.org/?_ga=2.183876774.1492974597.1636997541-951712783.1636997540#!/cancer-site/Oral%20cavity%20and%20pharynx.

American Cancer Society. (2022b). *Signs and symptoms of oral cavity and oropharyngeal cancer.* Available at https://www.cancer.org/cancer/oral-cavity-and-oropharyngeal-cancer/detection-diagnosis-staging/signs-symptoms.html.

American Cancer Society. (2022c). *Survival rates for nasopharyngeal cancer.* Available at https://www.cancer.org/cancer/nasopharyngeal-cancer/detection-diagnosis-staging/survival-rates.html.

American Cancer Society. (2022d). *Signs and symptoms of nasopharyngeal cancer.* Available at https://www.cancer.org/cancer/nasopharyngeal-cancer/detection-diagnosis-staging/signs-and-symptoms.html.

Andreasen, S., Kiss, K., Mikkelsen, L. H., Channir, H. I., Plaschke, C. C., Melchior, L. C., ... Wessel, I. (2019). An update on head and neck cancer: new entities and their histopathology, molecular background, treatment, and outcome. *APMIS, 127*(5), 240–264.

De Felice, F., Tombolini, V., Valentini, V., de Vincentiis, M., Mezi, S., Brugnoletti, O., & Polimeni, A. (2019). Advances in the management of HPV-related oropharyngeal cancer. *Journal of Oncology, 2019,* 9173729.

Fournier, D. (2020). Navigating long-term effects of radiation therapy in head and neck cancer survivors. *ORL—Head and Neck. Nursing, 39*(2), 5–12.

Grant, S. R., Williamson, T. D., Stieb, S., Shah, S. J., David Fuller, C., Rosenthal, D. I., ... Gunn, G. B. (2020). A dosimetric comparison of oral cavity sparing in the unilateral treatment of early stage tonsil cancer: IMRT, IMPT, and tongue-deviating oral stents. *Advances in Radiation Oncology, 5*(6), 1359–1363.

Joo, Y. H., Cho, J. K., Koo, B. S., Kwon, M., Kwon, S. K., Kwon, S. Y., ... Chung, P. S. (2019). Guidelines for the surgical management of oral cancer: Korean Society of Thyroid-Head and Neck Surgery. *Clinical and Experimental Otorhinolaryngology, 12*(2), 107–144.

Moreno, A. C., Frank, S. J., Garden, A. S., Rosenthal, D. I., Fuller, C. D., Gunn, G. B., ... Blanchard, P. (2019). Intensity modulated proton therapy (IMPT)—The future of IMRT for head and neck cancer. *Oral Oncology, 88,* 66–74.

National Cancer Institute. (2022a). *Cancer stat facts: Oral cavity and pharynx cancer.* Available at https://seer.cancer.gov/statfacts/html/oralcav.html.

National Cancer Institute. (2022b). *Lip and oral cavity cancer treatment (adult) (PDQ)–health professional version.* Available at https://www.cancer.gov/types/head-and-neck/hp/adult/lip-mouth-treatment-pdq.

National Cancer Institute. (2022c). *Oral cavity and nasopharyngeal cancers screening (PDQ)–health professional version.* Available at https://www.cancer.gov/types/head-and-neck/hp/oral-screening-pdq.

Salivary Gland Cancer

Definition

Salivary glands are exocrine glands located in the upper aerodigestive tract. They release saliva, which contains enzymes such as amylase that predigest dietary starches and fats. Salivary glands also produce electrolytes, mucus, glycoproteins, and antibacterial compounds that protect the teeth from bacterial decay, moisten food, and shield mucosal surfaces from desiccation.

Salivary glands are divided into minor and major types. Between 800 and 1000 minor salivary glands are in the upper aerodigestive tract and paranasal sinuses. They are found in the oral mucosa, palate, and uvula. They are also found in the floor of the mouth, posterior tongue, retromolar area, peritonsillar area, pharynx, and larynx. A minor salivary gland may have a common excretory duct with another gland or its own excretory duct.

The three types of major salivary glands are the parotid glands, submandibular glands, and sublingual glands, which occur in pairs. A parotid gland is located in front of and just below each ear. A submandibular gland is located just below the midline of the mandible on the right and left, and the sublingual glands are located under the tongue in the floor of the mouth and anterior to the submandibular glands.

Incidence

- The National Cancer Institute SEER data states that more than 50% of tumors found in salivary glands are benign. The parotid gland is the largest salivary gland and accounts for 70% to 80% of salivary gland abnormal growths. The palate is the most common site of minor salivary gland abnormalities (National Cancer Institute, 2022).
- The frequency of salivary gland malignancies varies according to location (National Cancer Institute, 2022):
  - Parotid glands: 20% to 25%
  - Submandibular glands: 35% to 40%
  - Palate: 50%
  - Sublingual glands: 90%
- The ACS (2022d) reports that the incidence of salivary gland cancers in the United States is not very common, making up 6% to 8% of all head and neck cancers. Each year, there are an estimated 2000 to 2500 cases in the United States. While these cancers can occur at any age, according to ACS (2022d), the average age at time of diagnosis is 55.

Etiology and Risk Factors

- The etiology of most salivary gland cancers cannot be determined. However, there are some risk factors that have been identified including:
  - Increased age
  - Exposure to ionizing radiation or previous radiation treatment to the head and neck
  - Diet high in animal fat and low in vegetables
  - Occupational exposure to rubber products manufacturing, asbestos mining, plumbing, and some types of woodworking

Signs and Symptoms

- A lump or swelling in the mouth, cheek, jaw, or neck
- Pain in the mouth, cheek, jaw, ear, or neck that does not go away
- A difference between the size and/or shape of the left and right sides of face or neck
- Numbness in a part or parts of the face
- Weakness of the muscles on one side of the face
- Trouble in opening mouth wide
- Fluid draining from an ear

Diagnostic Workup

- Physical examination and medical history
- Imaging studies: MRI, CT, PET, or ultrasonography
- FNA of suspicious lesions or adenopathy
- Incisional biopsy of suspected neoplasm

Histopathology

(Andreasen, 2019)

- There are almost 40 histologic types of salivary gland tumors.
- Although salivary gland neoplasms are histologically diverse, the more common types of carcinomas include the following:
  - Mucoepidermoid carcinoma
  - Adenoid cystic carcinoma
  - Adenocarcinoma, such as acinic cell carcinoma
  - Malignant mixed tumors

- The most common tumor of the salivary gland is a pleomorphic adenoma, which is a benign neoplasm. Carcinoma ex pleomorphic adenoma is a mixed tumor which is a carcinoma that has arisen from a benign pleomorphic adenoma.
- Histologic grading of salivary gland carcinomas aids in determining treatment. Grading is used primarily for mucoepidermoid carcinomas, adenocarcinomas not otherwise specified, adenoid cystic carcinomas, and SCCs. In most instances, the histologic type defines the grade (i.e., salivary duct carcinoma is high grade, and basal cell adenocarcinoma is low grade).

Clinical Staging

Staging of salivary gland cancers is based on clinical and radiographic information obtained before treatment and histologic grade once pathology has been confirmed and uses the AJCC guidelines based on the TNM classification system. According to the National Cancer Institute (2022), tumor size plays a more critical role in outcome determination than the tumor histologic grade.

- Early-stage tumors (stage I or II) are contained within the gland and are under 4 cm.
- Locally advanced disease (stage III) is defined when the tumor is greater than 4 cm and/or there is evidence of soft tissue invasion, or a smaller tumor with metastasis to a single lymph node.
- With moderately advanced disease (stage IV), the tumor invades the skin, mandible, ear canal, and/or facial nerve and may have metastasis to the lymph nodes. Stage IV also includes all tumors that present with distant metastasis.

Treatment

- The primary treatment of salivary gland cancer is surgical removal of the gland.
  - Neck dissection of the affected side lymph nodes may also be necessary depending on type of malignancy and location.
- Pathologic findings such as perineural invasion, vascular invasion, and extracapsular spread dictate the need for adjuvant treatment with radiation.
- Surgical resection with postoperative adjuvant radiation therapy is done for the following:
  - Large, bulky tumors or high-grade tumors
  - Lymph node involvement
  - When adequate clear margins cannot be achieved by surgical resection
  - For inoperable, unresectable, recurrent, or metastatic cancers.
- Primary radiation therapy may be considered. Fast neutron-beam radiation therapy or accelerated hyperfractionated photon-beam radiation therapy is more effective than conventional x-ray radiation therapy.
- According to the National Cancer Institute (2022), the use of chemotherapy as a treatment is under evaluation, although some data suggest that a portion of salivary gland cancers may be responsive to it. Chemotherapy may be considered if a patient refuses surgery and radiation therapy or for patients with metastatic disease. Doxorubicin, cisplatin, cyclophosphamide, and fluorouracil can be used as single agents or in various combinations.
- Clinical trials should also be considered, as these cancers may be responsive to aggressive combinations of chemotherapy and radiation.

Prognosis

Based on people diagnosed with salivary gland cancer between 2011 and 2017, about 75% of people diagnosed with salivary gland cancer are alive at least 5 years after diagnosis (ACS, 2022c). Several factors impact prognosis including:

- Salivary gland of origin
- Histologic features
- Grade
- Stage
- Involvement of the facial nerve
- Fixation to the skin or deep structures
- Spread to the lymph nodes or distant sites

Clinical stage, particularly tumor size, may be the crucial factor for determining treatment outcome, as it is for other head and neck cancers. Early-stage, low-grade malignant salivary gland tumors are usually curable with adequate surgical resection.

The prognosis is more favorable for major salivary gland tumors, as tumors of the parotid gland have the most favorable prognosis, followed by those of the submandibular gland. The least favorable sites are the sublingual and minor salivary glands.

Prevention and Surveillance

Because the cause of salivary gland malignancies is not understood, no specific recommendations for prevention are available. However, avoiding risk factors such as tobacco use, excessive alcohol use, unhealthy diets, and industrial hazards may lessen the risk for developing salivary gland cancer.

Surveillance for recurrent disease after treatment depends on clinical stage (most importantly tumor size). Physical exams will be required every few months and serial imaging may also be ordered to monitor for recurrent disease. Patients should also be instructed to inform their physician in between visits of any new masses or other new concerning symptoms.

References

American Cancer Society. (2022a). *Salivary gland cancer tests.* Available at https://www.cancer.org/cancer/salivary-gland-cancer/detection-diagnosis-staging/how-diagnosed.html.

American Cancer Society. (2022b). *Signs and symptoms of salivary gland cancer.* Available at https://www.cancer.org/cancer/salivary-gland-cancer/detection-diagnosis-staging/signs-and-symptoms.html.

American Cancer Society. (2022c). *Survival rates for salivary gland cancer.* Available at https://www.cancer.org/cancer/salivary-gland-cancer/detection-diagnosis-staging/survival-rates.html.

American Cancer Society. (2022d). *Key statistics about salivary gland cancer.* Available at https://www.cancer.org/cancer/salivary-gland-cancer/about/what-is-key-statistics.html.

Andreasen, S., Kiss, K., Mikkelsen, L. H., Channir, H. I., Plaschke, C. C., Melchior, L. C., ... Wessel, I. (2019). An update on head and neck cancer: new entities and their histopathology, molecular background, treatment, and outcome. *APMIS, 127*(5), 240–264.

National Cancer Institute. (2022). *Salivary gland cancer treatment (adult) (PDQ)–health professional version.* Available at https://www.cancer.gov/types/head-and-neck/hp/adult/salivary-gland-treatment-pdq.

Thyroid and Parathyroid Cancers

Definition

The thyroid gland is located in the base of the neck on both sides of the lower part of the larynx and upper part of the trachea. The thyroid gland is a butterfly-shaped gland that consists of two lateral lobes (a left lobe and a right lobe) connected by an isthmus. The thyroid gland produces three hormones: triiodothyronine (T_3), thyroxine (T_4), and calcitonin. These hormones help regulate metabolism, heart rate, blood pressure, and body temperature and can become imbalanced. The thyroid gland may increase in size or produce nodules and, although infrequent, may house or convert to a thyroid carcinoma, which is the most common endocrine carcinoma.

The parathyroid glands secrete a substance known as parathormone (PTH), which regulates calcium in the blood as well as calcium storage and phosphorus metabolism. The four parathyroid glands are usually located on the inferior and superior poles of each thyroid lobe on the posterior surface, and each is about the size of a grain of rice (3 to 5 mm) and weighs between 30 and 60 mg (see the figure below).

Incidence

- The ACS reports the incidence of laryngeal cancer in the United States annually and the 2022 statistics are as follows (ACS, 2022b). In 2022, there will be an estimated 43,800 new cases of thyroid cancer and an estimated 2230 deaths in the United States.
- According to SEER data, thyroid cancer makes up 2.3% of all newly diagnosed cancer cases in the United States and is the 12th most diagnosed cancer (National Cancer Institute, 2022b).
- Based on 2015 to 2019 SEER data, the annual incidence of thyroid cancer is 14.6 new cases per 100,000 men and women (National Cancer Institute, 2022b).
- Thyroid cancer affects more women than men and it is most frequently diagnosed among people between the ages of 45 and 54 years, with the median age at diagnosis of 51 (National Cancer Institute, 2022b).
- The incidence in thyroid cancer has been increasing in the United States, believed to be due to an increase in disease detection. This is related to diagnostic procedures such as CT or MRI scans ordered for unrelated conditions, and due to the increased sensitivity of the imaging, smaller, incidental thyroid nodules are detected that would not have been found previously.
- Parathyroid carcinoma is rare and is the least commonly seen endocrine cancer worldwide. It occurs in about 1% of individuals diagnosed with primary hyperparathyroidism (National Cancer Institute, 2022b).

Etiology and Risk Factors

- Gender
  - Thyroid cancers occur three times more in females than in males

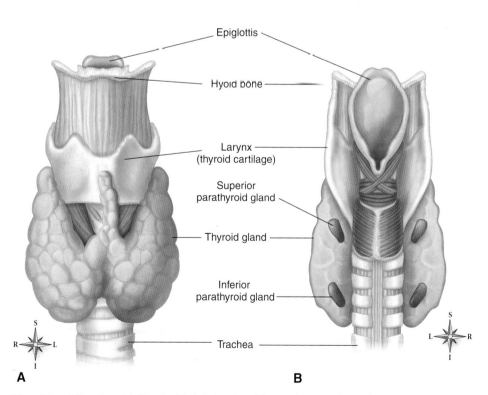

Thyroid and Parathyroid Glands. (A) Anterior view, (B) posterior view. (From Patton, K. T. [2024]. *The human body in health & disease* [8th ed.]. Elsevier.)

- Women are most often diagnosed in their 40s to 50s; men in their 60s or 70s
- Radiation exposure from certain medical treatments or radiation fallout in childhood
- Obesity
- Diet low in iodine
- History of goiter
- Asian race
- Family history of thyroid cancer
- Multiple endocrine neoplasia (MEN) syndromes
  - A family history of medullary carcinoma of the thyroid increases the risk for patients with MEN type 1 or 2. A mutation in the *RET* proto-oncogene has been identified in the familial form of medullary thyroid cancer.
  - In families with cases of MEN, screening for this mutation can be done as early as 5 or 6 years of age, and those testing positive are considered candidates for a prophylactic total thyroidectomy. Two out of 10 medullary thyroid cancers result from the inheritance of an abnormal gene.
  - MEN1 and MEN2 are disorders with an autosomal dominant pattern of inheritance. The genetic deficits produce hyperplasia or malignant tumors in several endocrine glands.
  - In MEN1, tumors occur in the parathyroids, pancreatic islet cells, adrenal cortex, and thyroid.
  - In MEN2, neoplasms include medullary thyroid cancer, pheochromocytoma, and parathyroid hyperplasia.
- Hyperparathyroidism occurs when a parathyroid gland produces excessive PTH resulting from gland overactivity. A benign tumor, called a parathyroid adenoma, may develop secondary to hyperparathyroidism. On rare occasions, parathyroid cancer can develop.

Signs and Symptoms

Thyroid Cancer
- Solitary thyroid mass
- Diffuse enlargement of the thyroid
- Enlarged neck node or mass
- Pain in the front of the neck
- Hoarseness or other voice changes that do not go away
- Dysphagia
- Dyspnea
- A constant cough that is not due to a cold

Parathyroid Cancer
- Hypercalcemia
- Fatigue
- Weight loss
- Forgetfulness
- Renal stones
- Low phosphorus levels
- High PTH serum levels
- Bone issues such as subcortical bone resorption, bone pain, or pathologic fractures
- Palpable neck mass
- Peptic ulcer
- Recurrent pancreatitis
- Muscle weakness

- Dehydration
- Nausea and vomiting

Diagnostic Workup

Thyroid Cancer
- Medical history and physical exam including palpation of thyroid gland and neck lymph nodes
- An FNA of the thyroid nodule(s) is done to screen for thyroid cancer. The Bethesda system is used to categorize the cytology of the FNA (Alshaikh et al., 2018). There are six categories:
  - Category I—nondiagnostic
  - Category II—benign
  - Category III—atypia of undetermined significance
  - Category IV—suspicious for follicular neoplasm
  - Category V—suspicious for malignancy
  - Category VI—malignant
- More information is needed to help to identify malignant thyroid tumors more accurately. Molecular markers (genetic testing) taken from the biopsied tissue are being studied to better screen for malignancy and therefore to reduce unnecessary thyroid surgeries with nodules in the Bethesda categories of III or IV (Alshaikh et al., 2018).
- Thyroid imaging: ultrasound, radioiodine scan, CT, MRI, or PET
- Laboratory tests: thyroid function, including T_3, T_4, TSH, and thyroglobulin levels; calcitonin for medullary thyroid cancer
- Flexible fiberoptic laryngoscopy to assess vocal cord function

Parathyroid Cancer
- Laboratory tests: serum calcium and PTH
  - Note: there is no definitive laboratory diagnosis to differentiate between hypercalcemia and parathyroid cancer.
- Neck ultrasound
- Sestamibi parathyroid scintigraphy: A small amount of radioactive material (technetium-99m) is given intravenously. If the parathyroid is overactive, ^{99m}Tc collects in the abnormal gland and is identified on the scan.
- High-resolution imaging such as a 4D CT may aid in gland identification.

Histopathology

Thyroid Cancer
The American Thyroid Association (ATA) describes the four types of thyroid cancers: papillary, follicular, medullary, and anaplastic.
- *Papillary carcinoma* is the most common, accounting for 70% to 80% of thyroid cancers (ATA, 2022). The primary tumors are often slow growing, multicentric, and can metastasize to lymph nodes.
- *Follicular carcinoma* is less common than papillary carcinoma and accounts for about 10% to 15% of thyroid cancers (ATA, 2022). It has a higher likelihood of vascular spread and distant metastases to the lungs and bones. A variant of follicular tumors, Hürthle cell tumors are carcinomas consisting of oncocytic cells in the thyroid and they carry a worse prognosis.

- *Medullary thyroid cancer* accounts for 1% to 2% of thyroid cancers (ATA, 2022). The tumors can manifest in a sporadic or familial form and arise from parafollicular cells or "C cells," which produce calcitonin instead of thyroid tumors like the other thyroid carcinoma types.
- *Anaplastic (undifferentiated) thyroid cancer* is fast-growing and aggressive. It accounts for less than 2% of thyroid cancers and the tumors often have lymph node and distant metastases at the time of diagnosis (ATA, 2022). The average survival rate is 6 months after diagnosis and one in five people are alive after 12 months. However, the cancers that are found incidentally tend to do better and have a much higher long-term survival rate.
- For clinical management, thyroid cancer is divided into two categories: well differentiated or poorly differentiated. The most common malignant tumors of the thyroid are well differentiated and include papillary, follicular, mixed, and Hürthle cell tumors.
- There are other types of carcinomas that can be found in the thyroid gland, such as lymphoma, sarcoma, or carcinosarcoma; however, those are much less common.

Parathyroid Cancer

Histologic criteria for parathyroid carcinoma are difficult to define. The distinction between benign and malignant parathyroid tumors is rarely made on the initial histologic analysis.

- A malignant parathyroid gland tumor is firm and has a stony-hard consistency and lobulation. They also tend to be surrounded by a dense, fibrous gray-white capsule that is invasive.
- A nonmalignant lesion, such as a parathyroid adenoma, usually manifests as a red-brown mass that is soft, round or oval, mobile, and noninvasive.
- Pathologic confirmation is determined by the frequency of mitoses, fibrosis, local invasion, vascular invasion, and nuclear pleomorphism.

Clinical Staging

Staging of both thyroid and parathyroid cancers are staged using the AJCC guidelines based on the TNM classification system. The National Cancer Institute lists the following:

Papillary (or Follicular) and Medullary Thyroid Cancers

(National Cancer Institute, 2022c)

Cancers that are defined as early stage (stage I) have disease limited to the thyroid gland. With locally advanced disease (stage II or III), there may be some disease outside of the thyroid and include some surrounding lymph nodes. Moderately advanced disease (stage IV) occurs when there is extrathyroidal extension into nearby tissues and may have distant metastasis.

Anaplastic Thyroid Cancer

(National Cancer Institute, 2022c)

Any patient diagnosed with anaplastic thyroid cancer is considered to have stage IV disease due to the aggressive nature of the tumor.

Parathyroid Cancer

There is no formal staging system that exists due to the limited data on tumor characteristics and prognosis (Machado & Wilhelm, 2019; National Cancer Institute, 2022a).

Treatment

Thyroid Cancer

- The primary treatment for thyroid cancer is surgery.
  - Lobectomy may be done to remove the lobe of the thyroid that contains the cancer.
  - Near total or total thyroidectomy may be indicated. In the event of a total thyroidectomy, a daily thyroid hormone medication is required indefinitely.
- A central neck dissection may be done if there is metastatic spread to the lymph nodes.
- The most common adjuvant therapy for thyroid cancer is radioactive iodine (RAI, or I-131). The thyroid gland absorbs the iodine found throughout the body, and RAI destroys the cells that take up iodine. RAI can be used to effectively destroy any thyroid tissue or cells that may remain after surgery, thus destroying any potential remaining thyroid cancer. RAI has little effect on the rest of the body. However, medullary and anaplastic thyroid cancers are not responsive to I-131 therapy, as they do not take up iodine (ACS, 2022c; National Cancer Institute, 2022c).
- External beam radiotherapy may be used for medullary or anaplastic thyroid cancers, extensive nodal or mediastinal disease, gross residual tumor after surgery, or for the management of bone or brain metastases.
- Chemotherapy is seldom used in most thyroid cancers and is usually reserved for anaplastic tumors or medullary thyroid cancer with metastatic disease (National Cancer Institute, 2022c).
- Targeted therapies for thyroid cancer, known as kinase inhibitors, are being investigated as potential treatment options. Those agents are sorafenib, lenvatinib, cabozantinib, selpercatinib, pralsetinib, larotrectinib, entrectinib, and vandetanib (NCI, 2022c).

Parathyroid Cancer

- The primary treatment for parathyroid cancer is surgery. PTH levels are drawn 10 minutes after removal of the gland and should drop to less than 50% of the preoperative level (Machado & Wilhelm, 2019).
- Parathyroid cancers are typically resistant to radiation, and chemotherapy is not used except in patients with widely metastatic disease.

Prognosis

Thyroid Cancer

- The 5-year relative survival rate for differentiated thyroid cancers from 2012 to 2018 was 98.4% (SEER, 2022).
- Overall survival depends on age at diagnosis and on tumor stage and histology. Age is the single most important prognostic factor in determining prognosis.
- Men who are younger than 40 years old and women younger than 50 years old without evidence of distant metastasis carry a low risk for recurrence.

- Lymph node status tends to be controversial in determining prognosis, as some studies show that regional lymph node disease has no effect on survival rates.
- There are several factors that contribute to a poorer prognosis for differentiated carcinomas (National Cancer Institute, 2022c):
  - Patients older than 45 years of age
  - Follicular histology
  - Primary tumor larger than 4 cm
  - Extrathyroidal extension
  - Distant metastases
- The median survival rate for anaplastic thyroid cancer is 3.16 months. Total thyroidectomy has been shown to reduce symptoms and improve overall survival rate with a median survival of 10 months and a 6-month survival rate of 59.3% (Lin et al., 2019).

Parathyroid Cancer

- Parathyroid cancer is a slow-growing cancer.
- Many patients are diagnosed after initial gland removal and therefore a complete resection is not typically done.
- Postsurgical recurrences occur typically 2 to 3 years after the initial resection and present with gradual rises in PTH and calcium levels.
- Machado and Wilhelm (2019) list the 5-year survival rate range to be 76% to 85%.
- Factors that have been identified with a shorter survival are large tumor size, male gender, and older age at time of diagnosis.
- Most patients die from complications related to hypercalcemia, not metastatic disease.

Prevention and Surveillance

There are no general prevention measures (ACS, 2022a).

- Genetic testing and counseling should be done for individuals with a family history of MEN1 syndrome.
  - Prophylactic thyroidectomy may be indicated for those with a family history of medullary thyroid cancer.
  - Patients with MEN1 should be closely monitored to ensure an early diagnosis.

- Surveillance for thyroid cancer includes periodic follow-up examinations as well as blood tests. Patients that undergo a total thyroidectomy need routine follow-ups with an endocrinologist or primary care provider to regulate the dose of thyroid replacement (levothyroxine).
- Parathyroid cancer surveillance calls for monitoring of calcium and PTH levels.

References

Alfouzan A. F. (2021). Radiation therapy in head and neck cancer. *Saudi Medical Journal*, *42*(3), 247–254. https://doi.org/10.15537/smj.2021.42.3.20210660.

Alshaikh, S., Harb, Z., Aljufairi, E., & Almahari, S. A. (2018). Classification of thyroid fine-needle aspiration cytology into Bethesda categories: An institutional experience and review of the literature. *CytoJournal*, *15*, 4.

American Cancer Society. (2021). Signs and symptoms of laryngeal and hypopharyngeal cancers. Available at https://www.cancer.org/cancer/types/laryngeal-and-hypopharyngeal-cancer/detection-diagnosis-staging/signs-symptoms.html.

American Cancer Society. (2022a). *Can thyroid cancer be prevented?*. Available at https://www.cancer.org/cancer/thyroid-cancer/causes-risks-prevention/prevention.html.

American Cancer Society. (2022b). *Key statistics for thyroid cancer*. Available at https://www.cancer.org/cancer/thyroid-cancer/about/key-statistics.html.

American Cancer Society. (2022c). *Radioactive iodine (radioiodine) therapy for thyroid cancer*. Available at https://www.cancer.org/cancer/thyroid-cancer/treating/radioactive-iodine.html.

American Thyroid Association. (2022d). *Cancer of the thyroid: Thyroid cancer (papillary and follicular)*. Available at https://www.thyroid.org/cancer-of-the-thyroid/.

Lin, B., Ma, H., Ma, M., Zhang, Z., Sun, Z., Hsieh, I. Y., … Lv, W. (2019). The incidence and survival analysis for anaplastic thyroid cancer: A SEER database analysis. *American Journal of Translational Research*, *11*(9), 5888–5896.

Machado, N. N., & Wilhelm, S. M. (2019). Parathyroid cancer: A review. *Cancers*, *11*(11), 1676.

National Cancer Institute. (2022a). *Parathyroid cancer treatment (PDQ)–health professional version*. Available at https://www.cancer.gov/types/parathyroid/hp/parathyroid-treatment-pdq.

National Cancer Institute. (2022b). *Cancer stat facts: Thyroid cancer*. Available at https://seer.cancer.gov/statfacts/html/thyro.html.

National Cancer Institute. (2022c). *Thyroid cancer treatment (PDQ)–health professional version*. Available at https://www.cancer.gov/types/thyroid/hp/thyroid-treatment-pdq#_313_toc.

National Organization of Rare Disease. (2019). Esophageal cancer. Available at https://rarediseases.org/rare-diseases/esophageal-cancer/#symptoms.

Leukemias

Kristen Hurley

Acute Lymphocytic Leukemia

Definition

Leukemias are malignant neoplasms that can occur across the life span of an individual. It is characterized by the production of increased numbers of immature leukocytes from the bone marrow and other blood-forming organs. These abnormal precursors proliferate and infiltrate the bone marrow, peripheral blood, and other organs suppressing the production of normal, mature cells.

Four types of leukemias are classified according to their cell type (i.e., lymphoid or myeloid) and whether they are acute or chronic. Acute leukemias are characterized by blocked lymphoid or myeloid progenitor cell differentiation, which results in a massive accumulation of immature cells or blasts; onset is acute.

Acute lymphocytic leukemia (ALL), also called *acute lymphoblastic leukemia,* is a cancer of lymphoblasts. Seventy-five percent of ALL patients have the B-cell subtype, and 25% of patients are diagnosed with the T-cell subtype (Terwilliger & Abdul-Hay, 2017).

Incidence

- An estimated 6660 new cases of ALL and 1560 deaths occurred in 2021 in the United States (National Cancer Institute Surveillance, Epidemiology, and End Results Program [NCI-SEER], 2022).
- ALL is the most common form of leukemia in children younger than 19 years of age. Adults have a low risk (1 in 1000), but 80% of ALL-related deaths occur among adults (NCI-SEER, 2022).
- ALL in children is the most common form of leukemia representing 75% to 80% of all leukemias diagnosed in childhood. Adult ALL represents 20% of all leukemias diagnosed in adults (Brown et al., 2021).
- Children under 5 years of age are at the greatest risk. The incidence then slowly rises again into the mid-20s. After the age of 50, the risk of developing leukemia increases slowly (American Cancer Society [ACS], 2018).
- More males than females have ALL (NCI-SEER, 2022).
- ALL is more common among Whites and Hispanics compared with other racial or ethnic groups (NCI-SEER, 2022).

Etiology and Risk Factors

- Radiation exposure is linked to the development of ALL, specifically those exposed to atomic bombs in Nagasaki and Hiroshima (ACS, 2015).
- An increased risk of ALL is associated with some genetic conditions, including Down syndrome, Klinefelter syndrome, Fanconi anemia, Bloom syndrome, ataxia-telangiectasia, and neurofibromatosis.
- Cytogenetic abnormalities are found, indicating the involvement of oncogenes such as *RAS, BCR/Abelson* gene (*ABL*), and B-cell lymphoma 2 (*BCL2*).
- Prior treatment with intensive immunosuppressive therapies is a risk factor.
- Exposure to the chemical benzene, which is used in many industries and can be found in cigarette smoke, glues, cleaning products, detergents, art supplies, and paint strippers (ACS, 2018).
- Additionally, infection with human T-cell lymphoma/leukemia virus-1 can cause a rare type of T-cell ALL, which is mostly found in Japan and the Caribbean (ACS, 2018).

Signs and Symptoms

- Signs and symptoms (usually manifest abruptly)
  - Malaise
  - Fatigue
  - Bony pain (especially sternal)
  - Sweats
  - Bleeding, easy bruising
- Physical findings
  - Pallor
  - Petechiae
  - Ecchymoses
  - Lymphadenopathy
  - Splenomegaly
  - Hepatomegaly
  - Mediastinal mass (usually a T-cell subtype)
  - Abdominal adenopathy (Burkitt type)

Diagnostic Work-up

- Medical history and physical examination
- Complete blood cell count (CBC) with differential count
  - Patients may have a high, normal, or low white blood cell count (WBC), but are usually neutropenic.
  - Pancytopenia resulting from marrow replacement by tumor may be identified.
  - Circulating blasts are usually observed in the peripheral smear; schistocytes can be found if the patient is experiencing disseminated intravascular coagulation (DIC) (Seiter, 2021).
- Serum chemistry panel: elevated lactate dehydrogenase and uric acid levels correlate with a large tumor burden and risk of tumor lysis syndrome. Potassium, phosphorus, and DIC panels may also be helpful.

- Cytogenetic analysis
  - Analysis permits identification of chromosomal and gene abnormalities. These occur in approximately 70% of adults. Additionally, abnormalities in chromosomal numbers can also be common in ALL (hyperdiploidy, hypodiploidy) (Seiter, 2021). The table below provides a summary of chromosomal and genetic abnormalities.
  - The t(9;22) transposition, called the Philadelphia (Ph) chromosome, is a common abnormality in adult ALL, occurring in 25% of cases, and carries a poorer prognosis (Brown et al., 2021).
  - The t(11q23) myeloid/lymphoid leukemia (MLL) is associated with poor prognosis found in adults and children less than 1 year.
  - The t(12;21) (p12;q22) translocation-ets-leukemia (TEL)/acute myelogenous leukemia 1 (AML1) is associated with a good prognosis in children.

Chromosomal and Genetic Abnormalities in Acute Lymphocytic Leukemia

Chromosome Abnormality	Genes Involved
• t(10;14) (q24;q11)	• HOX11/TCRA
• 6q	• Unknown
• 14q11	• TCRA/TCRD
• 11q23	• MLL
• 9p	• Unknown
• 12	• TEL
• t(1;19) (q23;p13)	• PBX1/E2A
• t(8;14) (q24;q32)	• c-myc/IGN
• t(2;8) (p12;q24)	• IGK/c-myc
• t(8;22) (q24;q11)	• c-myc/IGL
• t(9;22) (q34;q11)	• BCR-ABL
• t(4;11) (q21;q23)	• AF4-MLL

- Immunophenotyping enables the physician to determine the type of disease.
- Bone marrow aspiration to remove marrow fluid or a biopsy to remove a marrow sample is done to diagnose leukemic abnormalities.
- Lumbar puncture is done to identify malignant cells in the cerebrospinal fluid.
- Imaging: A chest radiograph is obtained to determine whether leukemia cells have formed a mass in the chest. Plain film findings also help to distinguish early-stage ALL from other diseases such as juvenile idiopathic arthritis. Computerized tomography (CT) neck/chest/abdomen/pelvis if indicated by symptoms.
- Hepatitis B/C, human immunodeficiency virus (HIV), CMV testing, and screen for opportunistic infections to rule out other etiologies.
- Echocardiogram should be considered since anthracyclines are important in treatment of ALL.
- Testicular exam, including scrotal ultrasound as indicated.

Histopathology

- Peripheral blood smear shows small lymphoblasts with scant cytoplasm, condensed nuclear chromatin, and indistinct nucleoli. Cytoplasmic granules may be present. There will not be Auer rods.
- In tissue sections, small to medium-sized tumor cells with scant cytoplasm; round, oval, or convoluted nuclei; fine chromatin; and indistinct small nucleoli. Antibody stains by flow cytometry is important. There will be expression of B-cell markers CD19, CD22, CD20, CD79a, CD45, and CD10.
- Additional antigens may define stages of differentiation from earliest to latest. Early precursors: B⁻ membrane $CD19^+$, $CD79a^+$, and cytoplasmic $CD22^+$.
- Common ALL-positive for CD10.
- Late Pre-B AA: positive for CD20.
- There may be coexpression of myeloid antigens in up to 30% of cases; the most common are CD13 and CD33.

Clinical Staging

- No clinical staging is performed for ALL except for assessment for central nervous system (CNS) involvement. Classification of CNS involvement determined by a lumbar puncture aspiration of cerebral spinal fluid (CSF) (Seiter, 2021):
  - CNS-1: No lymphoblasts in CSF regardless of WBC count.
  - CNS-2: WBC less than 5/µL in CSF with presence of lymphoblasts.
  - CNS-3 WBC ≥5/µL in CSF with presence of lymphoblasts.

Treatment

- The three phases of treatment for ALL usually require 1.5 to 3 years.
- Phase I is induction (i.e., remission induction), which typically requires hospitalization for approximately 4 weeks.
  - Many agents may be used
    - Prednisone
    - Vincristine
    - Anthracycline
    - Asparaginase
    - Cyclophosphamide
    - Etoposide
    - Methotrexate
    - Cytarabine
    - Tyrosine kinase inhibitors (TKIs) (for Ph chromosome–positive disease)
    - Mercaptopurine
    - Rituximab (for CD20+ disease)
- Complete remission (CR) rates range from 65% to 85% with these induction regimens (Seiter, 2021).

- Phase II is consolidation (i.e., intensification)
  - Patients must be in remission to begin the consolidation phase.
  - It usually lasts 1 to 3 months.
  - Many of the same agents administered during the induction phase are also used during consolidation.
  - High-risk patients may be considered for allogeneic stem cell or autologous stem cell transplantation.
- Phase III is maintenance
  - Maintenance therapy lasts approximately 2 years.
  - Several agents may be used
    - Methotrexate
    - 6-Mercaptopurine (6-MP)
    - Vincristine
    - Prednisone
  - The percentage of patients completing consolidation and maintenance therapy has declined as more patients are being referred for transplant while in first remission (Seiter, 2021).
- CNS prophylaxis is typically completed during the induction phase but may extend throughout therapy.
- Several agents are used.
  - Methotrexate
  - Hydrocortisone
  - Cytarabine
  - Cranial or spinal irradiation
  - High-dose intravenous methotrexate
  - Pegaspargase
- Patients who have relapsed after induction chemotherapy or maintenance therapy are unlikely to be cured by further chemotherapy alone. However, recent advances in immunotherapy, specifically T-cell therapies, provides new treatment options.
  - Blinatumomab, a bispecific, CD19-directed, CD3 T-cell engager immunotherapy, for use in relapsed and refractory B-cell ALL. This may also be used in first or second complete remission (CR) with minimal residual disease ≥0.1% (Brown et al., 2021).
  - Inotuzumab ozogamicin, CD22-directed antibody-drug conjugate, approved for treatment of adults with relapsed or refractory B-cell precursor ALL.
  - Tisagenlecleucel, CD19 chimeric antigen receptor (CAR) T-cell therapy, is indicated for patients up to age 25 with B-cell ALL that is refractory or in second or later relapse.
  - Brexucabtagene autoleucel, CD19 CAR T-cell therapy approved for adults (>18) relapsed or refractory B-cell ALL.
  - Reinduction chemotherapy followed by allogeneic bone marrow transplantation should be considered. For patients who do not have a human leukocyte antigen-matched donor and may be considered for an unrelated stem cell or bone marrow transplantation.
  - Clinical trials should also be considered.

Prognosis

- Overall, 5-year survival rates (Brown et al., 2021):
  - Adults: 20% to 40%.
  - Children and adolescents: 89% and 61%, respectively.
  - Although OS percentages can vary by how the age range is defined, it is clear the trend is lower OS as age increases (exception for infants younger than age 1, that age has not seen any improvement in OS in the past three decades and continues to have a 5-year OS of 55%).
- Long-term follow-up of childhood ALL survivors showed that many have late effects that dramatically affect their lives into adulthood. There are some that will have a secondary malignancy develop from the radiation and chemotherapy (1% to 6%), neurologic or neurocognitive disorders from cranial radiation or intrathecal chemotherapy (20% to 40%), cardiotoxicity due to anthracyclines or being overweight, endocrine disorders with obesity manifesting in 12% to 28%, bone disorders (osteoporosis, osteonecrosis), and social and psychological disorders (Kızılocak & Okcu, 2019).

Prevention and Surveillance

There are no known preventive measures for ALL. The National Comprehensive Cancer Network (NCCN) guidelines for 2022 recommend close surveillance after completion of therapy (NCCN, 2022a, 2022b).
- Year 1: follow-up every 1 to 2 months
  - Physical examination with CBC, differential count, and liver function tests.
  - Bone marrow aspirate as clinically indicated at a frequency of 3 to 6 months for at least 5 years.
  - Echocardiogram and CSF evaluation as indicated.
- Year 2: follow-up every 3 months
  - Physical examination (including a testicular examination), CBC, and differential count.
- Year 3: follow-up every 6 months
  - Physical examination (including a testicular examination), CBC, and differential count.
- Survivorship recommendations
  - Human papillomavirus (HPV) vaccine for men and women between 9 and 26 years of age.
  - Annual influenza vaccination.
  - Dental examination and cleaning every 6 months.
  - Neuropsychological testing as clinical indicated given increased risk of neurotoxicity in ALL survivors.
  - Monitor for healthy weight and encourage healthy lifestyle choices.
- Additional recommendations for children and young adults have also been developed by the Children's Oncology Group (COG) and the NCCN. The NCCN recommendations presented in the table on the next page are not ALL specific in contrast to the COG guidelines (2018), which are AML specific and provide guidance dependent on class

of chemotherapy used to treat AML. The COG guidelines can be found at http://www.survivorshipguidelines.org/pdf/2018/COG_LTFU_Guidelines_v5.pdf.

NCCN Screening Recommendations for Children and Young Adults

Treatment Exposures	Recommendations
Cranial or spinal radiation	• Neuroendocrine dysfunction screening • Neuropsychological evaluation
Chest radiation	• Females: breast cancer screening • Thyroid screening • Cardiovascular risk assessment and screening, including screening for cardiomyopathy and valvular heart disease • Pulmonary screening
Abdominal or pelvic radiation	• Colorectal cancer screening • Gonadal function assessment • Kidney and bladder function monitoring
Alkylating agents	• Gonadal function assessment • Pulmonary status monitoring • Therapy-related acute myeloid leukemia (t-AML) or myelodysplasia screening
Anthracyclines	• Cardiovascular function monitoring • t-AML or myelodysplasia screening
Bleomycin	• Pulmonary function monitoring
Cisplatin or carboplatin	• Cardiovascular function monitoring • Kidney and bladder function monitoring • Hearing evaluation • t-AML or myelodysplasia screening

Data from National Comprehensive Cancer Network (NCCN). (2022). NCCN Guidelines for adolescent and young adults, Version 2.2022. Available at http://www.nccn.org/professionals/physician_gls/pdf/aya.pdf.

References

American Cancer Society (ACS). (2015). *Do x-rays and gamma rays cause cancer?* Cancer.org. https://www.cancer.org/healthy/cancer-causes/radiation-exposure/x-rays-gamma-rays/do-xrays-and-gamma-rays-cause-cancer.html.

American Cancer Society (ACS). (2018). *Risk factors for acute lymphocytic leukemia (ALL).* Cancer.org. https://www.cancer.org/cancer/acute-lymphocytic-leukemia/causes-risks-prevention/risk-factors.html.

Brown, P. A., Shah, B., Advani, A., Aoun, P., Boyer, M. W., Burke, P. W., … Campbell, M. (2021). Acute lymphoblastic leukemia, version 2.2021, NCCN clinical practice guidelines in oncology. *Journal of the National Comprehensive Cancer Network, 19*(9), 1079–1109.

Children's Oncology Group (COG). (2018). Long-term follow up guidelines for survivors of childhood, adolescent and young adult cancers, Version 5.0. Retrieved January 3, 2022. http://www.survivorshipguidelines.org/pdf/2018/COG_LTFU_Guidelines_v5.pdf.

Kızılocak, H., & Okcu, F. (2019). Late effects of therapy in childhood acute lymphoblastic leukemia survivors. *Turkish Journal of Haematology: Official Journal of Turkish Society of Haematology, 36*(1), 1–11.

National Cancer Institute Surveillance, Epidemiology, and End Results Program (NCI-SEER). (2022). *SEER stat fact sheets: Acute lymphocytic leukemia (ALL).* http://seer.cancer.gov/statfacts/html/alyl.html.

National Comprehensive Cancer Network (NCCN). (2022a). NCCN clinical practice guidelines for acute lymphocytic leukemia, version 1.2022. http://www.nccn.org/professionals/physician_gls/pdf/all.pdf.

National Comprehensive Cancer Network (NCCN). (2022b). NCCN guidelines for adolescent and young adult, version 1.2023. http://www.nccn.org/professionals/physician_gls/pdf/aya.pdf.

Seiter, K. (2021) Acute lymphoblastic leukemia (ALL). Emedicine.medscape.com. https://emedicine.medscape.com/article/207631-overview.

Terwilliger, T., & Abdul-Hay, M. (2017). Acute lymphoblastic leukemia: a comprehensive review and 2017 update. *Blood Cancer Journal, 7*(6), e577.

Acute Myelogenous Leukemia

Definition

AML, also called *acute myeloid leukemia,* is a disease in which there are too many myeloid progenitor cells (i.e., immature granulocytes or monocytes) in the blood and bone marrow. Most cases of AML are distinguished from other blood disorders, such as myelodysplastic syndrome (MDS), by the finding of more than 20% blasts in the blood and bone marrow.

AML results from the failure of the myeloid progenitor cells to mature. The mechanism causing the arrest of cell maturation is not fully understood, but it involves the activation of abnormal genes through chromosomal translocations, deletions, duplications, or substitutions and genetic mutations leading to overexpression or underexpression of one or more proteins. Developmental arrest markedly decreases the production of normal blood cells, resulting in various degrees of anemia, thrombocytopenia, and neutropenia. The immature cells (i.e., blasts) accumulate in the blood, bone marrow, liver, and spleen as a result of their rapid proliferation and the reduction in apoptosis (i.e., programmed cell death).

Incidence

(National Cancer Institute [NCI], 2022)

- An estimated 20,050 new cases of AML (more than 90% are diagnosed in adults) and 11,540 deaths occurred in the United States in 2022.
- AML affects all age groups; the median age at diagnosis is 68 years.
- Prevalence increases with age. AML is the most common leukemia type in people between the ages of 75 and 84 years. The risk of AML increases 10-fold at age 30 compared with 70 years of age.
- AML is more common among Whites than other groups.
- AML is more common in men than women, particularly among older patients.

Etiology and Risk Factors

- The most common risk factor is an antecedent hematologic disorder, usually high-risk MDS.
- Compared with other leukemias, the increased risk of AML has the strongest link to prior radiation, cytotoxic chemotherapy, and toxin exposure.
  - Radiation exposure increases the risk, as seen in patients exposed to the atomic bomb explosion in Japan, in early radiologists (before appropriate shielding), and in patients irradiated for ankylosing spondylitis.
  - Prior chemotherapy, particularly with alkylating agents and topoisomerase II inhibitors, increases the risk of AML.
    - The period between an exposure and evidence of acute leukemia is approximately 3 to 5 years for alkylating agents or radiation exposure, but only 9 to 12 months for topoisomerase II inhibitors (Seiter, 2022).
- Smoking increases the relative risk of AML by 40% in active smokers, and by 25% in former smokers (King, 2019).
- Congenital disorders can result in AML during childhood, although some cases may develop in adulthood.

- Bloom syndrome, Down syndrome, congenital neutropenia, Fanconi anemia, and neurofibromatosis are risk factors.

Signs and Symptoms

- Presenting symptoms are related to bone marrow failure, including anemia, neutropenia, thrombocytopenia, and organ infiltration with leukemic cells.
- Patients may have signs and symptoms related to collection of leukemia cells in other organs such as the spleen, liver, CNS, testicular region, and gums. Organ infiltration occurs most commonly in patients with monocytic subtypes.
- Patient complaints
  - Fatigue
  - Weakness
  - Shortness of breath
  - Weight loss
  - Fever
  - Bleeding and easy bruising
  - Early satiety and fullness in right upper quadrant from splenomegaly
  - Bone pain resulting from a high leukemic cell burden and increased pressure in the marrow
  - Respiratory distress and altered mental status from leukostasis, which is a medical emergency that requires immediate treatment
  - Infections
- Physical findings
  - Pallor
  - Petechiae or ecchymoses
  - Hepatosplenomegaly
  - Signs of infection, including pneumonia
  - Gingivitis
  - Rash resulting from skin infiltration

Diagnostic Work-up

- Medical history and physical examination
- Laboratory tests
  - CBC with differential count
  - Serum chemistry panel: elevated lactate dehydrogenase and uric acid levels correlate with a large tumor burden.
  - Cytogenetics for the identification of chromosomal or genetic abnormalities—mandatory for AML patients as approximately 50% will have chromosomal abnormalities. Many of these mutations will assist in guiding treatment decisions and additional immune-chemotherapy regimens to use (NCI, 2022).
    - Detection of mutations such as NPM1, FLT3, CEPBA, and RUNX1 assists in providing the strongest information to predict outcomes of both remission induction and post remission therapy. Most commonly identified abnormalities occur t(8;21), inv(16), t(16;16), t(15;17), and translocations of the 11q23 breakpoint (NCI, 2022).
    - Mutations and/or deletions of the tumor suppressor gene *TP53* (located on the short arm of chromosome 17) occur in 2% to 20% of patients and are associated with older age, complex karyotypes, and therapy-related disease (Kantarjian et al., 2021).
- Additional studies
  - Bone marrow aspirate or biopsy

- Immunophenotyping to determine the type of proteins (e.g., mutated FLT3 receptor) expressed by cells through identification of antigens on the cell surface and the corresponding antibodies produced by the body.
- Imaging studies such as chest radiography

Histopathology

- The AML subtype helps to determine the prognosis and suggests treatment implications. However, the treatment is similar for all subtypes.
- The older French–American–British (FAB) classification of AML was revised by the World Health Organization (WHO) to incorporate and interrelate morphology, cytogenetics, molecular genetics, and immunologic markers and construct a classification system that is universally applicable and prognostically valid.
- Elements of the FAB classification that were specific to disease morphology have been retained. The WHO classification is outlined in the box below.

World Health Organization Classification of Myeloid Neoplasms and Acute Leukemia

- AML and related neoplasms
- AML with recurrent genetic abnormalities
- AML with t(8;21)(q22q22.1); RUNX1-RUNX1T1 (5%–12% of cases)
- AML with inv(16)(p13.1q22) or t(16;16)(p13.1;q22); CBFB-MYH11 (10%–12% of cases, predominantly in younger patients)
- APL with PML-RARA (5%–8% of cases, predominately adults in midlife; high CR rates and disease-free survival in APL can be obtained combining ATRA with chemotherapy)
- AML with t(9;11)(p21.3;q23.3); KMT2A-MLLT3 (5%–6% of cases and typically with monocytic features, more common in children or patients with therapy-related AML, typically associate with poor outcomes)
- AML with t(6;9)(p23;q34.1); DEK-NUP214 (1% of cases, associated with poor prognosis)
- AML with inv(3)(q21.3q26.2) or t(3;3)(q21.3;q26.2); GATA2, MECOM (1% of cases, associated with poor prognosis)
- AML (megakaryoblastic) with t(1;22) (p13.3;q13.1); RBM15-MKL1 (<1% of pediatric AML cases)
- Provisional entity: AML with BCR-ABL1
- AML with mutated NPM1 (confers improved prognosis in absence of the FLT3 [ITD] mutation)
- AML with biallelic mutation of CEBPA (in adults younger than 60, this represents 10%–15% of cases)
- Provisional entity: AML with mutated RUNX1
- AML with myelodysplasia-related changes (primarily in older patients)
- Therapy-related myeloid neoplasms (arise secondary to cytotoxic chemotherapy and/or radiation)
- AML, not otherwise specified (NOS)
  - AML with minimal differentiation
  - AML without maturation
  - AML with maturation
  - Acute myelomonocytic leukemia
  - Acute monoblastic and monocytic leukemia
  - Pure erythroid leukemia
  - Acute megakaryoblastic leukemia
  - Acute basophilic leukemia
  - Acute panmyelosis with myelofibrosis
- Myeloid sarcoma (also known as extramedullary myeloid tumor, granulocytic sarcoma, and chloroma)
- Myeloid proliferations associated with Down syndrome
  - Transient abnormal myelopoiesis (TAM) associated with Down syndrome
  - Myeloid leukemia associated with Down syndrome

AML, Acute myelogenous leukemia.
Modified from National Cancer Institute. (2023). Acute myeloid leukemia treatment (PDQ®) – Health professional version: Classification of AML. Available at www.cancer.gov/cancertopics/pdq/treatment/adultAML/healthprofessional.

Clinical Staging

- Clinical staging is not done for AML.
- Important adverse prognostic factors include:
  - Age at diagnosis—remission rates are inversely related to age with increased morbidity and mortality during induction directly related to age typically greater than 60.
  - CNS involvement with leukemia
  - Systemic infection at diagnosis
  - Elevated WBC greater than 100,0000 at diagnosis
  - Therapy-related myeloid neoplasms, from alkylating agents and radiation therapy
    - History of MDS or other hematologic disorder

Treatment

Treatment is typically administered in stages and will depend on whether the patient is newly diagnosed (previously untreated), in remission, or has recurrent disease. The cornerstone of AML treatment includes systemically directed chemotherapy to control both bone marrow involvement and systemic disease. CNS involvement is rare, so prophylactic treatment is typically not indicated.

Treatment for Newly Diagnosed Patients

- The initial treatment for newly diagnosed patients includes induction therapy, which aims to induce CR. The CR is defined as normal peripheral blood counts (absolute neutrophil count $>1000/mm^3$ and platelet count $>100,000/mm^3$) and normocellular marrow with less than 5% blasts and no symptoms of the disease. A CR can be further defined by with or without measurable residual disease (MRD) (MRD+ or MRD-, respectively).
- MRD is an important marker that can be prognostic and predictive and helps in monitoring and evaluating efficacy-response assessments.
  - MRD is determined using interphase fluorescence in situ hybridization (FISH) or multiparameter flow cytometry
- Cytogenic remission is determined when a previously abnormal karyotype reverts to normal (NCI, 2022).
- Some patients will respond to treatment but will not meet the strict criteria for CR and are then designated as one of the following:
  - CR with incomplete hematologic recovery (CRi)
  - Morphologic leukemia free state
  - Partial remission
- When selecting an agent for induction therapy, additional factors such as a patient's overall health status should be taken into consideration. Patients are typically divided into two categories: those that are eligible for intensive chemotherapy and those that are not eligible. Eligibility or ineligibility is determined by age and comorbidities as well as psychosocial factors, which would impact treatment compliance.

Induction Therapy—Intensive Remission Induction Chemotherapy

- The most common induction therapy is called "7 and 3"; 3 days of daunorubicin (short infusions) combined with cytarabine (i.e., cytosine arabinoside [ara-C]) as a 24-hour infusion over 7 days.
- Approximately 65% of patients achieve remission with one course of therapy (NCI, 2022).
- If there is a FLT3 mutation, the addition of a FLT3 inhibitor may be added to 7+3. Midostaurin, an FDA-approved FLT3 multikinase inhibitor, and quizartinib, an investigational selective type II FLT3-ITD inhibitor, have both shown improved overall survival in large phase 3 randomized clinical trials when combined with intensive chemotherapy for the treatment of newly diagnosed patients with FLT3+ AML (Erba et al., 2022; Stone et al., 2017).
- The addition of gemtuzumab ozogamicin (CD33-directed immunotoxin) to 7+3 is an option for those patients with CD33+ AML who are eligible for intensive chemotherapy. The addition of gemtuzumab ozogamicin has been linked to an increased risk of veno-occlusive disease and may render the patient ineligible for a stem cell transplant (Stanchina et al., 2020).
- Several clinical trials with targeted agents, vaccines, chimeric antigen receptor (CAR) T-cell therapies, bispecific T-cell engagers, and immune checkpoint blockade compounds are all currently in clinical trials for both newly diagnosed and relapsed/refractory AML and MDS (Stanchina et al., 2020).

Induction Therapy—Non-Intensive Chemotherapy
(Stanchina et al., 2020)

- Older adults or adults with significant comorbid conditions may decline or be too frail for intensive induction.
- Options for this group include:
  - Hypomethylating agents (azacytidine and decitabine)
  - Low-dose cytarabine
  - Liposomal daunorubicin and cytarabine are approved for patients with newly diagnosed therapy-related AML (t-AML) or AML with myelodysplasia-related changes (AML-MRC) (Chen et al., 2018).
  - Venetoclax plus azacytidine/decitabine or low-dose cytarabine for patients who are not eligible for intensive chemotherapy due to age (75 years of age and older) or for those who cannot undergo 7+3 induction because of comorbidities.
  - Glasdegib (hedgehog pathway inhibitor) plus low-dose cytarabine is approved in adults ≥75 years of age or who are unable to receive intensive chemotherapy.
  - Ivosidenib, an IDH1 targeted therapy, is approved for patients who are 75 and older with newly diagnosed AML or who have comorbidities that preclude the use of intensive induction chemotherapy.
  - Enasidenib, an IDH2 targeted therapy, is approved for patients who are 75 and older with newly diagnosed AML or who have comorbidities that preclude the use of intensive induction chemotherapy.
  - There are currently other agents under investigation, and clinical trials should be considered for all patients.

Post-Remission Therapy (Consolidation)

- Once patients finish induction and achieve remission, then post remission or consolidation therapy may be administered.
- The goal of post-remission therapy is to maintain and/or prolong remission by eliminating any residual leukemic cells and preventing relapse.
- Monitoring patients for MRD is helpful to identify patients at risk for relapse.
- NCCN guidelines for post-remission therapy are based on cytogenetic, molecular abnormalities, and age less than 60 years or greater than 60 years (see box below).

Summary of NCCN Post Remission Therapy

Age <60 Years With Favorable Risk
- HiDAC or cytarabine +/- gemtuzumab ozogamicin (CD33+ only)

Age <60 Years With Intermediate Risk
- Matched sibling or alternative donor stem cell transplant or
- HiDAC or cytarabine +/- gemtuzumab ozogamicin (CD33+ only)

Age <60 Years With Treatment Related Disease Other Than Core Binding Factor (CBF) and/or With Poor Risk
- Matched sibling or alternative donor stem cell transplant or
- HiDAC with/without HiDAC with midostaurin (FLT3+)
- Dual drug liposomal encapsulation with cytarabine and daunorubicin (for cytotoxic therapy-related AML or patients with MDS/CMML or cytogenetic changes consistent with MDS)

Age ≥60 Years With CR After Intensive Induction Therapy
- Reduced-intensity stem cell transplant or
- Standard dose cytarabine with/without anthracycline or
- Dual drug liposomal encapsulation cytarabine and daunorubicin (for cytotoxic therapy-related AML or patients with MDS/CMML or cytogenetic changes consistent with MDS) or
- Cytarabine + daunorubicin + gemtuzumab ozogamicin (CD33+) or
- Maintenance therapy with hypomethylating agent (azacytidine, decitabine) until disease progression

Age ≥60 Years With CR After Lower Intensity Therapy
- Reduced-intensity stem cell transplant or
- Hypomethylating agents (azacytidine, decitabine) until progression or
- Gemtuzumab ozogamicin up to eight continuation courses (CD33+)
- Continue enasidenib (IDH2+) or ivosidenib (IDH1+) until progression

AML, Acute myelogenous leukemia; *CR*, complete remission; *MDS*, myelodysplastic syndrome.
Data from the National Comprehensive Cancer Network. (2022). Acute myeloid leukemia v.2.2022. Available at https://www.nccn.org/guidelines/guidelines-detail?category=1&id=1411.

- The treatment regimens for post remission are typically short term for three to four cycles of relatively intensive chemotherapy.
- Stem cell transplantation can be used in select AML patients as part of the post-remission therapy.
  - Myeloablative allogeneic stem cell transplant has been traditionally used in younger and fit patients.
  - Older patients (>60 years) with minimal comorbidities may benefit from a reduced-intensity conditioning allogeneic stem cell transplant as part of consolidation therapy (NCCN, 2022).

Maintenance (Continuation) Therapy

- Maintenance therapy (longer period of therapy at lower doses) for patients in remission can be used in select patients with AML.

- Hypomethylating agents (azacytidine, decitabine) until progression following intensive chemotherapy and in patients who are ineligible for intensive chemotherapy.
- Gemtuzumab ozogamicin up to eight continuation courses (CD33+).
- IDH mutated patients: Continue enasidenib (IDH2+) or ivosidenib (IDH1+) until progression.
- FLT3 mutated patients: The NCCN recommends sorafenib as maintenance therapy for this patient type. Midostaurin is approved in Europe as a single-agent maintenance therapy for patients in remission; however, it is not recommended by the NCCN or approved by the FDA for this use in the United States (Medeiros et al., 2019; NCCN, 2022).
  - QuANTUM-First, a phase 3 study of quizartinib, an investigational FLT3 ITD selective inhibitor for newly diagnosed patients with FLT-3 ITD AML, included a continuation phase for patients in remission following consolidation or transplantation and as noted earlier overall survival was increased in this study. In time, this agent may be an option practices for this patient population across treatment phases (Erba et al., 2022).
- There are currently other agents under investigation, and clinical trials should be considered for all patients.

Treatment for Relapsed or Refractory Acute Myelogenous Leukemia

- Some patients, despite the intensive induction phase, are unable to reach remission and have refractory disease, and some may also relapse of disease after reaching an initial remission (NCI, 2022).
- No current standard treatment regimen exists for this group of patients
  - Options include intensive salvage chemotherapy, reduced-intensity therapy, including targeted therapy, allogeneic hematopoietic transplantation, and clinical trials.
  - Additionally, there are some treatment options that may be used post stem cell transplant in hopes of preventing relapse. Relapse after a stem cell transplant is typically associated with poor outcomes (Medeiros et al., 2019).
  - There are currently other agents under investigation, and clinical trials should be considered for all patients.

Prognosis

- The overall 5-year survival rate for AML ranges from 40% to 50% in patients aged ≤60 years and from 20% to 30% in those aged greater than 60 to 70, whole receive high-intensity chemotherapy regimens (Medeiros et al., 2019).
- Adverse prognostic factors include:
  - Age at diagnosis—remission rates are inversely related to age with increased morbidity and mortality during induction directly related to age typically greater than 60.
  - CNS involvement with leukemia
    - Systemic infection at diagnosis
    - Elevated WBC greater than 100,0000 at diagnosis

- Therapy-related myeloid neoplasms, from alkylating agents and radiation therapy
- History of MDS or other hematologic disorder
- Treatment-related death rates with consolidation therapy and no transplantation with cytarabine-containing regimens are usually less than 5% to 12%, and they have yielded disease-free survival rates of 30% to 50% (NCCN, 2022).
- Allogeneic bone marrow transplantation results in the lowest incidence of leukemic relapse.
  - Disease free rates with allogeneic transplantation in the first CR have ranged from 45% to 60% (Loke et al., 2021).
  - For those older than 60 years of age, reduced-intensity conditioning and allogeneic stem cell transplant have shown 40% to 60% 2-year overall survival with a 20% non-relapse mortality for those transplanted in remission (NCCN, 2022).
  - Allogeneic transplantation is limited by the need for a suitable donor, which can present some challenges for patients of older age or mixed lineage. Donor search should be done early in the treatment course if no sibling donor has been identified.
- Autologous bone marrow transplantation can be considered in select patients when no donor is suitable. However, efficacy (disease free survival, overall survival, and relapse rate) is higher disease with reduced-intensity allogeneic stem cell transplantation (NCCN, 2022).

Prevention and Surveillance

- The cause of AML is not fully understood, and specific measures to prevent AML have not been identified.
- Exposure to controllable risk factors such as toxins, radiation, and tobacco should be limited. Individuals with known exposures should be monitored, but most people with known risk factors do not get leukemia.
- Surveillance after consolidation therapy includes (NCCN, 2022):
  - CBC with platelets every 1 to 3 months for 2 years, then every 3 to 6 months up to 5 years.
  - Bone marrow aspirate and biopsy only if a peripheral smear is abnormal or cytopenia develops.
- MRD assessment should be done upon completion of induction before allogeneic transplantation and at any additional time point according to patient symptoms and prior detection of any abnormalities.
  - This can be done by real-time quantitative polymerase chain reaction (RQ-PCR) or multicolor flow cytometry (NCCN, 2022).

References

Chen, E. C., Fathi, A. T., & Brunner, A. M. (2018). Reformulating acute myeloid leukemia: Liposomal cytarabine and daunorubicin (CPX-351) as an emerging therapy for secondary AML. *OncoTargets and Therapy, 11*, 3425–3434.

Erba, H., Montesinos, P., Vrhovac, R., Patkowska, E., Kim, H. J., Zak, P., … Schlenk, R. (2022). Quizartinib prolonged survival vs placebo plus intensive induction and consolidation therapy followed by single-agent continuation in patients aged 18-75 years with newly diagnosed FLT3-ITD+ AML. *Hemasphere, 6*(S3), 1–2.

Hwang, S. M. (2020). Classification of acute myeloid leukemia. *Blood Research, 55*(S1), S1–S4.

Kantarjian, H. M., Kadia, T. M., DiNardo, C. D., Welch, M. A., & Ravandi, F. (2021). Acute myeloid leukemia: Treatment and research outlook for 2021 and the MD Anderson approach. *Cancer, 127*, 1186–1207.

King, J. (2019). Largest analysis to date examines link between smoking and outcomes in acute myeloid leukemia. *Cancer Network*. https://www.cancernetwork.com/view/largest-analysis-date-examines-link-between-smoking-and-outcomes-acute-myeloid-leukemia.

Loke, J., Buka, R., & Craddock, C. (2021). Allogeneic stem cell transplantation for acute myeloid leukemia: Who, when, and how? *Frontiers in Immunology, 12*, 659595.

Medeiros, B. C., Chan, S. M., Daver, N. G., Jonas, B. A., & Pollyea, D. A. (2019). Optimizing survival outcomes with post-remission therapy in acute myeloid leukemia. *American Journal of Hematology, 94*(7), 803–811.

National Cancer Institute (NCI). (2022). *Adult acute myeloid leukemia: Treatment—for health professionals (PDQ®)–Health Professional Version*. https://www.cancer.gov/types/leukemia/hp/adult-aml-treatment-pdq.

National Comprehensive Cancer Network (NCCN). (2022). NCCN clinical practice guidelines for acute myeloid leukemia, version 2.2022. https://www.nccn.org/guidelines/guidelines-detail?category=1&id=1411.

Seiter, K. (2022, May 31). Acute myeloid leukemia (AML). Emedicine.Medscape.com. https://emedicine.medscape.com/article/197802-overview.

Stanchina, M., Soong, D., Zheng-Lin, B., Watts, J. M., & Taylor, J. (2020). Advances in acute myeloid leukemia: Recently approved therapies and drugs in development. *Cancers, 12*(11), 3225.

Stone, R. M., Mandrekar, S. J., Sanford, B. L., Laumann, K., Geyer, S., Bloomfield, C. D., … Döhner, H. (2017). Midostaurin plus chemotherapy for acute myeloid leukemia with a FLT3 mutation. *The New England Journal of Medicine, 377*(5), 454–464.

Chronic Lymphocytic Leukemia

Definition

Chronic lymphocytic leukemia (CLL), an indolent cancer of the B cells, is the most common type of leukemia. It is characterized by lymphocytosis, lymphadenopathy, and splenomegaly. It results from an acquired injury to the deoxyribonucleic acid (DNA) of a lymphocyte in the bone marrow, causing uncontrolled growth of CLL cells in the marrow and increasing their concentration in the blood. Lymphocyte counts are usually greater than $5000/mm^3$, and cells have a characteristic immunophenotype (i.e., CD5- and CD23-positive B cells).

CLL cells in the marrow do not impede normal blood cell production to the extent that ALL cells do. This important distinction from acute leukemia accounts for the less severe early course of the disease.

Incidence

- An estimated 20,160 new cases (12,630 men and 7530 women) of CLL occurred with 4410 deaths in 2022 in the United States (American Cancer Society [ACS], 2022). CLL is the most prevalent adult leukemia in Western countries (Wierda et al., 2019).
- CLL affects middle-aged or elderly adults.
  - Median age at diagnosis is 70 years.
  - Most CLL patients are more than 55 years old.
  - CLL rarely affects children.
- CLL is more common in North America and Europe, and in men more often than women.
- The lifetime risk for CLL is 1 in 175 (0.57%) (American Cancer Society [ACS], 2022).

Etiology and Risk Factors

- It is not understood what induces the change in lymphocyte DNA.

- Risk factors include the following (ACS, 2022):
  - Age: the risk of development goes up as you age, 9 out of 10 people with CLL are over the age of 50.
  - Long-term exposure to herbicides or pesticides (e.g., Agent Orange during the Vietnam War).
  - Potentially radon exposure
  - Family history of CLL or cancer of the lymphatic system. First degree relatives of someone with CLL have more than twice the risk to develop CLL in their lifetime (parents, siblings, children).
  - Signs and Symptoms
- Symptoms usually exist with advanced disease.
- Diagnosis is typically made during routine blood work.
- Presenting symptoms
  - Fatigue
  - Shortness of breath with exertion
  - Weight loss
  - Night sweats
  - Frequent infections of the skin, lungs, kidneys, or other sites
- Physical findings
  - Ecchymosis
  - Lymphadenopathy
  - Splenomegaly

Diagnostic Work-up

(Hallek, 2019)
- Medical history and physical examination
- Laboratory tests
  - CBC with differential count
  - Presence of ≥5000 B lymphocytes/μL in peripheral blood sustained for at least 3 months
    - Anemia is found in 35% of patients.
    - Thrombocytopenia is found in 25% of patients.
  - Serum chemistry panel shows elevated lactate dehydrogenase and uric acid levels that correlate with a large tumor burden.
  - Evaluation of immunoglobulins (i.e., γ-globulins); CLL patients may not have enough of these proteins, which may lead to repeated infections.
  - Cytogenetics for identification of chromosomal or genetic abnormalities.
  - FISH to evaluate chromosome changes and to monitor response to treatment.
  - Immunophenotyping (i.e., flow cytometry) to identify whether the CLL began with a B lymphocyte or T lymphocyte; B-cell CLL is the most common form. A common panel used tests for CD19, CD5, CD20, CD23, κ and λ immunoglobulin light chains.
- Additional studies
  - Bone marrow aspirate or biopsy
  - Histochemical staining on sample
- Imaging studies
  - Chest radiography
  - CT
  - Magnetic resonance imaging (MRI)

Histopathology

(Hallek, 2019)
- The leukemic cell is a small mature lymphocyte with a narrow border of cytoplasm and a dense nucleus lacking any discernible nucleoli and having partially aggregated chromatin. There may be cleaved cells (prolymphocytes) up to 55% of the blood lymphocytes. Smudge cells are other characteristic morphologic features of CLL.
- Most leukemic cells are B cells with CD5 positivity. The T-cell variant is difficult to identify in marrow morphology alone.
- Bone marrow is hypercellular with nodules of neoplastic cells; the bone marrow becomes more filled as the leukemia progresses. Genetic mutations (either deletions or additions) are common in CLL. Some commonly seen deletions involve chromosome 13, chromosome 11, trisomy 12, chromosome 17 (17p), plus over 40 other mutated genes, and 11 recurrent somatic copy number variations have been identified in CLL. These include NOTCH1, MYD88, TP53, ATM, SF3B1, FBXW7, POT1, CHD2, RPS15, IKZF3, ZNF292, ZMYM3, ARID1A, and PTPN11.

Clinical Staging

- Staging is useful to predict prognosis and to stratify patients for treatment.
- Prognostic variables include certain gene mutations (i.e., TP53 or IgVH), bone marrow involvement, anemia, and thrombocytopenia as the major adverse variables.
- Typically, the use of Rai or Binet staging systems creates prognostic information by using the results of physical examination and blood counts but does not factor in any biologic or genetic markers (see table below).
- The international prognostic score (CLL-IPI) integrates the genetic, biologic, and clinical variables to identify distinct risk groups of CLL patients (see table on the next page) (Molica et al., 2016).

Rai and Binet Staging Systems

Rai System	Binet System
Stage 0 Lymphocytosis, lymphocytes in blood >5 × 10^9/L clonal B cells and >40% in bone marrow *Risk status = Low*	**Stage A** Hemoglobin ≥10 g/dL, and platelets ≥100,000/mm^3 and <3 enlarged areas
Stage I Stage 0 with enlarged node(s) *Risk Status = Intermediate*	**Stage B** Hemoglobin ≥10g/dL and platelets ≥100,000/mm^3 and ≥3 enlarged areas
Stage II Stage 0-I with splenomegaly, hepatomegaly, or both *Risk Status = Intermediate*	**Stage C** Hemoglobin <10 g/dL and/or platelets <100,000/mm^3 and any number of enlarged areas
Stage III Stage 0-II with hemoglobin <11 g/dL or hematocrit <33% *Risk Status = High*	
Stage IV Stage 0-III with platelets <100,000/mm^3 *Risk Status = High*	

Data from Hallek, M. (2019). Chronic lymphocytic leukemia: 2020 update on diagnosis. *American Journal of Hematology, 94*(11), 1266–1287.

The Chronic Lymphocytic Leukemia International Prognostic Score (CLL-IPI)

Variable	Adverse Factor	Grading
17p/TP53	Deleted and/or mutated	4
IGHV status	Unmutated	2
B_2M	>3.5 mg/L	2
Clinical stage	Binet B/C or Rai I–IV	1
Age	>65 years	1
	Prognostic score	0–10

Reprinted with permission from Elsevier, The Lancet Oncology. (2016). An international prognostic index for patients with chronic lymphocytic leukaemia (CLL-IPI): a meta-analysis of individual patient data. *The Lancet Oncology 17*(6),779–790.

Treatment

- CLL typically occurs in elderly patients, progresses slowly, and typically is not curable; therefore, treatment is often conservative.
- Treatment should be individualized and based on the clinical behavior of the disease.
- Treatment decisions depend on the patient's functional status, symptoms, prognostic factors, stage of disease, disease recurrence, and response to prior therapies.
- In asymptomatic patients, treatment may be deferred until the patient becomes symptomatic.
- Treatment may range from watchful waiting to treatment for complications as needed, applying a variety of therapeutic options, including steroids; chemotherapy with alkylating agents, purine analogs, or combinations; monoclonal antibodies; radiation; targeted immunotherapy agents or transplantation.
- The rate of disease progression is patient-specific, and there may be long periods of stable disease and sometimes spontaneous regressions; frequent and careful observation is required to monitor the clinical course.
- The decision for initiating treatment should commence when patients have progressed or present with symptomatic/active disease. Ways to define active or symptomatic disease have been outlined by the International Working Group for CLL (iwCLL) and should include one of the following (Hallek, 2019):
  - Worsening of anemia and/or thrombocytopenia suggesting progressive marrow failure
  - A very large spleen (i.e., ≥6 cm below the left costal margin) or progressive or symptomatic splenomegaly
  - Very enlarged lymph nodes (i.e., ≥10 cm in longest diameter) or progressive or symptomatic lymphadenopathy
  - Rapid lymphocytosis with an increase of ≥50% over a 2-month period
  - Autoimmune complications
  - Extranodal involvement that is either symptomatic or functional
  - Other symptoms related to CLL such as:
    - Unintentional weight loss of ≥10% in 6 months
    - Severe fatigue rendering the patient unable to work or perform usual activities
    - Fevers ≥100.5°F for ≥2 weeks without an infection
    - Night sweats for ≥1 month without an infection

Initiation of Treatment

- Patients should be evaluated for performance status prior to initiation of any therapy. Some patients should still be offered combination therapy such as fludarabine (F), cyclophosphamide (C), and rituximab (R) or FCR, while others may be offered more targeted agents up front as monotherapy (i.e., ibrutinib).
- Patients with deletion 17p or the TP53 mutation should have options of venetoclax and obinutuzumab, ibrutinib, or idelalisib plus rituximab offered along with discussion on stem cell transplant at the time of first or second relapse.

Relapsed/Refractory Disease

- Treatment of relapsed and refractory disease is based on the outcome of the front-line therapy and duration of the response (see table below).

Treatments for Relapsed and Refractory Chronic Myelogenous Leukemia

Response to 1st Line Therapy	Fitness	Therapy
Refractory or progresses within 3 years	Good fitness	Change to one of the following: ibrutinib, idelalisib + R, venetoclax + R, FCR or BR, lenalidomide (+R), alemtuzumab + dexamethasone, fludarabine + alemtuzumab. Discuss allogeneic stem cell transplant
	Poor fitness	Change to one of the following: ibrutinib, idelalisib + R, venetoclax + R, alemtuzumab + dexamethasone, FCR-lite, BR, lenalidomide (+R), high-dose rituximab
Progress after 3 years	ALL	Repeat 1L therapy if possible

ALL, Acute lymphocytic leukemia; *BR,* bendamustine + rituxan; *FCR,* fludarabine, cyclophosphamide, rituxan; *R,* rituximab.
Data from Hallek, M. (2019). Chronic lymphocytic leukemia: 2020 update on diagnosis, risk stratification and treatment. *American Journal of Hematology, 94*(11), 1266–1287.

Options for Chronic Lymphocytic Leukemia Treatment

- Agents considered for treatment in CLL may be used in combination or monotherapy depending on stage and status of the patient (Hallek, 2019).
- Cytostatic agents
  - Chlorambucil—low cost and oral therapy
    - Disadvantage—low rates of CR
    - Toxicities after extended use include prolonged cytopenia, myelodysplasia, and potentially secondary acute leukemia
    - May be used more today as palliation in elderly or unfit patients

- Purine analogs: fludarabine, pentostatin, and cladribine (2-CDA)
  - Fludarabine—superior overall response (OR) rates compared to other treatment regimen with alkylating agents or corticosteroids but does not improve survival when used as single agent.
  - Cladribine—produce higher CR rates than chlorambucil and steroids, but no survival benefit.
  - Bendamustine—higher OR rates than both fludarabine and chlorambucil, medical PFS better than both agents. Able to be given monotherapy.
- Monoclonal antibodies
  - Anti-CD20 antibodies
    - Rituximab—less active as a single agent in CLL, but in combination with chemotherapy is efficacious in CLL
    - Ofatumumab—some activity as single agent in CLL
- Other monoclonal antibodies
  - Alemtuzumab—fully humanized monoclonal antibody against CD52
  - Effective in chromosome deletions of 11, 17, and TP53 mutated patients
  - Currently only available on compassionate use program
- Targeted agents
  - Tyrosine kinases inhibitors
    - Bruton TKIs showed improvements in treating both newly diagnosed and relapsed CLL patients
      - Ibrutinib
      - Acalabrutinib
      - Zanubrutinib (pending FDA approval in CLL)
    - Spleen tyrosine kinase (Syk)
    - ZAP70
    - Src family kinases (Lyn)
- Phosphatidylinositol 3-kinases showed improvements in treating both newly diagnosed and relapsed CLL patients.
  - Idelalisib—In a phase 3 randomized double-blind study of relapsed or refractory CLL patients idelalisib + rituximab improved progression free survival and overall survival compared to rituximab plus placebo (Sharman et al., 2019). It is approved for use in combination with rituximab for those patients that rituximab alone would be an appropriate therapy due to comorbidities (Gilead, 2022).
    - Duvelisib—is another Pi3K inhibitor approved in relapsed/refractory CLL after two prior therapies (Secura Bio, 2021).
  - Thalidomide analogue
    - Lenalidomide
  - BCL2 inhibitors
    - Venetoclax
- Check point inhibitors
  - Programmed death 1 (PD-1) inhibitor
    - Pembrolizumab

- Clinical trials should always be considered for patients with relapsed and refractory CLL. Trials are ongoing for newer agents both in combination and in monotherapy, which may result in increased therapeutic efficacy and less toxicity. Clinical trials are also ongoing evaluating CAR T cells, NK cell for patients with CLL.

Prognosis

- There is a large variation in survival among individual patients, ranging from several months to a normal life expectancy.
- The overall 5-year survival rate for patients with CLL is 87% (National Cancer Institute, Surveillance, Epidemiology, and End Results Program [NCI-SEER], n.d.).

Prevention and Surveillance

- There are no prevention guidelines for CLL.
- Ongoing supportive care for people with CLL includes (National Comprehensive Cancer Network [NCCN], 2022):
  - Standard cancer screening guidelines for breast, cervical, colon, and prostate cancer
  - CLL patients are at an increased risk of developing nonmelanoma skin cancer.
    - Squamous cell carcinoma and basal cell carcinoma were 7 times and 14 times more likely in CLL patients, respectively.
    - CLL patients are more likely to die from or have metastatic squamous cell carcinoma than those without CLL.
      - Risk factors include Caucasian decent and history of intensive sun exposure at young age.
      - Yearly dermatologic evaluation is recommended.
  - Recurrent infections can occur patients should be monitored for infections ongoing as well as monitoring of serum IgG levels (if <500 mg/dL intravenous immunoglobulin replacement could be considered).
  - Annual flu vaccination is recommended.
  - Pneumococcal vaccination every 5 years.
  - COVID-19 vaccination is recommended for all CLL patients.

References

American Cancer Society (ACS). (2022). *About chronic lymphocytic leukemia.* https://www.cancer.org/cancer/chronic-lymphocytic-leukemia/about.html.

Gilead. (2022). *ZYDELIG® prescribing information.* https://www.gilead.com/-/media/files/pdfs/medicines/oncology/zydelig/zydelig_pi.pdf.

Hallek, M. (2019). Chronic lymphocytic leukemia: 2020 update on diagnosis, risk stratification and treatment. *American Journal of Hematology, 94*(11), 1266–1287.

Molica, S., Shanafelt, T. D., Giannarelli, D., Gentile, M., Mirabelli, R., Cutrona, G., … Morabito, F. (2016). The chronic lymphocytic leukemia international prognostic index predicts time to first treatment in early CLL: Independent validation in a prospective cohort of early stage patients. *American Journal of Hematology, 91*(11), 1090–1095.

National Cancer Institute, Surveillance, Epidemiology, and End Results Program. (n.d.). Cancer stat facts: Leukemia-chronic lymphocytic leukemia. Seer.cancer.gov. https://seer.cancer.gov/statfacts/html/clyl.html.

National Comprehensive Cancer Network. (2022). NCCN clinical practice guidelines for chronic lymphocytic leukemia/small lymphocytic lymphoma, version 3.2022. Available at: https://www.nccn.org/guidelines/guidelines-detail?category=1&id=1478.

Secura Bio. (2021). *COPIKTRA® prescribing information.* https://copiktra. com/pdf/COPIKTRA-PI-USCPR2007403.pdf.

Sharman, J. P., Coutre, S. E., Furman, R. R., Cheson, B. D., Pagel, J. M., Hillmen, P., … Stilgenbauer, S. (2019). Final results of a randomized, phase III study of Rituximab with or without Idelalisib followed by open-label Idelalisib in patients with relapsed chronic lymphocytic leukemia. *Journal of Clinical Oncology: Official Journal of the American Society of Clinical Oncology, 37*(16), 1391–1402.

Wierda, W. G., Byrd, J. C., Abramson, J. S., Bilgrami, S. F., Bociek, G., Brander, D., … Sundar, H. (2019). NCCN guidelines insights: Chronic lymphocytic leukemia/small lymphocytic lymphoma, version 2.2019. *Journal of the National Comprehensive Cancer Network, 17*(1), 12–20.

Chronic Myelogenous Leukemia

Definition

Chronic myelogenous leukemia (CML), also called *chronic myeloid leukemia*, is a cancer of granulocytes or monocytes. It is considered a myeloproliferative neoplasm and causes the rapid growth of myeloid precursors in the bone marrow, peripheral blood, and body tissues.

The Ph chromosome is identified in more than 95% of patients diagnosed with CML. It results from a reciprocal translocation between chromosomes 9 and 22, which is designated t(9;22), in a myeloid stem cell in the bone marrow (NCI, 2022). The transfer of DNA results in one chromosome 9 that is longer than normal and one chromosome 22 that is shorter than normal. The DNA removed from chromosome 9 contains most of the *ABL* gene. The break in chromosome 22 occurs in a gene in the middle of the breakpoint cluster region (BCR). Fusion of the two chromosome segments creates the BCR/*ABL* gene, which encodes an abnormal tyrosine kinase protein that causes CML.

Incidence

(American Cancer Society [ACS], 2022)
- In the United States, CML accounts for 15% of cases of leukemia.
- An estimated 8860 new cases of CML (5120 in men and 3740 in women) and 1220 estimated deaths occurred in 2022 in the United States.
- The median age at diagnosis is 67 years; 80% of patients diagnosed are older than 65 years of age.
- CML accounts for 2.6% of leukemias in children between the ages of 0 to 19 years.
- About 1 in 526 people will get CML in their lifetime in the United States.

Etiology and Risk Factors

(ACS, 2018)
- High-dose radiation exposure (such as a survivor an atomic bomb blast or nuclear reactor accident) increases the risk of CML.
- Age: the risk increases as age increases.
- Slightly more common in males than females.

Signs and Symptoms

(Emadi & Law, 2022)
- Symptoms typically develop gradually and are usually seen with advanced disease.
- The diagnosis is often made during a routine blood examination for other reasons.
- Patient complaints
  - Fatigue
  - Malaise
  - Fever
  - Weight loss
  - Night sweats
- Physical findings
  - Ecchymosis
  - Lymphadenopathy
  - Splenomegaly (about 60% to 70% of patients)

Diagnostic Work-up

- Medical history and physical examination
- Laboratory tests
  - CBC with differential count (may have anemia, leukopenia, neutropenia, and thrombocytosis may be present)
  - Serum chemistry panel
  - Elevated lactate dehydrogenase and uric acid levels correlate with a large tumor burden.
  - Cytogenetics to identify chromosomal or genetic abnormalities
  - Polymerase chain reaction (PCR), a highly sensitive test to detect as little as one *BCR/ABL*-positive cell in a background of about 500,000 normal cells
- Imaging studies
  - Chest radiography
  - CT
  - MRI
- Additional studies
  - Bone marrow aspirate or biopsy with cytogenetics to establish any additional chromosomal abnormalities in the Ph-positive cells (known as clonal cytogenetic evolution) (Deininger et al., 2020).

Histopathology

Peripheral Blood

(NCI, 2022)
- Leukocytosis with a median WBC in the 100,000 range usually composed of neutrophilic series, from myeloblasts to mature neutrophils, and an increased percent of myelocytes and segmented neutrophils. Blasts typically account for less than 2%.
- A greater proportion of myelocytes than metamyelocytes is a classic finding of CML, and dysplasia can develop in more advanced cases.
- Morphology will be normal but cytochemically abnormal. The cytochemical reaction called leukocyte alkaline phosphatase will be low. This is useful in determining a differential diagnosis of CML from a reactive leukocytosis due to infection or polycythemia vera.
- Absolute basophilia is a universal finding in CML blood smears.
- The platelet count can be normal or elevated.

Bone Marrow

(NCI, 2022)
- Immature forms of myeloid lineage will be observed in the biopsy sample. The marrow will be hypercellular, and

differential counts of the marrow and peripheral blood will show a degree of mature and immature granulocytes similar to what is seen in a normal marrow.

- Increased numbers of eosinophils or basophiles are usually present, and monocytosis can sometimes be discovered.
- Increased megakaryocytes are found in the marrow, while fragments of megakaryocytic nuclei are present in the peripheral blood, especially with highly elevated platelet counts.
- Although Ph chromosome translocation is the initiating event in CML, additional chromosomal or molecular changes are often found in accelerated or blast crisis phases of CML.
  - These can include trisomy 8, trisomy 19, duplication of the Ph chromosome, and isochromosome 17q (leading to loss of the P53 gene). When these occur, the prognosis is poorer.
  - Patients that are Ph-negative CML, which is a poorly defined entity that is less distinguished from other myeloproliferative syndromes. These patients generally have a poorer response to treatment TKI and shorter survival than Ph-positive patients.

Clinical Staging

- CML has three phases: chronic, accelerated, and blast. Transition from the chronic phase to the accelerated and blast phases may occur gradually over 1 year or longer, or it may occur abruptly (i.e., blast crisis).
  - Chronic-phase CML: Most patients (85%) are in the chronic phase of CML at diagnosis (Emadi & Law, 2022). It is characterized by cytogenetic findings of less than 10% blasts and promyelocytes in the peripheral blood and bone marrow (NCI, 2022).
  - Accelerated-phase CML: It is characterized by 10% to 19% blasts in the peripheral blood or bone marrow (NCI, 2022).
  - Blastic-phase CML: A total of 20% or more blasts may be found in the peripheral blood or bone marrow. A patient with fever, malaise, and splenomegaly with 20% or more blasts is considered to be in blast crisis (NCI, 2022).
- The annual rate of progression from chronic phase to blast crisis has significantly decreased after the introduction of the TKIs. Pre-imatinib, the progression rates were 1.5% to 3.7% per year. That has now decreased to 0.3% to 2.2% per year. The cumulative incidence of progression to blast phase at 2 years from diagnosis is 4.3%. Five percent to 10% in the first 2 years (Bonifacio et al., 2019).

Treatment

Chronic Phase

(Deininger et al., 2020)

- Determination of risk score using the Sokal, or Hasford (Euro), or European treatment and outcome study long-term survival (ELTS) scoring systems (mathematical calculations from physical exam findings, age, CBC results, and spleen size) prior to initiation of TKI therapy is recommended (see the table in the next column).

- Euro and Sokal Scoring systems are accessible online at https://www.leukemia-net.org/content/leukemias/cml/euro_and_sokal_score/index_eng.html
- Online ELTS score found at https://www.leukemia-net.org/content/leukemias/cml/elts_score/index_eng.html

Risk Classification Systems for Chronic Myelogenous Leukemia

Risk Score	Calculation	Risk Category
Sokal Score	$0.0116 \times (\text{age-43.4}) +$ (spleen-7.51) $+ 0.188 \times$ [(platelet count $\div 700)^2$- 0.563] $+ 0.0887 \times$ (blasts-2.10)	Low <0.8 Intermediate 0.8-1.2 High >1.2
Hasford (EURO) score	$(0.6666 \times \text{age}$ [0 when <50 years; 1 otherwise] $= 0.042 \times$ spleen size (cm below the costal margin) $+ 0.0584 \times$ percent blasts $+ 0.0413 \times$ percent eosinophils $+ 0.2039 \times$ basophils [0 when <3%; 1 otherwise] $= 1.0956 \times$ platelet count [0 when 1500×10^9/L; 1 otherwise] $\times 1000$	Low ≤780 Intermediate >780-≤1480 High >1480
EUTOS long-term survival (ELTS) score	$0.0025 \times (\text{age}/10)^3 + 0.0615 \times$ spleen size cm below costal margin $+ 0.1052 \times$ blasts in peripheral blood $+ 0.4104 \times$ (platelet count/1000)$^{-0.5}$	Low ≤1.5680 Intermediate >1.5680 but ≤2.2185 High >2.2185

- These scoring systems provide predictors of CML-related death in patients treated with first-line imatinib. Some basic principles of the scoring systems:
  - Higher age, higher peripheral blasts, bigger spleen, and low platelet counts were significantly associated with increased probabilities of dying of CML.
  - Intermediate and high-risk groups have a higher probability of dying of CML than the low-risk group (Deininger et al., 2020).

Low-Risk Chronic Phase Chronic Myelogenous Leukemia

(Deininger et al., 2020)

- Preferred regimens for initial treatment of low-risk score chronic phase CML
  - First-generation TKI (imatinib or generic imatinib), or second-generation TKI (bosutinib, dasatinib, nilotinib), or a clinical trial.

Intermediate or High-Risk Chronic Phase Chronic Myelogenous Leukemia

(Deininger et al., 2020)

- Allogeneic stem cell transplant is no longer recommended as first-line treatment in chronic phase CML.
- Disease progression is more frequent in intermediate or high-risk score CML, and prevention of disease progression to accelerated phase or blast phase is the primary goal of therapy.
- Second-generation TKIs have been associated with a lower risk of disease progression and have quicker molecular

responses as well as higher rates of major molecular responses than imatinib, thus they are preferred for intermediate or high-risk score CML patients.

- Preferred regimens for initial treatment of intermediate or high-risk score chronic phase CML
  - Second-generation TKI (bosutinib, dasatinib, nilotinib), or first-generation TKI (imatinib or generic imatinib), or a clinical trial.
- Asciminib is indicated for chronic phase CML with the T315I mutation and/or resistance or intolerance to at least two prior TKIs (Deininger et al., 2020).
  - The deep molecular response of second-generation TKIs may also allow discontinuation of TKI therapy in select patients.

Chronic Phase Chronic Myelogenous Leukemia Second Line/Relapsed or Tyrosine Kinase Inhibitor–Resistant Disease

- For patients with resistant disease to imatinib to an alternative TKI (second-generation TKIs are preferred).
- For those with an inadequate response to dasatinib, nilotinib, or bosutinib, switching to an alternate TKI except imatinib should be considered.
- For patients who fail two or more TKIs, omacetaxine is a treatment option. However, these patients have lower response rates and overall survival outcomes.

Accelerated Phase

- Patients with accelerated phase CML show signs and symptoms of progression but do not meet the criteria for blast crisis or acute leukemia. Symptoms include increasing fatigue and malaise, progressive splenomegaly, increasing leukocytosis and/or thrombocytosis, and worsening anemia.
- Bone marrow examination will have increasing blast percentage and basophilia. Additional cytogenetic abnormalities may occur during this phase. If there is additional cytogenetic abnormalities and progression of the hematologic findings this can predict for lower response rates and shorter time to treatment failure on imatinib (NCI, 2022).
- Treatment goals for the accelerated phase, or blast crisis phase, are to eliminate cells with the BCR/*ABL* gene and return the patient's disease to the chronic phase.
- Treatment options include:
  - TKI therapy
    - Bosutinib—FDA approval for first-line treatment in accelerate phase CML.
    - Imatinib
  - Interferon α; however, this no survival advantage has been seen.
  - Allogenic stem cell transplant after induction of remission using a TKI
  - High-dose cytarabine
  - Hydroxyurea or leukapheresis may be used to initially reduce WBC counts; however, they are not long-term treatments.

- Busulfan
- Clinical trials

Blast Phase

- Treatment options include:
  - Imatinib, dasatinib, nilotinib, and bosutinib have all have demonstrated activity in blast crisis
  - Allogeneic stem cell transplant after induction and achievement of return to chronic phase
  - Hydroxyurea is a palliative therapy
  - High-dose cytarabine
  - Other AML type induction therapy + TKI
  - Clinical trial—current trials include novel targeting drugs such as asciminib (ABL001), a selective allosteric inhibitor of BCR-ABL1, histone deacetylase inhibitors, BCL2 inhibitor (venetoclax), Janus kinase inhibitor 2 (JAK2), and aurora kinase inhibitors (tozasertib, danusertib, alisertib) (Bonifacio et al., 2019).

Tyrosine Kinase Inhibitor–Resistant Chronic Myelogenous Leukemia

- Omacetaxine mepesuccinate, a cephalotaxine is FDA-approved for patients who are in chronic or accelerated phases of CML and resistant to or intolerant of two or more TKIs. Omacetaxine mepesuccinate has shown activity independent of BCR/*ABL* with a hematologic response rate of 67% and a median PFS of 7 months in the study (Cortes et al., 2015).

Transplantation in Chronic Myelogenous Leukemia

- The use of allogeneic stem cell transplantation is reserved for those who fail TKI therapy, and those presenting with accelerated-phase disease, blast phase disease, and patients with T315I mutation resistant to ponatinib, and those with resistance or intolerance to the other pharmacologic options (NCI, 2022).
- Allogeneic transplantation is associated with significant morbidity and mortality rates, and because the typical age of CML patients is greater than 65 years, additional comorbidities may exclude its use (NCI, 2022).

Monitoring for Response

- Response to TKI therapy is the most important measurement for patients.
  - Analysis of marrow samples has been the preferred method for demonstrating CRs (i.e., clearance of BCR/ABL-containing cells), but because peripheral blood tests with FISH and PCR are highly sensitive and specific, most testing now uses peripheral blood samples for ongoing monitoring. Marrow testing should still be completed at regular intervals.
- FISH and PCR testing are often completed every 2 weeks until stable blood counts are achieved, and then testing is done every 3 months. If no hematologic response is seen (i.e., blood counts do not improve), the physician can consider switching agents.

- Achievement of molecular remission requires ongoing testing to ensure that the response is maintained. Bone marrow biopsies are typically done at 3-, 6-, and 12-month intervals and then annually.
- Those who achieve deep molecular remission (DMR) with undetectable BCR/ABL by quantitative polymerase chain reaction (qPCR) and continue in DMR for ≥2 or more years are the best candidates to consider discontinuation of TKI therapy.
  - Approximately 40% to 60% of these patients will relapse after the TKI is discontinued; however, almost all patients who progress can be successfully retreated and regain DMR with the previous TKI. It is essentially that patients who discontinue TKIs are monitored closely with frequent PCR peripheral blood and marrow testing. The monitoring interval has not been well defined but should be at least every 3 months after stopping therapy, as relapses have occurred even after one year off of a TKI. If BCR/ABL becomes detectable on two or more tests, the TKI should be resumed (Deininger et al., 2020).

Special Considerations

- Pregnancy and breastfeeding during CML management (Deininger et al., 2020)
  - Approximately 37% of patients are of reproductive age at the time of diagnosis.
  - TKIs can affect male hormones transiently but does not appear to affect fertility (the miscarriage or fetal abnormality rate is not elevated in female partners of men on TKI therapy).
  - TKI therapy during pregnancy, however, is associated with both a higher rate of miscarriage and fetal abnormalities
    - Consideration for prolonged washout or TKI prior to pregnancy.
    - Prompt consideration of holding TKI if pregnancy occurs while on a TKI.
    - Need for close monitoring during pregnancy and need to remain off the TKI for the duration of the pregnancy. Interferon alpha and hydroxyurea (outside the first trimester) have been used during pregnancy if treatment is necessary.
    - Monthly monitoring of qPCR is recommended with initiation of treatment if the BCR-ABL1 increases to greater than 1.0%.
  - Fertility preservation should be discussed prior to starting any TKI therapy.
  - Avoidance of the TKI must continue during the time of breastfeeding.

Prognosis

- Since the advent of TKI therapies, the median survival for most CML patients who are able to achieve DMR and stay on therapy for at least 2 years has reached the normal life expectancy of the general population (Deininger et al., 2020).

- The life expectancy is typically much shorter for those who continue to have BCR/ABL-positive cells, develop resistance to TKI agents, or progress to accelerated-phase CML or blast crisis. Those in blast crisis may live only a few months (Bonifacio et al., 2019).
- Ph-chromosome negative CML is a poorly defined entity that is less clearly distinguished from other myeloproliferative syndromes. The approximately 5% of patients with this form of CML usually have a poorer response to treatment and shorter survival than Ph chromosome–positive patients (NCI, 2022).

Prevention and Surveillance

- There are no prevention guidelines for CML.
- Children have a longer life expectancy than adults, thus they may need TKI therapy for decades; there are potential long-term complications such as delayed growth, changes in bone metabolism, thyroid abnormalities, and effects on puberty and fertility that should be monitored (National Comprehensive Cancer Network, 2022).
- Administration of the COVID-19 vaccine is recommended.
- Care providers should encourage a healthy lifestyle, including influenza vaccinations, tobacco abstinence, maintenance of a healthy weight and diet, and recommended cancer screening for other malignancies (ACS, 2022).
- CML patients are at higher risk for oral cavity cancer, lung cancer, CLL, small intestine cancer, thyroid cancer, melanoma, and prostate cancer. The risk is highest in the first 5 years after diagnosis (ACS, 2020).

References

American Cancer Society (ACS). (2018). *Risk factors for chronic myeloid leukemia.* Cancer.org. https://www.cancer.org/cancer/chronic-myeloid-leukemia/causes-risks-prevention/risk-factors.html.

American Cancer Society (ACS). (2020). *Second cancers after chronic myeloid leukemia.* Cancer.org. https://www.cancer.org/cancer/chronic-myeloid-leukemia/after-treatment/second-cancers.html.

American Cancer Society (ACS). (2022). *Key statistics for chronic myeloid leukemia.* Cancer.org. https://www.cancer.org/cancer/chronic-myeloid-leukemia/about/statistics.html.

Bonifacio, M., Stagno, F., Scaffidi, L., Krampera, M., & Di Raimondo, F. (2019). Management of chronic myeloid leukemia in advanced phase. *Frontiers in Oncology, 9,* 1132.

Cortes, J. E., Kantarjian, H. M., Rea, D., Wetzler, M., Lipton, J. H., Akard, L., & Nicolini, F. E. (2015). Final analysis of the efficacy and safety of omacetaxine mepesuccinate in patients with chronic- or accelerated-phase chronic myeloid leukemia: Results with 24 months of follow-up. *Cancer, 121*(10), 1637–1644.

Deininger, M. W., Shah, N. P., Altman, J. K., Berman, E., Bhatia, R., Bhatnagar, B., & Sundar, H. (2020). Chronic myeloid leukemia, version 2.2021, NCCN clinical practice guidelines in oncology. *Journal of the National Comprehensive Cancer Network, 18*(10), 1385–1415.

National Cancer Institute (NCI). (2022). *Chronic myelogenous leukemia treatment (PDQ*)—Health Professional Version.* Cancer.gov. https://www.cancer.gov/types/leukemia/hp/cml-treatment-pdq#cit/section_4.56.

National Comprehensive Cancer Network (NCCN). (2022). NCCN clinical practice guidelines for chronic myelogenous leukemia, version 3.2022. http://www.nccn.org/professionals/physician_gls/pdf/cml.pdf.

Emadi, A., & Law, J. Y. (2022). Chronic myeloid leukemia. Merck Manual Profession Version https://www.merckmanuals.com/professional/hematology-and-oncology/leukemias/chronic-myeloid-leukemia-cml.

Myelodysplastic Syndromes

Definition

MDSs are a group of acquired bone marrow stem cell malignancies that result in ineffective hematopoiesis in one or more myeloid lineages. Although technically not cancer, MDS may transform over time into leukemia and is often referred to as *preleukemia*. In patients with MDS, the marrow produces too few red blood cells (RBCs), WBCs, and platelets.

Incidence

(American Society of Clinical Oncology [ASCO], 2022)

- MDS is estimated to affect 200,000 persons in the United States.
- Between 10,000 new cases are diagnosed each year and numbers are expected to increase as the population continues to age.
- The median age at diagnosis is age 70 years; it is uncommon in people younger than 50 years of age.
- MDS occurs in men more often than women and affects Whites more often than other races (National Cancer Institute [NCI], 2022).
- Death from MDS is typically caused by bleeding and/or infection from low blood counts (ASCO, 2022).

Etiology and Risk Factors

- MDS can manifest de novo (i.e., primary MDS) or after treatment with chemotherapy or radiation therapy for other diseases, and rarely after environmental exposures. Primary MDS accounts for 90% of cases (NCI, 2022).
- Risk factors include the following: Almost 90% of MDS cases occur without an identifiable cause. Potential environmental risk factors include (NCI, 2022):
  - Cigarette smoking
  - Exposure to ionizing radiation
  - Immunosuppressive therapy/previous chemotherapy or radiation treatment: 20% of people with prior treatment with chemotherapy and radiation develop therapy-related MDS (ASCO, 2022)
  - Exposure to toxins (NCI, 2022):
    - Organic chemicals such as benzene, toluene, xylene, and chloramphenicol
    - Petroleum and diesel derivatives
    - Nitro-organic explosives
    - Exhaust gases
    - Stone and cereal dust
    - Heavy metals such as mercury or lead
    - Herbicides, pesticides, and fertilizers
    - Non-environmental risk factors include:
    - Age older than 60 years
    - Male sex
    - Some genetic disorders may pre-dispose people to development of MDS. These include: Fanconi anemia, familial MDS/AML, thrombocytopenia 2, thrombocytopenia 5, familial aplastic anemia, Shwachman-Diamond syndrome, Diamond–Blackfan anemia,

congenital neutropenia, familial platelet disorder, and myeloid neoplasms with germline predisposition (ASCO, 2022).

Signs and Symptoms

- Symptoms typically develop gradually and are usually seen with advanced disease.
- Disease usually manifests because of marrow failure in one or more cell lines. The diagnosis is often made during routine blood examination.
- Symptoms
  - Fatigue
  - Malaise
  - Fever
  - Shortness of breath with exertion
  - Weight loss
- Physical findings
  - Pallor
  - Ecchymosis or bleeding
  - Infection
  - Anemia
  - Splenomegaly

Diagnostic Work-up

- Medical history and physical examination
- Laboratory tests
  - CBC with differential count and reticulocyte count
  - RBC folate, serum B12, serum ferritin, iron, total iron-binding capacity, and TSH
  - Peripheral blood smear examination
  - Cytogenetics for identification of chromosomal or genetic abnormalities; 50% of MDS patients have chromosomal abnormalities, commonly deletion of all or part of chromosome 5 or 7 or trisomy 8 (NCI, 2022).
- Bone marrow aspirate or biopsy is essential for the diagnosis
- Imaging studies
  - Chest radiography
  - CT
  - MRI

Histopathology

(NCI, 2022)

- The bone marrow can be normocellular or hypercellular. The specimen yields megaloblastic erythroid hyperplasia with macrocytic anemia (despite normal vitamin B_{12} and folate levels).
- Ten percent of patients are hypoplastic, manifesting as profound cytopenias, which may respond well to immunosuppressant therapy.
- Small megakaryocytes may be seen in the marrow along with hypogranular or giant platelets in the peripheral blood.

Clinical Staging

(Greenberg et al., 2022)

- A variety of pathologic and risk classification systems have been developed to predict the overall survival of patients with MDS and the evolution from MDS to AML.

- Major prognostic classification systems include the International Prognostic Scoring System (IPSS), revised as the IPSS-R, and the WHO Prognostic Scoring System (WPSS).
- Clinical variables in these systems have included bone marrow and blood myeloblast percentages, specific cytopenias, transfusion requirements, age, performance status, and bone marrow cytogenetic abnormalities.
- IPSS incorporates bone marrow blast percentage, number of peripheral blood cytopenias, and cytogenetic risk group.
- IPSS-R updates and gives greater weight to cytogenetic abnormalities and severity of cytopenias while reassigning the weighting for blast percentages.
- In contrast to the IPSS and IPSS-R, which should be applied only at the time of diagnosis, the WPSS is dynamic, meaning that patients can be reassigned to categories as their disease progresses.
- The NCCN guidelines for MDS propose stratifying patients with clinically significant cytopenia(s) into two major risk groups: lower-risk and high-risk MDS:
  - Lower-risk MDS includes IPSS low and intermediate-1, IPSS-R very low, low, and intermediate, and WPSS very low, low, and intermediate patients.
  - High-risk MDS includes IPSS intermediate-2, high, IPSS-R intermediate-2, high, and very high, and WPSS high and very high patients.
- Treatment is then based on these categories along with the patient's age, comorbidities, performance status, and ability to tolerate certain intensive regimens.

Treatment

- MDS treatment individualizes therapy for each patient.
- Supportive care is an important aspect of MDS care and entails observation, clinical monitoring, psychosocial support, and quality of life assessment; it is also a mainstay of treatment (Greenberg et al., 2022).
  - Transfusions to correct symptomatic anemia and thrombocytopenia with bleeding, platelet transfusions should not be used routinely in the absence of bleeding unless platelet count less than 10,000/µL (irradiated products for transplant candidates).
  - Antibiotics as indicated for bacterial infections; no routine prophylaxis unless there are recurrent infections.
  - Aminocaproic acid or other antifibrinolytic agents may be considered for bleeding refractory to platelet transfusions or profound thrombocytopenia.
  - Erythropoiesis-stimulating agents (ESAs) may improve anemia, pretreatment serum erythropoietin levels and baseline transfusion needs should be assessed prior to beginning.
  - Clinically significant thrombocytopenia in lower-risk MDS with severe or life-threatening thrombocytopenia can consider use of thrombopoietin receptor agonist.
  - Iron chelation therapy should be considered for those receiving greater than 20 to 30 RBC transfusions.

- Daily chelation with deferoxamine is recommended subcutaneously or orally to decrease iron overload, especially with lower-risk MDS or those being considered for transplant.
- When serum ferritin levels are greater than 2500 ng/mL, the aim is to decrease them to less than 1000 ng/mL.
- Disease-modifying agents may also be used.
  - Lenalidomide is an immunomodulatory agent approved for low-risk, transfusion-dependent patients with del(5q) MDS (NCI, 2022).
  - Immunosuppression therapy with equine antithymocyte globulin with or without cyclosporine A and with or without eltrombopag is used in patients with hypoplastic marrow, paroxysmal nocturnal hemoglobinuria clone positivity, or STAT-3 mutant cytotoxic T-cell clones (Greenberg et al., 2022).
  - DNA methyltransferase inhibitors, which block the methylation of DNA and inhibit proliferation, include azacitidine and decitabine.
  - Decitabine/cedazuridine is a combination oral DNA methyltransferase inhibitor and cytidine deaminase inhibitor and can be substituted for intravenous decitabine in patients with IPSS Intermediate-1 and above.
  - Luspatercept-aamt is currently being studied in anemia and low-risk MDS without ringed sideroblasts—but is not yet FDA approved.
  - Imetelstat, a telomerase inhibitor currently under investigation for low-risk MDS patients that are ineligible or relapsed/refractory to ESAs and is not FDA-approved (Steensma et al., 2021).
  - AML induction-type chemotherapy may be tried but may be difficult for older patients to tolerate and is associated with higher infection rates when compared to observation (NCI, 2022).
  - Clinical Trials:
    - Targeted agents for IDH1 (ivosidenib) or IDH2 (enasidenib) mutations (which occur in 4% to 12% of MDS) have ongoing clinical trials.
- Venetoclax (BCL2 inhibitor) either monotherapy or in combination with hypomethylation agents (Greenberg et al., 2022).
- Higher-risk patients may also have some of the above therapies considered; however, these patients will also be evaluated for potential allogeneic transplantation.
  - The only curative treatment is intensive chemotherapy and allogeneic stem cell transplantation. Cure rates for selected patients range from 30% to 50% but are varied based on age and IPSS score at the time of transplant, and those with higher scores have inferior survival (NCI, 2022).
  - Reduced-intensity conditioning has also been used with some benefit when pretransplant disease burden is reduced.
  - Debulking therapy to reduce the marrow blasts to less than 5% is recommended to decrease post-transplant relapse, but an optimal regimen is yet to be determined.

Prognosis

- Secondary myelodysplasia usually has a poorer prognosis than de novo myelodysplasia.
- Prognosis is directly related to the number of bone marrow blast cells, to certain cytogenetic abnormalities, and to the amount of peripheral blood cytopenia.
- MDS transforms to AML in about one-third of patients (ASCO, 2022).
- By convention, the MDS is reclassified as AML with myelodysplastic features when blood or bone marrow blasts reach or exceed 20%.
- The risk of AML transformation for the five WPSS risk groups (very low, low, intermediate-1, high, and very high) was 3%, 14%, 33%, 54%, and 84% within 5 years, respectively. Median survival for the five groups was 11.8, 5.5, 4, 2.2 years, and 9 months, respectively (ACS, 2018).
- The acute leukemic phase is less responsive to chemotherapy than de novo AML.
- Many patients succumb to complications of cytopenias before progression to AML.

Prevention and Surveillance

There are no recommended measures for the prevention of MDS.

References

American Cancer Society (ACS). (2018). *Survival statistics for myelodysplastic syndromes.* Cancer.gov. https://www.cancer.org/cancer/myelodysplastic-syndrome/detection-diagnosis-staging/survival.html.

American Society of Clinical Oncology (ASCO). (2022). *Myelodysplastic syndromes—MDS guide.* https://www.cancer.net/cancer-types/myelodysplastic-syndromes-mds/introduction.

Greenberg, P. L., Stone, R. M., Al-Kali, A., Bennett, J. M., Borate, U., Brunner, A. M., … Hochstetler, C. (2022). NCCN Guidelines® Insights: Myelodysplastic syndromes, Version 3.2022. *Journal of the National Comprehensive Cancer Network: JNCCN, 20*(2), 106–117. https://doi.org/10.6004/jnccn.2022.0009.

National Cancer Institute. (2022). *Myelodysplastic syndromes treatment (PDQ®)—Health Professional Version.* Cancer.gov. http://www.cancer.gov/cancertopics/pdq/treatment/myelodysplastic/HealthProfessional.

Steensma, D. P., Fenaux, P., Van Eygen, K., Raza, A., Santini, V., Germing, U., … Platzbecker, U. (2021). Imetelstat achieves meaningful and durable transfusion independence in high transfusion-burden patients with lower-risk myelodysplastic syndromes in a phase II study. *Journal of Clinical Oncology, 39*(1), 48–56.

Malignant Lung Neoplasms

Elizabeth Maggio

Lung Cancer

Definition

Lung cancer results from uncontrolled growth of cells in the body and forms in the tissues of the lung, most commonly in the cells that line the bronchial endothelium (American Cancer Society [ACS], 2022).

Incidence

- Lung cancer remains the leading cause of cancer-related death in the United States and is the second most commonly diagnosed cancer in men and women. It accounts for about 13% of all cancer diagnoses (ACS, 2022).
- In 2022, the ACS estimates about 236,740 new cases of lung cancer and 130,180 deaths from the disease in the United States. In 2018, it was estimated that more than 500,000 people were living with lung and bronchus cancer in the United States (National Cancer Institute, Surveillance, Epidemiology, and End Results [NCI-SEER], 2021).
- The average age when diagnosed is about 70 years; however, it is less common in people younger than 45 years. Lung cancer diagnosed at a younger age, seen in mostly nonsmokers, may be attributed to a specific biomarker, anaplastic lymphoma kinase positive (ALK+), secondhand smoke, radon, air pollution, asbestos, or a family history of lung cancer (ACS, 2022).
- Although more than 80% of all lung cancers are thought to have been caused by cigarette, pipe, and cigar smoking, in the United States, approximately 10% to 20% happen in never smokers or those who smoked less than 100 cigarettes in their lifetime. More than 50% of lung cancer is diagnosed in former smokers (NCI-SEER, 2021).
- Among men and women, almost 25% of all cancer deaths are attributed to lung cancer. The current 5-year survival rate for all types of lung or bronchus cancer is 23%, up from the 1990s when the 5-year survival rate was around 13% (ACS, 2022).

Etiology and Risk Factors

- Exposure to cigarette smoke is the major risk factor for lung cancer, in fact, all types of tobacco products, including electronic cigarettes (also known as e-cigarettes, e-cigs, electronic nicotine delivery system [ENDS] or vapes) contain chemicals that can be harmful to your health. More than 300 harmful agents and over 40 known carcinogens are in tobacco smoke that can lead to heart and lung disease and can harm nearly every organ and organ system in the body (Cancer Genome Atlas Research, 2012).

- A person's risk increases with the number of years of smoking, the number of cigarettes smoked, exposure to secondhand smoke; radon and environmental and occupational exposures (arsenic, benzene, radon, asbestos [especially in smokers], copper, silica, lead, diesel exhaust, chromium). Air pollution can also increase the risk of lung cancer, as does radiation exposure from previous cancer treatment.
- A history of tuberculosis or chronic inflammatory diseases is a risk factor.
- Chronic obstructive pulmonary disease (COPD) is a risk factor for lung cancer.
- Most lung cancer cases do not have an inherited genetic change and are due mostly to somatic mutations that occur only in specific cells in the lung. However, there are several mutations that can occur, some of which are actionable biomarkers, meaning there is an approved targeted therapy versus nonactionable, without an approved targeted therapy (Cancer Genome Atlas Research, 2012).
- Currently, actionable biomarkers for lung cancer treatment (2021) include the following: epidermal growth factor receptor (EGFR) exon 19, 20 insertion, 21; ALK, ROS-1, PDL1 TPS 50%; *BRAF* V600E, NTRK, Her-2 (ERBB2); MET exon 14 skipping; RET; *KRAS* G12C; PDL1 TPS greater than 1%. There are multiple nonactionable mutations that have been identified; however, there are currently no approved therapies for them (Cancer Genome Atlas Research, 2012).
- Socioeconomic factors, serious psychological distress, adults with disabilities, and fewer years of education all affect current smoking rates (National Center for Chronic Disease Prevention and Health Promotion [US] Office on Smoking and Health, 2014).
- The incidence of a lung cancer diagnosis is 1.28 times greater in Black men with 1.22 times greater risk of lung cancer mortality compared to White men. Black men and women are more likely to be diagnosed at a later stage, are less likely to undergo invasive staging, and are more likely to refuse treatment when diagnosed, including surgery and clinical trial participation. Decades of research (Bach et al., 1999; Lathan et al., 2006; Cykert et al., 2015; Sineshaw et al., 2016; Taioli et al., 2017) have shown that Black patients undergo curative surgery less often than White patients, while comparable gaps are rising in the use of radiation (Corso et al., 2015). According to the National Comprehensive Cancer Network (NCCN) guidelines, both surgery and stereotactic radiation are viewed as appropriate curative treatments for early-stage NSCLC (NCCN, Version 1.2023-December 22,2022) https://www.nccn.org/professionals/physician_gls/pdf/nscl.pdf .

- Access to care, poverty, education level, and lack of insurance are all part of the structural barriers (O'Keefe et al., 2015).

Signs, Symptoms, and Screening

- There are few or no symptoms of early-stage lung cancer; however, early detection screening for lung cancer through low-dose computed tomography (LDCT) has significantly led to better survival and early diagnosis (Potter et al., 2022). The NCCN updated guidelines for lung cancer screening, and the United States Preventive Service Task Force (USPSTF) recommends annual screening for lung cancer with LDCT in adults aged 50 to 80 years who have a 20-pack-a-year smoking history and currently smoke or have quit within the past 15 years (Potter et al., 2021).
- In February 2022, the Centers for Medicare & Medicaid Services (CMS) announced expanded coverage for lung cancer screening with LDCT to improve health outcomes. Eligibility was expanded by lowering the starting age for screening from 55 to 50 years and reducing tobacco smoking history from at least 30 packs/year to at least 20 packs/year (Syrek Jensen, 2022).
- Early diagnosis is key to survival and is dictated by stage at diagnosis. This refers to the extent of cancer in the body. Only around 18% of lung cancer is diagnosed when the cancer is localized (stage 1). When the cancer is confined to the primary site, the 5-year relative survival rate is around 60%. With lung cancer diagnosed as regional (22%) or distant (56%), meaning the cancer has spread to the lymph nodes or different parts of the body, the 5-year survival is much less, 32% versus 6.3% (National Cancer Institute, 2021).
- Stigma, implicit bias, and nihilism contribute to barriers in early screening and detection, smoking cessation, and delays in seeking treatment. Studies have shown that subpopulations and people of color are more likely to experience stigma burden related to a health care provider implicit bias, differences in trust and physician perceptions. Stigma associated with lung cancer contributes to concealment of illness after diagnosis and threatens necessary coping mechanisms that may lead to decreased adherence to treatment, greater disability, and reduced quality of life (Carter-Harris et al., 2014). In addition to smoking stigma, these groups may also experience stigma because of their gender, sexual orientation, mental illness, disability, race, or ethnicity (Bergamo et al., 2013; Penner et al., 2016).
- Symptoms that occur as the cancer progresses include the following:
  - Persistent cough
  - Dyspnea
  - Hemoptysis
  - Pain in shoulder, back or chest
  - Hoarseness or wheezing
  - Recurrent pneumonia or bronchitis
- Late-stage symptoms include the following:
  - Pain possibly related to bone metastasis
  - Fatigue
  - Anorexia
  - Central nervous system changes from brain metastasis
  - Dysphagia
  - Weight loss

Diagnostic Work-up

To plan appropriate treatment, a diagnostic workup is necessary to differentiate non–small cell lung cancer (NSCLC) from small cell lung cancer (SCLC) or other conditions that may present with similar symptoms. The diagnostic workup will facilitate identifying the location of the primary cancer, the best site for a biopsy to identify tumor histology and subtype (i.e., non–small cell, small cell, or malignant pleural mesothelioma), and whether there are sites of metastatic disease.

- Key elements of the workup include the following:
  - History and physical examination, including weight loss, performance status, and smoking history.
    - Laboratory testing, including a complete blood cell count with differential, platelets, serum chemistry profile (calcium, sodium). Helpful to determine alkaline phosphatase (ALT), aspartate aminotransferase (AST) (liver involvement), smoking cessation advice/counseling, and pharmacotherapy.
  - Chest radiograph to identify pulmonary nodules, mass or infiltrates, mediastinal widening, atelectasis, hilar enlargement, and pleural effusion.
  - Standard for staging, computed tomography (CT) of the chest, abdomen, and pelvis with contrast to identify the location of the primary tumor and sites of metastatic disease (e.g., lymph nodes, liver, adrenal glands, bones). The findings may allow for presumptive differentiation between NSCLC and SCLC. Massive lymphadenopathy and direct invasion of the mediastinum are commonly associated with SCLC; and a mass in or close to the hilum is another SCLC characteristic in about 78% of cases (Ganti et al., 2021).
  - Positron emission tomography (PET) for evaluating solitary pulmonary nodules or assessing systemic spread. A bone scintigraphy (scan) to determine bone metastasis (Ganti et al., 2021).
- Diagnostic tools that should be routinely available include the following:
  - Sputum Cytologic Studies (SCC), specifically for centrally located endobronchial tumors (i.e., squamous cell carcinoma) which may shed malignant cells into sputum.
  - Bronchoscopy with biopsy and transbronchial needle aspiration (TBNA), needle thoracentesis (ultrasound guided) is both diagnostic and therapeutic in patients presenting with respiratory distress.
    - Image-guided transthoracic needle core biopsy (preferred) or fine-needle aspiration (FNA), thoracentesis, mediastinoscopy, video-assisted thoracic surgery (VATS), and open surgical biopsy
- Diagnostic tools that provide important additional strategies for biopsy include the following:
  - EBUS—endobronchial ultrasound-guided biopsy, EUS—endoscopic ultrasound-guided biopsy, navigational bronchoscopy, robotic bronchoscopy
  - Biopsy under CT guidance or bronchoscopy provides a means for direct visualization of tumor, allows collection

of specimens for direct biopsy, bronchial brushings and washings, and transbronchial biopsies. Bronchoscopy is the study of choice in patients with central tumors (88% combined sensitivity). Transthoracic needle biopsy is preferred for tumors located in the periphery of lungs if they are not accessible through bronchoscope.

- Thoracoscopy is reserved for tumors that remain undiagnosed after bronchoscopy and for the management of malignant pleural effusions. Mediastinoscopy is used to obtain tissue from cancer that has infiltrated into the mediastinum such as lymph nodes or surgical resection of the lung.
- Baseline brain magnetic resonance imaging (MRI) or CT if neurologic changes. MRI has a greater sensitivity than CT for CNS metastasis.
- If surgery is considered, pulmonary function tests should be obtained, and lymph node sampling by mediastinoscopy may be included in the initial workup (Ganti et al., 2021; Ettinger et al., 2022).

Genetic Testing for Targeted Therapies

- According to international evidence-based guidelines jointly published by the College of American Pathologists (CAP), International Association for the Study of Lung Cancer (IASLC), Association of Molecular Pathology (AMP) (Aisner and Riely, 2021), and The NCCN, unanimously recommends testing all eligible patients with advanced NSCLC (adenocarcinoma) or large cell carcinoma (Ettinger et al., 2022).
- Consideration for those with squamous cell, especially if a nonsmoker, for actionable mutations, including *KRAS* G12C mutation, EGFR exon 19,20,21, ALK, ROS-1, and RET rearrangements, *BRAF* V600E, NTRK1/2/3 gene fusions, MET exon 14 skipping, and pD-L1 expression. If there is insufficient tissue to allow for appropriate testing, it is recommended to obtain a repeat biopsy and/or plasma testing should be completed (Aisner and Riely, 2021).
- Numerous FDA-approved companion diagnostic tests and next-generation sequencing (NGS) are available.

Histopathology

There are two types of lung cancer: NSCLC and small cell lung cancer (SCLC).

Non–Small Cell Lung Cancer (NSCLC)

- The most common type of lung cancer is non–small cell lung cancer (NSCLC). NSCLC has three common histologic types: both adenocarcinoma and squamous cell account for about 84% of all lung cancers. Less common subcategories of adenocarcinoma, adenocarcinoma in situ (previously called bronchioloalveolar carcinoma [BAC]) may have a better long-term outlook (ACS, 2022).
  - Adenocarcinoma occurs in about 50% of NSCLC and stems from epithelial cells or glandular tissues that produce mucus. This histologic type has a strong association with previous smoking; however, it's the most common subtype diagnosed in people who have never smoked. Lung adenocarcinoma is commonly found in the periphery, in scars or areas of chronic inflammation (Meyers & Wallen, 2021).
  - Squamous cell carcinomas (SSCs) make up about 30% of NSCLCs and often occur in the central part of the lung or main airway, usually the left or right bronchus. Tobacco smoke is the main causative agent leading to cell transformation. This type tends to be slower growing than adenocarcinomas and stays localized for a longer period (ACS, 2022).
- Large cell carcinoma represents about 10% to 15% of NSCLCs. Because cells are typically undifferentiated, it tends to grow and spread quickly and can be difficult to treat. It usually arises as peripheral nodules within the lung and metastasizes early (ACS, 2022).

Small Cell Lung Cancer

- SCLC, previously known as oat cell carcinoma, is a neuroendocrine carcinoma that is less common, representing about 15% of all lung cancers (Ganti et al., 2021).
- It arises in peribronchial locations and infiltrates the bronchial submucosa. Widespread metastases occur early in the course of the disease, with common spread to the mediastinal lymph nodes, liver, bones, adrenal glands, and brain (Ganti et al., 2021).
- SCLC has an exceptionally high proliferative rate, a strong affinity for early metastasis, and a poor prognosis. In addition, production of various peptide hormones leads to a wide range of paraneoplastic syndromes; the most common of these are the syndrome of inappropriate secretion of antidiuretic hormone (SIADH) and the syndrome of ectopic adrenocorticotropic hormone (ACTH) production. An autoimmune phenomenon may lead to various neurologic syndromes, such as Lambert-Eaton syndrome (Ganti et al., 2021).
- Exposure to tobacco carcinogens is strongly associated with SCLC. Most patients have metastatic disease at diagnosis, with only one-third having earlier-stage disease when there is a chance for a curative multimodality therapy. Genomic profiling of SCLC reveals extensive chromosomal rearrangements and a high mutation burden, almost always including functional inactivation of the tumor suppressor genes TP53 and RB1 (Rudin et al., 2021).

Clinical Staging
Non–Small Cell Lung Cancer

- Lung cancer staging relies on the tumor-node-metastasis (TNM) system, an internationally accepted system used to characterize the extent of disease. The system is based on the spread of the primary tumor (T), lymph node involvement (N), and the presence or absence of cancer spread or metastasis (M). The TNM system is important in determining the appropriate stage of cancer and its implications for therapeutic and prognostic information (Amin et al., 2017).

Small Cell Lung Cancer

The staging workup for SCLC is to determine the prognosis and management as treatment differs between limited stage and extensive stage.

- Staging should be adequate before making the diagnosis of limited-stage SCLC. Any pleural effusion should be tested cytologically for malignant cells, and isolated liver or adrenal lesions should be sampled by FNA before a diagnosis of limited-stage disease is made. Some authorities suggest a bone marrow examination in the absence of any other evidence of spread (Ganti et al., 2021).
- Limited disease: Confined to the ipsilateral hemithorax, which can be safely encompassed within a tolerable radiation field (T any, N any, M0; except T3-T4 due to multiple lung nodules that do not fit in a tolerable radiation field (Ganti et al., 2021).
- Extensive disease: Beyond ipsilateral hemithorax, which may include malignant pleural or pericardial effusion or hematogenous metastases (T any, N any, M1a/b/c; T3-T4 due to multiple lung nodules that do not fit in a tolerable radiation field (Ganti et al., 2021).

Treatment

Non–Small Cell Lung Cancer

Surgery

- Surgery is the treatment of choice for patients with NSCLC stages I-IIIA if the patient is a low surgical risk and expected to have a good quality of life after removal of part of the lung.
- Surgical procedures include the following options:
  - Lobectomy and pneumonectomy—lobectomy that removes a lobe of the lung (most common), and pneumonectomy that removes the entire right or left lung.
  - Wedge resection/segmentectomy—removes small peripheral nodules (most conservative), segmentectomy that removes part of a lobe of the lung,
  - VATS is a minimally invasive surgical modality being used for both diagnostic and therapeutic lung cancer surgery.

Radiation Therapy

- Patients who are not surgical candidates but whose cancer is stage I or II can receive radiation therapy.
- Stereotactic body radiotherapy (SBRT) is another technique for nonoperative treatment of early-stage lung cancers that involves precise targeting of high-dose radiation to the tumor while minimizing toxicity to normal tissue.

- The role of adjuvant radiation therapy after resection of the primary tumor remains controversial. It may reduce local failures in completely resected (stages II and IIIA) NSCLC; however, it has not been shown to improve overall survival rates.
- Patients who cannot have surgery for a stage IIIA disease or those with a stage IIIB disease usually receive a combination of definitive chemotherapy and radiation therapy.
- Neoadjuvant therapy (i.e., chemotherapy with or without radiation therapy before surgery) has been an area of intense study as a way of shrinking the tumor to improve the chances of a successful resection and prolong survival.
- Although the survival rates have improved for stages IB through IIIA with neoadjuvant therapy, it does carry a greater risk of complications.
- Palliative radiation therapy is reserved for the treatment of symptomatic bone pain, spinal cord compression, brain metastasis, and postobstructive pneumonia (Azzoli et al., 2011).

Systemic Therapies

- First-line chemotherapy regimens for patients without actionable mutations include a choice of a platinum-based doublet (i.e., cisplatin or carboplatin) in combination with paclitaxel, pemetrexed in nonsquamous NSCLC, nab-paclitaxel, docetaxel, gemcitabine, or vinorelbine.
- The ability to target specific aspects of tumor development at the molecular level has improved patient survival and quality of life.
  - The toxicities of targeted therapies can be more tolerable than those of chemotherapy, including less severe effects caused by bone marrow suppression.
  - Despite the outstanding efficacy of targeted treatments, cancers ultimately develop resistance and resume growth. Continued research is needed to develop more treatments to combat disease resistance and improve overall survival of patients.
  - For patients with actionable mutations the appropriate targeted therapy should be used as outlined in the table below.
- Patients with poor performance status are usually treated with single agents or with supportive care.

Actionable Molecular Targets and Treatments

Target	Prevalence	Initial FDA Approval	Therapy
EGFR	10%–15%	2003	Gefitinib, erlotinib, afatinib, osimertinib
ALK	2%–7%	2011	Crizotinib, ceritinib, alectinib, lorlatinib, brigatinib
ROS-1	1%–2%	2016	Crizotinib, ontrectinib, ceritinib, lorlatinib
PD-L1 TPS 50%	30%	2016	Pembrolizumab, atezolizumab
B-RAF^{V600E}	2%	2017	Dabrafenib+trametinib, vemurafenib
NRAK	0.2%–3%	2018	Larotrectinib, entrectinib
HER-2 (ERBB2)	2%–5%	May 2020 March 2021	Trastuzumab deruxtecan (Enhertu); * poziotinib
MET $^{EXON\ 14\ skipping}$	3%–4%	May 2020	Capmatinib, tepotinib?, crizotinib

Actionable Molecular Targets and Treatments—cont'd

Target	Prevalence	Initial FDA Approval	Therapy
RET	1%–2%	September 2020	Salpercatinib, praisetinib, carbozantintib, vandetanib
EGFR**		December 2020	Osimertinib (adjuvant therapy for Stage 1B-IIIA)
EGFR exon 20 insertion	0.1%–4%	May 2021	*Amivantamab, *mobocertinib
		September 2021	
K-RAS G12C	12%	May 2021	Sotorasib
PDL1 TPS >1%		October 2021	Atezolizumab (adjuvant therapy for II-IIIA)

*Accelerated FDA approval; **Adjuvant therapy after curative intent resection; *** After platinum doublet therapy
Data from Lungevity (2021). *Biomarker testing.* Available at https://www.lungevity.org/for-patients-caregivers/navigating-your-diagnosis/biomarker-testing; Villalobos, P., & Ignacio, I. W. (2017). Lung cancer biomarkers. *Hematology/oncology clinics of North America, 31*(1), 13–29; Watson, S. (2021). *Lung cancer biomarkers: Testing, results, and more.* Available at https://www.healthline.com/health/lung-cancer/lung-cancer-biomarkers#biomarkers; American Cancer Society. (2022). *Immunotherapy for non-small cell lung cancer.* Available at https://www.cancer.org/cancer/lung-cancer/treating-non-small-cell/immunotherapy.html; American Lung Cancer Association. (2021). *Lung cancer biomarker testing: What do the results of the testing show?* Available at https://www.lung.org/lung-health-diseases/lung-disease-lookup/lung-cancer/symptoms-diagnosis/biomarker-testing; Boldt, C. (2019). *Lung cancer targeted therapy hits common HER2 variants across cancers.* Available at https://www.mdanderson.org/publications/cancer-frontline/lung-cancer-targeted-therapy-hits-common-her2-variants-across-cancers.h00-159306990.html; National Cancer Institute. (2021). *Tumor markers.* Available at https://www.cancer.gov/about-cancer/diagnosis-staging/diagnosis/tumor-markers-fact-sheet; Lung Cancer Foundation of America. (n.d). *What is ROS1-positive lung cancer and how is it treated?* Available at https://lcfamerica.org/lung-cancer-info/types-lung-cancer/ros1-positive-lung-cancer/); Riely, G. L. (2017). What, when, and how of biomarker testing in non-small cell lung cancer. *Journal of the National Comprehensive Cancer Network: JNCCN, 15*(5S), 686–688.

Treatment by Stage

(Ettinger et al., 2022)

- Stage IA—Surgery only; no adjuvant chemotherapy:
- Stage IB-IIIA—Surgery followed by adjuvant chemotherapy with four cycles of a cisplatin-based regimen followed by adjuvant atezolizumab improved disease-free survival (DFS) versus best supportive care (Felip and Altorki, 2021).
  - In cases with an *EGFR* exon 19 deletion or exon 21 L858R mutation, adjuvant osimertinib: amivantamab and mobocertinib have recently gained FDA-accelerated approval for EGFR exon 20 insertion. Poziotinib was granted FDA fast-track designation for use in previously treated patients with HER2 exon 20 mutations in March 2021 (Spectrum Pharmaceuticals, 2021).
- Stage IIA-IIB—Surgery with or without adjuvant or neoadjuvant therapy, surgery alone, adjuvant chemotherapy, adjuvant targeted therapy (EGFR mutations). Adjuvant immunotherapy, neoadjuvant chemotherapy, or radiation therapy for patients who are not surgery candidates.
- Stage IIIA—For resected/resectable, surgery, neoadjuvant or adjuvant therapy; unresectable stage IIIA—chemoradiation and radiation therapy.
- Stage IIIB and IIIC—Sequential or concurrent chemotherapy and radiation therapy or radiation therapy alone; consolidated immunotherapy—durvalumab is a selective human 1gG1 monoclonal antibody that inhibits PDL1.
- Stage IV—newly diagnosed, relapsed, or recurrent NSCLC will be based on history of molecular features, age, comorbidities, and performance status.
  - First-line treatment for patients without actionable mutations is cytotoxic combination chemotherapy, combination chemotherapy with monoclonal antibodies, and maintenance therapy after first-line chemotherapy (for patients with stable or responding disease after four cycles of platinum-based combination chemotherapy).
  - For patients with actionable molecular mutations, EGFR, ALK (ALK translocations), *BRAF* V600E and MEK, ROS1 rearrangement, NTRK fusions, RET fusions, MET exon 14 skipping mutations, and PDL-1. Targeted therapies for these mutations should be used.
- Stage IV, progressive, relapsed, and recurrent NSCLC. Standard treatment options for progressive stage IV, second-line therapy include (PDQ Adult Treatment Editorial Board, 2022):
  - Chemotherapy
  - Epidermal growth factor receptor (EGFR)-directed therapy
  - ALK-directed tyrosine kinase inhibitors (TKIs)
  - *BRAF* V600E and MEK inhibitors (for patients with *BRAF* V600E)
  - ROS1-directed therapy
  - NTRK inhibitors (for patients with NTRK fusions)
  - RET inhibitors (for patients with RET fusions)
  - MET inhibitors (for patients with MET exon 14 skipping mutations)
  - KRAS G12C inhibitor (for patients with *KRAS* G12C mutations)
  - Immunotherapy

Palliative Care

- In the setting of metastatic disease, the NCCN guidelines recommend the introduction of palliative care at the time of diagnosis, regardless of patient performance status (Mo et al., 2021).
- Research has shown that patients with metastatic NSCLC randomized to early palliative care had a better quality of life and, unexpectedly, longer median survival than those randomized to standard oncologic care alone. In the palliative care group, patients received less aggressive end-of-life care and experienced fewer depressive symptoms (Temel et al., 2022).
- Smoking cessation counseling should be offered during the initial visit, workup, and throughout treatment.

Small Cell Lung Cancer

Chemotherapy and radiation therapy have been shown to improve survival for patients with limited-stage disease (LD) or extensive-stage disease (ED) however, only a minority of patients have a possibility for cure as most are diagnosed in later stages of disease.

Systemic Therapy

- Incorporating current chemotherapy regimens into the treatment program has prolonged survival at least four- to fivefold in median survival compared to no therapy.
- Patients with SCLC tend to develop distant metastases, and surgical resection or radiation therapy rarely produces long-term survival, however, because the risk of recurrence is extremely high, patients undergoing surgery for SCLC usually have postoperative chemotherapy or radiation therapy (Ganti et al., 2021).
  - Combination of a platinum and etoposide chemotherapy is the most widely used standard chemotherapy regimen used in first-line therapy. Current dosing and schedules produce overall response rates (ORR) of 50% to 80% and complete response rates (CR) of 0% to 30% in patients with ED (Ganti et al., 2021).
- Factors influencing treatment with chemotherapy include performance status (PS) and age.
  - Impaired PS leads to a poorer prognosis and inability to tolerate aggressive chemotherapy regimens.
  - Age is another factor influencing treatment tolerability; however, older patients in good general condition (PS 0 to 1), with normal organ function, and with minimal comorbidities may have similar responses as younger patients (PDQ Adult Treatment Editorial Board, 2022).
- Genetic testing is not indicated for patients with SCLC, and there are no approved targeted therapies to treat the disease.
- Standard treatment options for recurrent SCLC include chemotherapy, immune checkpoint inhibitors, and palliative therapy.
  - Lurbinectedin for previously treated one-line chemotherapy-containing regimen, phase II basket trial, showed overall response rate of 35% with median response duration of 5.3 months (Patel et al., 2021).

Radiation Therapy

- SCLC is highly radiosensitive, and thoracic radiation therapy has been shown to improve survival in patients with LD and ED tumors.
- Cranial irradiation prophylactically prevents central nervous system recurrence and may improve the long-term survival of patients who have responded to chemoradiation and have a good performance status. This also offers palliation of symptoms related to metastases.
  - Potential toxicities include dementia, memory loss, and gait problems, which may be permanent.
  - Palliative radiation therapy is done for treatment of bone pain, superior vena cava syndrome, spinal cord compression, brain metastasis, and postobstructive pneumonia (PDQ Adult Treatment Editorial Board, 2022).

Treatment by Stage

- For patients with LD, definitive chemoradiation therapy is indicated. Chemotherapy and radiation therapy, combination chemotherapy, surgery followed by chemotherapy or chemoradiation therapy, prophylactic cranial irradiation.
- Patients usually receive four to six cycles of chemotherapy and are followed with CT or PET scans every 8 to 10 weeks.
  - If the patient relapses more than 6 months after completing first-line chemotherapy, the original regimen can be used again.
  - When the disease progresses in less than 6 months after completing first-line therapy, single-agent chemotherapy, such as topotecan, paclitaxel, docetaxel, oral etoposide, gemcitabine, vinorelbine, or irinotecan, is used.
  - Eventually, the tumor becomes resistant to chemotherapy.
- ED is treated with immunotherapy and combination chemotherapy.
  - Immune checkpoint inhibitors, atezolizumab and durvalumab programmed cell death-ligand-1 (PD-L1), are approved in frontline treatment of patients with extensive-stage SCLC. Both have demonstrated prolongation of overall survival (OS) when combined with platinum-based chemotherapy and etoposide, compared with same combination chemotherapy regimen alone.
  - Pembrolizumab PD-1, in combination with chemotherapy, did not meet statistical significance for the prespecified endpoint of OS (NCI-SEER, 2022).
- Radiation therapy to metastatic disease sites is standard treatment option for patients with ED SCLC. Brain metastasis is treated with whole brain radiation (WBR).
  - Chest radiation therapy is occasionally given for superior vena cava syndrome, however, chemotherapy alone, with radiation reserved for nonresponding patients, is also appropriate initial treatment.
  - Patients with ED and who respond to chemotherapy may be considered for thoracic radiation.
  - Prophylactic cranial irradiation (PCI) continues to be controversial. It may be done in patients with extensive-stage SCLC who have achieved a complete response with chemotherapy to help decrease the chance of brain metastasis (PDQ Adult Treatment Editorial Board, 2022).

Palliative Care

- The initiation of palliative care for these patients is indicated at the time of diagnosis.

Prognosis

Non–Small Cell Lung Cancer

- Lung cancer remains the leading cause of cancer-related death in the United States, and most patients are diagnosed with late-stage disease.
- The National Cancer Institute Surveillance, epidemiology, and end results program (NCI-SEER, 2021) report relative survival rates are the average percentages of people who are alive 5 years after diagnosis. These rates do not include people who died of something other than lung cancer.
  - Localized cancer that is confined to one lung has a 5-year survival rate of 60%.
  - Regional cancer that has spread outside the lung or to the lymph node has a 5-year survival rate of 33%.

- Distant cancer that has metastasized to other parts of the body has a 5-year survival rate of 6%.
- For all stages of lung cancer, the 5-year survival rate is 23%.
- The clinical stage of disease is the most important prognostic factor, with earlier stages having better responses to treatment and longer survival times. Survival rates based on clinical stage drop dramatically below stage I. A more detailed prognostic tool based on TNM system provides the actual percentage of a sampling of people who were diagnosed with either NSCLC or SCLC and were alive at 2 years and at 5 years (see table below).
- Poor prognostic factors include weight loss, poor performance status, alterations in serum hematology or chemistry results (including elevated lactate dehydrogenase levels), bone or liver metastases, and leptomeningeal disease (i.e., spreading to the cerebrospinal fluid and space).

Non–Small Cell Lung Cancer Survival Rates, 2-Year Versus 5-Year

Stage NSCLC	2-Year Survival Rate (%)	5-Year Survival Rate (%)
Stage IA1	97	90
Stage IA2	92	80
Stage IA3	92	80
Stage IB	89	73
Stage IIA	82	65
Stage IIB	76	56
Stage IIIA	65	41
Stage IIIB	47	24
Stage IIIC	30	12
Stage IVA	23	10
Stage IVB	10	0

From National Cancer Institute-Surveillance Epidemiology, and End Results Program. (2021). *Cancer stat facts: Lung and bronchus cancer*. Available at https://seer.cancer.gov/statfacts/html/lungb.html

Small Cell Lung Cancer

- Very few patients are cured of SCLC. The long-term survival rate for patients with extensive-stage SCLC is almost 0%.
- The median survival time for patients with limited-stage disease who complete definitive chemoradiation therapy is 15 to 26 months. For those with extensive-stage disease, it is 7 to 11 months. For untreated disease, the survival time is usually 6 to 12 weeks.
  - Limited-stage disease treated with combination chemotherapy plus chest radiation may have a complete response rate of 80% and survival of 17 months has been reported; 12% to 15% of patients are alive at 5 years.
- Approximately 60% to 70% of patients with SCLC have clinically advanced or ED at presentation. Extensive-stage SCLC is incurable.
  - Combination chemotherapy provides patients diagnosed with extensive-stage disease a complete response rate of more than 20% and a median survival longer than 7 months; however, only 2% are alive at 5 years.
- Genome-wide association studies have identified single-nucleotide polymorphisms (e.g., within the promoter region of YAP1 on chromosome 11q22) that may affect survival in patients with SCLC.

- Prognostic factors associated with improved outcomes include good performance status, female sex, and a normal lactate dehydrogenase level at diagnosis.
- Indicators of poor prognosis include the following (NCI-SEER, 2022):
  - Disease progression
  - Weight loss of greater than 10% of baseline body weight
  - Poor performance status
  - Hyponatremia

Prevention and Surveillance

- The number of new lung cancer cases is on the decline, in part, from prevention strategies include smoking cessation, tobacco treatment, and chemoprevention. Chemoprevention is defined as using natural or synthetic agents to prevent, delay, or reverse carcinogenetic progression to invasive cancer (Balata, 2019).
- There are ongoing studies in the field of chemoprevention that address the challenges of identifying candidates for primary, secondary, or tertiary approaches (New & Keith, 2018).
- Global initiatives encouraging smoking cessation and the continued expansion of smoke-free public policies, increase in tobacco prices, strong media campaigns, and early detection have largely influenced the drop in lung cancer incidence. As a result, the outlook for lung cancer has improved by lowering the risk and diagnosing people with earlier stage when a cure is possible (New & Keith, 2018).
- In February 2022, the Centers for Medicare & Medicaid Services (CMS) announced expanded coverage for lung cancer screening with LDCT to improve health outcomes. Eligibility was expanded by lowering the starting age for screening from 55 to 50 years and reducing tobacco smoking history from at least 30 packs/year to at least 20 packs/year (Syrek Jensen, 2022).
- Early diagnosis is key to survival and is dictated by stage at diagnosis. This refers to the extent of cancer in the body. Only around 18% of lung cancer is diagnosed when the cancer is localized (stage 1). When the cancer is confined to the primary site, the 5-year relative survival rate is around 60%. With lung cancer diagnosed as regional (22%) or distant (56%), meaning the cancer has spread to the lymph nodes or different parts of the body, the 5-year survival is much less, 32% versus 6.3% (NCI-SEER, 2021).
- The NCCN updated guidelines for lung cancer screening, and the USPSTF recommends annual screening for lung cancer with LDCT in adults aged 50 to 80 years who have a 20 pack-year smoking history and currently smoke or have quit within the past 15 years (Potter et al., 2021).
- The expansion of the screening criteria and the changes made are key to including more high-risk women and racial minorities in screening. This will enable over 14 million Americans to be eligible for screening. Screening for lung cancer with LDCT has been shown to reduce lung cancer mortality by 20% to 33% in high-risk populations and save an additional 10 to 20 thousand lives each year (Potter et al., 2021).

- The NCCN's recommended surveillance protocol includes the following (Potter et al., 2021):
  - A history, physical examination, and chest CT with contrast every 6 to 12 months for 2 years, decreasing to annual evaluations thereafter
  - Smoking cessation
  - Vaccinations, including influenza (annual), herpes zoster, and pneumococcal vaccines
  - Health promotion and wellness counseling

References

American Cancer Society. (2022). *Cancer facts & figures 2022*. Available at https://www.cancer.org/research/cancer-facts-statistics/all-cancer-facts-figures/cancer-facts-figures-2022.html.

Amin, M. B., Greene, F. L., Edge, S. B., Compton, C. C., Gershenwald, J. E., Brookland, R. K., … Winchester, D. P. (2017). The eighth edition AJCC cancer staging manual: Continuing to build a bridge from a population-based to a more "personalized" approach to cancer staging. *CA: A Cancer Journal for Clinicians, 67*(2), 93–99.

Aisner, D., & Riely, G. J. (2021). Non–small cell lung cancer: recommendations for biomarker testing and treatment. *Journal of the National Comprehensive Cancer Network, 19*(5.5), 610–613.

Azzoli, C. G., Temin, S., Aliff, T., Baker, S., Jr., Brahmer, J., Johnson, D. H., … American Society of Clinical Oncology. (2011). 2011 focused update of 2009 American Society of Clinical Oncology Clinical Practice Guideline Update on chemotherapy for stage IV non–small-cell lung cancer. *Journal of Clinical Oncology, 29*(28), 3825–3831.

Bach, P., Cramer, L., Warren, J., & Begg, C. B. (1999). Racial differences in the treatment of early-stage lung cancer. *New England Journal of Medicine, 341*, 1198–1205.

Balata, H., Fong, K. M., Hendriks, L. E., Lam, S., Ostroff, J. S., Peled, N., … Aggarwal, C. (2019). Prevention and early detection for NSCLC: Advances in thoracic oncology 2018. *Journal of Thoracic Oncology, 14*(9), 1513–1527.

Bergamo, C., Lin, J. J., Smith, C., Lurslurchachai, L., Halm, E. A., Powell, C. A., … Wisnivesky, J. P. (2013). Evaluating beliefs associated with late-stage lung cancer presentation in minorities. *Journal of Thoracic Oncology, 8*(1), 12–18.

Cancer Genome Atlas Research Network. (2012). Comprehensive genomic characterization of squamous cell lung cancers. *Nature, 489*(7417), 519–525.

Corso, C., Park, H., Kim, A., Yu, J. B., Husain, Z., & Decker, R. H. (2015). Racial disparities in the use of SBRT for treating early-stage lung cancer. *Lung Cancer, 89*, 133–138.

Cykert, S., Walker, P., Edwards, L., McGuire, F. R., & Dilworth-Anderson, P. (2015). Weighing projections of physical decline in lung cancer surgery decisions. *American Journal Medical Science, 349*, 61–66.

Dancey, J., Szabo, E., & Rajan, A. (2022, April). *Small cell lung cancer treatment (PDQ)—health professional version*. National Cancer Institute. Available at https://www.cancer.gov/types/lung/hp/small-cell-lung-treatment-pdq.

Ettinger, D. S., Wood, D. E., Aisner, D. L., Akerley, W., Bauman, J. R., Bharat, A., … Hughes, M. (2022). Non-small cell lung cancer, version 3.2022, NCCN Clinical Practice Guidelines in Oncology. *Journal of the National Comprehensive Cancer Network: JNCCN, 20*(5), 497–530.

Felip, E., & Altorki, N. (2021). Adjuvant atezolizumab after adjuvant chemotherapy in resected stage IB-IIIA non-small-cell lung cancer (IMpower010): a randomized, multicenter, open-label, phase 3 trial. Available at https://www.thelancet.com/journals/lancet/article/PIIS0140-6736(21)02098-5/fulltext.

Ganti, A. K. P., Loo, B. W., Bassetti, M., Blakely, C., Chiang, A., D'Amico, T. A., … Hughes, M. (2021). Small cell lung cancer, version 2.2022, NCCN clinical practice guidelines in oncology. *Journal of the National Comprehensive Cancer Network: JNCCN, 19*(12), 1441–1464.

Lathan, C., Neville, B., & Earle, C. (2006). The effect of race on invasice staging and surgery in non-small cell lung cancer. *Journal of Clinical Oncology, 24*, 413–418.

Meyers, D. J., & Wallen, J. M. (2021, September 21). *Lung adenocarcinoma*. StatPearls. Available at https://www.ncbi.nlm.nih.gov/books/NBK519578/#_NBK519570_pubdet_.

Mo, L., Urbauer, D. L., Bruera, E., & Hui, D. (2021). Recommendations for palliative and hospice care in NCCN guidelines for treatment of cancer. *The Oncologist, 26*(1), 77–83.

National Cancer Institute. (2021). *Tumor markers*. Cancer.gov. Available at https://www.cancer.gov/about-cancer/diagnosis-staging/diagnosis/tumor-markers-fact-sheet.

National Cancer Institute, Surveillance, Epidemiology, and End Results. (2021). *Cancer of the lung and bronchus—cancer stat facts. SEER*. Available at https://seer.cancer.gov/statfacts/html/lungb.html.

National Center for Chronic Disease Prevention and Health Promotion (US) Office on Smoking and Health. (2014). *The health consequences of smoking—50 years of progress: A report of the surgeon general*. US: Centers for Disease Control and Prevention. Available at https://pubmed.ncbi.nlm.nih.gov/24455788/.

New, M., & Keith, R. (2018). Early detection and chemoprevention of lung cancer. *F1000Research, 7*, 61.

O'Keefe, E. B., Meltzer, J. P., & Bethea, T. N. (2015). Health disparities and cancer: Racial disparities in cancer mortality in the United States, 2000–2010. *Frontiers in Public Health, 3*, 51.

Patel, S., Petty, W. J., & Sands, J. M. (2021). An overview of lurbinectedin as a new second-line treatment option for small cell lung cancer. *Therapeutic Advances in Medical Oncology, 13*, 17588359211020529.

PDQ Adult Treatment Editorial Board. (2022). *Small Cell Lung Cancer Treatment (PDQ®): Health professional version. In PDQ Cancer Information Summaries*. National Cancer Institute (US). Available at https://www.cancer.gov/types/lung/hp/small-cell-lung-treatment-pdq.

Penner, L. A., Dovidio, J. F., Gonzalez, R., Albrecht, T. L., Chapman, R., Foster, T., & Eggly, S. (2016). The effects of oncologist implicit racial bias in racially discordant oncology interactions. *Journal of Clinical Oncology, 34*(24), 2874–2880.

Potter, A. L., Bajaj, S. S., & Yang, C. J. (2021). The 2021 USPSTF Lung Cancer Screening Guidelines: A new frontier. *The Lancet Respiratory Medicine, 9*(7), 689–691.

Potter, A. L., Rosenstein, A. L., Kiang, M. V., Shah, S. A., Gaissert, H. A., Chang, D. C., … Yang, C. J. (2022). Association of computed tomography screening with lung cancer stage shift and survival in the United States: Quasi-experimental study. *BMJ (Clinical Research ed.), 376*, e069008.

Rudin, C. M., Brambilla, E., Faivre-Finn, C., & Sage, J. (2021). Small-cell lung cancer. *Nature reviews. Disease Primers, 7*(1), 3.

Sinceshaw, H., Wu, X., Flanders, W., Osarogiagbon, R. U., & Jemal, A. (2016). Variations in receipt of curative-intent surgery for early-stage non-small cell lung cancer by state. *Journal of Thoracic Oncology, 11*, 880–889.

Spectrum Pharmaceuticals. (2011, March 11). *Food and Drug Administration grants fast track designation to spectrum pharmaceuticals' Poziotinib. News Release*. Available at https://bwnews.pr/3IjwoNf.

Syrek Jensen, T. (2022). *Press release CMS expands coverage of lung cancer screening with low dose computed tomography*. CMS. Available at https://www.cms.gov/newsroom/press-releases/cms-expands-coverage-lung-cancer-screening-low-dose-computed-tomography.

Taioli, E., & Flores, R. (2017). Appropriateness of surgical approach in black patients with lung cancer-15 years later, little has changed. *Journal of Thoracic Oncology, 12*, 573–577.

Temel, J. S., Petrillo, L. A., & Greer, J. A. (2022). Patient-centered palliative care for patients with advanced lung cancer. *Journal of Clinical Oncology, 40*(6), 626–634.

Malignant Pleural Mesothelioma

Definition

Malignant pleural mesothelioma (MPM) is a type of rare cancer that develops in the pleura, the thin membrane that lines the lungs and chest cavity. It is often associated with exposure to asbestos that gets lodged in the lining of the lungs causing inflammation and scaring. The tumors that develop in the pleura are known as pleural mesothelioma (Tsao et al., 2009).

Incidence

(Tsao et al., 2009; National Cancer Institute, Surveillance, Epidemiology, and End Results Program [NCI-SEER], 2021)

- MPM is a rare cancer with about 3000 new cases being diagnosed each year.
- The incidence is higher among older men (>70 years).

- Although the most common site of mesothelioma is the pleural space, it can also be found in the lining of the pericardium, peritoneum, and testis.
- Although the incidence of MPM is leveling off due to decreased asbestos use, the United States continues to report more cases of MPM than anywhere else in the world.

Etiology and Risk Factors

(Tsao et al., 2009; NCI-SEER, 2021)

- Unlike other lung cancers, smoking is not a risk factor for MPM.
- Asbestos exposure is the leading risk factor, but the exposure typically occurs 20 to 40 years before the cancer diagnosis.
- Radiotherapy, exposure to erionite (i.e., mineral found in gravel roads), and genetic factors may also increase the risk of developing

Signs and Symptoms

(American Society of Clinical Oncology [ASCO], 2017)

- Most patients have advanced disease by the time they are diagnosed.
- Significant symptoms include the following:
  - Chest or lower back pain
  - Dyspnea and cough
  - Palpable chest wall masses
  - Weight loss and dysphasia
  - Swelling of the face and arms
  - Fever and sweating
- Pleural effusions may develop.

Diagnostic Workup

- The purpose of the diagnostic workup is to distinguish MPM from other pathologies, including benign pleural disease and primary lung cancer (compared with metastasis from another site), and to determine the extent of disease.
- The initial workup includes the following:
  - History and physical examination, including details of asbestos exposures which are reported in 70% to 80% of all cases of mesothelioma (Wyant, 2018).
  - Laboratory testing, including a complete blood cell count and kidney and liver function tests
- Imaging, chest x-ray, radioactive particles, ultrasound, CT scan, or MRI to assess the chest to identify the location of the primary tumor and sites of metastatic disease (e.g., lymph nodes, liver, adrenal glands, bones), which may then be followed by PET scans.
- Echocardiogram
- Pleural biopsy under CT guidance or using a thoracoscopic approach
- Thoracentesis is often required to diagnose and palliate pleural effusions, and it may need to be repeated several times.
- Blood work—specifically fibulin-3, soluble mesothelin-related peptides (SMRPs). High levels found in these substances can make the diagnosis more likely.

Histopathology

- There are three histologic subtypes of MPM: epithelioid is the most common and has the best prognosis. Mixed or biphasic have both epithelioid and sarcomatoid cells and sarcomatoid or fibrous occurs in about 10% to 20% of all mesotheliomas (PDQ Adult Treatment Editorial Board, 2022).

Clinical Staging

(Amin et al., 2017)

- The purpose of staging is to determine whether the patient is a surgical candidate and the patient's treatment options.
- Histology is not a factor in staging.
- There are two prognostic scoring systems developed for advanced unresectable mesothelioma that are used to stratify patients enrolling in clinical trials: the Cancer and Leukemia Group B (CALGB) index and the European Organization for the Research and Treatment of Cancer (EORTC) index.
- Clinical staging is based on the International Mesothelioma Interest Group (IMIG) staging system and uses the TNM system adopted by the AJCC

Treatment

(PDQ Adult Treatment Editorial Board, 2022)

- Standard treatment for all but localized mesothelioma is rarely curative.
- Management of MPM uses a multidisciplinary team approach.
- Treatment options based on disease stage, performance status, and risk of morbidity include surgery, radiation therapy, and chemotherapy. The best outcomes result from the use of all three.
- Surgical approaches can be quite extensive and include pleurectomy with decortication (i.e., lung-sparing approach if possible), extrapleural pneumonectomy (i.e., removal of the entire lung, pleura, ipsilateral diaphragm, and often pericardium), and nodal dissection.
- Surgery can be considered for patients with stage 1 through III disease, although patients with sarcomatoid histology are often considered inoperable.
- A trimodality approach refers to a combination of chemotherapy, definitive surgery, and radiation therapy. Pemetrexed-based chemotherapy is the treatment of choice in combination with cisplatin or carboplatin before or after surgery and for patients who have stage IV or inoperable disease.
  - On disease progression, patients can receive single-agent gemcitabine or vinorelbine.
  - First-line nivolumab and ipilimumab, and cisplatin plus pemetrexed with or without bevacizumab.
- Radiation therapy alone is not recommended as the primary treatment for MPM and is typically used for adjuvant treatment after surgery.
- Palliative radiation therapy is often used in smaller doses to treat painful chest wall or bone metastases.
- Multimodality clinical trials should be considered.
- Tumor Treating Fields (TTFields) is a treatment option utilizing a noninvasive application of low-intensity intermediate frequency of electric fields to disrupt mitosis.

This treatment option has been studied in combination with chemotherapy in a phase II clinical trial for front-line treatment of unresectable malignant pleural mesothelioma (Ceresoli et al., 2019). Further information on TTFields is provided in "Tumor Treating Fields" chapter.

Prognosis

Mesothelioma is incurable and carries a poor prognosis. The average life expectancy is 4–18 months from diagnosis and survival ranges between 12 and 18 months with treatment. Only about 12% of patients with pleural mesothelioma live for 5 years or longer (ACS, 2023).

Factors that may determine a patient's prognosis/life expectancy include:

- Age-younger (40 and under) tend to live longer versus older (over 40 years)
- Gender-women are less likely than men to be diagnosed with pleural mesothelioma and have been shown to live longer than men diagnosed with the same cell type. More men experience occupational exposure to asbestos (construction, firefighters), contributing to increase risk and diagnosis (Van Gerwen et al., 2019).
- Histology and the presence of prognostic and predictive markers.
  - Pleura epithelial tumor cells have a life expectancy average of 14.4 months (Verma, 2018).
  - Patients with pleural mesothelioma, epithelioid type, with loss of BAP1 by IHC and retained p16 expression by IHC have prolonged survival in both univariate and multivariate analyses (Chou et al., 2018).
  - Patients with germline BAP1 mutations have a prolonged survival (Baumann et al., 2015; Pastorino et al., 2018).
- Early diagnosis and stage at diagnosis: Early diagnosis with response to treatment increases life expectancy and averages 21 months; however, without treatment, life expectancy significantly decreases life expectancy to 6–8 months. Stage 4 is the most advanced and final stage. Patients diagnosed with stage 4 disease is less than 12 months (Verma, 2018).
- A person's overall health including lifestyle and health habits may also play an important role. Smoking significantly decreases life expectancy. Tobacco use does not cause pleural mesothelioma, however, it can worsen a person's general health. Chronic illness such as heart disease, COPD, obesity, and diabetes may also decrease life expectancy.

Prevention and Surveillance

- Avoiding exposure to airborne asbestos particles is the best prevention. The Environmental Protection Agency (EPA) has regulated the use of asbestos in building materials since the 1970s. Some buildings, homes, and products made prior to 1980s may still to have asbestos.
- Attention to early warning signs such as shortness of breath, chronic cough, pain in the side of the chest or lower back, fatigue, weight loss, dysphasia, or hoarseness, swelling of the face and arms.
- Surveillance for response to treatment imaging is recommended using contrast enhanced CT scans.

References

Adult Treatment Editorial Board. (2022). *PDQ adult cancer treatment summaries.* https://www.cancer.gov/types/mesothelioma/hp/mesothelioma-treatment-pdq.

American Cancer Society (ACS). (2023). *Survival Rates for Mesothelioma.* Retrieved from https://www.cancer.org/cancer/malignant-mesothelioma/detection-diagnosis-staging/survival-statistics.html.

American Society of Clinical Oncology. (2017). *Mesothelioma: Diagnosis.* Cancer.net. https://www.cancer.net/cancer-types/mesothelioma/diagnosis.

Amin, M. B., Edge, S., & Greene, F. (Eds.). (2017). *Malignant pleural mesothelioma: AJCC cancer staging manual* (8th ed.). Springer International Publishing, American Joint Commission on Cancer.

Baumann, F., Flores, E., Napolitano, A., Kanodia, S., Taioli, E., Pass, H., … Carbone, M. (2015). Mesothelioma patients with germline BAP1 mutations have 7-fold improved long-term survival. *Carcinogenesis, 36*(1), 76–81. https://doi.org/10.1093/carcin/bgu227.

Ceresoli, G. L., Aerts, J. G., Dziadziuszko, R., Ramlau, R., Cedres, S., van Meerbeeck, J. P., … Grosso, F. (2019). Tumour treating fields in combination with pemetrexed and cisplatin or carboplatin as first-line treatment for unresectable malignant pleural mesothelioma (STELLAR): A multicentre, single-arm phase 2 trial. *The Lancet Oncology, 20*(12), 1702–1709.

Chou, A., Toon, C. W., Clarkson, A., Sheen, A., Sioson, L., & Gill, A. J. (2018). The epithelioid BAP1-negative and p16-positive phenotype predicts prolonged survival in pleural mesothelioma. *Histopathology, 72*(3), 509–515. https://doi.org/10.1111/his.13392.

National Cancer Institute, Surveillance, Epidemiology, and End Results Program (NCI-SEER). (2021). *Cancer of the lung and bronchus—cancer stat facts Surveillance, Epidemiology, and End Results (SEER) 18 registries.* https://seer.cancer.gov/statfacts/html/lungb.html.

Pastorino, S., Yoshikawa, Y., Pass, H. I., Emi, M., Nasu, M., Pagano, I., … Carbone, M. (2018). A subset of mesotheliomas with improved survival occurring in carriers of BAP1 and other germline mutations. *Journal of Clinical Oncology: Official Journal of the American Society of Clinical Oncology, 36*(35). JCO2018790352. Advance online publication https://doi.org/10.1200/JCO.2018.79.0352.

Tsao, A. S., Wistuba, I., Roth, J. A., & Kindler, H. L. (2009). Malignant pleural mesothelioma. *Journal of Clinical Oncology, 27*(12), 2081–2090. https://doi.org/10.1200/jco.2008.19.8523.

Van Gerwen, M., Alpert, N., Wolf, A., Ohri, N., Lewis, E., Rosenzweig, K. E., … Taioli, E. (2019). *Prognostic factors of survival in patients with malignant pleural mesothelioma: An analysis of the National Cancer Database.* Retrieved from https://academic.oup.com/carcin/article/40/4/529/5288470.

Verma, V., Ahern, C. A., Berlind, C. G., Lindsay, W. D., Shabason, J., Sharma, S., … Simone, C. B. (2018). *Survival by histologic subtype of malignant pleural mesothelioma and the impact of surgical resection on overall survival.* Retrieved from https://www.sciencedirect.com/science/article/abs/pii/S1525730418302018.

Wyant, T. (Ed.). (2018). *How is malignant mesothelioma diagnosed?* American Cancer Society. https://www.cancer.org/cancer/malignant-mesothelioma/detection-diagnosis-staging/how-diagnosed.html.

Lymphomas

Laura J. Zitella

Overview of Lymphomas

Definition

Lymphomas are a group of diverse cancers of B lymphocytes, T lymphocytes, or, rarely, natural killer (NK) cells that originate in the lymph nodes or lymphatic tissue but can affect any organ (Linch, 2021). Lymphomas arise from a normal counterpart cell at various stages of differentiation (Bond & Baiocchi, 2021). For example, acute lymphoblastic lymphoma arises from an early precursor B-cell, whereas follicular lymphoma arises from a germinal center B-cell. Lymphomas have distinct patterns of cell growth, size and shape, immunologic, cytogenetic, and molecular features (Bond & Baiocchi, 2021). The disease may be localized or widespread at the time of diagnosis. The clinical behavior of lymphomas ranges from indolent to aggressive based on the characteristics of the disease and the patient's life expectancy if the disease is left untreated (Bond & Baiocchi, 2021). The probability of disease progression, survival, and/or response rates to standard therapies varies with each clinical entity (Bond & Baiocchi, 2021).

In general, most indolent lymphomas are incurable, yet they progress slowly with a relatively low symptom burden and are associated with prolonged survival (Batlevi et al., 2020). Indolent lymphomas often do not need immediate treatment. When treatment is indicated, they tend to have a high response rate to initial chemoimmunotherapy that achieves a remission for a period followed by a continuous relapsing pattern that requires multiple lines of therapy over time (Batlevi et al., 2020). Treatment generally focuses on minimizing symptom burden, maximizing quality of life, and producing durable remissions (Batlevi et al., 2020). In contrast, aggressive lymphomas are typically symptomatic at presentation with rapidly enlarging lymph nodes and may involve extranodal sites (Onaindia et al., 2021). Aggressive lymphomas are rapidly fatal if left untreated, yet they are often curable with combination chemotherapy or chemoimmunotherapy (Onaindia et al., 2021).

Lymphomas are divided into two major categories: Hodgkin lymphoma (HL) and all other lymphomas, called non-Hodgkin lymphomas (NHLs). There are two major subtypes of HL and more than 70 subtypes of NHL, so a complete review is beyond the scope of this chapter. Thus, for NHL, this chapter reviews the most common indolent lymphoma, follicular lymphoma; the most common aggressive lymphoma, diffuse large B-cell lymphoma (DLBCL); and the most common very aggressive lymphoma, Burkitt lymphoma.

Classification

- The World Health Organization Classification of Haematolymphoid Tumours (WHO-HAEM5) is the established global guideline for the diagnosis of malignant lymphomas (Alaggio et al., 2022).
- The major categories of lymphoid malignancies are precursor B-cell neoplasms, mature B-cell neoplasms, plasma cell neoplasms, precursor T-cell neoplasms, and mature T-cell and NK-cell neoplasms (Alaggio et al., 2022). These classifications can be found in the box below.
- The subtypes of lymphomas are based on pathologic, immunophenotypic, genetic, and clinical features (Alaggio et al., 2022). These classifications can be found in the box.
- Both lymphomas and lymphoid leukemias are included in this classification because both the solid and circulating phases are present in many lymphoid neoplasms and distinction between them is artificial.
- The more than 70 clinicopathological entities described by the WHO classification and these can be divided into the more clinically useful categories of indolent or aggressive lymphomas.
- Indolent or low-grade classifications account for approximately 35% of lymphomas, whereas the remaining 65% are aggressive lymphomas (Freedman & Jacobsen, 2020).
- In the United States, B-cell lymphomas account for about 90% of all NHL cases (de Leval & Jaffe, 2020).

World Health Organization Classification of Haematolymphoid Tumors

Tumor-Like Lesions With B-Cell Predominance	Precursor B-Cell Neoplasms *B-Cell Lymphoblastic Leukemias/Lymphomas*
- Reactive B-cell-rich lymphoid proliferations that can mimic lymphoma - IgG4-related disease - Unicentric Castleman disease - Idiopathic multicentric Castleman disease - KSHV/HHV8-associated multicentric Castleman disease	- B-lymphoblastic leukemia/lymphoma, NOS - B-lymphoblastic leukemia/lymphoma with high hyperdiploidy - B-lymphoblastic leukemia/lymphoma with hypodiploidy - B-lymphoblastic leukemia/lymphoma with iAMP21 - B-lymphoblastic leukemia/lymphoma with BCR::ABL1 fusion

Continued

World Health Organization Classification of Haematolymphoid Tumors—cont'd

- B-lymphoblastic leukemia/lymphoma with BCR::ABL1-like features
- B-lymphoblastic leukemia/lymphoma with KMT2A rearrangement
- B-lymphoblastic leukemia/lymphoma with ETV6::RUNX1 fusion
- B-lymphoblastic leukemia/lymphoma with ETV6::RUNX1-like features
- B-lymphoblastic leukemia/lymphoma with TCF3::PBX1 fusion
- B-lymphoblastic leukemia/lymphoma with IGH::IL3 fusion
- B-lymphoblastic leukemia/lymphoma with TCF3::HLF fusion
- B-lymphoblastic leukemia/lymphoma with other defined genetic abnormalities

Mature B-Cell Neoplasms

Pre-Neoplastic and Neoplastic Small Lymphocytic Proliferations

- Monoclonal B-cell lymphocytosis
- Chronic lymphocytic leukemia/small lymphocytic lymphoma

Splenic B-Cell Lymphomas and Leukemias

- Hairy cell leukemia
- Splenic marginal zone lymphoma
- Splenic diffuse red pulp small B-cell lymphoma
- Splenic B-cell lymphoma/leukemia with prominent nucleoli

Lymphoplasmacytic Lymphoma

- Lymphoplasmacytic lymphoma

Marginal Zone Lymphoma

- Extranodal marginal zone lymphoma of mucosa-associated lymphoid tissue
- Primary cutaneous marginal zone lymphoma
- Nodal marginal zone lymphoma
- Pediatric marginal zone lymphoma

Follicular Lymphoma

- In situ follicular B-cell neoplasm
- Follicular lymphoma
- Pediatric-type follicular lymphoma
- Duodenal-type follicular lymphoma

Cutaneous Follicle Centre Lymphoma

- Primary cutaneous follicle center lymphoma

Mantle Cell Lymphoma

- In situ mantle cell neoplasm
- Mantle cell lymphoma
- Leukemic non-nodal mantle cell lymphoma

Transformations of Indolent B-Cell Lymphomas

- Transformations of indolent B-cell lymphomas

Large B-Cell Lymphomas

- Diffuse large B-cell lymphoma, NOS
- T-cell/histiocyte-rich large B-cell lymphoma
- Diffuse large B-cell lymphoma/high-grade B-cell lymphoma with MYC and BCL2 rearrangements
- ALK-positive large B-cell lymphoma
- Large B-cell lymphoma with IRF4 rearrangement
- High-grade B-cell lymphoma with 11q aberrations
- Lymphomatoid granulomatosis
- EBV-positive diffuse large B-cell lymphoma
- Diffuse large B-cell lymphoma associated with chronic inflammation
- Fibrin-associated large B-cell lymphoma
- Fluid overload-associated large B-cell lymphoma
- Plasmablastic lymphoma
- Primary large B-cell lymphoma of immune-privileged sites (includes primary large B-cell lymphoma of the CNS, primary large B-cell lymphoma of the vitreoretinal, and primary large B-cell lymphoma of the testis)
- Primary cutaneous diffuse large B-cell lymphoma, leg type
- Intravascular large B-cell lymphoma
- Primary mediastinal large B-cell lymphoma
- Mediastinal grey zone lymphoma
- High-grade B-cell lymphoma, NOS

Burkitt lymphoma

- Burkitt lymphoma

KSHV/HHV8-Associated B-Cell Lymphoid Proliferations and Lymphomas

- Primary effusion lymphoma
- KSHV/HHV8-positive diffuse large B-cell lymphoma
- KSHV/HHV8-positive germinotropic lymphoproliferative disorder

Lymphoid Proliferations and Lymphomas Associated With Immune Deficiency and Dysregulation

- Hyperplasias arising in immune deficiency/dysregulation
- Polymorphic lymphoproliferative disorders arising in immune deficiency/dysregulation
- EBV-positive mucocutaneous ulcer
- Lymphomas arising in immune deficiency/dysregulation
- Inborn error of immunity-associated lymphoid proliferations and lymphomas

Hodgkin Lymphoma

- Classic Hodgkin lymphoma
  - Nodular sclerosis (NSCHL)
  - Mixed cellularity (MCCHL)
  - Lymphocyte rich (LRCHL)
  - Lymphocyte depleted (LDCHL)
- Nodular lymphocyte predominant Hodgkin lymphoma

Plasma Cell Neoplasms and Other Diseases With Paraproteins

Monoclonal Gammopathies

- Cold agglutinin disease
- IgM monoclonal gammopathy of undetermined significance
- Non-IgM monoclonal gammopathy of undetermined significance
- Monoclonal gammopathy of renal significance

Diseases With Monoclonal Immunoglobulin Deposition

- Immunoglobulin-related (AL) amyloidosis
- Monoclonal immunoglobulin deposition disease

Heavy Chain Diseases

- Mu heavy chain disease
- Gamma heavy chain disease
- Alpha heavy chain disease

Plasma Cell Neoplasms

- Plasmacytoma
- Plasma cell myeloma
- Plasma cell neoplasms with associated paraneoplastic syndrome
- POEMS syndrome
- TEMPI syndrome
- AESOP syndrome

Tumor-Like Lesions With T-Cell Predominance

- Kikuchi-Fujimoto disease
- Indolent T-lymphoblastic proliferation
- Autoimmune lymphoproliferative syndrome

Precursor T-Cell Neoplasms

- T-lymphoblastic leukemia/lymphoma
- T-lymphoblastic leukemia/lymphoma, NOS
- Early T-precursor lymphoblastic leukemia/lymphoma

Mature T-Cell and NK-Cell Neoplasms

Mature T-Cell and NK-Cell Leukemias

- T-cell prolymphocytic leukemia
- T-cell large granular lymphocytic leukemia
- NK-cell large granular lymphocytic leukemia
- Adult T-cell leukemia/lymphoma
- Sézary syndrome
- Aggressive NK-cell leukemia

Primary Cutaneous T-Cell Lymphomas

- Primary cutaneous CD4-positive small or medium T-cell lymphoproliferative disorder
- Primary cutaneous acral CD8-positive lymphoproliferative disorder
- Mycosis fungoides
- Primary cutaneous CD30-positive T-cell lymphoproliferative disorder: Lymphomatoid papulosis

World Health Organization Classification of Haematolymphoid Tumors—cont'd

- Primary cutaneous CD30-positive T-cell lymphoproliferative disorder: Primary cutaneous anaplastic large cell lymphoma
- Subcutaneous panniculitis-like T-cell lymphoma
- Primary cutaneous gamma/delta T-cell lymphoma
- Primary cutaneous CD8-positive aggressive epidermotropic cytotoxic T-cell lymphoma
- Primary cutaneous peripheral T-cell lymphoma, NOS

Intestinal T-Cell and NK-Cell Lymphoid Proliferations and Lymphomas
- Indolent T-cell lymphoma of the gastrointestinal tract
- Indolent NK-cell lymphoproliferative disorder of the gastrointestinal tract
- Enteropathy-associated T-cell lymphoma
- Monomorphic epitheliotropic intestinal T-cell lymphoma
- Intestinal T-cell lymphoma, NOS

Hepatosplenic T-Cell Lymphoma
- Hepatosplenic T-cell lymphoma

Anaplastic Large Cell Lymphoma
- ALK-positive anaplastic large cell lymphoma
- ALK-negative anaplastic large cell lymphoma
- Breast implant-associated anaplastic large cell lymphoma

T-Follicular Helper (TFH) Cell Lymphoma
- Nodal TFH cell lymphoma, angioimmunoblastic-type
- Nodal TFH cell lymphoma, follicular-type
- Nodal TFH cell lymphoma, NOS

Other Peripheral T-Cell Lymphomas
- Peripheral T-cell lymphoma, not otherwise specified

EBV-Positive NK/T-Cell Lymphomas
- EBV-positive nodal T- and NK-cell lymphoma
- Extranodal NK/T-cell lymphoma

EBV-Positive T- and NK-Cell Lymphoid Proliferations and Lymphomas of Childhood
- Severe mosquito bite allergy
- Hydroa vacciniforme lymphoproliferative disorder
- Systemic chronic active EBV disease
- Systemic EBV-positive T-cell lymphoma of childhood

Adapted from Alaggio, R., Amador, C., Anagnostopoulos, I., Attygalle, A. D., Araujo, I. B. O., Berti, E., … Xiao, W. (2022). The 5th edition of the World Health Organization classification of haematolymphoid tumours: Lymphoid neoplasms. *Leukemia*, *36*(7), 1720–1748.

Signs and Symptoms

(Cheson et al., 2014; Linch, 2021)
- Most common early symptom is painless lymphadenopathy (generally in the neck, armpit, groin, or abdomen)
- B symptoms are constitutional symptoms defined as:
- Unexplained loss of more than 10% of body weight in the 6 months before diagnosis.
- Unexplained fevers to more than 101°F (38.3°C)
- Drenching night sweats
- Fatigue
- Pruritus (especially HL)
- Given the heterogeneity of lymphomas, signs and symptoms can vary greatly depending on the areas of the body that are affected. For example:
- Mucosa-associated lymphoid tissue (MALT) lymphoma of the stomach may cause nausea, vomiting, and abdominal pain.
- Cutaneous T-cell lymphoma affects the skin and can cause redness, itching, or raised patches, nodules, or plaques on the skin.
- Patients with HL may experience pain in involved areas after ingestion of alcohol.

Diagnostic Workup

(Cheson et al., 2014; Linch, 2021)
- Malignant lymphomas are made up of a very large number of distinct clinicopathologic entities, and optimal therapy and outcomes depend on precise diagnosis.
- Therefore, the single most important test in a lymphoma patient is an adequate biopsy of affected tissue with morphology, immunohistochemistry, and flow cytometry reviewed by an experienced lymphoma pathologist and, where appropriate, molecular studies to accurately categorize the lymphoma.

- The optimal biopsy is an excisional lymph node biopsy of one of the largest nodes available or generous incisional biopsy of an extranodal site.
- Core biopsies ideally should be reserved for situations when the only sites of disease involvement are deep in the thorax or pelvis, rendering excisional node biopsy difficult.
- Fine-needle aspiration alone is inadequate and should never be used as the sole method of establishing the initial diagnosis of lymphoma.
- Pathologic confirmation of noncontiguous extra-lymphatic involvement is strongly suggested.
- Re biopsy is essential at time of relapse to confirm relapsed disease versus transformation to another sub-type of lymphoma.
- History and physical examination
  - Includes measurement of accessible nodal groups and the size of the spleen and liver in centimeters below their respective costal margins in the midclavicular line
- Complete blood count (CBC) with differential
- Metabolic panel, including renal and hepatic function
- Uric acid
- Lactate dehydrogenase (LDH) and/or β2 microglobulin (important prognostic markers)
- Hepatitis B and C serologies
- Human immunodeficiency virus (HIV) serology
- Tumor biopsy specimen with histopathology
- Flow cytometry of tumor specimen
- Immunohistochemistry of tumor specimen
- Cytogenetic analysis
- Fluorescence in situ hybridization (FISH) for lymphoma-associated translocations

- Positron emission tomography–computed tomography (PET-CT) scans of neck, chest, abdomen, and pelvis (for fluorodeoxyglucose [FDG]-avid lymphomas)
  - FDG-PET is critical as a baseline measurement and recommended for routine staging for FDG-avid, nodal lymphomas (essentially all histologies except chronic lymphocytic leukemia/small lymphocytic lymphoma, lymphoplasmacytic lymphoma/Waldenström macroglobulinemia, angioimmunoblastic lymphoma, mycosis fungoides, cutaneous B-cell lymphomas, and marginal zone NHLs, unless there is a suspicion of aggressive transformation) (Cheson et al., 2014)
- Contrast-enhanced CT scans of neck, chest, abdomen, and pelvis (for lymphomas that are not FDG avid)
- Additional studies (useful in selected cases)
  - Bone marrow aspiration and biopsy
    - PET-CT is adequate for determination of bone marrow involvement for HL and DLBCL. However, bone marrow biopsy and aspiration are recommended for staging other histologies (Cheson et al., 2014)
  - Pregnancy testing in women of childbearing potential.
  - Immunoglobulin and T-cell receptor (TCR) gene rearrangement studies.
  - Cardiac ejection fraction measurement (if anthracycline therapy planned).
  - Magnetic resonance imaging of brain if neurologic signs or symptoms.
  - Cerebrospinal fluid analysis (including flow cytometry) for high-risk aggressive lymphomas or if neurologic signs or symptoms are present.
  - Gastrointestinal studies (imaging and endoscopy) if Waldeyer ring involvement, mantle cell lymphoma, or enteropathy-associated lymphoma.

Clinical Staging

- The Lugano modification of the Ann Arbor staging system is the staging system for primary nodal lymphomas in adults (Cheson et al., 2014). The table on this page outlines this system.
- Initial staging criteria designed for HL were revised and ultimately led to the Ann Arbor staging system, which subdivided the disease into four stages based on the number and location of involved lymph node sites and extranodal involvement. It included the subclassifications "A," "B," and "E" (Linch, 2021).
  - A: Absence of B symptoms
  - B: Presence of B symptoms—fevers to greater than 101°F (38.3°C), weight loss, and/or drenching night sweats
  - E: Used for stages I-III and notes the presence of extralymphatic disease resulting from direct extension of an involved lymph node region.
- The Cotswold modification of the Ann Arbor staging system maintained the original four-stage clinical and pathologic staging framework of the Ann Arbor system and incorporated CT scans. It also introduced "X" for bulky disease and complete remission unconfirmed (CRu) to describe patients with a residual mass after treatment that was most likely represented by fibrous scar tissue (Linch, 2021).

- The Ann Arbor staging system was modified again in 2014 and is now referred to as the Lugano staging system. The Lugano staging system is the current staging system for primary nodal lymphomas (Cheson et al., 2014).
  - The Lugano staging system classifies lymphomas as limited (stages I and II, nonbulky) or advanced (stages III or IV) disease, with stage II bulky disease considered limited or advanced as determined by histology and several prognostic factors.
  - The designation "E" for extranodal disease is used for limited extranodal disease in the absence of nodal involvement (IE) or in patients with stage II disease and direct extension to a non-nodal site. E is not appropriate to use for patients with advanced-stage diseases.
  - The Ann Arbor classification "A" for those without B symptoms and "B" for those with defined B symptoms are no longer used except for patients with HL.
  - The previously used "X" subclassification to designate bulky disease is no longer necessary since there is no validated definition of bulky diseases.
  - The extent of disease is assessed by PET/CT imaging for FDG-avid lymphomas and by CT imaging for non-avid histologies (Cheson et al., 2014).
    - PET-CT is adequate for determination of bone marrow involvement and can be considered highly suggestive for involvement of other extralymphatic sites.
  - Biopsy confirmation of those sites can be considered if necessary.

Lugano Staging System for Primary Nodal Lymphomas

Stage	Involvement	Extranodal (E) Status
Limited		
I	One nodal group involved	Single extranodal lesions without nodal involvement
II	Two or more nodal groups involved on the same side of the diaphragm	Stage I or II nodal involvement with limited, contiguous extranodal involvement
II bulky	As in II above but with "bulky" disease	N/A
Advanced		
III	Involvement of nodal groups on both sides of the diaphragm	N/A
IV	Diffuse involvement of a visceral organ not contiguous with an involved nodal site	N/A

Note

Extent of disease is assessed by positron emission tomography/computed tomography (PET/CT) imaging for 2-fluorodeoxyglucose–avid lymphomas and by CT imaging for non-avid histologies. The tonsils, Waldeyer ring, and spleen are considered nodal tissue in this staging system.

Adapted from Cheson, B. D., Fisher, R. I., Barrington, S. F., Cavalli, F., Schwartz, L. H., Zucca, E., ... United Kingdom National Cancer Research Institutes. (2014). Recommendations for initial evaluation, staging, and response assessment of Hodgkin and non-Hodgkin lymphoma: The Lugano classification. *Journal of Clinical Oncology, 32*(27), 3059–3067.

Treatment

(PDQ Adult Treatment Editorial Board, 2022)

- Treatment for lymphoma depends on the stage, histologic type, and indolent or aggressive nature of the disease.
- Chemotherapy or chemoimmunotherapy are the most commonly used treatments.
- Other therapies include radiation, hematopoietic cell transplantation, targeted therapies, monoclonal antibodies, and chimeric antigen receptor T-cell therapy (CART).
- Radiation therapy may be used to treat localized diseases or symptomatic areas.
- Surgery is not generally used for treatment of lymphomas.

Treatment Response

- PET-CT scanning has become the standard for assessment of response for FDG-avid lymphomas, and CT scans are used for non–FDG-avid lymphomas (Cheson et al., 2014).
- In addition to PET-CT, all diagnostic studies that detected disease at baseline should be repeated at the completion of therapy (Linch, 2021).
- The Deauville 5-point scale is used to interpret the results of PET-CT (Barrington et al., 2014). The scale is a standard for radiologists to visually compare FDG uptake with the FDG uptake of the mediastinum (blood pool) and the liver of the individual patient, which have relatively constant uptake.
  1. No FDG uptake
  2. Slight FDG uptake, but equal to or below the mediastinum
  3. FDG uptake is above mediastinum but below or equal to uptake in the liver
  4. FDG uptake is moderately higher than liver
  5. Markedly increased FDG uptake or any new lesion
- The Lugano response criteria are used to determine complete response, partial response, stable disease, or progression disease (Cheson et al., 2014).
  - Complete metabolic response (CR): Deauville scores 1, 2, or 3, irrespective of a persistent mass on CT.
  - Partial response (PR): Deauville score 4 or 5 with decreased uptake compared with baseline and no evidence of progressive disease.
  - Stable disease (SD): Deauville score 4 or 5 without a significant change in FDG uptake from baseline.
  - Progressive disease (PD): Deauville score 4 to 5 with increasing intensity compared to baseline or any interim scan and/or any new FDG-avid lesions.

Supportive Care for B-Cell Lymphomas

- The risk of tumor lysis syndrome (TLS) should be assessed for all patients (NCCN, 2022a)
  - The risk of tumor lysis is highest with aggressive lymphomas (Dickinson & Seymour, 2021).
  - Elevated LDH and high tumor burden increase the risk of TLS (Dickinson & Seymour, 2021).
  - Patients at risk for TLS should be treated with prophylactic measures that include monitoring laboratory values, hydration, and management of uric acid by administration of allopurinol or rasburicase (NCCN, 2022a).

- Hepatitis B and hepatitis C and HIV testing are recommended for all patients. There is a risk of reactivation of viruses, particularly with the use of anti-CD20 antibodies. Prophylaxis for hepatitis B is recommended for chronic carriers of hepatitis B (Dickinson & Seymour, 2021).
- Infusion reactions can occur with monoclonal antibody therapy. Appropriate pre-medication and monitoring are recommended. For rituximab, if no infusion reaction was experienced with prior cycle of rituximab, a rapid 90-minute infusion or subcutaneous formulation may be used (NCCN, 2022a).
- Alternate forms of rituximab are now available, including biosimilars and an SQ formulation (NCCN, 2022a).
- Delayed-rituximab neutropenia may occur weeks or months after completion of therapy in up to 10% of patients. It usually resolves spontaneously, or a short course of G-CSF may be used (NCCN, 2022a).
- Patients at risk pneumocystis jirovecii pneumonia should receive prophylaxis, typically with trimethoprim–sulfamethoxazole. This includes patients treated with a prolonged course of high-dose glucocorticoids, bendamustine, hematopoietic stem cell transplantation, and CAR-T therapy (NCCN, 2022a, 2022b).
- Herpes zoster reactivation (shingles) and herpes reactivation are common, and prophylaxis with acyclovir or valacyclovir is commonly prescribed to at-risk patients, particularly those with a prior history of viral reactivation (Dickinson & Seymour, 2021).
- Patients treated with anti-CD20 monoclonal antibodies or anti-CD19 CAR-T therapy may experience hypogammaglobulinemia. Intravenous immune globulin (IVIG) replacement may be indicated, particularly if patients have recurrent infections (NCCN, 2022a).

Surveillance

- Patients with lymphoma in remission require ongoing survivorship care, which includes active surveillance for relapse and monitoring for late effects.
- For curable histologies such as HL and DLBCL, the likelihood of relapse decreases over time; thus, the frequency of follow-up is every 3 months for the first 2 years and then every 6 months for the next 3 years (Linch, 2021).
- For DLBCL, the risk of relapsing beyond 2 years after achieving a first CR is less than 10%, and only 1% to 2% of relapses are first detected by imaging (Linch, 2021). For that reason, the Lugano IWG guidelines discourage routine surveillance CT imaging for asymptomatic patients with HL and DLBCL who are in remission (Cheson et al., 2014).
- In contrast, for follicular lymphoma and other incurable histologies, the likelihood of recurrence continues or increases over time, and patients should be observed every 3 to 6 months. History, physical examination, and labs including a CBC, metabolic panel, and serum LDH are recommended at every follow-up visit (Cheson et al., 2014; Linch, 2021).

References

Alaggio, R., Amador, C., Anagnostopoulos, I., Attygalle, A. D., Araujo, I. B. O., Berti, E., … Xiao, W. (2022). The 5th edition of the World Health Organization classification of haematolymphoid tumours: Lymphoid neoplasms. *Leukemia, 36*(7), 1720–1748.

Barrington, S. F., Mikhaeel, N. G., Kostakoglu, L., Meignan, M., Hutchings, M., Müeller, S. P., … Cheson, B. D. (2014). Role of imaging in the staging and response assessment of lymphoma: Consensus of the International Conference on Malignant Lymphomas Imaging Working Group. *Journal of Clinical Oncology: Official Journal of the American Society of Clinical Oncology, 32*(27), 3048–3058.

Batlevi, C. L., Sha, F., Alperovich, A., Ni, A., Smith, K., Ying, Z., … Younes, A. (2020). Follicular lymphoma in the modern era: Survival, treatment outcomes, and identification of high-risk subgroups. *Blood Cancer Journal, 10*(7), 74.

Bond, D. A., & Baiocchi, R. A. (2021). Classification of malignant lymphoid disorders. In K. Kaushansky, J. T. Prchal, L. J. Burns, M. A. Lichtman, M. Levi, & D. C. Linch (Eds.), *Williams hematology* (10th ed.). McGraw-Hill Education. Available at http://accessmedicine.mhmedical.com/content.aspx?aid=1178750323.

Cheson, B. D., Fisher, R. I., Barrington, S. F., Cavalli, F., Schwartz, L. H., Zucca, E., … United Kingdom National Cancer Research Institutes. (2014). Recommendations for initial evaluation, staging, and response assessment of Hodgkin and non-Hodgkin lymphoma: The Lugano classification. *Journal of Clinical Oncology, 32*(27), 3059–3067.

de Leval, L., & Jaffe, E. S. (2020). Lymphoma classification. *The Cancer Journal, 26*(3), 176–185.

Dickinson, M., & Seymour, J. F. (2021). Diffuse large B-cell lymphoma and related diseases. In K. Kaushansky, J. T. Prchal, L. J. Burns, M. A., et al. (Eds.), *Williams hematology* (10th ed.). McGraw-Hill Education. Available at http://accessmedicine.mhmedical.com/content.aspx?aid=1178751274.

Freedman, A., & Jacobsen, E. (2020). Follicular lymphoma: 2020 update on diagnosis and management. *American Journal of Hematology, 95*(3), 316–327.

Linch, D. C. (2021). General considerations of lymphomas: incidence rates, etiology, diagnosis, staging, and primary extranodal disease. In K. Kaushansky, J. T. Prchal, L. J. Burns, et al. (Eds.), *Williams hematology* (10th ed.). McGraw-Hill Education. Available at http://accessmedicine.mhmedical.com/content.aspx?aid=1178750836.

National Comprehensive Cancer Network. (2022a). *NCCN Clinical Practice Guidelines in Oncology (NCCN Guidelines®): B-cell lymphomas (v. 4.2022)*. NCCN.org. Available at https://www.nccn.org/professionals/physician_gls/pdf/b-cell.pdf.

National Comprehensive Cancer Network. (2022b). *NCCN Clinical Practice Guidelines in Oncology (NCCN Guidelines®): Prevention and treatment of cancer-related infections (v. 1.2022)*. NCCN.org. Available at https://www.nccn.org/professionals/physician_gls/pdf/infections.pdf.

Onaindia, A., Santiago-Quispe, N., Iglesias-Martinez, E., & Romero-Abrio, C. (2021). Molecular update and evolving classification of large B-cell lymphoma. *Cancers, 13*(3), 3352.

PDQ Adult Treatment Editorial Board. (2022). *Adult non-Hodgkin lymphoma treatment (PDQ®): Health professional Version*. Available at https://www.cancer.gov/types/lymphoma/hp/adult-nhl-treatment-pdq#_993.

Hodgkin Lymphoma

Definition

HL is an uncommon neoplasm arising from malignant transformation of a mature B-cell at the germinal center stage of differentiation (Spinner et al., 2021). Two clinicopathologic entities are described: classical HL (cHL) and nodular lymphocyte predominant HL (NLPHL) (Alaggio et al., 2022). Approximately 95% of cases are cHL, and 5% are NLPHL (Spinner et al., 2021).

cHL is characterized by the presence of multinucleated Hodgkin and Reed-Sternberg (HRS) cells embedded within a mixed infiltrate of inflammatory cells. HRS cells are derived from B cells but have most of the B-cell–specific characteristics. Epstein-Barr virus (EBV) is an important environmental factor in the pathogenesis of cHL (Spinner et al., 2021). cHL disproportionately affects young adults and adolescents, with a second peak occurring in people older than 60 years (Momotow et al., 2021). Combination chemotherapy is the mainstay of treatment, and all stages of HL are potentially curable with a long-term survival rate that exceeds 85% (Spinner et al., 2021).

NLPHL is characterized by malignant lymphocyte-predominant (LP) cells, or "popcorn cells," embedded within B-cell-rich nodules (Spinner et al., 2021). In contrast to HRS cells, LP cells express typical B-cell markers. NLPHL commonly presents with early-stage disease and peripheral lymphadenopathy. Radiotherapy is an integral part of therapy for most patients. There is a tendency for late relapses as well as a risk of transformation into DLBCL (Spinner et al., 2021).

Incidence

- HL is estimated to represent 0.4% of all cancers diagnosed in the United States in 2022 (National Cancer Institute [NCI], 2022).
- It is estimated that there will be 8540 new cases of HL and 920 deaths from HL in the United States in 2022 (NCI, 2022).
- The median age of onset is 38 years, with bimodal incidence peaks at ages 20 to 29 and 60 to 69 (Spinner et al., 2021).

Etiology and Risk Factors

- The etiology of HL is uncertain.
- Males are slightly more likely to develop HL than females (NCI, 2022).
- A history of symptomatic infectious mononucleosis caused by the EBV is associated with three-fold increased risk of HL. EBV-positive HL accounts for 30% to 50% of cHL cases (Spinner et al., 2021).
- Infection with HIV is associated with 10 to 20 times increased risk than general population, and the incidence has increased despite effective HIV therapy (Spinner et al., 2021).
- Personal history of autoimmune conditions is associated with increased risk (Spinner et al., 2021).
- There is a familial predisposition and familial HL represents approximately 5% of new cases (Spinner et al., 2021).

Histopathology

- The World Health Organization classification of Lymphoid Neoplasms, 5th edition, is the current classification system (Alaggio et al., 2022). See the box in the Overview of this chapter.
- Two clinicopathologic entities are described: NLPHL and CHL (Alaggio et al., 2022).

Classic Hodgkin Lymphoma

- Accounts for 95% of cases (Spinner et al., 2021)
- Typical immunophenotypes are CD3−, CD15+, CD20−, CD30+, CD45−, CD79a−, PAX-5+ B-cell lymphocytes.

- The malignant cells of HL are multinucleated HRS cells, which are derived from germinal center-mature B cells but have lost typical B-cell markers. HRS cells account for less than 1% of cells in the affected tissue and are embedded within a mixed infiltrate of inflammatory cells (Spinner et al., 2021).
- HRS cells harbor near-universal genetic alterations of chromosome 9p24.1, leading to overexpression of the programmed death-1 (PD-1) ligands, PD-L1 and PD-L2 contributing to immune evasion (Spinner et al., 2021).
- Four subtypes of cHL (Alaggio et al., 2022):
- Nodular sclerosis
- Mixed cellularity
- Lymphocyte rich
- Lymphocyte depleted

Nodular Lymphocyte-Predominant Hodgkin Lymphoma

- Approximately 5% of HL cases (Spinner et al., 2021).
- Typically diagnosed in asymptomatic young men with cervical, axilla, or inguinal lymph nodes without mediastinal involvement.
- Typical immunophenotypes are CD3−, CD15−, CD20+, CD30−, CD45+, CD79a+, BCL6+, PAX-5+ B-cell lymphocytes (Spinner et al., 2021).
- Patients are usually diagnosed with an earlier-stage disease (75% of cases), longer survival, and fewer treatment failures (Spinner et al., 2021).

Clinical Staging

- The staging classification that is currently used is the Lugano modification of the Ann Arbor staging system as presented in table on page 146.
- cHL typically spreads in a predictable, contiguous manner and is classified into four stages, I to IV, based on the number and location of involved lymph nodes and extranodal involvement (Spinner et al., 2021).
- Stages I, II, III, and IV can be subclassified into A and B categories:
  - A for those without B symptoms, and B for those with defined B symptoms.
  - The E designation is also used in stages I-III.
    - The E designation notes the presence of extralymphatic disease resulting from direct extension of an involved lymph node region. It is not appropriate to use this designation in the presence of widespread disease or diffuse extralymphatic disease.
- There are several prognostic scoring systems used for early stages (stages I and II nonbulky disease). Unfavorable risk factors include bulky mediastinal disease (defined as mediastinal mass width greater than one-third of the maximum intrathoracic diameter), B symptoms, ESR ≥50, greater than 3 sites of disease, and any site greater than greater than 10 cm (Spinner et al., 2021).
- The International Prognostic Score-3 (IPS-3) is the prognostic scoring system for advanced stage HL (Hayden et al., 2020). Advanced stage is defined as Ann Arbor stages III or

IV, or stage II with B symptoms and stage I or II with bulky disease (≥10 cm diameter). The three variables associated with poorer survival are: age ≥45 years, stage IV disease, and hemoglobin less than 10.5 gdL. These are described in the table below.

International Prognostic Score for Advanced Hodgkin Lymphoma

	Risk Factors	% of pts	Freedom From Progression (%)	Overall Survival (%)
Risk Factors:	0	43	84	95
Age ≥45 years	1	37	76	87
Stage IV	2	16	72	80
Hemoglobin <10.5 g/dL	3	4	68	61
Assign one point for each risk factor				

Data from Hayden, A. R., Lee, D. G., Villa, D., Gerrie, A. S., Scott, D. W., Slack, G. W., ... Savage, K. J. (2020). Validation of a simplified international prognostic score (IPS-3) in patients with advanced-stage classic Hodgkin lymphoma. *British Journal of Haematology, 189*(1), 122–127.
Note: Advanced stage is defined as Ann Arbor stage III or IV, or stage II with B symptoms and stage I or II with bulky disease (≥10 cm diameter).

Treatment

- Treatment is based on stage and prognostic factors.
- Doxorubicin-containing chemotherapy plays a major role in the treatment of all stages of the disease, and the mainstay of treatment is doxorubicin, bleomycin, vinblastine, and dacarbazine (ABVD) chemotherapy (Spinner et al., 2021). See the table on the next page.
- PET after two cycles of chemotherapy is used to guide treatment decisions. If the interim PET is negative, the intensity of chemotherapy can be de-escalated. If the interim PET is positive, the intensity of chemotherapy can be escalated or involved-site radiation may be recommended (Spinner et al., 2021).
- Early-stage favorable disease is treated with ABVD for two cycles with PET performed after two cycles. If PET is negative, an additional one to two cycles of ABVD is recommended (National Comprehensive Cancer Network [NCCN], 2022).
- Early-stage unfavorable disease is treated with ABVD for two cycles with PET performed after two cycles. If PET is negative, an additional four cycles of ABVD are recommended (NCCN, 2022).
- Advanced stage HL is treated with ABVD for two cycles with PET performed after two cycles. If PET is negative, bleomycin is omitted and an additional four cycles of AVD are recommended (NCCN, 2022).
- High-risk advanced-stage HL may be treated with BV-AVD, which substitutes brentuximab vedotin for bleomycin. Brentuximab vedotin is a monoclonal antibody-drug conjugate targeting CD30 (NCCN, 2022).

- Early-stage NLPHL is treated with involved-site radiation therapy. Advanced-stage disease may be treated with rituximab and involved-site radiation, rituximab monotherapy, or with combination regimens (NCCN, 2022).
- Salvage treatments:
- In late recurrences, the same regimen used for front-line therapy may be effective. Early recurrence should be treated with different agents (NCCN, 2022).
- Relapsed HL can be cured with autologous stem cell transplantation for approximately half of patients with chemo-sensitive disease (Spinner et al., 2021).
- Several novel biologic agents are highly effective for relapsed or refractory cHL (Spinner et al., 2021).
  - Brentuximab vedotin (an anti-CD30 antibody–drug conjugate).
  - PD-1-blocking antibodies: nivolumab and pembrolizumab.
- Radiation to sites not previously irradiated (NCCN, 2022).

ABVD Chemotherapy

Doxorubicin	25 mg/m^2	IV	Days 1 and 15
Bleomycin	10 units/m^2	IV	Days 1 and 15
Vinblastine	6 mg/m^2	IV	Days 1 and 15
Dacarbazine	375 mg/m^2	IV	Days 1 and 15

Cycles are every 28 days × 4 to 6 cycles.
Delivering full-dose chemo on schedule is associated with improved survival and chemotherapy can be administered irrespective of the neutrophil count on the day of treatment. The routine use of filgrastim is not recommended with ABVD because it increases risk of bleomycin pulmonary toxicity.

Data from National Comprehensive Cancer Network. (2022). *NCCN Clinical Practice Guidelines in Oncology (NCCN Guidelines): Hodgkin lymphoma (v. 2.2022)*. NCCN.org. Available at https://www.nccn.org/professionals/physician_gls/pdf/hodgkins.pdf.

Prognosis

- HL is considered a curable disease, with an overall 5-year survival rate of 89% (NCI, 2022).
- A complete response by PET imaging performed after two cycles of chemotherapy is one of the most powerful prognostic factors for long-term survival (Spinner et al., 2021).

Prevention and Surveillance

- Patients with HL need surveillance for treatment-related toxicities and disease relapse.
- The risk of relapse is highest within the first 2 years of diagnosis (Spinner et al., 2021).
- A history and physical examination are performed every 3 to 6 months for the first 2 years, every 6 to 12 months in the third year, and then annually thereafter (Spinner et al., 2021).
- Long-term effects of therapy for HL include second cancers, cardiopulmonary disease, infertility, hypothyroidism, and peripheral neuropathy (Spinner et al., 2021).

References

Alaggio, R., Amador, C., Anagnostopoulos, I., Attygalle, A. D., Araujo, I. B. O., Berti, E., … Xiao, W. (2022). The 5th edition of the World Health Organization classification of haematolymphoid tumours: lymphoid neoplasms. *Leukemia, 36*(7), 1720–1748.

Hayden, A. R., Lee, D. G., Villa, D., Gerrie, A. S., Scott, D. W., Slack, G. W., … Savage, K. J. (2020). Validation of a simplified international prognostic score (IPS-3) in patients with advanced-stage classic Hodgkin lymphoma. *British Journal of Haematology, 189*(1), 122–127.

Momotow, J., Borchmann, S., Eichenauer, D. A., Engert, A., & Sasse, S. (2021). Hodgkin lymphoma—review on pathogenesis, diagnosis, current and future treatment approaches for adult patients. *Journal of Clinical Medicine, 10*(5), 1125.

National Cancer Institute [NCI]. (2022). *SEER cancer stat facts: Hodgkin lymphoma*. https://seer.cancer.gov/statfacts/html/hodg.html.

National Comprehensive Cancer Network. (2022). *NCCN Clinical Practice Guidelines in Oncology (NCCN Guidelines): Hodgkin lymphoma (v. 2.2022)*. NCCN.org. Available at https://www.nccn.org/professionals/physician_gls/pdf/hodgkins.pdf.

Spinner, M. A., Mou, E., & Advani, R. H. (2021). Hodgkin lymphoma. In K. Kaushansky, J. T. Prchal, L. J. Burns, et al. (Eds.), *Williams hematology* (10th ed.). McGraw-Hill Education. Available at http://accessmedicine.mhmedical.com/content.aspx?aid=1178751112.

Non-Hodgkin Lymphoma

Definition

NHL is a diverse group of cancers of the immune system. NHL can be divided into aggressive and indolent types and can be classified as either B-cell or T-cell NHL. B-cell NHLs include Burkitt lymphoma, DLBCL, follicular lymphoma, and mantle cell lymphoma. T-cell NHLs include mycosis fungoides, anaplastic large cell lymphoma, and peripheral T-cell lymphoma. The NHL subtype predicts the necessity of early treatment, the response to treatment, the type of treatment required, and the prognosis. The most common indolent lymphoma is follicular lymphoma, and the most common aggressive lymphoma is DLBCL.

Due to the diversity of NHL, this section will discuss incidence, etiology, and risk factors for all of NHL and discuss select types of NHL individually—the most common indolent lymphoma, follicular lymphoma; the most common aggressive lymphoma, DLBCL; and a very aggressive lymphoma, Burkitt lymphoma.

Incidence

- Seventh most common cancer in adults in the United States (NCI, 2022c).
- 80,470 new cases in the United States are expected to be diagnosed in 2022, with 20,250 deaths from the disease (NCI, 2022c).
- The median age at diagnosis is 67 years of age (NCI, 2022c).
- Incidence increases with age with a few exceptions. For example, acute lymphoblastic lymphoma occurs most commonly in children, Burkitt lymphoma in the 20- to 64-year-old age group, and primary mediastinal B-cell lymphoma develops at a median age of 35 years (Linch, 2021).
- More common among men than women (NCI, 2022c).
- The incidence is higher for those of European descent or Hispanic origin (Linch, 2021).

Etiology and Risk Factors

- The etiology of NHL is unknown.
- Environmental risk factors (Linch, 2021)
  - Exposure to pesticides, herbicides, dyes, engine exhausts, and solvents has been associated with increased risk.
  - Occupations associated with increased risk include crop farming but not animal farming, women's hairdressers, cleaners, spray painters, carpenters, and textile workers.
- Cigarette smoking
- Increased body mass index
- Radiation exposure

- Risk factors related to viral or bacterial exposure include the following (Linch, 2021):
- EBV is associated with 60% of Burkitt's lymphoma. It is also associated with post-transplantation lymphoproliferative disorders, HIV-associated lymphomas (immunodeficiency-related Burkitt lymphoma, primary central nervous system (CNS) lymphoma, primary effusion lymphoma, the immunoblastic-plasmacytoid type of DLBCL, and oral cavity plasmablastic lymphoma), and extranodal NK/T-cell lymphoma, nasal type.
- Human T-cell leukemia/lymphoma virus-1 is associated with adult T-cell leukemia/lymphoma (ATLL)
- Human herpes virus-8 is associated with Kaposi sarcoma, Castleman disease, and primary effusion lymphoma and is found most often in immunodeficient individuals infected with HIV.
- Hepatitis B and C viruses
- MALT lymphoma of the stomach is associated with *Helicobacter pylori* infection.
- *Chlamydophila psittaci* is associated with extranodal MALT lymphomas of the eye.
- *Campylobacter jejuni* has been associated with extranodal MALT lymphomas of the small intestine.
- *Borrelia burgdorferi* is associated with B-cell lymphoma of the skin.
- Increased risk factors resulting from immunosuppressed conditions (Linch, 2021):
  - HIV infection
  - Organ or bone marrow transplant (requiring immune suppression medications)
  - Inherited immune deficiencies
- Increased risk factors from autoimmune conditions, presumably due to chronic immune stimulation (Linch, 2021):
  - Rheumatoid arthritis
  - Primary Sjögren syndrome
  - Systemic lupus erythematosus
  - Hashimoto thyroiditis
- Familial Predisposition (Linch, 2021)
  - The observed risk (OR) is 1.5 in first-degree relatives of patients with NHL
- Increasing age; rates are much higher among persons over the age of 65 years (Linch, 2021)

Indolent Non-Hodgkin Lymphoma
- Indolent lymphomas are generally considered incurable yet highly treatable.
- Many patients with indolent lymphomas survive for decades, yet a subset of patients may have a clinically aggressive course (Freedman & Jacobsen, 2020).
- Indolent lymphomas are characterized by a continuous relapsing pattern that requires multiple lines of therapy over time, and the duration of response (DOR) decreases with each line of therapy.
- Indolent lymphomas can transform into a more aggressive histology such as DLBCL (Freedman & Jacobsen, 2020).
- Often a chronic disease that requires balancing quality of life (QoL) with sequencing of the available treatment options.

- Early initiation of therapy does not improve outcomes, so asymptomatic patients with low tumor burden initially can be observed with active surveillance and no specific therapy (Batlevi et al., 2020).
- A biopsy is recommended at every relapse to determine if the disease remains indolent or has transformed (NCCN, 2022a).
- Transformation should be suspected if there is rapid progression of lymphadenopathy, high standardized uptake value on PET scan, extranodal disease (besides the marrow), B symptoms, hypercalcemia, or elevated serum LDH (NCCN, 2022a).

Follicular Lymphoma
Incidence
- Follicular lymphoma is the most common indolent B-cell lymphoma and represents approximately 20% to 25% of all NHLs (Ngu et al., 2022).
- The median age at diagnosis is 64 years old (NCI, 2022b).
- Advanced (stage III/IV) disease is present at diagnosis in ~90% of patients (Batlevi et al., 2020).

Histopathology
- Follicular lymphoma (FL) is classified into three grades based on the percent of large cells present.
  - In grades 1 and 2, the malignant cells are mostly small lymphocytes (NCCN, 2022a).
  - Grade 3 FL is characterized by large lymphocytes and is divided into grades 3A and 3B.
    - Grades 1-3A FL exhibit indolent behavior, while grade 3B FL is a unique subtype of FL that has a worse prognosis; its natural history is more akin to that of DLBCL. For this reason, grade 3B FL is treated as a DLBCL (NCCN, 2022a).

Treatment
- Early initiation of therapy does not improve outcomes, so asymptomatic patients with FL and low tumor burden initially can be observed with no specific therapy (Batlevi et al., 2020).
- Initial treatment is indicated when FL becomes symptomatic or bulky (NCCN, 2022a). Nearly 50% of patients will require therapy within 3 years of diagnosis, but ~20% may not need therapy for up to 10 years (Batlevi et al., 2020).
- The Modified Groupe d'Etude des Lymphomes Folliculaires (GELF) criteria are widely accepted for therapy initiation in patients with advanced-stage disease (NCCN, 2022a). See the box on next page.
- Immunochemotherapy is recommended for most patients (NCCN, 2022a).
  - Preferred regimens include bendamustine and obinutuzumab or rituximab; cyclophosphamide, doxorubicin, vincristine, and prednisone (CHOP) and obinutuzumab or rituximab; cyclophosphamide, vincristine, and prednisone (CVP) and obinutuzumab or rituximab; and lenalidomide and rituximab (NCCN, 2022a).
  - For patients who are not expected to tolerate chemotherapy, rituximab alone is preferred for initial therapy.

Groupe d'Etude des Lymphomes Folliculaires Criteria for Initiating Therapy in Advanced Stage Follicular Lymphoma

- Involvement of ≥3 nodal areas, each with a diameter of ≥3 cm
- Any nodal or extranodal mass with a diameter of ≥7 cm
- Disease-related symptoms, including B symptoms
- Lymphoma-related cytopenias (white blood cell count <1000 cells/mcL or platelets <100/mcL)
- Leukemia (>5000 cells/mcL)
- Splenomegaly
- Pleural effusions or ascites

Data from National Comprehensive Cancer Network. (2022a). *NCCN Clinical Practice Guidelines in Oncology (NCCN Guidelines): B-cell lymphomas (v. 4.2022).* NCCN.org. Available at https://www.nccn.org/professionals/physician_gls/pdf/b-cell.pdf.

Treatment for Patients With Relapsed/Refractory Follicular Lymphoma

- A biopsy is recommended at every relapse to determine if the disease remains indolent or has transformed (NCCN, 2022a).
- Transformation should be suspected if there is rapid progression of lymphadenopathy, high standardized uptake value on PET scan, extranodal disease (besides the marrow), B symptoms, hypercalcemia, or elevated serum LDH (NCCN, 2022a).
- If the first remission was greater than 2 years, an alternative chemoimmunotherapy may be used. If bendamustine-rituximab was used for first-line treatment, it is not recommended for second-line therapy due to the risk of opportunistic infections and secondary malignancies. If the disease burden is low, rituximab monotherapy also can be considered (NCCN, 2022a). Treatments are outlined in the box below.
- A first remission lasting less than 2 years is associated with shorter overall survival (OS). In these cases, consider non-immunochemotherapy treatments such as lenalidomide-based regimens, novel therapies, or high-dose chemotherapy with autologous stem cell rescue (NCCN, 2022a).

Prognosis

- While advanced-stage FL is considered incurable, the median OS is more than 20 years old (Batlevi et al., 2020).
- Follicular lymphoma is characterized by an excellent response to initial treatment, and patients often enjoy a 5- to 8-year remission before requiring additional treatment. Even after second-line therapy, the median OS is more than 10 years (Batlevi et al., 2020).
- FL is a heterogeneous disease, and while many patients survive for decades, a subset of patients may have a clinically aggressive course with short DOR after treatment and recurrence of disease within 1 to 2 years after initial treatment (Freedman & Jacobsen, 2020).
- Progression of disease within 2 years after starting initial treatment is associated with a poor prognosis (Freedman & Jacobsen, 2020).
- Indolent FL can transform into a more aggressive histology, and ~15% of such cases transform to DLBCL within 10 years (Freedman & Jacobsen, 2020).

Aggressive Non-Hodgkin Lymphoma

- Aggressive lymphomas are highly sensitive to chemotherapy. All patients should be assessed for risk TLS prior to start of therapy. Risk factors for TLS include elevated LDH and high tumor burden (NCCN, 2022a).
- Aggressive NHL has a shorter natural history than indolent lymphomas, but more than 50% of patients can be cured (NCCN, 2022a).
- Most relapses will occur in the first 2 years after therapy (NCCN, 2022a).

Diffuse Large B-Cell Lymphoma

Incidence

- The most common aggressive lymphoma is DLBCL (NCI, 2022a).
- The median age at diagnosis is 66 years old (NCI, 2022a).
- Approximately 30% of patients with DLBCL present with limited-stage disease (Ngu et al., 2022).

Summary of Treatment Options for Relapsed/Refractory Follicular Lymphoma

Second Line	Third Line
• Active surveillance until symptoms or bulky disease • Bendamustine + obinutuzumab or rituximab (not recommended if treated with prior bendamustine) • CHOP + obinutuzumab or rituximab • CVP + obinutuzumab or rituximab • Lenalidomide + rituximab • Ibritumomab tiuxetan • Lenalidomide (if not a candidate for anti-CD20 monoclonal antibody therapy) • Lenalidomide + obinutuzumab • Obinutuzumab • Rituximab • Tazemetostat (only if patient is not candidate for other alternatives) • Chlorambucil ± rituximab (for elderly or frail) • Cyclophosphamide ± rituximab (for elderly or frail)	• Any second-line option not previously used • Tazemetostat if EZH2 mutation present, or if patient is not candidate for other alternatives • CAR-T

Data from National Comprehensive Cancer Network. (2022a). *NCCN Clinical Practice Guidelines in Oncology (NCCN Guidelines): B-cell lymphomas (v. 4.2022).* NCCN.org. Available at https://www.nccn.org/professionals/physician_gls/pdf/b-cell.pdf.

CAR-T, Chimeric antigen receptor T cell therapy; *CHOP,* cyclophosphamide, doxorubicin, vincristine, and prednisone; *CVP,* cyclophosphamide, vincristine, and prednisone

Histopathology

- DLBCL is biologically heterogeneous with two distinct cells of origin: germinal center B-cell–like and activated B-cell–like. There are inferior outcomes with the activated B-cell–like (or non–germinal center B-cell–like) subtype with 3-year progression-free survival (PFS) of approximately 45% compared with 75% with the germinal center B-cell–like subtype (Ngu et al., 2022).
- Double-expressor lymphomas are lymphomas with over-expression of both MYC and BCL2 proteins (measured by immunohistochemistry) and occur in approximately 30% of cases of DLBCL (Ngu et al., 2022). Double-expressor lymphomas have an inferior prognosis, yet the prognosis is better than that of double-hit lymphomas (Ngu et al., 2022).
- All patients with DLBCL should have FISH testing for MYC, BCL2, and BCL6 as this has prognostic and treatment implications (NCCN, 2022a).
- Approximately 12% of patients with DLBCL have MYC rearrangements, yet this does not by itself affect outcome or warrant alternative treatment.
- Diffuse large B-cell lymphoma DLBCL with MYC and BCL2 gene rearrangements is a high-risk, aggressive subtype with the poorest prognosis. It is commonly referred to as double-hit lymphoma and is treated with more intensive chemotherapy regimens (Alaggio et al., 2022; Ngu et al., 2022).

Staging

- The International Prognostic Index (IPI) for DLBCL uses five significant risk factors to predict overall survival and help to guide treatment decisions for patients with DLBCL (Ruppert et al., 2020). See the box on this page.
  - Age (<60 years vs. >60 years)
  - Performance status (ECOG 0 or 1 vs. 2 to 4)
  - Serum LDH level (normal vs. elevated)
  - Stage (I or II vs. III or IV)
  - Extranodal site involvement (0 or 1 vs. 2 or more areas)

Treatment

- Rituximab plus cyclophosphamide, doxorubicin, vincristine, and prednisone (R-CHOP regimen) is standard front-line treatment that achieves cure in ~60% of patients (Ngu et al., 2022)
  - R-CHOP is administered for four cycles for patients with limited-stage disease and six cycles for advanced-stage disease (NCCN, 2022a).

International Prognostic Index for Diffuse Large B-Cell Lymphoma

Unfavorable prognostic risk factors (mnemonic "APLES")
- Age >60 years
- Performance status ECOG ≥2
- Elevated serum LDH
- Extranodal site ≥2
- Ann Arbor stage III or IV

Risk Groups	Incidence	5-Year PFS	5-Year OS
Low risk: 0–1 factors	34%	81%	88%
Low-intermediate risk: 2 factors	23%	67%	76%
High-intermediate risk: 3 factors	23%	58%	67%
High risk: 4–5 factors	20%	46%	54%

Data from Ruppert, A. S., Dixon, J. G., Salles, G., Wall, A., Cunningham, D., Poeschel, V., … Schmitz, N. (2020). International prognostic indices in diffuse large B-cell lymphoma: A comparison of IPI, R-IPI, and NCCN-IPI. *Blood, 135*(23), 2041–2048.

- DA-EPOCH-R is a dose-intensive regimen a treatment option for certain high-risk DLBCLs. It consists of infusional chemotherapy, and the doses of doxorubicin, etoposide, and cyclophosphamide may be increased or decreased with each cycle guided by the neutrophil and platelet nadir (Dunleavy et al., 2013).
  - An overview of these treatment regimens and adverse event management are listed in the tables on the next page.
- Polatuzumab vedotin is an antibody-drug conjugate (ADC) directed against CD79b. Polatuzumab vedotin, rituximab, cyclophosphamide, doxorubicin, and prednisone (R-Pola-CHP) improved progression-free survival compared with R-CHOP and is a first-line treatment option (Ngu et al., 2022).
- CNS prophylaxis is recommended for patients with paranasal sinus involvement, testicular involvement, epidural involvement, bone marrow with large cell lymphoma, HIV-positive lymphoma, kidney or adrenal gland involvement, stage IE DLBCL of the breast, concurrent *MYC* and *BCL2* gene expression, or 2+ extranodal sites and elevated LDH levels (NCCN, 2022a).

R-CHOP and DA-EPOCH-R

R-CHOP	Dose-Adjusted EPOCH-R			
• Rituximab 375 mg/m² IV day 1	Rituximab	375 mg/m²	IV	day 1
• Cyclophosphamide 750 mg/m² IV day 1	Doxorubicin	10 mg/m²/day	CIV over 24 h	days 1-4
• Doxorubicin 50 mg/m² IV, day 1	Etoposide	50 mg/m²	CIV over 24 h	days 1-4
• Vincristine 1.4 mg/m² (max 2 mg) IV, day 1	Vincristine	0.4 mg/m² (no cap)	CIV over 24 h	days 1-4
• Prednisone 40 mg/m² PO, days 1-5	Cyclophosphamide	750 mg/m²	IV over 30-60 min	day 5
• Cycles are every 21 days	Prednisone	60 mg/m²/day	PO	days 1-5

Cycles are every 21 days

Filgrastim 5 mcg/kg SQ daily starting 24 h after the completion of chemotherapy × 7 days or until neutrophil recovery or pegfilgrastim 6 mg SQ given once 24–72 h after the completion of chemotherapy

CBC w/ diff two times per week

Dose adjustment paradigm: apply to etoposide, doxorubicin, and cyclophosphamide. Drug doses based on the previous cycle ANC nadir; Measurements of ANC nadir are based on twice weekly CBC only.
- If ANC nadir ≥500 on all measurements: increase 20% above last cycle
- If ANC nadir <500 on 1 or 2 measurements: same dose(s) as last cycle
- If ANC nadir <500 on 3 measurements: decrease 20% below last cycle
- If platelet nadir <25,000: decrease dose 20% below last cycle

Data from Coiffier, B., Thieblemont, C., Van Den Neste, E., Lepeu, G., Plantier, I., Castaigne, S., ... Tilly, H. (2010). Long-term outcome of patients in the LNH-98.5 trial, the first randomized study comparing rituximab-CHOP to standard CHOP chemotherapy in DLBCL patients: A study by the Groupe d'Etudes des Lymphomes de l'Adulte. *Blood, 116*(12), 2040–2045; Dunleavy, K., Pittaluga, S., Maeda, L. S., Advani, R., Chen, C. C., Hessler, J., ... Wilson, W. H. (2013). Dose-adjusted EPOCH-rituximab therapy in Primary mediastinal B-Cell lymphoma. *New England Journal of Medicine, 368*(15), 1408–1416.

Adverse Effects With R-CHOP and DA-EPOCH-R

Adverse Event	Intervention
Myelosuppression	• Median time to recovery varies • Delay dosing until counts recover • Dose-reduction protocols with DA-EPOCH-R • Hematopoietic growth factor support required with DA-EPOCH-R and for patients >60 years old with RCHOP
Steroid-induced hyperglycemia	• Dietary modifications • Glucose monitoring • Insulin and oral agents
Peripheral neuropathy	• Pt education and early detection • Vincristine dose reduction
Constipation	• Senna 2 tablets PO daily—BID as necessary for constipation
Nausea and vomiting	• Highly emetogenic • Requires routine, scheduled antiemetics every day of chemotherapy and for at least 2 days after the last day of chemotherapy
Stomatitis, mucositis	• Daily oral care; keep mouth moist; lip balm • Adequate hydration • Bland oral rinses (saline or sodium bicarbonate)
Infection	• PJP prophylaxis with DA-EPOCH-R regimen • Antiviral prophylaxis if VZV or HSV seropositive

Data from Brown, T. J., & Gupta, A. (2020). Management of cancer therapy–associated oral mucositis. *JCO Oncology Practice, 16*(3), 103–109; Dunleavy, K., Pittaluga, S., Maeda, L. S., Advani, R., Chen, C. C., Hessler, J., ... Wilson, W. H. (2013). Dose-adjusted EPOCH-rituximab therapy in Primary mediastinal B-Cell lymphoma. *New England Journal of Medicine, 368*(15), 1408–1416; Larkin, P. J., Cherny, N. I., La Carpia, D., Guglielmo, M., Ostgathe, C., Scotté, F., ... ESMO Guidelines Committee. (2018). Diagnosis, assessment and management of constipation in advanced cancer: ESMO Clinical Practice Guidelines. *Annals of Oncology, 29*(Suppl. 4), iv111-iv125; Loprinzi, C. L., Lacchetti, C., Bleeker, J., Cavaletti, G., Chauhan, C., Hertz, D. L., ... Hershman, D. L. (2020). Prevention and management of chemotherapy-induced peripheral neuropathy in survivors of adult cancers: ASCO Guideline Update. *Journal of Clinical Oncology, 38*(28), 3325–3348; National Comprehensive Cancer Network. (2022a). *NCCN Clinical Practice Guidelines in Oncology (NCCN Guidelines®): B-cell lymphomas (v. 4.2022).* NCCN.org. Available at https://www.nccn.org/professionals/physician_gls/pdf/b-cell.pdf ; National Comprehensive Cancer Network. (2022b). *NCCN Clinical Practice Guidelines in Oncology (NCCN Guidelines®): Prevention and treatment of cancer-related infections (v. 1.2022).* NCCN.org. Available at https://www.nccn.org/professionals/physician_gls/pdf/infections.pdf.
DA-EPOCH-R, Dose adjusted etoposide, prednisone, vincristine, cyclophosphamide, doxorubicin plus rituximab; *HSV,* herpes simplex virus; *PJP,* pneumocystis jiroveci pneumonia; *R-CHOP,* rituximab, cyclophosphamide, doxorubicin, vincristine, and prednisone; *VZV,* varicella zoster virus.

Treatment for Patients With Relapsed/Refractory Diffuse Large B-Cell Lymphoma

- At least 30% of patients with DLBCL will have refractory disease or experience relapse after standard frontline treatment, most commonly within 24 months of completion (Ngu et al., 2022).
- Patients with relapsed disease may be treated with high-dose chemotherapy and autologous stem cell rescue, CAR-T therapy, or novel agents (NCCN, 2022a).
- Relapsed disease in fit patients is treated with salvage combination chemotherapy with the goal of obtaining disease control (NCCN, 2022a).
- Consolidation with high dose chemotherapy and autologous stem cell transplantation can be curative in patients with chemosensitive disease (NCCN, 2022a). More information on stem cell transplantation can be found in "Hematopoietic Stem Cell Transplantation and Chimeric Antigen Receptor T-Cell Therapy" chapter.

- CAR-T therapy is also an option for relapsed disease and is associated with 50% complete response rate (NCCN, 2022a). Refer to "Hematopoietic Stem Cell Transplantation and Chimeric Antigen Receptor T-Cell Therapy" chapter for additional information on T-cell therapies including CAR-T cell therapy.
- Novel therapies for relapsed DLBCL include tafasitamab and lenalidomide, selinexor, and loncastuximab tesirine (NCCN, 2022a).

Prognosis

- The overall survival rate at 5 years is 74% (NCI, 2022a)
- However, subsets of patients have less favorable diseases. Factors that predict a poor prognosis with a median overall survival of 6 months include (Crump et al., 2017):
  - Primary refractory disease is defined as progressive or stable disease after at least four cycles of first-line therapy.
  - Refractory disease after two cycles of second-line or later therapy.
  - Relapse less than 12 months from autologous stem cell transplantation.

Burkitt Lymphoma

Burkitt lymphoma (BL) is a highly aggressive, B-cell, NHL with rapidly progressive tumors and high rates of central nervous system involvement. Approximately 20% of patients have CNS involvement at diagnosis (Crombie & LaCasce, 2021).

Incidence

- This is a rare lymphoma in adults, comprising ~1% of cases; it is more common in children, where it represents 20% to 30% of lymphomas (Crombie & LaCasce, 2021).

Histopathology

- The defining chromosomal translocation is t(8;14), which involves the *MYC* gene and the immunoglobulin heavy chain *(IGH)* (Crombie & LaCasce, 2021).

Diagnostic Workup

- Immunodeficiency, such as HIV, is a risk factor for BL and ~20% of BL are in the setting of immunodeficiency. All patients diagnosed with BL should be tested for HIV (Crombie & LaCasce, 2021).
- All patients need a lumbar puncture to assess for CNS involvement, which is typically leptomeningeal rather than parenchymal. If CNS disease is present, it is treated with CNS-directed therapy. If CNS disease is not present at diagnosis, CNS-directed therapy is recommended for prophylaxis because 30% to 50% will develop CNS disease without CNS-directed therapy (Crombie & LaCasce, 2021).
- Since BL grows so rapidly, spontaneous tumor lysis can occur. Tumor lysis labs (creatinine, potassium, phosphorus, uric acid, calcium, and LDH) should be obtained at diagnosis prior to the start of treatment. Tumor lysis precautions and continued monitoring are essential during the first cycle of chemotherapy (Crombie & LaCasce, 2021).

Treatment

- Treatment for Burkitt lymphoma consists of intensive chemotherapy with CNS prophylaxis.
- Two recommended regimens are DA-EPOCH-R and Modified Magrath as shown in the figure below.
- The number of cycles is guided by assessment of low-risk versus high-risk disease features as shown in the figure below.
- The table on next page provides an overview of adverse events of anti-CD20 antibodies including rituximab, obinutuzumab, and ofatumumab.

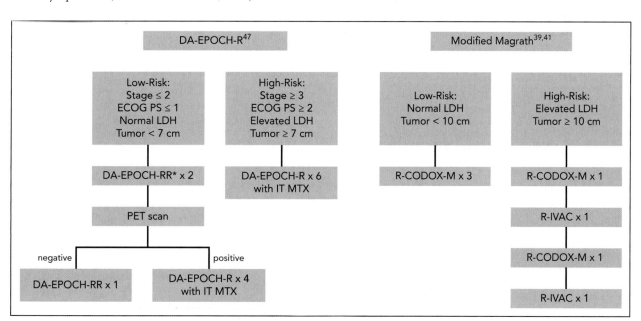

Recommended Treatment Regimens for Burkitt Lymphoma. *RR implies that patients were treated with rituximab on days 1 and 5. *CODOX-M*, cyclophosphamide, vincristine, doxorubicin, vincristine with intrathecal methotrexate and cytarabine followed by high-dose methotrexate plus rituximab; *DA-EPOCH-R*, dose-adjusted etoposide, prednisone, vincristine, cyclophosphamide, doxorubicin, and rituximab; *IT MTX*, intrathecal methotrexate; *PET*, positron emission tomography *R-IVAC*, rituximab, ifosfamide, cytarabine, etoposide, and intrathecal methotrexate. (From Crombie, J., & LaCasce, A. (2021). The treatment of Burkitt lymphoma in adults. *Blood, 137*(6), 743–750.)

Anti-CD20 Antibodies Adverse Events: Rituximab, Obinutuzumab, Ofatumumab

Infusion reaction (fever, chills, hypotension, and asthenia)	• Prophylaxis: antihistamine and acetaminophen (glucocorticoid with obinutuzumab and ofatumumab) before; withhold antihypertensives 12 h before infusion • Symptomatic treatment for infusion reactions
Hepatitis B virus (HBV) reactivation	• HBcAg and HBsAg prior to therapy • HBV antiviral therapy if HbsAg-positive and strongly consider if HBcAb-positive
Herpes simplex virus (HSV)/varicella zoster virus (VZV) reactivation	• Prophylaxis for seropositive patients with acyclovir 400 mg PO BID or valacyclovir 500 mg PO daily
Tumor lysis syndrome (high tumor burden, high circulating lymphocyte counts)	• Assess risk prior to treatment • Hydration and prophylaxis for hyperuricemia based on risk • Correct electrolyte abnormalities, monitor renal function, fluid balance
Progressive multifocal leukoencephalopathy (PML)	• Monitor for new onset or changes in preexisting neurologic symptoms • If suspected, discontinue treatment and consult a neurologist, perform brain MRI and lumbar puncture
Late-onset neutropenia	• Typically delayed in onset, occurring weeks to months after last dose • Occurs in up to 10% of patients • Can be severe, but usually not presenting with infections • May recover spontaneously or a short course of G-CSF can be used
Severe mucocutaneous reaction	• Onset 1–13 weeks following exposure • If suspected, discontinue anti-CD20 antibody

Data from National Comprehensive Cancer Network. (2022). *NCCN Clinical Practice Guidelines in Oncology (NCCN Guidelines®): B-cell lymphomas (v. 4.2022)*. NCCN.org. Available at https://www.nccn.org/professionals/physician_gls/pdf/b-cell.pdf; National Comprehensive Cancer Network. (2022). *NCCN Clinical Practice Guidelines in Oncology (NCCN Guidelines®): Prevention and Treatment of Cancer-related Infections (v. 1.2022)*. NCCN.org. Available at https://www.nccn.org/professionals/physician_gls/pdf/infections.pdf; Shimony, S., Bar-Sever, E., Berger, T., Itchaki, G., Gurion, R., Yeshurun, M., ... Wolach, O. (2021). Late onset neutropenia after rituximab and obinutuzumab treatment—characteristics of a class-effect toxicity. *Leukemia & Lymphoma, 62*(12), 2921–2927.

References

Alaggio, R., Amador, C., Anagnostopoulos, I., Attygalle, A. D., Araujo, I. B. O., Berti, E., ... Xiao, W. (2022). The 5th edition of the World Health Organization classification of haematolymphoid tumours: Lymphoid neoplasms. *Leukemia, 36*(7), 1720–1748.

Batlevi, C. L., Sha, F., Alperovich, A., Ni, A., Smith, K., Ying, Z., ... Younes, A. (2020). Follicular lymphoma in the modern era: Survival, treatment outcomes, and identification of high-risk subgroups. *Blood Cancer Journal, 10*(7), 74.

Crombie, J., & LaCasce, A. (2021). The treatment of Burkitt lymphoma in adults. *Blood, 137*(6), 743–750.

Crump, M., Neelapu, S. S., Farooq, U., Van Den Neste, E., Kuruvilla, J., Westin, J., ... Gisselbrecht, C. (2017). Outcomes in refractory diffuse large B-cell lymphoma: Results from the international SCHOLAR-1 study. *Blood, 130*(16), 1800–1808.

Dunleavy, K., Pittaluga, S., Maeda, L. S., Advani, R., Chen, C. C., Hessler, J., ... Wilson, W. H. (2013). Dose-adjusted EPOCH-rituximab therapy in Primary mediastinal B-cell lymphoma. *New England Journal of Medicine, 368*(15), 1408–1416.

Freedman, A., & Jacobsen, E. (2020). Follicular lymphoma: 2020 update on diagnosis and management. *American Journal of Hematology, 95*(3), 316–327.

Linch, D. C. (2021). General considerations of lymphomas: Incidence rates, etiology, diagnosis, staging, and primary extranodal disease. In K. Kaushansky, J. T. Prchal, L. J. Burns, et al. (Eds.), *Williams hematology* (10th ed.). McGraw-Hill Education. Available at http://accessmedicine.mhmedical.com/content.aspx?aid=1178750836.

National Cancer Institute. (2022a). *SEER cancer stat facts: Diffuse Large B-Cell Lymphoma (DLBCL)*. Available at https://seer.cancer.gov/statfacts/html/hodg.html.

National Cancer Institute. (2022b). *SEER cancer stat facts: Follicular lymphoma*. Available at https://seer.cancer.gov/statfacts/html/follicular.html.

National Cancer Institute. (2022c). *SEER cancer stat facts: Non-Hodgkin lymphoma*. Available at https://seer.cancer.gov/statfacts/html/nhl.html.

National Comprehensive Cancer Network. (2022a). *NCCN Clinical Practice Guidelines in Oncology (NCCN Guidelines®): B-cell lymphomas (v. 4.2022)*. NCCN.org. Available at https://www.nccn.org/professionals/physician_gls/pdf/b-cell.pdf.

National Comprehensive Cancer Network. (2022b). *NCCN Clinical Practice Guidelines in Oncology (NCCN Guidelines®): Prevention and treatment of cancer-related infections (v. 1.2022)*, NCCN.org. Available at https://www.nccn.org/professionals/physician_gls/pdf/infections.pdf.

Ngu, H., Takiar, R., Phillips, T., Okosun, J., & Sehn, L. H. (2022). Revising the treatment pathways in lymphoma: New standards of care—How do we choose? *American Society of Clinical Oncology Educational Book, 42*, 629–642.

Ruppert, A. S., Dixon, J. G., Salles, G., Wall, A., Cunningham, D., Poeschel, V., ... Schmitz, N. (2020). International prognostic indices in diffuse large B-cell lymphoma: A comparison of IPI, R-IPI, and NCCN-IPI. *Blood, 135*(23), 2041–2048.

Multiple Myeloma

Laura J. Zitella

Definition

Multiple myeloma (MM) is a plasma cell neoplasm characterized by excess paraprotein secretion with secondary organ effects including renal, bone, bone marrow, neurologic, and immune dysfunction. MM is highly treatable, yet incurable and inevitably relapses. Novel treatments have improved survival, and the number of people living with myeloma continues to increase.

- Myeloma cells continually produce abnormal immunoglobulin. There are at least three primary types of MM based on predominant component of abnormal protein (O'Donnell et al., 2021):
  - Heavy chain: IgG (most common—60%), IgA (20%), and IgD (rare); IgM is most often associated with Waldenstrom macroglobulinemia.
  - Light chain: can be represented by kappa or lambda light chain; represents ~20% of MM cases.
  - Nonsecretory: although the presence of an M protein is the hallmark of myeloma, 1% to 2% of patients have nonsecretory myeloma with no M protein detectable on serum or urine electrophoresis.

Incidence

- MM accounts for 1.8% of all cancers and 18.7% of hematologic malignancies; it is the second most prevalent hematologic cancer after non-Hodgkin lymphoma (Siegel et al., 2021).
- In 2022, 34,470 new cases of MM and 12,640 deaths from MM are projected (National Cancer Institute [NCI], 2022).

Etiology and Risk Factors

Risk factors for MM include advanced age, male gender, obesity, African American descent, family history, the presence of monoclonal gammopathy of undetermined significance (MGUS), and exposure to chemicals or radiation (O'Donnell et al., 2021).

- Age: Median age at diagnosis: 69 years.
  - 64% of patients are over the age of 65 (NCI, 2022).
  - 33.5% of patients are over the age of 75 (NCI, 2022).
- Ethnicity: The incidence of MM is highest in persons of African American descent (NCI, 2022):
  - In 2019, the incidence in African American males was more than double than that of White males estimated at 17/100,000, compared to 8.1/100,000.
  - African American females are more likely to develop MM compared to White females (12.9/100,00 vs. 5/100,000).
  - The cause of the increased incidence in the African American population has not been determined and emphasizes the need for continued investigation into genetic predisposition.

- Family history: Two- to fourfold increased risk if sibling or parent has disease (Clay-Gilmour et al., 2020)
- Obesity (Chang et al., 2016; Lauby-Secretan et al., 2016)
- MGUS: A unique feature of the MM disease continuum is that it is consistently preceded by a premalignant phase, termed MGUS.
  - The incidence of MGUS is 3% of the general population age greater than 50 years of age and 5% of the general population age greater than 70 years (Kyle et al., 2018).
  - The risk of progression from MGUS to a plasma cell or lymphoid cancer is 1% per year (Kyle et al., 2018).
- Exposure to chemicals, including pesticides, arsenic, cadmium, lead, and various cleaning solutions also has been linked to an increased risk of MM (Perrotta et al., 2013).
  - Vietnam veterans who conducted aerial herbicide spray missions of Agent Orange had a rate of 7/1% of MGUS compared with 3.1% of Vietnam veterans who had similar duties in Southeast Asia but were not involved with Agent Orange missions (Landgren et al., 2015).
  - A sample of White male firefighters involved with rescue and/or recovery work at the World Trade Center disaster site in 2001 had a MGUS prevalence rate of 7.63 per 100 persons, which is 1.8-fold higher than a reference population of White males (Landgren et al., 2018).
- Radiation exposure victims (e.g., survivors of atomic bomb explosions in Japan) have an increased risk, although this number is small.

Signs and Symptoms

- Most common symptoms at presentation are bone pain and fatigue (O'Donnell et al., 2021)
- Signs and symptoms result from an overproduction of monoclonal plasma cells and monoclonal immunoglobulins (O'Donnell et al., 2021)
  - Plasma cell invasion of the bone and increased osteoclast activity: bone pain, fractures, hypercalcemia, cord compression
  - Bone marrow involvement: fatigue, anemia, neutropenia, thrombocytopenia
  - Renal injury: fatigue, anemia, hematuria, frothy urine, elevated creatinine, hypercalcemia, urate nephropathy, acute renal failure
  - Abnormal immunoglobulin function: fever, infections, hypogammaglobulinemia (unaffected paraprotein), neurologic symptoms
  - Hyperviscosity: pain, paresthesia, immobility, peripheral neuropathy, stroke

Diagnostic Work-up

The diagnostic workup for MM requires laboratory, radiologic, and hematopathologic evaluation (National Comprehensive Cancer Network [NCCN], 2022).

- History and physical
- Labs:
  - Complete blood count (CBC) with differential
  - Serum blood urea nitrogen (BUN)/creatinine, electrolytes, albumin, calcium, serum uric acid, serum lactate dehydrogenase (LDH), and beta2-microglobulin
  - Creatinine clearance (calculated or measured directly)
  - Serum quantitative immunoglobulins (IgG, IgM, IgA), serum protein electrophoresis (SPEP), serum immunofixation electrophoresis (SIFE)
  - 24-hour urine for total protein, urine protein electrophoresis (UPEP), and urine immunofixation electrophoresis (UIFE)
  - Serum free light chain (FLC) assay (kappa, lambda)
- Bone marrow biopsy and aspiration including immunohistochemistry (IHC) and/or multi-parameter flow cytometry and plasma cell fluorescence in situ hybridization (FISH) panel on bone marrow [del 13, del17p13, t(4;14), t(11;14), t(14;16), t(14;20), 1q21amplification, 1p deletion]
- Imaging: All patients should have whole-body low-dose computed tomography (WBLDCT) scan to assess for bone lesions. If WBCLCT is not available, PET/CT is an acceptable alternative. Skeletal survey is no longer recommended due to low sensitivity (Hillengass et al., 2019).

Spectrum of Monoclonal Gammopathies

Monoclonal gammopathies are classified by increasing levels of monoclonal protein (M protein) and the presence of end-organ damage (Rajkumar et al., 2014). The International Myeloma Working Group updated guidelines for the diagnosis of MM in 2014 (see the table below).

- MGUS: benign, premalignant condition characterized by the presence of a M protein and no symptoms or end-organ damage.
- Smoldering multiple myeloma (SMM)
  - Increased M protein and more plasma cells are found in the bone marrow compared to MGUS. This is a stage of the disease where there is no evidence of symptoms or related organ disease. Patients with smoldering myeloma may have an indolent course for many years without therapy.
- Active (symptomatic) MM
  - Clonal bone marrow plasma cells (BMPCs) ≥10% or biopsy-proven plasmacytoma PLUS either a myeloma-defining event (MDE) or a biomarker of early progression.

Diagnostic Criteria for Monoclonal Gammopathy of Undetermined Significance, Smoldering Multiple Myeloma, and Active (or Symptomatic) Multiple Myeloma

Condition	MGUS	SMM	Active Myeloma
Clonal bone marrow plasma cells (BMPCs)	<10%	10%–60%	≥10% or biopsy-proven bony or extramedullary plasmacytoma *AND* one or more MDEs
Presence of myeloma-defining events (MDEs)	None	None	Yes
Monoclonal protein (M-protein)	<3 g/dL	≥3 g/dL serum protein (IgG or IgA) or ≥500 mg/24 h urinary protein	No specific level required. Active disease is defined by MDE

MYELOMA-DEFINING EVENTS

SLiM-CRAB Criteria

Malignancy Biomarker (SLiM Criteria)
S	Clonal bone marrow plasma cells ≥60%
Li	Uninvolved/involved serum FLC ratio ≥100 and involved FLC concentration ≥10 mg/dL
M	One or more focal lesions on MRI studies ≥5 mm

End-Organ Damage (CRAB Criteria)
C	Calcium elevation: Serum calcium >1 mg/dL higher than ULN or >11 mg/dL
R	Renal dysfunction: CrCl <40 mL/min or serum Cr >2 mg/dL
A	Anemia: Hemoglobin <10 g/dL or hemoglobin >2 g/dL below the LLN
B	Bone disease: One or more osteolytic lesions on skeletal radiography, CT, or PET/CT

BMPC, Bone marrow plasma cell; *CrCl,* creatinine clearance; *CT,* computed tomography; *FLC,* free light chain; *LLN,* lower limit of normal; *MDE,* myeloma-defining event; *MGUS,* myeloma of undetermined significance; *MRI,* magnetic resonance imaging; *PET/CT,* positron emission tomography/computed tomography; *SMM,* smoldering multiple myeloma; *ULN,* upper limit of normal.
Data from Rajkumar, S. V., Dimopoulos, M. A., Palumbo, A., Blade, J., Merlini, G., Mateos, M. V., ... Miguel, J. F. (2014). International Myeloma Working Group updated criteria for the diagnosis of multiple myeloma. *The Lancet Oncology, 15*(12), e538–e548.

Clinical Staging and Risk Classification

- The International Staging System (ISS) provides a measure of proliferative tumor and prognostic information based on multivariate analysis of clinical features. Using β2M and serum albumin, patients are categorized as stage I (median survival 62 months), stage II (median survival 44 months), or stage III (median survival 29 months) (Greipp et al., 2005). Refer to the Clinical Staging for Multiple Myeloma table below.
- The Revised International Staging System (R-ISS) incorporates lactate dehydrogenase (LDH) and chromosomal abnormalities based on bone marrow FISH studies (Palumbo et al., 2015a).

- High-risk cytogenetics: FISH: t(4;14), t(14;16), and del(17p)
- Standard risk: No high-risk chromosomal abnormality
- In addition to the high-risk cytogenetics used in the R-ISS staging system, there are additional high-risk features that are used to inform treatment decisions in clinical practice. The most common risk classification was developed at the Mayo Clinic and is called the mSMART 3.0 Classification of Active MM (see the mSMART 3.0: Risk Classification of Active Multiple Myleoma table below).

Clinical Staging for Multiple Myeloma

Stage	International Staging System (ISS)	Median Overall Survival	Revised-ISS (R-ISS)	Median Overall Survival
I	Serum beta2-microglobulin <3.5 mg/dL Serum albumin >3.5 g/dL	62 months	ISS stage I and standard-risk chromosomal abnormalities by FISH AND Serum LDH ≤ULN	NR
II	Not ISS stage I or III	44 months	Not R-ISS stage I or III	83 months
III	Serum beta2-microglobulin ≥5.5 mg/L	29 months	ISS stage III and either high-risk chromosomal abnormalities by FISH [del(17p), t94;14), and/or t(14;16)] OR Serum LDH >ULN	43 months

LDH, Lactate dehydrogenase; NR, not reached; ULN, upper limit of normal.
Data from Greipp, P. R., San Miguel, J., Durie, B. G., Crowley, J. J., Barlogie, B., Bladé, J., … Westin, J. (2005). International staging system for multiple myeloma. *Journal of Clinical Oncology, 23*(15), 3412–3420; Palumbo, A., Avet-Loiseau, H., Oliva, S., Lokhorst, H. M., Goldschmidt, H., Rosinol, L., … Moreau, P. (2015a). Revised international staging system for multiple myeloma: A report from International Myeloma Working Group. *Journal of Clinical Oncology, 33*(26), 2863–2869.

mSMART 3.0: Risk Classification of Active Multiple Myeloma

High-Risk	Standard-Risk
t(4;14) t(14;16) t(14;20) Del 17p p53 mutation Gain 1q R-ISS Stage 3 High plasma cell S-phase GEP: High-risk signature **Double Hit Myeloma:** Any two high-risk genetic abnormalities **Triple Hit Myeloma:** Three or more high-risk genetic abnormalities	All others including: Trisomies t(11;14) t(6;14)

GEP, Gene expression profile; R-ISS, Revised International Staging System.
From Dispenzieri, A., Rajkumar, S. V., Gertz, M. A., Fonseca, R., Lacy, M. Q., Bergsagel, P. L., … Stewart, A. K. (2007). Treatment of newly diagnosed multiple myeloma based on Mayo Stratification of Myeloma and Risk-adapted Therapy (mSMART): Consensus statement. *Mayo Clinic Proceedings, 82*(3), 323–341; Kumar, S. K., Mikhael, J. R., Buadi, F. K., Dingli, D., Dispenzieri, A., Fonseca, R., … Bergsagel, P. L. (2009). Management of newly diagnosed symptomatic multiple myeloma: Updated Mayo Stratification of Myeloma and Risk-Adapted Therapy (mSMART) consensus guidelines. *Mayo Clinic Proceedings, 84*(12), 1095–1110; Mikhael, J. R., Dingli, D., Roy, V., Reeder, C. B., Buadi, F. K., Hayman, S. R., … Mayo Clinic. (2013). Management of newly diagnosed symptomatic multiple myeloma: Updated Mayo Stratification of Myeloma and Risk-Adapted Therapy (mSMART) consensus guidelines 2013. *Mayo Clinic Proceedings, 88*(4), 360-376. Available at https://static1.squarespace.com/static/5b44f08ac258b493a25098a3/t/6244859445f2cf719cca6b93/1648657812271/RiskStrat+3.0_Mar2022_FINAI_REV.pdf.

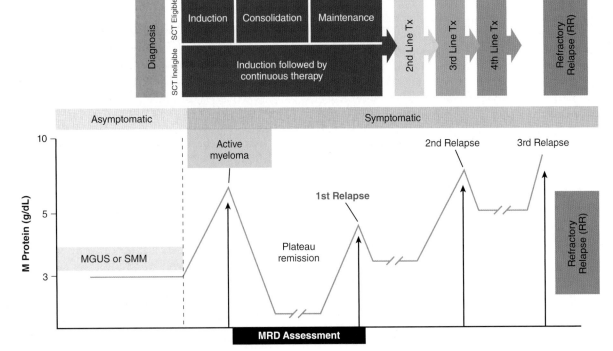

Natural History and Treatment Paradigm for Multiple Myeloma. (Data from Borrello, I. (2012). Can we change the disease biology of multiple myeloma? *Leukemia Research, 36*, S3–S12; Callander, N. S., Baljevic, M., Adekola, K., Anderson, L. D., Campagnaro, E., Castillo, J. J., … Kumar, S. K. (2022). NCCN Guidelines® insights: Multiple myeloma, version 3.2022: Featured updates to the NCCN Guidelines. *Journal of the National Comprehensive Cancer Network, 20*(1), 8–19.)

Treatment

- Treatment of MM is based on risk stratification (standard- vs. high-risk cytogenetics) and transplant eligibility.
- Patients are treated with a primary therapy, followed by prolonged maintenance therapy (see the figure above).
- Myeloma is a chronic disease with a succession of remissions and relapses that require treatment (see the figure above).
- Goals of therapy include disease control, improved quality of life, and prolonged survival
- Risk-adapted therapy selection is based on patient and disease characteristics.
  - Determine eligibility for autologous hematopoietic cell transplant (HCT)
  - Age
  - Comorbidities (e.g., diabetes, neuropathy, heart disease)
  - Fit versus Frail
    - The International Myeloma Working Group developed a scoring system to predict mortality and risk of toxicity in elderly myeloma patients. This frailty score is called the Myeloma Frailty Score Calculator and can be found at http://www.myelomafrailtyscorecalculator.net/ (Palumbo et al., 2015b)
  - Personal choice
  - Social support
  - Disease characteristics: renal failure, neurologic complications, extramedullary disease
  - Risk stratification based on R-ISS staging system and others
- General principles of choosing therapy:
  - Triplet regimens using two drug classes (usually proteasome inhibitor (PI) and an immunomodulatory drug [IMiD]) and steroids are preferred over two-drug regimens unless a patient is frail. If a two-drug regimen is used, a third drug can be added if the performance status improves. The benefit of adding a fourth drug for the primary treatment of transplant-eligible patients has been reported in clinical trials. Combination therapies have demonstrated improved response rates, PFS, and/or OS compared to single agents (Callander et al., 2022)
  - Consider frailty/fitness, age and comorbidities when selecting drug/doses
  - Logistics of drug administration (Route: IV, subcutaneous, oral as well as frequency)
- Primary myeloma therapy for transplant-eligible: Induction therapy × 4 cycles, then autologous transplant followed by maintenance therapy (see the figure on next page)
- Primary myeloma therapy for transplant ineligible: Induction therapy × 8 to 12 cycles followed by maintenance therapy (see the figure on next page)
- Early and sustained complete response (CR) after primary myeloma therapy leads to better overall survival (NCCN, 2022).
- Minimal residual disease (MRD) negativity by next-generation flow cytometry or next-generation sequencing with a minimum sensitivity of 1 in 10^5 nucleated cells or higher is associated with improved survival (NCCN, 2022).
- Major classes of drugs used to treat myeloma:
  - IMiDs: lenalidomide, pomalidomide, thalidomide
  - PIs: bortezomib, carfilzomib, ixazomib
  - Anti-CD38 monoclonal antibodies: daratumumab, isatuximab

Note: Clinical trial participation should be encouraged.

Transplant-Eligible		Transplant-Ineligible	
Standard Risk	**High Risk**	**Standard Risk**	**High Risk**
VRd × 4 cycles	Dara-VRd or KRd × 4 cycles	VRd × 12 cycles followed by lenalidomide maintenance OR DRd × 12 cycles followed by Dara-lenalidomide maintenance	VRd × 12 cycles
ASCT	ASCT		Bortezomib-lenalidomide maintenance
Lenalidomide maintenance	Bortezomib-lenalidomide maintenance		

Treatment Approach to Newly Diagnosed Multiple Myeloma. *ASCT,* Autologous stem cell transplant; *Dara-VRD,* daratumumab, bortezomib, lenalidomide, dexamethasone; *DRD,* daratumumab, lenalidomide, dexamethasone; *KRd,* carfilzomib, lenalidomide, dexamethasone; *VRd,* bortezomib, lenalidomide, dexamethasone. (Data from National Comprehensive Cancer Network. (2022). NCCN Clinical Practice Guidelines in Oncology (NCCN Guidelines®): Multiple myeloma (v.3.2022). Available at http://www.nccn.org/professionals/physician_gls/pdf/myeloma.pdf.)

Supportive Care

- MM is associated with one of the highest symptom burden and poorest quality of life of all cancers. In addition, many patients require continuous treatment that results in side effects that further compromise their quality of life (LeBlanc et al., 2022).
- All patients with MM should receive supportive care.
- Common toxicities reported with agents used to treat MM are outlined in the Immunomodulatory Agents (IMiDs) table on page 162, the Proteasome Inhibitors (PIs) table on page 162 and the Anti-CD38 Monoclonal Antibodies table on page 163.
- Treatment of bone disease
  - All newly diagnosed patients with bone disease or osteopenia should be treated with bisphosphonates (zoledronic acid or pamidronate) or denosumab monthly for up to 2 years (Anderson et al., 2018). The NCCN guidelines recommend a bone-modifying agent for all patients with myeloma regardless of documented bone disease given monthly or every 3 months for up to 2 years. Subsequently, bisphosphonates or denosumab should be resumed when there is a new-onset skeletal event (Anderson et al., 2018).
  - Dental exam and any needed dental work should be done prior to initiation of bisphosphonates or denosumab. Invasive dental procedures should be avoided while on bisphosphonates to minimize risk of osteonecrosis of the jaw (Anderson et al., 2018).
  - Monitor renal function and calcium.
  - Kyphoplasty or vertebroplasty may be beneficial for patients with vertebral compression fractures
  - Low-dose radiation may be used for treatment of uncontrolled bone pain, impending pathologic fracture, or impending spinal cord compression
- Treatment of hypercalcemia
  - Hydration, furosemide, bisphosphonates, steroids, or calcitonin may be used to treat symptomatic hypercalcemia
- Treatment of hyperviscosity

- Plasmapheresis may be helpful in treating symptomatic hyperviscosity. Concurrent anti-myeloma therapy is recommended.
- Treatment of anemia
  - Anti-myeloma treatment
  - Transfusion of packed red blood cells if indicated
  - Erythropoietin-stimulating agents may be used based on current safety guidelines
- Treatment of infections
  - Pneumococcal infections are common in patients with MM. Pneumococcal conjugate vaccination (PCV) should be given at the time of diagnosis, followed by the pneumococcal polysaccharide vaccine (PPSV) 1 year later.
  - Shingles (herpes zoster) reactivation is common in patients with MM. Shingles prophylaxis is recommended for all patients (even if they have received a shingles vaccine) receiving a proteosome PI, daratumumab, isatuximab, or elotuzumab (Callander et al., 2022)
  - *Pneumocystis jirovecii* pneumonia (PJP) prophylaxis, herpes zoster prophylaxis, and antifungal prophylaxis are recommended for patients receiving high-dose dexamethasone (Callander et al., 2022)
  - Live vaccines are not recommended
  - Reactivation of hepatitis B can occur in patients treated with carfilzomib or daratumumab so hepatitis B testing is recommended.
  - Patients with MM are at risk of hypogammaglobulinemia, and intravenous immune globulin (IVIG) can be used for severe hypogammaglobulinemia, especially in the setting of recurrent, life-threatening infections.
- Renal compromise is common in patients with MM (O'Donnell et al., 2021).
  - Less than 10% have end-stage renal disease requiring hemodialysis at diagnosis
  - 30% to 50% have renal dysfunction (creatinine >2.0 mg/dL or an estimated glomerular filtration rate <40 mL/min) at diagnosis

- The two major causes of renal insufficiency are myeloma cast nephropathy (also called light-chain cast nephropathy or myeloma kidney) and hypercalcemia.
- Treatment of renal dysfunction
  - Treat the MM
  - Treat hypercalcemia
  - Treat hyperviscosity
  - Avoid aggravating factors
    - Dehydration
    - Diabetes
    - HTN
    - Medications (NSAIDs, loop diuretics)
    - IV contrast
  - Dose adjustment may be required for selected active agents
- Prevention of coagulopathies/thrombosis
- Highest risk for VTE is in the first 6 months after MM diagnosis
- Prophylactic anticoagulation is recommended for all patients with MM based on risk stratification score such as IMPEDE-VTE (see the IMPEDE VTE Risk Stratification Algorithm and Choice of Thromboprophylaxis in Patients With Multiple Myeloma table on page 164)
- Immunomodulatory agents (IMiDs) significantly increase the risk of VTE, especially in combination with dexamethasone
- Full-dose anticoagulation is contraindicated if platelets are less than 50,000/mcL; prophylactic anticoagulation may be appropriate for high-risk patients if platelets are 25,000/mcL or higher

Immunomodulatory Agents (IMiDs)

	Thalidomide	Lenalidomide	Pomalidomide
Dosing and Administration	• 50–200 mg/day by mouth at bedtime at least 1 h after evening meal • Variable dosing in combination regimens • Dose modification for neuropathy, cytopenias, rash	• 25 mg/day by mouth days 1–21 of a 28-day cycle for induction • Take with or without food • Variable dosing in combination regimens • Dose modification based on renal function, cytopenias, rash	• 4 mg/day by mouth on days 1-21 of a 28–day cycle • Take with or without food • Dose modifications for cytopenias
Peripheral neuropathy	√		
Deep vein thrombosis	√ Increased risk with dexamethasone	√ Increased risk with dexamethasone	√ Increased risk with dexamethasone
Myelosuppression	√ Neutropenia	√ Neutropenia, thrombocytopenia, anemia	√ Neutropenia, thrombocytopenia, anemia
Fever		√	√
Fatigue, weakness	√	√	√
Sedation	√		
Rash	√	√	√
Cardiovascular	√ Peripheral edema	√ Peripheral edema	√ Peripheral edema
Gastrointestinal disturbance	√ Constipation	√ Constipation, diarrhea	√ Constipation, diarrhea
Renal/Hepatic		√ Hepatotoxicity Reduce dose for CrCL <60 mL/min	√ Increased creatinine
Thyroid	√ Hypothyroidism	√ Hypothyroidism Hyperthyroidism	√ Hypothyroidism Hyperthyroidism
Muscle spasms		√	√

All IMiDs are subject to REMS program for embryo-fetal toxicity

IMiD, Immunomodulatory drug; *REMS,* Risk Evaluation and Mitigation Strategy.
Data from Lexicomp Online. Available at https://online.lexi.com (accessed June 1, 2022).

Proteasome Inhibitors (PIs)

	Bortezomib	Carfilzomib	Ixazomib
Dosing and administration	• 1.3 mg/m^2 subcutaneously on days 1, 4, 8, 11, every 21 days • Variable dosing as a single agent and in combination regimens • Subcutaneous dosing has less peripheral neuropathy than IV • Dose modification for neuropathy, cytopenias	• 20 mg/m^2 IV (cycle 1), 27 mg/m^2 (cycles 2-12) on days 1, 2, 8, 9, 15, 16, every 28 days • Variable dosing as a single agent and in combination regimens • Dose modifications for cytopenias, cardiopulmonary symptoms	• 4 mg orally on days 1, 8, and 15 of a 28-day cycle • Dose should be taken at least 1 h before or at least 2 h after food • Dose modification for moderate or severe hepatic impairment, renal impairment, cytopenias, rash, peripheral neuropathy
Peripheral neuropathy	√		√

Proteasome Inhibitors (PIs)—cont'd

	Bortezomib	Carfilzomib	Ixazomib
Myelosuppression	√ • Thrombocytopenia Anemia Neutropenia	√ • Thrombocytopenia	√ • Thrombocytopenia Neutropenia
Cardio/pulmonary	√ • Heart failure Hypotension	√ • Hypertension, heart failure, cardiomyopathy, peripheral edema, pulmonary edema, myocardial infarction	√ • Peripheral edema
Rash	√		√
Fever	√	√	
Fatigue, weakness	√	√	√
Viral reactivation of herpes zoster	√	√	√
Gastrointestinal disturbance	√ • Nausea and vomiting, diarrhea, constipation	√ • Nausea and vomiting, diarrhea, constipation, mucositis/stomatitis	√ • Diarrhea, constipation, nausea
Renal/hepatic	√ • Hepatic	√ • Renal toxicity Hepatotoxicity	√ • Hepatotoxicity
Infusion reactions		√	
Ocular	√ • Stye, blepharitis		√ • Blurred vision • Cataract • Conjunctivitis • Dry eyes
Dietary considerations	• Green tea and green tea extracts • Grapefruit juice and ascorbic acid supplements may diminish the therapeutic effect of bortezomib and should be avoided		

IV, Intravenous
Data from Lexicomp Online. Available at https://online.lexi.com (accessed June 1, 2022).

Anti-CD38 Monoclonal Antibodies

	Daratumumab	Isatuximab
Dosing	• Weeks 1–8: 16 mg/kg IV once weekly for 8 doses. • Weeks 9–24: 16 mg/kg IV once every 2 weeks for 8 doses. • Weeks 25 and beyond: 16 mg/kg IV once every 4 weeks until disease progression. • Dosing varies in combination regimens • Dose adjustments for hepatic impairment	• Cycle 1: 10 mg/kg IV on days 1, 8, 15, and 22 of a 28-day cycle • Cycle 2 and beyond: 10 mg/kg IV on days 1 and 15 of a 28-day cycle
Pre-treatment	• Hepatitis B testing • Type and screen (interfere with blood bank tests)	• Hepatitis B testing • Type and screen (interfere with blood bank tests)
Adverse events	• Neutropenia, thrombocytopenia, anemia • Fatigue • Diarrhea • Vomiting • Arthralgia • Dyspnea, cough, upper respiratory tract infection • Fevers • Peripheral edema • Hypertension • Viral reactivaton: herpes zoster, hepatitis B reactivation • Infusion-related reactions	• Anemia, neutropenia, febrile neutropenia, thrombocytopenia • Infections • Infusion reactions • Hypertension • Diarrhea • Nausea • Fatigue • Cough • Cardiac failure • Secondary malignancy
Infusion-related reactions (IRRs)	• Pre-medication with steroid, acetaminophen, and antihistamine(s) • Infusion rate titration • Post-daratumumab steroid recommended for at least first 4 infusions to prevent delayed infusion reactions • Rapid infusion daratumumab may be considered over 90 min from day 15 onward if no IRRs	• Pre-medication with steroid, acetaminophen, and antihistamine(s) • Infusion rate titration

Continued

Anti-CD38 Monoclonal Antibodies—cont'd

	Daratumumab	Isatuximab

Subcutaneous dosing	• Dose: Daratumumab 1800 mg/hyaluronidase 30,000 units/15 mL
	  • Administration: Inject subcutaneously into the abdomen over 3–5 min
	  • Significantly reduced incidence of infusion reactions compared with IV
	    • Pre-medications: corticosteroid, acetaminophen, antihistamine
		None

Therapeutic monoclonal antibodies (daratumumab, elotuzumab, and isatuximab) may interfere with SPEP and IFE tests. mAbs are IgG antibodies and they can appear as another M spike.

IFE, Immunofixation electrophoresis; *IgG,* immunoglobulin G; *IV,* intravenous; *M spike,* monoclonal spike; *SPEP,* serum protein electrophoresis.
Data from Lexicomp Online. Available at https://online.lexi.com (accessed June 1, 2022).

IMPEDE VTE Risk Stratification Algorithm and Choice of Thromboprophylaxis in Patients With Multiple Myeloma

Risk Factor	Acronym	Score
Immunomodulatory drug (IMiD)	I	4
Body **M**ass index ≥25 kg/m²	M	1
Pelvic, hip, or femur fracture	P	4
Erythropoiesis-stimulating agent	E	1
Doxorubicin	D	3
Dexamethasone: High dose (≥480 mg/month)		4
Dexamethasone: Low dose		2
Ethnicity/Race = Asian or Pacific Islander	E	−3
History of **V**enous thromboembolism before MM	V	5
Tunneled line/central venous catheter	T	2
Existing thromboprophylaxis: therapeutic LMWH or warfarin	E	−4
Existing thromboprophylaxis: prophylactic LMWH or aspirin		−3

Risk Factors	6-Month Cumulative Incidence Without VTE Prophylaxis (%)	Recommended VTE Prophylaxis
≤3	3.3	• Aspirin 81–325 mg/day
4-7	8.3	• LMWH (equivalent to enoxaparin 40 mg subcutaneous daily)
≥8	15.2	• Rivaroxaban 10 mg daily
		• Apixaban 2.5 mg PO BID
		• Fondaparinux 2.5 mg subcutaneous daily
		• Warfarin with therapeutic dosing (INR 2-3)

IMiD, Immunomodulatory drug; *INR,* international normalized ratio; *IV,* intravenous; *LMWH,* low molecular weight heparin; *MM,* multiple myeloma; *VTE,* venous thromboembolism.
Data from Sanfilippo, K. M., Luo, S., Wang, T. F., Fiala, M., Schoen, M., Wildes, T. M., ... Gage, B. F. (2019). Predicting venous thromboembolism in multiple myeloma: Development and validation of the IMPEDE-VTE score. *American Journal of Hematology, 94*(11), 1176–1184.

Prognosis

- The 5-year relative survival has doubled since 1975, increasing from 26.3% in 1975 to an estimated 57.9% in 2018 (NCI, 2022)
- Complete remission is associated with improved PFS and OS (O'Donnell et al., 2021)
  - CR does not imply elimination of the malignant clone
- MRD negativity by next-generation flow cytometry or next-generation sequencing with a minimum sensitivity of 1 in 10^5 nucleated cells or higher is associated with improved survival (Callander et al., 2022; NCCN, 2022; O'Donnell et al., 2021)

Surveillance

MM inevitably relapses, and patients must be monitored at regular intervals for both toxicity of treatment and progression of disease.

- Laboratory assessments may include:
  - CBC with differential, metabolic panel
  - Serum quantitative immunoglobulins, SPEP, and SIFE
  - 24-hour urine for total protein, UPEP, and UIFE at baseline and as clinically indicated or if there is a significant change in FLC levels
  - Serum FLC assay

- Advanced imaging (i.e., whole-body FDG PET/CT, whole-body low-dose CT scan, whole-body MRI without contrast) as clinically indicated, ideally with the same technique used at diagnosis.
- Bone marrow aspirate and biopsy with multiparameter flow cytometry and MRD as clinically indicated.

Treatment for Relapsed Disease

- If there is only biochemical progression, the patient may not need immediate treatment and can continue active surveillance (e.g., standard-risk disease with slow increasing trend in myeloma markers)
- Treatment is indicated for patients with clinical progression or CRAB criteria (refer to table on page 158)
- Treatment indicated for high-risk disease with any progression, and progressive disease with renal or neurologic complications, or rapid doubling of M spike
- General principles of selecting therapy for relapsed/refractory disease:
  - Prior drug exposure: may re-treat with regimen used previously if disease is not refractory to it and more than 6 months have elapsed since last used
  - High risk versus standard risk
  - Age, frailty, and comorbidity
  - Toxicity with prior drugs
  - Transplant eligibility/prior transplant
  - Patient preference/goals of care
  - Logistics of drug administration
  - Triplet therapy is preferred over doublet therapy
- If refractory to the three main classes of drugs (IMiDs, PIs, and anti-CD38 monoclonal antibodies), there are novel agents that are approved for use.
  - Selinexor: first in class oral XPO1 inhibitor that induces nuclear retention and activation of tumor suppressor proteins and the glucocorticoid receptor in the presence of steroids and suppresses oncoprotein expression.
    - Side effects: thrombocytopenia, fatigue, decreased appetite, nausea, vomiting, weight loss, diarrhea, hyponatremia, neutropenia
  - Elotuzumab: monoclonal antibody directed against SLAMF-7 antigen
    - Side effects: infusion reactions
  - Venetoclax: oral BCL-2 inhibitor; only used for MM with t(11;14) translocation
    - Side effects: neutropenia, rash, diarrhea
  - B-cell maturation antigen (BCMA) targeted therapy: BCMA is expressed on plasma cells and is critical for survival of long-lived plasma cells
    - Belantamab mafodotin: anti-BCMA antibody drug conjugate
    - Side effects: ocular toxicity-blurry vision, dry eyes, photophobia, eye pain (Risk Evaluation and Mitigation Strategy [REMS] program requires eye exam at baseline and prior to each dose); infusion reactions, thrombocytopenia, anemia, infection, diarrhea
  - CART (chimeric antigen receptor T cells) targeting BCMA: idecabtagene vicleucel and ciltacabtagene autoleucel
- Side effects: cytokine release syndromes, cytopenias, infection, neurologic complications, hypogammaglobulinemia

References

Anderson, K., Ismaila, N., & Kyle, R. A. (2018). Role of bone-modifying agents in multiple myeloma: American Society of Clinical Oncology clinical practice guideline update summary. *Journal of Oncology Practice*, 14(4), 266–269.

Borrello, I. (2012). Can we change the disease biology of multiple myeloma? *Leukemia Research*, 36, S3–S12.

Callander, N. S., Baljevic, M., Adekola, K., Anderson, L. D., Campagnaro, E., Castillo, J. J., … Kumar, S. K. (2022). NCCN guidelines® Insights: Multiple myeloma, version 3.2022: Featured updates to the NCCN guidelines. *Journal of the National Comprehensive Cancer Network*, 20(1), 8–19.

Chang, S. H., Luo, S., Thomas, T. S., O'Brian, K. K., Colditz, G. A., Carlsson, N. P., & Carson, K. R. (2016). Obesity and the transformation of monoclonal gammopathy of undetermined significance to multiple myeloma: A population-based cohort study. *Journal of the National Cancer Institute*, 109(5). djw264.

Clay-Gilmour, A. I., Hildebrandt, M. A. T., Brown, E. E., Hofmann, J. N., Spinelli, J. J., Giles, G. G., … Vachon, C. M. (2020). Coinherited genetics of multiple myeloma and its precursor, monoclonal gammopathy of undetermined significance. *Blood Advances*, 4(12), 2789–2797.

Greipp, P. R., San Miguel, J., Durie, B. G., Crowley, J. J., Barlogie, B., Bladé, J., … Westin, J. (2005). International staging system for multiple myeloma. *Journal of Clinical Oncology*, 23(15), 3412–3420.

Hillengass, J., Usmani, S., Rajkumar, S. V., Durie, B. G. M., Mateos, M. V., Lonial, S., … Lentzsch, S. (2019). International myeloma working group consensus recommendations on imaging in monoclonal plasma cell disorders. *The Lancet Oncology*, 20(6), e302–e312.

Kyle, R. A., Larson, D. R., Therneau, T. M., Dispenzieri, A., Kumar, S., Cerhan, J. R., & Rajkumar, S. V. (2018). Long-term follow-up of monoclonal gammopathy of undetermined significance. *New England Journal of Medicine*, 378(3), 241–249.

Landgren, O., Shim, Y. K., Michalek, J., Costello, R., Burton, D., Ketchum, N., … Vogt, R. F. (2015). Agent orange exposure and monoclonal gammopathy of undetermined significance: an operation ranch hand veteran cohort study. *JAMA Oncology*, 1(8), 1061–1068.

Landgren, O., Zeig-Owens, R., Giricz, O., Goldfarb, D., Murata, K., Thoren, K., … Prezant, D. J. (2018). Multiple myeloma and its precursor disease among firefighters exposed to the world trade center disaster. *JAMA Oncology*, 4(6), 821–827.

Lauby-Secretan, B., Scoccianti, C., Loomis, D., Grosse, Y., Bianchini, F., Straif, K., & International Agency for Research on Cancer Handbook Working Group. (2016). Body fatness and cancer—viewpoint of the IARC Working Group. *The New England Journal of Medicine*, 375(8), 794–798.

LeBlanc, R., Bergstrom, D. J., Côté, J., Kotb, R., Louzada, M. L., & Sutherland, H. J. (2022). Management of myeloma manifestations and complications: the cornerstone of supportive care: recommendation of the Canadian Myeloma Research Group (formerly Myeloma Canada Research Network) consensus guideline consortium. *Clinical Lymphoma Myeloma and Leukemia*, 22(1), e41–e56.

National Cancer Institute. (2022). *SEER cancer stat facts: Myeloma*. Available at http://seer.cancer.gov/statfacts/html/mulmy.html (accessed June 1, 2022).

National Comprehensive Cancer Network. (2022). NCCN clinical practice guidelines in oncology (NCCN Guidelines®): Multiple myeloma (v.3.2022). Available at http://www.nccn.org/professionals/physician_gls/pdf/myeloma.pdf (accessed June 1, 2022).

O'Donnell, E. K., Bianchi, G., & Anderson, K. (2021). Myeloma. In K. Kaushansky, J. T. Prchal, L. J. Burns, M. A. Lichtman, M. Levi, & D. C. Linch (Eds.), *Williams hematology* (10th ed.). McGraw-Hill Education.

Palumbo, A., Avet-Loiseau, H., Oliva, S., Lokhorst, H. M., Goldschmidt, H., Rosinol, L., … Moreau, P. (2015a). Revised international staging system for multiple myeloma: A report from International Myeloma Working Group. *Journal of Clinical Oncology*, 33(26), 2863–2869.

Palumbo, A., Bringhen, S., Mateos, M. V., Larocca, A., Facon, T., Kumar, S. K., … Rajkumar, S. V. (2015b). Geriatric assessment predicts survival and toxicities in elderly myeloma patients: an International Myeloma Working Group report. *Blood*, *125*(13), 2068–2074.

Perrotta, C., Kleefeld, S., Staines, A., Tewari, P., De Roos, A. J., Baris, D., … Cocco, P. (2013). Multiple myeloma and occupation: A pooled analysis by the International Multiple Myeloma Consortium. *Cancer Epidemiology*, *37*(3), 300–305.

Rajkumar, S. V., Dimopoulos, M. A., Palumbo, A., Blade, J., Merlini, G., Mateos, M. V., … Miguel, J. F. (2014). International Myeloma Working Group updated criteria for the diagnosis of multiple myeloma. *The Lancet Oncology*, *15*(12), e538–e548.

Siegel, R. L., Miller, K. D., & Fuchs, H. E. (2021). Cancer statistics, 2021. *CA: A Cancer Journal for Clinicians*, *71*, 7–33.

Myelofibrosis

Kristen Hurley

Definition

Classified as a Philadelphia chromosome–negative myeloproliferative neoplasm, myelofibrosis (MF) can arise on its own (i.e., primary myelofibrosis [PMF]); or occur as a progression of polycythemia vera (post-PV-MF) or of essential thrombocythemia (post-ET-MF). The manifestations of PMF, post-PV-MF, and post-ET-MF are virtually identical, and treatment usually is the same for all three.

MF is a clonal disorder arising from the neoplastic transformation of early hematopoietic stem cells. The abnormal stem cells produce more mature cells that grow quickly and take over the bone marrow, causing fibrosis (i.e., scar tissue formation) and chronic inflammation. As a result, the bone marrow becomes less able to create normal blood cells, and blood cell production may move to the spleen, causing enlargement, or to other areas of the body. Many symptoms of MF are caused by insufficient numbers of normal blood cells or chronic inflammation.

Approximately 50% to 60% of patients with PMF have a gain in function in the Janus activated kinase 2 gene (*JAK2*), which normally encodes a protein that promotes the growth and proliferation of cells (Cervantes et al., 2009) The V617F *JAK2* mutation leads to the overproduction of abnormal myeloid cells, which results in excess collagen production leading to scar tissue formation in PMF. Additional mutations that are common but not essential for diagnosis are calreticulin (CALR) and MPL (Tefferi, 2021).

Incidence

(Leukemia and Lymphoma Society [LLS], 2012; National Cancer Institute-Surveillance, Epidemiology, and End Results Program [NCI-SEER], n.d.)

- Incidence: 0.5 to 1.5 per 100,000 persons per year.
- About 15,000 to 18,000 people are living with MF in the United States.
- Patients are typically middle-aged to elderly people. In published reports, the median age at diagnosis was 60 to 67 years, and 20% of patients were younger than 55 years at diagnosis.
- MF affects men and women equally.
- It is rare in children; young girls are twice as likely to be affected as boys.

Etiology and Risk Factors

(National Organization for Rare Disorders [NORD], 2018)

- About 50% of patients with PMF have the gain-of-function V617F *JAK2* mutation.
- Between 5% and 10% of patients have somatic mutations of *JAK2* exon 12 or activating mutations of the thrombopoietin receptor gene *MPL*. Between 5% and 15% of patients can have mutation of the TET2 gene.
- Mutations in the gene encoding *CALR* were found in *20% of patients.*
- There are no known modifiable risk factors for PMF, but secondary MF can result from disease or damage to the bone marrow through exposure to radiation, industrial solvents (e.g., benzene, toluene), fluoride, phosphorus, or viral infections.

Signs and Symptoms

- Patients at the time of diagnosis may have severe symptoms associated with advanced disease or may be asymptomatic.
- About one-third of patients do not have symptoms of MF due to the disease developing slowly in some patients. There may not be early signs or symptoms, but instead nonspecific symptoms of fatigue, weakness, shortness of breath, or pale skin (LLS, 2012).
- Symptoms (Cervantes et al., 2009; Mesa et al., 2016)
  - Splenomegaly is the hallmark of the disease in 90% of patients, usually with accompanying symptoms of abdominal pain and early satiety. The diagnosis typically is made during the work-up for splenomegaly.
  - Fatigue (up to 80% of patients)
  - Weight loss
  - Low-grade fever
  - Bone and joint pain (40%)
  - Night sweats (50%)
  - Hepatomegaly (40% to 70% of patients)
  - Skin itching or burning sensation (due to increased circulating cytokines) (40%)

Diagnostic Work-up

- MF is typically diagnosed through a process of exclusion of other diseases that cause bone marrow fibrosis, such as leukemia, infection, metastatic cancer, lymphoma, myelodysplastic syndrome, and hairy cell leukemia.
- Medical history and physical examination
- Laboratory tests
  - Complete blood count with differential count
  - Comprehensive metabolic panel
    - Aspartate transaminase and alanine transaminase
    - Alkaline phosphatase
    - Total bilirubin
    - Lactate dehydrogenase
    - Uric acid
- *JAK2* quantitative assay
- *CALR* and *MPL* mutational analysis are performed for prognostic purposes

- Bone marrow biopsy with cytogenetic testing may identify the following abnormalities that constitute an unfavorable karyotype: +8, −7/del(7q), i(17q), inv(3), −5/del(5q), del(12p), or 11q23 rearrangements.
  - The marrow specimen can be difficult to obtain, and the biopsy often results in a dry tap.

Histopathology

- Typically, analysis shows abnormal megakaryocytes and neutrophils (i.e., hyperplasia) in the marrow, hyperlobulation of granulocytes, and normal or increased erythroid precursors.
- The patient may have fibrosis, but the biopsy specimen may not reveal extensive replacement of the marrow by fibrosis.
- The World Health Organization (WHO) established criteria for the diagnosis of MF in 2008 (see box below)

World Health Organization Myelofibrosis Diagnostic Criteria

Major Criteria*

1. Presence of megakaryocyte proliferation and atypia, usually accompanied by reticulin and/or collagen fibrosis; or, in the absence of significant reticulin fibrosis, the megakaryocyte changes must be accompanied by increased bone marrow cellularity characterized by granulocytic proliferation and often decreased erythropoiesis (so-called prefibrotic cellular-phase disease).
2. Not meeting criteria for polycythemia vera, chronic myeloid leukemia, myelodysplastic syndrome, or other myeloid neoplasms.
3. Demonstration of *JAK2* 617V > F or other clonal marker; or, in the absence of a clonal marker, no evidence of bone marrow fibrosis caused by an underlying inflammatory disease or another neoplastic disease. About 60% of patients with primary myelofibrosis carry a *JAK2* mutation, and about 5%–10% of patients have activating mutations in the thrombopoietin receptor gene, *MPL*. Almost 90% of patients without *JAK2* or *MPL* mutations carry a somatic mutation of the calreticulin gene, which is associated with a more indolent clinical course than is seen with *JAK2* or *MPL* mutations.

Minor Criteria*

1. Leukoerythroblastosis
2. Increased serum level of lactate dehydrogenase
3. Anemia
4. Palpable splenomegaly

* To make the diagnosis, all three major criteria plus two minor criteria must be met.
From the National Cancer Institute. (2020). *Chronic myeloproliferative neoplasms treatment: Primary myelofibrosis disease overview*. Available at https://www.cancer.gov/types/myeloproliferative/hp/chronic-treatment-pdq#_9.

Clinical Staging

No clinical staging is performed for MF.

Treatment

- A watch-and-wait approach is often used for patients who are symptom free and have no signs of disease (e.g., no anemia, no splenomegaly). Patients may remain symptom free for many years, but they must be followed routinely to detect disease progression.
- Patients should be considered for clinical trials as appropriate.

Systemic Therapies

JAK2 Inhibitors

- Three agents, ruxolitinib, fedratinib, and pacritinib, are approved by the US Food and Drug Administration (FDA) to treat intermediate-risk and high-risk MF patients (Tefferi, 2021).
  - Ruxolitinib, a JAK2 inhibitor, is an oral agent that demonstrated significant reduction in spleen size, relief of constitutional symptoms, improved anemia, and improved survival.
    - Ruxolitinib can be effective for patients with or without the *JAK* mutation.
    - Ruxolitinib can be an effective alternative to hydroxyurea-refractory patients to help with constitutional symptoms and symptomatic splenomegaly.
    - Side effects include dizziness, anemia, thrombocytopenia, neutropenia, diarrhea, and edema.
    - Caution should be shown when discontinuing ruxolitinib due to severe withdrawal symptoms that can occur. This is characterized by acute relapse of disease symptoms, accelerated splenomegaly, worsening cytopenias, and occasional septic shock-like syndrome.
  - Fedratinib, a JAK2 and FLT3 inhibitor, is an oral agent that demonstrated higher inhibitory activity over JAK1, JAK3, and TYK2 pathways, and was shown to reduce spleen size, and provide relief of constitutional symptoms in clinical trials. FDA approved for patients who are intolerant or resistant to ruxolitinib.
    - Side effects include anemia, thrombocytopenia, gastrointestinal (GI) distress, elevations in serum liver function tests and pancreatic enzymes, as well as Wernicke encephalopathy.
  - Pacritinib, a JAK2, mutant JAK2v617F, and FLT3 inhibitor, is indicated for patients with intermediate- or high-risk primary or secondary MF.
    - Can be used in patients with platelets ≤100,000 × 10^9/L
    - Side effects include cardiac events, severe diarrhea, nausea, thrombocytopenia, anemia, and hemorrhage.
  - Another agent under current investigation is momelotinib, a JAK1/JAK2 inhibitor that inhibits hyperactivated ACVR1/ALK2 (activin receptor 1A/activin-like kinase 2) signaling (Rosa, 2022; Chifotides et al., 2022). This mechanism of action suppresses hepcidin expression in the liver, potentially allowing an increase in circulating iron and hemoglobin levels and restoration of erythropoiesis. This may lead to transfusion independence for patients along with decreasing splenomegaly and constitutional symptoms.
    - Side effects include peripheral neuropathy, thrombocytopenia, dizziness, nausea, hypotension, headache, and flushing (Tefferi, 2021),
- Allogeneic stem cell transplantation (SCT) may be used in high-risk patients who have two or more adverse features (e.g., hemoglobin <10 g/dL, constitutional symptoms, an isolated cytogenetic abnormality, or circulating blasts >1%) and are unresponsive to other therapies. SCT is considered

to be the only cure for MF. However, SCT carries significant morbidity and mortality and is limited to patients younger than 70 years of age.

- Newer forms of nonmyeloablative transplantation using reduced-intensity conditioning have been used to reduce the mortality rates and increase the long-term survival times for these patients.
- A variety of other agents have been used with various degrees of success in the treatment of MF (some of these agents provide response rates of 15% to 25% with response durations averaging 1 to 2 years) (Tefferi, 2021).
  - Alkylating agents such as busulfan have been used, but because they can cause prolonged, severe cytopenias even after discontinuation of therapy, they are rarely employed.
  - Hydroxyurea may assist in the reduction of spleen size (it may reduce the size in half in approximately 40% of patients), control of thrombocytosis and leukocytosis, and control of constitutional symptoms. Side effects can include myelosuppression and painful mucocutaneous ulcers.
  - Immunomodulatory drugs (IMiDs), such as thalidomide, lenalidomide, and pomalidomide, are oral agents that target cancer by affecting functions of the immune system. IMiDs can decrease spleen size, improve overall blood counts, and treat anemia.
    - Lenalidomide works best in presence of del(5q31).
    - Pomalidomide may alleviate anemia in a subset of JAK-2 mutated patients that do not have splenomegaly or excess circulating blasts.
    - Side effects include peripheral neuropathy (thalidomide), myelosuppression, and GI distress (lenalidomide). Pomalidomide may cause drowsiness and peripheral neuropathy.
  - Androgen therapy (testosterone enanthate IM, fluoxymesterone oral) does not treat the disease but can be used as supportive care to help with the symptoms of anemia. For some patients, it promotes red blood cell production. It can be extremely toxic to the liver and requires close monitoring. It may also cause facial hair growth and masculinizing effects in women.
  - Recombinant erythropoietin is used for treating the anemia by stimulating red blood cell production, but it does not treat the underlying disease. This can be ineffective in transfusion-dependent patients and could exacerbate splenomegaly.
  - Luspatercept, activin receptor-ligand trap-enhancing late-stage erythropoiesis, may be given to those who are not responding to erythropoietin agents but still require transfusions.
  - Anagrelide, an oral phospholipase A_2 inhibitor, has been used for MF patients with elevated platelet counts. Close monitoring is needed because it can cause significant pancytopenia.
  - Additional drugs under consideration alone or in combination, include PI3/AKT (phosphatidylinositol 3-kinase/protein kinase B) inhibitors (e.g., buparlisib), BET (bromodomain and extraterminal) inhibitor (e.g., CPI-0610), telomerase inhibitor (e.g., imetelstat), aurora kinase inhibitor (e.g., alisertib), BCL-2/BCL-X (B cell lymphoma 2/b cell lymphoma extra large) inhibitors (e.g., navitoclax, venetoclax), CD123 (IL3RA) directed cytotoxin (IL3 fused to diphtheria toxin) (e.g., tagraxofusp).

Radiation Therapy

- Radiation therapy is typically used to treat symptoms associated with an enlarged spleen. It can be difficult to get a long-standing response, and toxicity to underlying GI structures is common in MF patients with advanced disease and marked splenomegaly.

Surgery

- Splenectomy typically is not done late in the disease because spleen size and vascularity make surgical removal quite dangerous.
  - It may be considered if there is no response to other therapies.
  - It should be considered only by an experienced surgeon.
- Close monitoring after surgery is required to ensure complications do not arise.

Prognosis

- Median survival is 3 to 7 years for patients diagnosed in fibrotic stage; 10 to 15 years for patients diagnosed in early prefibrotic phase (NCI-SEER, n.d.).
- MF is a progressive disease with constitutional symptoms, splenomegaly, and cytopenias that worsen over time.
- Recent research has shown that patients with elevated circulating cytokine levels are a unique subset that carries a poorer prognosis; specifically, circulating CXCL8/IL-8 (C-X-C motif chemokine ligand 8/interleukin 8), IL-2R (interleukin-2R), IL-12 (interleukin-12), and IL-15 (interleukin-15) have been identified as negative prognostic indicators. However, this is still not fully understood and needs further research to determine its value and whether alternative therapies are necessary (Fisher et al., 2019).
- Transformation to acute myeloid leukemia occurs in 8% to 23% of patients with MF during the first decade after diagnosis (Quintás-Cardama et al., 2013).
- The International Prognostic Scoring System (IPSS), which was developed by the International Working Group for Myelofibrosis Research and Treatment (IWG-MRT), is used to estimate prognosis based on risk factors identified at diagnosis. The IPSS applies a one-point value to the following factors: age greater than 65 years old, presence of constitutional symptoms, hemoglobin less than 10 g/dL, white blood cell count greater than 25×10^9/L, and blood blasts ≥1%. Patients with a score of zero are considered (low risk), 1 (intermediate risk-1), 2 (intermediate risk-2), or ≥3 (high risk). Median survival times associated with the IPSS risk levels were 11.3, 7.9, 4, and 2.3 years, respectively (Cervantes et al., 2009).
- The Dynamic International Prognostic Scoring System (DIPSS) is used to reevaluate the prognosis as the disease

advances over time. The DIPSS differs from the IPSS as it assigns a two-point value to hemoglobin less than 10 g/dL. Survival is associated with the DIPSS score as follows:

- Risk score of 0: median survival not yet reached
- Risk score of 1 to 2: median survival is 14.2 years
- Risk score of 3 to 4: median survival is 4 years
- Risk score of 5 to 6: median survival is 1.5 years (Gangat et al., 2011)
- With the advancement in next-generation sequencing and karyotyping, the ability to predict outcomes based on presence of high risk or unfavorable karyotypes or mutations led to the additional development of the Mutation-enhanced International Prognostic Scoring System (MIPSS) for transplant age patients (age ≤70 or 70+ age), MIPSSv2 (karyotype enhanced MIPSS70) that utilized mutations, karyotype, and clinical variables, and the genetically inspired prognostic scoring system (GIPSS), which is based exclusively on mutations and karyotype. These newer systems allow for mutation profiles such as IDH1, IDH2, FLT3, and TP53 mutations to be taken into consideration when determining therapy for patients (Tefferi, 2021).

Prevention and Surveillance

- There is no known way to prevent PMF.
- Avoiding exposure to radiation, viruses, or industrial chemicals that damage the bone marrow may help to prevent secondary MF.

References

Cervantes, R., Dupriez, G., Pereiral, A., Passamonti, F., Reilly, J. T., Morra, E., & Rumi, E. (2009). New prognostic scoring system for primary myelofibrosis based on a study of the International Working Group for Myelofibrosis Research and Treatment. *Blood*, *113*(13), 2895–2901.

Chifotides, H. T., Bose, P., & Verstovsek, S. (2022). Momelotinib: An emerging treatment for myelofibrosis patients with anemia. *Journal of Hematology & Oncology*, *15*(1), 7.

Fisher, D., Miner, C. A., Engle, E. K., Hu, H., Collins, T. B., Zhou, A., … Oh, S. T. (2019). Cytokine production in myelofibrosis exhibits differential responsiveness to JAK-STAT, MAP kinase, and NFκB signaling. *Leukemia*, *33*(8), 1978–1995.

Gangat, N., Caramazza, D., Vaidya, R., George, G., Begna, K., Schwager, S., … Cervantes, F. (2011). DIPSS plus: A refined Dynamic International Prognostic Scoring System for primary myelofibrosis that incorporates prognostic information from karyotype, platelet count, and transfusion status. *Journal of Clinical Oncology*, *29*(4), 392–397.

Leukemia and Lymphoma Society (LLS). (2012). *Myelofibrosis facts*. Available at https://www.lls.org/sites/default/files/file_assets/FS14_Myelofibrosis_Fact%20Sheet_Final9.12.pdf.

Mesa, R., Miller, C. B., Thyne, M., Mangan, J., Goldberger, S., Fazal, S., … Boyle, J. (2016). Myeloproliferative neoplasms (MPNs) have a significant impact on patients' overall health and productivity: The MPN Landmark survey. *BMC Cancer*, *16*, 167.

National Cancer Institute. (2020). *Chronic myeloproliferative neoplasms treatment (PDQ®)—health professional version. Cancer.gov*. Available at https://www.cancer.gov/types/myeloproliferative/hp/chronic-treatment-pdq#_AboutThis_1.

National Cancer Institute-Surveillance, Epidemiology, and End Results Program (NCI-SEER). (n.d.). Primary myelofibrosis. *Seer.Cancer.gov*. Available at https://seer.cancer.gov/seertools/hemelymph/51f6cf57e3e27c3994bd5381/.

National Organization for Rare Disorders (NORD). (2018). *Primary myelofibrosis. Rarediseases.org*. Available at https://rarediseases.org/rare-diseases/primary-myelofibrosis/.

Quintás-Cardama, A., Kantarjian, H., Pierce, S., Cortes, J., & Verstovsek, S. (2013). Prognostic model to identify patients with myelofibrosis at the highest risk of transformation to acute myeloid leukemia. *Clinical Lymphoma, Myeloma & Leukemia*, *13*(3), 315–318.e2.

Rosa, K. (2022). FDA approval sought for momelotinib in myelofibrosis. *OncLive*. Available at https://www.onclive.com/view/fda-approval-sought-for-momelotinib-in-myelofibrosis.

Tefferi, A. (2021). Primary myelofibrosis: 2021 update on diagnosis, risk-stratification and management. *American Journal of Hematology*, *96*(1), 145–162.

Neuroendocrine Cancers

*Holly M. Reames**

Definition

Normal neuroendocrine cells have the characteristics of nerve and endocrine cells. The cells are diffusely spread throughout the body in various organs such as the gastrointestinal (GI) tract, pancreas, lung, and skin. They respond to neuronal stimuli by releasing peptide hormones that regulate normal function. The neuroendocrine system plays a specific role in each organ. For instance, the neuroendocrine cells in the GI tract regulate intestinal motility and the release of digestive enzymes, and islet cells in the pancreas release insulin.

Neuroendocrine tumors (NETs) are neoplasms that arise from cells of the endocrine (hormonal) and nervous systems. There are many types of NETs, but the neoplastic cells share common features such as morphology, special secretory granules, and the production of biogenic amines and polypeptide hormones.

In the United States, NETs, which most commonly occur in the intestine, have been traditionally referred to as *carcinoid tumors* and organized under the broad anatomic categories of foregut, midgut, and hindgut (see table below). However, the nomenclature has changed to reflect the fact that the tumors are cancer, not cancer-like lesions. Use of the terms *neuroendocrine tumor* (NET) and *neuroendocrine carcinoma* (NEC) more accurately portrays the malignant nature of the disease, although some NETs are benign.

Regional Classification of Neuroendocrine Tumors

Foregut neuroendocrine tumors	Stomach, first portion of the duodenum, pancreas, bronchus, lung, ovaries, and thymus
Midgut neuroendocrine tumors	Second portion of the duodenum, jejunum, ileum, appendix, and ascending colon
Hindgut neuroendocrine tumors	Transverse colon, descending colon, and rectum

NETs also are described by the anatomic site of origin and the degree of differentiation (see box in next column). They may be further classified as symptomatic due to hormonal syndromes resulting from the release of peptides (i.e., functional tumors) or as asymptomatic (i.e., nonfunctional tumors) NETs.

* Thanks to Nicole Korak for her contribution to the Neuroendocrine Cancers chapter.

In this chapter, the most common NETs are reviewed: gastrointestinal (GI NETs), pancreatic (pNETs), and bronchopulmonary or lung NETs.

Neuroendocrine Tumors (Carcinoids) of the Gastrointestinal Tract, Lung, and Thymus

Appendiceal carcinoid
Atypical lung carcinoid
Bronchopulmonary or thymus carcinoid
Duodenal carcinoid
Gastric carcinoid
Jejunal, ileal, and colon carcinoid
Rectal carcinoid
Neuroendocrine tumors of the pancreas (pNETs)
Gastrinoma
Nonfunctioning pancreatic tumors
Vasoactive intestinal peptide tumors (VIPoma)
Insulinoma
Glucagonoma
Somatostatinoma
Neuroendocrine tumor of the skin
Merkel cell carcinoma

Incidence

- The annual incidence of NETs is approximately 6.98 cases per 100,000 people, and based on the Surveillance, Epidemiology, and End Results (SEER) database (2012), and prevalence of individuals with NETs in the United States may exceed 170,000 (Dasari et al., 2017).
- The increasing incidence and prevalence can be attributed to a growing body of knowledge over the past two decades, improved pathologic distinction by immunohistochemical properties from other tumor types, evolving diagnostic capabilities such as unique imaging for NETs, improved treatment modalities, and increased rates of reporting to cancer registries.
- Grade 1 (G1) NET detection has increased more than any other grade group over time. Incidence of G1 NETs increased from 0.01 per 100,000 in 1973 to 2.53 incidences per 100,000 in 2012 (Dasari et al., 2017).
- pNETs are diagnosed in approximately 1000 people per year, accounting for 1% to 2% of pancreatic malignancies. They encompass all NET anomalies in the pancreas, including insulinomas, glucagonomas, and vasoactive intestinal peptide tumors (VIPomas; Ito et al., 2012).
- For bronchopulmonary NETs, 1.49 cases per 100,000 people occur each year. They account for only 1% to 2% of all lung cancers but account for 20% to 30% of all NETs (Dasari et al., 2017).

Etiology and Risk Factors

Gastrointestinal Neuroendocrine Tumors

- The exact causes of GI NETs are unknown, but there is a higher incidence among patients who have a first-degree family member with colon or prostate cancer.
- Most GI NETs are sporadic, but some cases are associated with familial syndromes. For example, there have been cases in which family members were diagnosed with midgut tumors.
- The risk of NETs is increased for the children of parents who have had a diagnosis of endometrial, kidney, or skin cancer or non-Hodgkin lymphoma.

Pancreatic Neuroendocrine Tumors

- When genetically linked, pNETs are most commonly associated with multiple endocrine neoplasia type 1 (MEN1) and MEN2 syndromes, von Hippel–Lindau (VHL) syndrome, and neurofibromatosis type 1.
- MEN1 confers a prevalence of over 80% in advanced age (Pieterman et al., 2021).
- Pancreatic NETs are found in 15% to 56% of patients with VHL, although mostly nonfunctional and rarely a cause for morbidity or mortality for affected patients (Chittiboina & Lonser, 2015).
- Insulinomas are associated with the MEN1 syndrome, and the tumors often express the mammalian target of rapamycin (mTOR), a protein kinase that is abnormally activated in a number of cancers.
- Glucagonomas, which result in overproduction of the peptide hormone glucagon, are associated with a family history of MEN1, but they also develop in people with no known risk factors.
- Gastrinoma is associated with MEN1 and Zollinger-Ellison syndromes.
- A meta-analysis found that diabetes and having a first-degree relative with cancer were associated with pNET.

Bronchopulmonary Neuroendocrine Tumors

- Although the exact causes of bronchopulmonary NETs are unknown, the frequency is reported to be from 3% to 13% in cases associated with MEN1 (Kamilaris & Stratakis, 2019).
- MEN1-associated bronchopulmonary NETs occur five times more often in women than in men (Kamilaris & Stratakis, 2019).

Signs and Symptoms

Nonfunctioning Neuroendocrine Tumors

The majority of NETs are nonfunctioning and therefore many patients will be asymptomatic.

- Signs and symptoms of a NETs are directly related to the cellular type and functional status of the tumor.
- If the NET is nonfunctional, symptoms are related to the location of the metastasis.
- Most NETs are diagnosed at an advanced stage, have metastasized to the liver, and produce symptoms such as jaundice, weight loss, and ascites.

Functional Gastrointestinal Neuroendocrine Tumors

Carcinoid Syndrome

- Carcinoid syndrome is the most common functional syndrome for GI NETs. It is a condition in which NETs release excessive amounts of serotonin (5-HT), prostaglandins, or other neuropeptides. Symptoms of carcinoid syndrome include chronic flushing, diarrhea, wheezing, pellagra due to niacin deficiency, and carcinoid heart disease. It occurs in about 30% of patients with GI NETs and most often in the setting of liver metastasis (Ahmed, 2020).
- Carcinoid crisis is a life-threatening complication of carcinoid syndrome. Symptoms include hemodynamic instability with a high propensity for hypotension, severe flushing, dyspnea, and confusion due to excess release of bioactive amines from the NET into the systemic circulation. The crisis can be triggered by exposure to anesthetics or manipulation of the tumor during a procedure (surgery or embolization).
- Symptoms of carcinoid syndrome include:
  - Chronic flushing occurs in 94% of patients with carcinoid syndrome (Ahmed, 2020).
    - Flushing can last minutes or hours and can be seen on the face, torso, and extremities.
    - Can be exacerbated by stress, exercise, or tyramine-containing foods such as cheese, wine, and chocolate.
  - Diarrhea affects approximately 80% of patients with carcinoid syndrome (Ahmed, 2020).
    - Described as urgency to defecate with watery stools which can be accompanied by colicky, abdominal cramping.
    - Differs from the symptoms of irritable bowel syndrome (IBS) in that patients with NETs are more often awakened in the middle of the night by the urge to have a bowel movement.
    - Diarrhea can continue when fasting.
  - Bronchoconstriction or carcinoid wheezing occurs in 10% to 20% of patients with carcinoid syndrome. The new-onset wheezing in adults is caused by overproduction of histamine, substance P, or 5-HT (Ahmed, 2020).
  - Right heart disease known as carcinoid heart disease is due to cardiac valve fibrosis results from 5-HT overproduction. The tricuspid and pulmonary valves are most affected, resulting in regurgitation, cardiac insufficiency, and dysrhythmias.
    - Carcinoid heart disease generally presents with symptoms consistent with right heart failure with systolic murmur along the left sternal edge.
    - Carcinoid heart disease should be managed with a multidisciplinary team including gastroenterologists, oncologists, endocrinologists, cardiologists, and surgeons.
    - Since the introduction of somatostatin analogs (SSAs), the risk for carcinoid heart disease has decreased.

Functional Pancreatic Neuroendocrine Tumors

- Functional pNETs have a variety of symptoms related to cell type and the hormone secreted.
- There are 10 commonly recognized pNETs, of which 9 are associated with a functional syndrome. The most common functional pNETs are discussed below.

Insulinomas

- Insulinomas secrete insulin and are most often benign pNET. Symptoms include the following:
  - Severe hypoglycemia (in the majority of patients)
  - Weakness
  - Sweating
  - Fainting
  - Confusion
  - Vision changes

Gastrinomas

- Gastrinomas are NETs of the pancreas or duodenum and secrete gastrin causing the following symptoms:
  - Severe peptic ulcer disease (i.e., Zollinger-Ellison syndrome) with decreased response to medical interventions
  - Abdominal pain
  - Bleeding
  - Vomiting
  - Diarrhea
  - Chronic reflux leading to complications normally seen with reflux disease
  - Vitamin B_{12} deficiency

Glucagonomas

- Glucagonomas are a type of pNET typically of the islet cells which secrete glucagon leading to the following symptoms:
  - Glucose intolerance
  - Migratory necrolytic erythema (80% of cases), characterized by a raised erythematous patch beginning in the perineum and spreading to the trunk
  - Weight loss
  - Diabetes mellitus (in the majority of patients)
  - Anemia
  - Stomatitis
  - High rate of thromboembolic events
  - Symptoms are also known as the *four Ds*: dermatosis, depression, deep vein thrombosis, and diarrhea.

VIPomas

- VIPomas also arise from the islet cells of the pancreas and secrete excessive quantities of vasoactive intestinal peptide, and symptoms include the following:
  - Profound secretory diarrhea (>3 L/day)
  - Hypokalemia
  - Achlorhydria

Functional Bronchopulmonary Neuroendocrine Tumors

- Carcinoid syndrome (described earlier for GI NETs) may occur in patients with bronchopulmonary NETs (described earlier for GI NETs), leading providers down the wrong path when looking for the primary tumor site.
- Presentation with hormonal fluctuations and paraneoplastic syndromes, such as those seen in small cell lung cancer, is possible.
- Patients with bronchopulmonary NETs may present with ectopic Cushing syndrome may be diagnosed with a bronchopulmonary NET.

Diagnostic Work-up

- NETs are rare and understandably due to the symptoms of carcinoid syndrome often mistaken for IBS.
- The subtle differences are outlined here, and a thorough investigation may lead providers to an earlier diagnosis, especially if the patient is not responding to IBS therapy.
  - IBS is typically diagnosed at a younger age, usually below 45 years.
  - Flushing, wheezing, or difficulty breathing may help differentiate carcinoid syndrome from IBS.
  - Patients with carcinoid syndrome are more likely to experience weight loss and should be considered a "red flag symptom" that there may be an underlying cause for diarrhea.
  - Those experiencing carcinoid syndrome often have various abdominal symptoms for many years without a confirmatory diagnosis (Nall, 2017).
- Laboratory evaluations
  - Test for 24-hour urinary 5-hydroxyindoleacetic acid (5-HIAA) level.
    - Foods to be avoided for 48 hours before testing include avocados, bananas or plantains, cantaloupe or honeydew melon, eggplant, pineapples, plums, tomatoes, kiwi, dates, grapefruit, and hickory nuts, pecans, or walnuts.
    - Coffee, alcohol, and smoking should be avoided.
  - Fasting serum 5-HIAA level (optional).
  - Chromogranin A is elevated in the majority of patients with NETs.
    - Can be elevated in functioning and nonfunctioning tumors.
    - Proton pump inhibitors should be withheld prior to testing because they can cause a false-positive result.
- Laboratory studies unique to specific functioning NETs.

Insulinoma

- Insulinomas for which a positive diagnosis is an inappropriately elevated level of insulin in the face of hypoglycemia during a 72-hour fast.
  - Serum insulin level of more than 10 µU/mL (normal <6 µU/mL)
  - Glucose level of less than 40 mg/dL
  - C-peptide level of more than 2.5 ng/mL (normal <2 ng/mL)
  - Plasma proinsulin level of more than 25% (up to 90%) that of immunoreactive insulin levels
  - Screening result for sulfonylurea is negative.

Gastrinoma

- Positive fasting hypergastrinemia of more than 150 pg/mL (for levels >1000, consider Zollinger-Ellison syndrome)
- Basal acid output of more than 10 mEq/h
- Intravenous secretin stimulation test result of more than 200 pg/mL in 2 minutes is positive for gastrinoma.
- Gastric pH of less than 3.0
- Elevated human chorionic gonadotropin levels

Glucagonoma

- Plasma glucagon levels of 500 to 1000 pg/mL
- Complete blood count and chemistry panel, including fasting blood sugar and liver enzyme levels

VIPoma

- Elevated plasma VIP level that is 2 to 10 times the normal range; patient must be symptomatic at the time of testing
- Secretory diarrhea volume of more than 700 mL/day
- Hypokalemia
- Achlorhydria
- Imaging evaluations
  - Octreotide scan or somatostatin receptor scintigraphy; the patient is injected with radiolabeled octreotide and evaluated for tumor uptake of the medication.
  - Abdominal/pelvic multiphasic computerized tomography or magnetic resonance imaging (MRI)
    - MRI with gadolinium contrast has been sensitive in finding insulinomas but not helpful for patients with glucagonomas.
  - Positron emission tomography
  - Bone scan if bone metastasis is suspected
  - Echocardiogram if carcinoid syndrome is identified
- Endoscopic procedures
  - Endoscopy
  - Bronchoscopy for the diagnosis of a lung carcinoid
  - Endoscopic ultrasound

Histolopathology

- Pathology reports should include unusual histologic features, such as clear cell, glandular, or oncocytic characteristics.
- The Ki-67 labeling index is useful for diagnosis, prognosis, and in the instance of an unusual presentation of aggressive NETs.

Pancreatic Neuroendocrine Tumors

- Most pNETs are well-differentiated islet cell or carcinoid-type tumors but in rare circumstances can be anaplastic.
- The tumor cells can be arranged in lobular acinar patterns.

Bronchopulmonary Neuroendocrine Tumors

- A well-differentiated, low-grade bronchopulmonary NET with fewer than two mitoses per 10 high-power fields (HPFs) and no necrosis is classified a typical carcinoid tumor of the lung.
- A well-differentiated, intermediate-grade NET with 2 to 10 mitoses per 10 HPFs and a focus of necrosis is an atypical carcinoid tumor of the lung.
- A poorly differentiated, high-grade NET with more than 10 mitoses per 10 HPFs is considered small cell carcinoma or a large cell NEC.

Clinical Staging

- After histologic identification of a NET, staging is based on the location of the tumor and applying the tumor size, lymph nodes, and metastasis system adopted by the American Joint Commission on Cancer.
- Grading of NETs is done according to the 2019 World Health Organization system.
  - G1: well-differentiated, low-grade NET with no necrosis, Ki-67 less than 3
  - G2: well-differentiated, intermediate-grade NET, Ki-67 from 3 to 20
  - G3: poorly differentiated, high-grade NET (rare), Ki-67 greater than 20
    - Appendix: 0.9%
    - Jejunum or ileum: 1.1%
    - Cecum: 14.2%
  - NEC, small cell type, poorly differentiated, high-grade, Ki-67 greater than 20
  - NEC, large cell type, poorly differentiated, high-grade, Ki-67 greater than 20
  - Mixed neuroendocrine-non-neuroendocrine neoplasm, well or poorly differentiated, variable Ki-67
- These are mostly seen in tumors of the appendix and cecum and are associated with poor prognosis.
- Clinical staging in combination with histopathology provide prognostic information that provides guidance in clinical therapy decision-making.

Treatment

- Treatment for NETs primarily depends on the location, grade, and stage of the tumor.
- Adjuvant therapy has not been beneficial.
- Current treatment options include surgical resection, SSA therapy, peptide receptor therapy, chemotherapy, and radiation.

Surgery

- For all NETs, surgical resection should be considered upfront if approximately 90% of the gross disease can be resected safely, per the 2013 North American Neuroendocrine Tumor Society (NANETS) consensus guidelines (Kunz et al., 2013).
- The National Comprehensive Cancer Network (NCCN) guidelines (2022) also confer that for locoregional NETs that are resectable, surgical excision is recommended.

Systemic Therapies

- SSAs have been used for decades to control symptoms of carcinoid syndrome, and in recent years were shown to improve progression-free survival as well. SSAs have been shown to induce tumor stabilization and may have some impact on tumor shrinkage in select cases.
  - Sandostatin LAR (long-acting release) and Somatuline Depot are injectable long-acting SSAs.

- Subcutaneous octreotide may be used for breakthrough symptoms such as excessive flushing or diarrhea.
- SSAs are generally well tolerated but common adverse events include nausea, abdominal pain, headache, dizziness, fatigue, and back pain. The drugs inhibit gallbladder contractions, which may result in gallbladder sludge or gallstones.
- The mTOR inhibitor, everolimus, is US Food and Drug Administration (FDA) approved for the treatment of progressive pNETs and progressive, well differentiated, nonfunctional GI NETs with unresectable locally advanced or metastatic disease.
- Sunitinib, an oral multi-targeted tyrosine kinase inhibitor is an antiangiogenic agent approved by the FDA for progressive, well differentiated pNETs with unresectable locally advanced or metastatic disease.
- Interferon-α is considered a second-line option for progressive NETs after SSAs. It has antiproliferative, pro-apoptotic, cytotoxic, and immunomodulatory effects, although data has not shown it to be highly effective. In addition, the agent induces several adverse events which has limited its use.
- Chemotherapy has a limited role for patients with NET. It is more likely to see utilization of chemotherapy in patients with midgut NETs with progressive disease (Herrera-Martinez et al., 2019).
  - Streptozocin plus 5-fluorouracil (5-FU)
  - Streptozocin plus doxorubicin
  - 5-FU, doxorubicin plus streptozocin
  - Temozolomide plus capecitabine

Peptide Receptor Radionuclide Therapy

- Peptide receptor radionuclide therapy (PRRT) is radioisotope therapy that uses radiolabeled octreotide. PRRT with lutetium 177 Lu dotatate (^{177}Lu-dotatate) is FDA approved for the treatment of somatostatin-receptor-positive NETs in the GI tract and pancreas in adults.
- When injected into the bloodstream, the radiopeptide travels to and binds to somatostatin receptors 2 and 5 on NET cells, delivering a high dose of radiation to the cancer cells. PRRT should be considered in the presence of disease progression.
- PRRT is generally well tolerated but adverse events including nausea, fatigue and abdominal pain have been reported. These symptoms are often related to an amino acid infusion that is given in combination with PRRT for kidney protection, and often resolve within 24 hours.

Local Therapies

- Hepatic embolization can be used for palliation of patients with bulky liver disease who are not candidates for surgery.
  - Embolization decreases hormone levels and side effects of the disease.

Prognosis

- While most NETs are known for their slowly progressive nature and well-differentiated histology, incidence and prevalence have increased in recent years.

- Nearly half of NET patients are not diagnosed until the disease has become advanced. The earlier the diagnosis and intervention, the better the outcome.
- The location of the primary tumor affects the extent of metastatic disease. For instance, NETs that start in the ileum or jejunum are more likely to have distant metastasis at diagnosis than those that start in the rectum.
- The 5-year survival rate for NETs varies by site of origin: 40.9% for colon, 44.2% for small intestine tumors, 38.3% for stomach tumors, 22.7% for pancreas, and 33.7% for lung and bronchus tumors (Man et al., 2018).

Prevention and Surveillance

- There are no preventative measures recommended by National Cancer Institute, American Cancer Society, or NCCN for NETs.
- Surveillance recommendations for NETs include recommendations for patients with resected disease follow-up every 3 to 6 months after curative resection and then every 6 to 12 months for at least 7 years. The maximum duration of follow-up has not been defined by NANETS (Kunz et al., 2013).
- Per the NCCN (2022), after potentially curative surgery, imaging surveillance is recommended for at least 10 years.
  - For patients with higher risk factors or greater risk of recurrence, this may be extended.
  - For patients with a hereditary cancer risk, such as MEN1/2 or VHL, surveillance is recommended at differing intervals based on the genetic mutation and prognostic risk.

References

Ahmed, M. (2020). Gastrointestinal neuroendocrine tumors in 2020. *World Journal of Gastrointestinal Oncology, 12*(8), 791–807.

Chittiboina, P., & Lonser, R. R. (2015). Von Hippel-Lindau disease. *Handbook of Clinical Neurology, 132*, 139–156.

Dasari, A., Shen, C., Halperin, D., Zhao, B., Zhou, S., Xu, Y., … Yao, J. C. (2017). Trends in the incidence, prevalence, and survival outcomes in patients with neuroendocrine tumors in the United States. *JAMA Oncology, 3*(10), 1335–1342.

Herrera-Martínez, A. D., Hofland, J., Hofland, L. J., Brabander, T., Eskens, F. A. L. M., Gálvez Moreno, M. A., … Feelders, R. A. (2019). Targeted systemic treatment of neuroendocrine tumors: current options and future perspectives. *Drugs, 79*(1), 21–42.

Ito, T., Igarashi, H., & Jensen, R. T. (2012). Pancreatic neuroendocrine tumors: Clinical features, diagnosis and medical treatment: Advances. *Best Practice and Research. Clinical Gastroenterology, 26*(6), 737–753.

Kamilaris, C., & Stratakis, C. A. (2019). Multiple endocrine neoplasia type 1 (MEN1): An update and the significance of early genetic and clinical diagnosis. *Frontiers in Endocrinology, 10*, 339.

Kunz, P. L., Reidy-Lagunes, D., Anthony, L. B., Bertino, E. M., Brendtro, K., Chan, J. A., … North American Neuroendocrine Tumor Society. (2013). Consensus guidelines for the management and treatment of neuroendocrine tumors. *Pancreas, 42*(4), 557–577.

Man, D., Wu, J., Shen, Z., & Zhu, X. (2018). Prognosis of patients with neuroendocrine tumor: a SEER database analysis. *Cancer Management and Research, 10*, 5629–5638.

Nall, R. (2017). Irritable bowel syndrome vs. carcinoid syndrome. *Healthline*. Available at https://www.healthline.com/health/carcinoid-syndrome/ibs-vs-carcinoid-syndrome.

Pieterman, C. R. C., van Leeuwaarde, R. S., van den Broek, M. F. M., van Nesselrooij, B. P. M., & Valk, G. D. (2021). Multiple endocrine neoplasia type 1. In K. R. Feingold, B. Anawalt, M.R. Blackman, et al. (Eds). Endotext. South Dartmouth, MA: MDText.com, Inc.

National Comprehensive Cancer Network (NCCN). (2022). Neuroendocrine and adrenal tumors (version 1.2022). Available at https://www.nccn.org/professinals/physician_gls/pdf/neuroendocrine.pdf.

Sarcomas

Rupa Ghosh-Berkebile

Bone Sarcomas

General Principles

Overview

Bone sarcomas are extremely rare, accounting for fewer than 0.2% of all cancers in the United States. The rate of new cases of bone and joint cancer was 1 per 100,000 men and women per year (National Cancer Institute [NCI], 2021). Approximately 0.1% of men and women will be diagnosed with bone sarcoma during their lifetime. Bone sarcomas tend to occur in males more than females and the non-Hispanic White and Black populations over other ethnicities (NCI, 2021).

- In 2021, an estimated 3610 new cases of bone sarcoma were diagnosed in the United States, and an estimated 2060 people died from the disease (Siegel et al., 2021).
- The 5-year relative survival is 66.8%. The most common types of bone sarcomas in adults are chondrosarcoma (40%), osteosarcoma (28%), Ewing sarcoma (8%), and undifferentiated pleomorphic sarcoma (UPS) of bone/fibrosarcoma (National Comprehensive Cancer Network [NCCN], 2022).
- In children and adolescents, the most common occurring types are osteosarcoma and Ewing sarcoma.

Management Considerations

Because bone sarcomas are so rare, it is important to seek treatment or refer patients to an established sarcoma center with a multidisciplinary team of physicians consisting of an orthopedic oncologist, sarcoma medical oncologist, sarcoma radiation oncologist, sarcoma or bone pathologist, and musculoskeletal radiologist. Having a team that includes plastic surgeons, vascular surgeons, physical therapists, and survivorship experts in sarcoma is also beneficial. Bone sarcomas frequently affect individuals of childbearing age, so fertility preservation options should be discussed prior to the beginning of treatment (Oktay et al., 2018; NCCN, 2022).

Biopsy Considerations

Biopsies of bone sarcomas are challenging because of the heterogeneity of the tumor. A complete imaging work-up for staging should be completed prior to biopsy (Liu et al., 2007). The biopsy should be directed at the most aggressive component of the tumor and should be performed at a sarcoma center where definitive treatment can be given.

Proper biopsy technique is crucial to avoid seeding the biopsy tract with tumor cells, which can lead to adverse patient outcomes and higher morbidity. Appropriate communication with the surgeon and radiologist is important in obtaining a suitable biopsy specimen.

- A core-needle biopsy or an open biopsy by an experienced sarcoma surgeon or sarcoma surgical pathologist are preferred.
- Typically, an incisional (rather than excisional) biopsy specimen is obtained from soft tissue extension of the tumor. Definitive surgery should include removal of the entire biopsy tract (Liu et al., 2007; NCCN, 2022).

References

Liu, P. T., Valadez, S. D., Chivers, F. S., Roberts, C. C., & Beauchamp, C. P. (2007). Anatomically based guidelines for core needle biopsy of bone tumors: Implications for limb-sparing surgery. *Radiographics: A Review Publication of the Radiological Society of North America, Inc, 27*(1), 189–206.

National Cancer Institute, Surveillance, Epidemiology and End Results (SEER) Program. (2021). SEER cancer statistics fact sheets: Bone and joint cancer. Available at https://seer.cancer.gov/statfacts/html/bones.html.

National Comprehensive Cancer Network. (2022). NCCN clinical practice guidelines in oncology: Bone cancer (version 2.2022). Available at http://www.nccn.org/professionals/physician_gls/pdf/bone.pdf.

Oktay, K., Harvey, B. E., & Partridge, A. H. (2018). Fertility preservation in patients with cancer: ASCO clinical practice guideline update. *Journal of Clinical Oncology: Official Journal of the American Society of Clinical Oncology, 36*(19), 1994–2001.

Siegel, R., Miller, K., Fuchs, H., & Jemal, A. (2021). Cancer statistics, 2021. *CA: A Journal for Cancer Clinicians, 71*(1), 7–33.

Chondrosarcoma

Definition

Chondrosarcomas are a group of malignant bone tumors that arise from the cartilage matrix. They are classified as primary or secondary lesions. They can range from low-grade tumors with a low risk of metastasis to high-grade tumors with a high risk of distant metastasis.

Incidence

- Chondrosarcoma is the most common bone sarcoma in adults and the second most common form of bone cancer overall, accounting for 20% to 27% of bone cancers in the United States (Lakshmanan, 2020).
- Chondrosarcoma can occur at any age, but it is usually diagnosed in middle-age (Lakshmanan, 2020).
- The most common primary sites of occurrence are the pelvis and the proximal femur (NCCN, 2022).

Etiology and Risk Factors

Chondrosarcomas characteristically produce cartilage matrices from neoplastic tissue.

Typically, no osteoid or bone-forming tissue is involved. Conventional chondrosarcomas account for about 90%

Major Cancers ②

of all chondrosarcomas and are divided into two groups (Weinschenk et al., 2021):

- Primary or central lesions, which arise from previously normal-appearing bone preformed from cartilage; and
- Secondary or peripheral tumors, which arise or develop from previously benign cartilage lesions, such as enchondromas, or osteochondromas (Suster et al., 2020).
- Secondary tumors resulting from the malignant transformation of typically benign bone lesions have been reported in patients with (Suster et al., 2020):
  - Ollier disease (enchondromatosis), a rare skeletal condition that results in abnormal bone development, leading to increased growth of the long bone cartilage resulting in cartilage masses (enchondromas) and thinning of cortical bone.
  - Maffucci syndrome, which describes enchondromatosis accompanied by soft tissue hemangiomas.
  - Malignant hereditary exostoses, a genetic condition in which multiple benign bone tumors (exostoses) develop primarily at the end of long bones and on flat bones such as the scapula and pelvis.
  - Isocitrate dehydrogenase (IDH1 or IDH2) mutations are associated with approximately 50% of all chondrosarcomas and almost all cases of secondary chondrosarcoma from Ollier disease or Maffucci syndrome (Amary et al., 2011). Typically these tumors are slower in onset and of low grade.
- In addition to conventional chondrosarcomas, there are other rare subtypes that account for 10% to 15% of all chondrosarcomas. These include clear cell, mesenchymal, juxtacortical, dedifferentiated, and myxoid types (NCCN, 2022).
- Risk factors also include Paget disease and radiation injury to the area.
- Alterations in the retinoblastoma (RB) pathway are present in a significant number of clear cell, mesenchymal, and dedifferentiated chondrosarcomas.

Signs and Symptoms

Symptoms of chondrosarcoma depend on tumor size and location. Patients with pelvic or axial lesions are typically diagnosed later in the disease course because the associated pain has a more insidious onset and often occurs when the tumor has reached a significant size. The mean interval from pain to diagnosis is 15 to 19 months (NCCN, 2022).

Clinical signs and symptoms of chondrosarcomas typically include the following:

- Pain: described as a deep, dull ache
- Night pain
- Decreased range of motion in the affected joint
- Paresthesias or nerve dysfunction if the tumor encroaches on the lumbosacral plexus or neurovascular bundle
- Pathologic fracture (primary symptom in 50% of dedifferentiated chondrosarcomas; Weinschenk et al., 2021)

Diagnostic Work-up

- Computed tomography (CT) of the chest, abdomen, and pelvis; bone scan; and positron emission tomography (PET) may be used for staging of the tumor and evaluation for systemic disease.

- Imaging of the primary lesion includes the following (Ollivier et al., 2003):
  - Plain radiography
    - Typically reveals large (>5 cm), cartilaginous lesions with evidence of discrete calcification ("stippled" appearance).
    - Lytic lesions are well defined, with endosteal scalloping and cortical thinning.
    - Shows cortical destruction and loss of medullary bone trabeculations, especially in high-grade or dedifferentiated lesions.
  - Serial radiography
    - Demonstrates a slow increase in size of the osteochondroma or enchondroma.
    - Demonstrates growth in a previously stable exostosis or enchondroma in an adult.
    - Reveals decreased calcification and increased lysis.
    - A cartilage "cap" measuring greater than 2 cm on a preexisting lesion or documented growth after skeletal maturity should raise the suspicion of sarcomatous transformation.
  - Magnetic resonance imaging (MRI)
    - Shows intramedullary involvement and extraosseous extension of the tumor.
    - Delineates extent of soft tissue involvement.
    - Is useful in preoperative planning.

Histopathology

The histologic grade and location of the chondrosarcoma are important in treatment decisions. There are three histologic grades based on cellularity, atypia, and pleomorphism (Weinschenk et al., 2021):

- Grade I (low grade): Intra-compartmental, cytologically similar to enchondroma with higher cellularity.
- Grade II (intermediate grade): Characterized by definitive increased cellularity, distinct nucleoli, and possible foci of myxoid change. Often treated as a high-grade tumor.
- Grade III (high grade): Characterized by high cellularity, prominent atypical nuclei, increased mitotic rate.
  - Dedifferentiated chondrosarcomas are high-grade lesions and should be treated as osteosarcoma; they exhibit bimorphic histology, with a low-grade chondroid component and a high-grade spindle cell component (NCCN, 2022).
  - Mesenchymal chondrosarcomas are treated as Ewing sarcoma according to their grade (NCCN, 2022).

Clinical Staging

- The American Joint Committee on Cancer (AJCC) TNM (Tumor, Nodes and Metastasis) staging system for bone sarcomas is used for all bone sarcomas (Amin et al., 2017).
- The Surgical Staging System (SSS) is also used for staging of musculoskeletal sarcomas (Enneking et al., 1980). Like the AJCC system, the SSS determines stage based on tumor, tumor grade, and the presence of metastasis (see table on the next page).

Surgical Staging System

Stage	Grade	Site
IA	Low (G1)	Intracompartmental (T1)
IB	Low (G1)	Extracompartmental (T2)
IIA	High (G2)	Intracompartmental (T1)
IIB	High (G2)	Extracompartmental (T2)
III	Any (G) and regional or distant metastasis	Any (T)

Data from Enneking, W. F., Spanier, S. S., & Goodman, M. A. (1980). A system for the surgical staging of musculoskeletal sarcoma. *Clinical Orthopaedics and Related Research, 153,* 106–120; National Comprehensive Cancer Network. (2022). *NCCN clinical practice guidelines in oncology: Bone cancer, version 2.* Available at http://www.nccn.org/professionals/physician_gls/pdf/bone.pdf.

Treatment

Surgery

(Lakshmanan, 2020)

- Surgery is the preferred primary treatment for chondrosarcoma.
- Patients with resectable low-grade or intracompartmental lesions are treated with intralesional excision or wide excision with negative surgical margins (R0 resection). This may be achieved by limb salvage or amputation.
- High-grade lesions (grade II, III, clear cell, or extracompartmental) are surgically treated with wide excision, obtaining negative surgical margins. This may be achieved by limb salvage or amputation.
- Re-resection may be necessary to achieve negative margins.

Radiation Therapy

- High-dose photons are used to treat high-grade, clear cell, or extracompartmental lesions and is a consideration for unresectable low-grade lesions (NCCN, 2022).
- Preoperative radiation therapy (RT) may be considered if microscopic residual disease (R1 resection) or positive margins (R2 resection) are likely, followed by postoperative RT.
- Postoperative RT may be considered after R1 or R2 resection for high-grade, dedifferentiated, or mesenchymal chondrosarcomas.
- For unresectable disease (low-grade or high-grade lesions), consider high-dose therapy, with specialized techniques such as intensity-modulated RT, stereotactic radiosurgery, or fractionated stereotactic RT, to maximize tissue sparing and limit toxicities.
- Proton beam RT is used to treat unresectable or recurrent disease in a previously radiated site (Hug & Slater, 2000).

Systemic Therapy

- Systemic therapy is considered for primary treatment in mesenchymal and dedifferentiated chondrosarcomas (van Maldegem et al., 2019).
- It can be considered for metastatic chondrosarcomas.
  - For oligometastatic sites, surgical excision or radiation are preferred.
  - For widespread disease:
    - Consider surgery, ablation, or radiation to specific sites for symptom control.
    - Use comprehensive genomic profiling with a US Food and Drug Administration (FDA)-approved assay to determine if targeted therapy, such as pazopanib or dasatinib, are options.
    - Consider testing for tumor mutational burden or programmed cell death protein 1 (PD-1) and programmed death-ligand 1 (PD-L1) expression for use of pembrolizumab.
- Clinical trial eligibility should always be a consideration.

Treatment for Recurrence

- Local recurrence (low and high grade)
  - Wide excision with surveillance if R0 resection.
  - Wide excision with RT if R1 or R2 resection.
  - Unresectable recurrences are treated with either conventional or specialized RT techniques (intensity-modulated, proton beam, stereotactic radiosurgery).

Prognosis

- The most important prognostic indicators are anatomic location, size of the lesion, and histologic grade.
- Late metastases and recurrences after 10 years are more common with chondrosarcoma than with other sarcomas.
- The 10-year survival rate is 83% for grade I and 64% for II tumors with a low potential for metastasis. The 10-year survival rate is reported to be 29% for grade III tumors, which have a 66% potential for metastasis (Weinschenk et al., 2021).
- The most common site for metastasis is the lungs.
- Dedifferentiated chondrosarcomas have the greatest metastatic potential, with a median survival of 11 months after diagnosis (NCCN, 2022).

Prevention and Surveillance

Prevention

- Many of the risk factors, such as race, age, or certain bone diseases or inherited conditions, cannot be changed.
- Other than prior RT, there is no known lifestyle or environmental factor that causes chondrosarcoma, so there is no way to prevent chondrosarcoma.
- For patients with Ollier disease, Maffucci syndrome, or multiple hereditary exostosis, close monitoring with serial images is indicated for earlier detection of secondary transformation into chondrosarcoma (Amary et al., 2011).

Surveillance

(NCCN, 2022)

- Low-grade lesions
  - Physical examination
  - Imaging of the lesion and chest radiography every 6 to 12 months for 2 years, then yearly as appropriate
- High-grade lesions
  - Physical examination
  - Primary site or cross-sectional imaging as indicated
  - Chest imaging every 3 to 6 months for the first 5 years and yearly thereafter for a minimum of 10 years

Bibliography

Amary, M. F., Damato, S., Halai, D., Eskandarpour, M., Berisha, F., Bonar, F., ... Aston, W. (2011). Ollier disease and Maffucci syndrome are caused by somatic mosaic mutations of IDH1 and IDH2. *Nature Genetics, 43*(12), 1262–1265.

Amin, M. B., Greene, F. L., Edge, S. B., Compton, C. C., Gershenwald, J. E., Brookland, R. K., ... Winchester, D. P. (2017). The Eighth Edition AJCC Cancer Staging Manual: Continuing to build a bridge from a population-based to a more "personalized" approach to cancer staging. *CA: A Cancer Journal for Clinicians*, 67(2), 93–99. https://doi.org/10.3322/caac.21388.

Bernstein-Molho, R., Kollender, Y., Issakov, J., Bickels, J., Dadia, S., Flusser, G., ... Merimsky, O. (2012). Clinical activity of mTOR inhibition in combination with cyclophosphamide in the treatment of recurrent unresectable chondrosarcomas. *Cancer Chemotherapy and Pharmacology*, 70(6), 855–860.

Enneking, W. F., Spanier, S. S., & Goodman, M. A. (1980). A system for the surgical staging of musculoskeletal sarcoma. *Clinical Orthopaedics and Related Research*, 153, 106–120.

Hug, E. B., & Slater, J. D. (2000). Proton radiation therapy for chordomas and chondrosarcomas of the skull base. *Neurosurgery Clinics of North America*, 11(4), 627–638.

Lakshmanan, P. (2020). Chondrosarcoma. In *Medscape*. http://emedicine.medscape.com/article/1258236-overview#a2.

Liu, P. T., Valadez, S. D., Chivers, F. S., Roberts, C. C., & Beauchamp, C. P. (2007). Anatomically based guidelines for core needle biopsy of bone tumors: Implications for limb-sparing surgery. *Radiographics: A Review Publication of the Radiological Society of North America, Inc*, 27(1), 189–206.

National Cancer Institute, Surveillance, Epidemiology and End Results (SEER) Program. (2021). SEER Cancer Statistics Fact Sheets: Bone and joint cancer. Available at https://seer.cancer.gov/statfacts/html/bones.html.

National Comprehensive Cancer Network. (2022). NCCN clinical practice guidelines in oncology: Bone cancer (version 2.2022). Available at http://www.nccn.org/professionals/physician_gls/pdf/bone.pdf.

Ollivier, L., Vanel, D., & Leclère, J. (2003). Imaging of chondrosarcomas. *Cancer Imaging: The Official Publication of the International Cancer Imaging Society*, 4(1), 36–38.

Siegel, R., Miller, K., Fuchs, H., & Jemal, A. (2021). Cancer statistics, 2021. *CA: A Journal for Cancer Clinicians*, 71(1), 7–33.

Suster, D., Hung, Y. P., & Nielsen, G. P. (2020). Differential diagnosis of cartilaginous lesions of bone. *Archives of Pathology & Laboratory Medicine*, 144(1), 71–82.

van Maldegem, A., Conley, A. P., Rutkowski, P., Patel, S. R., Lugowska, I., Desar, I. M., ... Gelderblom, H. (2019). Outcome of first-line systemic treatment for unresectable conventional, dedifferentiated, mesenchymal, and clear cell chondrosarcoma. *The Oncologist*, 24(1), 110–116.

Weinschenk, R. C., Wang, W. L., & Lewis, V. O. (2021). Chondrosarcoma. *The Journal of the American Academy of Orthopaedic Surgeons*, 29(13), 553–562.

Ewing Sarcoma Family of Tumors

Definition

Ewing sarcoma is a type of primary bone cancer that originates from a primordial, bone marrow–derived mesenchymal stem cell (National Cancer Institute [NCI], 2022). In 2020, the World Health Organization (WHO) modified its classification of bone and soft tissue tumors to include a separate chapter on undifferentiated small round cell tumors, which includes Ewing sarcoma, round cell sarcomas with EWSR1-non ETS fusions, CIC-rearranged sarcomas, and sarcomas with BCOR mutations (Choi & Ro, 2021). Ewing sarcoma, primitive neuroectodermal tumor (PNET), Askin tumor (Ewing sarcoma of the chest wall), PNET of bone, and extraosseous Ewing sarcoma are all included in the Ewing sarcoma family of tumors (Bernstein et al., 2006).

Incidence

- Ewing sarcoma is the third most common form of bone cancer and accounts for 16% of all bone cancer cases (NCCN, 2022).
- In 2022, the Surveillance, Epidemiology, and End Results (SEER) program reported an incidence of approximately one case per 1 million persons per year. This incidence has remained unchanged for the past 30 years. In children and adolescents, the incidence is 9 to 10 cases per 1 million people (NCI, 2021).
- Ewing sarcoma develops mainly in adolescents and young adults. The median age at diagnosis is 15 years, and 50% of patients are adolescents (NCI, 2022).

The incidence among non-Hispanic Whites is nine times that among Blacks, and the incidence is higher in males than females. Incidence is lower in Asians, possibly related to a polymorphism in the epidermal growth factor receptor 2 (*EGFR2*) gene (NCI, 2022).

- Most common primary sites are diaphysis of the femur (41%), pelvis (26%), and bones of the chest wall (16%) (NCI, 2022).
- For extraosseous Ewing sarcoma, the most common sites are the trunk (42%), extremities (26%), and head and neck (18%) (NCI, 2022).

Etiology and Risk Factors

- There are no clear risk factors specific to Ewing sarcoma; risk factors are generally similar to those of other bone sarcomas.
- Ewing sarcoma is characterized by fusion of the EWS gene (*EWSR1*) on chromosome 22q12 with the ETS gene family, which includes *FLI1*, *ERG*, *ETV1*, *ETV4*, and *FEV*. The fusion transcript is present in approximately 85% of Ewing sarcoma patients (NCI, 2022).

Signs and Symptoms

- There is localized pain or swelling, with a median duration of 2 to 5 months before diagnosis.
- It is sometimes accompanied by paresthesias or neuropathy.
- It is often mistaken for growing pains or a sports injury.
- Constitutional symptoms such as fever, weight loss, and fatigue are frequently observed on presentation.
- Approximately 25% of patients have metastatic disease at the time of diagnosis (NCI, 2022).
- Common sites of metastatic disease are lung, bone, and bone marrow.

Diagnostic Work-up

- If an Ewing family tumor is suspected as a diagnosis, the patient should undergo a complete staging before biopsy (NCCN, 2022).
- Imaging of the primary lesions includes the following modalities:
  - Plain radiographs of primary site
    - Destructive lesion with a "moth-eaten" appearance; may have reactive bone formation
    - Periosteal reaction is classic and is referred to as "onion skin" by radiologists
  - MRI of the entire involved bone or area
    - Identifies soft tissue extension and possible bone marrow involvement
    - Evaluates relationship of tumor to neurovascular structures and adjacent joints
  - CT of the chest
    - Identifies pulmonary metastasis
  - Bone scan
    - Evaluate for distant osseous metastasis

- PET scan
  - Initial staging of disease
  - Identification of lymph node disease
  - The combination of PET or PET/CT with conventional imaging has 96% sensitivity and 92% specificity (Treglia et al., 2012).
- MRI of the spine and pelvis should be considered to evaluate for distant metastasis if they are not the site of the primary tumor.
- Laboratory studies include the following:
  - Complete blood count: anemia, leukocytosis
  - Lactate dehydrogenase (LDH): elevated (prognostic value as a tumor marker)
  - Alkaline phosphatase (ALP): elevated
  - Erythrocyte sedimentation rate: elevated
- Cytogenetic analysis or comprehensive genomic profiling of the biopsy specimen to evaluate the t(11;22) translocation (NCCN, 2022)
  - Helpful if targeted polymerase chain reaction, fluorescence in situ hybridization (FISH) are negative to identify translocations as possible targets for treatment.
- Bone marrow biopsy should be considered to complete the work-up.
- Consider obtaining circulating tumor DNA (ctDNA) in blood (Shulman et al., 2018)

Histopathology

- The EWS-FLI1 fusion protein and its corresponding chromosomal translocation, t(11;22)(q24;q12), are identified in 85% of patients with Ewing sarcoma by FISH (Denny, 1996).
- Other fusion proteins occur in 5% to 10% of tumors, including some with *FUS* substitutions for the *EWS* gene (NCCN, 2022).
- There is strong expression of cell surface glycoprotein MIC2 (CD99).
- The tumor exhibits sheets of small round blue cells with prominent nuclei and minimal cytoplasm.
- "Rosettes" are present (tumor cells arranged in a circle around a necrotic center).

Clinical Staging

The American Joint Commission on Cancer (AJCC) staging system, which is based on tumor size, nodal involvement, and presence or absence of distant metastases, is used for all bone sarcomas (Amin et al., 2017).

The SSS is also used for staging musculoskeletal sarcomas. The SSS determines stage based on tumor, tumor grade, and the presence of metastasis (see Surgical Staging System table on page 178) (Enneking, 1980).

Treatment

(NCCN, 2022)

Surgery

- Surgery is the preferred approach but is rarely considered at initial diagnosis; preoperative chemotherapy is recommended (NCI, 2022).

- Surgery is used for local control. The surgical procedure includes wide excision after 12 weeks of multiagent chemotherapy if the patient had a good response or if there was disease progression.
- Amputation may be required in some cases.

Radiation Therapy

- RT is recommended for R1 or R2 resections; it is usually given concurrently with chemotherapy.
- Definitive RT for treatment of primary tumor is given after 12 weeks of primary systemic therapy (see "Systemic Therapy" below).
- RRT is given for unresponsive or progressive disease after 12 weeks of primary systemic therapy, with or without surgery for local control and palliation.

Systemic Therapy

(NCCN, 2022)

- Neoadjuvant and adjuvant chemotherapy are effective for localized disease at diagnosis and have improved outcomes for disease-free and progression-free survival.
- First-line chemotherapy for localized and metastatic disease typically includes a combination of the following drugs (known as VDC-IE): vincristine, doxorubicin, cyclophosphamide (usually alternating with ifosfamide), and etoposide.
  - Chemotherapy is administered over 49 weeks, including chemotherapy given before local therapy.
  - VDC-IE given every 2 weeks was found to be more effective than the traditional every-3-week schedule with no increase in toxicity in patients younger than 40 years of age.
    - Dactinomycin may be substituted for doxorubicin after the patient's maximum lifetime anthracycline dose is reached or if there is concern for cardiac toxicity.
- Second-line therapy for relapsed, refractory, or metastatic disease includes a combination of the following drugs: cabozatinib, docetaxel, gemcitabine, cyclophosphamide, topotecan, irinotecan, temozolamide, carboplatin, and etoposide, as well as ifosfamide (Italiano et al., 2020; NCCN, 2022).
- The dosing and drug combinations are typically myelosuppressive, and the use of myeloid growth factors is highly recommended.
- Patients are evaluated after 12 weeks of multiagent chemotherapy. If there is a good response to chemotherapy, the patient can proceed to one of the following:
  - Additional chemotherapy followed by definitive RT to the primary tumor and/or metastatic sites.
  - Wide excision of the tumor with adjuvant chemotherapy for negative margins (R0 resection) or adjuvant chemotherapy and concurrent RT for microscopic or gross positive margins (R1 or R2 resection).
  - Amputation in selected cases, followed by adjuvant chemotherapy and concurrent RT, depending on margin status.
- Fertility preservation should be discussed at the time of diagnosis because pelvic surgery, RT, and chemotherapy regimens can cause infertility.

Treatment of Recurrence

- The relapse rate is 30% to 40%. Relapse is associated with a poorer prognosis (Robinson et al., 2014).
- For early relapse (<2 years), second-line chemotherapies are recommended. Consider RT after chemotherapy if there is lung involvement.
- For late relapse (>2 years), rechallenge with the original chemotherapy regimen if the patient had a good response previously.
- Patients with late relapse, lung-only metastasis, local recurrence that is surgically resectable have a more favorable prognosis than those who have early relapse with multiple metastatic sites and an elevated LDH level (NCI, 2022).
- Clinical trials should be considered for patients with recurrent and metastatic disease.

Prognosis

- Previously, Ewing sarcoma was associated with a poor prognosis.
- The development of multiagent chemotherapy regimens for both neoadjuvant and adjuvant treatment has improved the prognosis greatly for patients with Ewing sarcoma:
  - The 5-year overall survival in patients with localized Ewing sarcoma is approximately 70% (NCI, 2022).
  - Even patients diagnosed with metastatic disease at presentation can achieve a cure.

Prevention and Surveillance

Prevention

- Many of the risk factors, such as race, age, or gender, cannot be changed.
- There is no known lifestyle or environmental factor that causes Ewing sarcoma, so there is no way to prevent Ewing sarcoma.

Surveillance

(NCCN, 2022)

- Physical examination and laboratory work.
- Chest imaging (CT scan or radiographs) and MRI or plain films of the extremity.
- Consider PET and/or bone scan.
- Evaluate every 3 months for the first 2 years, then every 4 months for the third year and every 6 months for the fourth and fifth years; then continue annually with chest radiographs and physical examination only.
- Long-term follow-up for late adverse effects is recommended. The most common late effects are cardiomyopathy, secondary cancers, permanent azoospermia, and renal impairment.

Bibliography

Amin, M., Gress, D., Meyer Vega, L., et al. (Eds.). (2017). *AJCC staging manual* (8th ed.). Springer.

Bernstein, M., Kovar, H., Paulussen, M., Randall, R. L., Schuck, A., … Juergensg, H. (2006). Ewing's sarcoma family of tumors: Current management. *The Oncologist*, 11(5), 503–519.

Choi, J. H., & Ro, J. Y. (2021). The 2020 WHO classification of tumors of soft tissue: Selected changes and new entities. *Advances in Anatomic Pathology*, 28(1), 44–58.

Denny, C. T. (1996). Gene rearrangements in Ewing's sarcoma. *Cancer Investigation*, 14, 83–88.

Enneking, W. F., Spanier, S. S., & Goodman, M. A. (1980). A system for the surgical staging of musculoskeletal sarcoma. *Clinical Orthopaedics and Related Research*, 153, 106–120.

Italiano, A., Mir, O., Mathoulin-Pelissier, S., Penel, N., Piperno-Neumann, S., Bompas, E., … Ray-Coquard, I. (2020). Cabozantinib in patients with advanced Ewing sarcoma or osteosarcoma (CABONE): A multicentre, single-arm, phase 2 trial. *The Lancet. Oncology*, 21(3), 446–455.

National Cancer Institute (NCI). (2022). *Ewing sarcoma and undifferentiated small round cell sarcomas of bone and soft tissue treatment (PDQ®)*. https://www.cancer.gov/types/bone/hp/ewing-treatment-pdq#_70.

National Cancer Institute, Surveillance, Epidemiology and End Results (SEER) Program. (2021). SEER cancer statistics fact sheets: Bone and joint cancer. Available at https://seer.cancer.gov/statfacts/html/bones.html.

National Comprehensive Cancer Network. (2022). NCCN clinical practice guidelines in oncology: Bone cancer (version 2.2022). Available at http://www.nccn.org/professionals/physician_gls/pdf/bone.pdf (accessed 26 March 2022).

Robinson, S. I., Ahmed, S. K., Okuno, S. H., Arndt, C. A., Rose, P. S., & Laack, N. N. (2014). Clinical outcomes of adult patients with relapsed Ewing sarcoma: A 30-year single-institution experience. *American Journal of Clinical Oncology*, 37(6), 585–591.

Shulman, D. S., Klega, K., Imamovic-Tuco, A., Clapp, A., Nag, A., Thorner, A. R., … Janeway, K. A. (2018). Detection of circulating tumour DNA is associated with inferior outcomes in Ewing sarcoma and osteosarcoma: A report from the Children's Oncology Group. *British Journal of Cancer*, 119(5), 615–621.

Siegel, R., Miller, K., Fuchs, H., & Jemal, A. (2021). Cancer statistics, 2021. *CA: A Journal for Cancer Clinicians*, 71(1), 7–33.

Treglia, G., Salsano, M., Stefanelli, A., Mattoli, M. V., Giordano, A., & Bonomo, L. (2012). Diagnostic accuracy of ^{18}F-FDG-PET and PET/CT in patients with Ewing sarcoma family tumours: A systematic review and a meta-analysis. *Skeletal Radiology*, 41(3), 249–256.

Womer, R. B., West, D. C., Krailo, M. D., Dickman, P. S., Pawel, B. R., Grier, H. E., … Weiss, A. R. (2012). Randomized controlled trial of interval-compressed chemotherapy for the treatment of localized Ewing sarcoma: A report from the Children's Oncology Group. *Journal of Clinical Oncology: Official Journal of the American Society of Clinical Oncology*, 30(33), 4148–4154.

Osteosarcoma

Definition

Osteosarcoma is a malignant bone tumor that produces malignant osteoid cells. It is thought to originate from primitive mesenchymal bone-forming cells. It is the oldest identified hominin cancer, dating back approximately 1.7 million years (Meltzer & Helman, 2021). Osteosarcomas can range from low-grade tumors with a low risk of metastasis to high-grade tumors with a high risk of distant metastasis.

Incidence

- Osteosarcomas is the most common form of bone cancer, accounting for 35% of bone cancers in the United States (NCCN, 2022).
- Osteosarcomas is the most common primary malignant bone tumor in children and young adults.
  - There is a bimodal age distribution pattern, with peaks in adolescence (10–14 years of age) and after 60 years of age (Zhao et al., 2021).
- Common sites for osteosarcoma are in the metaphysis of long tubular bones (such as the proximal humerus, the distal femur, and the proximal tibia). Rarely is osteosarcoma found in the spine, pelvis, or sacrum.

Etiology and Risk Factors

There are 11 known variants of osteosarcoma. High-grade intramedullary osteosarcoma, otherwise known as classic or conventional osteosarcoma, comprises 80% of all osteosarcomas. It is a high-grade spindle cell tumor that over-produces osteoid or immature bone. Other types include low-grade intramedullary, periosteal, and parosteal osteosarcomas.

The exact cause of osteosarcoma is unknown. Several risk factors have been identified, including the following:

- Rapid bone growth, as evidenced by the common occurrence of osteosarcoma in the metaphyseal area adjacent to the growth plate in long bones and increased incidence during the adolescent growth spurt
- Trauma, which has been implicated in the development of sarcoma, although a cause-and-effect relationship has not been identified
- Genetic predisposition also plays a role (Meltzer & Helman, 2021; NCI, 2022):
  - Bloom syndrome, a rare hereditary disorder with a mutation on the *BLM* gene, characterized by short stature and distinctive facial features
  - Li-Fraumeni syndrome, a familial syndrome that results in a germline mutation of the *TP53* gene, causing a cluster of cancers, including soft tissue sarcoma, osteosarcoma, premenopausal breast cancer, brain tumor, adrenocortical carcinoma, leukemia, and bronchoalveolar lung cancer diagnosed before age 46 years
  - Retinoblastoma (*RB*) gene mutation (risk is higher in patients with RB treated with RT)
  - Rothmund-Thomson syndrome, an autosomal recessive disorder with a mutation of the RECQL4 gene, associated with congenital bone defects, hair and skin dysplasias, hypogonadism, and cataracts
  - Diamond-Blackfan anemia, a defect in ribosomal proteins resulting in inherited pure cell aplasia, increased risk for myelodysplastic syndrome or acute myeloid leukemia; characterized by skeletal abnormalities
  - Werner syndrome, caused by a mutation on the *WRN* gene, characterized by features of premature aging and short stature
- Variants of osteosarcoma may be the result of the following:
  - Paget disease
  - Prior RT (radiation-induced osteosarcoma can occur 5–15 years after primary treatment for cancer)

Signs and Symptoms

- Clinical signs and symptoms of osteosarcoma include the following:
  - Pain, particularly with activity (in the beginning, pain is often described as intermittent and is often associated with an injury or diagnosed as a sprain or as growing pains)
  - Localized soft tissue swelling, with or without warmth or edema
  - Joint effusions
  - Limited range of motion
  - Pathologic fracture, usually with telangiectatic osteosarcoma
  - Rarely, constitutional symptoms (fevers, chills, night sweats)
- Osteosarcomas spread hematogenously with the lung being the most common metastatic site.

Diagnostic Work-up

Osteosarcoma usually manifests as a local lesion; however, there is concern for distant metastasis (NCCN, 2022).

Imaging of the primary lesion includes the following modalities:

- Plain radiographs:
  - Show cortical destruction, periosteal reaction, and irregular reactive bone formation (appearing as a "sunburst")
  - MRI
- Best study to define the extent of the lesion in the bone and in the soft tissues
  - Detects "skip" metastasis
  - Used to evaluate anatomic relationships with surrounding neurovascular structures
  - Essential for preoperative planning
- Bone scan
  - Usually uniformly abnormal at the lesion
  - May be useful in identifying any additional synchronous lesions
- CT scans
  - Useful in evaluating for metastatic disease
- PET scan
  - Pretreatment staging
  - Evaluation of response to chemotherapy
- Laboratory values
  - Complete blood count with differential and platelets (CBCD/P)
  - Comprehensive metabolic panel (CMP)
  - ALP and LDH—often elevated in osteosarcoma
- Biopsy of osteosarcoma lesions are challenging because of the heterogeneity of the tumor.
  - Failure to follow appropriate biopsy procedures may result in adverse patient outcomes and amputation of a potentially salvageable extremity (refer to Bone Sarcomas General Principles on page 176).

Histopathology

- Osteosarcoma is classified into two histopathologic subtypes: central and surface tumors (NCI, 2022)
  - Central, or intramedullary tumors, include conventional, telangiectatic, intraosseous well-differentiated, and small cell osteosarcomas.
    - Conventional osteosarcomas are the most common, characterized by areas of necrosis, atypical mitoses, and malignant osteoid formation (NCI, 2022).
    - Telangiectatic osteosarcomas can resemble nonmalignant bone lesions but are treated like conventional osteosarcomas.
    - Intraosseous well-differentiated and small cell osteosarcomas are very rare.
  - Surface or peripheral tumors including parosteal and periosteal variants.
  - Parosteal osteosarcomas are juxtacortical, low-grade, well-differentiated lesions arising from the bone surface. Most common in patients 20 to 30 years old (NCI, 2022).
  - Periosteal osteosarcoma is of intermediate to high grade in severity. It is a soft tissue mass with erosion of the bone cortex (NCI, 2022).

- High-grade surface osteosarcomas are rare, juxtacortical tumors that occur in 10% of osteosarcomas (NCCN, 2022).
- Extraskeletal osteosarcomas are considered soft tissue tumors and are treated as such.
- UPS of bone.

Clinical Staging

The AJCC TNM staging system for bone sarcomas is used for all bone sarcomas (Amin et al., 2017).

The SSS is also used for staging musculoskeletal sarcomas. Like the AJCC system, the SSS determines stage based on tumor, tumor grade, and the presence of metastasis (see Surgical Staging System table on page 178).

Treatment

(NCCN, 2022)

Surgery

- Surgery is the primary treatment modality for osteosarcoma and the best chance at long-term disease-free status and survival.
- The goal of wide excision is to achieve histologically negative surgical margins (R0 resection) for optimal local tumor control. To decrease the risk of distant metastasis. It often involves a multidisciplinary team of orthopedic, vascular, neurologic, and reconstructive plastic surgeons (NCCN, 2022).
- Local tumor control may be achieved by limb-sparing surgery or limb amputation.
  - Limb-sparing surgery is preferred if reasonable nerve and motor function can be preserved. It is used in 90% of surgical candidates. Limb sparing surgery is often preceded by neoadjuvant chemotherapy. It involves tumor resection with negative margins, followed by skeletal and soft tissue reconstruction (Meltzer & Helman, 2021).
  - Comparison of limb-sparing surgery versus amputation in patients with high-grade osteosarcoma has not shown a significant difference in overall survival or local recurrence rates.
  - However, there is a significant difference in functional outcomes, especially in patients who had a good histologic response to preoperative chemotherapy (Papakonstantinou et al., 2020).
- Low-grade intramedullary and surface osteosarcomas, such as parosteal lesions, are treated with wide excision as primary treatment.
- For intermediate and high-grade lesions (intramedullary and surface types), neoadjuvant chemotherapy is recommended before wide excision.

Radiation Therapy

- RT may be considered for high-grade osteosarcoma that remains unresectable after preoperative chemotherapy.
- RT may be considered for high-grade osteosarcoma that is resected with microscopic residual disease (R1 resection) or grossly positive surgical margins (R2 resection), followed by additional chemotherapy or surgical re-resection.

Systemic Therapy

- Neoadjuvant and adjuvant chemotherapy are effective for localized disease at diagnosis and have improved outcomes in disease-free and progression-free survival.
  - Neoadjuvant chemotherapy is preferred for high-grade osteosarcoma and can be considered in periosteal lesions. Selected elderly patients may benefit from immediate surgery.
  - Adjuvant chemotherapy should be used for patients with pathologic findings of high-grade disease after wide excision for suspected low-grade or periosteal sarcoma.
    - After wide excision, patients with high-grade osteosarcoma and a good histologic response (viable tumor is <10% of tumor area) should continue to receive several more cycles of the same chemotherapy.
    - Patients with a poor histologic response (viable tumor is $\geq$10% of tumor area) can be considered for adjuvant chemotherapy with a second-line regimen.
- First-line chemotherapy for primary, preoperative, adjuvant, and metastatic disease typically includes a combination of the following drugs: doxorubicin, cisplatin, ifosfamide, and high-dose methotrexate.
- Second-line therapy for relapsed, refractory, or metastatic disease includes a combination of the following medications: docetaxel, gemcitabine, cyclophosphamide, topotecan, carboplatin, etoposide, ifosfamide, and high-dose methotrexate.
- Regorafenib (category 1 evidence) and sorafenib are preferred targeted therapies, in relapsed/refractory and metastatic disease (Davis et al., 2019).
- Other recommended regimens include cabozatinib, sorafenib + everolimus (Grigani et al., 2012; Italiano et al., 2020).
- Dosing and drug combinations are typically myelosuppressive, and the use of myeloid growth factors is highly recommended.

Treatment for Metastatic Disease at Presentation

- Approximately 10% to 20% of patients present with metastatic disease at the time of diagnosis (NCCN, 2022).
- The number of metastases and the complete surgical resection of these lesions are predictive of prognosis in this group of osteosarcoma patients. Patients with lung-only metastasis have a better prognosis than those who have other areas of metastasis or multiple areas of disease at presentation (NCI, 2022).
- Preoperative chemotherapy followed by wide excision is recommended.
- Metastatectomy for lung-only recurrence is included in the treatment plan.
- Targeted therapy with regorafenib or sorafenib are also effective treatment options in lung-only metastasis.
- Management with systemic therapy and RT is recommended, as well as possible surgical resection of the primary lesion for local control.

Treatment for Recurrence

- The goal is palliation of symptoms and maintenance of quality of life.

- Patients should be considered for participation in a clinical trial.
- Systemic therapy with either first-line or second-line treatment options can be used as appropriate, followed by surgical resection.
- Manage relapse/progression or unresectable metastases with palliative RT, stereotactic radiosurgery, samarium-153 ethylene diamine tetramethylene phosphonate (^{153}Sm-EDTMP, Anderson et al., 2014) or best supportive care.

Prognosis

(Meltzer & Helman, 2021)

- In the past, osteosarcoma was associated with a poor prognosis.
  - All patients with extremity osteosarcomas were treated with amputation.
  - Before the routine use of systemic therapy, 80% to 90% of patients developed metastases despite local tumor control and died of their disease.
- The development of multiagent systemic therapy regimens for both neoadjuvant and adjuvant treatment has improved the prognosis greatly for patients with osteosarcoma.
- The 5-year disease-free survival rate is significantly higher in patients with localized disease (60%). The overall survival rate for patients who present with metastatic disease or develop metastasis is approximately 20% (Meltzer & Helman, 2021).

Prevention and Surveillance

Prevention

- Many of the risk factors, such as race, age, and certain bone diseases and inherited conditions, cannot be changed.
- Other than prior RT, there is no known lifestyle or environmental factor that causes osteosarcoma, so there is no way to prevent osteosarcoma currently.

Surveillance

- Physical examination and laboratory work if patient received chemotherapy.
- Chest imaging (CT scan or radiographs) and MRI or plain films of the extremity.
- Consider PET and/or bone scan.
- Evaluate every 3 months for the first 2 years, then every 4 months for the third year and every 6 months for the fourth and fifth years; then continue annually with chest radiographs and physical examination only.
- Long-term follow-up for late adverse effects is recommended. The most common late effects are cardiomyopathy, secondary cancers, permanent azoospermia, renal impairment, and ototoxicity/hearing impairment.

Bibliography

Amin, M., Gress, D., Meyer Vega, L., et al. (Eds.). (2017). *AJCC staging manual* (8th ed.). Springer.

Anderson, P. M., Subbiah, V., & Rohren, E. (2014). Bone-seeking radiopharmaceuticals as targeted agents of osteosarcoma: Samarium-153-EDTMP and radium-223. *Advances in Experimental Medicine and Biology, 804,* 291–304.

Davis, L. E., Bolejack, V., Ryan, C. W., Ganjoo, K. N., Loggers, E. T., Chawla, S., … Rushing, D. (2019). Randomized double-blind phase II study of regorafenib in patients with metastatic osteosarcoma. *Journal of Clinical Oncology: Official Journal of the American Society of Clinical Oncology, 37*(16), 1424–1431.

Enneking, W. F., Spanier, S. S., & Goodman, M. A. (1980). A system for the surgical staging of musculoskeletal sarcoma. *Clinical Orthopaedics and Related Research, 153,* 106–120.

Grigani, G., Palmerini, E., Dileo, P., Asaftei, S. D., D'Ambrosio, L., Pignochino, Y., … Ferrari, S. (2012). A phase II trial of sorafenib in relapsed and unresectable high-grade osteosarcoma after failure of standard multimodal therapy: An Italian Sarcoma Group study. *Annals of Oncology, 23,* 508–516.

Italiano, A., Mir, O., Mathoulin-Pelissier, S., Penel, N., Piperno-Neumann, S., Bompas, E., … Ray-Coquard, I. (2020). Cabozantinib in patients with advanced Ewing sarcoma or osteosarcoma (CABONE): A multicentre, single-arm, phase 2 trial. *The Lancet. Oncology, 21*(3), 446–455.

Mehlman, C. T. (2022, May 23). Osteosarcoma. *Medscape.* Available at http://emedicine.medscape.com/article/1256857-overview.

Meltzer, P. S., & Helman, L. J. (2021). New horizons in the treatment of osteosarcoma. *The New England Journal of Medicine, 385*(22), 2066–2076.

National Cancer Institute, Surveillance, Epidemiology and End Results (SEER) Program. (2021). SEER cancer statistics fact sheets: Bone and joint cancer. Available at https://seer.cancer.gov/statfacts/html/bones.html.

National Cancer Institute (NCI). (2022). *Soft tissue sarcoma treatment (PDQ)-health professional version.* https://www.cancer.gov/types/soft-tissue-sarcoma/hp/adult-soft-tissue-treatment-pdq.

National Comprehensive Cancer Network. (2022). NCCN clinical practice guidelines in oncology: Bone cancer (version 2.2022). Available at http://www.nccn.org/professionals/physician_gls/pdf/bone.pdf.

Papakonstantinou, E., Stamatopoulos, A., Athanasiadis, D. I., Kenanidis, E., Potoupnis, M., Haidich, A. B., & Tsiridis, E. (2020). Limb-salvage surgery offers better five-year survival rate than amputation in patients with limb osteosarcoma treated with neoadjuvant chemotherapy. A systematic review and meta-analysis. *Journal of Bone Oncology, 25,* 100319.

Siegel, R., Miller, K., Fuchs, H., & Jemal, A. (2021). Cancer statistics, 2021. *CA: A Journal for Cancer Clinicians, 71*(1), 7–33.

Zhao, X., Wu, Q., Gong, X., Liu, J., & Ma, Y. (2021). Osteosarcoma: A review of current and future therapeutic approaches. *Biomedical Engineering Online, 20*(1), 24.

Soft Tissue Sarcoma

Definition

Soft tissue sarcomas are a diverse group of rare solid tumors. Adult soft tissue sarcomas can occur anywhere in the body, but typically originate in the supporting structures and soft tissues of the body, including muscle, fat, blood vessels, lymphatic system, nerve/nerve sheath, ligaments, fibrous tissues, and tissue surrounding the joints. Typically, the distribution is (National Cancer Institute [NCI], 2022):

- Extremities: 45%
- Internal organs, viscera, or retroperitoneum: 38%
- Trunk: 10%
- Head and neck: 5%

There are more than 100 different subtypes of soft tissue sarcomas listed in the 2020 WHO classification (Bansal et al., 2021). Adult soft tissue sarcomas are classified by the types of tissue cells from which they arise.

Incidence

- Soft tissue sarcoma is a relatively rare cancer, accounting for about 0.7% of all adult cancers diagnosed and approximately 15% of pediatric malignancies (National Cancer Institute-Surveillance, Epidemiology, and End Results Program [NCI-SEER], 2021).
- In 2022, an estimated 13,190 new cases of soft tissue sarcoma were diagnosed in adults and children in the United States, and an estimated 5130 patients died of the disease (NCI, 2021).
- There is an increased prevalence in males.
- From 2003 to 2007, the median age at diagnosis was 58 years (NCI-SEER, 2021).

Etiology and Risk Factors

(NCI, 2022)

- Exposure to ionizing radiation accounts for fewer than 5% of all soft tissue sarcomas.
  - The most common form is RT for other primary cancers such as lymphoma, breast cancer, or cervical cancer.
  - The time between the exposure to radiation and diagnosis of soft tissue sarcoma is approximately 10 years.
- Family history: People with a family history of these inherited conditions or a strong family history of sarcomas may wish to discuss genetic testing with their health care providers. These genetic conditions are outlined in the table below.
- Chronic lymphedema: Lymphangiosarcoma can occur rarely in parts of the body where lymph nodes have been removed or damaged by radiation.
- Chemical exposure (Singer et al., 2019):
  - Agent Orange has been linked to soft tissue sarcoma and is covered under Veterans Administration (VA) benefits (Institute of Medicine, 1994).
  - There is a moderately strong association between exposure to vinyl chloride, arsenic, anabolic steroids, or thorium and hepatic angiosarcoma.
- There is no evidence to date that injury causes soft tissue sarcoma.

Genetic Conditions Associated With Soft Tissue Sarcomas

Condition	Characteristics
von Recklinghausen disease (Neurofibromatosis [NF] type 1; NF1 mutation)	Autosomal dominant Clinical manifestations: café au lait spots, benign neurofibromas, optic gliomas One in 10 will develop into a malignant peripheral nerve sheath tumor.
Werner syndrome (WRN mutation)	Autosomal dominant, less common Clinical manifestations: schwannomas, meningiomas, gliomas, neurofibromas Increased risk for radiation induced cancers
Gardner syndrome (APC mutation)	An inherited genetic disorder that leads to benign polyps, colon cancer, desmoid tumors in the abdomen, and benign bone tumors Variant of familial adenomatous polyposis
Li-Fraumeni syndrome (TP53 mutation)	Autosomal dominant syndrome that increases the risk for early-onset development of breast cancer, brain tumors, leukemias, adrenal cancer, and bone and soft tissue sarcoma Carriers have an approximately 50% chance of developing cancer by the age of 30 years and an approximately 57% risk of developing a second primary cancer. Approximately 2%–4% of sarcoma patients carry the TP53 mutation. Patients with Li-Fraumeni syndrome who have received radiation therapy for cancer are at very high risk for development soft tissue sarcoma in the area of the body where they received the radiation.
Retinoblastoma syndrome (RB tumor suppressor mutation)	Autosomal dominant syndrome Children with the inherited form of retinoblastoma are at increased risk for development of both bone and soft tissue sarcomas.

Signs and Symptoms

- Sarcomas that develop in the extremities usually begin as a painless lump that may be stable in size or may grow rapidly over a period of weeks to months.
- Sarcomas that manifest elsewhere in the body (e.g., chest, abdomen) may also begin as painless lumps.
- Masses may become painful if they grow to greater than 10 cm or compress neurologic structures (Mayerson et al., 2014).
- Retroperitoneal sarcomas or those that develop within the abdomen or chest begin with more vague symptoms, such as abdominal pain, bowel obstruction, or bleeding.
- About 72% of patients have lung metastasis on diagnosis. Respiratory symptoms vary depending on the extent of lung involvement (Hong et al., 2021).

Diagnostic Work-up

(NCCN, 2022)

- A comprehensive cancer center specializing in sarcoma is recommended to complete the work-up.
- Complete medical history and physical examination.
- Imaging
  - General considerations
    - Initial imaging usually includes the site of the primary tumor and the lungs, which are the primary site of metastasis.
    - CT of the abdomen and pelvis for myxoid/round cell liposarcoma, epithelioid sarcoma, angiosarcoma, and leiomyosarcoma.
    - Spine imaging for myxoid/round cell liposarcoma.
    - Brain MRI for alveolar soft part sarcoma and angiosarcoma.
  - Plain radiography
    - It is useful in assessment of bone tumors with associated soft tissue masses.
    - It can be useful in diagnosing lung metastasis with masses greater than 1 cm in size.
    - It is not useful in the primary evaluation of retroperitoneal sarcomas but is helpful in diagnosing complications that result from the tumor, such as bowel obstruction or perforation.
  - CT scans
    - A three-dimensional view of the mass and surrounding structures is recommended.
    - CT is the preferred modality for primary evaluation of intraabdominal and intrathoracic lesions.
    - CT can determine the size of the tumor and nodal involvement.
    - CT detects the presence of early metastasis on presentation, particularly in the lung.
    - Use of contrast is preferred.
  - MRI
    - MRI has better contrast resolution and a larger field of view than CT and is the preferred modality for extremity and trunk soft tissue lesions.
    - MRI is the best study to define the extent of the lesion in the bone and in the soft tissues.
    - MRI is used to evaluate anatomic relationships with surrounding neurovascular structures.

- MRI is essential for preoperative planning.
- Gadolinium contrast is essential to differentiate between soft tissue structures and tumor.
- A magnetic field strength of 1.5 Tesla or greater is necessary for adequate imaging.
- ^{18}F-Fluorodeoxyglucose positron emission tomography (FDG PET)
  - Assess metabolic activity in conjunction with CT. Malignant tumors tend to have higher metabolic activity than normal soft tissue. Intensity is measured in standard uptake values.
  - FDG PET can distinguish between benign tumors and high-grade sarcomas, but it cannot reliably distinguish between benign tumors and low- to intermediate-grade sarcomas.
  - Imaging includes the entire body from skull base to feet.
  - FDG PET is useful in initial staging, detecting occult metastases, and evaluating the response to chemotherapy.
- Biopsy of soft tissue sarcomas is challenging because of the heterogeneity of the tumor.
  - Fine-needle aspiration (FNA)
    - FNA is used when the mass is palpable and superficial.
    - It can be done as an office procedure but is best performed in selected institutions by a sarcoma pathologist with clinical expertise.
    - The advantage of FNA is that a rapid preliminary diagnosis can be determined.
    - The disadvantage is that there may not be enough cells to determine the exact type and grade of a sarcoma if one is present.
    - FNA is useful in ruling out other conditions such as other types of cancers, benign tumors, and infection.
    - If FNA leads to a diagnosis of sarcoma, usually another biopsy is needed to yield further information.
  - Core-needle biopsy
    - A larger tissue sample is obtained than with FNA.
    - The biopsy specimen usually contains enough tissue to adequately make a diagnosis of soft tissue sarcoma.
    - CT or ultrasound can be used to guide core-needle biopsies when the mass cannot be palpated.
  - Excisional biopsy
    - The entire tumor and a margin of surrounding normal tissue are removed, combining diagnostic biopsy and surgical treatment in one procedure.
    - Excisional biopsy is used when the tumor is small and not located next to any critical structures.
    - Excisional biopsy is used for a large mass that cannot be completely removed.

Histopathology

- Soft tissue sarcoma can occur anywhere in the body, and more than 100 subtypes have been identified. The most common ones are pleomorphic sarcoma (formerly malignant fibrous histiocytoma), leiomyosarcoma, liposarcoma, synovial sarcoma, and malignant peripheral nerve sheath tumor (MPNST) (Bansal et al., 2021).
- Cytogenetic, immunohistochemistry, and molecular genetic testing are useful in differentiating the subtype of soft tissue sarcoma and is highly recommended. Many of which have defined translocations, deletions, amplifications, and single-base-pair substitutions (NCCN, 2022).
- Skeletal muscle tumors
  - Rhabdomyosarcoma
    - Most common subtype in children; also affects adults
    - Embryonal, alveolar, and pleomorphic forms
    - Occur most frequently in the arms and legs but may also be found in the head and neck area and in reproductive or urinary organs (i.e., vagina or bladder)
    - Chromosomal translocation results in a fusion gene transcript
- Smooth muscle tumors
  - Leiomyosarcoma
    - Occurs primarily in older adults
    - Can occur anywhere in the body but is commonly found in the retroperitoneum, internal organs, and blood vessels; may develop in the deep soft tissues of the arms and legs
    - Leiomyosarcoma of the uterus is common.
- Adipocytic tumors
  - Liposarcomas
    - Commonly found in the thigh, behind the knee, or in the retroperitoneum but may develop almost anywhere in the body
    - Most prevalent in middle-aged adults
    - Range from slow-growing, atypical lipomatous tumors to very aggressive dedifferentiated liposarcomas
    - Other forms include myxoid/round cell and pleomorphic types.
    - The tumor can be heterogeneous, with areas of dedifferentiated liposarcoma arising from a well-differentiated tumor.
    - Gene amplification of region 12q14-15 is involved.
- Peripheral nerve tumors
  - MPNST includes the cells that surround the peripheral nervous system.
  - Neurofibrosarcomas involve degeneration of neurofibromatosis lesions.
- Connective tissue tumors
  - Fibrosarcomas
    - Affect adults, most commonly between the ages of 30 and 80 years (Singer et al., 2019).
    - Musculoaponeurotic fibromatoses are closely attached to skeletal tissue.
    - Other types include low-grade myxofibrosarcoma, low-grade fibromyxoid sarcoma, sclerosing epithelioid fibrosarcoma, and dermatofibrosarcoma protuberans.
  - Chondro-osseous tumors
  - Extraskeletal chondrosarcoma (mesenchymal and other variants)
  - Extraskeletal osteosarcoma
  - Fibrohistiocytic tumors

- UPS (formerly malignant fibrous histiocytomas)
  - Tends to grow locally but can metastasize; typically considered a high-grade tumor
  - Most commonly found in the arms and legs, less commonly in the retroperitoneum
  - Occurs most frequently in older adults
  - Other types include giant cell, myxoid/high-grade myxofibrosarcoma, and inflammatory forms
- Vascular tumors
  - Angiosarcoma
    - A rare, aggressive tumor arising from endothelium of blood vessels
    - Risk factors include chronic stasis, trauma, and previous site of irradiation
    - Occurs more often in males and in the elderly
    - Tends to metastasize to lymph nodes and lungs
  - Other types include lymphangiosarcoma, cutaneous angiosarcoma, and epithelioid hemangioendothelioma
- Tumors of uncertain differentiation: soft tissue sarcomas that cannot be linked to any specific type of soft tissue
  - Alveolar soft part sarcoma
    - Affects adolescents and young adults
    - Can metastasize to lung, liver, and brain
    - May resemble renal cell carcinoma or melanoma
  - Clear cell sarcoma
    - Develops primarily in the tendons of the arms or legs; can also develop in the gastrointestinal tract
    - Primarily affects young adults, ages 20 to 40 years (Singer et al., 2019)
    - Chromosomal translocation of EWSR1/ATF1 or a EWSR1/CREB1 is involved
    - It has some features of malignant melanoma
  - Desmoplastic small cell tumor
    - Characterized by small round blue cells surrounded by scar-like tissue
    - Found in the retroperitoneum and may metastasize to lung, liver, and lymph nodes; more than 40% of patients have distant metastasis at the time of presentation (NCCN, 2022)
    - Most often seen in adolescents and young adults of child-bearing age
    - Chromosomal translocation of t(11;22) (p13;q12) results in the EWS-WT1 fusion protein
  - Synovial sarcoma
    - Knees and ankles are the most common locations; may occur in shoulders or hips and may metastasize to lymph nodes, lung, and liver
    - Most common soft tissue sarcoma found in young adults, ages 15 to 40 years (Singer et al., 2019)
    - Chromosomal translocation of t(x,18) results in SYT-SSX1 fusion protein
- Other types: Epithelioid sarcoma, extraskeletal myxoid chondrosarcoma, PNET/extraskeletal Ewing tumor, extrarenal rhabdoid tumor, undifferentiated sarcoma.

Clinical Staging

- The AJCC TNM staging system based on tumor nodal involvement and presence or absence of metastasis is used for all soft tissue sarcomas. Staging has an important role in determining the most effective treatment of soft tissue sarcomas and estimating prognosis (Amin et al., 2017).
- FNCLCC histologic grade (NCI, 2022)
  - Grade is determined by three parameters: Histopathology specific tumor differentiation, extent of necrosis, and mitotic activity.
  - The purpose is to help determine which patients are more likely to develop metastasis and who can benefit the most from adjuvant chemotherapy.
  - Grading scale is GX to G3 (Enneking et al., 1980).
- Nodal involvement is rare and occurs in fewer than 3% of soft tissue sarcomas (NCCN, 2022).
- For complete staging, a thorough physical examination, radiographs, laboratory studies, and careful review of all biopsy specimens (including those from the primary tumor, lymph nodes, and other suspicious lesions) are essential.

Treatment

Surgery

- Surgery is standard primary treatment for most soft tissue sarcomas and stand-alone treatment for stage IA and stage IB tumors.
- Surgery is often preceded by RT and/or chemotherapy to downgrade and shrink large high-grade tumors to ensure negative surgical margins, avoid critical neurovascular structures, and preserve limb function.
- The biopsy site should be excised en bloc with the surgical specimen. Transverse incisions should be avoided because they can be considered areas that are contaminated with tumor.
- Hemostasis must be maintained; hematomas can contain tumor cells and can contaminate the site, increasing the risk of recurrence and the area of re-resection.
- Resection margins must be documented by the surgeon and the pathologist.
  - R0 resection: no residual microscopic disease
  - R1 resection: microscopic residual disease
  - R2 resection: gross residual disease
- If surgical margins are positive on pathology (except for bone, nerve, or major blood vessels), surgical re-resection should be considered if at all possible.
- Postoperative (adjuvant) RT should be considered for microscopically positive margin on a bone, nerve, or major blood vessel or for close surgical margins (<1 cm).
- Myxofibrosarcoma, dermatofibrosarcoma protuberans, and angiosarcoma are more infiltrative in nature, and it is more difficult to obtain an R0 resection.
- Abdominal surgery considerations:
  - If RT is to be considered, preoperative (neoadjuvant) radiation is preferred, with shielding of critical structures.
  - If R1 or R2 resection is anticipated, surgical clips should be left in place to identify high-risk areas for recurrence.
- Extremity surgery considerations:
  - Limb salvage surgery, with or without preoperative chemotherapy and RT, is the treatment of choice in more than 90% of sarcomas. Survival rates are 60% to 70%.

- Reconstructive plastic surgery with split-thickness skin grafts or muscle flaps is often required.
- Indications for amputation:
  - R0 resection would leave the patient with a nonfunctional limb and/or chronic pain
  - Infiltrative tumors of the hand or foot or regional (skip) metastasis
- Rehabilitation: Evaluate patient preoperatively for physical and occupational therapy and continue rehabilitation therapy postoperatively until maximal function is achieved.

Radiation Therapy

- Can be administered as preoperative (neoadjuvant) and postoperative (adjuvant) treatment
- Indicated for stage II, III, and IV tumors and as palliative treatment
- Recommended for R1 and R2 resections
- Total dose delivered depends on tissue tolerance and toxicity
- Four types:
  - External beam radiotherapy (EBRT), in which an external source of radiation is directed at the tumor bed using electron beams
  - Brachytherapy: direct application of radioactive seeds into the tumor bed through surgically placed catheters; can be given as low dose or high dose
  - Intensity-modulated radiotherapy (IMRT): conformal radiotherapy that shapes the radiation beams to closely fit the tumor or tumor bed
  - Intraoperative radiotherapy (IORT): radiation delivered during surgery using brachytherapy or EBRT techniques
- Preoperative RT: typically delivered over 5 weeks
  - Advantages:
    - Direct visualization of tumor
    - Smaller treatment field with less exposure of normal tissues to radiation toxicity
    - Lower dose requirement and lower rate of late toxicity
    - Increased sensitivity of tumor due to intact blood supply
    - Creation of a pseudocapsule, allowing for ease of resection and lower risk of recurrence
  - Disadvantage: wound healing complications, which can delay further treatment
- Postoperative RT: typically delivered over 6 to 7 weeks
  - Advantages:
    - Improves local control in patients with positive surgical margins
    - Allows for pathology review to determine whether postoperative RT is needed at all
    - Fewer wound complications, especially for thigh sarcomas
  - Disadvantages:
    - Larger treatment field required to include entire surgical bed and incision
    - Higher rate of treatment-related side effects

Systemic Therapy

- Chemotherapy can be administered as preoperative (neoadjuvant) and postoperative (adjuvant) treatment.

- It is a treatment option for stage IIB, III, and IV tumors and as palliative treatment for disseminated metastatic disease.
- Patient selection and optimal drug selection are important criteria to decrease risk of short- and long-term toxicities.
- Reserve use for large, high-grade, chemosensitive tumors.
- Patients need to have good performance status to withstand potential toxicities, including myelosuppression.
- The most used chemotherapeutic agents are ifosfamide and doxorubicin, or a gemcitabine combination.
- Other chemotherapeutic agents include docetaxel, gemcitabine, cyclophosphamide, dacarbazine, epirubicin, trabectedin (category 1 for liposarcoma), pegylated liposomal doxorubicin, eribulin (category 1 for liposarcoma),
- Chemotherapy agents can be given as monotherapy or combination therapy, depending on tumor histology and patient tolerance of regimen.
- Major side effects include myelosuppression, peripheral neuropathy, hepatic dysfunction, renal dysfunction, and cardiotoxicity. The use of myeloid growth factors is highly recommended.

Targeted Therapies

- Target angiogenesis of tumor cells by blocking growth factors that promote blood vessel formation, thus starving the tumor of nutrients and blood supply, leading to increased cell death.
- Target the cell cycle signaling cascade at multiple sites by blocking nutrient, oxygen, and energy level sensing mechanisms that contribute to oncogenesis.
- Not used as first-line (primary) therapy but usually in cases of recurrent, advanced, or metastatic disease.
- Best responses occur with specific histologic subtypes.
- Goal is stabilization of the tumor.
- Currently used agents:
  - Tyrosine kinase inhibitors: Pazopanib is approved by the FDA for soft tissue sarcoma, except liposarcoma.
- Clinical trials studying targeted therapies for sarcoma are ongoing.

Immunotherapy

(Ayodele & Razak, 2020)

- Unused in recurrent soft tissue sarcomas
- Pembrolizumab (for myxofibrosarcoma, UPS, undifferentiated sarcoma, cutaneous angiosarcoma)
- Other medications being studied: ipilumimab, nivolumab

Treatment for Recurring Disease

- The recurrence rate for high-grade tumors is about 50% during the first 3 years after diagnosis (NCCN, 2022).
- Local recurrence is treated as a primary lesion
  - Brachytherapy may be used if the area has previously been irradiated.
- Treatment of metastatic disease depends on the extent of metastasis
  - Limited
    - Surgery with or without chemotherapy or RT
    - Single organ, limited bulk: consider metastatectomy, radiofrequency ablation, embolization
    - Metastasized to the lung: the site of the metastasis can be surgically removed

- Disseminated
  - Palliative chemotherapy and/or RT
  - Debulking surgery for symptom management
  - Radiofrequency ablation or embolization
- Isolated regional disease or lymph node involvement
  - Regional node dissection with or without chemotherapy and/or RT
  - Metastatectomy

Prognosis

(NCCN, 2022)

- Tumor stage and location are prognostic factors in predicting survival.
- Patients with extremity sarcomas have a higher survival rate than those with retroperitoneal or head and neck sarcomas.
- Re-resection of tumors to obtain negative surgical margins is a significant predictor of local control and good long-term outcome.
- Overall, 5-year survival ranges from 60% to 80%, depending on age, tumor size, location and depth, histologic grade, and subtype.
- Estimated 5-year survival for localized sarcomas is 83% (54% if lymph node metastasis is present).
- Median overall survival time for patients with metastatic disease is 12 to 18 months.
- The 5-year survival rate with resectable metastasis is 25% to 40%; with unresectable distant metastasis, the estimated 5-year survival rate is 16%.
- Several predictive nomograms have been developed to help provide more accurate information to patients and providers. Future staging systems and nomograms are likely to include molecular markers and other biologic factors.

Prevention and Surveillance

Prevention

- Many of the risk factors, such as race, age, or gender, cannot be changed.

- Other risk factors and their associations with soft tissue sarcoma are still poorly understood.
- There are no current screening recommendations or effective preventative measures for soft tissue sarcoma.

Surveillance

- Low-grade lesions
  - Physical examination
  - Imaging of the lesion and chest radiography every 6 to 12 months for 2 years, then yearly as appropriate
- High-grade lesions
  - Physical examination
  - Primary site or cross-sectional imaging as indicated
  - Chest imaging every 3 to 6 months for the first 5 years and yearly thereafter for a minimum of 10 years

Bibliography

Amin, M., Gress, D., Meyer Vega, L., et al. (Eds.). (2017). *AJCC staging manual* (8th ed.). Springer.

Ayodele, O., & Razak, A. (2020). Immunotherapy in soft-tissue sarcoma. *Current Oncology (Toronto, Ont.), 27*(Suppl 1), 17–23.

Bansal, A., Goyal, S., Goyal, A., & Jana, M. (2021). WHO classification of soft tissue tumours 2020: An update and simplified approach for radiologists. *European Journal of Radiology, 143*, 109937.

Hong, Z., England, P., Rhea, L., Hirbe, A., McDonald, D., & Cipriano, C. A. (2021). Patterns of extrapulmonary metastases in sarcoma surveillance. *Cancers, 13*, 4669.

Institute of Medicine. (1994). *Veterans and Agent Orange: Health effects of herbicides used in Vietnam*. Washington, DC: National Academies Press.

Mayerson, J. L., Scharschmidt, T. J., Lewis, V. O., & Morris, C. D. (2014). Diagnosis and management of soft-tissue masses. *Journal of the American Academy of Orthopedic Surgeons, 22*, 742–750.

National Cancer Institute (NCI). (2022). *Soft tissue sarcoma treatment (PDQ)-health professional version*. https://www.cancer.gov/types/soft-tissue-sarcoma/hp/adult-soft-tissue-treatment-pdq.

National Cancer Institute (NCI). (2021). Surveillance, Epidemiology and End Results (SEER) Program. In *SEER cancer stat facts: Soft tissue including heart cancer*. https://seer.cancer.gov/statfacts/html/soft.html.

National Comprehensive Cancer Network. (2022). NCCN clinical practice guidelines in oncology: Soft tissue sarcoma (version 2.2022). Available at http://www.nccn.org/professionals/physician_gls/pdf/sarcoma.pdf

Siegel, R., Miller, K., Fuchs, H., & Jemal, A. (2021). Cancer statistics, 2021. *CA: A Journal for Cancer Clinicians, 71*(1), 7–33.

Singer, S., Tap, W. D., Kirsch, D. G., & Crago, A. M. (2019). Soft tissue sarcoma. In V. T. DeVita, T. S. Lawrence, & S. A. Rosenberg (Eds.), *Cancer principles and practice of oncology* (11th ed.) Philadelphia, PA: Wolters Kluwer.

Skin Cancers

Lisa Kottschade

The epidermis, which is the outermost layer of skin, contains cells that help the skin protect the body, including squamous cells, basal cells, and melanocytes. Skin cancers can arise from a variety of cells and are generally classified into melanoma and nonmelanoma cancers. There are four different varieties of skin cancer and include melanoma, basal cell carcinoma (BCC), squamous cell carcinoma, and Merkel cell carcinomas (MCC). BCCs arise from the basal cell, which is a round cell found in the lower epidermis (American Cancer Society [ACS], 2022a). The second most common type of skin cancer is cutaneous squamous cell carcinoma (cSCC). This subtype accounts for approximately 20% of all skin cancers diagnosed in the United States each year. Cutaneous SCC arises from epidermal keratinocytes, usually in areas of sun damaged skin (ACS, 2022a). MCC is a rare type of skin cancer generally thought to arise from Merkel cells found in the basal layer of the epidermis (Paulson et al., 2018). Malignant melanoma is a malignant tumor of melanocytes (ACS, 2022b). Melanocytes are the cells that make the pigment melanin, which gives skin its tan or brown color and helps protect the deeper layers of skin from damage due to exposure to ultraviolet (UV) light.

Melanoma

Definition

Melanoma is a malignancy of the melanocytes, which make the pigment melanin, which gives skin its color (ACS, 2022b). Melanin also helps to protect your skin from UV damage from the sun or other sources. Although most melanomas arise in the skin, they may develop on other parts of the body such as the eyes, mouth, anal area, or genitals.

Incidence

- The ACS (2022b) estimates that 99,780 cases of melanoma will be diagnosed in 2022.
- Melanoma incidence is slightly higher among men than women (ACS, 2022b).

Etiology and Risk Factors

- Melanomas are generally associated with exposure to UV light: sunlight, tanning beds, and sun lamps. However, there are two rare subtypes that involve the mucosal membranes or the eyes and may not be as directly related to UV damage.
- Risk factors include the following:
  - Prior melanoma (occurs in 5% of melanoma population)
  - Family history of melanoma (first-degree relative)

- Nevi (moles), particularly if numerous, large, or unusual (dysplastic nevus syndrome)
- Fair complexion, light hair, and light eyes
- History of unprotected or excessive sun exposure
- Severe sunburns as a child
- Use of tanning beds and sun lamps
- Residence in the southern latitudes of the Northern Hemisphere
- Exposure to coal tar, pitch, creosote, arsenic compounds, or radium
- History of radiation therapy (RT) or UV treatments
- Immune suppression from disease or medical treatment (ACS, 2022b)

Signs and Symptoms

- Suspicion of a melanoma can arise with either a new lesion or a change in the shape, size, diameter, or color of an existing skin lesion.
- Melanoma signs are generally referred to as "ABCDEs" (AIM at Melanoma, 2022):
  A: Asymmetry (one half of the mole does not match the other)
  B: Border (irregular)
  C: Color (blue, black, or variation in the same mole)
  D: Diameter (>6 mm)
  E: Evolution (changes of any sort in the lesion, including size, color, shape)

Diagnostic Work-up

- Identification of any suspicious lesions starts with thorough self-examination of the skin and clinical examination. It is often difficult to distinguish a benign pigmented lesion from an early melanoma. Dermatologists will often use dermoscopy to help guide whether a suspicious lesion to the naked eye should undergo biopsy.
- A definitive diagnosis is made based on biopsy, when possible, a biopsy should be done via punch or excisional method to allow accurate diagnostic depth.
- In patients with palpable disease (i.e., lymph nodes) that are biopsy proven to be melanoma, positron emission tomography/computed tomography (PET/CT), computed tomography (CT), and/or magnetic resonance imaging (MRI) are done to identify any potential sites of metastasis and complete staging.

Histopathology
(Swetter & Geller, 2021)

- Malignant melanoma is divided into clinicopathologic cellular subtypes. These subtypes are considered descriptive only; here they are listed in order of their diagnostic commonality:

- *Superficial spreading*, the most common melanoma subtype, commonly arises in preexisting nevi and usually manifests with irregular borders; with a scaly, crusty surface; and in a variety of colors. Pattern of spread is usually horizontal.
- *Nodular melanoma* is raised, usually blue-black in color, and has a rapid vertical growth phase.
- *Lentigo maligna melanoma* is a large, freckle-like lesion, tan to black in color, or a raised nodule with notched borders.
- *Acral lentiginous* is usually seen in the palmar/plantar regions and/or under nailbeds. It is flat and irregular in shape and varies in color; it may be smooth or ulcerated.
- *Desmoplastic* is a rare subtype of cutaneous melanoma that has very distinct histologic differences. Often it looks like a nodule, scar-like growth, and usually is lacking pigment.
- Miscellaneous unusual types (noncutaneous):
  - Mucosal—This is a very rare melanoma that presents clinically in the mucosal linings of internal structures. Most often is found in the sinonasal, anorectal, vulvar/vaginal tracts, but can also present other places as well.
  - Uveal—Primary melanoma of the eye that is usually found in the choroid structures of the eye but can also be seen in the retinal space.
- A number of functional somatic mutations have been identified in malignant melanoma including *BRAF*, *NRAS*, *cKIT*, *PTEN*, *TP53*, and *CDKN2A*.
  - The *BRAF* mutation is the most common and occurs in 50% of patients and affects a single amino acid, valine that is replaced with glutamic acid at position 600 (BRAF V600).

Clinical Staging

The current method for staging melanoma using the eighth edition of the American Joint Committee on Cancer (AJCC), involves a combination of pathologic findings, including vertical thickness (Breslow thickness), the presence or absence of ulceration, as well as lymph node involvement and distant metastasis (Gershenwald & Scolyer, 2018). The following systems are used:

- Breslow thickness: measures the actual vertical thickness of the lesion in millimeters.
- Clark level: scores the primary tumor as level I through level V to describe the penetration into the various layers of the skin. However, it should be noted that the Clark level is no longer figured into the staging process.
- Final stage is determined by the tumor (T), node (N), metastasis (M) (TNM) system: the system incorporates Breslow thickness, presence or absence of ulceration, involvement of lymph nodes, and presence or absence of distant metastasis to assign stages.

Treatment

Surgery

(Gershenwald & Keung, 2021)

- Wide local surgical excision (usually down to the muscle fascia) with a wide margin if possible (depending on tumor thickness) is the primary treatment for melanoma.
  - Margins are based on depth of lesion as well as anatomic location (i.e., ability to achieve such margins):
    - Melanoma in situ: 0.5 to 1 cm margins
    - T1 lesions: 1 cm margins
    - T2 lesions: 1 to 2 cm margins
    - T3 and T4 lesions: 2 cm margins. Because of the need for wider margins, as well as anatomic location skin grafting may be needed to close the wound.
- Depending on the depth of the primary lesion a sentinel lymph node biopsy (SLNB) may be indicated. An SLNB is done to identify lymph nodes in the primary drainage basin of the primary melanoma that may contain micrometastases in patients with primary melanomas greater than 1 mm (and in certain situations greater than 0.8 mm) in depth.
  - Lymphoscintigraphy is the technique used to identify the sentinel node(s) as the first lymph node(s) encountered in drainage from the primary tumor.
  - This surgical procedure became the standard of care and is used to determine the presence of disease in the draining lymph node basin and allows the surgeon to remove as few as possible lymph nodes, leading to maximum benefit and decreasing the side effects and complications from lymph node dissection.
- Regional lymph node dissection is done when there are macro metastatic lymph nodes present. These may be palpable or identified on pre-op imaging.
- Surgery may also be done in the metastatic setting either as a metastasectomy or for palliation of painful or draining lesions.

Radiation Therapy

(National Comprehensive Cancer Network [NCCN], 2022)

- RT may be used in a variety of settings for the treatment of melanoma, including both in the adjuvant and metastatic setting. There are a variety of methods that can be used to deliver RT.
- Stereotactic radiosurgery is high-intensity tumor-directed radiation. The most common use of this technique is for localized metastatic lesion (i.e., painful bone metastasis) or small brain metastases. This allows for increased amounts of radiation to be delivered to more precise areas with fewer side effects for the patient.

Systemic Therapy

(NCCN, 2022)

- There have been multiple improvements in systemic therapy for the treatment of melanoma in the last decade. In addition to traditional chemotherapy, there are now several immunotherapies as well as targeted therapies (i.e., BRAF/MEK inhibitors) that have proven to be of benefit to patients in both the adjuvant and metastatic settings (see table on the next page).

FDA-Approved Systemic Therapies for Malignant Melanoma

Chemotherapy	Immunotherapy	Targeted Therapy
DTIC (dacarbazine)	Pembrolizumab	Dabrafenib/trametinib
Temozolomide (compendium)	Nivolumab	Vemurafenib/ cobimetinib
Paclitaxel/carboplatin (compendium approved)	Interleukin 2 (IL-2)	Encorafenib/ binimetinib
	Ipilimumab	
	Ipilimumab/ nivolumab	
	Tebentafusp	
	Nivolumab and relatlimab-rmbw	

Immunotherapy

- Currently approved adjuvant therapies consist of three immune checkpoint inhibitors (ICI) (pembrolizumab, ipilimumab, and nivolumab). While not commonly used in the era of the ICI agents, interferon α-2B and peginterferon α-2B also remain approved for the treatment of melanoma in the adjuvant setting.
- In the metastatic setting, the first immunotherapy approved was interleukin-2. Additionally, the same three agents noted above are approved for patients with unresectable metastatic melanoma. Ipilimumab and nivolumab are approved in combination for the treatment of metastatic melanoma. Most recently the U.S. Food and Drug administration (FDA) has approved a bi-specific antibody known as tebentafusp specifically for the treatment of metastatic uveal melanoma for patients that are human leukocyte antigen 0201 positive. This is the first approval of its kind specifically for this disease. Up until now, the treatment of metastatic uveal melanoma was extrapolated from cutaneous data with poor response rates given its different biologic make-up.

Chemotherapy

- To date the only chemotherapy FDA approved for metastatic melanoma is dacarbazine. However, there are several chemotherapies that are compendium approved including temozolomide and the combination of carboplatin and paclitaxel.

Targeted Therapy

- For patients with *BRAF* mutations there are combinatorial therapies utilizing both a BRAF and MEK inhibitor to target the mutation. There are three combinations approved by the FDA: dabrafenib/trametinib; vemurafenib/cobimetinib; and encorafenib/binimetinib.

Prognosis
(ACS, 2022b)

- It is estimated that approximately 7650 people will die from melanoma in 2022.
- The 5-year survival rate for localized melanoma is 97%; for regional metastasis, it is 59%; and for distant metastatic stages, it is 15% to 20%.

- Several factors affect the prognosis, including the location of the lesion and, more important, the histopathologic features of the tumor: thickness or level of invasion of the melanoma, mitotic rate, presence of tumor infiltrating lymphocytes, number of regional or distant lymph nodes involved, and ulceration or bleeding at the primary site.

Prevention and Surveillance

- Skin screening, including monthly self-examination and examination of suspicious areas by a physician, should be done to identify lesions early (ACS, 2022b; AIM at Melanoma, 2022).
- High-risk individuals (those with multiple nevi, dysplastic nevus syndrome, or a personal or family history of melanoma) should perform monthly self-examinations and have annual full-body skin examination by a dermatologist (ACS, 2022b; AIM at Melanoma, 2022).
- The following should be used as guidance to help prevent overexposure to UV rays:
  - Limit exposure to the sun during midday (10 AM to 4 PM).
  - Use protection with a wide-brimmed hat shading the face, neck, and ears; long sleeves and pants; and sunglasses.
  - Use sunscreen with a sun protection factor (SPF) of 15 or higher; more important, apply it liberally and reapply at least every 2 hours.
  - Avoid tanning beds and sun lamps (ACS, 2022b; AIM at Melanoma, 2022).
- Common follow-up recommendations by the National Comprehensive Cancer Network (NCCN, 2022) include the following:
  - Skin examination at least annually for life.
  - Educate patient about regular self-examination of the skin and lymph node examination.
  - Regional lymph node ultrasonography may be considered for patients with a suspicious lymph node on clinical examination, and those with a positive SLNB who did not have a complete lymph node dissection.
  - The follow-up schedule is determined by risk of recurrence, prior primary melanoma or a family history of melanoma, and other factors such as atypical moles, dysplastic nevi, and patient or physician concern.

References

AIM at Melanoma. (2022). What are the ABCDE's of melanoma? *Aim at Melanoma.* Available at https://www.aimatmelanoma.org/melanoma-101/understanding-melanoma/moles-and-other-lesions/know-your-abcdes/.

American Cancer Society. (2022a). Basal and squamous cell carcinoma. *Cancer.org.* Available at https://www.cancer.org/cancer/basal-and-squamous-cell-skin-cancer.html.

American Cancer Society. (2022b). Melanoma skin cancer. *Cancer.org.* Available at https://www.cancer.org/cancer/melanoma-skin-cancer.html.

Gershenwald, J. E., & Scolyer, R. A. (2018). Melanoma staging. American Joint Committee on Cancer (AJCC) 8th edition and beyond. *Annals of Surgical Oncology, 25*(8), 2105–2110.

Gershenwald, J. E., & Keung, E. (2021). Surgical management of primary cutaneous melanoma or melanoma at other unusual sites. In *UpToDate.* Available at https://www.uptodate.com/contents/surgical-management-of-primary-cutaneous-melanoma-or-melanoma-at-other-unusual-sites?search=surgical%20management%20of%20melanoma&source=search_result&selectedTitle=1~150&usage_type=default&display_rank=1.

National Comprehensive Cancer Network. (2022). Clinical practice guidelines: Melanoma—cutaneous (version 3.2022). Available at https://www.nccn.org/professionals/physician_gls/pdf/cutaneous_melanoma.pdf.

Paulson, K. G., Park, S. Y., Vandeven, N. A., Lachance, K., Thomas, H., Chapuis, A. G., … Nghiem, P. (2018). Merkel cell carcinoma: Current US incidence and projected increases based on changing demographics. *Journal of the American Academy of Dermatology*, 78(3), 457–463.e2.

Swetter, S. G., & Geller, A. C. (2021). Melanoma: Clinical features and diagnosis. In *UpToDate*. Available at https://www.uptodate.com/contents/melanoma-clinical-features-and-diagnosis?search=melanoma%20histology&source=search_result&selectedTitle=2~150&usage_type=default&display_rank=2.

Merkel Cell Carcinoma

Definition

MCC is a nonmelanoma skin cancer but differs from BCC and cSCC and is felt to be of neuroendocrine origin. MCC is a very rare disease that carries with it a high risk of metastasis. There are two conflicting thoughts on the origin of MCC. Traditionally, it was felt to arise from Merkel cells located in the basal layer of the epidermis and hair follicles (Paulson et al., 2018). Alternatively, MCC may come from immature totipotential stem cells that acquire neuroendocrine features during their malignant transformation (Tai et al., 2021). Additionally, up to 80% of MCCs are thought to be directly caused by the Merkel cell polyomavirus (MCPyV) (Paulson et al., 2018).

Incidence

- It is estimated that approximately 2835 cases were diagnosed in 2020 with that number expected to rise to 3284 by 2025 (Paulson et al., 2018).

Etiology and Risk Factors
(Paulson et al., 2018; Tai et al., 2021)

As with other skin cancers a portion of MCC is thought to be caused by direct UV exposure, including patients who receive PUVA (psoralen plus UVA) treatments for other skin conditions.

- Light skin color
- Increasing age (mean age at diagnosis is 76)
- Male
- Immunosuppressed (transplant, autoimmune disease)
- Concurrent other malignancy, especially those with a hematologic malignancy (i.e., chronic lymphocytic leukemia (CLL))
- Positive for MCPyV

Diagnostic Work-up
(NCCN, 2022)

- MCC should be diagnosed with a tumor biopsy to confirm diagnosis.
- Due to high risk of metastasis, patients should undergo initial imaging to assess for metastatic disease either with PET/CT scanning or CT scans of the chest, abdomen, and pelvis. MRI imaging of the brain should be obtained for anyone with symptoms.
- Additionally, patients should undergo testing for MCPyV.

Clinical Staging
(American Joint Committee on Cancer, 2017; Tai et al., 2021)

Staging for MCC uses the eighth edition of AJCC staging recommendations applying the TNM.

- Stage I—Primary tumors ≤2 cm in maximum dimension, (T1) with no regional lymph node involvement.
- Stage II—Any primary tumor greater than 2 cm (T2 or T3) or a primary tumor with invasion into bone, muscle, fascia, or cartilage (T4), with no evidence of lymph node involvement.
- Stage III—Any primary tumor (any T) with in-transit metastasis or regional lymph node disease. This is further subdivided into subgroups based on extent of in-transit/lymph node involvement.
- Stage IV—Any metastasis beyond the regional lymph nodes.

Treatment
(NCCN, 2022)

Surgery

- For patients with no evidence of metastatic spread on initial staging, they should undergo surgical resection with an SLNB.
- For patients with a positive SLNB, a completion lymph node dissection is indicated.

Radiation

- Adjuvant radiation to the primary site and involved lymph node basins is generally recommended to help reduce the risk of local regional recurrence.
- Radiation can also be used as an initial treatment strategy for patients where surgical resection would be morbid or patients who are not surgical candidates.

Systemic Therapy
Chemotherapy

- The use of chemotherapy in the adjuvant setting with or without adjuvant radiation remains a topic of controversy. This is partly because there are no good, randomized trials looking at the role of chemotherapy or chemo/radiation in this patient population.
- Typical chemotherapy regimens whether given in the adjuvant or metastatic setting have usually involved carboplatin +/- etoposide.

Immunotherapy

- Currently there are two ICI agents approved for metastatic MCC. These include avelumab and pembrolizumab.
- There are no adjuvant ICI agents approved yet, but evaluation is ongoing in randomized clinical trials.
- ICI agents have also been evaluated in the neoadjuvant setting for patients with bulky disease or those whose tumors are considered to be of questionable surgical resectability. For patients that achieved a pathologic complete response at the time of surgery, there was significant improvement in the time until patients had recurrent disease.

Prognosis
(Tai et al., 2021)

- Overall survival (OS) is based on the stage of disease at initial presentation. For those with local disease the 5-year

OS rate is approximately 55% and survival progressively decreases for patients with larger primary disease.

- For those with regional disease, the 5-year OS rate is approximately 35.4%. Patients with in-transit disease fared better (41%) than those with clinically occult nodal disease (28.8%).
- Patients with metastatic MCC had the poorest OS with a 5-year survival rate of approximately 13.5%.
- Additionally, patients who are positive for the MCPyV tend to have a better prognosis in terms of improved disease-specific survival and decreased risk of recurrent disease.

Prevention and Surveillance

(ACS, 2022; NCCN, 2022)

- There are no current standards on prevention for MCC, but the ACS recommends limiting UV exposure as with other skin cancers.
- Current recommendations from NCCN include follow-up every 3 to 6 months for the first 3 years and then every 6 to 12 months thereafter.
- Patients should undergo a good physical exam including thorough skin and lymph node exams.
- For patients who are at high risk of recurrence, consideration should be given to cross-sectional imaging.
- For patients who have a positive MCPyV at time of diagnosis, there is some thought that patients should undergo routine MCPyV testing every 3 months for up to 5 years post diagnosis, especially if patients are not undergoing routine cross-sectional imaging. If there is a greater than 30% increase from the previous value, strong consideration for imaging should be done.

References

American Cancer Society. (2022). *Merkel cell skin cancer*. Available at https://www.cancer.org/cancer/merkel-cell-skin-cancer.html.

American Joint Committee on Cancer. (2017). AJCC cancer staging manual. In *AJCC cancer staging form supplement* (8th edition). Available at https://www.facs.org/quality-programs/cancer/ajcc/cancer-staging/manual.

National Comprehensive Cancer Network (NCCN). (2022). Merkel cell Carcinoma (version 2.2022). Available at https://www.nccn.org/professionals/physician_gls/pdf/mcc.pdf.

Paulson, K. G., Park, S. Y., Vandeven, N. A., Lachance, K., Thomas, H., Chapuis, A. G., … Nghiem, P. (2018). Merkel cell carcinoma: Current US incidence and projected increases based on changing demographics. *Journal of the American Academy of Dermatology, 78*(3), 457–463. e2.

Tai, P., Nghiem, P. T., & Park, S. Y. (2021). Pathogenesis, clinical features, and diagnosis of Merkel cell carcinoma. In *UpToDate*. Available at https://www.uptodate.com/contents/pathogenesis-clinical-features-and-diagnosis-of-merkel-cell-neuroendocrine-carcinoma?search=merkel%20cell%20carcinoma&topicRef=7609&source=see_link.

Nonmelanoma Skin Cancer: Basal Cell Carcinoma and Cutaneous Squamous Cell Carcinoma

Definition

The vast majority of the cells in the epidermis are keratinocytes, so named because they make the protein keratin. They form as basal cells in the lowest layer of the epidermis and then gradually migrate upward, becoming flat squamous cells before reaching the surface of the skin. Nonmelanoma skin cancers are mostly BCCs or cSCCs. Collectively these are the most diagnosed cancer type among non-Hispanic White Americans.

Incidence

(ACS, 2022)

- An estimated 5.4 million BCCs or SCCs of the skin are diagnosed each year in the United States in about 3.3 million Americans (allowing for multiple lesions in the same person).
- Exact numbers are unknown as BCCs and cSCC are not required to be reported to the national tumor registries.
- It is estimated that 2000 deaths occurred annually from nonmelanoma skin cancer. This rate has been dropping in recent years.
- cSCC account for approximately 20% of all nonmelanoma skin cancers.
- Nonmelanoma skin cancer is the most common type of cancer, yet it accounts for fewer than 0.1% of cancer deaths.

Etiology and Risk Factors

(Que et al., 2018)

- BCC and cSCC are generally associated with exposure to UV light from the sun and/or tanning beds.
- They are commonly found on sun-exposed areas of the skin, such as the face, ears, neck, lips, and backs of the hands. However, they can be found anywhere on the body, including the genitalia.
- Other risk factors
  - Fair complexion
  - Older age (possibly due to cumulative sun exposure over time)
  - History of unprotected or excessive sun exposure
  - Severe sunburns as a child
  - Use of tanning beds
  - Residence in the southern latitudes of the Northern Hemisphere
  - Exposure to coal tar, large amounts of arsenic, paraffin, or radium
  - History of RT or UV treatments for conditions such as psoriasis
  - Immune suppression due to disease or medical treatment (e.g., organ transplantation)
  - Family history of skin cancer
  - Gender: Males are twice as likely to develop BCCs and three times more likely to develop cSCCs than women
  - Smoking increases the risk of cSCC, especially on the lips
  - History of human papillomavirus (HPV) infection
  - Prior history of skin cancer: Approximately 35% of people with BCC develop a second BCC within 5 years
  - Basal cell nevus syndrome (also known as Gorlin syndrome, Gorlin-Goltz syndrome, or nevoid BCC syndrome) is a rare congenital condition in which people develop multiple basal cell lesions over their lifetime.

Signs and Symptoms

(Bader, 2021; Que et al., 2018)

- Key signs are a new growth, a spot or bump that is getting larger over time, or a sore that fails to heal within several months.

- cSCCs can occur anywhere, but they usually occur on sun-exposed areas that show evidence of sun damage (e.g., wrinkles, pigment changes, freckles, "age spots," loss of elasticity, broken blood vessels).
- cSCCs that arise in areas of non–sun-exposed skin or that originate de novo on areas of sun-exposed skin have a worse prognosis because these have a greater tendency to metastasize.
  - cSCCs usually manifest as a growing lump with a rough, scaly, or crusted surface or as a flat, reddish patch that grows slowly. They can manifest as a sore that does not heal, and they can develop in scars or skin sores elsewhere.
- BCCs may be nodular to flat, firm, pale areas or small, raised pink or red lesions. They are commonly found on the head and neck.
  - They may also manifest as a nodular ulcerative lesion; a translucent, shiny, pearly area that bleeds easily after a minor injury; or a sore that does not heal. The nose is the most frequent site. Large basal cell lesions may also have oozing or crusted areas.

Diagnostic Work-up

- Definitive diagnosis requires a biopsy of the suspicious lesion:
  - Excisional biopsy, in which the entire lesion is removed
  - Punch biopsy, in which a small portion of the lesion is lifted
  - Shave biopsy, in which a thin slice of the lesion is removed (not recommended if the lesion is suspicious for melanoma because it interferes with proper tumor depth measurement and staging)
- If the BCC or SCC primary lesion is pathologically aggressive, is large, or was neglected, full body imaging should be done to identify any sites of metastasis.

Histopathology

- Both BCCs and cSCCs are of epithelial origin.
- There are several histologic subtypes of cSCC (Que et al., 2018):
  - Those that are well-differentiated and therefore of low risk for metastasis including keratoacanthoma and verrucous carcinoma
  - Those that are of higher risk for metastasis include desmoplastic and adenosquamous cSCC.
- BCC is divided into two categories including undifferentiated and differentiated (Bader, 2021).
  - Undifferentiated subtypes include:
    - Pigmented, superficial, sclerosing, and infiltrative BCC
  - Differentiated subtypes include:
    - Keratotic, sebaceous, tubular, and noduloulcerative BCC

Clinical Staging

- Staging for BCC/cSCC is based on the eighth edition, AJCC Staging Manual (2017) applying TNM system.
  - Stage 0—Carcinoma *in situ* (Tis)
  - Stage I—Any primary tumor ≤2 cm in maximum diameter (T1) with no regional lymph node involvement (N0)

- Stage II—Any primary tumor greater than 2 cm but ≤4 cm in greatest diameter (T2) with no regional lymph node involvement (N0)
- Stage III—Any primary tumor greater than 4 cm in maximum dimension or minor bone erosion or perineural invasion, or deep invasion (T3) without lymph node involvement (N0) or any primary tumor (T1–T3) with metastasis in a single ipsilateral lymph node, ≤3 cm in greatest diameter and no extra nodal extension (ENE–) (N1)
- Stage IV—Any primary tumor (T1–T3) with metastasis in a single ipsilateral lymph node greater than 3 cm but less than 6 cm in diameter and ENE(–) or metastasis in multiple ipsilateral lymph nodes less than 6 cm in diameter and ENE(–) or metastasis in bilateral or contralateral lymph nodes less than 6 cm in diameter and ENE(–) (N2) OR any primary tumor with gross cortical bone/marrow, skull base invasion and/or skull base foramen invasion, and any lymph node involvement (N1–3) OR any primary tumor with metastasis in a lymph node greater than 6 cm in diameter and ENE(–) or in a single ipsilateral lymph node greater than 3 cm and ENE(+) or multiple ipsilateral, contralateral, or bilateral nodes with ENE(+) or a single contralateral node of any size and ENE(+) OR any primary tumor size, any lymph node involvement and distant metastasis (M1)

Treatment

(Aasi, 2021; Aasi & Hong, 2021; NCCN, 2022a, 2022b)

Surgery

- Localized BCCs and cSCCs can be treated with surgical excision alone and have high cure rates. There are several types of surgery that can be performed, depending on the location, and/or size of the primary lesion.
  - Mohs (pronounced "moes") micrographic surgery offers the highest cure rate for difficult-to-treat BCCs and cSCCs. Mohs micrographic surgery repeatedly removes thin layers of tissue. Each layer of tissue is examined for tumor cells. This procedure maximizes the greatest tumor control while maintaining cosmetic results.
- Simple excision is done with either frozen or permanent sectioning for evaluation and determination of clear margins ranging from 3 to 10 mm, depending on the diameter of the original tumor.
- Electrodesiccation and curettage should be limited to very small tumors. In this method, the tumor is scraped away, and electricity is used to destroy the remaining tumor cells; the process is then repeated. This method limits the visualization of the depth of tumor invasion.
- Cryosurgery may be used for clinically well-defined or in situ tumors. This procedure uses liquid nitrogen to freeze cancer cells, causing cell death.

Radiation

- For tumors that cannot be removed by surgery, or where negative margins cannot be achieved, radiation may be considered.

Tumor-Directed Therapy

- Photodynamic therapy (PDT) is a two-step process in which light is used to destroy cancer cells. A chemical is applied to the area and given time to absorb, after which a special light is used to promote cancer cell death.
- Topical chemotherapy with 5-fluorouracil can be used for premalignant lesions (actinic keratoses), recurrences, or cases in which surgery and RT cannot be done.

Systemic Therapy

Cutaneous Squamous Cell Carcinoma

- Chemotherapy options include carboplatin and paclitaxel.
- Cemiplimab and pembrolizumab are two FDA approved immunotherapies for unresectable or metastatic cSCC.
- Cetuximab, an EGFR inhibitor, can also be given as single agent or in combination with chemotherapy.

Basal Cell Carcinoma

- Hedgehog inhibitors have been approved as a targeted treatment target for BCC. There are two FDA-approved hedgehog inhibitors, sonidegib and vismodegib.

Prognosis

(Aasi, 2021; Aasi & Hong, 2021)

- Early diagnosis allows for the best outcomes in patients with BCC or SCC.
- The overall cure rate is directly related to the stage of disease and the treatment used for the primary lesion.
- Precise disease-free survival rates are not known because neither BCC nor SCC of the skin is a reportable disease.
  - It is estimated that the 5-year disease-free survival rate for BCC ranges from 85% to 95%.
  - Disease-free survival rates for SCC are dependent on the size and aggressiveness of the primary lesion.
    - For small lesions, it is about 90%.
    - For squamous cell lesions of the lip, ears, and palms of the hands or soles of the feet, there is an increased incidence of metastatic disease to regional lymph nodes and distant sites.
    - In 2012, an estimated 2% of US patients with SCC died of the disease.

Prevention and Surveillance

(ACS, 2022)

- The most important preventative measure is self-examination of the skin. Monthly skin examination allows patients to identify new or changing skin lesions, leading to early diagnosis and treatment.
- Patients who are at a higher risk of developing these skin cancers should have annual skin examinations by a dermatologist as part of their routine care.
- Guidelines help to prevent overexposure to UV rays include the following:

- Limit exposure to the sun during midday (10 AM to 4 PM).
- Use protection with a wide-brimmed hat shading the face, neck, and ears; long sleeves and pants; and sunglasses.
- Apply sunscreen containing an SPF of 15 or higher generously and reapply it at least every 2 hours.
- Do not use tanning beds or sun lamps.
- Protect children to minimize their sun exposure by using the Slip, Slop, Slap, and Wrap method: Slip on a shirt, Slop on sunscreen, Slap on a hat, and Wrap on sunglasses.
- NCCN (2022a) recommendations for follow-up of patients with BCC include:
  - History and physical examination, including a complete skin examination, every 6 to 12 months for life.
  - Patient education about sun protection and self-examination of the skin.
- NCCN (2022b) follow-up recommendations for patients with localized cSCC include:
  - A complete history and physical examination, including skin and lymph node examination, every 3 to 12 months (depending on risk) for 2 years, then every 6 to 12 months for 3 years, and then annually for life.
  - Patient education on sun protection and self-examination of the skin.
- Follow-up for patients with regional SCC according to NCCN (2022b) include:
  - A complete history and physical examination, including skin and lymph node examination for 1 year, then every 2 to 4 months for 1 year, then every 36 months for 3 years, then every 6 to 12 months for life.
  - Patient education on sun protection and self-examination of the skin.

References

Aasi, S. Z. (2021). Treatment and prognosis of basal cell carcinoma at low risk of recurrence. In *UpToDate*. Available at https://www.uptodate.com/contents/treatment-and-prognosis-of-low-risk-cutaneous-squamous-cell-carcinoma-cscc?search=cutaneous%20squamous%20cell%20carcinoma&topicRef=13714&source=see_link.

Aasi, S. Z., & Hong, A. M. (2021). Treatment and prognosis of low-risk cutaneous squamous cell carcinoma (cSCC). In *UpToDate*. Available at https://www.uptodate.com/contents/treatment-and-prognosis-of-low-risk-cutaneous-squamous-cell-carcinoma-cscc?search=cutaneous%20squamous%20cell%20carcinoma&topicRef=13714&source=see_link.

American Cancer Society. (2022). *Basal and squamous cell carcinoma*. Available at https://www.cancer.org/cancer/basal-and-squamous-cell-skin-cancer.html.

American Joint Committee on Cancer. (2017). AJCC cancer staging manual. In *AJCC cancer staging form supplement* (8th edition). Available at https://www.facs.org/quality-programs/cancer/ajcc/cancer-staging/manual.

Bader, R. (2021). Basal cell carcinoma workup. In *Medscape*. Available at https://emedicine.medscape.com/article/276624-workup#c1.

National Comprehensive Cancer Network. (2022a). Basal cell skin cancer (version 2.2022). Available at https://www.nccn.org/professionals/physician_gls/pdf/nmsc.pdf.

National Comprehensive Cancer Network. (2022b). Squamous cell skin cancer (version 2.2022). Available at https://www.nccn.org/professionals/physician_gls/pdf/squamous.pdf.

Que, S. K. T., Zwald, F. O., & Schmults, C. D. (2018). Cutaneous squamous cell carcinoma: Incidence, risk factors, diagnosis, and staging. *Journal of the American Academy of Dermatology, 78*(2), 237–247.

Surgical Therapy

Lisa S. Parks

In oncologic care of solid tumors, surgery remains the only curative treatment. Surgery for the oncology patient can have many goals including prevention, cure, reconstruction, and palliation. Nurses working in surgical oncology must possess knowledge of both oncology and surgical nursing.

Goals of Surgical Procedures

Prevention

A personal and/or family history of cancer often leads patients and family members to undergo genetic testing. Identified gene mutations predispose patients to a higher risk of developing cancer. These individuals often undergo surgery for precancerous situations or are treated with preventive therapy. For example, with breast cancer, patients with the *BRCA1* and *BRCA2* genes may be treated with selective estrogen receptor modulators or undergo a bilateral risk-reducing mastectomy reducing breast cancer risk by 90% (Thorat & Balasubramanian, 2020). Patients with unilateral breast cancer may opt to undergo contralateral mastectomy to eliminate the chance of developing breast cancer in the unaffected breast. Routine screening, as well as screening in high-risk individuals, may lead to discovery of precancerous lesions and removal prior to the development of cancer.

Diagnosis

Surgery is often performed for removal of tissue for histologic examination by various methods, including incisional biopsy, excisional biopsy, open approach, and diagnostic laparoscopy. After removal of lymph nodes or tissue, the specimen is examined with genetic assays. Besides the identification of individual targetable alterations, genomic methods can gauge mutational load, which may predict a therapeutic response to immune-checkpoint inhibitors or identify cancer-specific proteins (Berger & Mardis, 2018).

Staging

All solid cancers are clinically staged at diagnosis but are restaged after surgery which is called pathologic staging. Evaluation of lymph nodes which are removed during surgery as well as biopsies of distant sites creates a more accurate stage of the cancer. This information is essential in determining cancer treatment plans. Most cancers use the American Joint Committee on Cancer (AJCC) staging system which uses tumor size (T), number of lymph nodes (N), and presence or absence of distant metastasis (M).

Treatment

The goal of curative surgery is removal of the entire primary cancer, which includes a margin of normal tissue surrounding the tumor. The National Comprehensive Cancer Network (NCCN) recommendations may include treatment sequencing with specific modalities, such as, immunotherapy, chemotherapy, and radiation therapy before, during, or after surgery (Canter, 2016). NCCN guidelines determine the amount of surgical margin that is removed with the tumor during the procedure. If a positive margin is noted during pathologic analysis, the resection is incomplete or noncurative (Orosco et al., 2018). With a positive margin, re-excision of the margin or adjuvant chemo-radiation may be required.

Minimally invasive surgery has continued to evolve in surgical oncology. Robotic-assisted surgery has been revolutionary for oncologic surgery (Jara et al., 2020). Laparoscopic surgery is used for diagnostics, rather than treatment. Better outcomes have been reported due to a three-dimensional interface, tremor filtration, improved wrist motion, and improved ergonomics.

Reconstruction

Plastic surgeons are important members of the patient's surgical cancer team. Their expertise in reconstruction, microsurgery, and repair of defects prevents further postoperative complications. Reconstructive surgery decreases the patient's psychological stress by improving their body self-image. An example of this is breast reconstruction in breast cancer.

Palliation

Palliative surgery is undertaken to provide comfort for the patient, not a cure. It often is utilized in surgical oncologic emergencies, such as malignant bowel obstruction. A surgical diversion may be completed for an obstructed area to decrease pain and to provide comfort often allowing these patients to leave the hospital. An example of this is a patient with colon cancer who has numerous metastases blocking the bowel. A diverting ostomy allows this patient to live without the pain of a malignant bowel obstruction. Decompression by inserting gastrointestinal tubes is another method which allows the patient to pursue hospice care. A patient with a gastric outlet obstruction can have a nasogastric tube removed after a palliative gastrostomy tube is placed allowing the patient to return home.

Surgical Stress Response

Anesthesia and associated physiologic changes create the surgical stress response. This response is activated by afferent input to the hypothalamus from the site of surgical trauma, which results in inflammatory, endocrine, and metabolic responses (Bierle et al., 2020). The degree of surgical injury corresponds with the surgical stress response.

The endocrine stress response involves an increase in levels of antidiuretic hormone (ADH), growth hormone, catecholamines, cortisol, and renin (Bierle et al., 2020). ADH influences salt and water metabolism promoting free water retention and the production of concentrated urine (Bierle et al., 2020). Renin and aldosterone promote water and sodium resorption. Catabolism of carbohydrates, fat, and protein are some metabolic changes that provide increased energy for the production of glucose and acute-phase proteins (Bierle et al., 2020). The inflammatory response to surgery includes the release of cytokines (interleukin-1, interleukin-6, and tumor necrosis factor-α) from leukocytes, fibroblasts, and endothelial cells from the surgical trauma site (Bierle et al., 2020). Cytokines initiate both a local and systemic response producing acute-phase proteins from the liver (Bierle et al., 2020). This stress response has a variable duration. ADH effect can last 3 to 5 days and cytokine effect lasts 2 to 3 days.

Preoperative Risk Assessment

All patients scheduled for surgery should be considered for preoperative evaluation even for low-risk procedures and those without any comorbidities. It is recommended that a high-risk patient with poor functional status be assessed by an expert in evaluation of noninvasive testing (Cohn, 2016).

For many cancer centers, these patients are referred to a specialty clinic for preoperative evaluation. A preoperative history and physical should be performed by the clinic nurse and the nurse practitioner on the patient's initial visit. This should include:

1. Medication use, including dietary or herbal supplements
2. Exercise tolerance
3. Use of tobacco, alcohol, and illicit substances
4. Reaction to past surgeries, such as bleeding and experience with anesthesia
5. Cardiac risk—using the Revised Cardiac Risk Index (Cohn, 2016)

Surgical Preoperative Evaluation

Geriatric Assessment

Frailty assessment is recommended by the American College of Surgeons (ACS), but many surgeons still use age as the sole predictor for risk which is unreliable (Johnston et al., 2019). Frailty is a syndrome with a depleted physiologic reserve and diminished resistance to stressors (Hanna et al., 2019). The American Geriatric Society's gold standard for assessment is the Comprehensive Geriatric Assessment (CGA). This is a multidisciplinary evaluation including assessment of physical, mental, social, economic, functional, and environmental aspects of the elderly. Unfortunately, due to the time it takes to complete the CGA, the ACS endorses the modified Frailty Index (mFI). The mFI was created from data from the National Surgical Quality Improvement Program (NSQIP). Several factors should be taken into account regarding physiologic reserve including comorbidities and nutritional status.

Obesity

Anesthesia and paralysis cause major alterations in the respiratory function of the obese patient related to lung structure, mechanics, and gas exchange (Bazurro et al., 2018). In order to optimize the perioperative risk management, several tools have been developed. The Snoring, Tiredness, Observed apnea, Blood pressure, Body mass index, Age, Neck circumference, and Gender (STOP-Bang) is the most utilized scale to assess preoperative risk. Often referrals to cardiology and pulmonology for further evaluation are necessary. These patients need an electrocardiogram as they are high risk. The American College of Physicians recommends a chest x-ray for patients older than 50 years of age in preparation for abdominal or thoracic surgery (Bierle et al., 2020).

Pregnancy

Nonurgent surgery in the second trimester has a lower risk for preterm labor or spontaneous abortion and is therefore preferred (Brown & Holt, 2019). The surgery plan should be personalized and discussed with multiple disciplines. Pregnancy earlier than 24 weeks should have documentation of fetal heart tones before and after the procedure. A nonstress test and tocometry before and after surgery should also be performed (Brown & Holt, 2019). The obstetrical team should be involved throughout the planning process and for postoperative evaluation.

Endocrine

Studies have shown that patients with hyperglycemia and a hemoglobin A_{1C} higher than 8% should be optimized prior to elective surgery (Himes et al., 2020). This allows for revision of the diabetic treatment plan and improvement of perioperative glycemic control. Referrals to endocrinology or the patient's primary care physician should be made in the preoperative process.

Cardiac

There are several high-risk cardiac conditions which are contraindicated in noncardiac surgery. These include symptomatic, severe aortic stenosis; acute decompensated heart failure, tachyarrhythmias or bradyarrhythmias with hypotension; and acute coronary syndrome (Smilowitz & Berger, 2020). Patients who have undergone chemotherapy may require additional cardiovascular evaluation because of potential side effects of chemotherapy that may affect the cardiovascular system. Classification systems and risk scores assist in estimating perioperative risk. The most commonly used are the Revised Cardiac Risk Index, the NSQIP perioperative myocardial infarction and the universal surgical risk calculator (Smilowitz & Berger, 2020).

It is important to determine the bleeding risk of the procedure and weigh it against the risk of interrupting or withholding anticoagulation during the time leading up to surgery (Ford & Robertson, 2020). If the risk of withholding anticoagulation is higher than the procedure bleeding risk, the patient may be placed on low-molecular-weight heparin (LMWH). This patient may often be preadmitted prior to surgery and placed on a heparin drip (Mar et al., 2016). The table on the next page outlines further information regarding novel oral anticoagulants.

Peri-Procedural Management of Anticoagulates

CrCl (mL/min)	DABIGATRAN (PRADAXA) DAYS BEING HELD		RIVAROXABAN (XARELTO) DAYS BEING HELD		APIXABAN (ELIQUIS) DAYS BEING HELD		EDOXABAN (SAVAYSA) DAYS BEING HELD	
	Normal or Low Bleeding Risk	High Bleeding Risk	Normal or Low Bleeding Risk	High Bleeding Risk	Normal or Low Bleeding Risk	High Bleeding Risk	Normal or Low Bleeding Risk	High Bleeding Risk
>80	1	2	1	2	1	2	1	2
50–79	2	3	1	2	1	3	1	3
30–49	2	4	1	3	2	3	2	3
<30	3	5	2	3	2	4	2	4

Data from Doherty, J. U., Gluckman, T. J., Hucker, W. J., Januzzi, J. L., Jr., Ortel, T. L., Saxonhouse, S. J., & Spinler, S. A. (2017). 2017 ACC expert consensus decision pathway for periprocedural management of anticoagulation in patients with nonvalvular atrial fibrillation: A report of the American College of Cardiology Clinical Expert Consensus Document Task Force. *Journal of the American College of Cardiology, 69*(7), 871–898.

Principles of Cancer Management

③

The American Society of Anesthesiologists recommends obtaining hemoglobin and hematocrit levels for patients of advanced age and those undergoing blood loss surgery. Platelets should be obtained in patients with hepatic or hematologic disease.

Prehabilitation

Prehabilitation is the initiation of preoperative optimization strategies and is part of Enhanced Recovery After Surgery (ERAS). During the preoperative assessment, risk factors are identified that can be addressed and improved for a better surgical outcome. Prehabilitation involves three phases: screening and assessment; individualized needs-based interventions; and posttreatment evaluation (Tew et al., 2020). Improving the patient's nutritional state and exercise capacity, building muscle mass, and psychologically preparing patients for surgery are all part of the prehabilitation process (Boudreaux & Simmons, 2019).

Cigarette smoking is a risk factor associated with venous thrombosis, surgical site infections, pulmonary and cardiovascular complications. Incisional healing is impaired when peripheral vasculature is altered, and carboxyhemoglobin levels are increased. Patients who stop smoking preoperatively, even for a short time, may reduce these complications (Boudreaux & Simmons, 2019). Smoking cessation programs can be utilized to assist with smoking cessation. Nurses should assist with referral to these programs or offer the patient oral or dermal nicotine withdrawal tools.

Malnutrition is common among cancer and the frail elderly patient (Hanna et al., 2019). Low serum albumin and prealbumin levels are commonly used to assess malnutrition. Body mass index (BMI) is also used as a marker of nutritional status with reduced BMI associated impaired survival in a variety of cancers (Whittle et al., 2018). However, there are many screening tools to assess malnutrition, such as the Malnutrition Universal Screening Tool, the Nutrition Risk Screening 2002, and the Short Nutrition Assessment Questionnaire (Whittle et al., 2018). Frail patients often have sarcopenia, or reduced muscle mass and have poorer surgical outcomes. Preoperative nutritional intervention has been shown to reduce surgical site infections by 20% to 40% (Whittle et al., 2018). Nursing and dietary team members can educate the patient on a high-protein diet and protein supplementation. The best effect has been noted if dietary supplementation is started 7 to 10 days preoperatively (Gustafsson et al., 2019). If the patient is unable to achieve this goal with oral intake, the use of an enteral feeding tube may be utilized. If due to an anatomic condition, parenteral nutrition may need to be utilized for at least 7 to 14 days preoperatively (Whittle et al., 2018).

Poor physical fitness is a predictor of poor surgical outcome (Durrand et al., 2019). Adults age 60 or older can benefit from increased exercise capacity. Age is often associated with reduced lean muscle mass termed sarcopenia, which is a predictor of poor surgical outcome. Patients may be referred to a physical and/or occupational therapist for instruction and assistance in daily exercise time permitting. It is important that this activity is cost effective and increases aerobic capacity while being safe, time efficient, and acceptable to patients (Whittle et al., 2018). Walking, which is moderate exercise, is easier and effective in the long-term results, but may not achieve short term results.

The neuroendocrine response is enhanced by alcohol (Durrand et al., 2019). Alcohol consumption may affect up to 23% of surgical patients. These patients may have an elevated surgical risk without exhibiting alcohol dependence or organ dysfunction. Patients should be counseled to stop or reduce alcohol intake at least 6 weeks prior to surgery. This reduces the risk of developing alcohol withdrawal or delirium postoperatively.

Enhanced Recovery After Surgery

The ERAS Society is dedicated to enhancing recovery after surgery and publishes evidence-based guidelines and protocols from large prospective cohort studies, meta-analyses, and randomized control studies across all surgical subspecialties (Smith et al., 2020). All ERAS protocols in the surgical subspecialties share the same objectives: accelerated recovery time after surgery, decrease in perioperative stress, preoperative patient optimization, and maintenance of postoperative physiologic function (Kleppe & Greenberg, 2018; Smith et al., 2020). The goal of ERAS is to improve the value of the care provided to the patient and the healthcare system.

Health care is measured by the quality, patient-reported outcomes, safety, and the cost of the care delivered (Kleppe & Greenberg, 2018).

ERAS guidelines optimize perioperative nutritional status and fluid balance, promotion of opioid sparing analgesia, antiinflammatory interventions both pharmacologic and nonpharmacologic, early mobilization, and early feeding to prevent the body's response to surgical stress. The objectives are achieved by a multidisciplinary team which includes preoperative nurses, anesthesiologists, operative nurses, postoperative recovery nurses, medical-surgical nurses, dieticians, physical therapists, social workers, and surgeons. ERAS has demonstrated reduction in length of stay and complication rates without adversely affecting readmission rates and mortality (Senturk et al., 2017).

Perioperative Nursing Care

The basis for creating a safe and successful postoperative recovery begins with preoperative assessment and planning. The nurse assesses the patient's clinical and psychosocial status. Patient-centered care identifies the patient as a special being. The nurse should explain what is going to happen while providing support and reassurance. This allows for an environment of trust to develop (Nilsson et al., 2020).

Prophylactic antibiotics are broad spectrum and often determined by institutional protocol based on institutional bacterial resistance. Cephalosporins are the most commonly recommended antibiotic class due to their low cost, allergy potential, and broad spectrum. Antibiotics are administered intravenously within 30 minutes to 1 hour prior to the skin incision. Dosing should be increased in obese patients, and in prolonged surgeries should be repeated after one or two times the half-life of the antibiotic (Nelson et al., 2016a). For patients allergic to penicillin or cephalosporin, a combination of clindamycin and gentamicin IV or a quinolone may be used (Nelson et al., 2016a).

Skin preparation prior to surgery includes a shower with a skin antiseptic solution requiring nursing to teach prior to surgery. Chlorhexidine alcohol is preferred over aqueous povidone-iodine solution for skin cleansing (Nelson et al., 2016a).

Postoperative Nursing Care

If possible oral fluid and food intake should be started on the day of surgery. Intravenous (IV) fluids with oral intake should be maintained 12 to 24 hours. IV fluids should be an hourly volume of 1 to 2 mL/kg (Makaryus et al., 2018; Nelson et al., 2016b). Crystalloid solutions are preferred to normal saline due to the risk of hyperchloremic acidosis (Nelson et al., 2016b). Oliguria (20 cm^3/h) is a normal response to surgery due to ongoing postoperative neurohumoral stress response leading to renal vasoconstriction and the conservation of salt and water (Myles et al., 2017). The clinical situation should be assessed for the need for IV fluid boluses utilizing hemodynamics (Nelson et al., 2016b). Traditionally, a fluid bolus of 500 to 1000 mL was given as a fluid volume challenge. This increased cardiac output for 120 minutes and then cardiac output would return to normal (Gordon & Spiegel, 2020). Systemic inflammatory response syndrome may develop postoperatively causing hypotension and vasodilation without sepsis. Vasopressors may be required postoperatively in this situation.

Supplemental protein drinks should be offered three times daily to ensure protein and calorie intake early in the recovery process. These supplements also contain vitamins, minerals, and trace elements. Quicker return to bowel function and reduced length of stay have been demonstrated in randomized trials (Nelson et al., 2016b).

Bedrest is associated with venous thromboembolic events (VTEs). Early mobilization is important in prevention of VTEs. Pneumatic stockings are useful for prevention while the patient is immobile. Daily prophylaxis with LMWH has been shown by a Cochrane review to prevent VTEs and is extended for 28 days postoperatively upon discharge (Nelson et al., 2016b).

Encouraging patients to get out of bed as early as possible is effective in pain management (Schreiber, 2021). Health education is important particularly in the geriatric population including their family members. This group may believe that after cancer surgery, patients should stay in bed. These patients may refuse early postoperative ambulation leading to complications, delayed discharge, and even readmission (Li et al., 2018). On the day of surgery, the patient will be asked to sit up in the chair, and to ambulate short distances. The activity level is progressed within the patient's tolerance range. The urinary catheter is removed as soon as possible to assist in ambulation (Li et al., 2018).

Analgesia through the synergistic effects of various types of drugs that are nonnarcotic is the foundation of multimodal analgesia and a part of ERAS protocols. Nonsteroidal antiinflammatory drugs (NSAIDs) are effective in pain reduction, reduction in opioid use, and improved patient satisfaction. A combination of an NSAID and acetaminophen is more effective than either drug alone. Both drugs should be scheduled as an alternate. Gabapentin is also used in the multimodal approach and helps lessen neuropathic pain. The drug of choice in pregnancy is acetaminophen due to safety to the fetus and no dependency risk (Brown & Holt, 2019). NSAIDs are contraindicated in pregnancy due to the risk of alterations in fetal renal blood flow and premature closure of the ductus arteriosus (Brown & Holt, 2019). A short course of cyclobenzaprine can also be utilized. The shortest and lowest dose of opioids may be utilized for severe pain (Brown & Holt, 2019).

Conclusion

Care of the oncology patient with a solid tumor in an early stage will involve surgery at some point in their cancer journey. Surgical care undergoes constant revision with evidence-based guidelines, which has been developed in several surgical specialties. These evidence-based protocols are called ERAS. ERAS has changed surgical oncology nursing practice from tradition passed down over the years to evidence-based practice allowing a faster and safer recovery for the patient.

References

Bazurro, S., Ball, L., & Pelosi, P. (2018). Perioperative management of obese patient. *Current Opinions in Critical Care, 24*(6), 560–567.

Berger, M. F., & Mardis, E. R. (2018). The emerging clinical relevance of genomics in cancer medicine. *Nature Reviews. Clinical Oncology, 15*(6), 353–365.

Bierle, D. M., Raslau, D., Regan, D. W., Sundsted, K. K., & Mauck, K. F. (2020). Preoperative evaluation before noncardiac surgery. *Mayo Clinic Proceedings, 95*(4), 807–822. https://doi.org/10.1016/j.mayocp.2019.04.029.

Boudreaux, A. M., & Simmons, J. W. (2019). Prehabilitation and optimization of modifiable patient risk factors: The importance of effective preoperative evaluation to improve surgical outcomes. *AORN Journal, 109*(4), 500–507.

Brown, B. P., & Holt, R. (2019). Palliative care and the pregnant surgical patient: Epidemiology, ethics, and clinical guidance. *Surgical Clinics of North America, 99*(5), 941–953.

Canter, R. J. (2016). Chemotherapy: Does neoadjuvant or adjuvant therapy improve outcomes? *Surgical Oncology Clinics of North America, 25*(4), 861–872.

Cohn, S. L. (2016). Preoperative evaluation for noncardiac surgery. *Annals of Internal Medicine, 165*(11). ITC81–ITC96.

Durrand, J., Singh, S. J., & Danjoux, G. (2019). Prehabilitation. *Clinical Medicine, 19*(6), 458–464.

Ford, C., & Robertson, M. (2020). Care of the surgical patient-part 2: oral anticoagulants. *British Journal of Nursing, 29*(21), 1242–1246. https://doi.org/10.12968/bjon.2020.29.21.1242.

Gordon, D., & Spiegel, R. (2020). Fluid resuscitation: History, physiology, and modern fluid resuscitation strategies. *Emergency Medical Clinics of North America, 38*(4), 783–793.

Gustafsson, U. O., Scott, M. J., Hubner, M., Nygren, J., Demartines, N., Francis, N., … Ljungqvist, O. (2019). Guidelines for perioperative care in elective colorectal surgery: Enhanced recovery after surgery (ERAS®) society recommendations: 2018. *World Journal of Surgery, 43*(3), 659–695.

Hanna, K., Ditillo, M., & Joseph, B. (2019). The role of frailty and prehabilitation in surgery. *Critical Care, 25*(6), 717–722.

Himes, C. P., Ganesh, R., Wight, E. C., Simha, V., & Liebow, M. (2020). Perioperative evaluation and management of endocrine disorders. *Mayo Clinic Proceedures, 95*(12), 2760–2776.

Jara, R. D., Guerrón, A. D., & Portenier, D. (2020). Complications of robotic surgery. *Surgical Clinics of North America, 100*(2), 461–468.

Johnston, M. E., 2nd, Sussman, J. J., & Patel, S. H. (2019). Surgical oncology and geriatric patients. *Clinical Geriatric Medicine, 35*(1), 53–63.

Kleppe, K. L., & Greenberg, J. A. (2018). Enhanced recovery after surgery protocols: Rationale and components. *Surgical Clinics of North American, 98*(3), 499–509.

Li, K., Cannon, J. G. D., Jiang, S. Y., Sambare, T. D., Owens, D. K., Bendavid, E., & Poultsides, G. A. (2018). Diagnostic staging laparoscopy in gastric cancer treatment: A cost-effectiveness analysis. *Journal of Surgical Oncology, 117*(6), 1288–1296.

Makaryus, R., Miller, T. E., & Gan, T. J. (2018). Current concepts of fluid management in enhanced recovery pathways. *British Journal of Anaesthesia, 120*(2), 376–383.

Mar, P. L., Familtsev, D., Ezekowitz, M. D., Lakkireddy, D., & Gopinathannair, R. (2016). Periprocedural management of anticoagulation in patients taking novel oral anticoagulants: Review of the literature and recommendations for specific populations and procedures. *International Journal of Cardiology, 202*, 578–585.

Myles, P. S., Andrews, S., Nicholson, J., Lobo, D. N., & Mythen, M. (2017). Contemporary approaches to perioperative IV fluid therapy. *World Journal of Surgery, 41*(10), 2457–2463.

Nelson, G., Altman, A. D., Nick, A., Meyer, L. A., Ramirez, P. T., Achtari, C., … Dowdy, S. C. (2016a). Guidelines for pre- and intra-operative care in gynecologic/oncology surgery: Enhanced recovery after surgery (ERAS®) society recommendations—part I. *Gynecologic Oncology, 140*(2), 313–322.

Nelson, G., Altman, A. D., Nick, A., Meyer, L. A., Ramirez, P. T., Achtari, C., … Dowdy, S. C. (2016b). Guidelines for postoperative care in gynecologic/oncology surgery: Enhanced recovery after surgery (ERAS®) society recommendations—part II. *Gynecologic Oncology, 140*(2), 323–332.

Nilsson, U., Gruen, R., & Myles, P. (2020). Postoperative recovery: The importance of the team. *Anaesthesia, 75*(Suppl 1), e158–e164.

Orosco, R. K., Tapia, V. J., Califano, J. A., Clary, B., Cohen, E. E. W., Kane, C., … Nguyen, Q. T. (2018). Positive surgical margins in the 10 most common solid cancers. *Scientific Reports, 8*(1), 5686.

Schreiber, M. L. (2021). Mobility: A pathway to recovery. *MedSurg Nursing, 30*(4), 279–281.

Senturk, J. C., Kristo, G., Gold, J., Bleday, R., & Whang, E. (2017). The development of enhanced recovery after surgery across surgical specialties. *Journal of Laparoendoscopic & Advanced Surgical Techniques, 27*(9), 863–869.

Smilowitz, N. R., & Berger, J. S. (2020). Perioperative cardiovascular risk assessment and management for noncardiac surgery. *JAMA, 324*(3), 279–290.

Smith, T. W., Jr., Wang, X., Singer, M. A., Godellas, C. V., & Vaince, F. T. (2020). Enhanced recovery after surgery: A clinical review of implementation across multiple surgical subspecialties. *The American Journal of Surgery, 219*(3), 530–534.

Tew, G. A., Bedford, R., Carr, E., Durrand, J. W., Gray, J., Hackett, R., & Danjoux, G. (2020). Community-based prehabilitation before elective major surgery: The PREP-WELL quality improvement project. *BMJ Open Quality, 9*(1), e000898.

Thorat, M. A., & Balasubramanian, R. (2020). Breast cancer prevention in high-risk women. *Best Practice & Research Clinical Obstetrics and Gynaecology, 65*, 18–31.

Whittle, J., Wischmeyer, P. E., Grocott, M. P. W., & Miller, T. E. (2018). Surgical prehabilitation: Nutrition and exercise. *Anesthesiology Clinic, 36*(4), 567–580.

Radiation Therapy

Danielle M. Fournier

Definition

Radiation therapy is one of the cornerstones of cancer therapy and involves the use of high-energy x-rays or radioactive substances to treat local or regional areas of sites of disease. Radiation therapy utilizes electromagnetic radiation including x-rays, gamma rays, and particulate radiation such as electrons, protons, and neutrons to cause damage to cancer cells. Radiation therapy is designed to deliver targeted treatment to the tumor while simultaneously sparing the surrounding healthy tissue.

The Role of Radiation in Cancer Care

Approximately 60% of patients with cancer receive radiation therapy at some point during the treatment of their disease (Abshire & Lang, 2018). Radiation therapy may be used as a single modality, but it is often combined with surgery or systemic therapy. The following terms describe the use of radiation therapy as a treatment modality:

- *Definitive therapy* implies that treatment is used for curative intent. Radiation may be given as a single treatment modality but may also be administered with concomitant systemic therapy (chemotherapy, biotherapy, targeted therapy, immunotherapy) to enhance its effectiveness. Definitive radiation may also be considered for treatment of cancer in patients who are not surgical candidates due to comorbid conditions. Definitive radiation therapy is an option to treat head and neck, cervical, anal, prostate, and early-stage lung cancers.
- *Neoadjuvant therapy* is radiation administered before primary therapy (surgery) with the purpose of shrinking the tumor to improve the possibility of complete resection. In this situation, it is often administered with concurrent chemotherapy, which serves as a radiosensitizer. Neoadjuvant radiation therapy is commonly used to treat esophageal or rectal cancer.
- *Adjuvant therapy* is radiation therapy given after primary surgical therapy, with the intention of improving local control to reduce the risk for cancer recurrence. An advantage of adjuvant radiation therapy is there is a smaller target volume after resection. Adjuvant radiation therapy is commonly used to treat breast, lung, or head and neck cancers.
- *Prophylactic therapy* refers to radiation therapy administered when there is no clinical evidence of disease, but there is substantial risk for microscopic disease. One example of this is prophylactic cranial irradiation (PCI) in patients with small cell lung cancer.
- *Palliative therapy* is radiation treatment that is used to alleviate symptoms. Palliative radiation is not given with a curative intent and typically consists of a shorter treatment course (1 to 10 treatments). Examples include irradiation of bone metastases to relieve pain, irradiating tumors causing spinal cord compression, or radiation tumors with frequent bleeding.

Radiobiology

Radiobiology is the study of the effects of ionizing radiation on biologic systems (Zeman, 2021). While radiation therapy can cause a multitude of effects on biologic matter including DNA damage, chromosomal aberrations, and carcinogenesis, the most significant effect of radiation therapy is cytotoxicity or cell killing. Radiation therapy can cause damage and cell death either directly or indirectly. Direct damage results in single or double-strand DNA breaks, incorrect cross-linkages, or damage and/or loss of a nitrogenous base. Indirect damage is caused by interaction of the radiation with the surrounding environment fluid, leading to the creation of free radicals, which cause damage to the cell. The radiation dose must be sufficient to create tumor control, while also limiting damage to the surrounding tissue. This concept is known as the *therapeutic ratio*.

There are four stages in the radiobiology continuum leading to cell destruction: (1) the *physical stage*, which includes the ionization of atoms after radiation exposure; (2) the *physicochemical stage*, which includes the formation of free radicals; (3) the *biochemical stage,* when DNA damage occurs; and (4) the *biologic stage*, characterized by unrepaired or mis-rejoined DNA damage (Zeman, 2021). Cells are most sensitive to radiation damage during the late G_2 and M phases of the cell cycle and most resistant during the late S phase (Trifiletti & Zaorsky, 2019). Cells that have a more rapid rate of mitosis are more radiation sensitive.

The success or failure of radiation therapy depends on the five Rs of radiobiology: (1) reoxygenation of hypoxic areas of tumor, (2) repair of DNA damage, (3) redistribution of cells in the cell cycle, (4) repopulation of cells, and (5) radiosensitivity of the targeted tissue (Behrand, 2019). These factors are important to consider when determining the dose, timing, and fractionation of radiation therapy to help maximize the desired effects of treatment.

Both normal and cancerous cells are susceptible to radiation damage and may be injured or destroyed during treatment. *Fractionation* refers to the division of the total dose of radiation into several smaller doses, allowing normal cells time to repair sublethal damage and repopulate in the time between fractions. There is a maximum tolerated dose that can be administered without causing permanent, irreparable damage. The dose per fraction and dose per time period are factors in delivering effective doses of radiation to limit toxicities experienced by the patient.

Radiosensitizers

Radiosensitizers are pharmaceutical agents or chemicals that help to improve the tumor killing effect of radiation therapy. There are several mechanisms for how an agent may increase the effectiveness of radiation. Radiosensitizing agents such as cisplatin and fluorouracil help to increase radiation damage. These drugs damage the DNA in the cell, predisposing the DNA to further damage with concurrent radiation exposure (Willey et al., 2021). Some radiosensitizing agents, such as fluorouracil, gemcitabine, fludarabine, methotrexate, cisplatin, etoposide, and hydroxyurea, inhibit DNA damage repair in cancer cells, which also helps to amplify radiation damage. Some agents can help to maintain tumor cells in the radiation sensitive G2 and M phase of the cell cycle. These include taxanes, nucleoside analogs, and modified pyrimidines.

Chemotherapy agents with cytotoxic or cytostatic effects can reduce repopulation of cancer cells when given with radiation therapy.

A hypoxic environment protects cancer cells from radiation damage since radiation therapy relies on the generation of oxygen free radicals to cause cell damage. Antiangiogenic drugs such as bevacizumab normalize blood flow to the tumor to reduce hypoxia. Hypoxic radiosensitizers such as misonidazole, can reverse the radiation resistance of tumor cells and mimic the effects of oxygen in hypoxic areas (Willey et al., 2021).

Drugs Commonly Used as Radiosensitizers

Drug Class	Commonly Used Agents
Antimetabolites	Fluorouracil
	Capecitabine
	Gemcitabine
	Cytarabine
	Methotrexate
	Trimetrexate
	Pemetrexed
Alkylating agents	Chlorambucil
	Melphalan
	Cyclophosphamide
	Ifosfamide
	Procarbazine
	Dacarbazine
	Temozolomide
	Mitomycin C
Platinums	Cisplatin
	Carboplatin
	Oxaliplatin
Taxanes	Paclitaxel
	Docetaxel
	Albumin-bound paclitaxel
Vinca alkaloids	Vincristine
	Vinblastine
	Vinorelbine
Topoisomerase I inhibitors	Irinotecan
	Topotecan
Anthracyclines	Idarubicin
	Doxorubicin
	Epirubicin
	Daunorubicin
Podophyllotoxins	Etoposide
	Teniposide

Radiation Delivery

Radiation Units

There are several units used to measure radiation dose and exposure. The *absorbed dose* is the energy deposited in the tissue by the radiation beam. It is measured in joules/kilogram, and 1 joule/kilogram is known as a gray (Gy) (Trifiletti & Zaorsky, 2019). The *equivalent dose* is calculated for a specific organ and is based on the absorbed dose adjusted for the type of radiation given. Equivalent dose is measured in millisieverts (mSv). The *effective dose* is calculated for the whole body and is the sum of the equivalent doses to each organ, adjusted for the sensitivity of each organ to radiation. Effective dose is also measured in mSv.

Equipment

A linear accelerator (LINAC) is the machine used to deliver external beam radiation therapy. The LINAC accelerates electrons which collide with a heavy metal target to produce high-energy x-rays, which are then shaped by a *multileaf collimator* to conform to the patient's tumor. The beam comes out of the gantry, a large mechanical arm, which can rotate around the patient to deliver radiation therapy from multiple angles. The LINAC is used for various radiation delivery techniques including, intensity-modulated radiation therapy (IMRT), volumetric modulated arc therapy (VMAT), image-guided radiation therapy (IGRT), stereotactic body radiotherapy (SBRT), and stereotactic radiosurgery (SRS).

Proton therapy uses different technology to deliver treatment. A particle accelerator such as a synchrotron or cyclotron accelerates protons, which originate from hydrogen atoms to high velocities using magnets (LaRiviere et al., 2019). In doing so, this energizes the proton particle. The energized proton particles are transported to each of the proton facility's treatment rooms through a beam line. Within each room, an organized group of electromagnets focuses the proton beam towards the gantry, which can rotate 360 degrees around the patient to deliver treatment from multiple angles. Computed tomography (CT) imaging is built into the gantry to ensure accurate tumor location identification prior to delivering treatment.

Radiation Treatment Team

The radiation treatment team consists of a multidisciplinary team of health care professionals, oftentimes including:

- Radiation oncologist—A physician trained in radiation therapy delivery; responsible for prescribing therapy and overseeing patient care during treatment.
- Physicist and dosimetrist—Individuals who help to develop the radiation treatment plan in coordination with the radiation oncologist. They determine the best way to deliver the prescribed dose of radiation to the tumor safely to the patient to protect surrounding vital organs.
- Radiation technologist—The technologist operates the machinery that delivers the radiation dose to the patient.
- Mold and cast technician—A technician creates custom immobilization devices to ensure safe and consistent patient positioning.

- Registered nurse—The nurse provides ongoing support to the patient while they are undergoing radiation therapy treatment. This may include wound care, symptom assessment and management, and general support.
- Dietitian—The dietitian can provide guidance and support for patients who have trouble eating, drinking or experience significant weight loss during treatment.
- Speech language pathologist—The speech therapist can help patients with issues related to radiation therapy treatment, especially in the setting of head and neck cancer treatment.

Radiation Planning

Prior to beginning radiation therapy, the patient meets with the radiation oncologist and multidisciplinary treatment team for consultation, who will determine the type of radiation therapy that would be most beneficial to treat the cancer. The goal is to maximize the therapeutic ratio, delivering the maximum tolerated radiation dose to the tumor while sparing radiation dose to the surrounding tissue (Gardner et al., 2019). If radiation therapy is recommended, informed consent is obtained from the patient before proceeding.

Before the patient starts treatment, they must undergo radiation simulation, typically involving three-dimensional imaging with CT or magnetic resonance imaging to generate an image of the treatment field and determine target volume. Simulation helps to formulate a multidimensional treatment plan, taking into consideration external landmarks and any shielding of critical organs. The simulation process usually takes about 1 hour. Consistent patient positioning is crucial for the safe delivery of radiation therapy. In some cases, tattoos on the skin are needed to mark the treatment field and aid in alignment of the body. In other cases, immobilization devices are used to ensure consistent patient positioning throughout treatment. If necessary, tattoos or immobilization devices are created during the simulation.

After simulation is completed, the technical planning process begins. The radiation oncologist maps out the relevant organs and tissues on the imaging, known as *contouring*, which allows for treatment customization (Gardner et al., 2019). This process defines the gross tumor volume (GTV), or any visible tumor present on imaging. Once the GTV is defined, they can determine the radiation clinical target volume, which incorporates the GTV and any anatomic areas with suspected subclinical microscopic disease that will also require treatment. The radiation oncologist also reviews and delineates any organs at risk, which may be particularly susceptible to radiation therapy damage and need to be spared from excess radiation exposure. Based on this information, the medical physicists and dosimetrists review the imaging and design, generate, and measure radiation dose distributions to create a treatment plan. This process takes approximately 1 week.

Radiation Modalities

External Beam Radiation Therapy

External beam radiation therapy (EBRT) is the most common form of delivery of radiation treatment and involves the delivery of radiation from a unit outside of the body. Advances in technology have led to improved imaging techniques, which have contributed to better conformality of treatment. With EBRT, the patient is positioned on a treatment couch of the LINAC, with close attention to patient alignment to ensure consistent dose delivery. Each treatment will take 15 to 30 minutes, including set-up time.

With EBRT, the total dose of radiation is achieved through administering equal fractions of radiation. These are traditionally administered once a day, for 5 days per week, until the total dose is reached. EBRT is typically given over the course of several weeks and is an outpatient treatment. It is important for patients to understand that they will not become radioactive while receiving EBRT.

There are many forms of EBRT:

- *Three-dimensional conformal radiation therapy* uses static beams to best deliver the radiation dose to the target, while sparing surrounding tissues. This was the first conformal radiation therapy technique to utilize three-dimensional treatment planning (Feng et al., 2021).
- *Intensity-modulated radiation therapy* involves the use of multiple small beam arrangements and intensities to customize delivery of the optimal dose distribution. This allows for maximal conformation of the dose to the target.
- *Image-guided radiation therapy* can be used in addition to IMRT and utilizes imaging obtained prior to each radiation treatment session to ensure accurate dose delivery. On-board imaging uses images to confirm the radiation therapy set-up reflects their treatment plan. This technique helps to eliminate inconsistencies in patient set-up or motion due to respiration (Gardner et al., 2019).
- *Volumetric modulated arc therapy* is a type of IMRT which uses one or more arc beams as well as intensity modulation during the delivery of radiation. As opposed to IMRT which consists of static delivery with the LINAC rotating between beam deliveries, VMAT involves continuous delivery as the LINAC rotates around the patient (Gardner et al., 2019).
- *Proton therapy* is a form of EBRT that harnesses protons, which are heavy charged particles, delivered to the patient in a manner like conventional radiation therapy (LaRiviere et al., 2019). An advantage of proton therapy is that energy is deposited in the designated target without an exit dose, enhancing tumor destruction and limiting damage to the surrounding tissues.

Brachytherapy

Brachytherapy is the temporary or permanent placement of a radioactive source directly in or near the target tissue. An advantage of brachytherapy is that it can deliver a highly localized radiation dose that minimizes radiation exposure to the surrounding tissue, reducing toxicity to the patient (Otter et al., 2021). Brachytherapy utilizes radioisotopes to delivery treatment; the most used radioisotopes are iridium-192, cesium-137, iodine-125, palladium-103, and gold-198 (Mallick et al., 2020). The brachytherapy unit stores the radioisotope until the isotope is mobilized near the tumor during treatment delivery. Brachytherapy is commonly used in the treatment of cervical, endometrial, gastrointestinal, vaginal, prostate, breast, lung-endobronchial, head and neck, and skin cancers. Brachytherapy can be used alone or in conjunction with EBRT, which can help to treat bulky disease and improve local control (Behrand, 2019).

There are two main types of brachytherapy: high dose rate (HDR) brachytherapy and low dose rate (LDR) brachytherapy. HDR brachytherapy is delivered quickly and results in better cell kill due to higher radiation doses. In preparation for HDR brachytherapy, needles, catheters, or applicators are placed in or near the treatment site. Depending on the location, these may be left in place for the duration of treatment or removed and reinserted prior to each treatment (Miller & Scherbak, 2021). During HDR brachytherapy, the radioactive source, usually iridium-192, travels inside the catheter and is controlled by a device called a remote afterloader. The radioactive source is only in the patient for a few minutes. During this time, the patient is radioactive, and precautions are necessary until the source is removed. All HDR brachytherapy occurs in a treatment vault and staff remain outside the vault while the radiation source is out of its shielded housing to reduce exposure (Thomadsen, 2019). This procedure is done on an outpatient basis, and patients need to receive multiple treatments over several days to weeks. Benefits include increased safety for patients and staff, less patient discomfort, faster treatment, and no need for prolonged immobilization.

LDR brachytherapy involves placement of the radiation source in the tumor area, where it releases a continuous low dose of radiation over an extended period. This can span from several hours to several days. Effective treatment relies on the accurate placement of the radioactive source. LDR brachytherapy has a superior radiobiologic effect as the longer time course allows for cells to transition into the phase of the cell cycle where they are most susceptible to radiation damage while also allowing sufficient time for healthy tissues to repair sublethal damage (Mallick et al., 2020). As opposed to HDR which is done outpatient, patients receiving LDR brachytherapy are admitted as inpatients. To avoid dislodging the radioactive implant once it has been placed, prolonged bedrest may be needed.

LDR brachytherapy was developed prior to the availability of technology that allowed for remote after loading, and there is higher risk of radiation exposure to staff who are involved in the care of patients receiving LDR brachytherapy. Nurses caring for these individuals are instructed to observe the important precautions of time, distance, and shielding to protect themselves from radiation exposure. Radiation dosimetry monitors are worn by any staff members who enter the patient's room during this time. After the radiation source has been removed and returned to storage and the area shows no radiation contamination when surveyed, no further radiation protection is needed.

One form of LDR brachytherapy comes in the form of permanent implants or "seeds," which are small sources of radioactive materials that are inserted into the body and not removed. This therapy is often used in the treatment of low-risk, localized prostate cancer. Each seed is the size of a grain of rice and is implanted in the prostate gland, where it releases a steady dose of radiation over the course of 8 to 10 months.

The sources used are weak emitters of gamma radiation and yield low surface doses. The most source is iodine-125 or palladium-103. Patient education should include information on limiting close contact (<3 feet) with other people for the first 2 weeks after treatment to avoid prolonged close contact with pregnant women and children during the first 2 months after implantation.

Radioisotope Therapy

Radioisotope therapy uses unsealed sources of radiation in liquid or capsule form that are ingested by mouth. Radiopharmaceuticals are engineered to concentrate in specific areas of the body. Because of this, once the radioisotope has been ingested, there is selective uptake of the substance into the tumor cells. The radioisotope decays and produces alpha, beta, or gamma particles, which induce double-strand breaks that are cytotoxic to the tumor cell (van der Zande et al., 2021). Radioactive iodine-131 for thyroid cancer and radium-223 for prostate cancer that has metastasized to bone are two common applications of radioisotope therapy. Patient education should highlight that radiation can be present in body fluids for 1 week after treatment and precautions should be taken to minimize risk of exposure to caregivers or family. This includes thorough hand washing, sitting to urinate, double flushing the toilet, and wiping down the toilet seat after use. Other precautions include sleeping in a separate bed or at least 6 feet away from a partner, minimizing exposure to pregnant women or children, and avoiding public transportation or air travel for the first week.

Stereotactic Radiosurgery

Despite the name, SRS is a noninvasive procedure, designed to deliver a precise, high dose of external radiation to a small volume of tissue. SRS requires three-dimensional, high-resolution stereotactic imaging to maximize precision. This technique allows for destruction of the tumor, while minimizing radiation exposure to the surrounding healthy tissue. Treatment is typically completed in one session but may require up to five sessions. The high dose per fraction facilitates direct cytotoxic damage like the DNA damage seen in a course of low-dose fractionated radiation therapy. It is also effective in damaging the microvasculature of tumors, which helps to cut off blood supply to the tumor.

The most common indication for the use of SRS is treatment of brain metastases. When SRS is used to treat tumors in the head or spine, it may be referred to as Gamma Knife. Studies have suggested that SRS is a favorable alternative to whole brain radiation therapy (WBRT) in the treatment of brain metastases as WBRT does not lead to a survival benefit and causes accelerated cognitive decline (Abraham et al., 2021). There is also a role for SRS in treating arterial venous malformations, trigeminal neuralgia, and benign intracranial neoplasms such as meningiomas, acoustic neuromas, pituitary adenomas.

Stereotactic Body Radiation Therapy

In SBRT, high-dose fractions of radiation are delivered to extracranial tumors in a short timeframe typically not exceeding five fractions. Doses often range from 10 to 20 Gy per fraction. SBRT is used as a definitive treatment option for patients with medically inoperable early-stage non–small cell lung cancer (tumors <5 cm) and research has shown that it is associated with high rates of primary tumor control, low rates of treatment-related morbidity, and a rare need for salvage surgery in this population (Timmerman et al., 2018). SBRT can also be used to effectively treat primary hepatocellular, pancreatic, prostate, or renal cancers (Trifiletti & Zaorsky, 2019). There is also a role for SBRT in the treatment of oligometastatic tumors in the liver or lungs.

SBRT uses imaging guidance and immobilization devices to facilitate treatment precision. To achieve a high-dose distribution within the target, a combination of multiple beams and arcs is needed. Due to larger fractions, patient positioning, target localization and accounting for breathing-related motion is of utmost importance to ensure radiation delivery to the targeted tissue (Kavanagh & Timmerman, 2021). A single SBRT treatment may take up to 90 minutes.

Interoperative Radiation Therapy

Interoperative radiotherapy (IORT) is the delivery of radiation during surgery, with the goal of enhancing local tumor control. A LINAC is present in the operating room, and radiation can be delivered to an area of tumor while the area is opened for surgery. Utilizing radiation therapy during surgery allows for reducing the volume of the radiation "boost" through direct tumor visualization and conformational treatment. This allows for dose escalation. The National Comprehensive Cancer Network currently incorporates IORT in treatment guidelines for soft-tissue sarcomas, oligo-recurrent intraabdominal disease, resected pancreatic cancer, rectal cancer, and breast cancer (Czito et al., 2021). Current treatment approaches combine IORT with EBRT, with or without concurrent chemotherapy.

Patients who are potential candidates for IORT should be evaluated by the surgeon and radiation oncologist to allow for multidisciplinary decision making (Czito et al., 2021). Patients are good candidates for IORT when there is a high probability of incomplete resection leaving microscopic or gross residual disease, there are no evidence of distant metastases, EBRT doses needed for local control following resection exceed tissue-specific tolerances, and/or if surgical displacement or shielding of vital organs is possible during IORT administration. IORT dose is determined by the amount of residual disease, previous EBRT treatment and type and volume of healthy tissue irradiated. Based on these factors, IORT doses typically range from 10 to 20 Gy.

Radiation Side Effects

While technologic advances in radiation therapy delivery have helped to improve the delivery of radiation to the tumor, while sparing the surrounding tissue, incidental radiation exposure of the healthy tissue is unavoidable. This can lead to both acute and long-term side effects. The side effects the patient experiences correlate to the anatomic location, total radiation dose and fractionation, volume of tissue being irradiated, previous and concurrent therapies and treatment time (Palmer et al., 2020). Acute side effects of radiation therapy begin during treatment and may persist for up to several weeks after completing treatment. Chronic side effects of radiation therapy may take months to years to develop; these issues are typically related to the formation of fibrosis in the surrounding healthy tissues and damage to the microcirculation. The table below provides a list of common acute and chronic site-specific side effects of radiation treatment and the associated interventions to help manage these problems (Matta et al., 2019; Milano et al., 2021; Ozyigit & Selek, 2020; Sourati et al., 2017).

Site-Specific Side Effects of Radiation Therapy and Management

Site	Radiation Effect	Management
Bone	Chronic: • Radiation-induced bone fractures • Osteoradionecrosis (ORN)	Chronic: • Bisphosphonates for radiation-induced bone fractures • Surgery as warranted • Analgesia for fractures • Pentoxifylline and tocopherol for ORN • Hyperbaric oxygen therapy (HBO) for ORN
Brain	Acute: • Alopecia • Dermatitis • Dizziness • Headache • Nausea and vomiting • Fatigue Chronic: • Late cognitive changes • Radiation necrosis	Acute: • Mild moisturizing skin products • Sun protection measures such as sunscreen and wearing a hat • Teach energy conservation measures • Antiemetics as needed Chronic: • Assess neurocognitive function • May be a role for memantine, donepezil, and central nervous system stimulants (modafinil, methylphenidate) to treat cognitive decline • Dexamethasone for radiation necrosis • HBO for radiation necrosis • Surgical resection of necrotic tissue

Site-Specific Side Effects of Radiation Therapy and Management—cont'd

Site	Radiation Effect	Management
Breast	Acute: • Radiation dermatitis (dry and moist desquamation) Chronic: • Breast fibrosis • Breast atrophy • Edema • Hyperpigmentation • Chronic wounds • Telangiectasias	Acute: • Loose, comfortable clothing • Avoid friction to skin • Ongoing skin care including mild moisturizing soap and use of skin emollients (do not apply directly before therapy) • Topical steroids (mometasone, betamethasone) • Protective dressings over areas of moist desquamation • Treatment of secondary infections as needed Chronic: • Pentoxifylline and tocopherol for fibrosis • HBO • Pulsed dye laser for telangiectasias
Lung	Acute: • Cough • Shortness of breath • Fatigue • Nausea and vomiting • Skin changes Chronic: • Cough • Shortness of breath • Radiation pneumonitis (RP) • Radiation pulmonary fibrosis (RPF) • Radiation-induced cardiovascular disease (pericarditis, cardiomyopathy, congestive heart failure, coronary artery disease, valvular disease, myocardial ischemia, or infarction)	Acute: • Expectorants • Antiemetics as needed • Mild moisturizing skin products Chronic: • Monitor for signs and symptoms of pneumonitis including dyspnea, cough, low-grade fever • Corticosteroids for RP once infection or tumor progression ruled out • Nintedanib and pirfenidone under investigation to reduce/prevent RP and RPF • Role for lipid screening, transthoracic echocardiogram, noninvasive stress imaging to monitor for cardiac dysfunction • Cardiology involvement for patients with preexisting cardiac disease
Esophagus	Acute: • Esophagitis • Dysphagia • Odynophagia • Nausea and vomiting Chronic: • Esophageal stricture • Dysmotility • Odynophagia • Fistula	Acute: • Small, frequent meals • Avoid irritant foods (acidic, spicy) • Dietitian referral • Oral supplements or intravenous hydration for reduced oral intake • Possible temporary gastrostomy tube (G-Tube) placement to help maintain hydration and nutrition • Antacid and proton pump inhibitor (PPI) therapy • Analgesics for pain control Chronic: • Esophageal dilation for stricture; may need repeat dilations • Refer to surgeon if fistula develops
Head and Neck	Acute: • Xerostomia • Mucositis • Dysphagia • Loss of taste Chronic: • Xerostomia • Dental caries • ORN • Dysphagia • Trismus • Cervical fibrosis and dystonia • Lymphedema • Hypothyroidism	Acute: • Diligent oral hygiene • Saliva substitutes or pharmacologic therapy (pilocarpine, cevimeline) for xerostomia • Avoid tobacco and alcohol use • Acupuncture for xerostomia • Prophylactic dental care including extractions • Short-term G-Tube placement for enteral hydration and nutrition • Analgesics for mucositis Chronic: • Pentoxifylline and tocopherol for fibrosis • HBO therapy for early ORN • Surgical resection of necrotic bone with reconstruction for severe ORN • Rehabilitation: Physical, occupational and speech therapies • Possible G-Tube placement for severe, chronic dysphagia to reduce risk for aspiration events • Complete decongestive therapy for lymphedema management • Routine thyroid function tests (thyroid-stimulating hormone and Free T4) and thyroid hormone replacement if indicated

Continued

Site-Specific Side Effects of Radiation Therapy and Management—cont'd

Site	Radiation Effect	Management
Pelvis	Acute: • Diarrhea • Cystitis • Dysuria • Urinary frequency Chronic: • Urinary frequency • Dysuria • Hematuria • Proctitis • Rectal bleeding • Fistula • Infertility • Menopause • Sexual dysfunction • Lumbosacral plexopathy • Insufficiency fractures	Acute: • Antidiarrheal medications • Maintain oral hydration • Rule out and treat underlying urinary tract infection • Anticholinergics to reduce bladder spasms Chronic: • Pentoxifylline and tocopherol for chronic cystitis • Argon plasma coagulation (APC) or formalin installation for chronic rectal bleeding • Refer to a surgeon for surgical management of a fistula • Fertility counseling • Diet modification: low-fiber diet • Psychosocial support and patient education related to sexual function changes • Patient education on vaginal dilator use • Pharmacotherapy (sildenafil) for erectile dysfunction • Imaging work-up if suspected insufficiency fracture • Conservative management of fracture or surgery as warranted • Analgesia for fractures
Rectum	Acute: • Rectal pain • Increased frequency and urgency of defecation • Diarrhea • Skin reactions • Passing blood or mucus Chronic: • Rectal stricture • Decreased rectal compliance • Rectal bleeding • Fistula	Acute: • Antidiarrheal medications • Dietary modifications to increase fiber intake • Perianal skin care • Sitz baths several times daily Chronic: • Steroid or sulfasalazine suppositories for chronic proctitis or bleeding • APC or formalin installation for chronic bleeding • HBO for bleeding • Pentoxifylline and tocopherol for bleeding • Refer to a surgeon for surgical management of a fistula
Stomach	Acute: • Dyspepsia • Nausea and vomiting • Gastric cramping Chronic: • Hemorrhagic gastritis • Bowel obstruction • Fistula	Acute: • Antiemetics • Diet modification; avoid spicy and acidic foods • Maintain oral hydration • Histamine 2 (H_2) blockers or PPIs as needed for acid reflux symptoms • Antispasmodic agents for cramping Chronic: • Antisecretory agents and H_2 receptor blockers for hemorrhagic gastritis • APC for hemorrhagic gastritis • Refer to surgeon if fistula develops

With traditional EBRT, late effects are typically more severe when patients receive a higher dose per fraction of treatment. Hypofractionation schedules, in which patients are given higher doses of radiation in fewer fractions, are becoming more common. As a result of this abbreviated schedule, patients may not begin to experience side effects until after their course of radiation therapy is complete. Patient education and follow-up with these patients is critical to ensure side effects are appropriately managed.

The patient's treatment team will complete a survivorship care plan (SCP) once the patient has finished cancer treatment. The SCP includes information on the treatment the patient received, potential late effects of treatment, self-care measures to minimize these effects, primary cancer prevention measures (smoking cessation, balanced diet, regular exercise), and measures to enhance quality of life. This serves as a resource for the patient, their caregivers, and their primary care provider to help them identify and manage any side effects that may arise from their previous treatment and improve their health.

Nursing Implications

Oncology nurses play a critical role in providing comprehensive care for patients undergoing radiation therapy. Radiation therapy is oftentimes unfamiliar and scary, and nurses give vital information that can help to familiarize patients with what to expect while they undergo treatment. The nurse can determine what knowledge the patient has about radiation therapy before starting treatment and use this information to tailor information to their educational needs. Patient education should include information about what side effects to expect, when to expect the onset of symptoms, and their anticipated duration. Nurses should also educate patients on preventive and self-care techniques, such as skin care, that can empower patients to help manage side effects as they complete treatment. Nurses should educate patients on "red flag" symptoms that need to be reported to the physician promptly (see box below). Ideally this information is discussed with patients and provided in written form prior to the start of treatment. This is the best time to provide contact information for the radiation team as well.

Symptoms to Seek Care for Urgently While Undergoing Radiation Therapy

- Fever >100.4° F or chills
- Unmanaged diarrhea, constipation, nausea, or vomiting
- Unmanaged pain
- Signs of dehydration; dizziness, thirst, dark urine, less urine than normal
- Difficulty swallowing or mouth sores preventing oral intake
- Swelling, erythema, or pain in the extremities
- Shortness of breath or chest pain
- New onset productive cough or hemoptysis

Claustrophobia can be an issue for patients undergoing radiation therapy. Patients receiving radiation for head and neck cancer, brain cancer, or brain metastases will require the use of a thermoplastic mask, which serves as an immobilization device. The mask helps to ensure consistent patient set-up. Patients may experience claustrophobia during the mask-making process, which occurs during simulation, or with repeated use of the mask during treatment. The nurse's pretreatment assessment can include questioning about prior issues with claustrophobia. In some cases, patients will receive a prescription for anxiolytic medication, which they should be instructed to take at least 30 minutes prior to treatment. If the patient requires medication to help manage anxiety during treatment, they will require a caregiver to drive them home as these medications cause sedation. Complementary therapies such as music therapy, meditation, controlled breathing, and guided imagery can also help reduce patient anxiety during treatment (Miller & Scherbak, 2021).

While the patient is undergoing treatment and in the period after treatment, the nurse can help to assess for side effects of therapy. Radiation dermatitis is one of the most common side effects, characterized by damage to the basal layer of the skin. This treatment side effect can be amplified by concurrent use of chemotherapy or biotherapy agents. Radiation dermatitis is often progressive; patients may experience initial issues with transient and mild erythema at the start of treatment, which can progress to loss of skin integrity, erythema, peeling, or weeping over the next 3 to 6 weeks (Miller & Scherbak, 2021). Ongoing skin assessment is vital to identify and promptly address skin toxicity.

Other side effects the patient may experience depend on the treatment location, and the nurse should tailor assessment to the individual patient. Pain can also worsen over the course of treatment, and it is important to address this topic at every visit. Fatigue is a common side effect of radiation therapy and tends to be progressive as the patient undergoes treatment. Encouraging patients to continue to perform light exercise during radiation therapy can help to manage fatigue, enhance sleep, and maintain their appetite. Nurses should consider referring the patient to meet with a dietitian if they are struggling with oral intake or

persistent weight loss. In some cases, complementary therapies such as acupuncture, massage, or meditation can assist patients in managing symptoms such as pain, anxiety, fatigue, hot flashes, and nausea. Nurses can also help to connect patients with additional resources such as support groups, social workers, case managers, chaplains, or other community resources.

References

Abraham, C. D., Kavanagh, B. D., & Sheehan, J. P. (2021). Stereotactic irradiation: CNS tumors. In J. E. Tepper, R. L. Foote, & J. M. Michalski (Eds.), *Gunderson & Tepper's clinical radiation oncology* (5th ed.). Philadelphia, PA: Elsevier.

Abshire, D., & Lang, M. K. (2018). The evolution of radiation therapy in treating cancer. *Seminars in Oncology Nursing, 34*(2), 151–157.

Behrand, S. W. (2019). Radiation therapy. In J. M. Brant, D. G. Cope, & M. G. Saria (Eds.), *Core curriculum for oncology nursing* (6th ed.). St. Louis, MO, Elsevier.

Czito, B. G., Calvo, F. A., Haddock, M. G., Blitzblau, R., & Willett, C. G. (2021). Intraoperative radiation. In J. E. Tepper, R. L. Foote, & J. M. Michalski (Eds.), *Gunderson & Tepper's clinical radiation oncology* (5th ed.). Philadelphia, PA: Elsevier.

Feng, M., Matuszak, M. M., Ramirez, E., & Fraass, B. A. (2021). Intensity-modulated and image-guided radiotherapy. In J. E. Tepper, R. L. Foote, & J. M. Michalski (Eds.), *Gunderson & Tepper's clinical radiation oncology* (5th ed.). Philadelphia, PA: Elsevier.

Gardner, S. J., Kim, J., & Chetty, I. J. (2019). Modern radiation therapy planning and delivery. *Hematology/Oncology Clinics of North America, 33*(6), 947–962.

Kavanagh, B. D., & Timmerman, R. D. (2021). Stereotactic body irradiation: Extracranial tumors. In J. E. Tepper, R. L. Foote, & J. M. Michalski (Eds.), *Gunderson & Tepper's clinical radiation oncology* (5th ed.). Philadelphia, PA: Elsevier.

LaRiviere, M. J., Santos, P., Hill-Kayser, C. E., & Metz, J. M. (2019). Proton therapy. *Hematology/Oncology Clinics of North America, 33*(6), 989–1009.

Mallick, S., Rath, G. K., & Benson, R. (Eds.). (2020). *Practical radiation oncology*. Singapore: Springer.

Matta, R., Chapple, C. R., Fisch, M., Heidenreich, A., Herschorn, S., Kodama, R. T., … Nam, R. K. (2019). Pelvic complications after prostate cancer radiation therapy and their management: An international collaborative narrative review. *European Urology, 75*(3), 464–476.

Milano, M. T., Marks, L. B., & Constine, L. S. (2021). Late effects after radiation. In J. E. Tepper, R. L. Foote, & J. M. Michalski (Eds.), *Gunderson & Tepper's clinical radiation oncology* (5th ed.). Philadelphia, PA: Elsevier.

Miller, J., & Scherbak, C. (2021). Radiation therapy: Understanding the patient experience. *Clinical Journal of Oncology Nursing, 25*(6), 717–720.

Otter, S. J., Holloway, C. L., O'Farrell, D. A., Devlin, P. M., & Stewart, A. J. (2021). Brachytherapy. In J. E. Tepper, R. L. Foote, & J. M. Michalski (Eds.), *Gunderson & Tepper's clinical radiation oncology* (5th ed.). Philadelphia, PA: Elsevier.

Ozyigit, G., & Selek, U. (Eds.). (2020). *Prevention and management of acute and late toxicities in radiation oncology*. Switzerland: Springer.

Palmer, J. D., Hall, M. D., Mahajan, A., Paulino, A. C., Wolden, S., & Constine, L. S. (2020). Radiotherapy and late effects. *Pediatric Clinics of North America, 67*, 1051–1067.

Sourati, A., Ameri, A., & Malekzadeh, M. (2017). *Acute side effects of radiation therapy: A guide to management*. Switzerland: Springer.

Thomadsen, B. (2019). Radiation protection responsibility in brachytherapy. *Health Physics, 116*(2), 189–204.

Timmerman, R. D., Paulus, R., Pass, H. I., Gore, E. M., Edelman, M. J., Galvin, J., & Choy, H. (2018). Stereotactic body radiation therapy for operable early-stage lung cancer: Findings from the NRG Oncology RTOG 0618 trial. *JAMA Oncology, 4*(9), 1263–1266.

Trifiletti, D. M., & Zaorsky, N. G. (Eds.). (2019). *Absolute clinical radiation oncology review* Switzerland: Springer.

van der Zande, K., Oyen, W. J. G., Zwart, W., & Bergman, A. M. (2021). Radium-223 treatment of patients with metastatic castration resistant prostate cancer: Biomarkers for stratification and response evaluation. *Cancers, 13*(17), 4346.

Willey, C. D., Yang, E. S., & Bonner, J. A. (2021). Interaction of chemotherapy and radiation. In J. E. Tepper, R. L. Foote, & J. M. Michalski (Eds.), *Gunderson & Tepper's clinical radiation oncology* (5th ed.). Philadelphia, PA: Elsevier.

Zeman, E. M. (2021). The biological basis of radiation oncology. In J. E. Tepper, R. L. Foote, & J. M. Michalski (Eds.), *Gunderson & Tepper's clinical radiation oncology* (5th ed.). Philadelphia, PA: Elsevier.

Tumor Treating Fields

Laura Benson and Melissa Shackelford

Introduction

Tumor treating fields (TTFields) therapy is a unique locoregional treatment modality that disrupts division and proliferation processes critical for cancer cell viability and tumor progression (Mun et al., 2018). Patients with aggressive solid tumors are often faced with poor prognosis as a result of treatment challenges stemming from tumor heterogeneity, treatment resistance, delivery barriers, and systemic toxicities (Dagogo-Jack & Shaw, 2018). Multimodal therapeutic regimens are helpful strategies to overcome these limitations, but the effectiveness of combining systemic therapies may be compromised by additive systemic toxicities and the potential for drug-drug interactions (Gotwals et al., 2017). TTFields therapy is delivered noninvasively to the solid tumor site via a portable medical device. It is well tolerated with localized, mild-to-moderate skin irritation and no significant increase in systemic adverse effects. This favorable therapeutic profile makes TTFields a viable cancer treatment modality either as a monotherapy or concomitant with other standard-of-care regimens.

This chapter provides an overview of the science of TTFields including, (1) an overview of the multi-modal mechanism of action (MoA) of TTFields, (2) summary of the clinical development and evolving use in different solid tumors, (3) the devices used to deliver TTFields therapy, (4) guidance for proactive prevention and management of side effects, and (5) the importance of patient usage over time to optimize outcomes.

TTFields Therapy Is a Noninvasive Treatment for Treating Solid Tumors

Electric fields have diverse clinical applications depending on the specific frequency of the electric field (Omer, 2021). TTFields disrupt cancer cell division by delivering electric fields over a frequency range of 100 kilohertz (kHz, a unit of frequency equal to 1000 cycles per second) to 500 kHz. Frequencies within this range are unable to injure healthy tissue (Karanam & Story, 2021; Wenger et al., 2015). At the cellular level, cell division and motility are dependent on charged intracellular components for normal function (Kirson et al., 2004), and these charged molecules and structures can be influenced by electric fields. Within the range of 100 to 500 kHz, TTFields acting on charged intracellular components are known to selectively inhibit various biologic processes in cancer cells. This is due in part to the rate of replication associated with most cancer cells, as well as distinct morphologies, including size and electrical properties as compared to non-cancerous cells (Kirson et al., 2004, 2007). The specific frequency selected for delivery of TTFields (i.e., optimal frequency), depends on the cancer cell type and electrical properties, meanwhile sparing nondividing cells (see figure below) (Porat et al., 2017). Further, because normal cells and tissues have lower rates of replication and different conformations, they remain largely unaffected (Blatt et al., 2021).

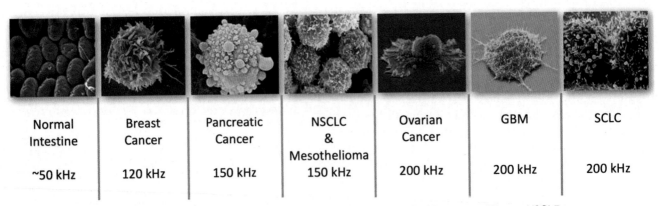

Normal Intestine	Breast Cancer	Pancreatic Cancer	NSCLC & Mesothelioma	Ovarian Cancer	GBM	SCLC
~50 kHz	120 kHz	150 kHz	150 kHz	200 kHz	200 kHz	200 kHz

TTFields Effect on Cancer Cells Are Frequency Specific. *GBM,* Glioblastoma multiforme; *NSCLC,* non–small cell lung cancer; *SCLC,* small cell lung cancer; *TTFields,* tumor treating fields. (Reused with permission from © 2023 Novocure GmbH—all rights reserved.)

In the clinical setting, TTFields therapy is delivered by two sets of paired arrays composed of disks, arranged on an adhesive bandage. These paired arrays are connected to a powered TTFields generator, which induces an alternating electric field at an optimal frequency to impact the targeted tumor within the region of interest of the body. Personalized placement of the paired arrays results in an increased field intensity at the site of the tumor, a critical aspect for the clinical benefit and an essential component of treatment planning. TTFields therapy (200 kHz) was approved by the Food and Drug Administration (FDA) as monotherapy for recurrent glioblastoma (rGBM) and in combination with temozolomide (TMZ) for the treatment of newly diagnosed glioblastoma (ndGBM) in 2011 and 2015, respectively. Additionally, TTFields therapy using the frequency of 150 kHz was approved by the FDA in 2019 for unresectable locally advanced or metastatic malignant pleural mesothelioma (MPM), when combined with platinum and pemetrexed chemotherapies. For GBM and MPM, and a growing number of solid tumor types, TTFields therapy is becoming a component of a multimodal treatment strategy. Understanding aspects of the MoA of TTFields therapy helps the nurse understand potential concomitant synergies.

TTFields Therapy Has Multiple Mechanisms of Action

Early and ongoing research indicates that TTFields therapy has a variety of MoAs related to their biophysical effects on the charged molecules and components of cancer cells. The objective of this section is to provide a summary of the current leading proposed MoAs for TTFields. TTFields treatment has been observed to disrupt mitosis, enhance antitumor immunity, interfere with cancer cell motility, downregulate DNA damage response, upregulate autophagy, and increase cancer cell permeability as well as other MoAs (see the figure on the next page) (Rominiyi et al., 2021). In addition to understanding the effects of TTFields on cellular processes, this evolving body of evidence lends insight and support for potential tumor treatment combinations.

The Antimitotic Effects of TTFields

The initial focus of preclinical research indicated that TTFields exposure exerts electric forces on polar components within a cell, causing them to align with the field direction and disrupting their regulated movement within the cell thus preventing normal function. The greatest effect is during cell division, especially during metaphase, anaphase, and telophase. During metaphase, TTFields application disrupts the process of tubulin polymerization and depolymerization and during anaphase prevent septin localization to the mitotic spindle and assembly of the septin complex at the site of cleavage (Gera et al., 2015; Kirson et al., 2004). During telophase, the late stages of cell division, the hour-glass shape of the dividing cell leads to a nonuniformity of the electric field distribution, which increases the intensity of the electric field at the site of the cleavage furrow. This causes polarizable molecules to aggregate toward this region—a phenomenon referred to as dielectrophoresis (Kirson et al., 2004, 2007). Ultimately, these cumulative disruptions of normal molecular processes during cell division result in abnormal chromosomal segregation and cell death. This effect is most prevalent with rapidly dividing cells and thus explains the much higher sensitivity of cancer cells to TTFields relative to normal cells and tissues.

Anti-migratory Effects of TTFields

TTFields treatment leads to disruptive changes in the cytoskeletal dynamics of cancer cell motility and focal adhesions due to changes in microtubule organization (Voloshin et al., 2020). To date, there is significant preclinical evidence that TTFields exposure disrupts cancer cell motility, migration, and invasion in vitro, and reduce the appearance of metastases in animal models, suggesting that TTFields may have antimetastatic effects on cancer cells and produce an abscopal effect (Kim, Song, et al., 2016; Kirson, Giladi, et al., 2009; Silginer et al., 2017; Voloshin et al., 2020).

TTFields Treatment Inhibits DNA-damage Repair

Experiments with glioma cells have shown that TTFields exposure enhances the sensitivity of cancer cells to the DNA damaging effects of radiation. Concurrent application of TTFields, either during radiation treatment or immediately after, has been shown to delay the repair of radiation damage to DNA, as well as reduce cell survival (Giladi et al., 2017; Kim, Kim, et al., 2016). The observed synergy between the two modalities at the cellular level has clinical implications for a combined anticancer regimen of radiation therapy and TTFields therapy.

TTFields Exposure Enhances Autophagy

Autophagy is a process by which the cell cleans out damaged cellular components. In cancer, autophagy plays a conflicting role in cancer progression. During the preliminary stages of cancer development, autophagy can inhibit tumor development; but during later stages, it can enhance tumor cell survival and treatment resistance (Rominiyi et al., 2021). TTFields treated cancer cells have shown that the cellular characteristics of upregulation of autophagy in in vitro experiments (Kim et al., 2019; Shteingauz et al., 2018).

TTFields Application Enhances Anti-tumor Immunity

Preclinical evidence suggests that TTFields may induce a systemic anticancer immune response. Cell culture experiments with multiple cancer cell lines show that treatment with TTFields produces hallmarks of immunogenic cell death (Voloshin et al., 2020). TTFields treatment has also been shown to induce the activation of dendritic cells *in vitro* and increase leukocyte recruitment and intra-tumor infiltration of T cells in animal models (Diamant et al., 2021; Kirson, Giladi, et al., 2009; Voloshin et al., 2020). Enhanced immunogenic response associated with TTFields application highlights potential synergies with immunotherapies currently used for tumor treatment.

TTFields Treatment Increases Cell Membrane Permeability

Electric fields and TTFields increase the permeability of the cell membrane through their effects on voltage-gated ion

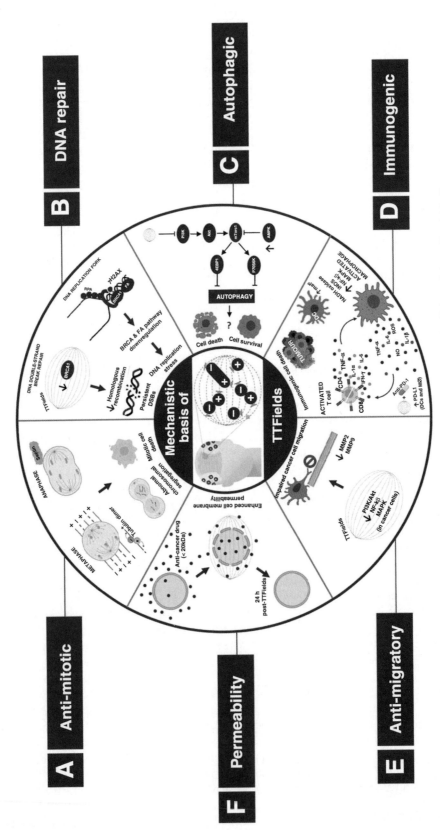

Mechanism of Action of TTFields. *TTFields*, Tumor treating fields. (Adapted from Rominiyi, O., Vanderlinden, A., Clenton, S. J., Bridgewater, C., Al-Tamimi, Y., & Collis, S. J. [2021]. Tumour treating fields therapy for glioblastoma: Current advances and future directions. *British Journal of Cancer, 124*[4], 697–709. https://doi.org/10.1038/s41416-020-01136-5. CC-BY, version 4.0.)

channels, electrorheological processes, and electroporation (Aguilar et al., 2021; Neuhaus et al., 2019). TTFields applied to human glioma cell lines affect membrane permeability in part by increasing the number and size of pores in the cell membrane; this was noted in glioma cells and not normal human fibroblasts (Chang et al., 2018). The clinical implication of this observation is that TTFields may potentiate the clinical efficacy of chemotherapies by assisting with cell permeability and subsequent increased drug delivery thus increasing concentration within cancer cells (Rominiyi et al., 2021).

Efficacy and Safety of TTFields Therapy

TTFields Therapy for Recurrent Glioblastoma

The initial clinical evaluation of TTFields therapy, at an optimal frequency of 200 kHz was for rGBM. Though rare, GBM tumors are the most common malignant brain tumor in adults and are associated with a poor prognosis for survival due to their propensity for recurrence and resistance to treatment (Barthel et al., 2022).

The phase III, multicenter, EF-11 clinical study compared the efficacy and safety of TTFields monotherapy with physician's choice of chemotherapy for the treatment of patients with rGBM (Stupp et al., 2012). The median overall survival (mOS) for patients treated with TTFields therapy was found to be comparable to physician's choice of chemotherapy (6.6 months vs. 6 months, respectively), and the 1-year survival rate was 20% for both treatment arms. Progression-free survival (PFS) at the 6-month assessment was greater for TTFields therapy (21%) compared to the standard-of-care treatment group (15%). The EF-11 study demonstrated that TTFields therapy was as effective as chemotherapy with fewer side effects. Patients treated with TTFields as a monotherapy reported better health-related quality of life (HRQoL) with improved cognitive and emotional functioning when compared to the chemotherapy group (Stupp et al., 2012). The primary adverse event (AE) observed with TTFields therapy was mild-to-moderate skin irritation on the scalp underneath the arrays. In 2011, these results provided evidence for the United States Food and Drug Association (FDA) to approve TTFields therapy for use in adults who have rGBM after receiving chemotherapy and whose disease is refractory to surgical and radiation treatment options.

TTFields Therapy for Newly Diagnosed Glioblastoma

Cell culture studies with glioma cells demonstrated that the combination of TMZ and TTFields applied to human glioma cells in vitro had an additive cytotoxic effect (Kirson et al., 2007; Kirson, Schneiderman, et al., 2009). These data suggested the combination of TTFields with maintenance TMZ therapy in ndGBM following surgical resection and chemoradiotherapy, might be a viable multimodal regimen (Kirson, Schneiderman, et al., 2009). These preclinical observations provided a foundation for the EF-14 study, a phase III study in patients with ndGBM who received standard-of-care therapy of maximum possible resection and chemoradiotherapy with TMZ. In the adjuvant setting, 695 patients were randomly

assigned (2:1) to receive either TMZ plus TTFields (200 kHz) or TMZ alone as maintenance therapy. At the preplanned interim analysis, 315 patients had enrolled in the study and reached a minimum time on study of 18 months. The interim analysis demonstrated that adding TTFields to maintenance TMZ significantly prolonged median PFS (mPFS), 7.1 versus 4.0 months and median OS of 20.5 versus 15.6 months in the per-protocol population (Stupp et al., 2015). In the Intent-to-treat (ITT) population, the mOS was 19.6 months in the TTFields + TMZ group compared with 16.6 months in the TMZ alone group ($P = .03$). Based on these interim results, in 2015, the FDA approved TTFields for use in combination with TMZ for the maintenance treatment of adult patients with ndGBM.

Analysis of the 5-year full data set (695 patients) confirmed the improvements in mPFS and mOS seen in the interim analysis. In the analysis of the 695 enrolled patients, the minimum follow-up was 24 months, and the median was 40 months. The study's primary endpoint of mPFS was 6.7 months for patients in the TTFields plus TMZ group compared to 4.0 months for patients treated with TMZ alone. The 2-year OS rates were 43% versus 31% for TTFields plus TMZ versus the TMZ alone treatment group, respectively. The 5-year OS rates were 13% versus 5% for TTFields plus TMZ versus the TMZ alone treatment group, respectively. TTFields device usage (amount of time receiving TTFields therapy) was a significant predictor of survival outcomes. In patients whose usage was 18 h/day (≥75%) or greater (usage is measured objectively by the device via internal log files), OS was significantly longer than patients receiving TTFields for less than 18 h/day (<75%) (Stupp et al., 2017). Mild-to-moderate skin irritation beneath the arrays occurred in 52% of patients who received TTFields plus TMZ (Stupp et al., 2017). The National Comprehensive Cancer Network (NCCN) guidelines recommend TTFields as a standard treatment category 1 option for ndGBM in patients with good functional status (NCCN, 2021).

In a secondary analysis of the EF-14 clinical study data, the addition of TTFields to TMZ during the TMZ maintenance phase of treatment for ndGBM patients did not adversely affect patients HRQoL apart from increased "itchy" skin with TTFields therapy. Further, TTFields plus TMZ resulted in significantly longer deterioration-free survival in global health status, physical and emotional functioning, pain, and weakness of legs. TTFields significantly increased mPFS and mOS (Stupp et al., 2017) while maintaining patient HRQoL (Taphoorn et al., 2018).

In a subgroup analysis of elderly patients (≥65 years of age) from the phase III EF-14 clinical study, TTFields plus maintenance TMZ improved PFS and OS outcomes compared to TMZ chemotherapy alone. Evidence from this sub-analysis of the EF-14 study confirms the safety and efficacy of TTFields in elderly patients with ndGBM, without added risk or systemic toxicity and no negative effect on HRQoL. Skin AEs (beneath the arrays) were mild to moderate in 51% of patients. No other AEs were reported that were more frequent in elderly patients treated with TTFields plus TMZ compared to TMZ alone. TTFields usage of ≥75%, based on recommendations, was associated with additional survival benefits in this typically high-risk elderly patient population (Ram et al., 2021).

TTFields Therapy in Clinical Practice

The Patient Registry Dataset (PRiDe) was a postmarketing registry compiling data from patients with rGBM ($N = 457$) who received TTFields therapy in a real-world, clinical practice setting in the United States between 2011 and 2013. Median OS was significantly longer with TTFields in clinical practice (PRiDe) than in the EF-11 study (9.6 vs. 6.6 months, respectively). The most frequent AEs reported in the PRiDe analysis were mild-to-moderate skin irritation (Mrugala et al., 2014). A larger, more recent retrospective safety analysis of TTFields usage in the real-world setting, utilized unsolicited, postmarketing surveillance data from greater than 11,000 TTFields-treated patients (October 2011-February 2019). This analysis included both ndGBM and rGBM patients and confirmed the low-toxicity profile of TTFields. Most skin AEs reported were mild-to-moderate and manageable with topical interventions. Other TTFields-related AEs (all $\leq11\%$) in patients with ndGBM and rGBM included under-array heat sensation (i.e., warmth), electric sensation (i.e., tingling), and headache (Shi et al., 2020). Both studies suggest that in noncontrolled, real-world settings, the rate of TTFields AEs are comparable to clinical studies and across age groups and demographics.

TTFields Therapy and Quality of Life

As part of the EF-14 study HRQoL was examined and results confirm quality of life was maintained in eight of the nine domains: global health status, physical functioning, cognitive functioning, role functioning, social functioning, emotional functioning, weakness of legs, and pain, apart from "itchy skin" (Taphoorn et al., 2018). These results were confirmed in a 2021 large survey study of patients in the United States and Europe (Palmer et al., 2021). Using validated and country-specific questionnaires (the EuroQol's EQ-5D-5L questionnaire and EuroQol's visual analogue scale [EQ-VAS]), the study compiled data from 1106 respondents. The progression of GBM and patient age both negatively affected measures of HRQoL. The results also indicated that the longer time between diagnosis and actively using TTFields therapy was associated with positive measures of HRQoL. The time on TTFields therapy had a positive effect on measures of mobility, self-care, and usual activities (Palmer et al., 2021).

TTFields Therapy for Malignant Pleural Mesothelioma

MPM is a rare cancer that is commonly a result of asbestos exposure. MPM is associated with a poor prognosis and limited treatment options. These options include surgery (though not an option for advanced MPM) and first-line chemotherapy combination of cisplatin/pemetrexed regimen (Vogelzang et al., 2003) and radiation therapy. In preclinical data, MPM cells treated with TTFields at a frequency of 150 kHz exhibited optimal antiproliferative effect and a reduction in clonogenicity. In addition, combining TTFields with different concentrations of either cisplatin or pemetrexed resulted in improved dose–response, suggesting synergies between these treatments (Mumblat et al., 2021). In 2015, a single-arm, phase II clinical study was conducted (STELLAR, EF-23) to examine the safety and efficacy of TTFields (150 kHz) concomitant with standard-of-care chemotherapy to treat unresectable, treatment-naïve MPM. The study enrolled 80 patients and showed favorable results. The mOS and mPFS were 18.2 months and 7.6 months, respectively, offering a substantive advance when compared to historical controls with mOS and mPFS of 12.1 months and 5.7 months, respectively (Ceresoli et al., 2019). These encouraging outcomes were achieved with no increase in systemic toxicity. Skin irritation was the only AE associated with TTFields therapy. Overall, TTFields (150 kHz) delivered to the thorax concomitant with pemetrexed and platinum chemotherapy were shown to be an active and safe combination for the front-line treatment of unresectable MPM (Ceresoli et al., 2019). Based on these data the FDA approved TTFields therapy with pemetrexed plus platinum-based chemotherapy for the first-line treatment of unresectable, locally advanced, or metastatic MPM in 2019.

TTFields Therapy for Other Tumors: Future Clinical Investigation

The clinical use of TTFields therapy for GBM and MPM underscore the potential for TTFields in the treatment of solid tumors in the cranium (other than GBM), thorax, and abdomen. Current and ongoing preclinical research has identified unique synergies for TTFields with new and existing therapies for future clinical investigation. Ongoing clinical research include investigations of TTFields therapy for brain metastases, non–small cell lung cancer, ovarian cancer, hepatocellular carcinoma, and pancreatic cancer.

Factors Impacting the Clinical Benefit of TTFields Therapy

TTFields therapy is noninvasive and is actively delivered only when the device field generator is powered on and connected to the arrays after placement on the skin. Optimal placement of the arrays and compliance with recommended duration of use is critical in achieving therapeutic intensities of TTFields at the site of the tumor. For patients with GBM, integrating magnetic resonance imaging (MRI) of the tumor combined with simulations of TTFields distributions in the brain have demonstrated that personalizing the placement of the arrays can result in an increased field intensity at the site of the tumor (Ballo, Urman, Bomzon, et al., 2019; Ballo, Urman, Lavy-Shahaf, et al., 2019; Sun, 2018) (see the figure on the next page). Treatment planning for TTFields therapy involves determining an optimal layout of the arrays on the head that can help maximize the field intensity at the tumor. This is performed using a sophisticated treatment planning software system that utilizes patient morphometric measurements and tumor dimensions made by a physician using the MRI images from the patient for more personalized precision medicine.

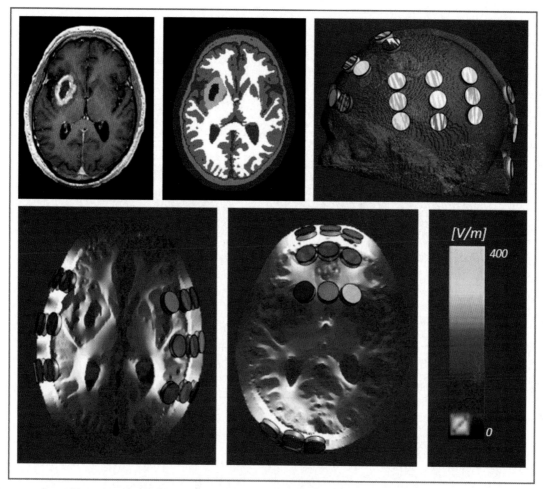

Array Placement Guided by MRI and Tumor *(upper panel)*. A T1c MRI of the patient is selected *(left)* and used to create a patient specific model *(middle)*. The virtual arrays used to deliver the field are shown in the right panel. Finite element simulations are used to calculate the field distribution within brain, which can be visualized using a colormap *(lower panel)*—left panel shows simulated TTFields intensity with left to right arrays active and the center panel shows TTFields intensity with anterior-posterior array placement. *TTFields,* Tumor treating fields. (Reused with permission from © 2023 Novocure GmbH—all rights reserved.)

Systems for Delivering TTFields Therapy

The earliest preclinical research has demonstrated that effects of TTFields application are direction dependent. The cells that divide parallel to the electric field show higher rates of damage than those dividing perpendicular to the field (Kirson et al., 2004). Therefore, TTFields therapy is delivered noninvasively via two orthogonal pairs of arrays that produce two perpendicular alternating electric fields. These arrays are applied directly on the surface of the skin such that the site of the tumor is within the body space between the arrays. The device comes preset to the optimal frequency used to target the specific tumor type. The alternating electric fields switch between the two pairs of arrays every second.

The NovoTTF-200A system (Optune, Novocure GmbH) is a wearable portable medical device approved for use as TTFields therapy for GBM, as monotherapy for rGBM and in combination with TMZ for ndGBM treatment. The NovoTTF-200T system (Optune Lua, Novocure GmbH) is a wearable portable device approved for TTFields therapy of MPM, while used concurrently with pemetrexed and platinum-based chemotherapy.

The TTFields therapy delivery system includes an electric field generator, arrays, portable rechargeable batteries, battery charger, plug-in power supply, connection cable, and carrying case (see the figure on the next page). This system is prescribed by a certified healthcare provider, who has received special certification training by the device manufacturer, as mandated by the U.S. FDA. TTFields therapy provides continuous therapy, through the wearable portable system and is used in the outpatient setting allowing patients to continue participating in their daily activities. The patient is seen in the outpatient clinic by the oncology team on a routine basis and individual patient usage reports are provided directly to the oncology team by the device manufacturer. The reports are uploaded approximately every month, via remote monitoring system (MyLink) (see the figure on the next page). Additional supplies, including educational resources and technical support

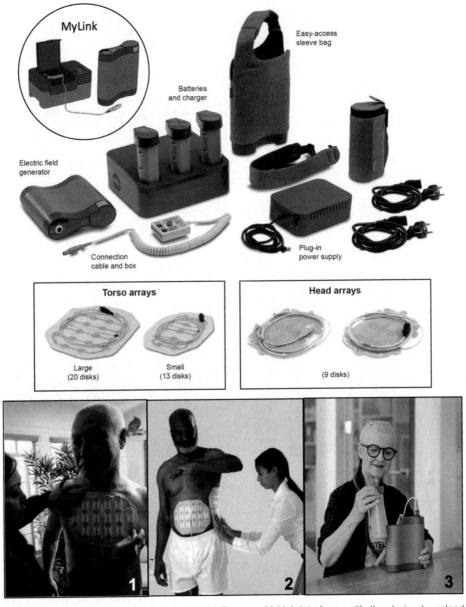

TTFields Therapy Device for Treating Solid Tumors. MyLink interfaces with the device to upload device usage data to help optimize treatment. Models shown wearing arrays for treating tumors of the torso (lung (1) and abdomen (2)) and head (3); models are actors and not patients. TTFields, Tumor Treating Fields. *TTFields,* Tumor treating fields. (Reused with permission from © 2023 Novocure GmbH—all rights reserved.)

are provided by the manufacturer. When therapy is discontinued, the system is returned to the manufacturer.

For GBM, TTFields are delivered by four arrays placed in sets on opposing sides of the head, correlating to the location of the tumor and each array has nine disks (see the figure on the next page). There are two array sizes for the treatment of MPM, with either 13 or 20 disks, to accommodate various body sizes and contours (see the figure on the next page). The insulated disks are separated from the skin by a layer of conductive hydrogel. To help keep the arrays in place on the scalp and in continuous direct contact with the skin, the ceramic disks, hydrogel, and circuitry are attached to a hypoallergenic medical adhesive bandage (Lacouture et al., 2014, 2020). A cord from each set of arrays plugs into the connection cable box, which then plugs into the field's generator device. Patients may describe a "warm sensation" under the arrays. Each array has multiple temperatures sensors; the device will shut off and sound an alarm if array temperature exceeds 41° C (105.8° F), well below the threshold for a skin burn injury (Lacouture et al., 2014, 2020). The portable device is designed to minimize the impact of treatment on the ADLs (see the figure on the next page).

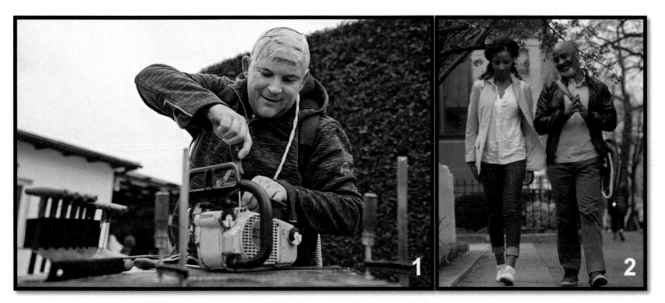

Devices for TTFields Therapy Are Designed to Minimize the Impact of Use on Activities of Daily Living. (*Figure on the left* [1] depicts a GBM patient: Reused with permission from © 2023 Novocure GmbH—all rights reserved. Permission for global image use was obtained from the patient. Models are depicted in the *figure on the right* [2], models are actors and not patients. Reused with permission from © 2023 Novocure GmbH—all rights reserved.)

Important considerations for inpatients with GBM with an active implanted medical device, a skull defect, or bullet fragments should be noted, as these are a contraindication for TTFields therapy. Similarly, patients should not use TTFields therapy for MPM, if they have implantable electronic medical devices including a pacemaker, implantable automatic defibrillator, etc. as it may lead to malfunctioning of the implanted device.

Oncology Nursing and the Role of Patient and Caregiver Education in Optimizing TTFields Therapy

A cancer patient's social, cognitive, psychological, and physical status are essential factors to consider when determining candidacy for TTFields therapy. Patients with more restrictive physical or cognitive limitations, combined with lack of a close support system of family or caregivers, may have difficulty navigating therapy or achieving recommended usage goals. Ideally a patient should have at least one support person who can assist the patient with device alarms, AEs, and help with removing and accurately replacing the arrays as part of the normal maintenance of TTFields therapy (Murphy et al., 2016).

Patient and caregiver education are pivotal milestones before initiating TTFields—each should have a basic understanding of the MoA, the components of the TTFields device systems, how they work, and the importance of achieving treatment usage goals. This training includes instructions in caring for and maintaining the system components, managing system alarms, and recommendations on how to proactively prevent and manage skin irritation when and if they manifest. The device manufacturer deploys a team of Device Support Specialists (DSSs) to educate the patient and caregiver prior to treatment initiation.

General recommendations are for patients to replace the arrays two times per week (approximately every 4 days) (Murphy et al., 2016). Patients and caregivers are instructed on the importance of shaving/re-shaving the scalp or chest and applying/reapplying new arrays. Some patients may require more frequent array changes depending on their individual hair growth, sweating, activity level, and weather. An important point to note is that TTFields therapy poses no danger to anyone near the patient, including children and pets.

The multidisciplinary healthcare team, including nurses supporting the patient and caregiver, can help develop strategies to optimize treatment outcomes and aid in integrating the device into the patient's lifestyle and ADLs (see the above figure). The multidisciplinary care team should have a shared decision-making approach to manage the patient's treatment journey and may include team members from: oncology, oncology nursing, specialty oncology, dermatology, etc. that are optimized to best support the patient needs, safety, and HRQoL. The role of nurse navigators and oncology social workers are crucial in coordinating the steps in the patient's treatment journey. The DSSs also have a role as part of this multidisciplinary team. Additionally, a therapist and/or patient support group can be instrumental for supporting the emotional and psychological needs of patients and caregivers as they attempt to cope with diagnosis and treatment.

Strategies to minimize the visibility of TTFields therapy for GBM, include selecting wigs and hats for covering the head while in public. Restrictive or tightly woven wigs or hats may trap heat and effect device operation; alternatively, scarves, and loosely woven or ventilated wigs that are appropriately sized for the patient while wearing the arrays, will help dissipate heat effectively and cover the arrays while not affecting device operation. Additionally, the cables connecting the power supply and fields generator to the arrays can be arranged under layers of breathable clothing to make them less obvious.

The device is designed to assist the patient, caregiver, and healthcare team achieve device usage goals and therapy goals. The device records the amount of time per day that the patient receives TTFields therapy. This information is captured on a monthly report, which provides an objective time on therapy, rather than subjectively relying on patient recall. An at home-based remote monitoring system (see the figure on page 216) allows patients to share usage data (time on therapy), privately and securely to the device manufacturer, so the monthly usage reports can be generated. Additionally, these reports provide key usage data for review and discussion, between the healthcare providers, healthcare team, and the patient and caregiver. Such discussions aid in addressing any issues so that strategies can be implemented in real-time to improve treatment duration and potentially improve clinical response. Usage data is combined with clinical data, including MRI imaging, to optimize treatment decisions for each individual patient.

The device manufacturer provides a team of field-based DSSs, who are trained to assist patients and caregivers with the daily operation of the TTFields delivery systems (Murphy et al., 2016). The DSS provides training and education during regularly scheduled encounters, either in person or via telehealth to the patient and their caregivers. The focus of the training is on the operation of the TTFields delivery device, as well as guidance on specific placement of the arrays and is part of the 24/7 device support portal. Prior to the COVID-19 pandemic, initiation of TTFields therapy and follow-up visits with the DSS were predominately in-person. As experienced in oncology clinics, the COVID-19 lockdown forced the amendment of patient support protocols. The rapid adoption of virtual platforms, including telehealth, allowed improved access to support services for TTFields therapy, while ensuring safe (virtual) education for patients, caregivers, and healthcare teams. One assessment of utilization of virtual training, demonstrated no observed differences between virtual versus in-person patient starts when analyzing demographics, time-to-start, treatment discontinuations, percentage continuing therapy, and overall complaints (Frongillo et al., 2021). The capacity to virtually start and manage TTFields therapy remotely opens treatment to patients that might have difficulties traveling and geographic restrictions, in general.

There are a variety of sponsored educational resources, accessible via emerging technologies, to enhance patient and caregiver understanding and use of TTFields therapy (Frongillo et al., 2020; Shackelford et al., 2019). These educational platforms are linked under the device web portal (Optune.com) and include educational videos, resources and support for patients and caregivers. Additionally, there are links to assist the healthcare team with education related to TTFields therapy. Awareness of such TTFields therapy resources, provide potential supplements for oncology nurses education in the use of TTFields therapy for cancer treatment (Shackelford et al., 2019). The figure on the next page summarizes elements of the oncology nurse's role in aiding and educating patients and caregivers to navigate their clinical journey.

Nurse Management and Prevention of Skin Irritation Resulting From TTFields Therapy

The most common AEs related to the use of TTFields therapy are mild-to-moderate skin irritation and headache (Stupp et al., 2012, 2015). Dermatologic AEs occurring under the arrays are summarized in the table on page 220, including their symptoms, causes, and management (Anadkat et al., 2023; Lacouture et al., 2014, 2020). TTFields therapy for tumors of the thoracic cavity present with skin AEs with unique exacerbations for the arrays associated with the motion of respiration and pressure from sitting or reclining (Anadkat et al., 2023). An example of contact dermatitis related to TTFields therapy is shown in the figure on page 221. Maintaining skin integrity through essential good hygiene and skin preparation, along with proper array placement, are critical components of maintaining long-term and effective contact between the arrays and skin (Murphy et al., 2016). Strategies for proactively preventing and managing skin irritation are summarized in the table on page 221. Most dermatologic AEs can be managed with topical treatments and frequent adjustment of the arrays to minimize skin irritation (Anadkat et al., 2023; Lacouture et al., 2014, 2020). Interrupting TTFields therapy may be necessary in the event of dermatologic AEs that are more severe or worsening despite management efforts. Treatment interruption would involve a period of 2 to 7 days without applying arrays and TTFields therapy to allow the skin to heal. It is important to note that prolonged interruption of therapy could affect the outcome of therapy (Lacouture et al., 2020).

Diagnosis

Assess:
- Identify and navigate the diagnostic process

Plan:
- Provide educational resources reflective of diagnosis

Evaluate:
- Educational needs

Key Nursing Resources:
- www.ONS.org
- www.nccn.org/
- www.cancer.gov/about-cancer/treatment/types
- www.cancer.org/cancer/brain-spinal-cord-tumors-adults/treating/alternating-electric-field-therapy
- www.optune.com/hcp
- www.optunelua.com/hcp
- https://www.frontiersin.org/articles/10.3389/fonc.2022.975473/full#supplementary-material (management of thoracic skin AEs)

Planning

Assess:
- Personalize treatment options

Plan:
- Educate patients and caregivers regarding TTFields therapy:
  - MOA & activity with other therapies
  - At home wearable-portable device
  - Treatment start (in-person vs virtual)
  - Daily life on therapy
  - Importance of daily usage goals
  - Management of side effects

Key Patient Resources:
- www.nccn.org/patientresources/patient-resources
- www.clinicaltrials.gov
- www.cancer.gov/about-cancer/treatment/types
- www.cancer.org/cancer/brain-spinal-cord-tumorsadults/treating/alternating-electric-field-therapy
- www.optune.com
- www.optunelua.com
- www.curemeso.org

Treatment

Assess:
- Help start and manage TTFields therapy to optimize outcomes and prevent/minimize localize skin AEs

Plan:
- Educate patients and caregivers on:
  - Proper skin care, array placement & change
  - Treatment integration into their daily lives
  - Time on treatment (usage goals)

Evaluate:
- Region (scalp/torso) for array application and care
- Establish treatment usage goals [(min. ≥75% (18 hours)] to maximize optimal outcomes

Nursing Role in Aiding and Educating Patients in Their TTFields Therapy Journey. *AEs,* Adverse events; *TTFields,* tumor treating fields. (Reused with permission from © 2023 Novocure GmbH—all rights reserved.)

TTFields Therapy—Summary of Cutaneous Adverse Events: Symptoms, Causes, and Treatment Recommendations

Symptom	Causes	Management
Hyperhidrosis • Excessive sweating	• Genetic predisposition • Heat/humidity environment • Intense activity • Medications	• Treat with aluminum chloride antiperspirant or topical glycopyrrolate at every array change • Avoid ointments/medications that may cause sweating (e.g., topical steroids, acne medications, antidepressants) • Consider referral to dermatologist for botulinum toxin injections
Pruritus • Dry skin (xerosis) • Itchy skin (pruritis) • Flaky skin (dandruff)	• Genetic predisposition • Cold/dry environment • Loss of skin moisture/oil • Medications (e.g., diuretics, statins, antihistamines) • Possibly due to contact dermatitis	• Advise use of fragrance-free or anti-dandruff shampoo • Limit skin contact with alcohol-based skin products • Topical corticosteroids may be prescribed if inflammation is present (e.g., betamethasone, clobetasol, fluocinonide)
Contact/irritant Dermatitis *Contact* • Skin rash with red, itching papules • May look like a burn • Rash may present with red bumps, forming moist, weeping blisters • Mostly localized *Irritant* • Skin redness • Mild edema • Scaling • Rash—may be itchy or painful • Dermatitis restricted locally to the area of irritant	• Allergy to specific exogenous allergens, such as adhesive tape and/or hydrogel, that come into contact with the skin • Nonspecific inflammation caused by direct cellular damage upon contact with an inherently harmful substance to cells (e.g., chemical irritation from hydrogel, moisture, and/or alcohol)	• Immediate removal of the irritant/allergen • Adjust array from area of concern • Topical corticosteroid application • Consider use of barrier film • Consider trimming array adhesive and use of surgilast, if reaction related to tape/adhesive • If blistering develops, cold, moist compress application (20 min; 3 times/day) • Consider systemic corticosteroids/treatment breaks if condition persists
Erosion and Ulceration *Erosion* • Breakdown of the outer epidermal layer • Skin discontinuity with incomplete loss of the epidermis • May present as a delineated moist or depressed lesion • Mild bleeding with pain or burning may be present • Typically, erosions do not result in scarring *Ulcer* • Open skin defects with potential for bleeding or oozing • Complete loss of epidermis and portions of the dermis, fat, or muscle, with increased risk of scarring • Pustules may develop when infected	• Mechanical trauma from shaving and/or array application/removal • May develop from inflammation or maceration due to sweat, rupture of vesicles, bullae from infection, or epidermal necrosis • Ischemic injury and/or decreased perfusion related to mechanical pressure of array (especially in areas overlying scars, hardware, and prior radiation exposure)	• Shift array from site of erosion/ulcer • Assess wound and treat with topical antibiotic (e.g., clindamycin, gentamicin) • Consider wound culture • Frequent skin surveillance
Dermatitis with Infection • Inflammation of skin or hair follicle (red pimple with hair in the center) • May have pus, itching, or burning	• Secondary bacterial infection • Ultimately, infection with or without pustules may occur when the skin is affected by pathogenic bacteria	• Assess wound and treat with topical antibiotic (e.g., clindamycin or gentamicin) • Warm compresses with saltwater or Burow's solution (5% aluminum subacetate) • Obtain culture of wound and consider dermatologist referral • Return to clinic in 2 weeks; if condition persists, consider oral antibiotic/treatment break
Regular array repositioning to minimize direct pressure to the scalp and ensure avoidance of surgical scar lines	• At each array change, shift array placement by ~2 cm, ensuring that pairs of arrays are moved together • Move arrays back to original position at subsequent change • Avoid placing an array disc immediately over scars or surgical screws • Wear breathable headwear to avoid overheating	

TTFields—Proactive Strategies to Minimize Cutaneous Adverse Events with TTFields Therapy

Intervention	Recommendations for Patients and Caregivers
Optimal shaving and preparation of the scalp to maximize array skin contact and minimize erosions and other factors increasing the risk of infection	• Perform thorough hand washing before preparing the scalp for array application • Shave the scalp every time arrays are changed using gentle but firm circular motions—complete hair removal is required for optimal adhesion • Use a clean, electric razor to avoid cuts • Mineral (baby) oil may be applied before shaving to allow for cleansing of the skin and facilitate removal of bacteria and scale
Removal of natural oils and any moisture (sweat) from the scalp prior to array placement	• Wash the scalp with mild, fragrance-free shampoo (e.g., baby shampoo) or dandruff shampoo • If no skin irritation is present, wipe the scalp with a gauze or cotton ball soaked in isopropyl alcohol (70%) • Ensure scalp is completely dry before array placement
Careful application and removal of arrays is crucial to decrease the risk of cutaneous irritation	• Change arrays at least every 3–4 days, or more frequently if they become wet or loosen (e.g., excessive sweating during warmer weather or after intense physical activity) • Apply mineral (baby) oil to the scalp to gently remove arrays; slowly and gently peel back the arrays from the skin—pulling the skin or forceful rubbing of the scalp to remove adhesive can contribute to skin irritation and potential breakdown • Alternatively, the arrays may be removed in a warm shower by rubbing in a body wash containing coconut oil causing them to slide off the scalp • Evaluate the skin and scalp for signs of irritation with every array change, and notify your healthcare provider if there are signs of irritation (taking a picture of the affected area is advised)
Regular array repositioning to minimize direct pressure to the scalp and ensure avoidance of surgical scar lines	• At each array change, shift array placement by ~2 cm, ensuring that pairs of arrays are moved together • Move arrays back to original position at subsequent change • Avoid placing an array disc immediately over scars or surgical screws • Wear breathable headwear to avoid overheating

Adapted from Lacouture, M. E., Anadkat, M. J., Ballo, M. T., Iwamoto, F., Jeyapalan, S. A., La Rocca, R. V., ... Glas, M. (2020). Prevention and management of dermatologic adverse events associated with tumor treating fields in patients with glioblastoma. Frontiers in Oncology, 10, 1045. https://doi.org/10.3389/fonc.2020.01045. CC-BY, version 4.0.

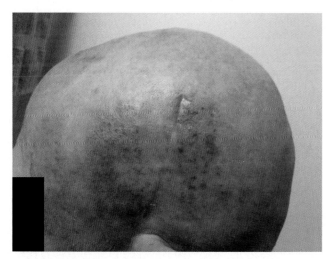

Example of Mild-to-Moderate Skin Irritation in a 60-Year-Old Man Who Had Been on TMZ and TTFields Therapy for 3 Months. *TMZ,* Temozolomide; *TTFields,* tumor treating fields. (Reprinted from Lacouture, M. E., Davis, M. E., Elzinga, G, Butowski, N., Tran, D., Villano, J. L., ... Wong, E. T. [2014]. Characterization and management of dermatologic adverse events with the NovoTTF-100A System, a novel anti-mitotic electric field device for the treatment of recurrent glioblastoma. *Seminars in Oncology, 41*[Suppl 4], S1–S14.)

Conclusion

Based on its complementary MoA and evidence of broad applicability to target difficult-to-treat solid tumors, TTFields therapy is emerging as part of new multimodal therapeutic strategies for treating various solid tumors. With efficacy and safety established for the treatment of GBM and MPM, including high-risk subgroups such as elderly patients, current studies are exploring the expanding role of TTFields therapy for other solid tumors. Consequently, oncology nurses are likely to encounter TTFields therapy in the clinic more and more frequently. The best clinical outcomes for TTFields therapy are directly correlated with an average daily or monthly usage ≥75% and optimal field intensity at the site of the tumor. Oncology nurses have an essential role in the patient journey by educating and streamlining information for the patient and their caregiver(s) concerning appropriate treatment options and guiding them to key resources. In the utilization of TTFields therapy, oncology nurses are critical in helping identify strategies to maximize usage and to minimize therapy limiting local skin AEs to maximize patient outcomes.

References

Aguilar, A. A., Ho, M. C., Chang, E., Carlson, K. W., Natarajan, A., Marciano, T., … Patel, C. B. (2021). Permeabilizing cell membranes with electric fields. *Cancers, 13*(9), 2283. https://doi.org/10.3390/cancers13092283.

Anadkat, M. J., Lacouture, M., Friedman, A., Horne, Z. D., Jung, J., Kaffenberger, B., … Grosso, F. (2023). Expert guidance on prophylaxis and treatment of dermatologic adverse events with Tumor Treating Fields (TTFields) therapy in the thoracic region. *Frontiers in Oncology, 12*, 975473. https://doi.org/10.3389/fonc.2022.975473.

Ballo, M. T., Urman, N., Bomzon, Z., Lavy-Shahaf, G., & Toms, S. (2019). Increasing tumor treating fields dose at the tumor bed improves survival: Setting a framework for TTFields dosimetry based on analysis of the EF-14 Phase III trial in newly diagnosed glioblastoma. *Cancer Research, 79*(13_Supplement), CT204. https://doi.org/10.1158/1538-7445.Am2019-ct204.

Ballo, M. T., Urman, N., Lavy-Shahaf, G., Grewal, J., Bomzon, Z., & Toms, S. (2019). Correlation of tumor treating fields dosimetry to survival outcomes in newly diagnosed glioblastoma: A large-scale numerical simulation-based analysis of data from the phase 3 EF-14 randomized trial. *International Journal of Radiation Oncology, Biology, Physics, 104*(5), 1106–1113. https://doi.org/10.1016/j.ijrobp.2019.04.008.

Barthel, L., Hadamitzky, M., Dammann, P., Schedlowski, M., Sure, U., Thakur, B. K., & Hetze, S. (2022). Glioma: Molecular signature and crossroads with tumor microenvironment. *Cancer Metastasis Reviews, 41*(1), 53–75. https://doi.org/10.1007/s10555-021-09997-9.

Blatt, R., Davidi, S., Munster, M., Shteingauz, A., Cahal, S., Zeidan, A., … Palti, Y. (2021). In vivo safety of tumor treating fields (TTFields) applied to the torso. *Frontiers in Oncology, 11*, 670809. https://doi.org/10.3389/fonc.2021.670809.

Ceresoli, G. L., Aerts, J. G., Dziadziuszko, R., Ramlau, R., Cedres, S., van Meerbeeck, J. P., … Grosso, F. (2019). Tumour treating fields in combination with pemetrexed and cisplatin or carboplatin as first-line treatment for unresectable malignant pleural mesothelioma (STELLAR): A multicentre, single-arm phase 2 trial. *The Lancet Oncology, 20*(12), 1702–1709. https://doi.org/10.1016/S1470-2045(19)30532-7.

Chang, E., Patel, C. B., Pohling, C., Young, C., Song, J., Flores, T. A., … Gambhir, S. S. (2018). Tumor treating fields increases membrane permeability in glioblastoma cells. *Cell Death Discovery, 4*, 113. https://doi.org/10.1038/s41420-018-0130-x.

Dagogo-Jack, I., & Shaw, A. T. (2018). Tumour heterogeneity and resistance to cancer therapies. *Nature Reviews Clinical Oncology, 15*(2), 81–94. https://doi.org/10.1038/nrclinonc.2017.166.

Diamant, G., Simchony Goldman, H., Gasri Plotnitsky, L., Roitman, M., Shiloach, T., Globerson-Levin, A., … Volovitz, I. (2021). T cells retain pivotal antitumoral functions under tumor-treating electric fields. *Journal of Immunology, 207*(2), 709–719. https://doi.org/10.4049/jimmunol.2100100.

Frongillo, P., Shackelford, M., & Certo, J. (2020). Abstract LB-255: Impact of innovative educational approaches to enhance patient and caregiver understanding of tumor treating fields (TTFields) for glioblastoma implications for outcomes. *Cancer Research, 80*(16_Supplement), LB-255. https://doi.org/10.1158/1538-7445.AM2020-LB-255.

Frongillo, P., Shackelford, M., & Rain, L. (2021). Abstract 717: Rapid transformation of TTFields care-delivery during COVID-19 pandemic to optimize treatment of patients with glioblastoma (GBM). *Cancer Research, 81*(13_Supplement), 717. https://doi.org/10.1158/1538-7445.AM2021-717.

Gera, N., Yang, A., Holtzman, T. S., Lee, S. X., Wong, E. T., & Swanson, K. D. (2015). Tumor treating fields perturb the localization of septins and cause aberrant mitotic exit. *PLoS One, 10*(5), e0125269. https://doi.org/10.1371/journal.pone.0125269.

Giladi, M., Munster, M., Schneiderman, R. S., Voloshin, T., Porat, Y., Blat, R., … Palti, Y. (2017). Tumor treating fields (TTFields) delay DNA damage repair following radiation treatment of glioma cells. *Radiation Oncology, 12*(1), 206. https://doi.org/10.1186/s13014-017-0941-6.

Gotwals, P., Cameron, S., Cipolletta, D., Cremasco, V., Crystal, A., Hewes, B., … Dranoff, G. (2017). Prospects for combining targeted and conventional cancer therapy with immunotherapy. *Nature Reviews Cancer, 17*(5), 286–301. https://doi.org/10.1038/nrc.2017.17.

Karanam, N. K., & Story, M. D. (2021). An overview of potential novel mechanisms of action underlying tumor treating fields-induced cancer cell death and their clinical implications. *International Journal of Radiation Biology, 97*(8), 1044–1054. https://doi.org/10.1080/09553002.2020.1837984.

Kim, E. H., Jo, Y., Sai, S., Park, M. J., Kim, J. Y., Kim, J. S., … Hwang, S. G. (2019). Tumor-treating fields induce autophagy by blocking the Akt2/miR29b axis in glioblastoma cells. *Oncogene, 38*(39), 6630–6646. https://doi.org/10.1038/s41388-019-0882-7.

Kim, E. H., Kim, Y. H., Song, H. S., Jeong, Y. K., Lee, J. Y., Sung, J., … Yoon, M. (2016). Biological effect of an alternating electric field on cell proliferation and synergistic antimitotic effect in combination with ionizing radiation. *Oncotarget, 7*(38), 62267–62279. https://doi.org/10.18632/oncotarget.11407.

Kim, E. H., Song, H. S., Yoo, S. H., & Yoon, M. (2016). Tumor treating fields inhibit glioblastoma cell migration, invasion and angiogenesis. *Oncotarget, 7*(40), 65125–65136. https://doi.org/10.18632/oncotarget.11372.

Kirson, E. D., Dbalý, V., Tovarys, F., Vymazal, J., Soustiel, J. F., Itzhaki, A., … Palti, Y. (2007). Alternating electric fields arrest cell proliferation in animal tumor models and human brain tumors. *Proceedings of the National Academy of Sciences of the United States of America, 104*(24), 10152–10157. https://doi.org/10.1073/pnas.0702916104.

Kirson, E. D., Giladi, M., Gurvich, Z., Itzhaki, A., Mordechovich, D., Schneiderman, R. S., … Palti, Y. (2009). Alternating electric fields (TTFields) inhibit metastatic spread of solid tumors to the lungs. *Clinical & Experimental Metastasis, 26*(7), 633–640. https://doi.org/10.1007/s10585-009-9262-y.

Kirson, E. D., Gurvich, Z., Schneiderman, R., Dekel, E., Itzhaki, A., Wasserman, Y., … Palti, Y. (2004). Disruption of cancer cell replication by alternating electric fields. *Cancer Research, 64*(9), 3288–3295. https://doi.org/10.1158/0008-5472.can-04-0083.

Kirson, E. D., Schneiderman, R. S., Dbalý, V., Tovarys, F., Vymazal, J., Itzhaki, A., … Palti, Y. (2009). Chemotherapeutic treatment efficacy and sensitivity are increased by adjuvant alternating electric fields (TTFields). *BMC Medical Physics, 9*, 1. https://doi.org/10.1186/1756-6649-9-1.

Lacouture, M. E., Anadkat, M. J., Ballo, M. T., Iwamoto, F., Jeyapalan, S. A., La Rocca, R. V., … Glas, M. (2020). Prevention and management of dermatologic adverse events associated with tumor treating fields in patients with glioblastoma. *Frontiers in Oncology, 10*, 1045. https://doi.org/10.3389/fonc.2020.01045.

Lacouture, M. E., Davis, M. E., Elzinga, G., Butowski, N., Tran, D., Villano, J. L., … Wong, E. T. (2014). Characterization and management of dermatologic adverse events with the NovoTTF-100A System, a novel antimitotic electric field device for the treatment of recurrent glioblastoma. *Seminars in Oncology, 41*(Suppl 4), S1–S14. https://doi.org/10.1053/j.seminoncol.2014.03.011.

Mrugala, M. M., Engelhard, H. H., Dinh Tran, D., Kew, Y., Cavaliere, R., Villano, J. L., … Butowski, N. (2014). Clinical practice experience with NovoTTF-100A™ system for glioblastoma: The Patient Registry Dataset (PRiDe). *Seminars in Oncology, 41*(Suppl 6), S4–S13. https://doi.org/10.1053/j.seminoncol.2014.09.010.

Mumblat, H., Martinez-Conde, A., Braten, O., Munster, M., Dor-On, E., Schneiderman, R. S., … Palti, Y. (2021). Tumor treating fields (TTFields) downregulate the Fanconi Anemia-BRCA pathway and increase the efficacy of chemotherapy in malignant pleural mesothelioma preclinical models. *Lung Cancer, 160*, 99–110. https://doi.org/10.1016/j.lungcan.2021.08.011.

Mun, E. J., Babiker, H. M., Weinberg, U., Kirson, E. D., & Von Hoff, D. D. (2018). Tumor-treating fields: A fourth modality in cancer treatment. *Clinical Cancer Research: An Official Journal of the American Association for Cancer Research, 24*(2), 266–275. https://doi.org/10.1158/1078-0432.CCR-17-1117.

Murphy, J., Bowers, M. E., Barron, L. (2016). Optune®: Practical nursing applications. *Clinical Journal of Oncology Nursing, 20*(5 Suppl), S14–S19. https://doi.org/10.1188/16.CJON.S1.14-19. PMID: 27668385.

National Comprehensive Cancer Network (NCCN). (2021). Central nervous system cancers (version 2.2021). https://www.nccn.org/professionals/physician_gls/pdf/cns.pdf.

Neuhaus, E., Zirjacks, L., Ganser, K., Klumpp, L., Schüler, U., Zips, D., … Huber, S. M. (2019). Alternating electric fields (TTFields) activate Cav1.2 channels in human glioblastoma cells. *Cancers, 11*(1), 110. https://doi.org/10.3390/cancers11010110.

Omer, H. (2021). Radiobiological effects and medical applications of non-ionizing radiation. *Saudi Journal of Biological Sciences, 28*(10), 5585–5592. https://doi.org/10.1016/j.sjbs.2021.05.071.

Palmer, J. D., Chavez, G., Furnback, W., Chuang, P. Y., Wang, B., Proescholdt, C., & Tang, C. H. (2021). Health-related quality of life for patients receiving tumor treating fields for glioblastoma. *Frontiers in Oncology, 11*, 772261. https://doi.org/10.3389/fonc.2021.772261.

Porat, Y., Giladi, M., Schneiderman, R. S., Blat, R., Shteingauz, A., Zeevi, E., … Palti, Y. (2017). Determining the optimal inhibitory frequency for cancerous cells using tumor treating fields (TTFields). *Journal of Visualized Experiments: JoVE, 123*, 55820. https://doi.org/10.3791/55820.

Ram, Z., Kim, C. Y., Hottinger, A. F., Idbaih, A., Nicholas, G., & Zhu, J. J. (2021). Efficacy and safety of tumor treating fields (TTFields) in elderly patients with newly diagnosed glioblastoma: Subgroup analysis of the phase 3 EF-14 clinical trial. *Frontiers in Oncology, 11*, 671972. https://doi.org/10.3389/fonc.2021.671972.

Rominiyi, O., Vanderlinden, A., Clenton, S. J., Bridgewater, C., Al-Tamimi, Y., & Collis, S. J. (2021). Tumour treating fields therapy for glioblastoma: Current advances and future directions. *British Journal of Cancer*, 124(4), 697–709. https://doi.org/10.1038/s41416-020-01136-5. Epub 2020 Nov 4. Erratum in: British Journal of Cancer. 2021 Aug;125(4), 623. PMID: 33144698; PMCID: PMC7884384

Shackelford, M., Frongillo, P., & Certo, J. (2019). INNV-17. Innovative educational approaches to enhance patient and caregiver understanding of ttfields for glioblastoma. *Neuro-Oncology*, 21(Supplement_6), vi134. https://doi.org/10.1093/neuonc/noz175.560.

Shi, W., Blumenthal, D. T., Oberheim Bush, N. A., Kebir, S., Lukas, R. V., Muragaki, Y., … Glas, M. (2020). Global post-marketing safety surveillance of tumor treating fields (TTFields) in patients with high-grade glioma in clinical practice. *Journal of Neuro-Oncology*, 148(3), 489–500. https://doi.org/10.1007/s11060-020-03540-6.

Shteingauz, A., Porat, Y., Voloshin, T., Schneiderman, R. S., Munster, M., Zeevi, E., … Palti, Y. (2018). AMPK-dependent autophagy upregulation serves as a survival mechanism in response to tumor treating fields (TTFields). *Cell Death & Disease*, 9(11), 1074. https://doi.org/10.1038/s41419-018-1085-9.

Silginer, M., Weller, M., Stupp, R., & Roth, P. (2017). Biological activity of tumor-treating fields in preclinical glioma models. *Cell Death & Disease*, 8(4), e2753. https://doi.org/10.1038/cddis.2017.171. PMID: 28425987; PMCID: PMC5477589.

Stupp, R., Taillibert, S., Kanner, A., Read, W., Steinberg, D., Lhermitte, B., … Ram, Z. (2017). Effect of tumor-treating fields plus maintenance temozolomide vs maintenance temozolomide alone on survival in patients with glioblastoma: A randomized clinical trial. *JAMA*, 318(23), 2306–2316. https://doi.org/10.1001/jama.2017.18718.

Stupp, R., Taillibert, S., Kanner, A. A., Kesari, S., Steinberg, D. M., Toms, S. A., … Ram, Z. (2015). Maintenance therapy with tumor-treating fields plus temozolomide vs temozolomide alone for glioblastoma: A randomized clinical trial. *JAMA*, 314(23), 2535–2543. https://doi.org/10.1001/jama.2015.16669.

Stupp, R., Wong, E. T., Kanner, A. A., Steinberg, D., Engelhard, H., Heidecke, V., … Gutin, P. H. (2012). NovoTTF-100A versus physician's choice chemotherapy in recurrent glioblastoma: A randomised phase III trial of a novel treatment modality. *European Journal of Cancer*, 48(14), 2192–2202. https://doi.org/10.1016/j.ejca.2012.04.011.

Sun, Y. S. (2018). Direct-current electric field distribution in the brain for tumor treating field applications: A simulation study. *Computational and Mathematical Methods in Medicine*, 2018, 3829768. https://doi.org/10.1155/2018/3829768.

Taphoorn, M., Dirven, L., Kanner, A. A., Lavy-Shahaf, G., Weinberg, U., Taillibert, S., … Stupp, R. (2018). Influence of treatment with tumor-treating fields on health-related quality of life of patients with newly diagnosed glioblastoma: A secondary analysis of a randomized clinical trial. *JAMA Oncology*, 4(4), 495–504. https://doi.org/10.1001/jamaoncol.2017.5082.

Vogelzang, N. J., Rusthoven, J. J., Symanowski, J., Denham, C., Kaukel, E., Ruffie, P., … Paoletti, P. (2003). Phase III study of pemetrexed in combination with cisplatin versus cisplatin alone in patients with malignant pleural mesothelioma. *Journal of Clinical Oncology: Official Journal of the American Society of Clinical Oncology*, 21(14), 2636–2644. https://doi.org/10.1200/JCO.2003.11.136.

Voloshin, T., Schneiderman, R. S., Volodin, A., Shamir, R. R., Kaynan, N., Zeevi, E., … Palti, Y. (2020). Tumor treating fields (TTFields) hinder cancer cell motility through regulation of microtubule and acting dynamics. *Cancers*, 12(10), 3016. https://doi.org/10.3390/cancers12103016.

Wenger, C., Salvador, R., Basser, P. J., & Miranda, P. C. (2015). The electric field distribution in the brain during TTFields therapy and its dependence on tissue dielectric properties and anatomy: A computational study. *Physics in Medicine and Biology*, 60(18), 7339–7357. https://doi.org/10.1088/0031-9155/60/18/7339.

Principles of Cancer Management

3

Hematopoietic Stem Cell Transplantation and Chimeric Antigen Receptor T-Cell Therapy

Terry Wikle Shapiro

Introduction

Nearly six decades ago, the concept of using bone marrow (i.e., hematopoietic stem cell transplantation [HSCT]) to treat humans with inherited diseases of immune function, marrow failure syndromes, and leukemia was met with much skepticism and varying degrees of enthusiasm. Transferring what was known from experimental animal models to humans was fraught with many challenges and disappointments. When the first HSCTs were performed six decades ago, they were used as a last-resort therapy in an attempt to deliver high doses of radiation and chemotherapy to patients with incurable malignancies (Granot & Storb, 2020; Norkin & Wingard, 2017). Considered radicals in the early 1970s, HSCT pioneers E. Donall Thomas and Robert Goode were able to demonstrate in humans that diseased or poorly functioning bone marrow could be replaced by a central venous infusion of bone marrow from a healthy donor after cytotoxic doses of chemoradiotherapy (Granot & Storb, 2020).

HSCT is no longer a treatment modality only for lethal diseases such as primary immunodeficiency diseases or hematologic malignancies. It is also a valid approach of cellular engineering for treating solid tumors, hemoglobinopathies, marrow failure syndromes, autoimmune diseases, inherited disorders of metabolism, histiocytic disorders, and other nonmalignancies.

Advances in histocompatibility matching; reduced-intensity conditioning (RIC) regimens; better techniques for determining minimal residual malignant disease; state-mandated newborn screening for diseases such as severe combined immunodeficiency (SCID) and Hurler syndrome; improvements in stem cell collection and cryopreservation techniques; development of pharmacologic agents to accelerate the recovery of hematopoiesis; advances in infectious disease monitoring and detection; development of effective antimicrobial agents; refinements in the prevention, diagnosis, and management of acute and chronic graft-versus-host disease (GVHD); a better understanding of the biology of the graft-versus-tumor (GVT) effect has contributed to the evolving success of HSCT (Norkin & Wingard, 2017). In addition to these medical advances, astute nursing care of transplant recipients continues to be the cornerstone for the prevention and treatment of HSCT-related complications and death.

In addition to the expanding use of HSCT, there is also the use of chimeric antigen receptor (CAR) therapies. CAR cell therapy involves re-engineering a patient's own autologous T cells to recognize and eradicate certain cancers. These T cells are genetically altered to express artificial receptors that enable the T cells to bind to a specific antigen on the patient's tumor cells and kill them. Unlike T-cell receptor-mediated immune reactions, CAR T-cell-mediated immune reactions lead to direct recognition of extracellular tumor-associated antigens (Herrick, 2021).

This chapter reviews the principles of caring for patients undergoing autologous and allogeneic HSCT as well as patients receiving CAR T-cell therapies.

Rationale for High-Dose Therapy With Stem Cell Transplantation

HSCT involves replacing diseased, destroyed, or nonfunctioning hematopoietic cells with healthy hematopoietic progenitor cells (i.e., stem cells). Stem cells are primitive hematopoietic cells that are capable of self-renewal, and they are pluripotent, meaning that they can mature into a red blood cell (RBC), white blood cell (WBC), or platelet. Stem cells may be collected directly from the bone marrow spaces by a bone marrow harvest procedure, from the peripheral blood by apheresis, or from the umbilical cord of newborns by cannulation of the large vessels of the umbilical cord and placenta after delivery.

For adult allogeneic HSCT, peripheral blood stem cells (PBSCs) have become the preferred source for grafting. Collection of PBSCs through apheresis is easier and less costly, and it may also result in a more rapid recovery of neutrophil and platelet counts. For pediatric allogeneic HSCT, bone marrow remains the preferred source of stem cells due to the long-term risk of chronic GVHD associated with PBSCs. In both related and unrelated donor allogeneic HSCT, the source of stem cells may be bone marrow, PBSCs, or umbilical cord blood (UCB). PBSCs are used almost exclusively in autologous HSCT.

Types of Hematopoietic Stem Cell Transplantations

The various types of HSCTs can be differentiated in terms of the hematopoietic stem cell donor, the method used to collect the cells, and the intensity of the conditioning regimen. Each source of stem cells has advantages and disadvantages, as summarized in the table on the next page. In autologous HSCT, the patient serves as his or her own donor of stem cells, whereas for allogeneic HSCT, the donor is related (sibling or a parent) or unrelated. Identical twin or *syngeneic transplant* donors were once considered when available (*syngeneic transplantation*); however, given the lack of therapeutic GVT effect when using identical twin donors, choosing such a donor is no longer common practice when HSCT is pursued for a malignant condition (Kurosawa et al., 2021). Stem cells may be collected from the peripheral bloodstream (i.e., PBSCs), from the bone marrow spaces (i.e., bone marrow stem cells), or from the umbilical cord and placenta of newborns (i.e., UBC stem cells).

Comparison of Hematopoietic Stem Cell Sources

Technique	Advantages and Disadvantages
Bone marrow harvest	Harvest-related pain General anesthesia required Longer postcollection recovery time No growth factor mobilization required Lower incidence of chronic GVHD
PBSCs	Less invasive Higher cell procurement for autologous procedures Shorter recovery time May be more cost-effective and more convenient for donors Incidence of chronic GVHD may be higher Improved graft-versus-tumor effect More than 1 day of collection may be required Requires mobilization with chemotherapy (autologous) or hematopoietic growth factors, or both
Cord blood	Inexpensive to collect Excellent source to increase pool of unrelated donors Associated with less GVHD Full HLA-compatibility not required More than one cord blood unit may be necessary in adults Increased risk of graft rejection Delayed posttransplantation immune recovery No donor available for posttransplantation DLI, HSCT boost, or CTLs

CTLs, Cytotoxic T lymphocytes; *DLI*, donor lymphocyte infusion; *GVHD*, graft-versus-host disease, *HLA*, human leukocyte antigen.

HSCTs can also be differentiated based on the intensity of the conditioning regimen. Myeloablative transplantation involves the use of high doses of chemotherapy with or without total body irradiation (TBI) to treat the underlying disease, ablate the bone marrow, and cause myelosuppression that would be irreversible without the infusion of hematopoietic stem cells.

RIC during allogeneic HSCT reduces transplantation-related mortality (TRM) and morbidity by relying more on the GVT effect than the conditioning regimen to eradicate disease. RIC regimens can provide a curative option for patients who may otherwise not be candidates for myeloablative (intensive) transplantation because of age or poor performance status (Song et al., 2021). RIC transplants are often used when there is increased concern about fatal or debilitating TRM and morbidity.

Indications for and Outcomes of Hematopoietic Stem Cell Transplantation

HSCT represents an important advance in restoring or replacing hematopoietic or immune function in patients whose bone marrow has been destroyed by the cytotoxic effects of radiation therapy and high-dose chemotherapy to treat an underlying disease. Many factors influence the indications and patient eligibility for transplantation. HSCT is used when the bone marrow or immune system is diseased, defective, or destroyed as a result of prior treatment. The table below lists the diseases treated with autologous or allogeneic HSCT.

Factors that may affect the outcomes of HSCT include the type and stage of disease at the time of transplantation, type of procedure (i.e., allogeneic or autologous), degree of human leukocyte antigen (HLA) matching for allogeneic transplants, intensity of the conditioning regimen, ages of the donor and recipient, cytomegalovirus (CMV) status compatibility of the donor and recipient, and experience of the transplantation center (Chao, 2021; Styczyński et al., 2020). The TRM risk for allogeneic HSCT improved from 30% to 50% in the 1990s to about 5% to 10% (given the above factors) in 2021 (Chao, 2021; Styczyński et al., 2020). The improved rate most likely resulted from the increasing use of RIC regimens, agents that avoid hepatic and renal toxicity, and better infection control methods (Chao, 2021; Styczyński et al., 2020). At most transplantation centers, the acceptable TRM rate for autologous HSCT is less than 5%.

Disease-free survival at 5 years can range from 10% to 75% after HSCT, depending on the age of the recipient, underlying disease, disease status at the time of transplantation, type of HSCT procedure, and extent of prior treatment. The table on next page lists 5-year disease-free survival rates for the most common malignant diseases treated with HSCT.

Diseases Treated With Hematopoietic Stem Cell Transplantation

AUTOLOGOUS TRANSPLANTATION		ALLOGENEIC TRANSPLANTATION	
Malignant Disorders	**Nonmalignant Disorders**	**Malignant Disorders**	**Nonmalignant Disorders**
Neuroblastoma Non-Hodgkin lymphoma Hodgkin disease		Acute myeloid leukemia (AML) Non-Hodgkin lymphoma Hodgkin disease	Aplastic anemia Fanconi anemia Severe combined immunodeficiency
Brain tumors (type specific) Medulloblastoma Germ cell tumors Multiple myeloma*	Autoimmune disorders Amyloidosis	Acute lymphoblastic leukemia (ALL) Chronic myeloid leukemia (CML) Myeloproliferative disorders Multiple myeloma* Chronic lymphocytic leukemia (CLL)*	β-Thalassemia major Diamond-Blackfan anemia Sickle cell anemia Wiskott-Aldrich syndrome Osteopetrosis Inborn errors of metabolism Autoimmune disorders Chronic congenital neutropenia

*Uncommon in children but a common reason for transplantation in adults.

Data from Brown, V. (Ed.). (2018). *Hematopoietic stem cell transplantation for the pediatric oncologist.* Switzerland: Springer International Publishing AG; Duarte, R. F., Labopin, M., Bader, P., Basak, G. W., Bonini, C., Chabannon, C., ... European Society for Blood and Marrow Transplantation (EBMT). (2019). Indications for haematopoietic stem cell transplantation for haematological diseases, solid tumours and immune disorders: Current practice in Europe. *Bone Marrow Transplantation, 54*(10), 1525–1552; Fraint, E., Holuba, M. J., & Wray, L. (2020). Pediatric hematopoietic stem cell transplant. *Pediatrics in Review, 41*(11), 609–611.

Five-Year Disease-Free Survival Rates

| | | | SURVIVAL RATE (%) | | |
| | | | ALLOGENEIC TRANSPLANTATION | | |
Disease	Stage	Autologous Transplantation	Sibling Donor	Unrelated Donor	Pediatric (All Donor Types)
Acute lymphoblastic leukemia (ALL)	CR 1	NA	65	60	80
	CR2	NA	50	45	65
Acute myeloid leukemia (AML)	CR1	NA	60	50	65
	CR2	NA	50	50	
	No remission	NA	30	30	
Chronic myeloid leukemia (CML)	Chronic phase <1 year	NA	70	55	
	Chronic phase >1 year	NA	60	50	
Hodgkin disease	85	80	NA	NA	
	Chemosensitive	70	NA	NA	
	Chemoresistant	45	NA	NA	
Diffuse large cell lymphoma	CR1	70	50	45	
Mantle cell lymphoma		75	50	NA	
Stage IV neuroblastoma		40	NA	NA	
Severe aplastic anemia		85	75	95	

CR, Complete response; *NA*, not applicable.
Data from Auletta, J. J., Kou, J., Chen, M., & Shaw B. E. (2021). Current use and outcome of hematopoietic stem cell transplantation: CIMBTR US summary slides. Available at https://cibmtr.org/CIBMTR/Resources/Summary-Slides-Reports.

Overview of the Process and Implications for Nursing Care

Pretransplantation Evaluation of the Recipient and Donor

The pretransplantation evaluation of the recipient includes a thorough physical and psychosocial evaluation, assessment of the adequacy of insurance coverage, and evaluation of the adequacy of family and caregiver support. Before transplantation, the patient and family should receive extensive education about the risks, benefits, and process of transplantation to permit informed consent for the procedure. For allogeneic HSCT, the selection of an appropriate donor includes confirmatory high-resolution tissue typing, an assessment of specific viral serologies, a donor health assessment, and a physical examination.

Donors must be carefully evaluated and fully informed before the donation of PBSCs or bone marrow (Connelly-Smith, 2020). Legal and ethical aspects should be considered, especially when using minors as donors. Although the selection of an appropriate donor should be performed by the HSCT team, the donor evaluation should be performed by a provider who is not directly involved in the recipient's care during the transplantation process (Foundation for the Accreditation of Cellular Therapy, 2021). Evaluation for autologous and allogeneic HSCT includes an assessment of the patient's overall performance status, disease status, and organ function; evaluation of specific viral serologies; and exclusion of active infection. The components of the evaluation of recipient and donor are summarized in the box below.

Pretransplantation Evaluation of Recipient and Donor

Evaluation of the Autologous and Allogeneic Hematopoietic Stem Cell Transplant Recipient

Pretreatment testing and evaluation of the patient undergoing HSCT includes the following:
- History of current illness, including presenting signs and symptoms, previous therapies, initial diagnosis, pathology and staging, complications, relapses or progressions, current disease status, and transfusion history.
- Medical history, including major illnesses, chronic illnesses, recurring illnesses, surgical history, childhood illnesses, and infectious disease exposure. For women, the medical history should also include menarche, onset of menopause or date of last menstrual period, pregnancies, and outcomes.
- Current medications
- Allergies
- Social and family history, including identified caregiver and alternate.
- Performance status
- Complete blood cell count (CBC), which must be obtained within a 24-h period before the first PBSC collection and within 24 h of each subsequent collection.
- Current laboratory studies, including liver and renal function studies; 24-h urine test for creatinine clearance or nuclear glomerular filtration rate (GFR), if there is a history of renal dysfunction or nephrotoxins; prothrombin time (PT), partial prothrombin time (PTT), or international normalized ratio (INR); blood grouping and Rh typing (ABO and Rh).
- Infectious disease serologies, including human immunodeficiency virus type 1 (HIV-1) antibody, HIV-2 antibody, HIV antigen, human T-cell lymphotropic virus (HTLV), hepatitis B surface antigen, hepatitis B core antigen, hepatitis C antibodies, human T-cell leukemia/lymphoma virus type 1 (HTLV-1), West Nile virus, and *Trypanosoma cruzi* (Chagas disease) within 30 days of collection.
- Infectious disease serologies specific to allogeneic recipients, such as CMV antibodies (immunoglobulin G [IgG] and immunoglobulin [IgM]), herpes simplex virus (HSV) antibodies (IgG and IgM), toxoplasmosis IgG and IgM antibodies, and Epstein-Barr virus (EBV) nuclear antibodies.
- Polymerase chain reaction (PCR) test for COVID-19
- HLA typing (allogeneic)

Continued

Pretransplantation Evaluation of Recipient and Donor—cont'd

- Pretransplantation chimerism studies (by PCR or by short tandem repeat [STR] method if the donor and recipient are the same sex or XY DNA analysis if the donor and recipient are different sexes).
- Chest radiograph
- Electrocardiogram and echocardiogram
- Multiple gated acquisition (MUGA) scan for adult patients or echocardiogram for children
- Pulmonary function tests, including single-breath diffusing capacity
- A 24-h urine test for creatinine clearance or nuclear GFR testing
- Computed tomography (CT) of chest and sinuses for pretransplantation infection surveillance if there are symptoms, a history of repeated infections, or periods of prolonged neutropenia.
- Disease restaging, including radiographic studies (e.g., CT), nuclear medicine studies, bone marrow aspirate and biopsy (hematologic malignancies, Hodgkin lymphoma, and neuroblastoma), cytogenetics, molecular diagnostics, and measures of minimal residual disease.
- Dental evaluation, including full-mouth x-ray record and cleaning
- Sperm, oocyte, or fertilized embryo banking when clinically possible
- Informed consent for treatment, transfusion support, clinical trials
- Nutritional evaluation, if appropriate
- Consultations with radiation therapy, infectious disease, pulmonary, cardiology, or renal services if clinically indicated.
- Financial screening
- Psychosocial evaluation
- The following must be documented:
  - Suitability to undergo transplantation
  - Abnormal findings and rationale for proceeding to transplantation
  - Counseling of patient regarding abnormal findings
  - Patient informed of tests performed to protect the health of the patient
  - Patient informed of right to review test results

Evaluation of the Hematopoietic Stem Cell Donor

Pretreatment testing and evaluation of the hematopoietic stem cell donor usually includes the following:

- Human leukocyte antigen A (HLA-A), HLA-B, HLA-DR, and HLA-DQ typing
- History and physical examination, documenting serious or chronic illnesses, hematologic problems (including bleeding tendencies), cancer history, prior transfusions, current medications, allergies, and pregnancy history for females.

- Presence of risk factors for HIV or viral hepatitis infection and other communicable diseases.
- Physical examination for abnormalities and assessment of the adequacy of peripheral veins.
- CBC with differential count, chemistry panel, liver and renal function tests, coagulation studies, pregnancy test (within 7 days of starting growth factors).
- ABO group and Rh type (red cell phenotype, RBC crossmatch between donor and recipient, and anti-A and anti-B titers as appropriate).
- Hemoglobinopathy assessment
- Confirmatory HLA typing
- Pretransplantation chimerism studies (by PCR if the donor and recipient are the same sex or XY DNA analysis if the donor and recipient are different sexes).
- Infectious disease serologies, including human HIV-1 antibody, HIV-2 antibody, HIV antigen, HTLV, hepatitis B surface antigen, hepatitis B core antigen, hepatitis C antibodies, HTLV-1, CMV antibodies (IgG and IgM), EBV nuclear antibodies, West Nile virus, and *Trypanosoma cruzi* (Chagas disease) within 30 days of collection.
- PCR test for COVID-19
- Electrocardiogram based on age and history if undergoing general anesthesia for bone marrow harvest.
- The following must be documented:
  - Suitability of the donor to undergo stem cell or bone marrow collection
  - Vaccination history
  - Travel history
  - Blood transfusion history
  - Risk of disease transmission, including a targeted screening history, physical examination, and laboratory testing (as previously described)
  - Abnormal findings and rationale for proceeding to transplantation
  - Counseling of donor regarding abnormal findings and planned follow-up
  - Recipient informed of abnormal findings and findings documented in his or her chart
  - Patient informed of tests performed to protect the health of the patient
  - Patient informed of the right to review test results

Data from Foundation of Cellular Therapy (FACT). (2021). *Patient care and laboratory procedures.* Available at http://www.factwebsite.org/.

In selecting an individual to serve as an allogeneic HSCT donor, histocompatibility testing (i.e., tissue typing) is performed to evaluate the HLA match between the tissue antigens of the donor and those of the recipient. HLAs are expressed on the surface of various cells, particularly WBCs. The genes that encode these antigens are known as the major histocompatibility complex (MHC) in nonhuman vertebrates. Most HLA genes occupy the short arm of chromosome 6. This genetic region has been subdivided into chromosomal regions called classes I, II, and III. The role of class III antigens in HSCT remains unclear.

Class I antigens are encoded by *HLA-A, HLA-B,* and *HLA-C* genes, as well as genes that are less frequently discussed (e.g., *HLA-E, HLA-F, HLA-G*). Class II antigens are encoded by *HLA-DR, HLA-DP,* and *HLA-DQ* genes, as well as variations of these genes. Traditionally, the loci critical for matching in HSCT are *HLA-A, HLA-B,* and *HLA-DR. HLA-C* and *HLA-DQ* are also sometimes considered when determining the appropriateness of a donor (Negrin, 2021). A person's tissue type is determined by these genes, which contain information for cell surface antigens that all T lymphocytes use to differentiate themselves from nonself. To ensure the best possible acceptance of donor stem cells and to prevent significant GVHD, it is best to match all HLA sites.

Each person has two *HLA-A, HLA-B, HLA-C, HLA-DR,* and *HLA-DQ* genes that are inherited as a haplotype (i.e., DNA segment containing closely linked gene variations that are inherited as a single unit) from each parent. Many genetic variations can occur at each locus, resulting in a large number of HLA combinations. The higher the number of antigens that match between donor and transplant recipient, the higher the likelihood of compatibility and the lower the risk of severe acute and chronic GVHD and graft rejection.

Donor selection is critical to the success of allogeneic HSCT (Dehn et al., 2019; Negrin, 2021). Selection of an appropriate HLA-matched donor for allogeneic HSCT is based on a number of factors, the most important of which is the degree of HLA matching between the donor and recipient. Other factors are the CMV serologic status of the donor and recipient, type and stage of the recipient's underlying disease, urgency to move ahead with transplantation, speed of engraftment, need for a subsequent graft or donor lymphocyte infusion (DLI), donor and recipient ages, and recipient comorbidities.

Related donors are usually siblings because they have the greatest chance of matching HLA major and minor antigens. Because one half of an HLA type is inherited from each parent, patients statistically have a one in four chance of having a sibling that is a full HLA match. In some clinical circumstances, half-matched, or haploidentical, transplant may be pursued using a family member if the patient lacks a fully HLA-matched donor (McCurdy & Luznik, 2019). If more than one donor is being considered, donor selection is based on sex of the donor, CMV serologic status of recipient and the donor, ABO compatibility, donor age, recipient-donor body size difference, and donor (if female) parity. All of these factors are associated with improved outcomes of HSCT (Dehn et al., 2019; Negrin, 2021).

A mismatch in ABO blood group between patient and donor does not preclude successful HSCT. Depending on the direction of the incompatibility (i.e., major or minor incompatibility), the hematopoietic stem cell product may have to be depleted of RBCs to prevent a hemolytic reaction at the time of infusion caused by ABO antibodies. After engraftment of the donor hematopoietic stem cells, donor-derived RBCs are then produced approximately 100 days after transplantation, and the recipient of an ABO-mismatched transplant seroconverts to the ABO type of the donor.

Alternative Donor Sources of Hematopoietic Stem Cells

Matched Unrelated Donor

The average patient in the United States in need of an allogeneic HSCT has about a 25% chance of finding an HLA-matched family donor (Negrin, 2021). For the 75% of patients who do not have an HLA-compatible donor, an unrelated donor is sought through the bone marrow donor registries and placental cord blood registries, the largest of which is the National Marrow Donor Program (NMDP). The NMDP was established in 1986 to allow patients without a related donor to find an HLA-matched unrelated donor or a matched unrelated source of UCB.

The same factors that are considered when choosing a matched sibling donor also apply when choosing among multiple matched unrelated donors (MUDs). Nineteen million potential bone marrow or PBSC donors and 472,000 UCB units have been typed for the NMDP, giving a patient in need of allogeneic HSCT transplantation a 91% to 99% chance of finding an appropriate donor. Minority patients (i.e., non-white groups) have a significantly lower chance of finding a well-matched donor due to the limited donor pool. Finding an appropriate, well-matched, healthy adult volunteer donor may take weeks or months. The recipient's transplantation physician may request PBSC or bone marrow collection. The overall risk of GVHD, graft rejection, and TRM is higher with MUD transplantation than with matched sibling donor transplants.

Umbilical Cord Blood

UCB transplantation refers to the use of hematopoietic stem cells collected from the umbilical cord and placenta at the time of birth. About 40 to 70 mL of fetal cord blood is collected immediately after the cord is clamped and cut. Worldwide, these units are cryopreserved and then stored in a public or private cord blood bank for future use. This type of collection has no risk to the donor if the cord is appropriately clamped. Recipients of UCB stem cells may be related (i.e., cells from a family member) or unrelated (i.e., cells donated to a UCB registry) (National Marrow Donor Program [NMDP], 2021).

Because of the relative immaturity of the immune system in cord samples, stem cells from UCB allow crossing of immunologic barriers that would otherwise be prohibitive. The degree of tolerable HLA disparity is much greater in cord blood transplants. A match of four to six of the six HLA-A, HLA-B, and HLA-DRB1 antigens is sufficient for transplantation because the degree and severity of GVHD are lower after cord blood transplantation (Gupta & Wagner, 2020). Unfortunately, the lack of GVHD may also result in a diminished GVT effect and higher rates of posttransplantation relapse compared with MUD transplantations using PBSCs or bone marrow.

Advantages of a UCB transplant are that cord units are readily available and can be shipped to the recipient's transplantation center immediately on request; it carries less risk of viral contamination (e.g., CMV and EBV); and it is transplantable across HLA barriers with diminished risk of GVHD compared with similarly mismatched stem cells from peripheral blood or bone marrow (Ballen, 2017). UCB stem cells have historically been thought of as immunologically naïve and are typed and matched for HLA-A, HLA-B, and HLA-DRB1 only, without consideration of HLA-C. Some data suggest that mismatch of HLA-C is an independent risk factor for TRM, and it is being further reviewed (Ballen, 2017).

A major limitation of UCB HSCT is the relatively small number of stem cells obtained from each collection. This approach is difficult for transplantation in older (larger) children and adults because the small stem cell volume may result in delayed or poor engraftment and an increased risk of infections and TRM. Many adult patients require more than one cord blood unit to achieve adequate engraftment (Ballen, 2017). Other limitations include a decreased GVT effect and an inability to obtain additional cells from the donor if a DLI or graft boost is needed (Ballen, 2017).

Haploidentical Hematopoietic Stem Cell Transplantation

Haploidentical (i.e., four-antigen or half-matched family member) HSCT may provide an opportunity for most patients to benefit from HSCT when an HLA genotypically matched sibling or MUD donor is not available. Early, mismatched allograft results from the late 1980s and 1990s were disappointing because of unacceptable TRM and morbidity, such as fatal GVHD and infectious complications.

Haploidentical stem cell grafts require the removal of T lymphocytes because they are responsible for the immunologic response of GVHD. Advances with effective T-cell depletion (TCD), including the use of posttransplantation cyclophosphamide for in vivo depletion and the use of megadoses of stem cells, have lowered the risk of acute and chronic GVHD, produced acceptable TRM rates, and improved overall survival (Fuchs & Luznik, 2021). However, the problems related to delayed immune reconstitution causing posttransplantation infectious complications and posttransplantation relapse remain.

Ongoing studies are comparing the effectiveness of haploidentical bone marrow donated by family members with two partially matched unrelated donor UCB units in adult patients with high-risk leukemia or lymphoma (National Library of Medicine, 2021). Studies such as these offer HSCT to selected patients who lack a well-matched HLA sibling or unrelated donor.

Stem Cell Harvesting, Mobilization, and Collection

Although the bone marrow spaces contain more pluripotent stem cells than blood, a significant number of them circulate in the peripheral blood and are used in autologous and allogeneic HSCT. The process of harvesting and collecting hematopoietic stem cells depends on the type of transplantation. Progenitor (pluripotent) stem cells may be obtained by bone marrow harvest or collected from the peripheral blood by apheresis. The third option for obtaining pluripotent stem cells is the use of umbilical cord and placental blood. These cells are harvested immediately after delivery and cryopreserved for subsequent use.

Bone Marrow Harvest

Bone marrow is the most common stem cell source in pediatric allogeneic transplantation because of the long-term risk of chronic GVHD associated with PBSCs. When stem cells

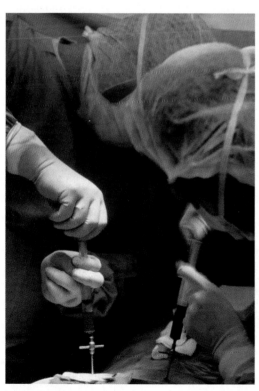

Bone Marrow Harvest Procedure. (Courtesy BSIP Boucharlat/Science Photo Library.)

are obtained from the donor's bone marrow, the harvesting procedure is performed in the operating room under spinal or general anesthesia. The figure on this page shows a bone marrow harvest procedure. Multiple aspirations are obtained from each posterior iliac crest with large-bore bone marrow harvest needles until a total of 1 to 4×10^8 nucleated cells per kilogram of the recipient's body weight or ideal body weight is achieved (Arora et al., 2017). The total volume of harvested bone marrow usually is 10 mL/kg of the recipient's actual or ideal body weight.

The marrow is placed in a heparinized tissue culture medium and filtered for the removal of fat and bone particles and then is infused at the recipient's bedside. Marrow is ideally harvested from the donor on the same day it is infused into the patient. Rarely, the bone marrow may be cryopreserved until the recipient is ready for transplantation. The bone marrow harvest procedure usually takes 1 to 2 hours, and most donors are discharged the same day. Postoperative pain after a bone marrow harvest is mild to moderate and usually lasts 2 to 7 days after the procedure.

Complications of bone marrow harvest are rare, but donors may experience infection, hypovolemia, hematoma, and general anesthesia side effects. Bone marrow donors may also become anemic and require an RBC transfusion. The bone marrow donor may elect to bank his or her blood for autotransfusion after the bone marrow harvest. It is recommended that bone marrow donors take 5 to 7 days off from work or school. Typically, the bone marrow cells removed from the donor are repopulated within a few weeks following marrow harvest.

Peripheral Blood Stem Cell Collection

Hematopoietic stem cells may be collected from the peripheral blood for autologous and allogeneic HSCT. Collecting stem cells from the blood compared with harvesting them from the bone marrow has demonstrated several advantages for the transplant recipient. The greatest advantage is that PBSCs provide a more rapid hematopoietic recovery (Auletta et al., 2021; Singhal et al., 2000).

Because stem cells are not abundant in the peripheral blood, chemotherapy (for autologous transplant recipients providing their own stem cells), or colony-stimulating factors (for autologous transplant recipients and healthy donors providing an allogeneic stem cell transplant) must be given before collecting PBSCs. Chemotherapy, granulocyte colony-stimulating factor (G-CSF), and granulocyte-macrophage colony-stimulating factor (GM-CSF) are commonly used before collection because they stimulate the stem cells that originate in the bone marrow to move into the peripheral blood circulation. This process is called *mobilization*. Chemotherapy given before autologous stem cell collection stimulates stem cell mobilization and provides an antitumor effect. Chemokine antagonists such as plerixafor have been used in combination with G-CSF to mobilize stem cells into the bloodstream of patients who have difficulty mobilizing cells with CSFs alone or with chemotherapy (Bilgin, 2021). Stem cell collection usually begins after 4 or 5 days of daily G-CSF or GM-CSF injections, depending on the donor's WBC count.

After stem cell mobilization, hematopoietic progenitor cells are collected from the peripheral blood by a method called apheresis. The patient's (autologous) or donor's (allogeneic) blood is withdrawn through a wide-bore, double-lumen central venous catheter or large-bore, antecubital angiocath intravenous catheter. An apheresis machine, a commercial cell separator, is used to centrifuge the blood and separate the components by density into various layers (Be the Match, n.d.). The WBC and platelet layer is located between the RBC and plasma layers. Pluripotent stem cells are located in the WBC layer. The stem cell layer is transferred into a collection bag, and the remaining blood components are returned to the patient. The figure below shows a donor undergoing PBSC collection. The procedure takes approximately 3 to 6 hours, and the number of leukapheresis procedures required is determined by the number of stem cells harvested at each session. The goal is to collect 5×10^6 CD34$^+$ cells per kilogram of the recipient's body weight (Singhal et al., 2000). The CD34$^+$ antigen is expressed on the surface of early progenitor cells.

Side effects during and immediately after PBSC collection are usually minimal but include transient headache, hypocalcemia, chills, fatigue, vertigo, and tingling in the lips and extremities. Hypocalcemia is relatively common and is caused by the sodium citrate solution that is used to prevent blood clotting in the machine during the collection procedure. Symptoms may be averted by administering an oral calcium carbonate supplement during the collection. Intravenous calcium supplementation may be required if the serum calcium level is low or hypocalcemia symptoms are severe.

Conditioning Therapy and Preparative Regimen

The treatment course begins with the preparative or conditioning regimen. The combination of chemotherapy, radiotherapy,

and biologic therapy in preparation for HSCT is referred to as the preparative regimen. Because evidence has not shown that one conditioning regimen is superior to another, the choice is often based on the transplantation team's experience and preference and the patient's clinical situation. Selection of the ideal regimen for the patient should consider the following: stem cell source (i.e., autologous or allogeneic), diagnosis, disease stage at the time of transplantation, prior therapies, and comorbidities (Lum et al., 2019; Metheny et al., 2021).

The preparative regimen usually includes high doses of chemotherapy with or without TBI, which is administered over the days preceding stem cell infusion. The doses and schedule of the preparative regimen depend on the patient's underlying disease, type of transplantation (i.e., autologous or allogeneic), underlying comorbidities, and goal of therapy (Gagelmann & Kröger, 2021). In allogeneic transplantation, the purpose of the preparative regimen is to eradicate malignant disease, ablate the existing bone marrow to create space for the donor stem cells to engraft, and provide sufficient immunosuppression to allow the recipient to accept the transplanted stem cells. The goal of the preparative regimen in autologous transplantation is to deliver high-dose, intensive myeloablative therapy. Subsequent infusion of autologous stem cells rescues the patient from myeloablation. Posttransplantation immunosuppression is not required for autologous transplantation because the patient receives his or her own hematopoietic stem cells, avoiding the risk of graft rejection and GVHD.

Myeloablative Preparative Regimen

The rationale for selecting agents for a myeloablative preparative regimen is that a greater degree of tumor cell death can improve disease response and overall survival. High-dose chemotherapy preparative regimens are combinations of the most effective agents for a particular disease given at high doses

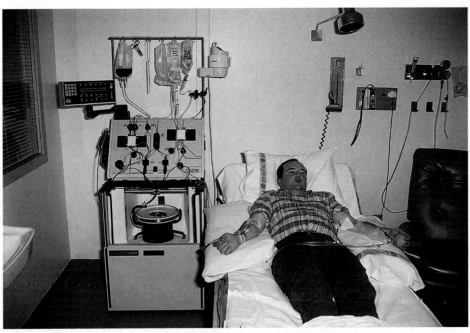

Patient Undergoing Peripheral Blood Stem Cell Collection. (From Hoffbrand A. V., Pettit J. E., & Vyas P. (2010). *Color atlas of clinical hematology* [4th ed.]. Mosby.)

with the goal of myeloablation. Drugs with different (i.e., non-overlapping) nonhematologic dose-limiting toxicities are typically combined and given at maximal doses. Alkylating agents such as cyclophosphamide, carboplatin, busulfan, thiotepa, cisplatin, melphalan, and carmustine are used in combination with other agents such as etoposide, fludarabine, and cytarabine, and sometimes with TBI, to destroy the bone marrow and eradicate disease.

The tables below list common preparative regimens, their indications, and the adverse effects of individual drugs used in combination in the preparative regimen for transplantation, respectively.

Common Preparative Regimens and Indications

Regimen	Indication
Total body irradiation, etoposide, cyclophosphamide (TBI/CY/VP)	Lymphoid malignancies
Cyclophosphamide, total body irradiation (CY/TBI)	Hematologic malignancies, non-Hodgkin lymphoma, myelodysplastic syndromes
Busulfan, cyclophosphamide (Bu/CY)	Myeloid leukemias, metabolic disorders, myelodysplastic syndromes
Busulfan, fludarabine (Bu/Flu) ± rabbit antithymocyte globulin or alemtuzumab	Hematologic malignancies, myelodysplastic syndromes, nonmalignant allogeneic hematopoietic stem cell transplantation
Carmustin, etoposide, cytarabine, melphalan ± rituximab (BEAM ± R)	Hodgkin lymphoma, non-Hodgkin lymphoma
Cyclophosphamide, carmustine, etoposide ± rituximab (CBV ± R)	Hodgkin lymphoma, non-Hodgkin lymphoma
Cyclophosphamide, antithymocyte globulin (CY/ATG)	Marrow failure syndromes (severe aplastic anemia), hemoglobinopathies
Carboplatin, thiotepa (Carbo/Thio)	Brain tumors
Melphalan ± bortezomib	Multiple myeloma
Reduced-Intensity Regimens	
Busulfan, fludarabine (Bu/Flu)	Hematologic malignancies (poor performance status)
Fludarabine, melphalan (Flu/Mel)	Multiple myeloma
Low-dose total body irradiation, fludarabine	Multiple myeloma, hemoglobinopathies

Data from Gagelmann, N., & Kröger, N. (2021). Dose intensity for conditioning in allogeneic hematopoietic cell transplantation: can we recommend "when and for whom" in 2021? *Haematologica, 106*(7), 1794–1804; Jethava, Y. S., Sica, S., Savani, B., Socola F, Jagasia M, Mohty M. … Bacigalupo A. (2017). Conditioning regimens for allogeneic hematopoietic stem cell transplants in acute myeloid leukemia. *Bone Marrow Transplantation, 52*(11), 1504–1511; Lum, S. H., Hoenig, M., Gennery, A. R., & Slatter MA. (2019). Conditioning regimens for hematopoietic cell transplantation in primary immunodeficiency. *Current Allergy and Asthma Reports, 19*(11), 52; Negrin, R. S. (2022). Preparative regimens for hematopoietic cell transplantation. *UptoDate*. Available at https://www.uptodate.com/contents/preparative-regimens-for-hematopoietic-cell-transplantation.

Nonhematologic Adverse Effects of Agents Used in Preparative Regimens and Conditioning Therapy

Therapeutic Agent	Side Effects
Antithymocyte globulin (ATG) and alemtuzumab	Fever, chills, and hypersensitivity during infusion (reaction may worsen with each subsequent dose), prolonged immunosuppression
Busulfan	Seizures, interstitial pulmonary fibrosis, hepatic dysfunction (including veno-occlusive disease [VOD]), acute cholecystitis, mucositis, skin hyperpigmentation, desquamation, and acral erythema
Carmustine	Hepatic, pulmonary, central nervous system (with BCNU), cardiac effects (arrhythmias and hypotension), nausea, and vomiting
Carboplatin	Nausea and vomiting, nephrotoxicity, liver function abnormalities (including VOD), ototoxicity
Cisplatin	Nausea and vomiting, neurotoxicity (peripheral neuropathy, ataxia, visual disturbances), ototoxicity, renal dysfunction
Clofarabine	Nausea and vomiting, myelosuppression, infection, liver dysfunction, and capillary leak
Cyclophosphamide	Cardiac effects (cardiomyopathy, congestive heart failure, hemorrhagic cardiac necrosis, pericardial effusion, electrocardiographic abnormalities), interstitial pulmonary fibrosis, hemorrhagic cystitis, elevated liver enzyme values, nausea and vomiting, and metabolic (syndrome of inappropriate antidiuretic hormone secretion [SIADH])
Cytosine arabinoside (Ara-C)	Cerebellar toxicity, encephalopathy, seizures, conjunctivitis, skin (rash, acral erythema), nausea and vomiting, diarrhea, renal insufficiency, liver function abnormalities, pancreatitis, noncardiogenic pulmonary edema, fever, arthralgias
Etoposide (Etopophos)	Hypersensitivity reactions, hypotension, liver function abnormalities and chemical hepatitis, renal dysfunction, nausea and vomiting, metabolic acidosis, mucositis, stomatitis, painful rash on the palms, soles, and periorbital area
Fludarabine	Mucositis, diarrhea, pulmonary fibrosis, pneumonitis, hypersensitivity reaction during infusion, neuropathy, central nervous system toxicity, coma
Ifosfamide	Hemorrhagic cystitis at high doses, encephalopathy, coma, hallucinations, confusion, mental status changes
Melphalan	Acute hypersensitivity, renal toxicity, mucositis, nausea and vomiting, hepatic toxicity (including VOD)
Thiotepa	Hyperpigmentation, acute erythroderma, dry desquamation, liver function abnormalities (including VOD), mucositis, esophagitis, dysuria, hypersensitivity reaction during infusion
TBI	Nausea, vomiting, diarrhea, parotitis, xerostomia, stomatitis, erythema, pneumonitis, VOD
Treosulfan	Myalgias, hepatic dysfunction (including VOD), acute cholecystitis, mucositis, skin hyperpigmentation, myelosuppression

Data from Mehdizadeh, M., Parkideh, S., Salari, S., Hajifathali, A., Rezvani, H., & Mabani, M. (2021). Adverse effects of busulfan plus cyclophosphamide versus busulfan plus fludarabine as conditioning regimens for allogeneic bone marrow transplantation. *Asian Pacific Journal of Cancer Prevention, 22*(5), 1639–1644; Wikle Shapiro, T. J. (2019). Hematopoietic stem cell transplantation. In J. Brant, D. Cope, M. Saria (Eds.). *Core curriculum for oncology nursing* (6th ed.). Philadelphia, PA: Elsevier; Hochberg, J., Zahler, S., Geyer, M. B., Chen, N., Krajewski, J., Harrison, L., … Cairo, M. S. (2019). The safety and efficacy of clofarabine in combination with high-dose cytarabine and total body irradiation myeloablative conditioning and allogeneic stem cell transplantation in Children, Adolescents, and Young adults (CAYA) with poor-risk acute leukemia. *Bone Marrow Transplant, 54*(2), 226–235.

Monoclonal and polyclonal agents such as ATG or alemtuzumab are added to the preparative regimen to provide the additional immunosuppression needed to prevent graft rejection and acute GVHD when an unrelated adult donor, an unrelated cord blood unit, or a haploidentical donor is used.

Reduced-Intensity Conditioning Regimens

GVHD can be a serious complication (described later), but it also controls the underlying malignancy by causing a GVT effect. The immunologic response is mediated by donor immunocompetent T cells that recognize the host tumor cells as foreign and destroy them. The GVT effect was recognized over time as contributing to the success of allogeneic HSCT.

To exploit the benefit of GVT, many investigators lowered the dose of radiation and chemotherapeutic agents in the conditioning regimen. This approach caused a major paradigm shift, and the pool of eligible patients for allogeneic HSCT was greatly expanded. However, not all malignancies are equally susceptible to the GVT effect. Myeloid leukemias, CLL, Hodgkin lymphoma, neuroblastoma, and low-grade indolent lymphomas (i.e., follicular lymphoma and mantle cell lymphoma) appear to be particularly responsive to the GVT effect.

A RIC regimen followed by allogeneic HSCT provides treatment options for older patients and those who have undergone a prior transplant or have comorbidities such as heart, lung, kidney, or liver disease and would therefore not tolerate a high-dose conditioning regimen. RIC regimens typically use combinations of chemotherapy drugs, such as fludarabine, busulfan, and melphalan, at reduced doses with or without low-dose TBI. Combinations of potent immunosuppressive medications such as ATG or alemtuzumab are also commonly added to the RIC chemoradiotherapy regimen.

The RIC regimens are not without risk. Patients undergoing transplantation after a RIC regimen experience many of the same complications as those undergoing conventional, fully myeloablative allogeneic transplantation regimens. Problems encountered in the early posttransplantation period, such as infection, bleeding, and regimen-related toxicities, may be less after a RIC regimen for HSCT, but the risk of GVHD and the long-term risk of infection continue to be problems.

Stem Cell Infusion

The infusion of stem cells is a relatively simple procedure, much like a blood transfusion. In allogeneic HSCT, the stem cells (i.e., bone marrow or PBSCs) are usually infused immediately after they are collected. Autologous stem cells and UCB units are cryopreserved with dimethylsulfoxide (DMSO) and must be thawed in a warm solution bath at the bedside or in the cellular therapy lab just before reinfusion.

The cells are typically infused through a central venous catheter over 30 to 90 minutes, depending on the total volume of the product and the size of the recipient. Cryopreserved stem cells (i.e., autologous PBSCs and UCB cells) are usually preserved in smaller volumes and are usually aspirated from the cryopreservation bag into a large syringe and slowly pushed through the central venous catheter. A leukocyte-depleting (leukopoor) filter should never be used when infusing HSCTs. An infusion pump should not be used to administer stem cells, and only normal saline solution should be used to prime and flush the tubing.

Premedication with acetaminophen and diphenhydramine is often recommended, and patients may also require hydration before and after the procedure to maintain renal perfusion and dilute the DMSO. Sodium bicarbonate may be given IV when a large number of DMSO cryopreserved cells are given. Patients who receive a cryopreserved product should be premedicated with an antiemetic to combat nausea from the DMSO or residual nausea from the chemotherapeutic preparatory regimen. Vital signs and pulse oximetry are monitored closely before, during, and at intervals after stem cell infusion. Some centers also use cardiac monitoring during, and for a brief period following the infusion of stem cells.

Complications of stem cell infusion are rare but may include pulmonary edema, hemolysis, infection, and anaphylaxis. Infrequently, DMSO can cause an infusion reaction that may include bradycardia (and rarely heart block) or hypertension, and an acute hypersensitivity reaction may occur. DMSO-associated RBC hemolysis may require vigorous hydration to prevent renal toxicity. Throughout the infusion, patients should be monitored for volume overload and complaints suggesting pulmonary embolism, such as chest pain, dyspnea, and cough.

Early Complications of Stem Cell Transplantation

After stem cell infusion, the hematopoietic stem cells migrate to the bone marrow spaces, where they are attracted by chemotactic factors. Engraftment occurs when the transplanted progenitor cells begin to grow and manufacture new hematopoietic cells in the bone marrow. After stem cell infusion but before completing hematopoietic cell engraftment, patients have severe pancytopenia that results in a heightened risk of infection and bleeding. Other early toxicities include mucositis, skin breakdown, renal dysfunction, and VOD of the liver. Examples of early and late complications arising from autologous and allogeneic stem cell transplantation can be found in the box on the next page.

Nonhematologic adverse effects depend on the agents used for the preparative regimen. The nonhematologic adverse effects that are associated with the agents that typically comprise stem cell transplant conditioning regimens are outlined in the table on the previous page.

Early and Late Complications of Autologous and Allogeneic Stem Cell Transplantation

Early (Before Day 100)
- Regimen-related toxicity
  - Hemorrhagic cystitis
  - Hepatic VOD
  - Pulmonary complications
  - Renal complications
  - Neurologic complications
  - Severe immunosuppression/myelosuppression
- Nutritional deficiencies
- Idiopathic pneumonitis
- Graft failure
- Infection
  - Viral
  - Bacterial
  - Fungal
  - Protozoal
- Acute GVHD
- Early posttransplant relapse

Late (After Day 100)
- Regimen-related toxicity
  - Cataracts
  - Neurologic conditions (peripheral and autonomic neuropathies)
  - Gonadal dysfunction
  - Endocrine dysfunction
- Immunodeficiency
- Infection
  - Encapsulated bacteria
  - Viruses (CMV, varicella-zoster virus [VZV])
  - Fungal (*Aspergillus* spores)
- EBV posttransplantation lymphoproliferative disorder (PTLD)
- Musculoskeletal problems
  - Osteoporosis
  - Avascular necrosis
- Chronic GVHD
- Bronchiolitis obliterans
- Relapse of malignancy
- Secondary relapse

Pancytopenia

Hematopoietic growth factors (e.g., G-CSF, GM-CSF) are given after transplantation to accelerate neutrophil recovery, reduce the period of neutropenia, and decrease the risk of early posttransplant infection. Transfusion support is provided by platelets and packed RBCs.

Except for hematopoietic stem cell grafts and donor lymphocytes, all blood products given to HSCT recipients should be leukoreduced to remove WBCs, which may transmit CMV, and irradiated with 2500 cGy to prevent transfusion-associated GVHD. Most centers recommend that allogeneic stem cell recipients receive irradiated blood products for the rest of their lives, and they are encouraged to purchase a MedicAlert bracelet that specifies their need for irradiated blood products.

Infection

Infections have constituted a major threat since the introduction of HSCT. They remain a significant obstacle to the success of HSCT, along with relapsed malignancy and GVHD. Most posttransplantation infections are divided into three phases.

Phase I is the pre-engraftment phase, phase II is the post-engraftment phase, and phase III is the late infection phase. During phase I (day 0 to 15), prolonged neutropenia and breaks in the mucocutaneous barrier result in a substantial risk of bacteremia and fungal infections, including those by *Candida* species and, as prolonged neutropenia continues, *Aspergillus* species. HSV reactivation occurs during this phase as well.

During phase II (days 15 to 100), infections are primarily associated with impaired cell-mediated immunity. The scope and impact of this defect are determined by the extent of GVHD and the immunosuppressive therapy used to control it. Herpesviruses, particularly CMV, are common infectious agents during this period. Other dominant pathogens include *Pneumocystis jirovecii* and *Aspergillus* species.

During phase III (day 100+), persons with chronic GVHD and recipients of alternative-donor allogeneic transplants remain most at risk for infection due to delayed or prolonged immunosuppression. Common pathogens include CMV, VZV, and encapsulated bacteria (e.g., *Streptococcus pneumoniae*).

The risk of disease from community-acquired respiratory viruses is elevated during all three phases. In phase III, the outpatient status of hematopoietic stem cell recipients can complicate efforts to reduce exposure and provide timely intervention. The figure on the next page shows the three posttransplantation phases of infections and contributory factors. The risk of infection is primarily determined by the time since transplantation, degree of immune reconstitution, and presence or absence of GVHD. Other factors include donor/host histocompatibility, disease status, type of transplantation (e.g., marrow, PBSCs, or UCB), marrow conditioning intensity, and neutrophil engraftment (Centers for Disease Control and Prevention et al., 2000; Pereira et al., 2019).

The table on the next page outlines the factors affecting the HSCT patient's risk of infection. Strategies to limit exposure to infectious organisms are essential for transplant recipients who are neutropenic and those receiving immunosuppressive medications.

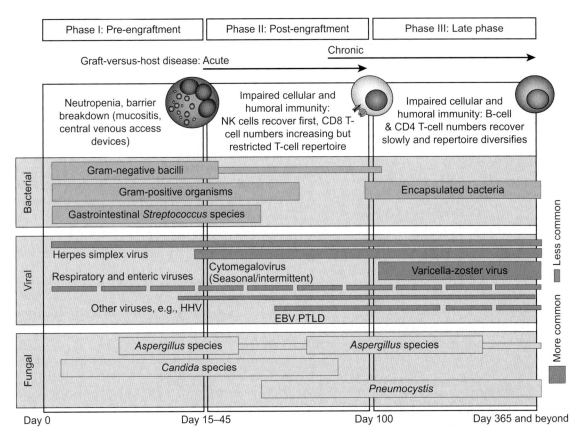

Three Posttransplantation Phases of Infections and Contributory Factors. (From Tomblyn, M., Chiller, T., Einsele, H., Gress, R., Sepkowitz, K., Storek, J., ... Centers for Disease Control and Prevention. (2009). Guidelines for preventing infectious complications among hematopoietic cell transplantation recipients: A global perspective. *Biology of Blood Marrow Transplantation, 15*(10), 1143–1238.)

Factors Affecting the Risk of Infection

Factor	Risk of Infection
Type of transplantation	Higher risk with allogeneic; lower risk with autologous or syngeneic, depending on graft manipulation and the clinical setting, including previous therapies
Time from transplantation	Lower risk with more time elapsed from transplantation (see the figure above)
Pretransplantation factors	Higher risk with extensive pretransplantation immunosuppressive therapy (e.g., fludarabine, clofarabine), prolonged pretransplantation neutropenia or pretransplantation infection
GVHD	Higher risk with grades III and IV acute GVHD or extensive, chronic GVHD requiring systemic immunosuppression
HLA match	Higher risk with HLA-mismatched donors, particularly with haploidentical donors
Disease (e.g., leukemia)	Higher risk with more advanced disease at the time of transplantation (heavy pretreatment chemotherapy or radiotherapy), hematologic malignancy
Donor type	Higher risk with unrelated donor marrow or UCB than with a fully matching sibling donor
Graft type	Highest risk with TCD and UCB, intermediate risk with bone marrow, and lowest risk with colony-stimulating factor—mobilized blood stem cells; higher risk with T-cell-depleted grafts, depending on method used
Immunosuppression after transplantation	Higher risk with immunosuppressive drugs, particularly with corticosteroids, antithymocyte globulin, alemtuzumab, delayed immune recovery (UCB, TCD), chronic GVHD
Conditioning intensity	Lower risk in the first 1–3 months after transplantation with reduced-intensity regimen; higher with TBI regimens

Data from Centers for Disease Control and Prevention, Infectious Disease Society of America, American Society of Blood and Marrow Transplantation. (2021). Guidelines for preventing opportunistic infections among hematopoietic stem cell transplant recipients, *Morbidity and Mortality Weekly Report Recommendations and Reports, 49*(RR-10), 1–125, 1CE7. Available at https://www.cdc.gov/mmwr/preview/mmwrhtml/rr4910a1.htm; Ford, A. M., Cushing Haugen, K. L., Boeckh, M., Carpenter, P. A., Flowers, M. E. D., Lee, S. J. ... Chow, E. J. (2020). Late infectious complications in hematopoietic cell transplantation survivors: A population-based study. *Blood Advances, 4*(7), 1232–1241; Pereira, M. R., Pouch, S. M., & Scully, B. (Eds.). (2019). Infections in allogeneic stem cell transplantation. *Principles and practice of transplant infectious diseases*. New York, NY: Springer.

Infection Prophylaxis and Treatment

Most post-HSCT infections are predictable and surmountable with the use of tailored preventative and early-detection strategies. Infectious disease prophylaxis and vaccinations can be used to prevent infections. Changes in transplantation procedures and the implementation of effective supportive care strategies have decreased the incidence and severity of infectious complications in each posttransplantation phase (Pereira et al., 2019).

The Centers for Disease Control and Prevention (CDC) in its *Morbidity and Mortality Weekly Report* provides guidelines for preventing opportunistic infections in patients undergoing HSCT (Centers for Disease Control and Prevention et al., 2000). Hospitals that perform HSCT should have appropriately designed facilities that have rooms with more than 12 air exchanges per hour and point-of-use high-efficiency particulate air (HEPA) filtration. HEPA filters should be able to remove particles at least as small as 0.3 μm in diameter. Rooms should have positive air pressure compared with the hallway unless they are housing a patient who has active disease with a pathogen that has airborne transmission (e.g., VZV); in such cases, a negative-pressure room is recommended.

Policies and procedures should be in the hospital infection-control manual to address issues of construction and renovation, cleaning, and isolation and barrier precautions. Barriers between patient care and renovation or construction areas (e.g., sealed plastic) should be provided that prevent dust from entering patient care areas and that are impermeable to *Aspergillus* species.

Handwashing should be strongly emphasized to prevent nosocomial transmission of infection. Most transplantation centers recommend that plants and dried or fresh flowers should not be allowed in HSCT patient rooms, although exposure has not been conclusively shown to cause fungal infections. Health care workers should follow a policy and CDC guidelines with regard to their immunizations and vaccinations. Health care workers with symptoms of viral illness should not care for HSCT patients.

Strict adherence to visitor policies is required, particularly for children with potentially infectious conditions (e.g., varicella, community-acquired respiratory viruses [e.g., COVID-19, RSV, parainfluenza]). Oral and skin care should be stressed to patients throughout the bone marrow transplantation process. All patients undergoing HSCT should receive a dental evaluation before initiation of the preparative phase of transplantation. Patients with mucositis during conditioning or after transplantation should maintain a regimen of proper oral care per institutional standards (Centers for Disease Control and Prevention, Infectious Disease Society of America, & American Society of Blood and Marrow Transplantation, 2000).

Strategies for safe living after discharge from the hospital are important to discuss with HSCT recipients. Many centers provide controlled patient housing for HSCT recipients who are in the early posttransplantation phase. Patient education at discharge should include a discussion of how to avoid environmental infectious exposures, safe sexual practices, pet safety, food and water safety, travel safety, and the need for posttransplantation vaccinations (CDC et al., 2000; Pereira et al., 2019).

Bacterial Infection Prophylaxis

The use of prophylactic antibiotic therapy in HSCT remains controversial (CDC et al., 2000; Pereira et al., 2019). Prophylactic antibiotics (antibacterials) should only be used following the review of hospital and HSCT center antibiotic-susceptibility profiles, particularly when using a single antibiotic for antibacterial prophylaxis. The emergence of fluoroquinolone-resistant coagulase-negative *Staphylococcus* and *Escherichia coli* vancomycin-intermediate *Staphylococcus aureus* and vancomycin-resistant *Enterococcus* (VRE) are increasing concerns (Centers for Disease Control and Prevention et al., 2000). Vancomycin should not be used as an agent for routine bacterial prophylaxis. During the pre-engraftment phase, fluoroquinolones are often used in HSCT recipients to decrease the incidence of gram-negative bacteremia. B-lactam and macrolide prophylactic antibiotics have also been used prophylactically to reduce the incidence of gram-positive bacteremia (CDC et al., 2000; Pereira et al., 2019). However, the use of prophylactic antibiotics may lead to the development of resistant organisms. Another concern is the increased risk of *Clostridium difficile* infection associated with the used of antibacterial antimicrobials.

Mucosal injury, which results from the conditioning regimen, leads to translocation of bacteria, with approximately 40% of infections due to gram-negative organisms such as *Pseudomonas, Enterobacter, E. coli,* and *Klebsiella.* Gram-positive bacteria, especially *Staphylococcus epidermidis, Streptococcus viridians,* and *S. aureus*, colonize central venous catheters, leading to bacteremia that requires prompt initiation of appropriate antibiotics (Dykewicz et al., 2001; Pereira et al., 2019). The treatment of bacterial infections before engraftment is usually empiric, with broad-spectrum antibiotic therapy started at the onset of any fever. Treatment is then tailored with the isolation of organisms but remains broad spectrum for continued coverage of all pathogens that are likely in HSCT patients who are profoundly neutropenic for a prolonged period. Treatment with empiric antibiotics usually continues until the engraftment of neutrophils.

Empiric coverage usually consists of one or more antipseudomonal agents alone or in combination with an anti-staphylococcal/streptococcal antibiotic. Common choices include a cephalosporin, such as cefepime and ceftazidime, or when there is concern for resistant gram-negative infection, a carbapenem, such as imipenem or meropenem. Gram-positive coverage such as vancomycin or linezolid should also be considered for empiric antibiotic coverage when there is concern for a high risk of gram-positive bacteremia in these patients (Ahmad et al., 2019). Local antimicrobial resistance patterns at the transplantation center should be considered when choosing specific antimicrobial agents.

The use of hematopoietic colony-stimulating factors, such as G-CSF, can reduce the period of neutropenia, but the incidence of bacteremia and overall HSCT outcomes have not been influenced (Ahmad et al., 2019; CDC et al., 2000; Dykewicz et al., 2001). Granulocyte transfusion does not appear to be beneficial, even in the setting of profound neutropenia, but it may be used for the treatment of severe, documented, gram-negative bacterial, and fungal infections in HSCT patients with anticipated prolonged neutropenia (Ahmad et al., 2019).

In the late posttransplantation phase, because of the increased risk of infection with encapsulated organisms, some centers suggest the use of penicillin prophylaxis and vaccination with the 23-valent polysaccharide *S. pneumoniae* vaccine (CDC et al., 2000).

Fungal Infections

Factors that increase the HSCT patient's risk of invasive fungal infection include prolonged neutropenia, an indwelling central venous catheter, empiric antibiotic therapy, potent immunosuppressive agents, corticosteroids, GVHD, total parenteral nutrition, and severe mucositis (CDC et al., 2000; Rahi et al., 2021). The risk of fungal infection is particularly increased after 5 to 7 days of continuous neutropenia, and most centers begin prophylactic therapy for fungi around this time. More than 80% of HSCT patients who develop fungal infection after transplantation are infected with *Candida* or *Aspergillus* species (CDC et al., 2000; Rahi et al., 2021).

Fluconazole prophylaxis has been effective in reducing the number of infections with *Candida albicans* and is used as prophylaxis in HSCT patients who are at lower risk of developing invasive *Aspergillus* infection (i.e., autologous and matched sibling donor transplants) because fluconazole possesses no significant activity against *Aspergillus*. With improved control of CMV infection, *Aspergillus* species have become the most common cause of infectious mortality after HSCT (Rahi et al., 2021).

For high-risk patients, such as those undergoing unrelated donor, haploidentical, or UCB HSCT, fungal prophylaxis is broadened to include prophylaxis against fungi and molds that are resistant to fluconazole. The newer antifungal agents (e.g., isavuconazole, posaconazole, voriconazole, caspofungin) are the most common and effective prophylactic agents against most species and are active against the more resistant fungi such as *Aspergillus* and *Fusarium* and the mucormycetes (invasive mold species) class of organisms. In HSCT patients with documented invasive fungal infection, a combination of these pharmacologic agents along with liposomal amphotericin may be used due to the associated severity and high mortality rates.

Viral Infections

Herpes Simplex Virus. Reactivation of HSV infection can occur at any time after HSCT. The use of prophylactic acyclovir has been very effective in reducing the rate of HSV reactivation from 80% to less than 5% to 10% for HSV-seropositive recipients (Anton-Vazques et al., 2020; Centers for Disease Control and Prevention et al., 2000). Prophylactic acyclovir should be started during the conditioning regimen, and it should continue until the HSCT patient's immune system is reconstituted. Higher-dose acyclovir is the treatment of choice if HSV reactivation occurs (Anton-Vazques et al., 2020). When patients do not respond to acyclovir, foscarnet is used until the infection resolves. If foscarnet is unsuccessful, therapy with cidofovir or brincidofovir should be attempted (Anton-Vazques et al., 2020; CDC et al., 2000). Patients who do not demonstrate clinical

improvement for HSV lesions with antiviral therapy should undergo testing of HSV resistance to antivirals.

Cytomegalovirus. Allogeneic HSCT recipients should be tested before transplantation for serum anti-CMV IgG antibodies before transplantation to determine the risk of primary CMV infection and reactivation after HSCT. Before the advent of early detection techniques and the use of ganciclovir prophylaxis in the mid-1990s, CMV was the leading cause of morbidity and mortality among HSCT recipients.

CMV infection can cause fatal pneumonia, enteritis, and retinitis. In addition to organ involvement, CMV reactivation can exert indirect effects such as immunosuppression or graft failure that may result in the development of concurrent infectious complications. Up to 60% to 70% of allogeneic HSCT patients who are seropositive for CMV or who receive a graft from a seropositive donor will reactivate CMV after transplantation (Barlow, 2021; Cho et al., 2019; Einsele et al., 2020). Risk factors for CMV reactivation and disease include acute or chronic GVHD, steroid use, graft failure, low CD4 counts ($<50/mm^3$), CMV-seronegative donors for CMV seropositive recipients, and unrelated, haploidentical, UCB, or TCD HSCTs. To minimize the risk of CMV primary infection, all blood products (except stem cell and granulocyte products) should be leukocyte filtered.

Two approaches are used when treating patients at risk for CMV disease. The older approach is to administer prophylaxis with ganciclovir to every patient at risk for CMV disease. A common approach is to perform routine CMV surveillance by viral PCR in patients at high risk for CMV reactivation (Barlow, 2021; Cho et al., 2019). Because of the potential harmful side effects of prophylactic ganciclovir and the advances in viral testing for CMV on which to base early therapy, the preference at most transplantation centers is to use a preemptive approach (Barlow, 2021; Cho et al., 2019).

Preemptive therapy is based on at least weekly CMV surveillance of allogeneic HSCT patients who are CMV seropositive or who have a CMV seropositive donor. The trend in CMV diagnostics is to use the PCR-determined viral load instead of the antigenemia assay. PCR has better quantitation, less assay variability, and increased sensitivity. After CMV is detected, early preemptive therapy with intravenous ganciclovir is initiated for a minimum of 3 weeks after clearance of the virus. Oral ganciclovir (i.e., the prodrug valganciclovir) is then used for the maintenance phase of CMV therapy. Foscarnet and cidofovir are also used in patients with apparent or documented ganciclovir-resistant CMV disease or in patients who suffer from significant myelosuppression (pre- or early engraftment) (Barlow, 2021; Cho et al., 2019; Shoham & Marr, 2017). Both drugs have significant nephrotoxicity and must be used with caution in patients on other nephrotoxic medications or with a history of renal dysfunction.

The newer antiviral drug, letermovir, can also significantly reduce the rate of clinically significant CMV infection. Recent studies have found reductions in clinically significant CMV infection and all-cause mortality in patients at high risk for CMV reactivation (e.g., patients undergoing an HCT from a haploidentical or mismatched donor or those receiving ATG for GvHD prophylaxis) (Einsele et al., 2020). CMV-specific immunoglobulin

(CMVIG) is often used in addition to ganciclovir in HSCT patients who show signs of CMV reactivation (Barlow, 2021; Cho et al., 2019; Einsele et al., 2020; Shoham & Marr, 2017). Supplemental intravenous immune globulin (IVIG) can also be administered to assist in the prevention and treatment of CMV infection in allogeneic HSCT patients. IVIG is usually administered to allogeneic HSCT patients who have hypogammaglobulinemia (i.e., quantitative IgG level <400 mg/dL). IVIG is also used as prophylaxis against a myriad of other viral infections.

Treatment of CMV viremia with antivirals does not improve virus-specific immunity, and CMV reactivation and infection can often recur. Cellular immunotherapy for patients with deficient or absent CMV-specific immune system function can be an effective means to provide immediate and long-term protection from CMV. Several small, phase I/II studies have been published using adoptive transfer of donor CMV-specific CD4$^+$ and CD8$^+$ T cells, especially in patients developing repeated episodes of CMV disease. However, none of these adoptive T-cell transfer techniques are used in routine clinical practice (Einsele et al., 2020; Kaeuferle et al., 2019).

Recipients of autologous HSCT can develop CMV viremia, but they are much less likely to develop clinical CMV infection because they are less immunocompromised. Patients undergoing autologous HSCT are not routinely screened or administered prophylactic ganciclovir therapy (CDC et al., 2000; Einsele et al., 2020).

Varicella-Zoster Virus. Varicella-zoster infections can occur in the late posttransplantation phase. Delayed immune reconstitution after transplantation due to immunosuppression, posttransplant therapies, poor engraftment, and GVHD leave many patients at risk for herpes zoster (shingles) and its highly morbid complications. Although prophylaxis with acyclovir or valacyclovir has reduced the incidence of VZV reactivation if prophylaxis is continued, the incidence of disease in the late posttransplant period or after stopping prophylaxis occurs in 20% to 50% of patients with these risk factors (Lee, Savani, et al., 2018).

Although prophylaxis is not recommended during the late posttransplant period, prevention should be attempted after exposure to chickenpox or shingles. Varicella-zoster immunoglobulin (VZIG) should be given to patients who are less than 24 months out from an allogeneic HSCT and to those more than 24 months out from an allogeneic HSCT who are on immunosuppressive therapy or have chronic GVHD (CDC et al., 2000; Lee, Savani, et al., 2018). For at-risk patients, VZIG is ideally administered within 48 to 96 hours after exposure to a person with chickenpox or shingles. Patients who have undergone HSCT who develop varicella should also be treated for 7 to 10 days with high-dose intravenous acyclovir and then placed on suppressive oral dosing (Lee, Savani, et al., 2018).

Community-Acquired Respiratory Viruses and Adenoviruses. Treatment for respiratory viruses and adenoviruses in patients who have undergone HSCT is not standardized. Respiratory virus infections in HSCT recipients are increasingly recognized as a cause of significant morbidity and mortality. The often overlapping clinical presentation makes molecular diagnostic strategies imperative for rapid diagnosis and to inform understanding of the changing epidemiology of each of the respiratory viruses. Most respiratory virus infections are managed with supportive therapy, although there is effective antiviral therapy for COVID-19, influenza, and adenovirus. The primary focus should remain on primary prevention of infection, isolation precautions, avoidance of ill contacts, and vaccination for influenza and COVID-19 (Fontana & Strasfeld, 2019). At-risk HSCT recipients with respiratory symptoms should have diagnostic testing for respiratory viruses via nasopharyngeal swab and testing by PCR. Such testing offers more rapid turnaround time, higher sensitivity, and the ability to test for multiple viruses (e.g., adenovirus, RSV, COVID-19, parainfluenza, rhinovirus, human metapneumovirus, and others) in a single test.

Adenoviral infections, including hemorrhagic cystitis, gastroenteritis, and pneumonitis, have been managed with some degree of success with cidofovir or brincidofovir therapy and supplemental IVIG. Adenovirus is more common in pediatric HSCT recipients and is often fatal after HSCT. High-risk HSCT recipients should have weekly screening for adenovirus by quantitative PCR (blood) for purposes of early detection and implementation of early preemptive antiviral therapy.

Most of the respiratory viruses, apart from influenza and, in some circumstances, respiratory syncytial virus (RSV) and adenovirus, are managed supportively. Many respiratory viruses (e.g., RSV, influenza, parainfluenza, rhinovirus) do not have a standard treatment protocol. These community-acquired viral infections can be life threatening after HSCT. Ribavirin treatment has been attempted using the intravenous or inhalation forms, but results have been inconclusive. In some studies, the addition of RSV immune globulin in conjunction with a traditional oral, intravenous, or inhalation form of ribavirin therapy has shown promise in preventing the progression of RSV upper respiratory infection to the lower respiratory tract and in the treatment of RSV pneumonia. HSCT recipients under the age of 2 or eligible for prophylactic monoclonal antibody therapy against RSV with palivizumab.

Autologous and allogeneic stem cell transplant recipients who are more than 6 months beyond transplantation should receive an annual influenza vaccine. Allogeneic HSCT patients more than 6 months but less than 1 year after transplantation should receive an influenza vaccine plus a booster vaccination. For individuals unlikely to receive benefit from influenza vaccine (i.e., <6 months after transplantation, IVIG dependent, or on corticosteroids), all household contacts should consider immunization. Oseltamivir is safe when given to HSCT patients and appears to play an important role in the prevention of the complications of influenza infection in those who test positive for influenza A and B viruses. Patients who test positive for influenza should receive treatment with this medication (Fontana & Strafeld, 2019).

Severe acute respiratory syndrome caused by coronavirus 19 (SARS-CoV-2) was declared a pandemic by the World Health Organization in March of 2020. HSCT recipients who are early posttransplant and on immunosuppression have at least a two-times higher risk of COVID-19-associated intensive care unit admission, invasive ventilation, and death compared with the general population (Sharma et al., 2021). To date, data on the outcomes of HSCT recipients with COVID-19 are limited to small case series and single-center experiences. Early studies suggest that overall survival 30 days after diagnosis was 68% for recipients of allogeneic HSCT and 67% for recipients of autologous HSCT. Among allogeneic HSCT recipients, risk factors associated with a higher mortality included being age (>50 years), male, and development of COVID-19 within 12 months of transplantation (Nierengarten, 2021).

Because of the rapidly changing nature of the COVID-19 pandemic, recommendations regarding vaccination and management of HSCT patients who test positive for COVID-19 (SARS-CoV-2) are evolving. HSCT patients greater than 5 years of age should be vaccinated against SAR-CoV-2. Patients could be given whatever vaccine is made available to them as long as it is not live-attenuated or contains replicating viral vectors. Since the only studies so far reported have been performed with mRNA vaccines, these vaccines seem preferable based on the currently existing information. Response rates to vaccines are lower than in healthy individuals, especially if patients are vaccinated soon after HSCT. Vaccination could be initiated as early as three months after HSCT. Whether an earlier start would have any protective effect is currently unknown. There is a risk for worsening/eliciting GVHD after allogeneic HSCT from vaccines. This risk needs to be considered when deciding about time for vaccination. Although side effects are expected as with any vaccine, side effects other than GVHD have not been reported to be more common in HSCT recipients than compared to healthy individuals. If an HSCT recipient has received COVID-19 vaccine before transplant or chimeric antigen receptor T-cell (CAR T) therapy, the procedures will most likely wipe out all immune memory of previous vaccines. Therefore, any previous COVID-19 vaccination should be considered discounted, and it is recommended that individuals are re-vaccinated as if they had never received a COVID-19 vaccine. Vaccination against COVID-19 should take priority over the regular post-HSCT vaccination program. Reasonable criteria to postpone COVID-19 vaccination based on our current knowledge are severe, uncontrolled grades III-IV acute GVHD, recipients of rituximab or obinutuzumab during the previous six months, or other B-cell depleting therapy such as inotuzumab or blinatumomab, CAR T-cell-treated patients with B-cell aplasia, or recent therapy with ATG or alemtuzumab.

HSCT donors should be vaccinated prior to donation. Health care workers caring for HSCT recipients should be vaccinated to protect their patients. Household contacts above the age of 5 years should be vaccinated, especially when the HCT recipient is early after transplant or receiving intensive immunosuppression. Since protection against COVID-19 wanes with time, and it is probable that it will be shorter in immunocompromised HSCT patients, a third dose of vaccine is recommended. The best timing of a third dose is currently unknown but can be considered 4 weeks to 5 months after the second dose of vaccine. No recommendation for post-vaccination determination of antibody level can be given at this time. However, it can be indicated in certain subgroups of patients, such as CAR T-cell treated patients, patients vaccinated early after HCT, or patients with unstable GVHD (Khawaja et al., 2022; Ljungman et al., 2020). HSCT recipients who are less than 90 days post-transplant or still on immunosuppressive therapy for GVHD

are now eligible for *pre-exposure* prophylaxis using COVID-19 dual monoclonal antibody therapy, which should be administered per institutional and FDA guidelines. Clinicians should follow the guidelines for evaluating and managing COVID-19 in nontransplant patients when treating transplant and CAR T-cell-treated patients.

Human herpes virus 6 (HHV-6) infection in the HSCT patient is a consequence of viral reactivation. HHV-6 reactivation affects 40% to 60% of allogeneic HSCT patients and usually occurs 2 to 4 weeks after transplantation. Multiple risk factors are associated with HHV-6 reactivation, including mismatched transplants, UCB transplants, younger age, conditioning regimens, acute GVHD, and use of corticosteroids (Wang et al., 2021; Ward et al., 2019).

HHV-6 reactivation has been associated with graft failure, prolonged pancytopenia, and encephalitis after HSCT. HHV-6–associated meningoencephalitis has been treated with ganciclovir, cidofovir, and foscarnet with limited success. Ganciclovir has also been used as prophylaxis to prevent HHV-6 disease. There are no randomized, controlled trials to prove treatment or prophylaxis with ganciclovir is effective against HHV 6.

Epstein-Barr Virus and Posttransplantation Lymphoproliferative Disorder. Stem cell donors and candidates for transplantation should be tested for serum anti-EBV IgG antibodies before transplantation to determine the risk for EBV reactivation after HSCT. The recommendation is stronger for pediatric patients than for adults. Although fever and mononucleosis can occur in primary EBV infection, the most significant clinical syndrome associated with EBV replication is PTLD. It is the result of EBV-infected B cells, resulting in clonal abnormalities and the resultant proliferation of lymphoid tissue (i.e., EBV-related lymphoma).

PTLD occurs principally in recipients who have profound T-lymphocyte cytopenia (e.g., after TCD, use of anti–T-cell antibodies, UCB transplants, haploidentical transplants). Early recognition in high-risk patients is important because PTLD tends to be rapidly progressive, and weekly surveillance with PCR may have a role in preventing progression. EBV DNA loads rise as early as 3 weeks before PTLD onset. Monitoring blood loads of EBV DNA allows preemptive reduction in immunosuppression as the first phase of managing PTLD.

Because of the variability of PCR techniques and the difference in risk for EBV-related PTLD (due to the degree of T-cell lymphopenia), no firm recommendation can be made about the threshold for initiation of preemptive therapy. If there is no response to a reduction in immunosuppression, preemptive treatment with immune-based therapies such as rituximab can prevent the progression to PTLD. Infusion of donor-derived, EBV-specific cytotoxic lymphocytes (CTLs) has demonstrated promise in the prophylaxis of EBV lymphoma. Expanded, donor-derived, EBV-specific T cells have also been used to control blood loads of EBV DNA in this setting, but the procedure remains experimental. Immunotherapies for EBV-related PTLD are offering promising results (Ru et al., 2020).

Managing the Risk of Infection

HSCT is characterized by a variable period of early infectious complications caused largely by neutropenia and mucosal damage because of the preparative regimen. The complications are predictable based on clinical findings of mucositis and absolute neutrophil count. Allogeneic HSCT patients experience a prolonged period of immunosuppression characterized by profound defects in cell-mediated and humoral immunity. Unfortunately, there are no readily available markers with which to accurately measure the relative risk for individual patients. Patients must be monitored carefully and receive early intervention for signs or symptoms of an infectious disease. For most patients, immunocompetence improves progressively with increasing time after transplantation. However, many hematopoietic stem cell recipients remain immunocompromised far beyond 2 years after transplantation, especially those with chronic GVHD, for whom infection remains the most important cause of morbidity and mortality. Work is needed to augment immune reconstitution, for early pathogen detection, and to identify accurate surrogate markers of immunocompetence to guide the long-term treatment of this high-risk population.

Important nursing responsibilities include maintaining a protective environment, practicing consistent and thorough provider hand hygiene, delivering meticulous oral and skin care, monitoring vital signs frequently, and conducting a thorough review of systems and a physical examination to identify potential locations (e.g., alimentary tract, skin, lungs, sinuses, intravascular access device sites) of infection. Although there is limited evidence to support their effectiveness, most transplantation centers provide additional protective measures that may include low-microbial diets, protective isolation with masks and gloves, laminar air filtration, gowning, and gut and skin decontamination.

Sinusoidal Obstructive Syndrome of the Liver

Sinusoidal obstructive syndrome (SOS), also called hepatic VOD, is part of a spectrum of organ injury syndromes that occur after HSCT. The incidence of VOD/SOS after

transplantation varies substantially from 2% to 60% (Bonifazi et al., 2020; Lai et al., 2021) because of the heterogeneity of transplant procedures that are center-specific and of application of differing diagnostic criteria. The box below outlines risk factors for developing hepatic SOS. The incidence of SOS is lower after autologous HSCT and with RIC regimens (Mohty et al., 2015).

Risk Factors for Hepatic Veno-Occlusive Disease

- Pretransplantation preparative regimen with busulfan or TBI
- Previous abdominal irradiation
- Pretransplantation hepatotoxic drug therapy (amphotericin)
- Abnormal liver function study results before transplantation
- Hepatic iron overload
- HLA-mismatched or unrelated donor
- Active infection
- Metastatic liver disease
- Poor pretransplantation performance status
- Second transplantation
- Older recipient age
- Female gender
- Prior exposure to gemtuzumab

Data from Bonifazi, F., Barbato, F., Ravaioli, F, Sessa, M., Defrancesco, I., Arpinati, M., … Colecchia, A. (2020). Diagnosis and treatment of VOD/SOS after allogeneic hematopoietic stem cell transplantation. *Frontiers in Immunology, 11*, 489.

SOS results from tissue injury to sinusoidal endothelial cells and hepatocytes caused by the transplant conditioning regimen, cytokines from injured tissue, calcineurin inhibitors (CNIs), microbial products (from active infection), and engraftment/alloreactivity (Bonifazi et al., 2020; Lai et al., 2021). Endothelial injury to the liver activates cytokine and tumor necrosis factor, which stimulate coagulation (procoagulative state) and thrombosis in the hepatic sinusoids and eventually in the venules. The resulting impairment of blood flow through the hepatic sinusoids leads to VOD/SOS. The figure below shows the pathophysiology that leads to the development of SOS.

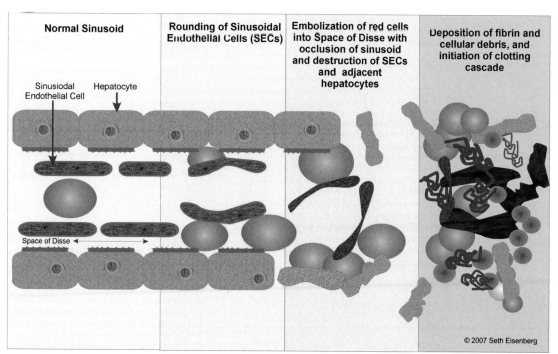

Pathophysiology of Hepatic Veno-Occlusive Disease. (Courtesy Seth Eisenberg, RN, OCN. Used with permission.)

Clinical manifestations of SOS usually begin within the first 2 weeks after transplantation and include hyperbilirubinemia, rapid weight gain, ascites, right upper quadrant pain, hepatomegaly, splenomegaly, jaundice, coagulopathy, and increased platelet consumption. There are three different VOD/SOS criteria that can be used when managing HSCT recipients. The table below summarizes the Seattle, Baltimore, and the European Bone Marrow Transplant (EBMT) diagnostic criteria used in the diagnosis of VOD/SOS.

Progression of SOS can lead to fatal liver failure. Treatment usually is supportive and focuses on maintaining intravascular volume and renal perfusion while minimizing fluid accumulation. Astute nursing care of these patients is critical. Nurses provide much of the supportive care essential to successful treatment of patients with SOS (see the Nursing Management of Hepatic Veno-Occlusive Disease or Sinusoidal Obstructive Syndrome table below).

Defibrotide is the medication of choice in managing SOS/VOD, and the only agent with proven efficacy for the treatment of severe/very severe SOS/VOD, with complete response rates of 30% to 60% (Bonifazi et al., 2020; Brown, 2018; Lai et al., 2021; Mohty et al., 2020). Defibrotide, a polydisperse oligonucleotide mixture of single-stranded oligonucleotides that has protective effects for vascular hepatic endothelium and is now FDA approved for use in the United States. Studies have demonstrated that defibrotide is also an effective agent for SOS prophylaxis after transplantation in patients at high risk for this complication (Mohty et al., 2023). The drug has antithrombotic, anti-ischemic, and anti-inflammatory effects. Systemic anticoagulants or thrombolytics have been studied but are associated with excessive bleeding complications and have not improved overall survival.

Diagnostic Criteria of Veno-Occlusive Disease/Sinusoidal Obstructive Syndrome

Adults

Baltimore criteria	Within first 21 days post HSCT with total bilirubin ≥2 mg/dL and at least two or more of the following: • Painful hepatomegaly • >5% weight gain over baseline • Ascites
Modified Seattle criteria	Presentation within first 20 days post HSCT with two or more of the following: • Total bilirubin >2 mg/dL • Hepatomegaly, right upper quadrant tenderness • Weight gain >2% over baseline
EBMT criteria	Classical presentation before or beyond 21 days post HSCT OR: • Biopsy proven VOD/SOS • >2 of the classical criteria AND • Ultrasound or hemodynamic evidence of VOD/SOS

Children

The presence of at least two or more of the following:
• Unexplained refractoriness to platelet transfusions defined as ≥1 weight-adjusted platelet transfusion/day
• Weight gain for 3 consecutive days diuretics or weight gain >5% above baseline
• Painful hepatomegaly best confirmed by imaging
• Ascites confirmed by imaging
• Increase in total bilirubin above baseline on 3 consecutive days or total bilirubin ≥2 mg/dL

Adapted from Bonifazi, F., Barbato, F., Ravaioli, F., Sessa, M., Defrancesco, I., Arpinati, M., ... Colecchia, A. (2020). Diagnosis and treatment of VOD/SOS after allogeneic hematopoietic stem cell transplantation. *Frontiers in Immunology, 11*, 489.

Nursing Management of Hepatic Veno-Occlusive Disease or Sinusoidal Obstructive Syndrome

Management	Procedures
Laboratory monitoring	Perform liver function studies, coagulation studies (e.g., PT, partial thromboplastin time, INR, fibrinogen D-dimer), frequent platelet counts, renal function tests, ammonia level assessment, complete blood count
Fluid management	Frequent weights, strict input and output measurements, daily abdominal girths, fluid restriction, concentrated medications in minimal fluid
Medication and transfusion administration	Administer colloid, blood productions (e.g., packed RBCs, platelets, fresh frozen plasma), defibrotide, ursodiol; monitor for overuse of hepatotoxic medications
Renal function	Review medications for renal adjustments based on change in renal function, monitor during dialysis
Pain management	Frequent pain assessment, position patient to alleviate stress on liver capsule
Patient safety	Evaluate for mental status changes and provide a safe environment
Patient/family education	Educate regarding VOD or SOS risks, signs, and symptoms
Identification of risk factors	Review patient's risk factors (e.g., busulfan- or TBI-containing regimen), posttransplantation infection, history of liver function abnormalities, second transplantation, unrelated or haploidentical donor

Data from Bonifazi, F., Barbato, F., Ravaioli, F., Sessa, M., Defrancesco, I., Arpinati, M., ... Colecchia, A. (2020). Diagnosis and treatment of VOD/SOS after allogeneic hematopoietic stem cell transplantation. *Frontiers in Immunology, 11*, 489; Brown, V. (Ed.). (2018). *Hematopoietic stem cell transplantation for the pediatric oncologist.* Switzerland: Springer International Publishing AG.

The prognosis for VOD/SOS depends on the extent of hepatic injury, liver dysfunction, and existence of multiorgan failure. Seventy percent of patients diagnosed with SOS spontaneously recover, but severe VOD/SOS is associated with an all-cause mortality rate of more than 90% by day 100 after HSCT (Bernasconi et al., 2019; Mothy et al., 2020). Standard therapy for mild VOD/SOS (no secondary organ involvement) in North America continues to be supportive care measures only.

Options for preventing SOS in patients who are at highest risk for the complications include anticoagulation with low-dose heparin, low-molecular-weight heparin, antithrombin III concentrates, prostaglandin E, and ursodeoxycholic acid (Bernasconi et al., 2019; Brown, 2018; Lai et al., 2021; Mothy et al., 2020). Despite many studies evaluating VOD/SOS prophylaxis, none has found a dramatic improvement in the overall incidence and severity of SOS (Brown, 2018; Bonifazi et al., 2020; Lai et al., 2021; Mothy et al., 2020).

Pulmonary Complications

Research suggests that pulmonary complications are the leading cause of posttransplantation morbidity and death in 25% to 50% of HSCT patients (Kapadia & Wikle Shapiro, 2018). The rate of significant pulmonary complications is lower for autologous transplant recipients than for allogeneic transplant recipients because of the absence of GVHD and posttransplantation immunosuppression. Few autologous HSCT preparative regimens include TBI, a significant factor for the development of pulmonary issues after transplantation. Posttransplantation pulmonary complications are classified as infectious or noninfectious and follow a predictable timeline after transplantation (see the table below).

Timeline of Typical Onset of Pulmonary Complications After Hematopoietic Stem Cell Transplantation

Cause	Pulmonary Complications
Day 0–30	
Infectious and noninfectious causes related to the preparative regimen and neutropenia	Pulmonary edema Pleural effusion Transfusion-related lung injury Idiopathic pneumonia syndrome (IPS) Engraftment syndrome Diffuse alveolar hemorrhage Aspergillosis Candidemia or candidal infection Respiratory viruses (community-acquired RSV, parainfluenza, or influenza) Bacterial pneumonia ARDS due to sepsis Chemotherapy-associated lung injury
Day 31–100	
Opportunistic infections due to impairment of cellular and humoral immunity and delayed lung injury from the preparative regimen. Community-acquired respiratory viruses	Diffuse alveolar hemorrhage CMV Adenovirus reactivation Aspergillosis *Pneumocystis jirovecii* pneumonia Respiratory viruses (community-acquired RSV, COVID-19, parainfluenza, or influenza) Toxoplasmosis ARDS due to many infections Idiopathic pneumonia syndrome Radiation-induced pneumonitis Busulfan-induced pneumonitis
Day 100+	
Infection from encapsulated bacteria and opportunistic infections due to delayed immune recovery, continued immunosuppressive therapy, and chronic GVHD	Aspergillosis Respiratory viruses (community-acquired RSV, COVID-19, parainfluenza, or influenza) Varicella zoster CMV *Pneumocystis jirovecii* pneumonia PTLD ARDS Bronchiolitis obliterans due to chronic GVHD Bronchiolitis obliterans organizing pneumonia Busulfan-induced chronic lung injury Radiation-induced chronic lung injury

Data from Kapadia, M., & Wikle Shapiro, T. J. (2018). Pulmonary complications associated with HSCT. In Brown, V. (Ed.). (2018). *Hematopoietic stem cell transplantation for the pediatric oncologist*. Cham, Germany: Springer; Haider, S., Durairajan, N., & Soubani, A. O. (2020). Noninfectious pulmonary complications of haematopoietic stem cell transplantation. *European Respiratory Review, 29*(156), 190119.

Common pulmonary complications seen in the first 30 days after transplantation include pulmonary edema, bacterial or fungal pneumonia, pulmonary hemorrhage, diffuse alveolar hemorrhage, and acute respiratory distress syndrome (ARDS) associated with septic shock. Through day 100, patients remain at risk for these complications and for viral pneumonia, *Pneumocystis jirovecii* pneumonia, and idiopathic interstitial pneumonitis due to TBI.

Late pulmonary complications that can occur after day 100 include bronchiolitis obliterans syndrome as a result of chronic GVHD, idiopathic interstitial pneumonitis from TBI, PTLD involving the lung, infectious pneumonias due to encapsulated bacteria (e.g., pneumococcus), fungal disease due to *Aspergillus* or viral pneumonias caused by CMV, VZV, or community-acquired viruses (e.g., COVID-19, RSV, parainfluenza, human metapneumovirus, adenovirus).

Early detection and prompt investigation of pulmonary symptoms are essential for successful management of pulmonary complications. Early diagnosis and prompt intervention can reduce disease progression and premature death. Patients at risk can be screened weekly with viral PCRs for adenovirus, CMV, and EBV; a serum galactomannan immunoassay for early *Aspergillus* detection; and a comprehensive respiratory viral panel for a broad range of viruses before transplantation. Periodic chest radiographs, chest CT for persistent fever, and intermittent evaluations of pulmonary function are obtained.

HSCT patients should have frequent assessments for new symptoms such as rhinorrhea, cough, shortness of breath, fever, or a change in activity tolerance. Prophylactic measures include frequent incentive spirometry, encouraging activity, compliance with prophylactic antimicrobials, influenza vaccination, isolation from community, and avoidance of sick contacts.

Engraftment and Recovery

Complete engraftment after HSCT is usually defined as an absolute neutrophil count greater than 0.5×10^9/L for 3 consecutive days and a platelet count greater than 20×10^9/L achieved without transfusion support. The rate of engraftment depends on the source of the progenitor cells. For patients who receive bone marrow or PBSCs, neutrophil engraftment can occur as early as 10 days after transplantation, but it is more common between days 14 and 20. Patients who receive UCB cells typically take about 25 days after transplantation for engraftment, but it can take as long as 42 days (Auletta et al., 2021). The total number of progenitor cells transplanted, the use of colony-stimulating factors to prevent GVHD, strength of conditioning regimen, and infection or other posttransplantation complications may affect the patient's time to engraftment (Hutt, 2018).

Graft Failure

A significant obstacle to the success of allogeneic HSCT is graft failure, defined as a lack of initial engraftment of donor cells (i.e., primary graft failure) or loss of donor cells after initial engraftment (i.e., secondary graft failure). Graft failure caused by the immune cells of the recipient attacking the donor stem cells before they have the opportunity to engraft is called *graft rejection*. Factors associated with graft failure and rejection include HLA disparity between the donor and recipient, ABO disparity between the donor and recipient, the patient's underlying disease, viral infections, type of conditioning regimen, and stem cell source (Hunt, 2018).

The overall incidence of graft failure is less than 5%. It occurs most often in patients with aplastic anemia who are chemotherapy naïve or those receiving unrelated donor UCB transplants. The cause is multifactorial and may include primary diagnosis, HLA disparity, ABO mismatching, graft manipulation, insufficient dose intensity of the conditioning regimen, inadequate stem cell dose, insufficient posttransplantation immunosuppression, posttransplantation administration of medications with myelosuppressive side effects, viral infection, and folate or vitamin B12 deficiency (Hunt, 2018).

Medications with myelosuppressive side effects (e.g., cotrimoxazole, ganciclovir) should be administered with caution after HSCT as they may affect the health of the stem cell graft. Treatment of graft failure may include larger doses of hematopoietic growth factors and administration of additional donor-derived hematopoietic stem cells, also called a *stem cell boost*. If graft failure persists, a second transplantation with additional immunosuppressive drugs may be indicated.

Engraftment Syndrome

During neutrophil recovery after HSCT, a constellation of signs and symptoms, including fever, erythrodermatous rash, weight gain, and noncardiogenic pulmonary edema, often occur. These clinical findings are usually referred to as *engraftment syndrome* or *capillary leak syndrome*, which reflect the manifestations of increased capillary permeability. Although this syndrome was first described after autologous HSCT, a more severe manifestation has been observed after allogeneic HSCT.

Distinguishing engraftment syndrome from hyperacute GVHD in the allogeneic setting can be difficult. In some cases, engraftment syndrome may be a manifestation of graft rejection by the host. Experience with nonmyeloablative conditioning for stem cell transplantation revealed that engraftment syndrome may occur independent of GVHD. Although cellular and cytokine interactions are thought to be responsible for these clinical findings, a distinct effector cell population and cytokine profile have not been identified. Engraftment syndromes have been associated with increased TRM, mostly from pulmonary and associated multiorgan failure.

Corticosteroid therapy and supportive measures are often dramatically effective for engraftment syndrome, particularly for the treatment of pulmonary manifestations.

A more uniform definition of engraftment syndrome is being developed to allow reproducible reporting of complications and evaluation of prophylactic and therapeutic strategies (Hunt, 2018).

Graft-Versus-Host Disease

GVHD is a complication unique to allogeneic HSCT. GVHD results when the infused donor stem cells (i.e., graft) recognize the recipient (i.e., host) as foreign tissue. The attack of donor-derived T lymphocytes damages recipient (host) tissues. GVHD is classified as acute or chronic. Classically, this determination has been made based on the time at which GVHD occurs after transplantation. Clinical manifestations that occur before day 100 after transplantation are often designated as acute GVHD. Chronic GVHD is a set of clinical manifestations that occur 100 or more days after transplantation. Historically, a clear distinction was drawn between an early (acute) GVHD and a delayed (chronic) form of GVHD. However, recent observations of patients receiving UCB transplants, RIC regimens, and DLIs after transplantation confirmed that acute GVHD can occur several months after transplantation and that the classic characteristics of chronic GVHD can occur as early as 2 months after transplantation (Hamilton, 2018; Schoemans et al., 2018). There is growing recognition that acute and chronic GVHD are best differentiated by their features rather than the time at which they occur.

A new paradigm for identifying acute and chronic GVHD and for diagnosing and staging chronic GVHD (Lee, 2017) includes classic acute GVHD (i.e., maculopapular rash, nausea, vomiting or diarrhea, and elevated liver function test results); persistent, recurrent, or late acute GVHD (i.e., features of acute GVHD occurring beyond 100 days, often during withdrawal of immune suppression); classic chronic GVHD without features of acute GVHD; and an overlap syndrome that includes the diagnostic or distinctive features of chronic GVHD and acute GVHD.

The incidence of acute and chronic GVHD is 30% to 60% in cases involving histocompatible, sibling-matched allografts, with more GVHD occurring with greater HLA mismatches between the donor and recipient. The mortality rate directly or indirectly related to GVHD may reach 50% (Schoemans et al., 2018; Wikle Shapiro & Kapadia, 2018). Risk factors other than histoincompatibility include sex mismatching, donor parity, older age at the time of transplantation, posttransplantation infection (i.e., viral infections), the use of DLIs after transplantation, and the type of GVHD prophylaxis used.

Acute Graft-Versus-Host Disease

The reported incidence of acute GVHD varies from 20% to 80%, depending principally on the degree of HLA mismatch and donor type (i.e., matched or mismatched, sibling or unrelated donor), stem cell source (i.e., bone marrow, peripheral blood, or UCB), and to a lesser extent, donor age (i.e., older adult donors are associated with a higher risk of acute GVHD) and sex (i.e., multiparous female donor) (Schoemans et al., 2018).

In order of frequency, acute GVHD predominantly affects the skin, gastrointestinal tract, and liver. Skin involvement commonly starts as an erythematous maculopapular rash on the palms and soles but can involve any part of the skin, and when severe, it can lead to bullae formation. The figure below illustrates the typical findings of the various severities of acute GVHD skin manifestations. The differential diagnosis of cutaneous acute GVHD includes engraftment syndrome rash, infections (especially viral), and drug reactions, and it may require pathologic identification through a skin biopsy.

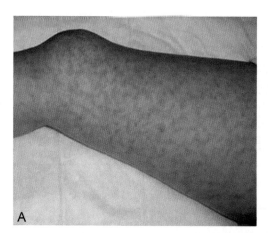
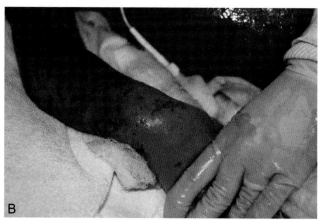

Acute Graft-Versus-Host Disease of the Skin.

Gastrointestinal acute GVHD manifests with secretory diarrhea (i.e., copious and sometimes bloody in severe cases) and may cause abdominal pain, nausea, vomiting, and anorexia. The differential diagnosis includes treatment-related mucositis or enteritis and infection. Endoscopies of the upper and lower gastrointestinal tract with biopsies of multiple sites may be needed to differentiate infection from acute GVHD.

Hepatic acute GVHD usually manifests with cholestatic jaundice and raised levels of liver enzymes (typically γ-glutamyl transpeptidase). Differential diagnoses include VOD/SOS, viral infection, sepsis, and drug toxicity. Hepatic acute GVHD with prominent transaminitis is rare but well described. Transjugular liver biopsy may be necessary, but the risk of bleeding from this procedure must be considered (Penack et al., 2020).

The Glucksberg grading and staging of acute GVHD are shown in the table below. This system assesses the degree of skin, liver, and gut involvement with the staging of each organ system, and the sum total provides the overall grade.

With the significant improvements in post-HSCT supportive care in the past 2 to 3 decades, particularly the reduction of infection-related mortality, there is a greater focus on preventing and managing GVHD. Guidelines for the diagnosis and management of acute GVHD were published in 2012 by the American Society of Blood and Marrow Transplantation (Martin et al., 2012) in an attempt to standardize the care of patients. The strategies used for prophylaxis of acute GVHD depend on the nature of the conditioning regimen, donor type, stem cell source, and degree of HLA mismatch.

Glucksberg Staging and Grading System for Acute Graft-Versus-Host Disease

CLINICAL STAGING OF INDIVIDUAL ORGAN MANIFESTATIONS

Organ[*]	Stage	Description
Skin[†]	0	No evidence of GVHD
	1	Maculopapular eruption over <25% of body area
	2	Maculopapular eruption over 25%–50% of body
	3	Generalized erythroderma
	4	Generalized erythroderma with bullous formation and often with desquamation
Liver	0	Bilirubin <2.0 mg/dL
	1	Bilirubin 2.0–3.0 mg/dL
	2	Bilirubin 3.1–6.0 mg/dL
	3	Bilirubin 6.1–15 mg/L
	4	Bilirubin >15 mg/dL
Gut	0	Diarrhea Adult: <500 mL/day Child: 10 mL/kg/day
	1	Diarrhea (adult: 500–999 mL/day and child: 10–19.9 mL/kg/day) OR persistent nausea, vomiting, or anorexia with histologic evidence of GVHD in the stomach or duodenum
	2	Diarrhea Adult: 1000–1499 mL/day Child: 20–30 mL/kg
	3	Diarrhea ≥1500 mL/day Child: >30 mL/kg/day
	4	Severe abdominal pain with or without ileus or grossly bloody stool

OVERALL GRADE

Grade	Skin Stage[‡]	Liver Stage	Gut Stage
0	None	None	None
I	1–2	0	0
II	1–3	1 and/or Gut GVHD	1
III	2–3	2–3 and/or Gut GVHD	2–3
IV	2–4	2–4 and/or Gut GVHD	2–4

[*] Criteria for staging minimum degree of organ involvement required to confer that stage.

[†] Use rule of nines or burn chart to determine extent of rash.

[‡] If no skin disease is present, the overall grade is the highest isolated liver or gut stage.

Data from Martin, P. J., Rizzo, J. D., Wingard, J. R., Ballen, K., Curtin, P. T., Cutler, C., ... Carpenter, P. A. (2012). First- and second-line systemic treatment of acute graft-versus-host disease: Recommendations of the American society of blood and marrow transplantation. *Biology of Blood and Marrow Transplantation, 19*(8), 1150–1163; Wikle Shapiro, T. J. (2019). Hematopoietic stem cell transplantation. In J. Brant, D. Cope, & M. Saria (Eds.). *Core curriculum for oncology nursing* (6th ed.). Philadelphia, PA: Elsevier.

Acute Graft-Versus-Host Disease Prophylaxis

Prophylaxis for acute graft-versus-host disease (aGVHD) post-HSCT usually includes cyclosporine or tacrolimus for approximately 2 to 12 months (depending on the underlying disease) with or without a short course of intravenous methotrexate (usually three to four doses). Tacrolimus is preferred to cyclosporine in many transplantation centers, although published evidence comparing these two CNIs is lacking (Hamilton, 2018; Martin et al., 2012). Pre-HSCT anti–T-cell serotherapy with ATG or alemtuzumab is usually added for the use of unrelated donor transplants (i.e., PBSC, bone marrow, or UCB), and it provides additional prophylaxis against graft rejection (Penack et al., 2020). Prophylaxis for reduced-intensity HSCTs usually includes cyclosporine and mycophenolate mofetil (MMF), although some centers prefer a corticosteroid to MMF. Serotherapy (i.e., ATG or alemtuzumab) is usually added for nonmalignant conditions or when an unrelated donor or UCB donor is used. Despite these common regimens, there are wide variations in drug scheduling and dosing for acute GVHD prophylaxis (Hamilton, 2018; Martin et al., 2012; Schoemans et al., 2018).

For some patients, not suitably matched related or unrelated donor can be found. A haploidentical graft (i.e., using a parent or sibling) is feasible, and various TCD strategies have been used to minimize GVHD and maximize sustained engraftment and early immune reconstitution. TCD techniques are used by some centers regardless of donor matching.

Historical methods to remove viable T lymphocytes include in vitro alemtuzumab, antilymphocyte antibodies, soy lectin, and sheep red cell rosette. Newer TCD techniques using CD34+ stem cell selection devices (e.g., Miltenyi Biotech's CliniMACS system) are showing promise (Roldan et al., 2019). Other techniques that focus on preserving the GVT effect while removing the T cells responsible for acute GVHD are being explored.

Posttransplant cyclophosphamide (PTCy) alone or in combination with other immunosuppressive agents has also emerged as an effective pharmacologic approach to GVHD prevention. This strategy was pioneered by investigators at Johns Hopkins in the haploidentical setting based on experimental models showing cyclophosphamide's potent and selective activity against alloreactive donor T cells, resulting in low incidences of GVHD and TRM. This approach has revolutionized our ability to cross the HLA barrier by performing mismatched transplants, greatly expanding donor availability (Hamilton, 2018). The table on this page reviews prophylaxis and first-line, second-line, and third-line treatment options for acute GVHD. The modified Glucksberg clinical grades correlate with overall survival and are usually used to stratify treatment for acute GVHD (Martin et al., 2012). The components of first-line management have changed little over the past 30 years. Grade I acute GVHD is managed by continuing the prophylactic CNI and applying topical steroids (and sometimes topical tacrolimus) to affected skin. Systemic immunosuppression with intravenous methylprednisolone (1 to 2 mg/kg/day) is added for grades II through IV. Higher steroid doses (>2 mg/kg/day) appear to offer no additional benefit and contribute to increased toxicity and the risk of fatal infection (Martin et al., 2012). In gastrointestinal acute GVHD, the addition of nonabsorbable steroids (i.e., budesonide and beclomethasone) may facilitate reduction of systemic steroid doses.

Management Options for Acute Graft-Versus-Host Disease

Options	Applications
Prophylaxis	• Myeloablative HSCT: cyclosporine (or tacrolimus) ± short-course methotrexate • Reduced intensity HSCT: cyclosporine (or tacrolimus) + MMF or a corticosteroid • Unrelated donor (or UCB) HSCT: serotherapy (ATG or alemtuzumab) + cyclosporin (or tacrolimus) + methotrexate • Haploidentical donor HSCT: TCD or CD34$^+$ selection ± cyclosporine
First-line treatment for acute GVHD	• Continue cyclosporine (or tacrolimus) to optimize blood level • Add corticosteroid (usually intravenous methylprednisolone, 1–2 mg/kg/day) • Add topical corticosteroid ± topical tacrolimus for skin acute GVHD • Consider enteral administration of nonabsorbable corticosteroids (e.g., budesonide) for gastrointestinal acute GVHD
Second-line treatment for steroid-refractory acute GVHD	Consider addition of one or more of anti- • TNF-α antibodies (e.g., infliximab, etanercept), • MMF, • mTOR inhibitor (e.g., sirolimus), • IL-2 receptor antibodies (e.g., basiliximab, daclizumab, inolimomab), • selective Janus kinase (JAK1 and JAK2) inhibitor (e.g., ruxolitinib), OR • extracorporeal photopheresis
Third-line treatment: after failure of at least two second-line treatments	Consider • Alemtuzumab • Methotrexate • Pentostatin • Human fecal transplant, and • Mesenchymal stem cells

ATG, Antithymocyte globulin; *GVHD,* graft-versus-host disease; *HSCT,* hematopoietic stem cell transplantation; *IL-2,* interleukin-2; *MMF,* mycophenolate mofetil; *mTOR,* mammalian target of rapamycin; *TNF,* tumor necrosis factor; *UCB,* umbilical cord blood.
Data from Brown V. (Ed). (2018). *Hematopoietic stem cell transplantation for the pediatric oncologist.* Switzerland: Springer International Publishing AG; Martin, P. J., Rizzo, J. D., Wingard, J. R., Ballen, K., Curtin, P. T., Cutler, C., … Carpenter, P. A. (2011). First- and second-line systemic treatment of acute graft-versus-host disease: Recommendations of the American Society of Blood and Marrow Transplantation, *Biology of Blood and Marrow Transplantation, 18*(8), 1150–1163.

Unfortunately, a complete response to steroid treatment is seen in only about 70% of cases of acute GVHD (Malard et al., 2020; Martin et al., 2012). However, newer treatments have been introduced for steroid-refractory acute GVHD, which is usually defined as failure to respond to 5 days of intravenous methylprednisolone and a CNI or deterioration after 3 days. Acute GVHD refractory to initial treatment is associated with a survival rate of less than 25% over 1 to 2 years due to the adverse consequences of GVHD itself (i.e., organ damage or subsequent development of chronic GVHD) and of its treatment (i.e., infectious complications due to severe immunosuppression) (Bride et al., 2018; Malard et al., 2020; Martin et al., 2012).

Chronic Graft-Versus-Host Disease

Chronic GVHD typically occurs 100 to 400 days after transplantation, although it can begin as early as 45 days after transplantation. It can be a debilitating, chronic condition that mimics an autoimmune disease. Chronic GVHD usually occurs in patients who have had acute GVHD, although it can occur in the absence of acute GVHD. Among patients who survived 150 days after allogeneic HSCT, chronic GVHD was observed in 35% to 50% of HLA-identical related transplantations and in 67% of matched unrelated donor transplantations (Sarantopoulos et al., 2019).

Risk factors for chronic GVHD include previous acute GVHD, older recipient age, and sex mismatching (i.e., female donor and male recipient). The incidence of chronic GVHD is also higher among recipients of PBSCs than recipients of bone marrow–derived stem cells. Clinical manifestations of chronic GVHD are graded and may be mild, moderate, or severe. They are commonly observed in the skin, liver, eyes, oral cavity, lungs, gastrointestinal system, neuromuscular system, and other body systems (Sarantopoulos et al., 2019; Wikle Shapiro & Kapadia, 2018). Sclerodermatous cutaneous and oral manifestations of chronic GVHD are seen in the figure on this page.

The NIH Consensus: Grading of Chronic Graft Versus Host Disease Severity table on the next page outlines the first National Institutes of Health (NIH) consensus publication with proposed diagnostic criteria and an improved classification for chronic GVHD. For assessing the severity of chronic GVHD, each organ or site is assigned a grade between 0 and 3 according to the clinical manifestations and resultant disability, and an overall grade of mild, moderate, or severe is assigned according to the extent of involvement of each organ. The grade has clinical relevance because moderate chronic GVHD implies at least one organ with clinically significant features but without major disability, whereas severe chronic GVHD (with a score of 3 in at least one organ) reflects major disability.

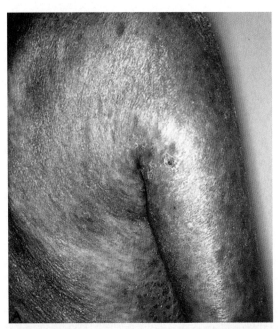

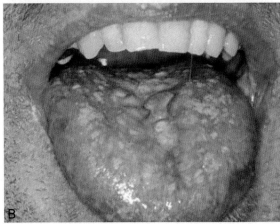

Chronic Graft-Versus-Host Disease of the Skin

NIH Consensus: Grading of Chronic Graft-Versus-Host Disease Severity

Severity	Definition*
Mild	Involves one or two organs or sites (except the lung), with no clinically significant functional impairment (maximum score of 1 in all affected organs or sites)
Moderate	At least one organ or site with clinically significant impairment but no major disability (maximum score of 2 in any affected organ or site) *or* 3 or more organs or sites with no clinically significant functional impairment (maximum score of 1 in all affected organs or sites) *or* lung with a score of 1
Severe	Major disability caused by chronic GVHD (score of 3 in any affected organ or site) *or* a lung score of ≥2

* Each organ is scored between 0 and 3 depending on physical manifestations and disabilities caused by GVHD (0, no symptoms/signs; 1–3, increasingly severe symptoms, signs, or abnormal studies). These scores and the number of organs or sites involved are used to grade the overall severity.
Data from Wikle Shapiro, T. J., & Kapadia, M. Chronic graft versus host disease. In Brown, V. (Ed.) (2018). *Hematopoietic stem cell transplantation for the pediatric oncologist*. Cham, Germany: Springer International Publishing.

The clinical features, screening, evaluation, and recommended interventions for patients with chronic GVHD are summarized in the table below. Because other conditions can mimic chronic GVHD, a systematic, multidisciplinary evaluation of the patient with chronic GVHD is essential.

Standard of care in the treatment of chronic GVHD depends on the organ(s) or site(s) that are affected, and adopted treatments can be topical or systemic. Nevertheless, about 50% to 60% of patients with chronic GVHD will require a second-line treatment within 2 years, but currently there is no consensus on the optimal choice of agents for second or further lines of therapy. Common agents used in combination with steroids include cyclosporine, tacrolimus, rapamycin, MMF, rituximab, pentostatin, hydroxychloroquine, ruxolitinib, imatinib, bortezomib, ibrutinib, nilotinib, pomalidomide, methotrexate, and extracorporeal photopheresis, with a wide range of cost-effectiveness (Saidu et al., 2020; Sarantopoulos et al., 2019; Wikle Shapiro & Kapadia, 2018). Early recognition and treatment of chronic GVHD before disability ensues is critical. First-line therapy for mild chronic GVHD includes topical and oral steroids, cyclosporine or tacrolimus, and azathioprine. Patients refractory to first-line therapies or those with moderate to severe chronic GVHD may be placed on azathioprine alternating with cyclosporine, steroids, or thalidomide. Clofazimine, an antileprosy agent, has been effective in treating cutaneous and oral lesions of chronic GVHD and may be useful as a steroid-sparing agent.

MMF is the most commonly used agent to treat steroid refractory chronic GVHD. Responses of 90% and 75% in first- and second-line settings are seen when MMF is added to standard tacrolimus, cyclosporine, and prednisone treatments (Saidu et al., 2020). MMF does not seem to increase the rate of infection or relapse posttransplant.

Psoralen and ultraviolet A (PUVA) radiation therapy plays a role for patients with refractory cutaneous chronic GVHD. In one study, it resulted in a 40% to 78% response rate and improvement in a few extracutaneous sites. Extracorporeal photopheresis, a modification of PUVA treatment, has also shown benefit, with the best responses in the skin, liver, eye, and oral mucosa. Studies using ECP in the prevention of chronic GVHD are emerging (Drexler et al., 2020).

Chronic Graft-Versus-Host Disease: Clinical Manifestations, Screening, and Interventions

Organ or System	Clinical Manifestations	Screening Studies or Evaluation	Interventions
Dermal	• Dyspigmentation, • Xerosis (dryness), • Hyperkeratosis, • Pruritus, • Scleroderma, • Lichenification, • Onychodystrophy (nail ridging or nail loss), • Alopecia	• Clinical examination • Skin biopsy: 3-mm punch biopsy	• Immunosuppressive therapy • Psoralen and ultraviolet A radiation (PUVA) • ECP • Topical with steroid creams, moisturizers, or emollients, antibacterial ointments to prevent superinfection • Avoid sunlight exposure, use sunblock lotion with a large hat that shades the face when outdoors
Oral	• Lichen planus, • Xerostomia, • Ulceration	• Oral biopsy	• Steroid mouth rinses • PUVA, pilocarpine, and anethole trithione for xerostomia • Fluoride gels or rinses • Careful attention to oral hygiene; regular dental evaluations
Ocular	• Keratoconjunctivitis • Sicca syndrome	• Schirmer test, • Ophthalmic evaluation, • Slit-lamp test	• Regular ophthalmologic follow-up • Preservative-free artificial tears and moisturizing lotions • Temporary or permanent lacrimal duct occlusion • System-specific interventions • Pancreatic enzyme supplementation
Hepatic	• Jaundice, abdominal pain	• Liver function tests	• Actigall orally • ECP

Continued

Chronic Graft-Versus-Host Disease: Clinical Manifestations, Screening, and Interventions—cont'd

Organ or System	Clinical Manifestations	Screening Studies or Evaluation	Interventions
Pulmonary	• Shortness of breath, • Cough, • Dyspnea, • Wheezing, • Fatigue, • Hypoxia, • Pleural effusion	• Pulmonary function studies, peak flow, • Arterial blood gas, • High-resolution CT of chest	• Prevent and treat pulmonary infections • Aggressively investigate changes in pulmonary function because they may represent GVHD of lung or bronchiolitis obliterans • Inhaled or systemic steroids • Prophylactic azithromycin
Gastro-intestinal	• Nausea, • Odynophagia, • Dysphagia, • Anorexia, • Early satiety, • Malabsorption, • Diarrhea, • Weight loss	• Esophagogastro-duodenoscopy, • Colonoscopy, • Nutritional assessment, • Fecal studies	• Referral to gastroenterologist • nutrition support
Nutritional	• Protein and calorie deficiency, • Malabsorption, • Dehydration, • Weight loss, • Muscle wasting	• Weight, • Fat store measurement, • Prealbumin	• Nutritional monitoring, • Supplementation, • Symptom-specific interventions
Genitourinary	• Vaginal sicca, • Vaginal atrophy, • Stenosis, • Inflammation	• Pelvic examination • Referral to GYN Medicine	• Intravaginal steroid cream
Immunologic	• Hypogammaglobulinemia, • Autoimmune syndromes, • Recurrent infections, including • CMV, • HSV, • VZV, fungi, • *P. jirovecii,* • Encapsulated bacteria	• Quantitative immunoglobulin levels, CD4/CD8 lymphocyte subsets • Antibody titer response to vaccines	• Intravenous immunoglobulins, prophylactic antimicrobials for prophylaxis against *P. jirovecii* pneumonia and encapsulated organisms, • Surveillance for CMV reactivation
Musculoskeletal	• Contractures, • Debility, • Muscle cramps	• Performance status, • Formal quality of life evaluation, • Rehabilitation needs • Orthopedic Medicine	• Physical therapy

Data from Lee, S. J. (2017). Classification systems for chronic graft-versus-host disease. *Blood, 129*(1), 30-37; Wikle Shapiro, T. J., & Kapadia, M. (2018). Chronic graft versus host disease. In Brown, V. (Ed.). *Hematopoietic stem cell transplantation for the pediatric oncologist.* Cham, Germany: Springer International Publishing.

The immunosuppressive agents commonly used in patients undergoing HSCT and the associated nursing implications are presented in the table on the next page. Drug levels of cyclosporine or tacrolimus should be monitored at regular intervals and dosing adjusted to maintain levels within the therapeutic range. Because many drug-drug interactions are associated with cyclosporine and tacrolimus, it is important to regularly review the patient's medication profile to identify potentially deleterious interactions. Patients should be instructed to take their immunosuppressive medications exactly as instructed and to contact their transplant provider before starting new medications. Because sun exposure may activate or exacerbate GVHD of the skin, patients should be advised about appropriate methods for minimizing exposure.

Chronic GVHD is a cause of significant morbidity after allogeneic stem cell transplantation. Supportive care measures such as infection prophylaxis, nutritional management (Saidu et al., 2020; Sarantopoulos et al., 2019; Wikle Shapiro & Kapadia, 2018), and coordinated multidisciplinary care are essential to improving the length pnand quality of life for patients with chronic GVHD. Antiviral prophylaxis against

HSV, VZV, and CMV can prevent oropharyngeal infection and interstitial pneumonia in patients with refractory GVHD on long-term immunosuppression. Antifungal agents that cover mold species are also needed to prevent and treat fungal infections in patients with chronic GVHD on active treatment.

Pain control with analgesics for patients with mouth sores allows oral intake. Oral beclomethasone can improve oral intake, nausea, and diarrhea without causing systemic or local toxicity. Retinoic acid is used for ocular sicca syndrome, and pilocarpine (Salagen) is used for oral sicca manifestations. Clonazepam may be used to treat neuromuscular manifestations (e.g., muscular aches, cramping, carpal spasm). Patients receiving chronic corticosteroid therapy are at increased risk for osteoporosis and fractures. For patients on long-term steroids or female patients, estrogen replacement, calcium supplements, and antiosteoporosis agents (e.g., alendronate, calcitonin) should be considered. A skin care specialist may be needed for moderate to severe cutaneous chronic GVHD (Lee, 2017).

Specialists in dentistry or oral medicine, dermatology, endocrinology, gynecology, ophthalmology, pulmonology, nutrition, orthopedics, physical therapy, and occupational therapy are essential in caring for patients with acute or chronic GVHD. Chronic GVHD is a primary factor in late transplantation-related morbidity, including abnormalities of growth and development in children, functional performance status, somatic symptoms, and decreased quality of life, psychological functioning, sexual satisfaction, and employment of adults. Support groups, individual and family psychotherapy, physical therapy, occupational therapy, and preventive and preemptive rehabilitation may help to prevent functional decline and emotional distress, thereby improving quality of life (Lee, Onstad, et al., 2018). Complicating care is the fact that by the time chronic GVHD develops, many patients have returned to their local community and are at a distance from health care providers with expertise in the identification and management of the diverse manifestations of chronic GVHD.

Alternative approaches to the prevention, treatment, and control of GVHD are being developed and evaluated preclinically and clinically. They include the application of cytokine shields to decrease the inflammatory tissue responses thought to promote acute GVHD, identification of GVHD biomarkers, and more selective TCD and other graft engineering strategies. Gene transfer technologies are promising tools for manipulating donor T-cell immunity to enforce GVT or graft-versus-infection while preventing or controlling acute GVHD (Gooptu & Koreth, 2020).

Nursing Implications of Selected Immunosuppressants Used in Allogeneic Stem Cell Transplantation

Agent	Nursing Implications
Cyclosporine	• Bioavailability differs for the oral solution and capsule formulation. After a regimen is established, patients should be instructed not to change their formulation or brand. • Take with food. • Capsules have a foul odor: open to air before taking. • Instruct the patient to notify the health care team immediately if unable to take because of gastrointestinal side effects. • Monitor serum creatinine, blood urea nitrogen, potassium, magnesium, glucose, and triglyceride levels. • Monitor levels carefully in patients with renal or hepatic dysfunction. • Doses should be adjusted for renal dysfunction, as ordered. • Replete electrolytes as indicated. • Avoid grapefruit juice or grapefruit-containing products due to interference with pharmacokinetics. • Drug-drug interactions can lead to subtherapeutic or toxic cyclosporine levels. Patients should advise their health care providers of changes made in concurrent medications. • Cyclosporine trough levels should be drawn before administration of morning dose. • Tacrolimus should be discontinued for at least 24 h before cyclosporine is started.
Tacrolimus (Prograf)	• Take on an empty stomach. • Instruct patient to notify the health care team immediately if unable to take because of gastrointestinal side effects. • Monitor serum creatinine, blood urea nitrogen, potassium, magnesium, phosphorus, glucose, and triglyceride levels. • Monitor levels carefully in patients with renal or hepatic dysfunction. • Doses should be adjusted for renal dysfunction, as ordered. • Replete electrolytes as indicated. • Avoid grapefruit juice or grapefruit-containing products due to interference with pharmacokinetics. • Drug-drug interactions can lead to subtherapeutic or toxic tacrolimus levels. Patients should advise their health care providers of changes made in concurrent medications. • Tacrolimus trough levels should be drawn before administration of morning dose. • Cyclosporine should be discontinued for at least 24 h before tacrolimus is started.
Corticosteroids	• Consult physical therapy for proximal muscle-strengthening exercise program. • Monitor serum chemistries. • Instruct patient in strategies to prevent or treat hyperglycemia and in diabetic self-management. Consult with diabetes educator, as indicated. • Administer oral corticosteroids with food or milk to minimize gastrointestinal upset. • Administer H_2-blockers or proton pump inhibitors to decrease gastric acidity. • Consider need for antiviral, antibacterial, and antifungal prophylaxis. • May increase tacrolimus or cyclosporine levels. • Report complaints of visual changes and consult ophthalmology. • For patients on long-term steroids at risk for osteopenia, ensure regular dual-energy x-ray absorptiometric scans, calcium and vitamin D supplementation, and specific treatment for osteopenia with antiresorptive agents such as alendronate (Fosamax). • A tapering calendar specifying the dosage to be taken each day can help facilitate adherence by patients who are on tapering doses of steroids or an alternate-day steroid regimen.
MMF	• Take on an empty stomach. • Monitor CBC at regular intervals, and adjust dosage for pancytopenia, as ordered. • Monitor liver function tests (i.e., bilirubin and serum transaminases) at regular intervals, and adjust dosage for liver function abnormalities, as ordered. • Monitor plasma levels of mycophenolic acid (i.e., metabolite of MMF) to guide treatment of patients with renal dysfunction. • There may be decreased absorption when coadministered with magnesium oxide, aluminum- or magnesium-containing antacids, or cholestyramine.

Continued

Principles of Cancer Management

3

Nursing Implications of Selected Immunosuppressants Used in Allogeneic Stem Cell Transplantation—cont'd

Agent	Nursing Implications
Azathioprine	• Dose reduction required when given with allopurinol. • May lead to anemia and leukopenia when given with angiotensin-converting enzyme inhibitors; synergistic with other bone marrow suppressants. • Use with caution in patients with hepatic or renal impairment. • Teratogenic; advise patient and partner about the need for contraception.
Methotrexate	• Dose and schedule for methotrexate prophylaxis for GVHD varies by institution. • A common regimen is 5–15 mg/m^2 on days 1, 3, 6, and 11 after transplantation. • Dose may be adjusted or held for severe mucositis and renal or liver insufficiency. Dose may need to be adjusted for hypoalbuminemia. • Use with caution in patients with ascites or pleural or pericardial effusion due to risk of drug accumulation. • Consider the need to monitor methotrexate levels. • Wait until at least 24 h after stem cell infusion to give day +1 dose.
Infliximab (Remicade®)	• Monitor patient for development of infusion-related toxicities. • Consider premedication with acetaminophen and diphenhydramine. • Medications for treating hypersensitivity reactions (e.g., acetaminophen, antihistamines, corticosteroids, epinephrine) and supplemental oxygen should be available for immediate use in the event of a reaction. • Incompatible with polyvinyl chloride equipment or devices. Use glass infusion bottles and polyethylene-lined administration sets.
• Ruxolitinib • (Jakafi)	• Monitor CBC at regular intervals, and adjust dosage for pancytopenia, as ordered. • Monitor liver function tests (i.e., bilirubin and serum transaminases) at regular intervals, and adjust dosage for liver function abnormalities, as ordered. • Consider need for antiviral, antibacterial, and antifungal prophylaxis. • Monitor serum cholesterol and triglycerides every 4–6 weeks.
Antithymocyte globulin (Atgam [equine], Thymoglobulin [rabbit])	• Monitor patient closely during and after infusion for signs of serum sickness and anaphylaxis. • Consider premedication with corticosteroids, acetaminophen, and H$_1$- and H$_2$-blockers. • Medications for treating hypersensitivity reactions (e.g., acetaminophen, antihistamines, corticosteroids, epinephrine) and supplemental oxygen should be available for immediate use in the event of a reaction. • Evaluate need for blood pressure support (e.g., fluid boluses, dopamine, dobutamine). • Because transient and sometimes severe thrombocytopenia may occur after antithymocyte globulin administration in patients with platelet counts less than 100,000/µL, the platelet count should be evaluated 1 h after administration and as ordered and platelets transfused as indicated. • Produces rapid and prolonged lymphopenia; patients require broad antifungal, antibacterial, antiviral, and antiprotozoal prophylaxis for at least 4 months after treatment and continuing surveillance for CMV reactivation.
Alemtuzumab (Campath)	• Premedicate patient with acetaminophen and diphenhydramine. • Medications for treating hypersensitivity reactions (e.g., acetaminophen, antihistamines, corticosteroids, epinephrine) and supplemental oxygen should be available for immediate use in the event of a reaction. • Consider treatment with meperidine to control infusion-related rigors. • Administer fluid bolus as ordered to treat hypotension. • Produces rapid and prolonged lymphopenia; patients require broad antifungal, antibacterial, antiviral, and antiprotozoal prophylaxis for at least 4 months after treatment and continuing surveillance for CMV reactivation.
Rapamycin (Sirolimus)	• May suppress hematopoietic recovery if used in patients who have recently undergone high-dose therapy. • Oral bioavailability is variable and may be improved when administered with a high-fat meal. • Like tacrolimus and cyclosporine, it is metabolized through the cytochrome P450-3A system; anticipate drug-drug interactions.
Thalidomide	• Thalidomide is a potent teratogen and is contraindicated in patients who are or who are likely to become pregnant. A systematic counseling and education program, written informed consent, and participation in a confidential survey program at the start of treatment and throughout treatment are required for all patients receiving thalidomide. Men and women who are of childbearing potential must practice protected sex while on this drug. • Perform pregnancy test before initiating treatment and periodically throughout treatment course. • Obtain baseline electrocardiogram before treatment. • Thalidomide should not be started if the absolute neutrophil count is less than 750/mm^3, and therapy should be reevaluated if the absolute neutrophil count drops below this level. • Administer doses in the evening to minimize impact of drowsiness on lifestyle and safety. • Teach patient to use caution when taking thalidomide with other drugs that can cause drowsiness or neuropathy. • Teach patient to rise slowly from a supine position to avoid lightheadedness. • Teach patient to report immediately signs or symptoms suggesting peripheral neuropathy, including numbness or tingling in the hands or feet or the development of rash or skin ulcerations. These may require immediate cessation of the drug until the patient can be evaluated. • Teach patient to use protective measures (e.g., sunscreens, protective clothing) against exposure to ultraviolet light or sunlight. • Prevent constipation with a stool softener or mild laxative.
Methoxsalen (Oxsoralen)	• Patients who have received cytotoxic chemotherapy or radiation therapy and who are taking methoxsalen are at increased risk for skin cancers. • Toxicity increases with concurrent use of phenothiazines, thiazides, and sulfanilamides. • Instruct patient to take methoxsalen with milk or food and to divide the dose into two portions, taken approximately ½ h apart. • Severe burns may occur from sunlight or ultraviolet A exposure. • Pretreatment eye examinations are indicated to evaluate for cataracts. Repeat eye examinations should be performed every 6 months while patients are undergoing psoralen and ultraviolet A therapy.

Data from Sarantopoulos, S., Cardones, A. R., & Sullivan, K. M. (2019). How I treat refractory chronic graft versus host disease. *Blood, 133*(11), 1191–1200; Wikle Shapiro, T. J., & Kapadia, M. (2018). Chronic graft versus host disease. In Brown, V. (Ed.). *Hematopoietic stem cell transplantation for the pediatric oncologist*. Cham, Germany: Springer International Publishing.

Posttransplantation Relapse

Because HSCT is an intensive curative treatment for many high-risk malignancies, its failure to prevent relapse leaves few options for successful salvage treatment. Although the mortality rate due to relapse is high, some patients respond to transplantation and have sustained remissions, and some may have another chance of cure after DLI or a second HSCT.

The prognosis for relapsed hematologic malignancies after stem cell transplantation depends on four factors: the time elapsed between HSCT and relapse (i.e., relapses within 6 months have the worst prognosis); the disease type (i.e., chronic leukemias and some lymphomas have a possibility of cure with further treatment); the disease burden and site of relapse (i.e., improved success if disease is treated early); and the conditions of the first transplantation (i.e., superior outcomes for patients with an opportunity to increase the GVT effect or the intensity of conditioning in a second transplantation). These features guide further treatment toward modified second transplantations, chemotherapy, targeted antileukemia therapy, immunotherapy using DLI, or palliative care (Bazarbachi et al., 2020; Zhan, 2019).

Treatment of relapsed diseases continues to evolve. A classic approach is to rapidly withdraw immunosuppressive agents in an attempt to trigger a GVT effect. DLIs are also an option for patients without rapidly progressing relapses, whose donors are readily available to donate lymphocytes. DLIs may be given alone or following chemotherapy. GVT effect can reverse relapse when given early following allogeneic HSCT. Second myeloablative or reduced-intensity HSCT after allogeneic HSCT carries significant TRM, and few patients are candidates due to organ dysfunction, inability to achieve remission (or near remission) status, or poor performance status. More clinical trials are needed to determine which patients might benefit from a second transplantation.

Ongoing clinical trials are under way using cellular adoptive immunotherapy after allogeneic HSCT to harness the powerful GVT effect of the donor's immune system against residual tumor cells. Some of these trials include ex vivo activated T cells (i.e., activated DLI given as consolidation to prevent relapse), cytokine-induced killer cells, natural killer cells, and antigen-specific cytotoxic T cells (Bazarbachi et al., 2020; Zhan, 2019).

Patients with relapse after HSCT who are not eligible for DLI, CAR T-cell therapy, or clinical trials, may choose palliative supportive care. This can be a difficult decision. Information should be provided to patients and their families so that informed decisions regarding end-of-life care can be made. If patients desire to receive no further treatment, nurses can help facilitate their transition to palliative and hospice care (Zhan, 2019).

Chimeric Antigen Receptor T-Cell Therapy

Patients with certain subtypes (CD19 positive) of refractory or relapsed ALL are difficult to treat but have benefited over the past 5 to 10 years from the use of adoptive transfer of T cells engineered to express a CAR. CAR T-cell therapy has emerged as a powerful, targeted immunotherapy, showing striking responses in patients with highly refractory diseases. CAR T-cell therapy is also yielding positive outcomes now in various hematologic malignancies, beyond B-cell acute lymphoblastic leukemia, that includes CLL, lymphoma, and multiple myeloma. CAR T-cell therapy uses gene transfer to reprogram the patient's own autologous T cells to recognize and eliminate cancerous cells by targeting and interacting with tumor-associated antigens. The CAR T-cell therapy process is illustrated in the figure below.

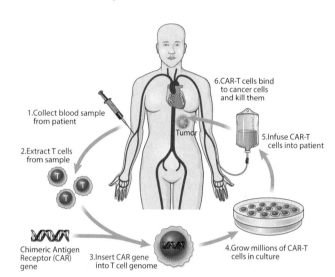

Autologous CART T-Cell Therapy Process. (From Chabner, D. (2021). *The language of medicine* (12th ed.). Elsevier.)

The process begins with the collection of the patient's autologous T cells via leukapheresis. The cells are then sent to an institutionally designated CAR T-cell manufacturing facility for "reprograming." CAR-coded viral DNA is incorporated into the patients T cells at the manufacturing facility, transforming them into CAR-T cells. The modified T cells are then allowed to multiply before reinfusion back into the patient. Patients are treated with a short course of preparatory chemotherapy aimed at making space for the cells to expand, and then reinfused. The receptors on these modified cells are attracted to CD19 antigen-positive (cancer) cells and destroy them.

The use of CAR T-cell therapies is on the rise, and nursing plays an integral role in the care of these patients. Like patients who undergo HSCT, specialized training in the care of these complex patients is necessary for successful patient outcomes. These patients require high levels of close monitoring and vigilant nursing care during their treatment courses. Prompt toxicity intervention is key to improved patient outcomes (Baer, 2021). The most common adverse events associated with CAR T-cell treatment are cytokine release syndrome (CRS), severe neurologic symptoms, and permanent B-cell aplasia.

CRS is an acute complication of CAR T-cell therapy that can be life-threatening and therefore requires hospitalization. CRS initially manifests with fever and can progress to life-threatening capillary leak with hypoxia and hypotension. The clinical signs of CRS correlate with T-cell activation and high levels of cytokines, especially IL-6 (Frey & Porter, 2019). CRS can either be self-limited (requiring only supportive care with antipyretics and intravenous fluids) or it may require intervention with anticytokine-directed therapy such as corticosteroids or tocilizumab. CRS occurs within 1 to 14 days after infusion depending on the product, clinical trial design, and population being treated. The duration of CRS is variable and dependent on intervention, with full resolution typically by 2 to 3 weeks after CAR-T infusion (Frey & Porter, 2019).

Fevers are a hallmark of CRS and can range from low to high grade and may persist for days or weeks. Acetaminophen is used for comfort but does not usually relieve fever. Associated symptoms are tachycardia, chills, anorexia, nausea, and vomiting, which can be managed with supportive care. If patients develop myalgia or headaches, intermittent IV opioids can be used.

More severe symptoms are capillary leak syndrome and hypotension, which can lead to pulmonary inflammation and hence the need for oxygen support and, in severe cases, mechanical ventilation. Management of hypotension generally includes IV fluid boluses but may move quickly to vasopressor support to minimize the risk of massive pulmonary edema and poor organ perfusion (Baer, 2021). Patients with severe CRS are generally managed in the critical care setting. CRS may also lead to severe coagulopathy, often requiring transfusion with cryoprecipitate and fresh frozen plasma. Inflammation from CRS and increased cytokine production can change hemodynamics, decreasing renal and liver blood flow and resulting in acute kidney injury and sometimes liver failure.

Because CRS inflammation is reversible, the treatment goal is to control symptoms without interfering with the T cells' ability to destroy cancer cells. First-line treatment is always supportive, such as antipyretics, pain medications, antiemetics, vasopressor support, and oxygen supplementation.

Patients who demonstrate signs of early multisystem organ failure require more aggressive anti-inflammatory interventions. Tocilizumab is a monoclonal antibody used in moderate to severe cases of CRS that binds to the IL-6 receptor, thereby preventing further acute inflammation. Tocilizumab does not seem to affect the efficacy of the infused CAR T cells and tends to quickly resolve symptoms. Institutions that perform CAR T-cell therapy are required to have an ample supply of tocilizumab on hand before CAR T cells can be infused back into patients.

Systemic IV steroids directly block T-cell activation and dampen the tumor-destroying benefits of CAR T-cell therapy. Use of systemic steroids is only indicated for severe cases of CRS when other interventions, including tocilizumab, are unsuccessful (Frey & Porter, 2019).

CAR T cells have also been found in the cerebral spinal fluid (CSF) and may cause some patients to develop encephalopathy. Symptoms include confusion, hallucination, delirium, and seizures. Encephalopathy cannot be reversed by any specific therapy, but it is usually self-resolving and is not associated with long-term neurologic effects. Patients at risk for seizures should receive prophylactic anticonvulsant therapy.

Since CAR T-cell therapy targets antigens found on the surface of B cells, these cells destroy not only cancerous B cells but also the patient's normal B cells. Therefore, B cell aplasia (low numbers of B cells or absent B cells) is an expected result of successful CD19-specific CAR T-cell treatment and has served as a useful indicator of ongoing CAR T-cell activity. This effect results in the inability to make the necessary antibodies that protect against infection. Lifelong antibody replacement with either intravenous or subcutaneous immunoglobulin replacement is expected for survivors of successful CAR T-cell therapy.

Complete remission rates as high as 40% to 90% have been reported in children and adults with relapsed and refractory B-cell ALL and B-cell lymphoma treated with CAR-modified T cells targeting the B-cell–specific antigen CD19 (Safarzadeh Kozani et al., 2021). Research that focuses on other antigens is ongoing. The role of CAR therapy beyond CD19 is also ensured by the ongoing development and early promise of CARs targeting other antigens and malignancies. Studies examining the use of CAR technology are ongoing for relapsed or refractory AML, T-cell malignancies, metastatic melanoma, and various other solid tumor are ongoing and expanding the therapeutic benefits of "self-derived" immunocellular therapies to cure certain cancers.

Long-Term Complications of Hematopoietic Stem Cell Transplantation: Assessment, Prevention, and Management

Long-term disease-free survival after HSCT has greatly improved, resulting in an expanding number of long-term survivors. Continuous changes in the transplantation process and in the types of patients selected are responsible for the evolving pattern of late effects after HSCT over time. Relevant changes include the avoidance of TBI conditioning when possible, older patients receiving transplants, the increasing use of unrelated and haploidentical donors, and the introduction of RIC. The detection of an increasing number of late effects should not be considered a drawback in HSCT. Late complications may be experienced months or years after HSCT.

Although patients often are cured of their initial disease, several malignant and nonmalignant late effects can cause substantial morbidity and have a considerable impact on the health status and quality of life of long-term HSCT survivors. Management of late effects after transplantation is increasingly important for a growing number of long-term survivors, which is estimated to be nearly one million worldwide. Many studies have shown that transplant survivors suffer from significant late effects that adversely affect morbidity, mortality, working status, and quality of life. Late effects include diseases of the cardiovascular, pulmonary, and endocrine systems, dysfunction of the thyroid gland, gonads, liver and kidneys, infertility, iron overload, bone diseases, infection, solid tumors, and neuropsychological effects. The box below demonstrates the late effects seen in HSCT survivors. The leading causes of late mortality include recurrent malignancy, lung diseases, infection, secondary cancers, and chronic GVHD.

The potential for fragmentation of care exists based on the significant number of specialists required to care for HSCT patients who suffer from late effects. The multidisciplinary team often consists of the transplant team, primary oncologist, and many medical specialists, such as dentistry, gynecology, reproductive endocrinology, pulmonary medicine, cardiology, endocrinology, and orthopedics/physical medicine. Counseling should include self-examination for early cancer detection, compliance with routine testing or screening, and advice for healthy lifestyle behaviors.

Beyond immediate survival, allogeneic HSCT is a lifelong commitment between long-term survivors and the transplantation team, involving the recipient's family and general health care providers. Proper information about life after HSCT should be provided to the whole community, which plays a key role in the social reinsertion of long-term survivors. HSCT patients require lifelong surveillance and preventive care for some complications, including second malignancies, cardiovascular and pulmonary effects, and relapse. Most transplantation centers have protocol-specific requirements for continued follow-up care, and the frequency of clinic visits is determined by the nature of the patient's complications (Bhatia et al., 2017). The table on the next page summarizes guidelines for screening for and evaluation of the potential late effects of HSCT. Guidelines for surveillance and follow-up are available to direct long-term supportive care, fertility preservation, healthy nutrition, and physical activity for HSCT patients (Dandekar, 2018; Inamoto & Lee, 2017). Routine follow-up should include the promotion of a healthy lifestyle and risk reduction strategies, including nutrition, exercise, safe sexual practices, breast and colorectal screening, avoidance of sun exposure, and smoking cessation.

Late Effects of Blood and Marrow Transplantation

Eyes/Ears
- Cataract
- Diminished hearing
- Microvascular retinopathy Sicca syndrome

Endocrine
- Abnormal glucose metabolism
- Adrenal insufficiency
- Growth retardation
- Hypothyroidism
- Obesity
- Ovarian failure
- Hypogonadism

Cardiovascular
- Cardiac arrhythmias
- Cardiac valve abnormalities
- Coronary artery, cerebrovascular and peripheral arterial disease
- Hypercholesterolemia/lipidemia
- Hypertension
- Pericarditis
- Reduction in ejection fraction/heart failure
- Thromboembolic event

Genital/Sexual
- Anorgasmia (females)
- Dyspareunia/vaginal dryness (females)
- Ejaculation disorders (males)
- Erectile dysfunction (males)

Secondary Cancers
- Hematologic malignancies
- Cancers of the head, neck and esophagus
- Upper gastrointestinal and colorectal cancers
- Thyroid cancer
- Gynecological cancer

Musculoskeletal
- Arthritis
- Osteopenia/osteoporosis
- Osteonecrosis
- Peripheral neuropathy

Pulmonary
- Asthma
- Bronchiolitis obliterans
- Pulmonary hypertension

Psychosocial
- Anxiety
- Depression
- Posttraumatic stress disorder

Renal
- Chronic kidney disease
- Thrombotic microangiopathy
- BK virus nephropathy

Data from Diesch-Furlanetto, T., Gabriel. M., Zajac-Spychala, O., et al. (2021). Late effects after haematopoietic stem cell transplantation in ALL, long-term follow-up and transition: A step into adult life. *Frontiers in Pediatrics, 9*, 773895; Park, S. S., Park, S. H., & Han, S. (2022). Risk of secondary nonhematologic malignancies after allogeneic stem cell transplantation: A nationwide case-control cohort study. *International Journal of Cancer, 151*(7), 1024–1032; Smeland, K., Holte, H., Fagerli, U. M., et al. (2022). Total late effect burden in long-term lymphoma survivors after high-dose therapy with autologous stem-cell transplant and its effect on health-related quality of life. *Haematologica, 107*(11), 2698–2707.

Evaluation and Screening of Late Effects of Hematopoietic Stem Cell Transplantation

System or Dimension	Possible Late Effects	Evaluation or Screening
Disease status	Relapse or recurrence	Determined on the basis of the site of original disease (CBC, periodic imaging) Evaluation for minimal residual disease as indicated
Engraftment	Graft failure or marrow dysfunction with cytopenias	CBC with differential count Bone marrow aspirate and biopsy Engraftment/chimerism studies Viral studies (CMV, human herpesvirus 6, parvovirus PCR)
Immunologic function or recovery	Disorders of B- and T-lymphocyte quantity and function Hypogammaglobulinemia	CD4 and CD8 lymphocyte subsets Mitogen stimulation studies Quantitative immunoglobulin levels Vaccination titers
Cardiopulmonary	Interstitial pneumonitis Bronchiolitis obliterans Hypertension, cardiomyopathy, pericardial damage, peripheral vascular disease	Chest radiograph Pulmonary function tests with single-breath diffusing capacity Electrocardiogram Echocardiogram History and physical examination
Neurologic	Peripheral and autonomic neuropathies Cognitive changes (shortened attention span, difficulty with concentration) Leukoencephalopathy Ototoxicity	Health history Neurologic examination Neuropsychological testing Rehabilitation medicine Audiologic testing
Gastrointestinal	Liver dysfunction Chronic GVHD Malabsorption syndromes	Liver function tests Hepatitis B serologies, hepatitis C PCR, qualitative Upper and lower gastrointestinal endoscopies Transjugular liver biopsy
Genitourinary	Renal dysfunction Radiation nephritis Hematuria, proteinuria Cancer of the bladder	Blood urea nitrogen, creatinine levels Urinalysis with microscopy 24-h urine for creatinine clearance and total protein, if indicated
Thyroid function	Hypothyroidism	Thyroid-stimulating hormone, triiodothyronine, thyroxine, free thyroxine
Gonadal function	Decreased production of gonadal hormones	Luteinizing hormone, follicle-stimulating hormone, estradiol (women) Pelvic examination Luteinizing hormone, follicle-stimulating hormone, testosterone (men)
Hypothalamic-pituitary	Abnormal pituitary gland function	Prolactin, follicle-stimulating hormone, luteinizing hormone, thyroid-stimulating hormone, growth hormone levels (children)
Metabolic syndrome	Increased blood pressure Elevated glucose level Central obesity Abnormal cholesterol levels	Fasting glucose, lipid profile
Ophthalmic	Cataracts	Ophthalmologic examination that includes slit-lamp examination and Schirmer test
Dental or oral cavity	Sicca syndrome Caries Periodontal disease Xerostomia Oral malignancy	Regular dental evaluations Meticulous attention to oral hygiene Fluoride gels or rinses
Musculoskeletal	Osteoporosis Avascular necrosis Myopathy	Dual-energy x-ray absorptiometry (DEXA) scan Magnetic resonance imaging (MRI) if pain in a joint, limited range of motion, or a limp Neurologic examination Electromyelogram

Evaluation and Screening of Late Effects of Hematopoietic Stem Cell Transplantation—cont'd

System or Dimension	Possible Late Effects	Evaluation or Screening
Second malignancy	Nonmelanoma skin cancer	Complete physical examination with biopsy of suspicious lesions Skin photographs may help to monitor status
	Breast cancer (especially in patients with history of chest irradiation)	Breast MRI, mammogram, self-examination
	Thyroid cancer	History and physical examination Ultrasonography Iodine-131 scan
	Treatment-related acute leukemia	CBC with differential count Bone marrow aspirate and biopsy
	Myelodysplastic syndrome	Bone marrow aspirate and biopsy (if CBC abnormal), cytogenetics
	PTLD	CT if PTLD is suspected Epstein-Barr viral load by PCR weekly in first few months after allogeneic hematopoietic stem cell transplantation CD4 count >200 cells/mm^3
	Cancer of the uterine cervix	Gynecologic examination with Papanicolaou smear
	Cancer of the bladder	Urinalysis with microscopy to detect microhematuria, urine cytology, follow-up cystoscopy
Integumentary	Increased incidence of benign and malignant nevi	Complete physical examination Skin biopsy of suspicious lesions
Psychologic or rehabilitation quality of life	Changes in body image, roles, family relationships, lifestyle, occupation, discrimination, overcoming stigma, living with compromises, coping with symptoms	Assessment of individual adjustment, achievement of normal developmental tasks, marital stress, sexual function, body image, rehabilitation needs, symptom distress through systematic, and structured evaluation

From Deeg, H. J. (2007). How I treat refractory acute graft versus host disease. *Blood, 109,* 4119–4126; Tierny, D. K., & Robinson, T. (2013). Long-term care of hematopoietic cell transplant survivors. In S. A. Ezzone (Ed.). *Hematopoietic stem cell transplantation: A manual for nursing practice* (2nd ed., pp. 251–267). Oncology Nursing Society; Roziakova, L., & Mladosievicova, B. (2010). Endocrine late effects after hematopoietic T stem cell transplantation. *Oncology Research, 18*(11–12), 607–615.

References

Ahmad, N., Pillinger, K., & Shahid, Z. (2019). Prophylaxis and management of infectious complications after hematopoietic cell transplantation. In Q. Bashir, & M. Hamadani (Eds.), *Hematopoietic cell transplantation for malignant conditions* (pp. 349–367). Amsterdam, The Netherlands: Elsevier.

Anton-Vazquez, V., Mehra, V., Mbisa, J. L., Bradshaw, D., Basu, T. N., Daly, M. L., … Zuckerman, M. (2020). Challenges of aciclovir-resistant HSV infection in allogeneic bone marrow transplant recipients. *Journal of Clinical Virology, 128,* 104421.

Arora, D., Tiwari, A. K., Misra, R., Dara, R. C., Aggarwal1, G., Sood, N., & Bhardwaj, G. (2017). Total leukocyte count-based predictor tool for calculating hematopoietic progenitor cell dose in bone-marrow harvest. *Global Journal of Transfusion Medicine, 2*(2), 97–101.

Auletta, J. J., Kou, J., Chen, M., & Shaw, B. E. (2021). *Current use and outcome of hematopoietic stem cell transplantation: CIBMTR US summary slides, 2021.* CIBMTR Summary Slides - HCT Trends and Survival Data.

Baer, B. (2021). CAR T-Cell therapy: Updates in nursing management. *Clinical Journal of Oncology Nursing, 25*(3), 255–258.

Ballen, K. (2017). Update on umbilical cord blood transplantation. *F1000Research, 6,* 1556.

Barlow, A. (2021). Cytomegalovirus management in allogeneic hematopoietic stem cell transplant recipients. *U.S. Pharmacist, 46*(4), HS2–HS9. https://www.uspharmacist.com/article/cytomegalovirus-management-in-allogeneic-hematopoietic-stem-cell-transplant-recipients.

Bazarbachi, A., Schmid, C., Labopin, M., Beelen, D., Wolfgang Blau, I., Potter, V., … Mohty, M. (2020). Evaluation of trends and prognosis over time in patients with AML relapsing after allogeneic hematopoietic cell transplant reveals improved survival for young patients in recent years. *Clinical Cancer Research, 26*(24), 6475–6482.

Bernasconi, P., Colombo, A. A., Caldera, D., & Borsani, O. (2019). Veno-occlusive disease (VOD) after hematopoietic stem cell transplant (HSCT): Always a catastrophic illness? *Blood, 134*(Suppl_1), 5649.

Be the Match. (n.d.). *Donating peripheral blood stem cells.* Be the Match. Available at https://bethematch.org/support-the-cause/donate-bone-marrow/donation-process/donating-pbsc/ (accessed June 17, 2022).

Bhatia, S., Armenian, S. H., & Landier, W. (2017). How I monitor long-term and late effects after blood or marrow transplantation. *Blood, 130*(11), 1302–1314.

Bilgin, Y. M. (2021). Use of plerixafor for stem cell mobilization in the setting of autologous and allogeneic stem cell transplantations: An update. *Journal of Blood Medicine, 12,* 403–412.

Bonifazi, F., Barbato, F., Ravaioli, F., Sessa, M., Defrancesco, I., Arpinati, M., Cavo, M., & Colecchia, A. (2020). Diagnosis and treatment of VOD/SOS after allogeneic hematopoietic stem cell transplantation. *Frontiers in Immunology, 11,* 489.

Bride, K. L., Patel, N. S., & Freedman, J. L. (2018). Acute graft versus host disease: Diagnosis, prophylaxis, and treatment. In V. Brown (Ed.), *Hematopoietic stem cell transplantation for the pediatric oncologist* (pp. 257–267). Cham, Germany: Springer International Publishing.

Brown, V. (2018). Hepatotoxicity in the peri-HSCT period. In V. Brown (Ed.), *Hematopoietic stem cell transplantation for the pediatric oncologist* (pp. 215–233). Springer International Publishing.

Centers for Disease Control and Prevention, Infectious Disease Society of America, American Society of Blood and Marrow Transplantation. (2000). Guidelines for preventing opportunistic infections among hematopoietic stem cell transplant recipients. *Morbidity and Mortality Weekly Report. Recommendations and Reports, 49*(RR-10), 1–125, CE1-7 https://www.cdc.gov/mmwr/preview/mmwrhtml/rr4910a1.htm.

Chao, N. J. (2021, July 14). In R. S. Negrin, & A. G. Rosmarin (Eds.), *Survival, quality-of-life, and late complications after hematopoietic cell transplantation in adults.* UpToDate https://www.uptodate.com/contents/survival-quality-of-life-and-late-complications-after-hematopoietic-cell-transplantation-in-adults.

Cho, S. Y., Lee, D. G., & Kim, H. J. (2019). Cytomegalovirus infections after hematopoietic stem cell transplantation: Current status and future immunotherapy. *International Journal of Molecular Sciences, 20*(11), 2666.

Connelly-Smith, L. (2020). Donor evaluation for hematopoietic stem and progenitor cell collection. In S. A. Abutalib, A. Padmanabhan, H. P. Pham, & N. Worel (Eds.), *Best practices of apheresis in hematopoietic cell transplantation* (pp. 23–49). Springer.

Dandekar, S. (2018). Life after HSCT: survivorship, and long-term issues. In V. Brown (Ed.), *Hematopoietic stem cell transplantation for the pediatric oncologist* (pp. 385–401). Springer International Publishing.

Dehn, J., Spellman, S., Hurley, C. K., Shaw, B. E., Barker, J. N., Burns, L. J., … Pidala, J. (2019). Selection of unrelated donors and cord blood units for hematopoietic cell transplantation: Guidelines from the NMDP/CIBMTR. *Blood, 134*(12), 924–934.

Drexler, B., Buser, A., Infanti, L., Stehle, G., Halter, J., & Holbro, A. (2020). Extracorporeal photopheresis in graft-versus-host disease. *Transfusion Medicine and Hemotherapy, 47*(3), 214–225.

Dykewicz, C. A., & Centers for Disease Control and Prevention (U.S.), Infectious Diseases Society of America, American Society of Blood and Marrow Transplantation. (2001). Summary of the guidelines for preventing opportunistic infections among hematopoietic stem cell transplant recipients. *Clinical Infectious Diseases, 33*(2), 139–144.

Einsele, H., Ljungman, P., & Boeckh, M. (2020). How I treat CMV reactivation after allogeneic hematopoietic stem cell transplantation. *Blood, 135*(19), 1619–1629.

Fontana, L., & Strasfeld, L. (2019). Respiratory virus infections of the stem cell transplant recipient and the hematologic malignancy patient. *Infectious Disease Clinics of North America, 33*(2), 523–544.

Foundation for the Accreditation of Cellular Therapy (FACT). (2021). *Patient care and laboratory procedures.* Available at http://www.factwebsite.org/.

Frey, N., & Porter, D. (2019). Cytokine release syndrome with chimeric antigen receptor T cell therapy. *Biology of Blood and Marrow Transplantation: Journal of the American Society for Blood and Marrow Transplantation, 25*(4), e123–e127.

Fuchs, E. J., & Luznik, L. (2021). *HLA-haploidentical hematopoietic cell transplantation.* UpToDate. Available at https://www.uptodate.com/contents/hla-haploidentical-hematopoietic-cell-transplantation.

Gagelmann, N., & Kröger, N. (2021). Dose intensity for conditioning in allogeneic hematopoietic cell transplantation: Can we recommend "when and for whom" in 2021? *Haematologica, 106*(7), 1794–1804.

Granot, N., & Storb, R. (2020). History of hematopoietic cell transplantation: Challenges and progress. *Haematologica, 105*(12), 2716–2729.

Gupta, A. O., & Wagner, J. E. (2020). Umbilical cord blood transplants: Current status and evolving therapies. *Frontiers in Pediatrics, 8*, 570282.

Gooptu, M., & Koreth, J. (2020). Translational and clinical advances in acute graft-versus-host disease. *Haematologica, 105*(11), 2550–2560.

Hamilton, B. K. (2018). Current approaches to prevent and treat GVHD after allogeneic stem cell transplantation. *Hematology. American Society of Hematology. Education Program, 2018*(1), 228–235.

Herrick, A. (2021). Introduction to CAR T cell therapy part 1: Background & Current Development Landscape. *Premier Research.* https://premier-research.com/blog-a-brief-introduction-to-car-t-cell-therapy.

Hutt, D. (2018). Engraftment, graft failure, and rejection. In M. Kenyon, & A. Babic (Eds.), *The European blood and marrow transplantation textbook for nurses: Under the auspices of EBMT* (pp. 259–270). Cham, Germany: Springer.

Inamoto, Y., & Lee, S. J. (2017). Late effects of blood and marrow transplantation. *Haematologica, 102*(4), 614–625.

Kaeuferle, T., Krauss, R., Blaeschke, F., Willier, S., & Feuchtinger, T. (2019). Strategies of adoptive T-cell transfer to treat refractory viral infections post allogeneic stem cell transplantation. *Journal of Hematology & Oncology, 12*(1), 13.

Kapadia, M., & Wilke Shapiro, T. (2018). Pulmonary complications associated with HSCT. In V. Brown (Ed.), *Hematopoietic stem cell transplantation for the pediatric oncologist* (pp. 301–325). Cham, Germany: Springer.

Khawaja, F., Chemaly, R. F., Dadwal, S., Pergam, S. A., Wingard, J., Auletta, J., … Papanicolaou, G. (2022). *ASH-ASTCT COVID-19 Vaccination for HCT and CAR T Cell recipients: Frequently asked questions.* American Society of Hematology. Available at https://www.hematology.org/covid-19/ash-astct-covid-19-vaccination-for-hct-and-car-t-cell-recipients.

Kurosawa, S., Mizuno, S., Arai, Y., Masuko, M., Kanda, J., Kohno, K., … Yanada, M. (2021). Syngeneic hematopoietic stem cell transplantation for acute myeloid leukemia: A propensity score-matched analysis. *Blood Cancer Journal, 11*(9), 159.

Lai, X., Liu, L., Zhang, Z., Shi, L., Yang, G., Wu, M., … Li, Q. (2021). Hepatic veno-occlusive disease/sinusoidal obstruction syndrome after hematopoietic stem cell transplantation for thalassemia major: Incidence, management, and outcome. *Bone Marrow Transplantation, 56*(7), 1635–1641.

Lee, C. J., Savani, B. N., & Ljungman, P. (2018). Varicella Zoster Virus reactivation in adult survivors of hematopoietic cell transplantation: How do we best protect our patients? *Biology of Blood and Marrow Transplantation, 24*(9), 1783–1787.

Lee, S. J. (2017). Classification systems for chronic graft-versus-host disease. *Blood, 129*(1), 30–37.

Lee, S. J., Onstad, L., Chow, E. J., Shaw, B. E., Jim, H. S. L., Syrjala, K. L., … Flowers, M. E. (2018). Patient-reported outcomes and health status associated with chronic graft-versus-host disease. *Haematologica, 103*(9), 1535–1541.

Ljungman, P., Mikulska, M., de la Camara, R., Basak, G. W., Chabannon, C., Corbacioglu, S., … European Society for Blood and Marrow Transplantation. (2020). The challenge of COVID-19 and hematopoietic cell transplantation; EBMT recommendations for management of hematopoietic cell transplant recipients, their donors, and patients undergoing CAR T-cell therapy. *Bone Marrow Transplantation, 55*(11), 2071–2076.

Lum, S. H., Hoenig, M., Gennery, A. R., & Slatter, M. A. (2019). Conditioning regimens for hematopoietic cell transplantation in primary immunodeficiency. *Current Allergy and Asthma Reports, 19*(11), 52.

Malard, F., Huang, X. J., & Sim, J. (2020). Treatment and unmet needs in steroid-refractory acute graft-versus-host disease. *Leukemia, 34*(5), 1229–1240.

Martin, P. J., Rizzo, J. D., Wingard, J. R., Ballen, K., Curtin, P. T., Cutler, C., … Carpenter, P. A. (2012). First- and second-line systemic treatment of acute graft-versus-host disease: recommendations of the American Society of Blood and Marrow Transplantation. *Biology of Blood and Marrow Transplantation, 18*(8), 1150–1163.

McCurdy, S. R., & Luznik, L. (2019). How we perform haploidentical stem cell transplantation with posttransplant cyclophosphamide. *Blood, 134*(21), 1802–1810.

Metheny, L., Politikos, I., Ballen, K. K., Rezvani, A. R., Milano, F., Barker, J. N., … American Society for Transplantation and Cellular Therapy Cord Blood Special Interest Group. (2021). Guidelines for adult patient selection and conditioning regimens in cord blood transplant recipients with hematologic malignancies and aplastic anemia. *Transplantation and Cellular Therapy, 27*(4), 286–291.

Mohty, M., Blaise, D., Peffault de Latour, R., Labopin, M., Bourhis, J. H., Bruno, B., … Dalle, J. H. (2023). Real-world use of defibrotide for veno-occlusive disease/sinusoidal obstruction syndrome: The DEFIFrance Registry Study. *Bone Marrow Transplantation, 58*(4), 367–376. https://doi.org/10.1038/s41409-022-01900-6.

Mohty, M., Malard, F., Abecassis, M., Aerts, E., Alaskar, A. S., Aljurf, M., … Carreras, E. (2015). Sinusoidal obstruction syndrome/veno-occlusive disease: Current situation and perspectives—A position statement from the European Society for Blood and Marrow Transplantation (EBMT). *Bone Marrow Transplantation, 50*(6), 781–789. https://doi.org/10.1038/bmt.2015.52.

Mohty, M., Malard, F., Abecasis, M., Aerts, E., Alaskar, A. S., Aljurf, M., … Carreras, E. (2020). Prophylactic, preemptive, and curative treatment for sinusoidal obstruction syndrome/veno-occlusive disease in adult patients: A position statement from an international expert group. *Bone Marrow Transplantation, 55*(3), 485–495.

National Library of Medicine. (2021). *Double cord versus haploidentical (BMT CTN 1101). ClinicalTrails.gov.* Available at https://clinicaltrials.gov/ct2/show/NCT01597778.

National Marrow Donor Program (NMDP). (2021). *Marrow donor program.* Be The Match. Available at https://bethematchclinical.org/about-us/what-we-do/our-registry/.

Negrin, R. S. (2021, January 12). *Donor selection for hematopoietic cell transplantation.* In N. J. Chao, & A. G. Rosmarin (Eds.), UptoDate. Available at https://www.uptodate.com/contents/donor-selection-for-hematopoietic-cell-transplantation.

Nierengarten, M. B. (2021). Poor overall survival in bone marrow transplant patients with COVID-19. *Cancer, 127*(21), 3919.

Norkin, M., & Wingard, J. R. (2017). Recent advances in hematopoietic stem cell transplantation. *F1000Research, 6*, 870.

Pereira, M. R., Pouch, S. M., & Scully, B. (2019). Infections in allogeneic stem cell transplantation. In A. Safdar (Ed.), *Principles and practice of transplant infectious diseases.* New York, NY: Springer.

Penack, P. O., Marchetti, M., Ruutu, T., Aljurf, M., Bacigalupo, A., Bonifazi, F., … Basak, G. W. (2020). Prophylaxis and management of graft versus host disease after stem-cell transplantation for haematological malignancies: Updated consensus recommendations of the European Society for Blood and Marrow Transplantation. *The Lancet. Haematology, 7*(2), 157–167.

Rahi, M. S., Jindal, V., Pednekar, P., Parekh, J., Gunasekaran, K., Sharma, S., … Jaiyesimi, I. A. (2021). Fungal infections in hematopoietic stem-cell transplant patients: A review of epidemiology, diagnosis, and management. *Therapeutic Advances in Infectious Disease, 8.* 20499361211039050.

Roldan, E., Perales, M. A., & Barba, P. (2019). Allogeneic stem cell transplantation with CD34+ cell selection. *Clinical Hematology International*, *1*(3), 154–160. https://doi.org/10.2991/chi.d.190613.001. PMID: 34595425; PMCID: PMC8432362.

Ru, Y., Zhang, X., Song, T., Ding, Y., Zhu, Z., Fan, Y., … Wu, D. (2020). Epstein-Barr virus reactivation after allogeneic hematopoietic stem cell transplantation: Multifactorial impact on transplant outcomes. *Bone Marrow Transplantation*, *55*(9), 1754–1762. https://doi.org/10.1038/s41409-020-0831-7.

Safarzadeh Kozani, P., Safarzadeh Kozani, P., & Rahbarizadeh, F. (2021). CAR-T cell therapy in T-cell malignancies: Is success a low-hanging fruit? *Stem Cell Research & Therapy*, *12*(1), 527.

Saidu, N. E. B., Bonini, C., Dickinson, A., Grce, M., Inngjerdingen, M., Koehl, U., … Galimberti, S. (2020). New approaches for the treatment of chronic graft-versus-host disease: Current status and future directions. *Frontiers in Immunology*, *11*, 578314.

Sarantopoulos, S., Cardones, A. R., & Sullivan, K. M. (2019). How I treat refractory chronic graft-versus-host disease. *Blood*, *133*(11), 1191–1200.

Schoemans, H. M., Lee, S. J., Ferrara, J. L., Wolff, D., Levine, J. E., Schultz, K. R., … EBMT (European Society for Blood and Marrow Transplantation) Transplant Complications Working Party and the "EBMT–NIH (National Institutes of Health)–CIBMTR (Center for International Blood and Marrow Transplant Research) GvHD Task Force". (2018). EBMT-NIH-CIBMTR Task Force position statement on standardized terminology & guidance for graft-versus-host disease assessment. *Bone Marrow Transplantation*, *53*(11), 1401–1415.

Sharma, A., Bhatt, N. S., St Martin, A., Abid, M. B., Bloomquist, J., Chemaly, R. F., … Shah, G. L. (2021). Clinical characteristics and outcomes of COVID-19 in haematopoietic stem-cell transplantation recipients: An observational cohort study. *Lancet Haematology.*, *8*(3), 185–193.

Shoham, S., & Marr, K. (2017). Viral infections after bone marrow transplant. *Cancer Therapy Advisor*. Available at https://www.cancertherapyadvisor.com/home/decision-support-in-medicine/hematology/viral-infections-after-bone-marrow-transplant/.

Singhal, S., Powles, R., Kulkarni, S., Treleaven, J., Sirohi, B., Millar, B., … Mehta, J. (2000). Comparison of marrow and blood cell yields from the same donors in a double-blind, randomized study of allogeneic marrow *vs* blood stem cell transplantation. *Bone Marrow Transplantation*, *25*(5), 501–505.

Song, Y., Yin, Z., Ding, J., & Wu, T. (2021). Reduced intensity conditioning followed by allogeneic hematopoietic stem cell transplantation is a good choice for acute myeloid leukemia and myelodysplastic syndrome: A meta-analysis of randomized controlled trials. *Frontiers in Oncology*, *11*, 708727.

Styczyński, J., Tridello, G., Koster, L., Iacobelli, S., van Biezen, A., van der Werf, S., … Infectious Diseases Working Party EBMT. (2020). Death after hematopoietic stem cell transplantation: Changes over calendar year time, infections and associated factors. *Bone Marrow Transplantation*, *55*(1), 126–136.

Wang, X., Patel, S. A., Haddadin, M., & Cerny, J. (2021). Post-allogeneic hematopoietic stem cell transplantation viral reactivations and viremias: A focused review on human herpesvirus-6, BK virus and adenovirus. *Therapeutic Advances in Infectious Disease*, *8*, 1–20.

Ward, K. M., Hill, J. A., Hubacek, P., de la Camara, R., Crocchiolo, R., Einsele, H., … 2017 European Conference on Infections in Leukaemia (ECIL). (2019). Guidelines from the 2017 European Conference on Infections in Leukaemia for management of HHV-6 infection in patients with hematologic malignancies and after hematopoietic stem cell transplantation. *Haematologica*, *104*(11), 2155–2163.

Wikle Shapiro, T. J. (2019). Hematopoietic stem cell transplantation. In J. Brant, D. Cope, & M. Saria (Eds.), *Core curriculum for oncology nursing* (6th ed.). Philadelphia, PA: Elsevier.

Wikle Shapiro, T. J., & Kapadia, M. (2018). Chronic graft versus host disease. In V. Brown (Ed.), *Hematopoietic stem cell transplantation for the pediatric oncologist*. Cham, Germany: Springer International Publishing.

Zhan, H. (2019). Leukemia relapse after transplantation—a consensus on monitoring, prevention, and treatment in China. *BMC Medicine*, *17*(1), 34.

Principles of Cancer Management

③

Chemotherapy

Savanna Gilson

This chapter provides basic principles related to chemotherapy and its mechanisms of action in the treatment of patients with cancer. Additionally, standards related to safe handling, administration, patient and family education, and special populations are reviewed.

Biologic and Pharmacologic Bases for Chemotherapy in Cancer Treatment

Cancer is characterized as a growth of abnormal cells, stemming from genetic alterations, that lead to unregulated cell growth, invasion into neighboring tissues, and metastasis to distant sites. Chemotherapy is the use of chemical agents to prevent cancer cells from multiplying, invading, or metastasizing (Dickens & Ahmed, 2018). Chemotherapy can be a systemic or regional treatment that combats primary disease sites, areas of known metastasis, and possibly microscopic spread of disease.

The biologic basis of cancer chemotherapy is grounded in the cell cycle, which is reviewed in Section One: Cancer Pathophysiology of this book. Briefly, the cell cycle is the mechanism by which all cells divide and replicate, including both normal and neoplastic cells (see the figure below). In general, the cell is most vulnerable during active division. Most chemotherapeutic agents are classified according to when and how they affect cell cycle activity (Olsen et al., 2019).

The goals of chemotherapy are cure, control, or palliation (American Cancer Society, 2019). Factors that determine the appropriate goal of cancer treatment for each patient are the extent of disease at diagnosis, functional status of the patient, and physiologic presentation. It is very important that patients and family members be informed of the goal of treatment before the initiation of therapy so they can set realistic expectations in their personal lives. The information also likely needs to be repeated throughout the course of planned treatments.

- **Cure** is the desired outcome for all patients, but its likelihood depends on several factors at the time of diagnosis and throughout the planned treatment course. Cure may be further defined as a prolonged absence of disease. The term *remission*, which is the absence of detectable disease, may be used instead of cure because some cancers, such as adult leukemia and lymphoma, are likely to recur.
- **Control** is the goal of most chemotherapy when a cure is unrealistic. Control focuses on shrinking the tumor or stopping the spread of cancer to extend life and maintain or improve functional status in the presence of known disease without complete elimination of disease.
- **Palliation** is the goal of chemotherapy when neither cure nor control is possible because of the extent of disease. Quality of life and disease symptom management are primary concerns when palliation is the goal.

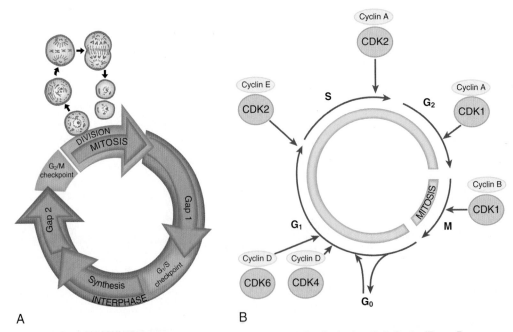

A   B

(A) Phases of the Cell Cycle. (B) The Role of CDK and Cyclin in the Cell Cycle (From Rogers, J. [2024]. *McCance & Huether's pathophysiology* [9th ed.]. Elsevier.)

Chemotherapy may be given as a primary, adjuvant, neoadjuvant, or chemopreventative treatment (Dickens & Ahmed, 2018).

- Primary chemotherapy is used as the sole treatment—for example, with leukemia and lymphomas.
- Adjuvant therapy is given after a primary treatment (e.g., surgery or radiation); the goal is to reduce the chance of recurrence by targeting remaining disease after primary treatment for patients at high risk of recurrence—for example, with breast or colorectal cancer.
- Neoadjuvant therapy is given before another treatment (e.g., surgery, radiation) to shrink tumor burden, provide cosmesis, and/or improve outcomes—for example, breast cancer and head and neck cancer. Neoadjuvant therapy also helps to reduce morbidity and mortality from treatment and to treat micrometastasis.
- Chemoprevention is used to prevent cancer from occurring in high-risk individuals, such as those with inherited cancer syndromes, a family history of cancer, or a previous diagnosis of cancer. One example of chemoprevention is the use of aspirin to prevent colorectal cancer (Umezawa et al., 2019).

Chemotherapy is usually given as combination therapy—that is, two or more agents are used together in an effort to combat drug resistance and increase therapeutic effect. The different agents affect the cell at different points in the cell cycle, allowing for maximum cell kill while minimizing toxicities. Chemotherapeutic agents for combination therapy include drugs that:

1. are effective when used singly against the specific cancer
2. have differing mechanisms of action
3. do not pose the same toxicity or have similar dose-limiting toxicities
4. do not have the same time of onset of toxicity (Olsen et al., 2019)

Tumor cells exposed to chemotherapy sometimes develop mechanisms to protect themselves against the drugs' effects; this is termed *drug resistance*. Resistance may result from drug exclusion, drug metabolism, or alteration of the target for the drug by mutation or overexpression. The most significant mechanism of drug resistance is the P-glycoprotein efflux pump, which is associated with overexpression of the multidrug resistance gene, *MDR1*. Drug resistance may involve many factors that affect response to therapy. Resistance may be inherent or acquired, single-agent or multidrug, temporary or permanent. Prevention of drug resistance is another justification for combination chemotherapy (Tortorice, 2018).

Cell Cycle Specificity and Chemotherapy

Chemotherapy principles leverage knowledge of the cell cycle in the attempt to destroy or disrupt the growth of cancer cells. Chemotherapeutic agents can be classified according to their phase of action in the cell cycle (Olsen et al., 2019).

- **Cell cycle–specific** agents exert effect during a specific phase in the cell cycle (i.e., G_1, S, G_2, or M phases).
  - These agents tend to be schedule dependent because the greatest tumor kill is obtained when the drug is given in frequent divided doses or in continuous infusions to capture the cancer cells in a specific phase.
  - Examples of cell cycle–specific agents include antimetabolites, plant alkaloids, and miscellaneous agents.

- **Cell cycle–nonspecific** agents are effective in all cell cycle phases, including the resting phase (G_0).
  - These agents may be effective treating in tumors with slowly dividing cells.
  - Cell cycle–nonspecific agents also exhibit a steep dose-response curve, meaning that the higher the dose, the greater the response.
  - These agents are given intermittently to allow the individual time to recover from dose-limiting toxicities.
  - Examples of cell cycle–nonspecific agents include alkylating agents, anti-tumor antibiotics, and nitrosoureas.

Chemotherapy Classifications

Chemotherapeutic agents are classified by mechanism of action and specificity. See the figure on the next page for a diagram of the various chemotherapeutic agents' mechanisms of action. Each drug class contains agents that have similar characteristics and side effect profiles.

Alkylating Agents

- Classification: Cell cycle–nonspecific
- Mechanism of action: Bind with DNA and protein molecules, resulting in DNA strand breakage
- Common toxicities: Myelosuppression, hypersensitivity, renal impairment, gastrointestinal (GI) toxicities (e.g., nausea and vomiting, diarrhea), and cutaneous toxicities (e.g., alopecia, skin rashes)
  - Side effects are dose dependent and may be cumulative
  - Also strongly associated with secondary malignancies (usually different malignancies from the original disease), which can occur months to years after treatment for a primary cancer
- Common alkylating agents: altretamine, bendamustine, busulfan, carboplatin, chlorambucil, cisplatin, cyclophosphamide, dacarbazine, ifosfamide, mechlorethamine, oxaliplatin, temozolomide, and thiotepa

Nitrosoureas

- Classification: Cell cycle–nonspecific
- Mechanism of action and toxicity profile similar to those of alkylating agents
- They have a high lipid solubility, which enables them to pass freely the blood-brain barrier
  - Blood-brain barrier penetration allows nitrosoureas to be prominently used in the treatment of brain tumors and other central nervous system (CNS) diseases
- Common nitrosoureas: carmustine, lomustine, and streptozocin

Antimetabolites

- Classification: Cell cycle–specific agents that work during the S phase of the cell cycle.
- Mechanism of action: Interfere with DNA synthesis by imitating the chemical structure of essential enzymes needed for DNA replication or by becoming incorporated into the structure of the DNA molecule. These agents are most effective against cancers that have a high growth fraction or rapidly dividing cells.

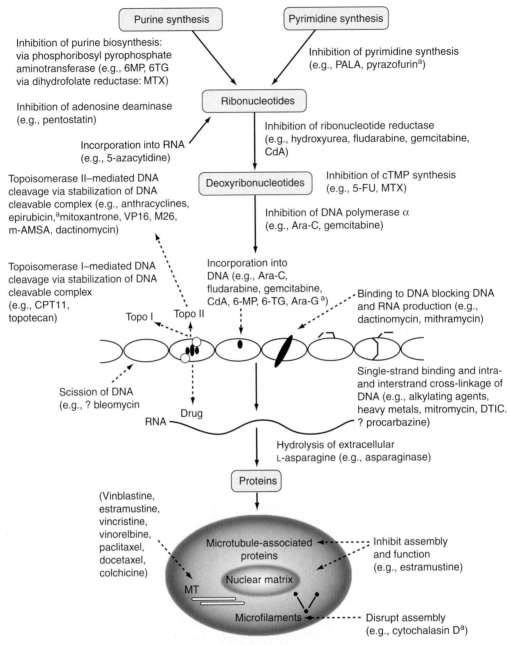

Overview of Sites and Mechanisms of Action of the Most Useful Chemotherapeutic Agents.
5-FU, 5-Fluorouracil; *6-MP,* 6-mercaptopurine; *ara-C,* cytarabine; *ara-G,* 9′-β-D-arabinofuranosylguanine; *DTIC,* dacarbazine; *Topo,* topoisomerase. (From Gerson, S. L., Caimi, P. F., Malek, E., & Tomlinson, B. [2023]. Pharmacology and molecular mechanisms of antineoplastic agents for hematologic malignancies. In R. Hoffman, E. J. Benz, L. E. Silberstein, et al. [Eds.], *Hematology: Basic principles and practice* [8th ed., pp. 900–936]. Elsevier.)

- Common toxicities: Myelosuppression, GI toxicities (e.g., nausea and vomiting, mucositis, diarrhea), and cutaneous toxicities (e.g., rash, alopecia, photosensitivity, hyperpigmentation).
- Common antimetabolites: capecitabine, cytarabine, fludarabine, fluorouracil, gemcitabine, methotrexate, and pemetrexed.

Antitumor Antibiotics

- Classification: Cell cycle–nonspecific
- Mechanisms of action: Interfere with DNA synthesis by binding with DNA at various points, preventing RNA synthesis

- Common toxicities: Myelosuppression and GI, cutaneous, and primary organ (e.g., cardiac, pulmonary) toxicities
- Common antitumor antibiotics: Bleomycin, dactinomycin, daunorubicin, doxorubicin, epirubicin, idarubicin, and mitomycin.

Plant Alkaloids

- Classification: Cell cycle–specific agents
- Mechanism of action: Bind to specific cell proteins that cause mitotic arrest, resulting in depletion of amino acids that are necessary for cell replication and apoptosis

- Plant alkaloids are naturally occurring alkaloids isolated from plant material or synthetic and semisynthetic compounds originally extracted from plants
- Common toxicities: Myelosuppression, GI toxicities (e.g., constipation, diarrhea), hypersensitivity reactions, cutaneous toxicities (alopecia), and autonomic and peripheral neurologic toxicities
- Plant alkaloids are divided into four categories:
  1. Camptothecins (e.g., irinotecan, topotecan)
  2. Epipodophyllotoxins (e.g., etoposide, teniposide)
  3. Taxanes (e.g., paclitaxel, docetaxel)
  4. Vinca alkaloids (e.g., vinblastine, vincristine)

Miscellaneous Agents

Additional miscellaneous agents exist that are cell cycle nonspecific and have different mechanisms of action. They inhibit protein synthesis, block DNA replication, or trigger mechanisms that mediate cell death. Side effects are drug specific. Routes of administration include intravenous (IV), subcutaneous, intramuscular (IM), and oral (PO). Commonly used miscellaneous agents include arsenic trioxide, asparaginase, bortezomib, mitotane, and pegaspargase.

Antibody Drug Conjugates

Antibody drug conjugates (ADCs) are agents comprised of a monoclonal antibody attached to a chemotherapeutic agent. The monoclonal antibody binds to specific antigens or receptors on the outside of the cancer cell, delivering the chemotherapy directly to the cancer cell. The advantage of ADCs is that the chemotherapy is able to act directly on the cancer cells, therefore minimizing its cytotoxic effects on normal tissue (Olsen et al., 2019).

See the table below for a list of chemotherapy agents, their classifications, mechanisms of action, routes of administration, and common uses.

Chemotherapy Drug Classes and Agents

Drug Class and Mechanism of Action	Drug Name	Route	Oncologic Indications
Alkylating Agents Cell cycle nonspecific Break DNA helix strand, thereby interfering with DNA replication	Altretamine (Hexalen)	PO	Ovarian cancer
	Bendamustine (Treanda, Bendeka, Belrapzo)	IV	Chronic lymphocytic leukemia (CLL) Non-Hodgkin lymphoma (NHL)
	Busulfan (PO: Myleran, IV: Busulfex)	PO, IV	Chronic myelogenous leukemia (CML) Hematopoietic stem cell transplant preparation
	Carboplatin (Paraplatin)	IV	Ovarian cancer Germ cell tumors Head and neck cancer Small cell lung cancer (SCLC) and non–small cell lung cancer (NSCLC) Bladder cancer Relapsed and refractory acute leukemia Endometrial cancer
	Chlorambucil (Leukeran)	PO	CLL NHL Hodgkin disease Waldenström macroglobulinemia
	Cisplatin (Platinol, CDDP)	IV Intraperitoneal (IP)	Testicular cancer Ovarian cancer Bladder cancer Head and neck cancer SCLC and NSCLC Esophageal cancer NHL Trophoblastic neoplasms
	Cyclophosphamide (Cytoxan, CTX)	IV, PO	Breast cancer NHL CLL Ovarian cancer Bone and soft tissue sarcoma Rhabdomyosarcoma Neuroblastoma and Wilms tumor
	Dacarbazine (DTIC-Dome, DIC, Imidazole Carboxamide)	IV	Metastatic malignant melanoma Hodgkin lymphoma Soft tissue sarcomas Neuroblastoma

Continued

Chemotherapy Drug Classes and Agents—cont'd

Drug Class and Mechanism of Action	Drug Name	Route	Oncologic Indications
	Ifosfamide (Ifex)	IV	Testicular cancer Soft tissue sarcoma Ewing sarcoma Osteogenic sarcoma NHL Hodgkin lymphoma SCLC and NSCLC Bladder cancer Head and neck cancer Cervical cancer
	Mechlorethamine (Nitrogen Mustard, Mustargen)	IV, Topical	Hodgkin lymphoma NHL Cutaneous T-cell lymphoma
	Melphalan (Alkeran, Phenylalanine mustard, L-PAM)	IV	Multiple myeloma Ovarian cancer Polycythemia vera Breast cancer Bone marrow/stem cell transplant setting
	Oxaliplatin (Eloxatin)	IV	Metastatic colorectal cancer Colon cancer Metastatic pancreatic cancer Metastatic gastric cancer
	Procarbazine (Matulane)	PO	Hodgkin lymphoma NHL Brain tumor Cutaneous T-cell lymphoma
	Temozolomide (Temodar)	PO	Anaplastic astrocytoma Glioblastoma multiforme
	Thiotepa (Thioplex)	IV Intravesical	Breast cancer Ovarian cancer NHL Hodgkin lymphoma Bladder cancer
	Trabectedin (Yondelis)	IV	Liposarcoma Leiomyosarcoma
Antitumor Antibiotics Cell cycle nonspecific Varying mechanisms Antimicrobial and cytotoxic	Bleomycin (Blenoxane)	IV, subcutaneous, IM, intrapleural	Squamous cell cancers Testicular cancer Hodgkin lymphoma and NHL Germ cell tumors Head and neck cancer
	Dactinomycin	IV	Wilms tumor Rhabdomyosarcoma Germ cell tumors Gestational trophoblastic disease Ewing sarcoma
	Daunorubicin (Cerubidine, Daunomycin, Rubidomycin)	IV	Acute myelogenous leukemia (AML) Acute lymphoblastic leukemia (ALL)
	Daunorubicin Liposome (DaunoXome)	IV	HIV-associated advanced Kaposi sarcoma
	Doxorubicin (Adriamycin, Hydroxydaunorubicin)	IV	Breast cancer Hodkin's and NHL Soft tissue sarcoma Ovarian cancer SCLC and NSCLC Bladder cancer Thyroid cancer Hepatoma Gastric cancer Wilms tumor Neuroblastoma ALL
	Doxorubicin Liposome (Doxil)	IV	Kaposi sarcoma in AIDS Ovarian cancer Multiple myeloma
	Epirubicin (Ellence)	IV	Breast cancer Gastric cancer

Chemotherapy Drug Classes and Agents—cont'd

Drug Class and Mechanism of Action	Drug Name	Route	Oncologic Indications
	Idarubicin (Idamycin PFS)	IV	AML ALL CML Myelodysplastic syndrome (MDS)
	Mitomycin (Mutamycin)	IV	Gastric cancer Pancreatic cancer Breast cancer NSCLC Cervical cancer Head and neck cancer Bladder cancer Anal cancer
	Mitoxantrone (Novantrone)	IV	Prostate cancer AML Breast cancer NHL
	Valrubicin (Valstar)	Intravesical	Bladder cancer
Plant Alkaloids: Camptothecins, Epipodophyllotoxins, Taxanes, and Vinca Alkaloids			
Cell cycle specific Bind to certain cell proteins to initiate mitotic arrest	Camptothecins: Irinotecan (Camptosar, CPT-11)	IV	Colorectal cancer SCLC and NSCLC
	Topotecan HCl (Hycamtin)	IV, PO	Ovarian cancer SCLC Cervical cancer
	Epipodophyllotoxins: Etoposide (Toposar, Etopophos, VP-16, VePesid)	IV, PO	Testicular cancer Prostate cancer SCLC and NSCLC Gastric cancer Hodgkin lymphoma NHL
	Teniposide (Vumon)	IV	ALL
	Taxanes: Cabazitaxel (Jevtana)	IV	Prostate cancer
	Docetaxel (Taxotere)	IV	Breast cancer NSCLC Gastric cancer Prostate cancer Head and neck cancer
	Paclitaxel (Taxol)	IV	Breast cancer Ovarian cancer SCLC and NSCLC Bladder cancer Prostate cancer Esophageal cancer AIDS-related Kaposi sarcoma
	Paclitaxel protein-bound particles (Abraxane)	IV	Breast cancer NSCLC Pancreatic cancer
	Vinca Alkaloids: Vinblastine (Velban)	IV	Hodgkin's and NHL Testicular cancer Breast cancer Kaposi sarcoma Renal cell carcinoma
	Vincristine (Oncovin, VCR)	IV	ALL Hodgkin lymphoma and NHL Neuroblastoma Rhabdomyosarcoma Ewing sarcoma Wilms tumor Multiple myeloma Chronic leukemias Thyroid cancer Brain tumors
	Vinorelbine (Navelbine)	IV	NSCLC Breast cancer Ovarian cancer Hodgkin lymphoma

Continued

Chemotherapy Drug Classes and Agents—cont'd

Drug Class and Mechanism of Action	Drug Name	Route	Oncologic Indications
Antimetabolites Cell cycle specific Act in S phase; interfere with DNA and RNA function	Azacitidine (Vidaza)	Subcutaneous, IV	Chronic myelomonocytic leukemia (CMML) MDS
	Capecitabine (Xeloda)	PO	Metastatic breast cancer Metastatic colorectal cancer
	Cladribine (Leustatin, 2-CDA, 2-Chlorodeoxyadenosine)	IV	Hairy cell leukemia CLL NHL
	Clofarabine (Clolar)	IV	Relapsed or refractory ALL (aged 1-21 years)
	Cytarabine (Arabinosylcytosine, ARA-C, Cytosar-U)	IV, IT, subcutaneous	AML CML ALL NHL Meningeal leukemia and lymphoma
	Decitabine (Dacogen)	IV	MDS
	Floxuridine (FUDR)	IV Intraarterial	Colorectal cancer Metastatic GI adenocarcinoma
	Fludarabine (Fludara)	IV, PO	CLL NHL Cutaneous T-cell lymphoma
	5-Fluorouracil (5-FU, Adrucil)	IV, topical	Breast cancer GI malignancies—colorectal, anal, esophageal, gastric, and pancreatic cancer Head and neck cancer Hepatoma Ovarian cancer Basal cell cancer of the skin (topical)
	Gemcitabine (Gemzar)	IV	Pancreatic cancer NSCLC Breast cancer Ovarian cancer Bladder cancer Soft tissue sarcoma Hodgkin lymphoma NHL
	Hydroxyurea (Droxia, Hydrea, Mylocel)	PO	CML Essential thrombocytosis Polycythemia vera Head and neck cancer Ovarian cancer
	Mercaptopurine (6-MP, Purinethol)	PO	ALL
	Methotrexate (Rheumatrex, Trexall)	IM, IT, IV, PO, subcutaneous	Breast cancer Head and neck cancers ALL Sarcomas NHL Primary CNS lymphoma Meningeal leukemia Bladder cancer Gestational trophoblastic cancer
	Nelarabine (Arranon)	IV	T-cell acute lymphoblastic leukemia T-cell lymphoblastic leukemia
	Pemetrexed (Alimta)	IV	Mesothelioma Nonsquamous NSCLC
	Pentostatin (Nipent)	IV	Hairy cell leukemia
	Pralatrexate (Folotyn)	IV	Peripheral T-cell lymphoma
	Thioguanine (Thioguanine Tabloid, 6-thioguanine, 6-TG)	PO	AML ALL CML
Nitrosoureas Cell cycle nonspecific Bind with DNA protein molecules, cross the blood-brain barrier	Carmustine (BCNU, BiCNU)	IV	Brain tumors Multiple myeloma Hodgkin lymphoma NHL

Chemotherapy Drug Classes and Agents—cont'd

Drug Class and Mechanism of Action	Drug Name	Route	Oncologic Indications
	Lomustine (CCNU, CeeNU)	PO	Brain tumors Hodgkin lymphoma NHL
	Streptozocin (Zanosar)	IV	Islet cell carcinoma of the pancreas Carcinoid tumors
Miscellaneous			
Varying mechanisms	All-*trans* retinoic acid (ATRA, tretinoin, Vesanoid)	PO	Acute promyelocytic leukemia (APL)
	Arsenic trioxide (Trisenox)	IV	APL
	Asparaginase (Elspar, L-Asparaginase)	IV, IM	ALL
	Bexarotene (Targretin)	PO	Cutaneous T-cell lymphoma
	Eribulin (Halaven)	IV	Breast cancer Liposarcoma
	Estramustine (Emcyt)	PO	Prostate cancer
	Ixabepilone (Ixempra)	IV	Breast cancer
	Mitotane (Lysodren)	PO	Adrenocortical cancer
	Romidepsin (Istodax)	IV	Cutaneous T-cell lymphoma
	Pegaspargase (Oncaspar, PEG-L-asparaginase)	IM, IV	ALL NHL
	Vorinostat (Zolinza)	PO	Cutaneous T-cell lymphoma

From Chu, E., & DeVita, V. T. (Eds.). (2021). *Physicians' cancer chemotherapy drug manual*. Jones and Bartlett Learning; Olsen, M. M., LeFebvre, K. B., & Brassil, K. J. (Eds.). (2019). *Chemotherapy and immunotherapy guidelines and recommendation for practice*. Oncology Nursing Society.
CNS, Central nervous system; *GI,* gastrointestinal; *IM,* intramuscular; *IV,* intravenous; *PO,* oral.

Chemotherapy Administration

Patient and Family Assessment and Preparation

Nurses administering chemotherapy should conduct a pretreatment assessment of the patient, considering individual characteristics of the patient and comorbidities that can affect the response to and toxicities of treatment. The needed preparation for chemotherapy should be individualized per patient and is affected by preconceived ideas of cancer, cultural and ethnic background, learning style, educational background, socioeconomic status and other social determinants of health, past coping mechanisms, and numerous other influences. Inclusion of family, significant others, and existing support systems is critical when preparing for chemotherapy initiation, including the patient education process (see the box below).

Patient Chemotherapy Education

1. Assess baseline knowledge of the disease and treatments.
   a. Clarify misconceptions
   b. Provide education and written resources on disease and treatments
2. Discuss goals of care.
3. Review each drug in the treatment plan—chemotherapy, targeted therapy, immunotherapy as applicable.
   a. Generic and brand name
   b. Specific side effects and their prevention/management
   c. Potential long-term effects
4. Reinforce the need to seek care for adverse side effects, with emphasis on those that may be serious or life-threatening.
5. Provide information on how to seek help during and after hours.

Safe Handling

Chemotherapy agents are hazardous drugs (HDs) and any healthcare professional involved in their administration must be knowledgeable in safe handling practices. Recommendations for practice have been established by the Oncology Nursing Society (ONS), the Occupational Safety and Health Administration (OSHA), and the National Institute for Occupational Safety and Health (NIOSH) for safe handling of chemotherapy agents. Safety guidelines must be used in storage and labeling, transportation, preparation, administration, and disposal of HDs.

For an agent to be classified as an HD, one or more of the following criteria must be met (NIOSH, 2020):

- Carcinogenicity—the ability or tendency to produce cancer
- Developmental toxicity (including teratogenicity)—adverse toxic affects to a developing embryo or fetus
- Reproductive toxicity—adverse effects on sexual function and fertility
- Genotoxicity—the ability to damage genetic information in cells
- Organ toxicity at low doses
- Structure and toxicity profile that mimics existing drugs determined hazardous by exhibiting any one of the previous five toxicity types

A complete list of HDs can be found at www.cdc.gov/niosh/topics/hazdrug. Health care professionals involved in preparation, administration, and disposal of HDs and waste face potential work-related exposure (NIOSH, 2020). Potential routes of exposure are:

- **Absorption** through skin or mucous membranes, including direct contact with the agent or a contaminated surface
- **Injection** from needlesticks
- **Ingestion** including via contaminated food or beverages
- **Inhalation** of drug aerosols or droplets

Recommended guidelines focus on eliminating or minimizing these routes of possible exposure (Olsen et al., 2019).

Environmental

Environmental safety is an important component of any institution's safety guidelines. The compounding and preparation of HDs should be performed in a controlled area, with access limited to authorized personnel specially trained in handling requirements. The following considerations should be addressed in the HD safety and health plan for drug preparation areas:

- Establishment of a designated HD handling area
- Use of containment devices such as biologic safety cabinets or compounding aseptic containment isolators
  - This provides a means for safe preparation of chemotherapy agents, minimizing airborne exposure of the healthcare worker
- Procedures for safe removal of contaminated waste
- Decontamination procedures

Additional guidelines for chemotherapy preparation and administration are presented in the box below.

Prevention of Hazardous Drug Exposure

- Consider reassignment if pregnant, considering pregnancy, or nursing
- Don personal protective equipment (PPE) as needed to prevent exposure
- Use double gloves
- Work over an absorbent pad to avoid spills and to contain any exposure
- Prime IV tubing with saline rather than chemotherapy
- Use Leur-loks to securely fit tubing and syringes
- Consider the use of drug transfer devices which offer a closed system and prevent leakage
- Dispose of PPE following administration; remove one pair of gloves at a time—outside gloves and then inside gloves
- Wash hands before leaving chemotherapy administration area

Personal Protective Equipment

To protect the health care worker, personal protective equipment (PPE) should be utilized anytime HDs are released into the environment. This may include:

- Handling HD vials, ampules, or packaging materials
- Introducing or withdrawing needles from HD vials
- Administering HDs by any route
- Handling HD leakage from tubing, syringe, and connection sites
- Discontinuing infusions of HDs
- Disposing of HDs and items contaminated by HDs
- Cleaning HD spills

HD PPE may include gloves, gowns, respirators, and eye and face protection. NIOSH recommends that gowns and gloves are worn for all HD handling, except when administering an intact tablet or capsule, in which case a single pair of

chemotherapy-tested gloves is sufficient. Respirators or eye or face protection should be used when there is risk for splashing or inhalation exposure (Olsen et al., 2019).

See the box below for specific PPE recommendations on the use of HDs.

Appropriate Personal Protective Equipment With Hazardous Drugs

Gloves
- Meet testing standards set by the American Society for Testing and Materials for use with hazardous drugs (designated "chemotherapy gloves")
- Inspect for defects before donning
- Powder free
- Disposable
- Double-glove
- Nitrile or neoprene material if latex sensitivity
- Change after 30–60 min or immediately if there is visible contamination or damage

Gowns
- Disposable, lint-free, low-permeability fabric
- Solid front with back closure
- Long sleeves with tight cuffs
- Single use
- Discard if visibly contaminated, before leaving drug preparation areas, and after handling hazardous drugs

Respirators
- NIOSH-approved respirator mask
- Used when cleaning an hazardous drug spill
- Surgical masks *do not* provide respiratory protection

Eye and Face Protection
- Wear protection whenever there is a possibility of splash
- Goggles or face shield should be available wherever hazardous drugs are prepared, mixed, or administered

---

Storage and Labeling in the Clinical Setting

Agents should be stored in a location that permits appropriate temperature and safety inspections and meets regulations. Labeling should indicate the contents as an HD. Standardized instructions (e.g., Material Safety Data Sheet) on what to do in the event of accidental exposure should be readily available in all areas where HDs are stored, prepared, transported, administered, or disposed of.

In the Home

When chemotherapy is given in the home setting, standardized safety guidelines must be followed, and the patient and family should be instructed about proper handling. Education should include the following:

- Keep drugs out of the reach of children and pets.
- Protect drugs and packages from puncture or breakage.
- Do not remove labels.
- Store in an area that is free of moisture and temperature extremes.
- Have a spill kit in the home with detailed instructions on appropriate use.
- Both verbal and written instructions about handling and storage of HDs, disposing of HD waste, and what to do with any unused drug.

Transportation

The following principles should be practiced when transporting HDs:

- Transported in a sealed leak-proof container.
- Always Luer-Lok the end of the syringe, and never transport with needles in place.
- The outermost container should have a "hazardous drug" label.
- Transporters should receive education on hazardous risk, safety precautions, and spill kit use in the event of a spill or contamination.

Spill Kit

An HD spill kit should be available wherever HDs are stored, transported, prepared, or administered. All staff members who work with HDs should be trained in spill cleanup. Spill kits may be purchased commercially or prepared by the individual institution if they meet approved guidelines. The following are ONS guidelines to manage an HD spill (Olsen et al., 2019):

1. Post signs to warn others of the spill.
2. Don two pairs of chemotherapy-safe gloves, a disposable gown, and a face shield.
3. Wear a respirator.
4. Contain the spill with plastic-backed absorbent pads.
5. Pick up glass fragments using scoop or utility gloves worn over chemotherapy gloves. Place glass in a puncture-proof container.
6. Place the puncture-proof container inside a bag and seal it. Double-bag all material, and label outermost bag as hazardous waste.
7. Remove PPE as previously instructed, place it in disposable waste bag, and seal.
8. Place all items in a puncture-proof container.

Documentation of a spill should include the name of the drug, the approximate volume spilled, how the spill occurred, spill management procedures followed, as well as the names of personnel and/or patients exposed and a list of personnel notified of the spill (see the table below).

Contents of Antineoplastic Spill Kit

Number	Item
Two pairs	Disposable chemical-protective gloves (optional pair of utility gloves)
1	Low-permeability, disposable protective garments (coveralls or gown and show covers)
1	Face shield
1	Respirator
1	Absorbent, plastic-backed sheets or spill pads
3-4	Disposable towels
2	Sealable thick plastic hazardous waste disposal bags with an appropriate warning label
1	Disposable scoop for collecting glass fragments
1	Puncture-resistant container for glass fragments

Data from American Society of Health-System Pharmacists. (2006). ASHP guidelines on handling hazardous drugs. *American Journal of Hospital Pharmacy, 63,* 1172–1193.

Waste and Disposal

Safe handling precautions should be used when handling body fluids (i.e., blood, emesis, or excreta) of a patient who has received chemotherapy within the past 48 hours.

- Wear double chemotherapy-tested gloves and a disposable gown.
- A face shield should be worn if splashing is possible.
- Flush the toilet with the lid down. If a lid is not present, open toilet with a plastic-backed pad to prevent splashing.
- For incontinent patients, a protective barrier ointment should be applied to the skin with each diaper change to decrease the chance of skin irritation.
- All linen with exposure to chemotherapy should be handled with proper PPE (Olsen et al., 2019).

Follow institutional policy when disposing of HDs. Contaminated materials should be placed in a sealable, leakproof bag with a label indicating it as hazardous. Syringes and needles should be disposed of intact, without breaking or recapping needles. Proper designated containers for HD disposal should be readily available in every area where HDs are administered.

Routes of Administration

Chemotherapeutic agents are administered by various routes to achieve systemic or regional delivery to the tumor.

- The goal of **systemic therapy** is to attain a drug concentration that is sufficient to achieve a therapeutic toxic effect against the disease without causing excessive toxicity to normal tissue.
  - The major routes for systemic administration are oral, IV, subcutaneous, and IM.
- **Regional chemotherapy** involves delivering the agent directly into the blood supply of the tumor or into the cavity or area in which the tumor is located.
  - Regional administration often allows for higher concentrations of the drug to be delivered to the area of the tumor with fewer systemic side effects.
  - Regional routes include intrathecal (IT), intraarterial, and intracavity.

Oral Route

The use of oral chemotherapeutic agents has greatly increased in recent years with the developments of targeted agents. Advantages of oral chemotherapeutic agents include ease of use, portability, and patient independence as these drugs can be managed at home. Several factors need to be evaluated before oral therapy is initiated:

1. Availability of the drug in an oral formulation
2. Functional status of the patient's GI tract (presence of nausea, vomiting, or dysphagia)
3. Patient's willingness and ability to adhere to the dosing schedule
4. Cost and reimbursement issues for oral preparations

Oral agents require special consideration and planning. Extensive patient/family education may be necessary and adherence to the treatment plan is critical. More information on this can be found in "Oral Adherence" chapter in Section Three of this book.

Subcutaneous and Intramuscular Routes

As with the oral agents, administration of chemotherapy by subcutaneous or IM routes allows for increased patient independence when administered in the home. Education of the patient and family regarding self-injection, disposal of sharps, site rotation, and monitoring should be incorporated into the teaching plan, along with safe handling in the preparation, administration, and disposal of waste in the home setting. Disadvantages include pain or discomfort at site of injection, possible infection at injection sites, and bleeding.

When administering subcutaneous or IM chemotherapy in the clinical setting, consider the following:

- Assess for adequate subcutaneous tissue or muscle.
- Review coagulation values or other risks for bleeding or bruising.
- The drug may be divided into multiple syringes based on the total volume to be administered.
- PPE should be worn including two pairs of gloves and a disposable gown. Face protection should be utilized if splashing is possible.
- Rotate sites.
- Post administration, monitor for pain, swelling, induration, hemorrhage, erythema, pruritus, or rash.

Topical Route

The topical route of chemotherapy is not frequently used aside from treatment for skin cancers. Safe handling guidelines should be adhered to when applying topical chemotherapy. Adherence to PPE is critical, as is environmental control during application and disposal of waste.

Intravenous Route

IV is one of the most common routes of administration of chemotherapy. Methods of IV administration include the following:

- Push—agent administered through syringe directly into vein
- Free-flow with a direct push—agent administered with syringe into the side port of a free-flowing IV
- Piggyback—use of a secondary bag or bottle and tubing connected to a primary infusion of IV fluids
- Continuous infusion—usually given over 12 hours for up to 5 to 7 days

IV chemotherapy may be administered via peripheral venipuncture or a central venous access device (CVAD) such as a peripherally inserted central catheter, percutaneous subclavian catheters (e.g., Hickman, Groshong, Broviac), or implanted devices and ports (e.g., chemoport, Passport, Infuse-a-Port).

- When utilizing a CVAD, correct placement is verified by aspirating for a blood return before each use.
  - Manufacturer or institutional guidelines should be closely followed for care, maintenance, and use of the CVAD.
  - Infection prevention should be a primary focus of nursing care.

- In peripheral sites, several factors must be considered including the patient's age and vein status, the drugs to be infused, and the expected period of infusion. See the table below for vein selection guidelines.

Vein Selection

- Select distal veins sites before proximal
- Avoid veins where damage to underlying tendons or nerves can occur
  - Antecubital
  - Wrist
  - Dorsal hand
- Avoid damaged or sclerosed veins
- Avoid mastectomy side or areas of lymphedema

Infusion-Related Reactions. Infusion reactions can occur with the administration of IV chemotherapy, and the risk varies between agents. Though infusion reactions typically occur with the patient's first or second exposure to the drug, 10% to 30% of reactions occur after the second exposure (Olsen et al., 2019). Nurses who administer chemotherapy should be knowledgeable in the background, identification, and management of these reactions. The table below presents the various types of infusion reactions, their etiology, and signs and symptoms.

Types of Infusion Reactions

Reaction Type	Etiology	Signs and Symptoms
Standard infusion reaction	Release of cytokines Irritant effect of chemotherapy	Flushing, itching, change in heart and blood pressure, dyspnea, back pain, fever, chills, rash, throat tightening, hypoxia, seizures, and dizziness
Hypersensitivity reaction and anaphylaxis	IgE mediated, considered an allergic reaction	Urticaria, angioedema, itching, cough, shortness of breath, wheeze, throat tightness, flushing, dizziness, hypotension, loss of consciousness

Adapted from Olsen, M. M., LeFebvre, K. B., & Brassil, K. J. (Eds.). (2019). *Chemotherapy and immunotherapy guidelines and recommendation for practice.* Oncology Nursing Society.

Cytokine release syndrome (CRS) is another infusion reaction seen specifically with agents that target the immune system and does not occur with chemotherapy. For more information on CRS, refer to "Targeted and Immunotherapy" chapter in Section Three of this book.

Management of infusion reactions requires prompt identification and intervention to prevent progression of symptoms and patient harm.

Steps to manage an infusion reaction (Olsen et al., 2019):

- Preadministration:
  - Administer premedications as ordered.

- Obtain orders for emergency medications in case of reaction. Standing orders for management of infusion reactions are recommended.
- Ensure emergency equipment and medications are readily available.
- Educate the patient on signs of infusion reaction to report immediately.
- At first sign of infusion reaction:
  - Stop the infusion immediately and maintain IV access with normal saline.
  - Stay with the patient and obtain help.
  - Monitor vital signs frequently.
  - Maintain airway and administer oxygen if needed.
  - Administer emergency medications as ordered based on symptoms. This will typically involve antihistamine, corticosteroid, and epinephrine for severe anaphylaxis.
- Following an infusion reaction:
  - Document the reaction and interventions taken.
  - Patients with a severe reaction may be hospitalized for monitoring of delayed reaction effects.
  - Administering subsequent doses of the drug should be avoided unless referred to an allergist for desensitization.

Vesicants and Irritants. Prevention of extravasation should be carefully considered when administering IV chemotherapy agents identified as vesicants or irritants.

- Vesicants: agents that have the ability to cause blistering or tissue necrosis.
- Irritants: agents that have the ability to cause aching, tightness, and phlebitis with or without a local inflammatory reaction but do not cause tissue necrosis.
- Extravasation: the passage of chemotherapeutic agents into tissue. Necrosis or sloughing may occur.

Risk factors for extravasation include the following:

- Small or fragile veins
- Poor vascular integrity
- Peripheral neuropathy
- Obesity
- Multiple venipunctures
- Disseminated skin diseases in the area of placement (e.g., eczema)
- Patient movement
- Limited vein availability due to other conditions (e.g., lymphedema)
- Sensory deficits resulting in patient inability to sense IV problems (e.g., paralysis)
- Cognitive impairment or somnolence
- Use of rigid IV devices such as steel-winged or butterfly catheters
- Site of venous access (avoid veins in hand, wrist, and antecubital fossa whenever possible)
- Inadequately secured catheter
- Probing the skin during insertion of a vascular access device (VAD)

- Long dwell time of the VAD (e.g., >6 months)

It is important to note that, though less common than peripheral sites, extravasation can occur in CVADs. Factors related to potential extravasation in a CVAD include catheter damage, displacement, and migration.

Prevention and early detection are of primary importance to avoid extravasation. Signs and symptoms of extravasation include the following:

- Swelling
- Stinging, burning, or intense pain
- Redness
- Loss of blood return
- Ulceration, blistering, sloughing (may be delayed up to 1 to 2 weeks after extravasation)

Nurses must know which chemotherapy agents can cause this damage and be aware of the symptoms for which to monitor. If extravasation does occur, nursing management is critical to patient outcome. Initial management includes the following measures:

- Stop infusion.
- Disconnect IV tubing from site or device. Do not remove device or catheter.
- Attempt to aspirate residual drug from device with a small (1 to 3 mL) syringe.
- Initiate appropriate measures in accordance with institutional policies. This may include use of hot or cold compress, elevate the extremity, and/or antidote administration (not every vesicant has a known antidote) (see the table below).
- Notify physician.

After extravasation, the following measures should be taken:

- Photograph the extravasation site and repeat weekly if appropriate.
- Give written instructions regarding what symptoms to report—fever, chills, blistering, skin sloughing, and worsening pain.
- Instruct patients to protect the area from sunlight.
- Arrange for return appointment.
- Consult plastic surgeon, if applicable.

Vesicant Treatments and Antidotes

Vesicant	Warm Versus Cool Therapy	Pharmacologic Antidote
Alkylating Agents	Cool	Sodium thiosulfate indicated for mechlorethamine only—local injection
Anthracyclines	Cool	Dexrazoxane—systemic
Antitumor Antibiotics	Cool	No known antidotes
Taxanes	Cool	No known antidotes
Vinca Alkaloids	Warm	Hyaluronidase—local injection

Data from Olsen, M. M., LeFebvre, K. B., & Brassil, K. J. (Eds.). (2019). *Chemotherapy and immunotherapy guidelines and recommendation for practice.* Oncology Nursing Society.

Intrathecal Route

IT chemotherapy is the direct installation of chemotherapy into the CNS by lumbar puncture or through an implanted intraventricular device (e.g., Ommaya reservoir). This method allows the therapeutic agent to bypass the blood-brain barrier and enter directly into the CNS, resulting in a direct and consistent drug concentration in the cerebrospinal fluid. Therapy administration requires a physician, specially trained registered nurse, or nurse practitioner to access and administer chemotherapy by the IT route. Post administration, patients should be monitored for signs of increased intracranial pressure, such as headache, blurred vision, vomiting, or changes in level of consciousness.

Intraarterial Route

Intraarterial chemotherapy involves cannulation of the artery that provides a tumor's blood supply or administration directly into an organ by way of an artery. This route can be used for management of brain cancers, hepatocellular carcinoma, and retinoblastoma. The chemotherapy agent can be delivered via percutaneous catheters, intraarterial ports or pumps, or in surgery or interventional radiology (transarterial hepatic chemoembolization). Nursing considerations involve monitoring for drug side effects and potential complications, such as infections or hematoma (Olsen et al., 2019).

Intracavity Route

Intracavity administration is the direct instillation of a chemotherapy agent into a body cavity. Examples include intrapleural (lung), intraperitoneal (abdomen), and intravesical (bladder) administration. This route allows direct exposure of a known area of disease to the chemotherapy drugs. Side effects are directly related to the cavity receiving instillation.

- Intrapleural instillation is usually aimed at sclerosing the pleural lining to prevent reoccurrence of effusions and requires placement of a thoracotomy (chest) tube.
- The intraperitoneal route requires installation into a peritoneal catheter or intraperitoneal port, most commonly used for ovarian cancer.
- The intravesical route requires the instillation of chemotherapy through a Foley catheter. This may be done intraoperatively, postoperatively, or in an outpatient area.
- Each of these methods carries the risk of infection along with other site-specific complications. The use of PPE is same as general chemotherapy safe handling guidelines (Olsen et al., 2019).

Administration in Special Populations

Several special populations require additional consideration when treating with chemotherapy. The National Comprehensive Cancer Network (NCCN) provides guidelines for adolescent and young adult (AYA) oncology, older adults, and cancer in people with HIV (PWH). Additionally, cancer in pregnant women is reviewed here. Nurses should be equipped with the knowledge to provide care and education to these groups.

Adolescent and Young Adults

The NCCN defines AYAs as those ages 15 to 39 at the time of a cancer diagnosis. In 2020, the incidence of cancer in AYAs was estimated at 89,500 (NCCN, 2023a, 2023b, 2023c). It is recognized that this group has distinct physical and psychosocial needs from pediatric and older adult groups. Common concerns for the AYA population include:

- Fertility preservation
- Parenting
- Education
- Employment attainment and retention
- These concerns will vary between patients and should be considered when treatment planning.
Chemotherapy considerations for AYAs:
- Fertility and sexual health must be addressed prior to chemotherapy treatments.
- Dose reductions may be made to avoid severe, irreversible organ damage.
- Establish a survivorship plan including specific screenings based on the agents the individual received (e.g., pulmonary function screening for bleomycin, cardiomyopathy screening for anthracyclines).

Considerations for Older Adults

Cancer is a disease associated with aging; 80% of all cancers in the United States are diagnosed in people 55 years of age and older (American Cancer Society, 2021). Although age 65 is often used to define an "older adult," the NCCN states the older adult oncology population is based on functional status rather than chronologic age. As such, physiologic and functional status, not chronologic age, should determine treatment options for this group.

Issues that may affect treatment options for older adults include:

- Impaired immune system
- Inadequate nutritional status
- Polypharmacy
- Poor or limited support systems
- Limited financial resources. Although consideration of these issues must be incorporated into the plan of care for an elderly patient, they do not eliminate the possibility of productive treatment for a cancer diagnosis.
Chemotherapy considerations for the older adult include (NCCN, 2023a, 2023b, 2023c):
- Biologic characteristics of the cancer and its responsiveness to chemotherapy may differ for older adults compared to younger individuals.
- Collaboration with a geriatric-trained clinician may be appropriate.
- Screening tools exist to help predict chemotherapy toxicity risk, such as the Cancer and Aging Research Group Chemo Toxicity Calculator, or the Chemotherapy Risk Assessment Scale for High-Age Patients (CRASH).
- Supportive care medications should be considered carefully. Certain drugs that are commonly used to manage chemotherapy side effects, such as corticosteroids,

benzodiazepines, or antihistamines, may not be appropriate for older adults due to adverse effects.

Considerations for People With HIV

PWH and AIDS have a higher incidence of many cancers compared to the general population. AIDS-defining cancers are non-Hodgkin lymphoma, Kaposi sarcoma, and invasive cervical cancer. Other common malignancies seen in this population are anal cancer, non–small cell lung cancer, and Hodgkin lymphoma.

Considerations for PWH (NCCN, 2023a, 2023b, 2023c):

- PWH who develop cancer should be co-managed by an oncologist and HIV specialist.
- PWH should receive cancer treatment according to standard guidelines.
- HIV therapy should continue during cancer treatment, though modifications to anti-retroviral therapy (ART) may be needed to minimize drug-drug interactions.

Pregnancy Considerations

A new cancer diagnosis during pregnancy is uncommon, estimated at 1 in 1000 women. About half of cancers associated with pregnancy are cervical or breast cancer, about one-quarter is hematologic malignancies, and the remainder can vary among melanoma, ovarian, thyroid, or colon cancers. Cancer treatment during pregnancy can be complicated, as the health of both the mother and the unborn fetus must be considered. Multidisciplinary care, involving oncologists, gynecologic oncologists, obstetricians, and perinatologists, and referral to tertiary cancer centers with expertise in treatment of cancer during pregnancy is recommended (NCCN, 2023a, 2023b, 2023c).

Chemotherapy considerations for pregnant women:

- It is possible to administer chemotherapy during pregnancy.
- Chemotherapy during the first trimester should be avoided if possible, as this period holds the highest risk for teratogenic effects or intrauterine fetal death.
- Chemotherapy may be given in the second or third trimester of pregnancy with careful monitoring of mother and fetus.
- Selection of the agent used is dependent on the cancer type, stage, gestational age of the fetus, the agent's ability to cross the placental barrier, and side-effect profile.

- Nursing interventions include incorporation of standardized education and emotional support for the patient and family in a nonjudgmental, professional manner.

Conclusion

Although cancer treatment continues to evolve, chemotherapy remains a mainstay of therapy. The number of drugs continues to expand, along with new side effects and toxicities experienced by the patient. Oncology nurses must stay knowledgeable about newly developed agents, and continue to provide expert care in patient assessment, education, chemotherapy administration, and management of treatment toxicities.

References

American Cancer Society. (2019, November 22). *How is chemotherapy used to treat cancer?*. Available at https://www.cancer.org/treatment/treatments-and-side-effects/treatment-types/chemotherapy/how-is-chemotherapy-used-to-treat-cancer.html.

American Cancer Society. (2021). *Cancer facts & figures 2021*. Available at https://www.cancer.org/research/cancer-facts-statistics/all-cancer-facts-figures/cancer-facts-figures-2021.html.

American Society of Health-System Pharmacists. (2006). ASHP guidelines on handling hazardous drugs. *American Journal of Hospital Pharmacy, 63,* 1172–1193.

Dickens, E., & Ahmed, S. (2018). Principles of cancer treatment by chemotherapy. *Surgery (Oxford), 36*(3), 134–138.

National Comprehensive Cancer Network (NCCN). (2023a). Older adult oncology guidelines, version 1.2023. Available at https://www.nccn.org/professionals/physician_gls/pdf/senior.pdf (accessed January 2, 2022).

National Comprehensive Cancer Network (NCCN). (2023b). Cancer in people with HIV guidelines, version 2.2023. Available at https://www.nccn.org/guidelines/guidelines-detail?category=4&id=1487 (accessed January 2, 2022).

National Comprehensive Cancer Network (NCCN). (2023c). Adolescent and young adult oncology guidelines, version 3.2023. Available at https://www.nccn.org/professionals/physician_gls/pdf/aya.pdf (accessed January 2, 2021).

NIOSH. (2020). *NIOSH list of hazardous drugs in healthcare settings, 2020.* Available at https://www.cdc.gov/niosh/docket/review/docket233c/pdfs/DRAFT-NIOSH-Hazardous-Drugs-List-2020.pdf.

Olsen, M. M., LeFebvre, K. B., & Brassil, K. J. (Eds.). (2019). *Chemotherapy and immunotherapy guidelines and recommendation for practice.* Oncology Nursing Society.

Tortorice, P. V. (2018). Cytotoxic chemotherapy: Principles of therapy. In C. H. Yarbro, D. Wujcik, & B. H. Gobel (Eds.), *Cancer nursing: Principles and practice* (pp. 375–416). Jones & Bartlett Learning.

Umezawa, S., Higurashi, T., Komiya, Y., Arimoto, J., Horita, N., Kaneko, T., … Nakajima, A. (2019). Chemoprevention of colorectal cancer: Past, present, and future. *Cancer Science, 110*(10), 3018–3026.

Targeted and Immunotherapy

Emily Groves

Targeted Therapy

In the rapidly changing world of cancer therapies, targeted therapies offer an alternative or adjunct therapy to traditional cytotoxic chemotherapy agents by identifying unique molecular targets within cancer cells to block cancer growth, progression, and metastasis (Lee et al., 2018). Multiple classes of novel targeted agents have been developed, and as translational research has brought targeted therapies into clinical practice, nurses must understand the implications of these therapies to provide comprehensive nursing care for patients and their families. This section will review the mechanism of action, classes, adverse effects, and nursing considerations of target therapy. A list of terms specific to targeted therapy is presented in the box below.

Targeted Therapy Terminology

Angiogenesis: Process by which new blood vessels form, sprouting from existing blood vessels.

Apoptosis: Programmed cell death. The normal process by which damaged cells are eliminated. Apoptosis is a tightly controlled process of normal cell function.

Cell-signaling cascades: Groups of factors that are linked and pass on messages from the cell surface to the inside of the cell.

Chromosomes: Thread-like structures inside the nucleus of cells. Each chromosome is made of protein and a single molecule of DNA. Passed from parents to offspring, DNA contains the specific instructions that make each type of living creature unique.

Conjugated antibody: A tagged, loaded, or labeled antibody used as a honing device to direct treatment toward a specific cancer cell.

Cross-talk: Activation of a cell signaling pathway without growth factor binding; activation of a receptor by another activated receptor in the absence of ligand binding.

Cytokine: A small protein or biologic factor that is released by cells and has a specific effect on cell-cell interactions, communication, and behavior of other cells.

Cytoplasm: The intracellular portion of a cell where biochemical reactions take place.

Degradation: The breaking down of a substance.

Dimerization: Joining two molecular subunits into a single dimer; results in little structural change.

DNA: A molecule called deoxyribonucleic acid (DNA), which contains the biologic instructions that make each species unique. DNA, along with the instructions it contains, is passed from adult organisms to their offspring during reproduction.

Domain: Functional region or component of a protein.

Downstream regulation: Changes that take place below the site of a signaling inhibition.

Endothelial cells: Cells that line the vascular system. They act as a barrier between the bloodstream and target cells that hormones must pass through to reach their receptors and exert their biologic action.

Enzyme: A protein that speeds up chemical reactions in the body. Enzymes take part in many cell functions, including cell signaling, growth, and division.

Enzyme inhibitor: A substance that blocks the action of an enzyme. In cancer treatment, enzyme inhibitors may be used to block certain enzymes that cancer cells need to grow.

Epidermal growth factor (EGF): One of a family of ligands (growth factors) that bind to receptors, resulting in stimulation of cell growth.

Epidermal growth factor-like domain 7: A secreted angiogenic factor that is highly conserved in vertebrates; it is almost exclusively expressed by, and acts on, endothelial cells.

Epidermal growth factor receptor (EGFR): A member of a family of receptors, each composed of four similarly structured transmembrane receptor–tyrosine kinases; activation of these tyrosine kinases is usually dependent on ligand binding to the external portion of the receptor. ErbB1 is also called human EGF receptor 1 (HER1) and is commonly referred to as EGFR. Other members of this receptor family are ErbB2 (HER2/neu), ErbB3 (HER3), and ErbB4 (HER4). These receptors are large proteins residing in the cell membrane.

Epidermal growth factor receptor–tyrosine kinase (EGFR-TK): The intracellular (cytoplasm) portion of the EGFR protein; essential for signaling transduction.

Expression: Production of proteins by messenger ribonucleic acids that result from transcription and translation of specific genes.

Extracellular matrix (ECM): The material that surrounds cells; important regulatory molecules in the ECM promote, inhibit, or guide growth of cells.

Genetic alteration: Changes in the instruction makeup of a cell that can cause a disruption in its signaling process so that the cell no longer grows and divides normally or dies when it should.

Genome: The complete set of DNA in a cell. DNA carries the instructions for building all of the proteins that make each living creature unique.

Growth factors: Function to regulate cell division and cell survival; produced by normal cells during embryonic development, tissue growth, and wound healing.

Hallmarks of cancer: Six distinctive and complementary capabilities that enable tumor growth and metastatic spread, providing a solid foundation for understanding the biology of cancer.

Heterodimerization: Pairing of two different (hetero) receptors.

Homodimerization: Pairing of two of the same (homo) receptors.

Integrins: Cell surface proteins that bind to components of the extracellular matrix.

Kinase: An enzyme that catalyzes transfer of a phosphate molecule from adenosine triphosphate (ATP) to an acceptor molecule, resulting in a cascade of kinase-mediated activation reactions.

Ligand: A molecule that binds to another molecule and activates receptors on the cell surface.

Targeted Therapy Terminology—cont'd

Ligand binding: The process by which the ligand attaches itself to a specific receptor on the cell surface and activates the receptor, initiating the signaling pathway.

Malignant: Cancerous; a cell or mass that divides and grows without control and order.

Matrix metalloproteinases (MMPs): Family of proteins that degrades the extracellular matrix ahead of sprouting vessels.

Monoclonal antibody: Genetically engineered protein designed to attach itself to a specific protein to recruit other parts of the immune system to destroy the cells containing the antigen.

Monomer: Single receptor in an inactivated state; also, a molecule of protein that can join with other identical monomers to form a polymer.

Naked monoclonal antibody: Antibody that works by itself, binding to antigens, free-floating proteins, or other noncancerous cells to boost the immune system response by targeting immune system checkpoints.

Oncogene: Mutated or overexpressed version of a normal gene that can release the cell from normal restraints on growth and promote or allow continuous growth and division, converting it into a tumor cell.

Pericytes: Cells associated with the walls of small blood vessels that are neither smooth muscle cells nor endothelial cells.

P-glycoprotein: A protein that pumps substances out of cells. Cancer cells that have too much p-glycoprotein may not be killed by anticancer drugs.

Phosphorylation: Creation or generation of free phosphorus that results from binding of a molecule of ATP to the tyrosine receptor site on the intracellular portion of the receptor.

Proteases: Enzymes that aid in the breakdown of proteins in the body.

Protein: A molecule made up of amino acids; the basis of body structures, such as skin and hair, and of other substances such as enzymes, cytokines, and antibodies.

Receptor: A structure on the outside or inside of a cell (cell membrane protein) that selectively binds to a specific drug, hormone, or chemical mediators to alter cell function.

Signaling pathway: Series of interdependent proteins responsible for transmitting signals to the nucleus of the cell.

Small molecules: Targeted drugs that work inside the cell; generic names for most of these drugs end in -*ib* (e.g., imatinib, dasatinib).

Targeted therapy: Anticancer agent used to block a specific cellular cycle or pathway with the goal of preventing replication or invasion while preserving normal cellular function.

Transcription: Process by which DNA passes genetic information to RNA. Transcription is the first step in producing proteins.

Translational research: The process by which the results of research done in the laboratory are used to develop new ways to diagnose and treat disease.

Transmembrane: Refers crossing or passing through the cell membrane.

Tumorigenesis: The change of a normal cell into tumor cells.

Tumor suppressor gene: A normal gene that signals a cell to slow down growth and division.

Tyrosine kinase (TK): Enzyme that catalyzes the transfer of a phosphate molecule from ATP to a tyrosine residue in proteins.

Tyrosine kinase receptor: Intracellular portion of the EGFR; activation of the TK receptor stimulates proliferation, invasion, angiogenesis, metastasis, and inhibition of apoptosis.

Upstream regulation: Changes that take place above the site of a signaling inhibition.

Vascular endothelial growth factor (VEGF): Growth factor essential to angiogenesis; binds to receptors on endothelial cells.

Targeted Therapy 101

One of the basic principles of the etiology of cancer is the alteration of the genetic profile, which leads to mutations or other changes in cell structure that regulate cell survival and proliferation (Røsland & Engelson, 2015). These genetic alterations that differentiate cancer cells from healthy cells become the molecular targets of the drugs classified as targeted therapies. Targeted therapies are also referred to as *precision medicine*.

Multiple targets for these therapies exist; however, primary targets include specific proteins in cancer cells, chromosomal abnormalities, and altered proteins that drive cancer progression National Cancer Institute (NCI). Most targeted therapies are small-molecule compounds that are designed to easily enter cells to bind to or deactivate proteins. Larger compounds are generally monoclonal antibodies, discussed later in this chapter.

As the U.S. Food and Drug Administration (FDA) continues to approve targeted therapies at a rapid rate, it is imperative to remain up to date on the types of therapies available. The table below lists the most recent FDA-approved targeted treatments, by cancer type.

List of Targeted Therapy Drugs Approved for Specific Types of Cancer

Cancer Type	FDA-Approved Targeted Treatments
Bladder cancer	Atezolizumab (Tecentriq), nivolumab (Opdivo), avelumab (Bavencio), pembrolizumab (Keytruda), erdafitinib (Balversa), enfortumab vedotin-ejfv (Padcev), sacituzumab govitecan-hziy (Trodelvy)
Brain cancer	Bevacizumab (Avastin), everolimus (Afinitor), belzutifan (Welireg)
Breast cancer	Everolimus (Afinitor), tamoxifen (Nolvadex), toremifene (Fareston), trastuzumab (Herceptin), fulvestrant (Faslodex), anastrozole (Arimidex), exemestane (Aromasin), lapatinib (Tykerb), letrozole (Femara), pertuzumab (Perjeta), ado-trastuzumab emtansine (Kadcyla), palbociclib (Ibrance), ribociclib (Kisqali), neratinib maleate (Nerlynx), abemaciclib (Verzenio), olaparib (Lynparza), talazoparib tosylate (Talzenna), alpelisib (Piqray), fam-trastuzumab deruxtecan-nxki (Enhertu), tucatinib (Tukysa), sacituzumab govitecan-hziy (Trodelvy), pertuzumab, trastuzumab, and hyaluronidase-zzxf (Phesgo), pembrolizumab (Keytruda), margetuximab-cmkb (Margenza)
Cervical cancer	Bevacizumab (Avastin), pembrolizumab (Keytruda), tisotumab vedotin-tftv (Tivdak)
Colorectal cancer	Cetuximab (Erbitux), panitumumab (Vectibix), bevacizumab (Avastin), ziv-aflibercept (Zaltrap), regorafenib (Stivarga), ramucirumab (Cyramza), nivolumab (Opdivo), ipilimumab (Yervoy), encorafenib (Braftovi), pembrolizumab (Keytruda)

Continued

List of Targeted Therapy Drugs Approved for Specific Types of Cancer—cont'd

Cancer Type	FDA-Approved Targeted Treatments
Dermatofibrosarcoma	Imatinib mesylate (Gleevec)
Endocrine/neuroendocrine tumors	Lanreotide acetate (Somatuline Depot), avelumab (Bavencio), lutetium Lu 177-dotatate (Lutathera), iobenguane I 131 (Azedra)
Endometrial cancer	Pembrolizumab (Keytruda), lenvatinib mesylate (Lenvima), dostarlimab-gxly (Jemperli)
Esophageal cancer	Trastuzumab (Herceptin), ramucirumab (Cyramza), pembrolizumab (Keytruda), nivolumab (Opdivo), fam-trastuzumab deruxtecan-nxki (Enhertu)
Head and neck cancer	Cetuximab (Erbitux), pembrolizumab (Keytruda), nivolumab (Opdivo)
Gastrointestinal stromal tumor	Imatinib mesylate (Gleevec), sunitinib (Sutent), regorafenib (Stivarga), avapritinib (Ayvakit), ripretinib (Qinlock)
Giant cell tumor	Denosumab (Xgeva), pexidartinib hydrochloride (Turalio)
Kidney cancer	Bevacizumab (Avastin), sorafenib (Nexavar), sunitinib (Sutent), pazopanib (Votrient), temsirolimus (Torisel), everolimus (Afinitor), axitinib (Inlyta), nivolumab (Opdivo), cabozantinib (Cabometyx), lenvatinib mesylate (Lenvima), ipilimumab (Yervoy), pembrolizumab (Keytruda), avelumab (Bavencio), tivozanib hydrochloride (Fotivda), belzutifan (Welireg)
Leukemia	Tretinoin (Vesanoid), imatinib mesylate (Gleevec), dasatinib (Sprycel), nilotinib (Tasigna), bosutinib (Bosulif), rituximab (Rituxan), alemtuzumab (Campath), ofatumumab (Arzerra), obinutuzumab (Gazyva), ibrutinib (Imbruvica), idelalisib (Zydelig), blinatumomab (Blincyto), venetoclax (Venclexta), ponatinib hydrochloride (Iclusig), midostaurin (Rydapt), enasidenib mesylate (Idhifa), inotuzumab ozogamicin (Besponsa), tisagenlecleucel (Kymriah), gemtuzumab ozogamicin (Mylotarg), rituximab and hyaluronidase human (Rituxan Hycela), ivosidenib (Tibsovo), duvelisib (Copiktra), moxetumomab pasudotox-tdfk (Lumoxiti), glasdegib maleate (Daurismo), gilteritinib (Xospata), tagraxofusp-erzs (Elzonris), acalabrutinib (Calquence), avapritinib (Ayvakit), brexucabtagene autoleucel (Tecartus), asciminib hydrochloride (Scemblix)
Liver and bile duct cancer	Sorafenib (Nexavar), regorafenib (Stivarga), nivolumab (Opdivo), lenvatinib mesylate (Lenvima), pembrolizumab (Keytruda), cabozantinib (Cabometyx), ramucirumab (Cyramza), ipilimumab (Yervoy), pemigatinib (Pemazyre), atezolizumab (Tecentriq), bevacizumab (Avastin), infigratinib phosphate (Truseltiq), ivosidenib (Tibsovo)
Lung cancer	Bevacizumab (Avastin), crizotinib (Xalkori), erlotinib (Tarceva), gefitinib (Iressa), afatinib dimaleate (Gilotrif), ceritinib (LDK378/Zykadia), ramucirumab (Cyramza), nivolumab (Opdivo), pembrolizumab (Keytruda), osimertinib (Tagrisso), necitumumab (Portrazza), alectinib (Alecensa), atezolizumab (Tecentriq), brigatinib (Alunbrig), trametinib (Mekinist), dabrafenib (Tafinlar), durvalumab (Imfinzi), dacomitinib (Vizimpro), lorlatinib (Lorbrena), entrectinib (Rozlytrek), capmatinib hydrochloride (Tabrecta), ipilimumab (Yervoy), selpercatinib (Retevmo), pralsetinib (Gavreto), cemiplimab-rwlc (Libtayo), tepotinib hydrochloride (Tepmetko), sotorasib (Lumakras), amivantamab-vmjw (Rybrevant), mobocertinib succinate (Exkivity)
Lymphoma	Ibritumomab tiuxetan (Zevalin), denileukin diftitox (Ontak), brentuximab vedotin (Adcetris), rituximab (Rituxan), vorinostat (Zolinza), romidepsin (Istodax), bexarotene (Targretin), bortezomib (Velcade), pralatrexate (Folotyn), ibrutinib (Imbruvica), siltuximab (Sylvant), belinostat (Beleodaq), obinutuzumab (Gazyva), nivolumab (Opdivo), pembrolizumab (Keytruda), rituximab and hyaluronidase human (Rituxan Hycela), copanlisib hydrochloride (Aliqopa), axicabtagene ciloleucel (Yescarta), acalabrutinib (Calquence), tisagenlecleucel (Kymriah), venetoclax (Venclexta), mogamulizumab-kpkc (Poteligeo), duvelisib (Copiktra), polatuzumab vedotin-piiq (Polivy), zanubrutinib (Brukinsa), tazemetostat hydrobromide (Tazverik), selinexor (Xpovio), tafasitamab-cxix (Monjuvi), brexucabtagene autoleucel (Tecartus), crizotinib (Xalkori), umbralisib tosylate (Ukoniq), lisocabtagene maraleucel (Breyanzi), loncastuximab tesirine-lpyl (Zynlonta)
Malignant mesothelioma	Ipilimumab (Yervoy), nivolumab (Opdivo)
Microsatellite instability-high or mismatch repair-deficient solid tumors	Pembrolizumab (Keytruda), dostarlimab-gxly (Jemperli)
Multiple myeloma	Bortezomib (Velcade), carfilzomib (Kyprolis), daratumumab (Darzalex), ixazomib citrate (Ninlaro), elotuzumab (Empliciti), selinexor (Xpovio), isatuximab-irfc (Sarclisa), daratumumab and hyaluronidase-fihj (Darzalex Faspro), belantamab mafodotin-blmf (Blenrep), idecabtagene vicleucel (Abecma), ciltacabtagene autoleucel (Carvykti)
Myelodysplastic/myeloproliferative disorders	Imatinib mesylate (Gleevec), ruxolitinib phosphate (Jakafi), fedratinib hydrochloride (Inrebic), pacritinib citrate (Vonjo)
Neuroblastoma	Dinutuximab (Unituxin), naxitamab-gqgk (Danyelza)
Ovarian epithelial/fallopian tube/primary peritoneal cancers	Bevacizumab (Avastin), olaparib (Lynparza), rucaparib camsylate (Rubraca), niraparib tosylate monohydrate (Zejula)
Pancreatic cancer	Erlotinib (Tarceva), everolimus (Afinitor), sunitinib (Sutent), olaparib (Lynparza), belzutifan (Welireg)
Plexiform neurofibroma	Selumetinib sulfate (Koselugo)
Prostate cancer	Cabazitaxel (Jevtana), enzalutamide (Xtandi), abiraterone acetate (Zytiga), radium 223 dichloride (Xofigo), apalutamide (Erleada), darolutamide (Nubeqa), rucaparib camsylate (Rubraca), olaparib (Lynparza), lutetium Lu 177 vipivotide tetraxetan (Pluvicto)
Skin cancer	Vismodegib (Erivedge), sonidegib (Odomzo), ipilimumab (Yervoy), vemurafenib (Zelboraf), trametinib (Mekinist), dabrafenib (Tafinlar), pembrolizumab (Keytruda), nivolumab (Opdivo), cobimetinib (Cotellic), alitretinoin (Panretin), avelumab (Bavencio), encorafenib (Braftovi), binimetinib (Mektovi), cemiplimab-rwlc (Libtayo), atezolizumab (Tecentriq), tebentafusp-tebn (Kimmtrak), nivolumab and relatlimab-rmbw (Opdualag)
Soft tissue sarcoma	Pazopanib (Votrient), alitretinoin (Panretin), tazemetostat hydrobromide (Tazverik), sirolimus protein-bound particles (Fyarro)
Solid tumors—TMB-H	Pembrolizumab (Keytruda)
Solid tumors with NTRK gene fusion	Larotrectinib sulfate (Vitrakvi), entrectinib (Rozlytrek)
Stomach (gastric) cancer	Pembrolizumab (Keytruda), trastuzumab (Herceptin), ramucirumab (Cyramza), fam-trastuzumab deruxtecan-nxki (Enhertu), nivolumab (Opdivo)
Systemic mastocytosis	Imatinib mesylate (Gleevec), midostaurin (Rydapt), avapritinib (Ayvakit)
Thyroid cancer	Cabozantinib (Cometriq), vandetanib (Caprelsa), sorafenib (Nexavar), lenvatinib mesylate (Lenvima), trametinib (Mekinist), dabrafenib (Tafinlar), selpercatinib (Retevmo), pralsetinib (Gavreto)

National Cancer Institute (NCI). (2022). *List of targeted therapy drugs approved for specific types of cancers.* Available at https://www.cancer.gov/about-cancer/treatment/types/targeted-therapies/approved-drug-list.

Angiogenesis

Although multiple classes and examples of targeted therapies approved by the FDA exist, one of the most widely utilized therapies is angiogenesis inhibitors (NCI, 2022). Angiogenesis is a normal physiologic process by which blood vessels are formed and maintained, beginning in utero and continuing throughout adult life. The lifelong process of angiogenesis of the vascular system is generally associated with maintenance controlled by angiogenesis inhibitors and activators.

In adults, new vessel formation is infrequent and is generally associated with repair of tissue during wound healing or cardiovascular injury (Teleanu et al., 2019). However, cancer cells exploit angiogenesis to form a blood supply capable of sustaining tumor growth, as well as metastasizing cancer cells throughout the body (NCI, 2022). Absorption of oxygen and nutrients is possible only within 1 to 2 mm of tumor borders, and further growth requires formation of new vessels through the recruitment of circulating endothelial cells (Li et al., 2018). Endothelial cells are the primary building blocks of vessels, lining the walls of blood vessels and possessing the extraordinary ability to divide and migrate; however, most of the time, the endothelial cell remains dormant until recruited for angiogenesis.

Many factors activate angiogenesis; for example, hypoxia is an important stimulator of tumor angiogenesis (Geindreau et al., 2021; Lugano et al., 2020). When a tumor can no longer obtain an adequate supply of oxygen and nutrients, its cellular environment upregulates large amounts of vascular endothelial growth factor (VEGF) into the surrounding tissue, at the same time downregulating proteins that inhibit angiogenesis within the tumor and its microenvironment. This activation is referred to as the *angiogenic switch* (Shaik et al., 2020). VEGF then binds to the appropriate receptor on the endothelial cell surface, activating the tyrosine kinase (TK) enzyme inside the cell, initiating the signaling pathway. The signaling pathway transmits a series of molecules (proteins) to the nucleus, where gene transcription is altered, stimulating new endothelial cell growth. The extracellular matrix is degraded so that the endothelial cells can invade the matrix and begin to divide and proliferate. As they divide, a string of endothelial cells is produced, eventually forming a hollow tube which is the basis of a new blood vessel. Eventually, a new network of blood vessels is created, making tumor tissue growth and repair possible (Li et al., 2018; Teleanu et al., 2019).

It is important to note that tumor angiogenesis involves the development of blood vessels that are structurally and functionally abnormal. Tumor vessels are irregular, distended, leaky capillaries with sluggish blood flow (Lugano et al., 2020). These new structures are tortuous, less organized, and less stable than normal blood vessels—resulting in enhanced vascular permeability. These "leaky vessels" enhance the migration and proliferation of endothelial cells, opening a pathway for metastasis (Jiang et al., 2020).

Targeted angiogenesis inhibitors can disrupt this entire process of tumor angiogenesis by binding with VEGF, or binding to the receptors on cell walls for VEGF, blocking blood vessel formation at multiple stages. Moreover, blocking VEGF may lead to apoptosis of the endothelial cells and a decrease in tumor vessel diameter, density, and permeability (NCI, 2022). The targeted therapy agents, which work by inhibiting angiogenesis within the tumor, include axitinib, pamalidomide, lenalidomide, and thalidomide, among others (Bejarano et al., 2021; Ribeiro et al., 2018). The monoclonal antibody bevacizumab also inhibits angiogenesis by binding to VEGF in the extracellular region and disrupting the angiogenic pathway (Bejarano et al., 2021).

Additional Targeted Therapies

In addition to antiangiogenic therapies, targeted therapies include hormone therapies, signal transduction inhibitors, gene expression modulators, apoptosis inducers, immunotherapies (discussed later), and monoclonal antibodies (NCI, 2022).

Monoclonal Antibodies

An antibody is a protein that attaches itself to another specific protein called an *antigen*. Antibodies circulate in the body until they find and attach to their specific antigen and then recruit other parts of the immune system to destroy the cells containing that antigen. Monoclonal antibodies (mAbs or MoAbs) are genetically engineered (man-made) antibodies that are produced by identical immune cells cloned from a unique parent cell; as such, they have known affinity for a specific part of a particular antigenic protein (Hafeez et al., 2020; NCI, 2022).

Monoclonal antibodies were developed out of historical work conducted across multiple centuries to develop understanding of virology, genetics, and the immune system (Packer, 2021).

In the Nobel Prize–winning work of Kohler and Milstein in 1975 to 1984, monoclonal antibodies were produced from a fusion of immunized rat spleen cells & a line of mouse myeloma cells. However, introduction of these antibodies into the human body was ineffective with each subsequent injection due to the development of a human anti-mouse antibody (HAMA) response. Recombinant-DNA technology eventually solved this problem by substituting the murine antibodies with chimeric, humanized, or human antibodies (Kimiz-Gebologlu et al., 2018).

Each monoclonal antibody that has been developed is named according to the World Health Organization international nomenclature standards to ensure universal identification of each mAB (see the box on the next page).

Monoclonal Antibody Nomenclature

Group 1: -tug for unmodified immunoglobulins

Monospecific full-length and Fc unmodified* immunoglobulins of any class. Molecules which might occur as such in the immune system. Including:

- IgG, IgA, IgM, IgD, IgE
- only allelic variants
- Glycoengineering without mutation
- C-terminal lysine deletion without any other mutation in the Fc region

Group 2: -bart for antibody artificial

Monospecific full-length immunoglobulins with engineered constant domains (CH1/2/3).

Monospecific full-length immunoglobulins that contain any point mutation introduced by engineering for any reason anywhere (hinge, new glycan attachment site, mixed allelic variants which would not occur in nature, altered complement binding, altered FcRn binding, altered Fc-gamma receptor binding, etc.).

- e.g., IGHG4 with S>P mutation, stabilized IgA

Group 3: -mig for multi-immunoglobulin

Bi- and multispecific immunoglobulins regardless of the format, type, or shape (full length, full length plus, fragments)

Group 4: -ment for fragment

All monospecific domains, fragments of any kind, derived from an immunoglobulin variable domain (all monospecific constructs that do not contain an Fc domain)

Infix Definition

-ami-	serum amyloid protein (SAP)/amyloidosis (pre- substem)	-ki-	cytokine and cytokine receptor2
-ba-	bacterial	-ler-	allergen
-ci-	cardiovascular	-sto-	immunostimulatory
-de-	metabolic or endocrine pathways	-pru-	immunosuppressive
		-ne-	neural
-eni-	enzyme inhibition	-os-	bone
-fung-	fungal	-ta-	tumour
-gro-	skeletal muscle mass-related growth factors and receptors (pre-substem)1	-toxa-	toxin
		-vet-	veterinary use (sub-stem)
		-vi-	viral

From World Health Organization. (2021). *New INN monoclonal antibody (mAB) nomenclature scheme.* Available at https://cdn.who.int/media/docs/default-source/international-nonproprietary-names-(inn)/new_mab_nomenclature-_2021.pdf

*Do not contain any amino acid differences with the native sequence (constant region amino acid changes by comparison with the closest genomic C gene and allele).

Mechanism of Action. Monoclonal antibody target cells are marked with a specific cell surface antigen. Two types of mAbs are used in cancer treatment: unconjugated and conjugated. Unconjugated mAbs are not fused to a toxin and therefore are called *naked* mAbs; they attach to a specific antigen on the cancer cell and prevent it from becoming active, then induce apoptosis and destroy the cell. Conjugated antibodies are attached to a radioisotope or chemotherapeutic agent. The mAb acts as a homing device, circulating in the body until it finds its targeted antigen, cytotoxic agent into the cancer cell. Conjugated antibodies are also called *labeled, loaded,* or *tagged* antibodies. Because they target cell surface markers instead of killing both tumor cells and normal, healthy cells, systemic side effects may be reduced (NCI, 2022).

Nursing Considerations. The side effect profile for mAbs differs from that of chemotherapy. Acute effects include infusion-related reactions, whereas chronic effects include significant fatigue and flu-like symptoms. Cytokine release syndrome is the primary cause for most infusion reactions to monoclonal antibodies. When the mAb binds to the antigen on the targeted cell, specific cytokines called *chemokines* recruit immune-effector cells (e.g., monocytes, macrophages, cytotoxic T cells, natural killer cells) and complement molecules. The immune-effector cells bind to the constant portion of the antibody (Fc region), targeting that cell for destruction. When they are destroyed, both target and immune-effector cells release cytokines into the circulation, further contributing to a group of symptoms. Immediate infusion-related events are common with the administration of mAbs. The intensity of the event depends on the specific mAb administered and whether other treatment modalities are concomitantly used. The following symptoms are described as an infusion reaction: chills, fevers, rigors, myalgias, arthralgias, urticaria, nausea, diarrhea, mucosal congestion, hypotension, fatigue, headache, tachycardia, and dyspnea (Freyer & Porter, 2020; Morris et al., 2022).

Cytokine release syndrome is widely documented, particularly in associated with CAR-T cell therapy for hematologic malignancies. The reaction can be observed typically during the first infusion and may occur within the first 2 hours of initiation, with subtle to severe symptoms. Pretreatment with acetaminophen and diphenhydramine 30 to 60 minutes before infusion is recommended to alleviate symptoms associated with and minimize cytokine release syndrome. Should symptoms develop during the infusion despite premedication, the infusion should be interrupted, and normal saline administered. Airway, breathing, and circulation should be assessed immediately, along with vital signs. Administration of meperidine and additional histamine blockers may be warranted for rigors. Most reactions will subside on their own, and the infusion may then be reinitiated at a slower rate (Freyer & Porter, 2020; Morris et al., 2022). Severe reactions may require supplemental oxygen, steroids, bronchodilators, or emergency medications. Most patients who experience moderate infusion reactions may be considered for rechallenge, because most reactions are likely caused by cytokine release and are not true anaphylaxis.

In summary, targeted therapies work best as combination therapies, as over time cancer cells may become resistant as they find alternative pathways to achieve tumor growth or mutations alter the targeted proteins all together. Combination therapies include using two targeted therapies together, or a targeted therapy in combination with traditional chemotherapy agents.

Nurses should be aware of the compounding side effects and potential toxicities associated with all therapies—especially adverse effects which can exacerbate underlying health considerations and impact patient quality of life. The most common side effects of targeted therapies are diarrhea and hepatic complications, such as elevated liver function tests (LFTs) and hepatitis. Skin problems, hypertension, impaired wound healing, and prothrombotic conditions are also associated with the use of targeted therapies.

References

Bejarano, L., Jordão, M. J. C., & Joyce, J. A. (2021). Therapeutic targeting of the tumor microenvironment. *Cancer Discovery*, 11(4), 933–959. https://doi.org/10.1158/2159-8290.CD-20-1808.

Freyer, C. W., & Porter, D. L. (2020). Cytokine release syndrome and neurotoxicity following CAR T-cell therapy for hematologic malignancies. *Journal of Allergy and Clinical Immunology*, 146(5), 940–948.

Geindreau, M., Ghiringhelli, F., & Bruchard, M. (2021). Vascular endothelial growth factor, a key modulator of the anti-tumor immune response. *International Journal of Molecular Sciences*, 22(9), 4871.

Hafeez, U., Parakh, S., Gan, H. K., & Scott, A. M. (2020). Antibody-drug conjugates for cancer therapy. *Molecules*, 25(20), 4764.

Jiang, X., Wang, J., Deng, X., Xiong, F., Zhang, S., Gong, Z., … Xiong, W. (2020). The role of microenvironment in tumor angiogenesis. *Journal of Experimental and Clinical Cancer Research*, 39(1), 204.

Kimiz-Gebologlu, I., Gulce-Iz, S., & Biray-Avci, C. (2018). Monoclonal antibodies in cancer immunotherapy. *Molecular Biology Reports*, 45(6), 2935–2940.

Lee, Y. T., Tan, Y. J., & Oon, C. E. (2018). Molecular targeted therapy: Treating cancer with specificity. *European Journal of Pharmacology*, 834, 188–196.

Li, T., Kang, G., Wang, T., & Huang, H. (2018). Tumor angiogenesis and anti-angiogenic gene therapy for cancer. *Oncology Letters*, 16(1), 687–702.

Lugano, R., Ramachandran, M., & Dimberg, A. (2020). Tumor angiogenesis: causes, consequences, challenges and opportunities. *Cellular and Molecular Life Sciences*, 77(9), 1745–1770.

Morris, E. C., Neelapu, S. S., Giavridis, T., & Sadelain, M. (2022). Cytokine release syndrome and associated neurotoxicity in cancer immunotherapy. *Nature Reviews Immunology*, 22(2), 85–96.

National Cancer Institute (NCI). (2022). *Targeted cancer therapies*. Available at https://www.cancer.gov/about-cancer/treatment/types/targeted-therapies/targeted-therapies-fact-sheet. Updated April 27, 2022.

Packer, D. (2021). The history of the antibody as a tool. *Acta Histochemica*, 123(4), 151710.

Ribeiro, A., Abreu, R. M. V., Dias, M. M., Barreiro, M. F., & Ferreira, I. C. F. R. (2018). Antiangiogenic compounds: Well-established drugs versus emerging natural molecules. *Cancer Letters*, 415, 86–105.

Røsland, G. V., & Engelsen, A. S. (2015). Novel points of attack for targeted cancer therapy. *Basic and Clinical Pharmacology and Toxicology*, 116(1), 9–18.

Shaik, F., Cuthbert, G. A., Homer-Vanniasinkam, S., Muench, S. P., Ponnambalam, S., & Harrison, M. A. (2020). Structural basis for vascular endothelial growth factor receptor activation and implications for disease therapy. *Biomolecules*, 10(12), 1673.

Teleanu, R. I., Chircov, C., Grumezescu, A. M., & Teleanu, D. M. (2019). Tumor angiogenesis and anti-angiogenic strategies for cancer treatment. *Journal of Clinical Medicine*, 9(1), 84.

Immunotherapy

Immunotherapy, also known as biotherapy, focuses on the use of the body's own immune system to fight cancer.

The body is protected from pathogens by physical barriers such as the skin and mucous membranes, as well as physiologic barriers such as temperature and acidity of the stomach. The immune system is composed of many cell types that collectively protect the body from infections and the growth of tumor cells and is generally broken down into two main branches: innate versus adaptive immunity. Cells of the innate system recognize and respond to pathogens in a generic way to provide immediate defense against infection, but they do not confer long-lasting or specific immunity. Each time an antigen is encountered in the body, the innate immune system will mount a generic response (e.g., elevate the body's temperature, cause inflammation) (NCI, 2022).

The adaptive system consists of specialized cells (e.g., lymphocytes) that eliminate or prevent pathogen growth, and provide long-lasting protection due to the presence of memory cells, leading to subsequent immune responses that are faster and stronger after an initial exposure to a foreign antigen. Like the innate system, the adaptive system includes two broad classes of responses: humoral (antibody) immunity and cell-mediated immunity (Tan et al., 2020).

- *Humoral immunity:* The immune response is mediated by specialized proteins and antibodies (i.e., immunoglobulins). Antibodies are secreted by activated B lymphocytes that are found in bone marrow. Antibodies travel through the bloodstream and bind to specific foreign antigens. Binding signals phagocytes or other immune cells to attack and inactivate the foreign antigen, preventing it from binding to the host.
- *Cell-mediated immunity:* The immune response is controlled by T cells and involves the activation of lymphocytes and release of cytokines in response to an antigen. T cells are made in the bone marrow, and most continue development in the thymus. T cells specifically bind to antigens recognized on foreign or nonself cells and can eliminate tumor cells before they have a chance to grow and spread (Abbott & Ustoyev, 2019).

Stimulatory and inhibitory factors in the immune response to cancer are shown in the figure on page 280. The nomenclature for immunotherapy is extensive (see the box on next page).

Principles of Cancer Management 3

Terms Used in Immunotherapy

Antibody: An immunoglobulin that is produced by B cells and that tightly binds to the surface antigen of a cell, tagging it for attack or directly neutralizing it.

Antigen: Any substance that induces an immune response, especially the production of antibodies.

Bacillus Calmette-Guérin (BCG): A weakened form of the bacterium *Mycobacterium bovis* (i.e., bacillus Calmette-Guérin) that does not cause disease. It is used in a solution to stimulate the immune system in the treatment of bladder cancer and as a vaccine to prevent tuberculosis.

B lymphocytes: White blood cells that produce antibodies specific to the antigen that stimulated their production.

Basophils: White blood cells that release histamine (i.e., substance involved in allergic reactions) and produce substances to attract other white blood cells (i.e., neutrophils and eosinophils) to an antigen.

Biologic response modifiers (BRMs): Substances made from living organisms to treat disease. They may occur naturally in the body, or they may be made in the laboratory. Some BRM therapies stimulate or suppress the immune system to help the body fight cancer, infection, and other diseases. Other BRM therapies attack specific cancer cells to prevent their growth or kill them.

BRCA1: A gene on chromosome 17 that normally helps to suppress tumor cell growth. Inherited mutations of *BRCA1* confer a higher risk of breast, ovarian, prostate, and other types of cancers.

BRCA2: A gene on chromosome 13 that normally helps to suppress tumor cell growth. Inherited mutations of *BRCA2* confer a higher risk of breast, ovarian, prostate, and other types of cancers.

Cell: The smallest unit of a living organism, composed of a nucleus and cytoplasm surrounded by a plasma membrane.

Center for Biologics Evaluation and Research (CBER): Organization within the FDA that regulates biologic products for human use and provides information to promote their appropriate use.

Chemotaxis: Process of using a chemical substance to attract cells to a particular site.

Complement system: Group of proteins that are involved in a series of reactions (i.e., the complement cascade) that help kill bacteria and other foreign cells by making them easier for macrophages to identify and ingest and by attracting macrophages and neutrophils to a foreign or nonself antigen.

Cytokines: Cell-signaling proteins that are secreted by immune and other cells and act as messengers to help regulate immune responses.

Cytotoxic T cells: T lymphocytes that attach to and kill cancer cells or cells that are otherwise infected or damaged; also known as *CD8+ T cells* or *killer T cells*.

Dendritic cells: Specialized white blood cells that reside in tissues and help T cells to recognize foreign antigens.

Effector T cells (Teffs): Mature T cells released into the bloodstream that are considered to be immunologically naïve until they encounter antigens for which their receptors have a high affinity; recognition of antigen leads to extensive T-cell proliferation and differentiation into effector cells.

Endogenous: Produced inside an organism or cell; the opposite of external (exogenous) production.

Eosinophils: White blood cells containing granules readily stained by eosin that can kill bacteria and other foreign cells too big to ingest, help immobilize and kill parasites, participate in allergic reactions, and help destroy cancer cells.

Ex vivo: A process performed or taking place outside of a living organism, such as genetic modification performed by taking tissue from an organ, modifying it in a controlled environment, and returning it to the original organ for therapeutic purposes.

Fibroblast: Connective tissue cell that makes and secretes collagen proteins.

Glycopeptide: A short chain of amino acids (i.e., building blocks of proteins) that has sugar molecules attached to it. Some glycopeptides have been studied for their ability to stimulate the immune system.

Glycoprotein: A protein that has sugar molecules attached to it.

Granulocyte-macrophage colony-stimulating factor (GM-CSF): Cytokine that promotes the growth of white blood cells, especially granulocytes, macrophages, and megakaryocytes (i.e., cells that become platelets); also called colony-stimulating factor 2. The pharmaceutic analogs of naturally occurring GM-CSF are sargramostim and molgramostim.

Helper T cells: T lymphocytes that carry the CD4 glycoprotein receptor on their surface; when stimulated by foreign antigens, they release cytokines that promote the activation and function of B cells and killer T cells.

Histocompatibility: Molecular profile of tissue defined by human leukocyte antigens and used to determine whether a transplanted tissue or organ will be accepted by the recipient.

Human leukocyte antigens (HLAs): Genetically determined system of proteins on the surface of cells that is almost unique for each person and thereby enables the body to distinguish self from nonself; the human version of the major histocompatibility complex (MHC) system found in most vertebrates.

Human papillomavirus (HPV): DNA virus with more than 100 HPV subtypes, some of which cause diseases in humans ranging from common warts to cervical cancer.

IDH1: A gene (isocitrate dehydrogenase 1) that is associated with a form of acute myeloid leukemia, chondrosarcomas, and brain tumors called gliomas. Recurrent point mutations affecting codon 132 of *IDH1*, located on chromosome locus 2q33, play a unique role in the pathogenesis of gliomas. Mutated *IDH1* is a strong prognostic factor in diffuse gliomas: Patients whose tumors harbored the wild-type gene had a median overall survival time of 1 year, compared with more than 2 years for those with tumors of the same grade and *IDH1* mutations.

Immune complex: Combination of an antibody and its corresponding antigen.

Immune modulators: Active agents of immunotherapy, such as natural or synthetic monoclonal antibodies and cytokines, or processes such as plasmapheresis, that are used to activate cell-mediated or humoral immunity.

Immune-related response criteria (irRC): Set of rules that define tumor responses during treatment with a drug being evaluated; based on new understanding of efficacy and the timing of response after initial treatment with an immunotherapeutic agent.

Immune response: The reaction of the immune system to an antigen.

Immunoglobulin: An antibody.

Immunosuppression: The immune system may be deliberately downregulated with drugs to prepare for bone marrow transplantation or to prevent rejection of donor tissue. It may also result from diseases such as acquired immunodeficiency syndrome and lymphoma or from the use of anticancer drugs.

Interleukins: Glycoproteins produced by white blood cells; a type of cytokine that regulates immune responses by communicating with and affecting other white blood cells.

Investigational new drug (IND) application: Federal law requires that a drug be the subject of an approved marketing application before it is transported or distributed across state lines. Before a laboratory or other sponsor ships the investigational drug to clinical investigators in other states, it must seek an exemption from the legal requirement by submitting an IND application to the U.S. Food and Drug Administration.

In vivo: A process performed or taking place inside a living organism, such as a genetic modification done within a cell.

Lentivector: *Lentivirus* is a genus in the Orthoretrovirinae subfamily of the Retroviridae family. Lentiviral vectors (LVs) include pathogens of bovine, equine, feline, ovine, and primate origin. Like other retroviruses, lentiviruses are enveloped particles that bud from an infected cell's plasma membrane. The particles bind to a target cell by an interaction between the cell's receptor and the viral glycoprotein.

Leukocytes: White blood cells, such as monocytes, neutrophils, eosinophils, basophils, B lymphocytes, and T lymphocytes.

Terms Used in Immunotherapy—cont'd

Lymphocytes: White blood cells responsible for adaptive (acquired) immunity. B cells produce antibodies, T cells distinguish self from non-self, and cytotoxic T cells kill infected cells and cancer cells.

Macrophages: Large cells that develop from white blood cells called monocytes. They ingest bacteria and other foreign cells, help T cells to identify microorganisms and other foreign substances, and are normally present in the lungs, skin, liver, and other tissues.

Major histocompatibility complex (MHC): System of genes that encode cell-surface proteins responsible for regulation of the immune system in vertebrates; in humans, these proteins are called *human leukocyte antigens* (HLAs).

Mast cells: Cells (i.e., granulocytes) found in connective tissues that release histamine and other substances during inflammatory and allergic reactions.

Mesenchymal cells: Loosely organized, mainly mesodermal embryonic cells that develop into connective and skeletal tissue, blood vessels, and lymphatic tissue.

MGMT: Gene that encodes O^6-methylguanine-DNA methyltransferase, which is a DNA repair enzyme that confers resistance to the effects of chemotherapy with nitrosourea derivatives (e.g., Carmustine— BCNU) or temozolomide in some tumors such as glioblastomas and astrocytomas.

Moiety: One-half or any significant portion of a molecule that may include a functional group.

Molecule: A group of electrochemically bonded atoms that represent the smallest fundamental unit of a chemical compound that can take part in a chemical reaction.

Monoclonal antibody: An antibody produced by cloning of a single cell line in the laboratory that binds to only one antigen. They are used to treat some types of cancers and can be designed to carry drugs, toxins, or radioactive substances directly to cancer cells.

Monocytes: Large, phagocytic white blood cells that are made in the bone marrow and travel through the bloodstream to other sites, where they can differentiate into macrophages and dendritic cells. Macrophages surround and kill microorganisms, ingest foreign material, remove dead cells, and boost immune responses.

Myeloid growth factor: Natural substances that stimulate the bone marrow to make blood cells and can be used prophylactically to reduce the severity and duration of neutropenia.

Natural killer (NK) cells: White blood cells that recognize, bind to, and kill virus-infected cells and cancer cells without having to be stimulated by antigens.

Nanoparticles: A microscopic particle that behaves as a whole unit in terms of its transport and other properties and can be designed to carry a drug to tiny metastatic tumors. They are further classified as ultrafine particles (1 to 100 nm), fine particles (100 to 2500 nm), and coarse particles (2500 to 10,000 nm).

Neutrophils: White blood cells that form an essential part of the innate immune system and are among the first responders to acute inflammation. They ingest and kill bacteria and other foreign cells.

Pathogen-associated molecular patterns (PAMPs): Molecules associated with groups of pathogens that activate innate immune responses, protecting the host from infection by identifying some nonself molecules.

Peptide: A molecule that contains two or more amino acids, which join to form proteins. Peptides that contain many amino acids are called *polypeptides* or *proteins.*

Peripheral blood stem cells (PBSCs): A small number of stem cells have escaped the bone marrow before maturation into red blood cells, white blood cells, or platelets and circulate in the bloodstream.

Phagocyte: A type of cell (e.g., neutrophil, macrophage) that is capable of engulfing and absorbing invading microorganisms, other small cells, and cell fragments.

Phagocytosis: The process of engulfing and ingesting invading microorganisms, other small cells, or cell fragments.

Pleiotropic cytokines: A cytokine that affects the activity of multiple cell types. Cytokines are small proteins that have specific effects on the interactions between cells and the behavior of cells.

Polypeptide: A substance that contains many amino acids, which join together to form proteins.

Receptors: Proteins embedded in surface membranes of cells and organelles to which complementary molecules, such as hormones, neurotransmitters, antigens, or antibodies, may become bound.

Regulatory T cells (Tregs): White blood cells that modulate the immune system, maintain tolerance to self-antigens, and abrogate autoimmune disease; formerly known as suppressor T cells.

Ribonucleic acid (RNA): Single-stranded molecule that is transcribed from DNA and assembled from long chains of nucleotides. Each nucleotide contains a nitrogenous base, a ribose sugar, and a phosphate group. RNA has roles in regulation and expression of genes.

RNA interference (RNAi): A process by which RNA molecules inhibit gene expression, as when microRNA (miRNA) or small interfering RNA (siRNA) molecules bind to specific messenger RNA (mRNA) molecules and increase or decrease their activity.

Signal transduction: Process by which a signal, such as a hormone or a change in the concentration of an ion, is converted into a biochemical response by activation of a receptor on the surface or interior of a cell.

Signal transduction pathways: Groups of molecules in a cell that transmit molecular signals, in a cascading fashion, to control cell functions. Some pathway components serve as markers of tumor activity or provide therapeutic targets, such as the PI3K/AKT/mTOR pathway, which plays a central role in cell growth and proliferation.

T lymphocytes: White blood cells that are involved in adaptive immunity ($\alpha\beta$ T cells) and innate immunity ($\gamma\delta$ T cells). Subpopulations include helper, killer (cytotoxic), and regulatory T cells.

Toll-like receptors (TLRs): A class of proteins that play a key role in the innate immune system. They are single, membrane-spanning, noncatalytic receptors, usually expressed in sentinel cells (e.g., macrophages, dendritic cells), that recognize structurally conserved molecules expressed by microbial pathogens.

TP53: A tumor suppressor gene that normally inhibits the growth of tumors and is mutated in many types of cancers. It is called the *guardian of the genome* because of its role in conserving stability by preventing genomic mutations.

Transcription: In biology, the first step of gene expression, in which a segment of DNA (gene) is copied (transcribed) into RNA by the enzyme RNA polymerase.

Transfer RNA (tRNA): A small RNA molecule that participates in protein synthesis. Each tRNA molecule has two important areas: a trinucleotide region called the *anticodon* and a region for attaching a specific amino acid. During translation, each time an amino acid is added to the growing chain, a tRNA molecule forms base pairs with its complementary sequence on the mRNA molecule, ensuring that the appropriate amino acid is inserted into the protein.

Tumor microenvironment: The normal cells, molecules, and blood vessels that surround and feed a tumor cell. A tumor can change its microenvironment, and the microenvironment can affect how a tumor grows and spreads.

U.S. Food and Drug Administration (FDA): The federal agency in the Department of Health and Human Services that is responsible for protecting and promoting public health.

Vaccine: One or more substances that are prepared from the causative agent of a disease and treated to act as an antigen (i.e., stimulate the immune system) without inducing the disease. A vaccine helps the body recognize and destroy cancer cells or microorganisms.

Vaccine adjuvant: A substance that is added to a vaccine to improve the immune response so that less vaccine is needed.

Vaccine therapy: Treatment that uses one or more substances to stimulate the immune response against tumor cells or infectious microorganisms such as bacteria or viruses.

Vector: In molecular cloning, a vehicle (e.g., virus, plasmid) whose DNA is used to carry a desired foreign DNA sequence into a host cell (also called *recombinant DNA*). Depending on the purpose of the cloning procedure, the vector may assist in multiplying, isolating, or expressing the foreign DNA insert.

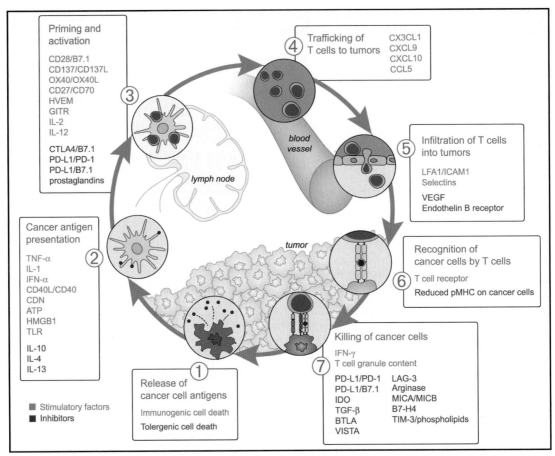

Stimulatory and Inhibitory Factors in the Cancer-Immunity Cycle. Each step of the cancer-immunity cycle requires the coordination of numerous factors, both stimulatory and inhibitory in nature. Stimulatory factors promote immunity, whereas inhibitors regulate immunity by reducing immune activity and/or preventing autoimmunity. (From Chen, D. S., & Mellman, I. [2013]. Oncology meets immunology: The cancer-immunity cycle. *Immunity, 39*[1], 1–10, 25.)

Cytokines

Cytokines are secreted by lymphocytes and monocytes, and they activate or deactivate downstream cellular function, activity, and division (NCI, 2022). They include the colony-stimulating factors, interferons, and interleukins.

Colony-Stimulating Factors

Colony-stimulating factors are a family of glycoproteins that help to regulate differentiation, proliferation, and activation of hematopoietic cell lineages. They act on different cells of the hematopoietic cascade at different times during the differentiation and proliferation phases.

Six colony-stimulating growth factors are approved for use in the United States:
1. Granulocyte colony-stimulating factor (G-CSF)
2. Granulocyte-macrophage colony-stimulating factor (GM-CSF)
3. Erythropoietin (EPO)
4. Interleukin-11 (IL-11)
5. Keratinocyte growth factor
6. Thrombopoietin (TPO) receptor agonists

Examples of FDA-Approved Immunotherapies

Agents	Drug Class	Oncologic Indications
Filgrastim Filgrastim-sndz Tbo-filgrastim Pegfilgrastim	Granulocyte colony-stimulating factor (G-CSF)	Tbo-filgrastim and pegfilgrastim are approved for use in patients with nonmyeloid malignancies receiving anticancer therapy. Filgrastim and filgrastim-sndz can be used in patients with acute myelogenous leukemia (AML), those undergoing peripheral blood progenitor cell collection, those undergoing bone marrow transplantation, and those with severe chronic neutropenia
Sargramostim	Granulocyte-macrophage colony-stimulating factor (GM-CSF)	Used after induction therapy for AML and for stem cell transplantation
Epoetin alfa Erythropoietin	Erythropoiesis-stimulating agent (ESA)	Treatment of anemia in patients with nonmyeloid malignancies for anemia due to myelosuppressive chemotherapy and when there are at least 2 more months of planned chemotherapy

Examples of FDA-Approved Immunotherapies—cont'd

Agents	Drug Class	Oncologic Indications
Oprelvekin	Thrombopoietic growth factor	Recombinant interleukin-11 prevents severe thrombocytopenia and reduces the need for platelet transfusions after myelosuppressive chemotherapy in adult patients with nonmyeloid malignancies
Romiplostim Eltrombopag	Thrombopoietin (TPO) receptor agonists	Immune thrombocytopenia
Palifermin	Keratinocyte growth factor	Decreases incidence and duration of severe inflammation and ulceration of the lining of the mouth and throat (i.e., mucositis) in patients with bone marrow cancer who are receiving chemotherapy and radiotherapy to prepare the bone marrow for stem cell transplantation
Interferon alfa	Interferon	Chronic hepatitis B and C Kaposi sarcoma related to acquired immunodeficiency syndrome (AIDS) Condyloma acuminatum Malignant melanoma Follicular lymphoma Predominantly clear cell stage IV renal cell carcinoma
Human papillomavirus quadrivalent vaccine	Vaccine	Prevention of cervical, vulvar, vaginal, and anal cancer in women Prevention of anal and penile cancer in men
Interleukin-2	Interleukin	Renal carcinoma Melanoma
Ipilimumab	Monoclonal antibody and checkpoint inhibitor	Targets the CTLA4 receptor and stimulates the immune system Unresectable or metastatic melanoma
Nivolumab	Monoclonal antibody and immunomodulator	Targets the programmed cell death protein 1 (PD1) receptor on T cells Unresectable or metastatic melanoma Metastatic squamous non–small cell lung cancer

Granulocyte Colony-Stimulating Factor. G-CSF is a myeloid growth factor that regulates cell proliferation, maturation, and function of the neutrophil cell lineage of the myeloid cell line. G-CSF's primary role is to reduce the incidence of neutropenia and aid hematopoietic recovery from cytotoxic and radiotherapeutic treatments. G-CSF can be secreted by a variety of cells in the body (Crawford et al., 2021). Circulating G-CSF levels and secretion are directly affected by inflammatory responses to toxins and tissue damage and are inversely affected by the total number of circulating neutrophils. In severely neutropenic subjects, detectable serum levels of G-CSF can be more than 2000 mg/dL (DeVita et al., 2015).

GCS-F agents allow patients receiving marrow toxic chemotherapeutic regimens to have earlier neutrophil recovery, which in turn decreases the risk of opportunistic and potentially life-threatening infections which can severely impact patient outcomes.

Four G-CSFs are in use in the United States (see table above):

1. Filgrastim (Neupogen)
2. Pegfilgrastim (Neulasta)
3. Tbo-filgrastim (Granix)
4. Filgrastim-sndz (Zarxio).

Use of these agents has reduced the incidence of febrile neutropenia and decreased the length of hospital stays (Cerchione et al., 2021; Crawford et al., 2021).

Granulocyte-Macrophage Colony-Stimulating Factor. GM-CSF is potent cytokine that directly affects hematopoiesis and has many implications for the care of patients with cancer. GM-CSF can increase circulating numbers of neutrophils, eosinophils, and macrophages (Petrina et al., 2021). The only form of GM-CSF approved by the FDA is sargramostim; however, accelerated approval is underway for additional thera-

pies. GM-CSF is used primarily after autologous or allogeneic hematopoietic cell transplantation (HCT) and is also used to chemotherapy-induced neutropenia in AML, after transplantation of autologous peripheral blood progenitor cells, and in the setting of bone marrow transplant failure and engraftment delay (Petrina et al., 2021).

Erythropoiesis-Stimulating Agents. Erythropoiesis-stimulating agents (ESAs), unlike other CSFs, act directly on pluripotent stem cells and in the later stages of hematopoietic development, targeting myeloid progenitor cells and erythrocytes. Erythropoietin (EPO) is also unique among cytokines in that it is almost exclusively secreted by the liver and kidneys rather than the bone marrow (Kidanewold et al., 2021).

EPO production and secretion are inversely affected by the oxygen-carrying capacity of the circulating red blood cells (Kidanewold et al., 2021). This negative feedback loop decreases EPO secretion when levels of oxygen-binding capacity are high and increases EPO secretion when levels are low, balancing the numbers of circulating red blood cells with the body's oxygen demands without overproduction of red blood cells. In some instances, EPO overproduction resulting in erythrocytosis is observed in patients with primary renal tumors that cause local renal hypoxic conditions or tumors that intrinsically oversecrete EPO (Bohlius et al., 2019).

In patients with cancer, ESAs are indicated for the effects of concomitant myelosuppressive but noncurative chemotherapy when at least two additional months of therapy are planned. Historically, ESAs have been widely used for the treatment of chemotherapy-associated anemia, but data have revealed that the agents may shorten overall survival time or increase the risk of tumor progression in some patients. When using ESAs, the lowest dose is recommended to avoid red blood cell transfusions, and the agent should be used only in patients with noncurative disease where physicians can also monitor patients closely during and after treatment (Bohlius et al., 2019).

Keratinocyte Growth Factor. Keratinocyte growth factor (KGF) is a cytokine originating from mesenchymal cells, fibroblasts, and microvascular endothelial cells. It activates epithelial cell repair and provides protection in response to inflammatory cytokines and steroidal hormones. Evidence suggests that the addition of KGF to chemotherapy for myeloid malignancies can prevent gastrointestinal graft-versus-host disease by acting as a cytokine protectant and by reducing the generation of proinflammatory cytokines. KGF can promote T-cell engraftment and reconstitution, indicating that KGF may play an important role in the prevention of epithelial toxicity in the treatment of myeloid malignancies (Sadeghi et al., 2021).

For patients with hematologic malignancies, trials have demonstrated a direct correlation between KGF administration and a reduction in the severity and duration of oral mucositis due to intense chemotherapy regimens. In vitro and in vivo studies have shown KGF to be an important cytoprotectant through its ability to positively affect epithelial cell differentiation, proliferation, and migration and because of having beneficial effects on epithelial cell survival, repair, and detoxification after exposure to cytotoxins (Sadeghi et al., 2021).

Thrombopoietin Agonists. Thrombopoietin (TPO) agonists increase platelet production through the regulation of thrombopoiesis. They are indicated for patients with chronic immune thrombocytopenia (ITP) and are activated by TPO receptors on the megakaryocyte cell surface. Two TPO receptor agonists, romiplostim and eltrombopag, are approved (Mahat et al., 2020).

Virology and Immunotherapy

Genetic material cannot be directly inserted into cells, requiring a vector to transport gene therapies into the cells. Viruses are commonly used as vectors as they recognize specific cells and can insert genetic material inside, as they would if infecting a cell. To make the process safer for humans, viruses are altered by inactivating genes that enable them to reproduce or cause disease, and enhancement of their ability to recognize and enter the target cell.

Oncolytic adenoviruses offer another therapeutic option. Adenoviruses are double-stranded DNA viruses that normally cause mild respiratory, digestive, and ocular infections in humans and can directly infect and kill tumor cells when genetically engineered to do so. Advances have been seen in the use of oncolytic virotherapy in brain tumors, and multiple myeloma as oncolytic adenoviruses demonstrate a tremendous capacity for tumor cell lysis and immune response stimulation (Peter & Kühnel, 2020; Zhao et al., 2021).

Interferons

Interferon alfa-2b, an antiviral drug, first received FDA approval for the treatment of hairy cell leukemia; however, it went on to receive approval for treating chronic hepatitis B and C, AIDS-related Kaposi sarcoma, condyloma acumina-

tum, malignant melanoma, follicular lymphoma, Philadelphia chromosome–positive chronic myelogenous leukemia (CML), and advanced renal cell carcinoma. Interferon-alpha (IFN-α) remains the only approved interferon for the treatment of malignancies in the United States. IFN-β has received approval for use in multiple sclerosis, and IFN-γ is approved for use in chronic granulomatous disease. Approved interferons include the following: interferon alfa-2a (Roferon-A), interferon alfa-2b (Intron-A), interferon alfa-n3 (Alferon-N), peginterferon alfa-2a (Pegasys), peginterferon alfa-2b (PegIntron), interferon beta-1a (Avonex), interferon beta-1b (Betaseron), interferon alfacon-1 (Infergen), interferon gamma-1b (Actmmune) (NCI, 2019).

All type I IFNs bind to type I receptors on cell surfaces (i.e., IFNAR1 and IFNAR2), which then bind to the Janus-activated kinase (JAK), where the receptor undergoes oligomerization, with transphosphorylation of JAKs followed by phosphorylation of the cytoplasmic tails of the receptor molecules. This provides a docking site for the signal transducers and activators of transcription. After binding, IFN exerts its effect by suppressing proliferation, inducing cell apoptosis, inhibiting angiogenesis, increasing the immunogenicity of tumor cells, and activating cytotoxicity against tumor cells. IFN plays an essential role in anticancer therapy through its immunomodulatory effects such as the upregulation of natural killer cells (key players in antibody-dependent cellular cytotoxicity), macrophages, dendritic cells, neutrophils, and T and B cells (Conlon et al., 2019).

Interleukins

Interleukins are the class of cytokines which play a significant role in the maintenance of hematopoiesis and response to foreign body invasion. Interleukins are a key component in the inflammatory response and attract effector cells to the point of origin of infection. They play an important role in the stimulation and proliferation of effector and immune cell lines during the infection process. Of the 18 interleukins discovered, those with the greatest potential for anticancer use are IL-1, IL-2, IL-3, IL-6, IL-7, IL-11, IL-12, and IL-16 (NCI, 2019).

IL-1 has a main role in inflammatory responses, is primarily produced by the macrophages in response to stimulation by toxins and other cytokines, and helps lymphocytes fight infection. It also helps leukocytes pass through blood vessel walls to sites of infection and causes fever by affecting areas of the brain that control body temperature. Two subtypes of IL-1 (IL-1α and IL-1β) share the same receptor site on cell surfaces, but each type affects cells in different ways. IL-1 locally affects cells by increasing production of adhesion molecules, prostaglandins, and chemokines. A systemic response to invading toxins occurs through the production of fever and hypotension in the host (Majidpoor & Mortezaee, 2021).

Interleukin-2. IL-2 has been the focus of clinical research in the treatment of malignancies and is the only interleukin to receive FDA approval for use in cancer. In 1992, the FDA approved its use in renal cell cancer, and it was approved for melanoma in 1997 because of its ability to upregulate proliferation and differentiation of natural killer cells and T lymphocytes. IL-2 also works with a cofactor to activate macrophages and B cells (Majidpoor & Mortezaee, 2021).

Adverse effects of IL-2 present the primary complication of the use of IL-2 immunotherapy, and include severe flulike symptoms, fever, chills, nausea, vomiting, diarrhea, capillary leak syndrome, rash, anemia, thrombocytopenia, neutropenia, myalgias, arthralgias, exfoliative dermatitis, and confusion. Life-threatening side effects include hypotension, cardiac arrhythmia, pulmonary edema with dyspnea and severe respiratory distress, renal insufficiency with decreased renal perfusion causing acute oliguric and anuric renal failure, hepatic toxicity with hyperbilirubinemia or transaminitis, hemostatic changes in thromboplastin and prothrombin times, encephalopathy, primary delirium, depression, somnolence, and anxiety (Majidpoor & Mortezaee, 2021; NCI, 2022).

Due to the significant impact of these adverse effects, IL-2 must be administered in carefully selected patients in a closely controlled hospital setting with optimal supportive care and prophylactic medications to prevent exacerbation of toxicities. Corticosteroids should not be used with IL-2 because they may blunt the immune response to IL-2, negating the therapeutic immunostimulatory effects against the cancer (Wrangle et al., 2018).

CAR T-Cell

In the last 6 years, CAR T-cell therapy has been approved by the FDA for the treatment of lymphomas, some forms of leukemia, and multiple myeloma—especially progressive disease (NCI, 2022). Unlike other gene therapies or immunotherapies, CAR T-cells are derived from collecting a patient's own T-cells and then re-engineering them to produce chimeric antigen receptors (CARs) while binding to specific cancer cell proteins. They are then reinfused to the patient (see the figure below). Although CAR-T continues to be refined as a therapy, the treatment has offered hope to patients with aggressive disease that was previously untreatable—and therapies beyond the six currently FDA-approved agents are anticipated in the coming years (see the table on the next page) (NCI, 2022).

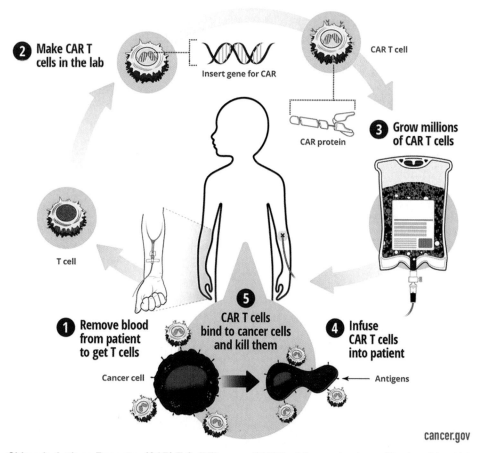

Chimeric Antigen Receptor (CAR) T-Cell Therapy. CAR T-cell therapy is a type of treatment in which a patient's T cells are genetically engineered in the laboratory so they will bind to specific proteins (antigens) on cancer cells and kill them. (1) A patient's T cells are removed from their blood. Then, (2) the gene for a special receptor called a CAR is inserted into the T cells in the laboratory. The gene encodes the engineered CAR protein that is expressed on the surface of the patient's T cells, creating a CAR T cell. (3) Millions of CAR T cells are grown in the laboratory. (4) They are then given to the patient by intravenous infusion. (5) The CAR T cells bind to antigens on the cancer cells and kill them. (From National Cancer Institute. [2022]. *CAR T cells: Engineering patients' immune cells to treat their cancers*. Available at https://www.cancer.gov/about-cancer/treatment/research/car-t-cells.)

FDA-Approved CAR T-Cell Therapies

Generic Name	Brand Name	Target Antigen	Target Disease	Patient Population
Tisagenlecleucel	Kymriah	CD19	B-cell acute lymphoblastic leukemia (ALL)	Children and young adults with refractory or relapsed B-cell ALL
			B-cell non-Hodgkin lymphoma (NHL)	Adults with relapsed or refractory B-cell NHL
Axicabtagene ciloleucel	Yescarta	CD19	B-cell NHL	Adults with relapsed or refractory B-cell NHL
			Follicular lymphoma	Adults with relapsed or refractory follicular lymphoma
Brexucabtagene autoleucel	Tecartus	CD19	Mantle cell lymphoma (MCL)	Adults with relapsed or refractory MCL
			B-cell ALL	Adults with refractory or relapsed B-cell ALL
Lisocabtagene maraleucel	Breyanzi	CD19	B-cell NHL	Adults with relapsed or refractory B-cell NHL
Idecabtagene vicleucel	Abecma	BCMA	Multiple myeloma	Adults with relapsed or refractory multiple myeloma
Ciltacabtagene autoleucel	Carvykti	BCMA	Multiple myeloma	Adults with relapsed or refractory multiple myeloma

From National Cancer Institute. (2022). *CAR T cells: Engineering patients' immune cells to treat their cancers*. Available at https://www.cancer.gov/about-cancer/treatment/research/car-t-cells.

Bibliography

Abbott, M., & Ustoyev, Y. (2019). Cancer and the immune system: The history and background of immunotherapy. *Seminars in Oncology Nursing*, 35(5), 150923.

Bohlius, J., Bohlke, K., Castelli, R., Djulbegovic, B., Lustberg, M. B., Martino, M., … Lazo-Langner, A. (2019). Management of cancer-associated anemia with erythropoiesis-stimulating agents: ASCO/ASH clinical practice guideline update. *Blood Advances*, 3(8), 1197–1210.

Cerchione, C., Nappi, D., & Martinelli, G. (2021). Pegfilgrastim for primary prophylaxis of febrile neutropenia in multiple myeloma. *Support Care in Cancer*, 29(11), 6973–6980.

Conlon, K. C., Miljkovic, M. D., & Waldmann, T. A. (2019). Cytokines in the Treatment of Cancer. *Journal of Interferon and Cytokine Research*, 39(1), 6–21.

Crawford, J., Moore, D. C., Morrison, V. A., & Dale, D. (2021). Use of prophylactic pegfilgrastim for chemotherapy-induced neutropenia in the US: A review of adherence to present guidelines for usage. *Cancer Treatment and Research Communications*, 29, 100466.

DeVita, V. T., Hellman, S., & Rosenberg, S. A. (2015). *Cancer principles and practice of oncology* (10th ed.). Philadelphia: Lippincott Williams & Wilkins.

Kidanewold, A., Woldu, B., & Enawgaw, B. (2021). Role of erythropoiesis stimulating agents in the treatment of anemia: A literature review. *Clinical Laboratory*, 67(4).

Mahat, U., Rotz, S. J., & Hanna, R. (2020). Use of thrombopoietin receptor agonists in prolonged thrombocytopenia after hematopoietic stem cell transplantation. *Biology of Blood and Marrow Transplantation*, 26(3), e65–e73.

Majidpoor, J., & Mortezaee, K. (2021). Interleukin-2 therapy of cancer-clinical perspectives. *International Immunopharmacology*, 98, 107836.

National Cancer Institute (NCI) (2019, April 24). Immune system modulators. Available at https://www.cancer.gov/about-cancer/treatment/types/immunotherapy/immune-system-modulators.

National Cancer Institute (NCI). (2022, March 10). CAR T cells: Engineering patients' immune cells to treat their cancers. Available at https://www.cancer.gov/about-cancer/treatment/research/car-t-cells.

Nessa, M. U., Rahman, M. A., & Kabir, Y. (2020). Plant-produced monoclonal antibody as immunotherapy for cancer. *BioMed Research International*, 2020, 3038564.

O'Donnell, J. S., Teng, M. W. L., & Smyth, M. J. (2019). Cancer immunoediting and resistance to T cell-based immunotherapy. *Nature Reviews. Clinical Oncology*, 16(3), 151–167.

Peter, M., & Kühnel, F. (2020). Oncolytic Adenovirus in cancer immunotherapy. *Cancers (Basel)*, 12(11), 3354.

Petrina, M., Martin, J., & Basta, S. (2021). Granulocyte macrophage colony-stimulating factor has come of age: From a vaccine adjuvant to antiviral immunotherapy. *Cytokine Growth Factor Rev*, 59, 101–110.

Sadeghi, S., Kalhor, H., Panahi, M., Abolhasani, H., Rahimi, B., Kalhor, R., … Rahimi, H. (2021). Keratinocyte growth factor in focus: A comprehensive review from structural and functional aspects to therapeutic applications of palifermin. *International Journal of Biological Macromolecules*, 191, 1175–1190.

Tan, S., Li, D., & Zhu, X. (2020). Cancer immunotherapy: Pros, cons and beyond. *Biomedicine and Pharmacotherapy*, 124, 109821.

Wrangle, J. M., Patterson, A., Johnson, C. B., Neitzke, D. J., Mehrotra, S., Denlinger, C. E., … Rubinstein, M. P. (2018). IL-2 and beyond in cancer immunotherapy. *Journal of Interferon and Cytokine Research*, 38(2), 45–68.

Zhao, Y., Liu, Z., Li, L., Wu, J., Zhang, H., Zhang, H., … Xu, B. (2021). Oncolytic Adenovirus: Prospects for Cancer Immunotherapy. *Frontiers in Microbiology*, 12, 707290.

Hormonal Therapy

Kristin M. Ferguson and Elizabeth Anderson Strand

Introduction

The importance of hormonal suppression in the treatment of breast cancer was recognized as early as the 19th century. In 1896, George Beatson observed an association between surgical removal of the ovaries and a reduction in some breast tumors (Beatson, 1896). Since that time, estrogen suppression has been attempted through many different mechanisms including surgical, chemical, and radiation. Because hormonal therapies are highly specific in their ability to block specific receptors and various feedback loops, they were the first form of targeted therapy. While hormone therapy was first used in the treatment of breast cancer, it was quickly added to the treatment regimens for prostate, endometrial, and ovarian cancers (Li et al., 2021). Tumor growth that is stimulated by testosterone or estrogen can be suppressed by blocking these hormones, inhibiting cancer cell communication and growth.

Adrenocorticosteroids

Adrenocorticosteroids are primarily responsible for the control of glucose metabolism, gluconeogenesis, and immune system regulation. The major forms of adrenocorticosteroids are glucocorticoids (e.g., cortisol, corticosterone), mineralocorticoids (e.g., aldosterone), and androgens. Adrenocorticosteroids are synthesized in the adrenal cortex and regulated through the action of adrenocorticotropic hormone (ACTH), which is produced in the anterior pituitary. The regulation of ACTH depends on a precise and sensitive balance between serum levels and stimulation from the central nervous system (Anandabaskar, 2021).

The most used corticosteroids in clinical practice are cortisone acetate, hydrocortisone, prednisolone, methylprednisolone, and dexamethasone. Because lymphoid cells are sensitive to glucocorticoids, which inhibit lymphocyte proliferation by encouraging apoptosis, adrenocorticosteroids are used commonly in treating lymphocyte-rich cancers such as acute lymphoblastic leukemia, chronic lymphocytic leukemia, Hodgkin disease, non-Hodgkin lymphoma, and multiple myeloma (Clarisse et al., 2020). The hormones also may be used as adjuvant treatment with routine antiemetics and analgesics, and to reduce cerebral edema due to central nervous system metastasis.

Potential side effects from this class of drugs include fluid retention, the appearance of Cushing syndrome, peptic ulcer disease, hypertension, bone loss leading to osteoporosis, diabetes mellitus, muscle weakness, and profound immune system suppression. Additional side effects can include facial flushing, headache, euphoria, anxiety, insomnia, and steroid psychosis. While glucocorticoids are essential in the treatment of many cancers, gradual resistance can develop over time (Clarisse et al., 2020).

Hormonal Therapy for Prostate Cancer

Antiandrogens

Androgens are the major sex steroids in males. The primary functions of the androgens are male development, spermatogenesis, inhibition of fat deposition, increased muscle mass, and brain development. The best-known adrenal androgen is testosterone, which is produced by the testes. Antiandrogens comprise a group of hormonal therapies used in men with castration-resistant prostate cancer for androgen-deprivation therapy (ADT). These medications block binding of dihydrotestosterone to the androgen receptor, inhibiting tumor growth that depends on these hormones (Dawson, 2021). ADT options include bilateral orchiectomy or luteinizing hormone–releasing hormone, also known as gonadotropin-releasing hormone (GnRH) agonist, or a combination of GnRH with antiandrogen. Abiraterone (an inhibitor of androgen synthesis) and enzalutamide (a selective inhibitor of androgen receptors) are two new agents that now prolong overall survival. They are considered first line system therapies when endocrine therapy is indicated (Dawson, 2021).

Antiandrogen agents include bicalutamide, nilutamide, and flutamide (see table below). Side effects of antiandrogens can include hot flashes, loss of libido, impotence, bone loss, and gynecomastia.

Hormonal Therapy for Prostate Cancer

Drug	Trade Names	Dose	Common Side Effects	Serious Side Effects
GnRH agonist: leuprolide (Lupron)	Eligard Lupron Depot Viadur	7.5 mg for 1 month, 22.5 mg for 3 months, 30 mg for 4 months, and 45 mg for 6 months	Hot flashes, pain, testicular atrophy, flu-like syndrome, decreased libido	Urinary retention, increased cholesterol, depression, weakness (loss of strength)
Antiandrogen: bicalutamide	Casodex	50 mg by mouth daily	Hot flashes, decreased libido, impotence	Diarrhea, elevated liver function tests, loss of fertility

Continued

Hormonal Therapy for Prostate Cancer—Cont'd

Drug	Trade Names	Dose	Common Side Effects	Serious Side Effects
Antiandrogen: nilutamide	Nilandron Anandron	300 mg by mouth daily for 30 days, then 150 mg by mouth daily	Vision changes—blurred, nausea	Pneumonitis (2%), osteoporosis, increase in LFTs
Antiandrogen: flutamide (not commonly used)	Eulexin	250 mg by mouth every 8 h for total daily dose of 750 mg	Diarrhea, nausea and vomiting, fatal hepatotoxicity, hot flashes, gynecomastia, decreased libido	Hepatotoxicity
Androgen receptor inhibitor: enzalutamide	Xtandi	160 mg by mouth daily; check website for modification options	Fatigue, back pain, decreased appetite, hot flashes, edema, hypertension	Upper respiratory tract infection, low white blood cell count, dizziness, seizure
CYP17 inhibitor: abiraterone	Zytiga	1000 mg by mouth daily 1 h before or 2 h after meals With prednisone 5 mg by mouth twice daily	Fatigue, edema, hot flashes, diarrhea, hypertension	Increased triglycerides, increased liver enzymes (AST)

AST, Aspartate transaminase; *GnRG,* gonadotropin-releasing hormone; *LFTs,* liver function test results.
Please refer to most updated guidelines from National Comprehensive Cancer Network on prostate cancer. Available at http://nccn.org/professionals/physician_gls/pdf/prostate.pdf (accessed January 28, 2022).

Hormonal Therapy for Breast Cancer

Antiestrogens: Breast Cancer

More than a century ago, estrogen was found to play an important role in the pathophysiologic mechanisms of breast cancer. As discussed earlier, in 1896, Dr. George Beatson showed evidence that oophorectomies in premenopausal women with inoperable breast cancer could improve survival (Kumar et al., 2022). In the same way, some postmenopausal women responded to adrenalectomy or hypophysectomy. With the discovery of the estrogen receptor (ER), the mechanism of action for estrogen on the various target tissues became better understood. Drugs were then developed to target these receptors. The two most common drug classes used for their antiestrogen-like effects are selective estrogen receptor modulators (SERMs) and aromatase inhibitors (AIs).

Estrogen Production. Current knowledge reveals two major routes for estrogen production: ovarian production and peripheral aromatization. In premenopausal women, both routes are active. In postmenopausal women, only the peripheral aromatization pathway is active because the ovaries have decreased production of estrogen. This difference has significant implications for the use of hormonal therapy in women with breast cancer, depending on their premenopausal or postmenopausal status. In most postmenopausal women, androstenedione is released from the adrenal glands. This adrenal steroid goes through several metabolic steps before interacting with the aromatase enzyme and being converted to estrogen. This process is known as aromatization. The enzymatic conversion occurs in sites such as breast tissue, liver, muscles, and fat cells and is catalyzed by the aromatase enzyme complex. Blocking or inhibiting the aromatase enzyme makes the conversion to estrogen impossible. AIs work in this way.

Selective Estrogen Receptor Modulators

SERMs work by occupying the estrogen receptors inside cells to block the action of estrogen in breast and other estrogen-sensitive tissues. When a receptor is blocked, the malignant cells cannot grow and divide. SERMs do not block all estrogen receptors. As the name suggests, they selectively inhibit certain estrogen receptors, such as those in breast tissue, while allowing stimulation of estrogen receptors in other organs, such as bone and uterus in postmenopausal women (although this is not the case for premenopausal women). Tamoxifen (Nolvadex) is the most commonly used SERM. Initially approved in the UK in 1973, tamoxifen became the first "targeted" therapies in the treatment of cancer helping establish the larger principles of chemoprevention (Quirke, 2017). Unlike tamoxifen, raloxifene (Evista) is only used in postmenopausal women (American Society of Clinical Oncology [ASCO], 2019). It has fewer side effects than tamoxifen and is not associated with an increased risk of uterine cancer although it has been shown to not be quite as effective as tamoxifen. It is sometimes used to treat osteoporosis for its benefit to bone health. Toremifene (Fareston) is another option, but it is not widely used in the United States.

Tamoxifen has been the mainstay of care, regardless of menopausal status, reducing both distant and locoregional recurrence by 40% to 50%, and is initiated after local therapy (adjuvant) for 5 years (Burnstein, 2020). In estrogen receptor positive early breast cancer, tamoxifen is the standard of care for premenopausal women. When estrogen receptor expression is high, it can also be used in postmenopausal women depending on a review of risk factors and the side effect profile (American Society of Clinical Oncology [ASCO], 2019).

Aromatase Inhibitors

Since the late 1990s, options for adjuvant endocrine therapy have widened beyond tamoxifen to include aromatase inhibitors (anastrozole, exemestane, and letrozole) and the injectable estrogen receptor antagonist fulvestrant. However, these agents are contraindicated in premenopausal women who are not undergoing ovarian suppression (OS) (Burnstein, 2020). Aminoglutethimide was the first drug used to block the aromatase enzyme in women with metastatic breast cancer. Since that time, several other agents have become available. Two major classes of AIs currently exist: nonsteroidal AIs and steroidal AIs.

Nonsteroidal aromatase inhibitors, also known as competitive AIs, bind reversibly to the receptor site on the enzyme and prevent the formation of estrogen for as long they occupy the site. These medications include anastrozole and letrozole.

Steroidal aromatase inhibitors, also called noncompetitive AIs, are derivatives of androstenedione. This class of AIs retain the androgenic properties. Because these agents bind irreversibly to the aromatase enzyme, they are also called *suicide inhibitors.* New enzymes must be synthesized to overcome this inhibitor even after the drug has been cleared from the body. Hypothetically, these agents should have improved efficacy compared with the reversible inhibitors, although it has been shown to be slightly less effective than tamoxifen. Exemestane is the steroidal AI currently used. Therefore, there are currently three AIs widely used in the postmenopausal setting. All three drugs have been shown to be equally efficacious and all three have similar side effects. For reasons we do not understand, some women may tolerate one AI better than another. The most common side effects of AIs include muscle and joint pain, hot flashes, vaginal dryness, and bone loss. Unlike tamoxifen, the AIs tend to speed up bone loss which can lead to osteoporosis. In early breast cancer, whether with a SERM or an AI, the minimum length of treatment is 5 years and may be up to 10 depending on the extent of disease and prognostic features at diagnosis (Richman and Dowsett, 2019). For those with high-risk disease who undergo adjuvant chemotherapy prior to starting oral endocrine therapy, it is important for patients to understand that although chemotherapy is typically more toxic and felt to be "aggressive," adherence to their pill is the mainstay of risk reduction in estrogen receptor positive breast cancer (Burnstein, 2020). AIs are contraindicated in premenopausal women who are not undergoing OS.

Hormonal Therapy in Metastatic Breast Cancer

SERMs and AIs are also given to women with metastatic breast cancer. In addition, fulvestrant (Faslodex), an injection can take the place of oral therapies if a patient has difficulty adhering to a pill every day. Treatment for metastatic breast cancer needs to be patient centered and tailored to the patient's preferences and disease state. If a woman does not present with acute visceral crisis, end-organ damage, or aggressive, immediately life-threatening disease, letrozole or fulvestrant given with a CDK 4/6 inhibitor (abemaciclib, palbociclib, or ribociclib) is the current standard of care in first line metastatic, estrogen positive, HER2-negative breast cancer. OS or ablation is added for premenopausal women (NCCN, 2022). CDK 4/6 inhibition causes cell cycle arrest and is felt to work synergistically with endocrine therapy. AIs in combination with CDK 4/6s have increased progression-free survival relative to an AI alone (Lauro et al., 2020). After disease progression on first-line endocrine therapy, second-line endocrine therapy options should be evaluated and offered. This may include switching to fulvestrant (Faslodex) or to an alternative AI (NCCN, 2022). Women with HER2-positive tumors may be given endocrine therapy along with other HER2 targeted therapies (NCCN, 2022) (see table below).

Hormonal Therapy for Breast Cancer

Drug	Dose	Side Effects	Use
SERMs: tamoxifen (toremifene and raloxifene are rarely used)	20 mg PO daily	Hot flashes, vaginal discharge, menstrual irregularities, stroke (low risk), thromboembolic risk (low risk), uterine cancer (low risk),	Premenopausal and postmenopausal DCIS; Adjuvant and metastatic therapy; Used also as chemoprevention in high-risk *BRCA*-positive patients; Can be used with GnRH ovarian suppression; Avoid using in patients w/hx of blood clots, stroke, PE, DVT
AIs: (1) Anastrozole (2) Letrozole (3) Exemestane (Aromasin)	1 mg PO daily 2.5 mg PO daily 25 mg PO daily	Osteoporosis, joint pain, arthralgias, hot flashes, decreased sexual interest, vaginal dryness	Postmenopausal; Premenopausal with ovarian suppression or ablation; Adjuvant and metastatic therapy; Used also in DCIS as chemoprevention in high-risk *BRCA*-positive patients
GnRH agonists: (1) Lupron (2) Goserelin	Varies: every 1, 3, or 6 months (subQ or IM)	Hot flashes, mood changes, weight gain, injection reaction	Premenopausal; Can be used with tamoxifen or an AI; Metastatic breast cancer
Estrogen receptor downregulator (antagonist): fulvestrant	500 mg IM on day 1, 15, and 29 and then monthly	Hot flashes, increased LFTs, arthralgias, injection site discomfort	Metastatic breast cancer; Adjuvant treatment; May be beneficial in nonadherent patients because of IM injection
Progestin: megestrol acetate	40 mg PO qid	Increased appetite, weight gain, diarrhea, rash	Metastatic breast cancer

AI, Aromatase inhibitor; *DCIS,* ductal carcinoma in situ; *DVT,* deep vein thrombosis; *GnRH,* gonadotropin-releasing hormone; *HER2,* human epidermal growth factor receptor 2; *hx, history*; *IM,* intramuscular; *LFTs,* liver function test results; *PE,* pulmonary embolus; *PO,* oral; *qid,* four times daily; *SERM,* selective estrogen receptor modulators; *subQ,* subcutaneous.
Please refer to the most recent data on breast cancer from National Comprehensive Cancer Network. Available at http://nccn.org/professionals/physician_gls/pdf/breast.pdf (accessed January 28, 2022).

Gonadotropin-Releasing Hormone Agonists

Ovarian ablation has been recognized as an effective means for treating breast cancer for more than a century in the same way that orchiectomy has been used to treat prostate cancer. Historically, surgical removal or irradiation of the ovaries or testes has been used to ablate hormonal stimulation, which can cause proliferation of cancer cells to tissues (Kumar et al., 2022).

The development of GnRH agonists has allowed chemical ovarian or testicular ablation rather than surgical ablation. The use of a GnRH agonist may minimize morbidity, providing a preferable, reversible alternative to other, more invasive procedures. The GnRH agonist mimics the naturally occurring substance in the body and produces the same physiologic effects. By mimicking the normal GnRH, the agonists fill the receptor in the pituitary; they also occupy the receptors for a longer time compared with endogenous GnRH.

GnRH agonists suppress ovarian production of estrogen by binding to the GnRH pituitary receptors. This results in downregulation of the receptors. With continued administration, estrogen and progesterone production are greatly reduced, although estrogen initially surges because of the primary stimulating effects on the receptors. After 2 to 4 weeks of treatment, the negative feedback mechanism is activated, and the desired inhibition of luteinizing hormone (LH) and follicle-stimulating hormone (FSH) can be achieved. Estrogen and progesterone levels then begin to fall. This exact process happens the same way in males, resulting in decreased LH and FSH stimulation on the testicles and ultimately in a decrease in testosterone production (Li et al., 2021).

Lupron and Zoladex

For women who have high enough risk of recurrence to warrant chemotherapy, the Adjuvant Exemestane with Ovarian Suppression in Premenopausal Breast Cancer studies demonstrated the benefit of adding OS to tamoxifen in young women who remained premenopausal after chemotherapy. Further improvement was then seen in OS plus an AI (Pagani et al., 2014).

Gonadotropin-Releasing Hormone Antagonists

GnRH antagonists are a class of peptide analogs with important oncologic and gynecologic applications. The antagonists act on the same receptor site as GnRH, causing immediate inhibition of the release of gonadotropins and sex steroids. The *flare response* is prevented because the antagonists induce immediate suppression. Just as with GnRH agonists, the ovaries are no longer stimulated to produce estrogen, and the testes are not stimulated to release testosterone. Degarelix is an example of this group of medications (National Cancer Institute, 2022).

Conclusion

The past century has brought many changes and advances in hormonal therapy for the treatment of cancer. One type of treatment that remains consistent is hormonal manipulation and hormonal blockade. Tumors that are stimulated to grow by hormones attached to specific receptor sites frequently respond to treatment that interrupts the communication between the hormone and receptor. Exciting advances in high risk and metastatic disease combining hormonal therapies with novel agents have advanced the field. Hormonal treatment has been used successfully since the 19th century and will continue to be a mainstay of treatment into the future.

References

Anandabaskar, N. (2021). Adrenocorticosteroids and their antagonists. In A. Paul, N. Anandabaskar, J. Mathaiyan, et al. (Eds.), *Introduction to basics of pharmacology and toxicology*. Singapore: Springer.

American Society of Clinical Oncology (ASCO). (2019). *ASCO Guidelines*. Available at https://www.asco.org/sites/new-www.asco.org/files/content-files/practice-and-guidelines/documents/2019-BCRR_Summary-of-Recs-Table.pdf.

Beatson, G. T. (1896). On the treatment of inoperable cases of carcinoma of the mamma: Suggestions for a new method of treatment, with illustrative cases. *Lancet, 2*, 104–107.

Burnstein, H. J. (2020). *Systemic therapy for estrogen receptor-positive, HER2-negative breast cancer*. Available at https://www.nejm.org/doi/pdf/10.1056/NEJMra1307118.

Clarisse, D., Offner, F., & De Bosscher, K. (2020). Latest perspective on glucocorticoid-induced apoptosis and resistance in lymphoid malignancies. *Biochica et Ciophysica Acta (BBA)-Reviews on Cancer, 1874*(2), 188430. Available at https://www.sciencedirect.com/science/article/pii/S0304419X20301499 (accessed March 4, 2022).

Dawson, N. A. (2021). *Alternative endocrine therapies for castration-resistant prostate cancer*. Available at https://www.uptodate.com/contents/alternative-endocrine-therapies-for-castration-resistant-prostate-cancer (accessed December 27, 2021).

Kumar, S., Gupta, S., Maurya, A. P., Singh, R., & Nigam, S. (2022). Hormonal and targeted treatments in breast cancer. In S. M. Bose, S. C. Sharma, A. Mazumdar, et al. (Eds.), *Breast cancer*. Singapore: Springer. https://doi.org/10.1007/978-981-16-4546-4_21.

Lauro, V., Rella, F. D., Fusco, G., Iodice, G., Nuzzo, F., Pacilio, C., Pensabene, M., & De Laurentiis, M. (2020). Progression-Free Survival and Overall Survival of CDK 4/6 Inhibitors Plus Endocrine Therapy in Metastatic Breast Cancer: A Systematic Review and Meta-Analysis. *International journal of molecular sciences, 21*(17), 6400. https://doi.org/10.3390/ijms21176400 (accessed on March 5, 2022).

Li, H., Liu, Y., Wang, Y., Zhao, X., & Qi, X. (2021). Hormone therapy for ovarian cancer: Emphasis on mechanisms and applications (Review). *Oncology Reports, 46*, 223.

National Cancer Institute. (2022). *Clinical trials using degarelix*. Available at https://www.cancer.gov/about-cancer/treatment/clinical-trials/intervention/degarelix (accessed March 5, 2022).

National Comprehensive Cancer Network (NCCN). (2022). *Breast cancer*. (accessed March 5, 2022). https://www.nccn.org/guidelines/category_1.

Pagani, O., Regan, M. M., Walley, B. A., Fleming, G. F., Colleoni, M., & Láng, I. (2014). Adjuvant exemestane with ovarian suppression in premenopausal breast cancer. *The New England Journal of Medicine, 371*(2). https://www.nejm.org/doi/full/10.1056/nejmoa1404037#article_citing_articles (accessed March 5, 2022).

Richman, J., & Dowsett, M. (2019). Beyond 5 years: Enduring risk of recurrence in oestrogen receptor-positive breast cancer. *Nature Reviews Clinical Oncology, 16*, 296–311.

Quirke, V. M. (2017). Tamoxifen from failed contraceptive pill to best-selling breast cancer medicine: A case-study in pharmaceutical innovation. *Frontiers in Pharmacology*. https://doi.org/10.3389/fphar.2017.00620. PMID: 28955226; PMCID: PMC5600945.

Oral Adherence

Martha Polovich

Introduction

The use of oral agents for the treatment of cancer is not new; many traditional agents such as methotrexate and cyclophosphamide have been available in oral dosage forms for decades. What has changed is the number of agents available for oral administration, the frequency of their use, and the number of patients taking them. In the last 2 years, 39% of Food and Drug Administration approvals for oncology and hematology drugs was oral agents. Because patients assume daily responsibility for managing their own therapy, medication adherence is an important aspect of treatment with oral agents. Nurses working in oncology settings must provide safe, efficient, and consistent quality care for patients receiving oral therapy. This chapter focuses on the role of the nurse in supporting patients to achieve a level of adherence that results in the best possible outcomes. Common terminology can be found in the box below.

Definition of Terms

Adherence: Extent to which a person's behavior corresponds with the agreed recommendations from a healthcare professional.

Medication adherence: Taking a drug as prescribed in relation to timing, dose, frequency, and appropriately as related to food, other prescribed medications, and over-the-counter medications, herbs, and vitamins.

Persistence: Duration of time from the initiation of a medication to discontinuation of therapy.

The Current Landscape of Oral Oncology-Hematology Therapies

Oral cancer therapies are on the rise. Oral cancer drugs have several advantages over intravenous (IV) drugs in that they allow patients to take a more active role in their care, feel more in control of their therapy, and experience greater independence and less chemotherapy chair time. For these reasons, most patients prefer an oral drug over IV therapy if treatment outcomes are equal or better. Oncology practices must evaluate how they currently manage patients receiving oral therapies and determine safe, efficient, and consistent processes for providing this service.

Oral regimens require patients to take responsibility for their treatment. Before the surge in oral chemotherapy, community oncology practices focused on delivering IV chemotherapy; minimal attention and resources were allocated for patients receiving oral cancer therapy regimens. Creating an oral therapy delivery model that can be used in tandem with the IV delivery model is now a necessity, and nursing expertise is critical in this redesign. Nurses assess and educate patients, provide symptom management, and coordinate the processes of care. Nurses are challenged to develop the necessary skills to meet the needs of the patients receiving oral cancer therapies.

Why Adherence Is Important?

Medication adherence means that patients take their medications exactly as prescribed and appropriately in relation to food and other medications. There are potentially serious consequences of nonadherence to oral cancer therapies. Missed doses, incorrect doses, or early discontinuation of oral agents can result in altered efficacy of treatment. Either nonadherence (taking less than the prescribed dose or altering the schedule) or overadherence (taking more than the prescribed dose) can result in increased toxicity, more physician visits, increased hospitalizations, and longer lengths of stay. Nonadherence to oral agents may have a negative effect on overall survival, disease-free survival, progression-free survival, and disease recurrence. Studies have shown that a molecular response to targeted agents is decreased by a lower dose, early discontinuation, and dose interruptions. Providers who evaluate treatment response may decide that a regimen is not effective when the reason for a lack of response is that the patient did not take the drug as prescribed.

Adherence and the reasons for nonadherence vary over time. The time from prescription to first dose is called the initiation phase, during which time a patient decides to start therapy or not. This decision may be affected by belief in the seriousness of the diagnosis, attitudes toward medication taking, and cost. The implementation phase, from first dose to last, is affected by the ongoing challenges associated with continuing therapy, including interruption in daily routine or undesirable side effects. The final phase is discontinuation that may occur by patient choice due to side effects, or thoughts that treatment is no longer necessary.

There is ample evidence for the complex nature of medication adherence. Nonadherence can be unintentional due to forgetfulness, which is one of the most common reasons patients give for missing doses. Sometimes nonadherence is intentional, such as when patients decide not to take their medication to avoid adverse effects. Another type of medication nonadherence is related to cost, which may be a reason for delays in starting a drug or obtaining refills due to out-of-pocket expenses.

In some studies, taking fewer medications was associated with better adherence; while in others, taking more medications was. Both older age and younger age have been associated with worse adherence, as have a higher education level and a lower education level. Studies suggest that racial or cultural factors and comorbid conditions can affect medication adherence. Several factors are not modifiable but must be considered when assessing patients' potential for nonadherence and developing a treatment plan that includes oral cancer drugs.

Assessment of Factors Affecting Adherence

Because adherence to oral cancer therapy can affect treatment outcomes, nurses must assess all patients for potential barriers and facilitators of adherence prior to the start of a regimen that includes oral drug(s). The World Health Organization describes adherence as multidimensional, including patient-related, socioeconomic-related, condition-related, treatment-related, and healthcare-system or provider-related factors. This challenges the bias that patients are solely responsible for taking their treatment as prescribed and recognizes that many factors influence a person's medication taking behavior. Nurses must collaborate with patients or their caregivers to identify any barriers to and facilitators of medication adherence when formulating a plan of care that is specific to an individual's needs.

Patient-related barriers that can affect medication adherence are memory issues, impaired cognition, depression, functional impairment, and comorbidities. Socioeconomic-related factors comprise out-of-pocket costs for treatment, lack of social support, and low health literacy. Examples of condition-related factors include diagnosis-related demands on the patient and the severity of the disease. Treatment-related factors to consider are side effects of treatment, duration of treatment, complexity of the regimen, and the immediacy of expected response. Finally, healthcare-system or provider-related factors such as how healthcare services are coordinated, the workload of the providers, and the quality of the patient-provider relationship can have a negative effect on adherence.

Several facilitators of medication adherence have been suggested. Individual factors include a perceived poor state of health and therefore a perceived need for the medication. Socioeconomic facilitators are affordable out-of-pocket costs, perceived social support and health literacy. Good healthcare provider communication and proactive symptom management can facilitate medication adherence and persistence. There is currently no validated assessment tool that collects information about factors that predispose a patient to nonadherence, although some are being evaluated. Assessment data from the physical assessment, psychosocial assessment, and distress inventory should be reviewed for potential barriers and facilitators of adherence such as those listed above.

Planning

Treatment plans typically include the goals of therapy; timing and dose of the medications, monitoring plans (e.g., frequency of office visits, laboratory testing, imaging procedures); foods, drugs, or lifestyle activities to avoid (e.g., smoking or alcohol); expected side effects and symptom management strategies. When patients are self-administering oral therapy, the plan needs to address strategies that will enhance the ability of the patient to be successful in following the regimen.

Motivational interviewing (MI) has been studied as a technique to promote medication adherence for patients with several types of illnesses, including cancer. Although most often described as an intervention, MI involves determining what motivates an individual's medication-taking behavior so that the most effective interventions are planned. MI focuses on patients' right to determine their own care approach and emphasizes a partnership with the healthcare team rather than telling them what to do. It involves listening to patients with empathy, understanding their values, and collaborating with them to identify and overcome the barriers to medication adherence. Recent evidence suggests that this patient-centered approach improves adherence with oral anticancer agents.

Interventions for Medication Adherence

There is no one-size-fits-all intervention that is effective in promoting medication adherence. There have been many systematic reviews about medication adherence, but most have been based on a small number of studies. Most recent research has found that no tested intervention is successful in improving adherence with all patients. This suggests the need for tailored interventions based on recognizing the specific barriers and facilitators for an individual patient. Multifactorial approaches are more likely to be successful than any single strategy.

Patient Education and Counseling Interventions

Education has often been described as the most important intervention for adherence with oral anticancer drugs. While knowledge about oral agents is necessary, it is insufficient to overcome many barriers to taking medication. Ongoing support from nurses, pharmacists, and other healthcare providers is also needed.

Patient Education

Education is the provision of information that is intended to help patients understand their therapy. Basic education regarding oral anticancer therapy includes information about the drug, dose, storage requirements, drug–drug and drug–food interactions, refill policies, what to do with leftover medication, and expected side effects. Providing information about symptom management has a high priority, since patients may choose not to take their drug due to unacceptable side effects. Nurses who provide drug-related information must ensure that patients are able to determine whether side effects can be self-managed or require timely reporting to the provider. Patient teaching is not a one-time occurrence but an ongoing process. Information is best provided in both verbal and written form so that patients can review the material in the future. Soliciting feedback from patients about their therapy allows healthcare providers to identify issues that may arise due to misunderstanding.

Counseling

Counseling provides guidance for patients on how to manage their care. Nurses, pharmacists, or other healthcare providers can influence some of the potentially modifiable factors for medication adherence such as positive attitudes toward medications, concerns about side effects, and self-efficacy for managing their treatment. Providing ongoing interactions in a supportive environment strengthens patient-provider relationships, which has been found to improve adherence.

Reminder Interventions

Patients with identified memory issues, impaired cognition, or who report having trouble remembering to take medications may benefit from some of the following interventions. Keep in mind that reminder interventions may be effective when forgetfulness is the reason that patients miss a dose but are ineffective for other barriers.

Calendars or Diaries

Calendars or diaries can be used for daily tracking of doses taken and can help the patient to remember whether a scheduled dose was taken. They can be especially helpful if the regimen is complex. Patients can check-off or record a dose after they take it.

Mobile Applications

Smart phone applications provide electronic reminders for patients to take their medications. Several programs are available for download to mobile devices, which can be personalized for the type of "alarm" used for the reminder. Short message service (SMS) uses reminders sent by text message. Emails or voicemails with tailored messages are other types of electronic reminders that may be helpful for some patients. These kinds of interventions depend on patients' ability to use technology. SMS, emails, and voicemails are not routinely available in all settings.

Life-style Interventions

Nurses can help patients improve adherence by assisting them to incorporate medication taking into their daily routine. Tying medication to a habit, such as brushing teeth or making coffee can help overcome forgetting a dose. Storing medications in a place where patients will see them may be helpful if storage requirements allow.

System Interventions

Individual-level interventions are not enough to improve medication adherence for all patients on oral anticancer agents. Many factors associated with health systems and how care is coordinated can affect patients' ability to access and take their medications. Several system-level interventions have been suggested for their impact on adherence with variable success.

Specialty Pharmacies

Oral anticancer drugs are often provided by specialty pharmacies rather than retail or hospital-based pharmacies. These provide a combination of services that may include prior authorization, financial assistance, drug-specific patient education, access to a pharmacist or nurse by telephone, and home delivery of medications by mail. There is some evidence for improved adherence with this type of service.

Prescription Refill Synchronization

Patients may be taking several medications for noncancer conditions and therefore need to make multiple trips to a pharmacy to fill their prescriptions. There is evidence that a cancer diagnosis can affect patients' adherence to medication for their comorbid conditions. Some pharmacies have attempted to synchronize refills to make this process less burdensome for patients and potentially improve adherence for all medications.

Call Centers and Programs

Call centers may be supported by pharmaceutical companies, insurance companies, or specialty pharmacies. They provide an opportunity for interaction with patients and caregivers, which can be used to remind patients to take their medications and allow for the evaluation of side effects. Each call center differs in terms of what information is collected, how the encounter is documented, and who receives the information.

Evaluation

As with any nursing intervention, the measures used to promote medication adherence must be evaluated for their effectiveness. This means that adherence should be assessed and documented at every patient encounter. One challenge in assessing interventions to improve adherence is that it is difficult to measure accurately. Measuring clinical response, physiologic markers, and blood levels of drugs or their metabolites are poor ways of examining adherence for oral anticancer agents, although these methods may be useful in other chronic conditions. The most accurate technique is direct observation—watching a patient take each dose and making sure it is swallowed. This is impractical outside of a healthcare setting when patients must take medication daily or for an extended time.

A second challenge is characterizing "adequate" adherence. Often in research, adherence is defined as patients taking their medication as prescribed 80% of the time. That level of adherence equates to missing 6 doses in a month or over 70 doses in a year for a drug prescribed once a day. Dose-response may vary so that some patients achieve disease response at a lower dose than prescribed; however, with some drugs a molecular response may depend on patients taking every dose as prescribed without fail.

Despite the measurement challenges, nurses need to evaluate patients' success in taking their medications as prescribed so that adjustments can be made to promote the best possible treatment outcomes. Some of the most-used methods to measure adherence are described in the following section. The applicability of some measures to clinical practice varies.

Patient Self-Report

Asking patients to report their medication-taking behavior is the most common and easiest method for measuring medication adherence. When done in a nonjudgmental manner in the context of a trusting nurse-patient or provider-patient relationship, self-report is fairly accurate. Open-ended questions, such as "What problems, if any, are you having taking your medication as prescribed?" Patients tend to report better adherence than that obtained using objective measures; therefore, if patients report a problem taking their medications, the reasons should be explored. When patients use diaries or calendars as reminders for taking their drugs, nurses can ask them to bring these records to a visit for review.

Questionnaires

Patient questionnaires are standardized forms of self-report that can be used to assess medication adherence. They are usually completed at a patient visit rather than on an ongoing basis. Questionnaires are more often used in research settings.

Prescription Refill Counts

Specialty pharmacies can provide information about whether a prescription was filled on time or not. This method measures the medication supply divided by the observed days and is reported as a proportion of days covered, or medication possession ratio. Refill counts are secondary measures of adherence because they do not measure taking drugs as prescribed.

Medication Count

A medication count is used most often in research as an objective measure of adherence but can also be used in clinical settings. Patients are asked to bring their medication bottles to the clinic and staff count the remaining pills. This is an objective measure but does not reflect dose interruption or patients' taking the medication.

Electronic Medication Monitors

Electronic pill caps track and record when a prescription bottle is opened. Some devices also provide timed reminders such as alarms or flashing lights. This technology is used most often in research and can be expensive. This is described as an objective measure but does not reflect patients' taking the medication.

Conclusion

Medication adherence is critical for the best outcomes when patients receive oral agents for the treatment of cancer. Concern for adherence begins with the initial assessment of the patient at the start of therapy and is ongoing when therapy is required long-term. Identifying barriers and facilitators that impact patients' ability to adhere to a regimen is essential to determining the most successful interventions, since each patient is unique. Nurses play a key role in building the right environment for support and monitoring during oral drug therapy and can positively influence patients' success in taking their medications as prescribed (Bosworth et al., 2018; Bryant et al., 2020; Dean et al., 2020; Fennimore & Ginex, 2017; Gönderen Çakmak & Kapucu, 2021; Inotai et al., 2021; Konstantinou et al., 2020; Li & Bounthavong, 2021; Lund et al., 2021; Sabate, 2003; Skrabal Ross et al., 2020; Washburn & Thompson, 2020).

References

Bosworth, H. B., Blaylock, D. V., Hoyle, R. H., Czajkowski, S. M., & Voils, C. I. (2018). The role of psychological science in efforts to improve cardiovascular medication adherence. *American Psychologist, 73*(8), 968–980.

Bryant, A. L., LeBlanc, T. W., Albrecht, T., Chan, Y. N., Richardson, J., Foster, M., … Wujcik, D. (2020). Oral adherence in adults with acute myeloid leukemia (AML): Results of a mixed methods study. *Supportive Care in Cancer, 28*(11), 5157–5164.

Dean, L. T., George, M., Lee, K. T., & Ashing, K. (2020). Why individual-level interventions are not enough: Systems-level determinants of oral anticancer medication adherence. *Cancer, 126*(16), 3606–3612.

Fennimore, L. A., & Ginex, P. K. (2017). Oral agents for cancer treatment: Effective strategies to assess and enhance medication adherence. *Nursing Clinics of North America, 52*, 115–131.

Gönderen Çakmak, H. S., & Kapucu, S. (2021). The effect of educational follow-up with the motivational interview technique on self-efficacy and drug adherence in cancer patients using oral chemotherapy treatment: A randomized controlled trial. *Seminars in Oncology Nursing, 37*(2), 151140.

Inotai, A., Ágh, T., Maris, R., Erdősi, D., Kovács, S., Kaló, Z., & Senkus, E. (2021). Systematic review of real-world studies evaluating the impact of medication non-adherence to endocrine therapies on hard clinical endpoints in patients with non-metastatic breast cancer. *Cancer Treatment Reviews, 100*, 102264.

Konstantinou, P., Kassianos, A. P., Georgiou, G., Panayides, A., Papageorgiou, A., Almas, I., … Karekla, M. (2020). Barriers, facilitators, and interventions for medication adherence across chronic conditions with the highest non-adherence rates: A scoping review with recommendations for intervention development. *TBM, 10*, 1390–1398.

Li, M., & Bounthavong, M. (2021). Cancer history, insurance coverage, and cost-related medication nonadherence in Medicare beneficiaries, 2013-2018. *Journal of Managed Care & Specialty Pharmacy, 27*(12), 1750–1756.

Lund, J. L., Gupta, P., Amin, K. B., Meng, K., Urick, B. Y., Reeder-Hayes, K. E., … Trogdon, J. G. (2021). Changes in chronic medication adherence in older adults with cancer versus matched cancer-free cohorts. *Journal of Geriatric Oncology, 12*(1), 72–79.

Sabate, E. (Ed.). (2003). *Adherence to long-term therapies: Evidence for action.* Geneva, Switzerland: World Health Organization.

Skrabal Ross, X., Gunn, K. M., Suppiah, V., Patterson, P., & Olver, I. (2020). A review of factors influencing non-adherence to oral antineoplastic drugs. *Support Care Cancer, 28*(9), 4043–4050.

Washburn, D. J., & Thompson, K. (2020). Medication adherence barriers: Development and retrospective pilot test of an evidence-based screening instrument. *Clinical Journal of Oncology Nursing, 24*(2), E13–E20.

Complementary and Alternative Therapies

Tahani Al Dweikat

Introduction

"Complementary," "alternative," and "integrative" therapies are often used to describe therapies outside of *conventional medicine*. The National Health Interview Survey (NHIS) reveals a significant increase in the use of complementary and alternative medicine (CAM) (National Institutes of Health [NIH], 2017). The center for Complementary and Integrative Health (National Center for Complementary and Integrative Health [NCCIH], 2016) categorized complementary therapies as psychological and physical approaches, which will be discussed in detail in this chapter.

Interest in using complementary therapies exists worldwide, and the interest in therapies is not limited geographically or to a particular population or disease type. The prevalence of CAM usage among patients with cancer is widely used as part of oncologic treatment. Estimates indicate more than 30% of American adults and about 12% of children use health care approaches that are not typically part of conventional medical care or that may have origins outside of usual Western practice (National Center for Complementary and Integrated Health [NCCIH], 2021a). The most recent NHIS report for 2017 showed the use of yoga, meditation, and chiropractic has significantly increased compared to the 2012 NHIS report (Clarke et al., 2018).

Professionals in clinical practice, education, and research contribute to the practice of CAM; therefore, it is imperative that they have knowledge and understanding of these various types of therapies. Assessing for the use of CAM and including these interventions in nursing practice can promote holistic nursing care.

Complementary and Alternative Medicine Definitions and Classifications

- *Conventional* or *traditional* medicine is an approach provided by the health care professional who holds a medical doctor, doctor of osteopathy, nurse practitioner, or other qualified degree; known as Western, mainstream, or allopathic medicine.
- *Complementary* medicine is used "in addition or in conjunction" with conventional medicine.
- *Alternative* medicine is used "instead of" conventional approaches.
- *Integrative* (or *integrated*) medicine, the more contemporary term, refers to combining evidence-based CAM therapies with evidence-based conventional therapies.
- A therapy can be both complementary and alternative; it is the *intent* with which a therapy is used that defines it (National Cancer Institute [NCI], 2022).

NCCIH and Centers for Disease Control and Prevention (CDC) define CAM as a group of medicines and health practices that are not usually used by doctors to treat cancer or any other disease (Centers for Disease Control and Prevention [CDC], 2022).

CAM in cancer care may be used:

- To help alleviate side effects of cancer treatments, such as nausea, pain, and fatigue
- For emotional distress from the cancer experience
- To help patients feel that they are doing something to help and participate with their own care
- As a belief that involvement of CAM will strengthen their immunity to fight the cancer and relieve side effects
- To support cancer therapy
- To treat or cure their cancer

Background

- Before the 19th century, unconventional methods of treatment were considered folk medicine or quackery.
- The Biologics Control Act of 1902 and the Food and Drug Act of 1906 formed the foundation of the present-day U.S. Food and Drug Administration (FDA).
- The Food, Drug, and Cosmetic Act, passed in 1938, required that new drugs provide evidence of safety before being placed on the market.
- In 1994, because of increasing interest in CAM therapies, the Dietary Supplement Health and Education Act was passed. This act defined dietary supplements as food, established regulations under the FDA, and created the Office of Dietary Supplements within the National Institutes of Health (NIH) to promote, conduct, compile research, and maintain a database on supplements and individual nutrients (Food and Drug Administration [FDA], 2018).
- In 1998, the Office of Alternative Medicine (OAM), which had been established 6 years earlier, became the National Center for Complementary and Alternative Medicine (NCCAM). In December 2014, its name was changed to the NCCIH. What is important to note is that the new title states integrative health and eliminates medicine and it also recognizes the increasing use of complementary therapies in health care (National Center for Complementary and Integrated Health [NCCIH], 2022b) (see table on the next page).
- Also in 1998, the National Cancer Institute (NCI) instituted an Office of Cancer Complementary and Alternative Medicine (OCCAM) to increase high-quality cancer research and information about CAM use. The table on the next page describes the various CAM modalities.

National Cancer Institute OCCAM Domains of Complementary and Alternative Medicine

Domain	Description	Examples
Alternative medical systems	Systems built upon completed systems of theory and practice	Traditional Chinese medicine, Ayurvedic medicine, homeopathy, naturopathy, acupuncture
Manipulative and body-based methods	Methods based on manipulation and/or movement of parts of the body	Chiropractic, therapeutic massage, osteopathy, reflexology
Energy therapies	Therapies involving the use of energy fields: biofield therapies and bioelectromagnetic-based therapies	Reiki, therapeutic touch, pulsed fields, magnet therapy
Mind-body interventions	Techniques designed to enhance the mind's capacity to affect body function and symptoms	Meditation, hypnosis, art therapy, biofeedback, mental healing, imagery, relaxation therapy, support groups, music therapy, cognitive-behavioral therapy, prayer, dance therapy, aromatherapy, animal-assisted therapy
Movement therapy	Modalities used to improve patterns of body movement	Tai chi, Feldenkrais method, Hatha yoga, Alexander technique, dance therapy, qi gong, Rolfing, Trager method
Nutritional therapeutics	The use of nutrients and nonnutrients, bioactive food components as chemopreventive agents and the use of specific foods or diets as cancer prevention or treatment strategies	Dietary regimens such as macrobiotics, vegetarian, Gerson therapy, Kelley/Gonzalez regimen, vitamins, dietary macronutrients, supplements, antioxidants, melatonin, selenium, coenzyme Q10, ephedrine, orthomolecular medicine
Pharmacologic and biologic therapies	Includes drugs, vaccines, off-label use of prescription drugs, and other biologic interventions not yet accepted in mainstream medicine	Vaccines, off-label use of drugs, antineoplastons, products from honeybees, 714-X, low-dose naltrexone, mephentermine, immunoaugmentative therapy, laetrile, hydrazine sulfate, Newcastle virus, melatonin, ozone therapy, thymus therapy, enzyme therapy, high-dose vitamin C
Complex natural products	Subcategory of pharmacologic and biologic treatments consisting of an assortment of plant samples (botanicals), extracts of crude natural substances, and unfractionated extracts from marine organisms used for healing and treatment of disease	Herbs and herbal extracts, mixtures of tea polyphenols, shark cartilage, Essiac tea, Sun's Soup, MGN-3

OCCAM, Office of Cancer Complementary and Alternative Medicine.
From Bauer-Wu, S., & Decker, G. M. (2012). Integrative oncology imperative for nurses. *Seminars in Oncology Nursing, 28*(1), 2–9.

- In 2000, the White House Commission on Complementary and Alternative Medicine Policy (WHCCAMP) was established to address issues of access to and delivery of CAM, priorities for research, and the need to educate consumers and health care professionals about these therapies; their final report was published 2 years later.
- In 2003 and 2004, the Institute of Medicine (IOM) of the National Academies sponsored meetings to explore scientific, policy, and practice questions related to increasing use of CAM by the American public; the committee's final report was released in 2005 (Institute of Medicine [IOM], 2005).

Use of Complementary and Alternative Medicine
(FDA, 2018; NCCIH, 2016; NCI, 2022)

Use of CAM and the reasons for its use vary among the general US population. Overall, the use of CAM therapy among cancer patients has steadily increased over the past decades, those with recurrent or refractory disease are seeking ways to "boost" their immune system to help fight their disease. Others report a preference for "natural" or nontoxic therapies to provide a sense of hope and control (Buckner et al., 2018).

Recent studies reported the use of CAM by approximately 85% of patients with cancer, most commonly with diet or vitamins, mind-body practices, and biologic products (e.g., green tea, ginger, curcumin, chaga mushrooms, and flaxseed oil), which are the most common in the United States (Greenlee et al., 2016; Judson et al., 2017). A recent systematic review of pooled studies found a lower prevalence of use in that 51% of patients with cancer used CAM. Being younger, female, and having a higher income were predictors of CAM use. The most common reason for CAM use was for cure (Keene et al., 2019).

While the use of CAM is high, less than 40% of all patients disclose their use of CAM to their primary care physician and other health care team members. A variety of reasons for nondisclosure include medical skepticism to CAM therapy, no one asked, and fear of disapproval or being dismissed by the provider or practice.

Multicultural orientation and establishing CAM use are essential to understanding the broad range of patients' personal, cultural, spiritual, and motivational factors for CAM use. It is most helpful for the health care team to open a nonjudgmental dialogue to build trust and cultural humility. Cultural humility has been defined as "the ability to maintain an interpersonal stance that is other-oriented (or open to the other) in relation to aspects of cultural identity that are most important to the client" (Hook et al., 2013).

Health care professionals report that they do not always ask about CAM use because they believe they lack the knowledge to appropriately counsel patients regarding efficacy and safety. It is essential that nurses become informed and are prepared to initiate and participate in these conversations with patients.

Contributing to the appeal of CAM therapies is displeasure with decreased personal attention from conventional medical practitioners and feelings of depersonalization with increased technology in conventional medicine. Embedded in this are patients' beliefs that if a product is proclaimed to be *natural*, it must be *safe*. Dr. David Eisenberg coined the phrase, *safety trumps efficacy*, meaning that even if a particular product or treatment is effective for the reason it is sought, it may not be safe for patients to use under their particular set of circumstances. For example, an important safety consideration with CAM is the potential for product contamination, as not all products are regulated by the FDA (Eisenberg et al., 1993).

Complementary and Alternative Medicine Approaches

The NCCIH described the main categories of complementary approaches including nutritional, psychological, and physical approaches (see table below).

- Nutritional approach/Natural product (e.g., special diets, dietary supplements, herbs, probiotics, and microbial-based therapies).

- Psychological approach (e.g., meditation, hypnosis, music therapy, relaxation, guided imagery, aromatherapy, and reflexology therapies).
- Physical approach (e.g., acupuncture, massage, spinal manipulation).
- Combination approach such as psychological and physical (e.g., yoga, Tai chi, dance therapies, some forms of art therapy), or psychological and nutritional (e.g., mindful eating).

NCCIH categorized nutritional approaches as natural products, whereas psychological and/or physical approaches as mind and body practices (National Center for Complementary and Integrated Health [NCCIH], 2021a). Nutritional approaches include "natural products," or substances produced by plants, microbes, and other living organisms, whereas "dietary supplements" have ingredients that include vitamins, minerals, amino acids, and herbs or other substances that can be used to supplement the diet.

Nutritional approaches or natural products are most widely used in complementary therapy by both adults and children (National Center for Complementary and Integrated Health [NCCIH], 2021a). An NHIS revealed almost 18% of American adults used a dietary supplement other than vitamins and minerals (e.g., special diets, dietary supplements, herbs, probiotics, and microbial-based therapies).

National Institutes of Health NCCIH Categories

Category	Therapies	Examples
Nutritional/ Natural products	Probiotics, prebiotics, vitamins, minerals, phytochemicals, dietary spices/herbs/spices, any special diets, "natural products," medicinal plants	Herbal medicines (botanicals), vitamins, minerals, and other natural products; some are sold as dietary supplements, including probiotics
Psychological	Mindfulness, spiritualism, psychotherapy, guided imagery	Meditation, hypnosis, music therapies, relaxation therapies
Physical	Manual therapies, cryotherapy, thermodynamic modalities, surgical
Mind and body practices focus on the interactions among brain, mind, body, and behavior, with the intent to use the mind to affect physical functioning and promote health
Manipulative and body-based methods focus on the structures and systems of the body: bones, joints, soft tissues, and circulatory and lymphatic systems	Meditation techniques, spinal manipulation, massage, various types of yoga, acupuncture, deep-breathing exercises, guided imagery, hypnotherapy, progressive relaxation, and Tai chi
Physical and/or Psychological	Can be incorporated into the combined approach	Acupuncture, osteopathic and chiropractic manipulation, devices (virtual reality), light, electrical, and magnetic stimulation, movement therapies, breathing and relaxation techniques, art, music, dance, yoga, Tai chi, qi gong, Feldenkrais method, Alexander technique, Pilates, Rolfing structural integration, Trager psychophysical integration
Combined	Homeopathy, ayurvedic medicine, Chinese medicine, acupuncture (component of Chinese medicine), naturopathy, functional medicine, traditional healers
Practices of traditional healers
Energy field manipulation to affect health	May include a component of nutritional, psychological, and physical aspects to diagnose and treat patients holistically
Native American healer/medicine man
Magnet and light therapies, qi gong, Reiki, healing touch, therapeutic touch

NCCIH, National Center for Complementary and Integrated Health.
From National Center for Complementary and Integrative Health. (2021). *Complementary, alternative, or integrative health: What's in a name?* Available at https://www.nccih.nih.gov/health/complementary-alternative-or-integrative-health-whats-in-a-name (accessed March 17, 2022).

Levels of Evidence

NCCIH focuses on gathering rigorous data on the safety, usefulness, and efficacy of natural products. The consumption of dietary supplements continues to increase globally year after year, with little evidence regarding their safety or efficacy. The NCCIH supports a broad range of research on dietary supplements, including clinical trials. These trials can be used to shape current policies and priorities for clinical research.

Sorting through scientific evidence is intimidating to the clinician as well as the patient and family. The "gold standard" for clinical research is evidence from double-blind, randomized controlled trials (RCTs). However, some researchers contend that this is not the best approach to study some CAM therapies (e.g., mind-body interventions) because of the complexity of the therapy. They hold that qualitative research provides opportunities to reach a greater understanding of the patient's well-being and gather information that can be helpful for future CAM research.

Although there remains much to be learned about CAM therapies, we now know far more than when the earliest surveys were conducted in the early 1990s. Clinical trials determine the safety and efficacy of a particular product or intervention and provide the foundation of evidence-based medicine and the accepted evidence of efficacy. Effectiveness, as opposed to efficacy, incorporates the evaluation of a clinically meaningful effect and whether the risks outweigh the benefits.

Levels of evidence are used by researchers and clinicians to assess the degree to which interventions meet preestablished criteria. A frequent outcome of level-of-evidence data is clinical practice guidelines that can be used as a basis for recommendations for the care of patients with specific conditions. The Society for Integrative Oncology published the first edition of its *Integrative Oncology Practice Guidelines* in 2007. The 2009 edition updated and expanded on the previous version and provided practical recommendations for the use of complementary therapies in the supportive care of cancer patients. In 2017, clinical practice guidelines were published enhancing the importance of utilizing evidence-based practice, importance of communication to strengthen patient-physician trust, rapport relationship, and improve patient's quality of life.

The table below provides examples of descriptions of levels of evidence. Large amounts of CAM information are available online, in the media, and in lay literature.

The American Society of Clinical Oncology website has a list of 71 comprehensive cancer centers. CAM centers are established at many major cancer centers to help manage both immediate and delayed cancer-related symptoms and side effects, support lifestyle changes, and improve quality of life for patients (Latte-Naor & Mao, 2019).

Levels of Evidence in Cancer Complementary and Alternative Medicine

Data Source	Strength of Study Design	Strength of End Points Measured	Level of Evidence Score
Centre for Evidence-Based Medicine Database, 2009	1a SR of RCTs 1b Individual RCT with narrow confidence interval 1c All or none 2a SR of cohort studies 2b Individual cohort study (including low-quality RCT) 2c Outcomes research, ecological studies 3a SR of case-controlled studies 3b Individual case-control study 4 Case-series (and poor-quality cohort and case-control studies) 5 Expert opinion without explicit critical appraisal or based on physiology, bench research, or "first principles"	A Consistent level 1 studies B Consistent level 2 or 3 studies or extrapolation from level 1 studies C Level 4 or extrapolation from level 2 or 3 studies D Level 5 evidence or troublingly inconsistent or inconclusive studies of any level	1 A, B, C 2 A, B, C 3 A, B 4 5
Physician Data Query, National Library of Medicine, 2023	1 RCT (DB/NB) 2 Non-RCT 3 Case series 4 Best case series	A Total mortality B Cause-specific mortality C Quality of life D Indirect surrogates	1–4 (study design score) joined with A–D (strength of end points measured)
Natural Medicines, 2023	A Strong scientific evidence B Good scientific evidence C Unclear or conflicting scientific evidence D Fair negative scientific evidence F Strong negative scientific evidence Lack of evidence; unable to evaluate efficacy due to lack of adequate human data	Quality of study 0–2 Poor 3–4 Good 5 Excellent	A B C D F Lack of evidence
Oncology Nursing Society, 2014	Nursing experts summarize and synthesize the evidence	*Green level:* Recommended for practice/likely to be effective *Yellow level:* Effectiveness not established *Red level:* Effectiveness unlikely/not recommended for practice	

DB, Double blind; *NB*, not blinded; *NCI*, National Cancer Institute; *RCT*, randomized controlled trial; *SR*, systematic review.

The Internet

The Internet is increasingly used by patients and families to gain knowledge about specific diagnoses, treatment choices, and CAM and supportive care. Distinguishing high-quality information from poor-quality information is essential. According to the NCI, websites that volunteer medical resources should openly discuss who visits the site, who pays for the site, the purpose of the site, the source of information, how information is selected for inclusion, how recent the information is, how links to other sites are selected, and what information the site collects about visitors. Recently, 71 NCI Designated Cancer Centers, located in 36 states were funded by the NCI to deliver cancer treatments to patients; however, their websites have not yet been evaluated regarding CAM therapies and information (National Cancer Institute [NCI], 2019) Some of the reputable websites that do exist are included in table below.

Complementary and Alternative Medicine Resources

Organization	Website
American Cancer Society	http://www.cancer.org/treatment/ treatmentsandsideeffects/ complementaryandalternativemedicine/ complementary-and-alternative-medicine-landing
Food and Drug Administration	https://www.fda.gov/regulatory-information/ search-fda-guidance-documents/ complementary-and-alternative-medicine-products-and-their-regulation-food-and-drug-administration
Medline Plus	https://www.nlm.nih.gov/medlineplus/ druginfo/herb_All.html
National Cancer Institute (NCI) Office of Cancer Complementary and Alternative Medicine (OCCAM)	http://cam.cancer.gov/
National Center for Complementary and Integrative Health (NCCIH)	https://nccih.nih.gov/ https://www.nccih.nih.gov/research/ clinicaltrials
National Institutes of Health (NIH) National Center for Complementary and Alternative Medicine	https://nccih.nih.gov/health/supplements
NIH Office of Dietary Supplements	https://ods.od.nih.gov/
National Library of Medicine	https://www.nlm.nih.gov/medlineplus/ complementaryandintegrativemedicine. html
National Library of Medicine for CAM Clinical Trials	https://clinicaltrials.gov/ct2/results?cond=&t erm=Complementary+&cntry=&state=&c ity=&dist=
Natural Medicine Comprehensive Database	http://naturaldatabase.therapeuticresearch. com/home.aspx?cs=CEPDA&s=ND&Aspx AutoDetectCookieSupport=1
Physician's Data Query	http://www.cancer.gov/publications/pdq/ information-summaries/cam

Alternative Medical Systems

Alternative medical systems are built on complete systems of theory and practice that typically developed before the conventional medical approaches used in the United States. Examples include traditional Chinese medicine, acupuncture, and homeopathy.

Traditional Chinese Medicine

- Traditional Chinese medicine has been used for thousands of years, and it is widely accepted as an alternative treatment for cancer (Xiang et al., 2019).
- Clinical diagnosis and treatment are typically based on the *yin-yang* and *five elements'* theories. These theories apply the occurrence and laws of nature to the study of the physiologic activities and pathologic changes of the human body and their interrelationships.
- Health is a balance of yin and yang (opposite forces present in everyone).
- Disease or any medical condition is a result of imbalance, usually a blockage or deficiency of energy.
- Typical Chinese medicine therapies include acupuncture, herbal medicine, Tai chi, and qi gong exercises.
- These therapies share the same underlying set of assumptions and insights on the nature of the human body and its place in the universe.

Acupuncture

- Acupuncture is a component of ancient Asian traditional medicine in which practitioners (Chinese, Korean, and Japanese) use thin, metallic needles to stimulate specific points on the body to relieve pain and other symptoms (Bao et al., 2018; Eaton & Hulett, 2019).
- Acupuncture has been found to be minimally invasive and generally safe when provided by trained acupuncturists.
- Acupuncture is supported as an adjunct to drug therapy for cancer pain management by the National Comprehensive Cancer Network (NCCN).
- Acupuncture has been increasingly used in treating cancer treatment-related symptoms and side effects such as chronic pain, hot flashes, musculoskeletal system problems, fatigue, neuropathy, headaches, nausea and vomiting, xerostomia, and dysphagia, as well as other health conditions, including stress, ear-nose-throat conditions (e.g., sinusitis, tinnitus, vertigo), allergies, dental pain, addictions, and immune system support.
- Acupuncture usually involves the insertion of needles into the skin at specific sites (acupoints) for therapeutic purposes.
- There are three different types of acupuncture:
  1. Electroacupuncture: refers to the small electric current applied to the acupuncture needles; for stronger stimulation this may also be achieved via electrical current, laser, moxibustion, pressure, ultrasound, or vibration.
  2. Pharmacopuncture: refers to the injection of a herbal extract via syringe at acupoints.
  3. Auricular acupuncture: refers to acupuncture applied on the external ear.

- The underlying principle is that *qi* (pronounced "chee" and translated as *energy*) is present at birth and maintained throughout life. *Qi* flows throughout the body via 12 major paths, or meridians.
- There are approximately 350 acupoints along the 12 meridians, and additional acupoints lie outside the meridian pathways.
- Acupuncture theory holds that stimulation of the appropriate acupoints aids the body in correcting any imbalance in the flow of energy, thus restoring balance. Moreover, it is believed that changes in the balance of energy and flow of *qi* may be identified before disease has developed and therefore that acupuncture has a role in the prevention of illness and maintenance of health.
- Common adverse effects include minimal bleeding at the injection sites, subcutaneous bruising, needling pain at the insertion site, and fainting.
- Serious adverse effects are rare.
- Prevention of skin infection is a noted concern for oncology patients undergoing active treatment.
- Special considerations exist for individuals on anticoagulant medications and those with underlying hematologic abnormalities (e.g., thrombocytopenia and/or coagulation disorder).
- Acupuncture sessions and services provided vary between 20 and 45 minutes.

Level of Evidence

- Insufficient evidence exists to make recommendations regarding the effectiveness of acupuncture in treating adult cancer pain.
- One systematic review suggests that acupuncture may be an appropriate adjunct therapy for managing chronic pain, including joint pain and stiffness. Moreover, combination of acupuncture and analgesics may provide effective and optimal pain control compared to each treatment alone (Deng et al., 2018).
- Systematic reviews by the Society of Integrative Oncology (SIO) Clinical Practice Guidelines (Greenlee et al., 2017) and the American Society of Clinical Oncology (ASCO) (Deng et al., 2018) suggested that although the evidence is low in quality, the benefits of acupuncture appear to outweigh the harms and offer a weak recommendation with moderate certainty due to less supportive scientific evidence for acupuncture in improving cancer pain.
- Efficacy is considered inconclusive by some authors, whereas others suggest that the evidence is equivocal and/or promising for some indications, including addiction, stroke rehabilitation, postoperative and chemotherapy-related nausea and vomiting, tennis elbow, carpal tunnel syndrome, and asthma.
- The impact of acupuncture on chemotherapy-induced nausea and vomiting has been studied for 2 decades, and the results have been mostly favorable. Acupuncture has been used as an adjunctive approach to alleviate the severity of chemotherapy-induced nausea and vomiting (Li et al., 2020).

Contraindications

- The "needling" technique is contraindicated in those patients who have severe bleeding disorders or are at increased risk for infection (e.g., neutropenia).
- Acupuncture is contraindicated during the first trimester of pregnancy, with the exception of treatment for nausea.
- Patients with cardiac pacemakers should not be treated with electrical stimulation.
- Caution is advised for the first acupuncture treatment because some patients may become drowsy. Care should be taken if driving or operating machinery after treatment. Needles should not be reused, and strict asepsis should be mandatory. Potential side effects include bleeding, bruising, pain with needling, and worsening of symptoms. Reported adverse events are rare but include pneumothorax and death.
- People on warfarin or other anticoagulants, people with a history of bleeding disorders or pregnancy are not contraindications to acupuncture (Kwon et al., 2018).

Practitioners

- Certification as an acupuncturist can be achieved in two ways: completion of a formal, full-time educational program that includes both classroom and clinical hours or participation in an apprenticeship program. Practitioners must also complete a "Clean Needle Technique" approved course. Medical doctors with training in acupuncture may also become board certified.
- Some states require licensure. The National Certification Commission for Acupuncture and Oriental Medicine has established standards for certification that are accepted by some states for licensure (www.nccaom.org). Medical doctors must possess a valid medical license and be certified through the American Academy of Medical Acupuncture (www.medicalacupuncture.org).
- Some states require medical referral, while others allow nonmedical practitioners to see patients without referral (www.nccaom.org).
- A comparison of licensed versus certified acupuncturists is available on the web site of the Acupuncture Society of New York (www.asny.org).

Homeopathy

- Homeopathic remedies have been used orally and topically for a range of conditions, including the common cold, flu (influenza), allergic rhinitis, asthma, diarrhea, dermatitis, fibromyalgia, chronic fatigue syndrome, anxiety, depression, fatigue, migraine headache, osteoarthritis, muscle pain, motion sickness, otitis media, and many others.
- Homeopathy was started by the German physician Samuel Hahnemann in 1796, when he presented the paper, *A New Principle of Healing*. This new principle was *homeopathy*.
- The word *homeopathy* means "similar disease" (Greek origin).
- Hahnemann believed that *like cures like*. For example, if a substance in large amounts causes a certain disease, then the same substance in small amounts could cure the disease. This is known as the *Law of Similars*.

- In order to find homeopathic treatments, *provings* were conducted in which substances such as herbs or minerals were tested in healthy people to see what kind of reaction occurred. These reactions were then documented in detail. For example, if a substance caused fever, then that substance would be identified as a treatment for conditions involving fever.
- Homeopathic treatment consists of small doses of the *proven* substance, based on the *Law of Infinitesimals*. It is believed that the more dilute the substance, the more potent its effect; this is known as *potentiation through dilution.*
- Commonly used homeopathic remedies include arnica, belladonna, chamomile, nux vomica, and poison ivy (Donelli & Antonelli, 2021).

Level of Evidence
- Homeopathic theories and principles are inconsistent with the current understanding of pharmacology, chemistry, and physics.
- The efficacy of homeopathy is scientifically unproven.
- Many clinical trials have found no benefit for homeopathic preparations compared with placebo; other research has found statistically significant benefits.
- Homeopathy's assumptions are not supported by scientific evidence; however, homeopathy exists, and it is even supported by the health care systems of many countries.
- When all evidence is pooled, regardless of study quality, findings often suggest that homeopathic preparations might offer some benefit.
- Homeopathic remedies are likely safe when used orally or topically and appropriately. Most preparations contain little or no active ingredients. Therefore, it is unlikely that they have any beneficial or harmful effects (Grams, 2019).

Contraindications
- Homeopathic treatments are contraindicated in pregnant or lactating women.
- There are no known interactions with drugs, herbs, foods, laboratory tests, diseases, or conditions.

Practitioners
- A Certificate of Classical Homeopathy is awarded by the Council for Homeopathic Certification (CHC). Information can be found on their web site (http://www.homeopathicdirectory.com/).
- This practitioner certificate program is open to anyone who is interested in studying professional-level homeopathy. This program is appropriate for physicians or health care practitioners.

Manipulative and Body-Based Methods

Several methods based on manipulation and/or movement of body parts exist. Examples include chiropractic, therapeutic massage, osteopathy, and reflexology.

Therapeutic Massage
- Therapeutic massage includes various forms of therapeutic manipulation of muscles and soft tissues through rubbing, kneading, stroking, and stretching (Eaton & Hulett, 2019).
- Massage has a variety of methods (e.g., Swedish and reflexology) for muscle pain and stiffness.
- Massage modalities could include aromatherapy and acupressure.
- Average massage session averages 30 minutes; one to three times weekly for 4 to 6 weeks.
- Massage therapy is considered as a safe practice, noninvasive, with few adverse effects, primarily include muscles soreness.
- Massage should be used with caution for oncology patients with impaired skin integrity, devices in place, open wounds, and those undergoing chemotherapy as well as radiation therapy.
- An important concern regarding massage in cancer care is whether massage could contribute to metastasis (based on the concept that increased blood and lymph circulation might encourage the spread of cancer). Evidence-based practices reveal the speed of circulation does not influence cancer spread (Eaton & Hulett, 2019; Gentile et al., 2018).

Levels of Evidence
- Six systematic reviews show inconclusive evidence, citing weak study designs and low levels of evidence; therefore, no recommendations have been issued regarding the use of massage for cancer pain.
- NCCN suggests massage may be considered as an adjunct therapy to drug therapy for pain relief.
- ASCO clinical practice guidelines offer a weak recommendation for the use of massage for reducing cancer pain, observing that the benefits of massage outweigh potential harm.
- Most recently, several RCTs offered favorable findings to support massage as a pain management therapy for chronic cancer pain.

Contraindications
- Contraindications are based on the most common element of massage, pressure, which needs to be modified in patients with cancer.
- Examples include the following:
  - Solid tumors
    - Avoid pressure on a solid tumor in any area that is accessible to the hands. It is OK to touch, hold, or stroke using soft hands. Use moderate pressure elsewhere.
    - For patients with palmar plantar erythrodysesthesia (PPE), use soft touch only.
  - Known or suspected bone metastasis, including the spine
    - Avoid pressure on the area or jostling or moving the joints. It is OK to use moderate pressure elsewhere.
  - Tendency toward bruising or bleeding
    - Avoid pressure or aggressive kneading or gliding. It is OK to use gentle kneading or light stroking with just enough pressure to apply lotion, "holding" the body with soft hands.

- Removal or irradiation of lymph nodes in the armpit, groin, neck, or jaw
  - Avoid pressure on the limb and the area drained by those lymph nodes. Touch or hold the area with soft hands (no pressure). It is OK to use moderate pressure elsewhere in the body.

Practitioners

Consensus exists that licensed or certified massage therapists should have additional knowledge, skill, and experience in oncology massage to provide safe and effective therapy for cancer patients. More information is available on the web site of the Society for Oncology Massage (http://www.s4om.org/).

Reflexology

Reflexology is the application of pressure to the feet and hands with specific thumb, finger, and hand techniques in specific zones or reflex areas, without the use of oil or lotion, to cause a physical change in the corresponding area or the body.

Level of Evidence

Systematic reviews of RCTs concluded that the evidence to date does not demonstrate reflexology as an effective treatment for any medical condition.

Contraindications

No contraindications have been reported.

Practitioners

- In the United Kingdom, reflexology is coordinated on a voluntary basis by the Complementary and Natural Healthcare Council (CNHC). Registrants are required to meet standards of proficiency outlined by profession-specific boards. CNHC registration is voluntary; therefore, anyone can describe himself or herself as a reflexologist.
- In Canada, reflexology is not regulated in any province, and the expenses incurred are not eligible as medical claims for income taxes. The Reflexology Association of Canada has reflexology therapists in all provinces, and British Columbia, Ontario, and Quebec have other associations.

Energy Therapies

Energy therapies involve the use of energy fields. There are two types of energy therapies: biofield and electromagnetic-based. *Biofield therapies* are intended to affect energy fields that purportedly surround and penetrate the human body. The existence of such fields has not yet been scientifically proven. Examples of biofield therapies include qi gong, Reiki, and therapeutic touch. *Electromagnetic-based therapies* involve the nontraditional use of electromagnetic fields, such as pulsed fields, magnetic fields, and alternating current or direct current fields. Examples include pulsed electromagnetic fields and magnet therapy.

Biofield Therapies (Reiki, Therapeutic Touch, Healing Touch)

- Biofield therapies consist of Reiki, therapeutic touch, and/or healing touch.

- Reiki is an ancient form of healing that in Japanese means "universal life energy." Furthermore, it is an ancient Japanese tradition intended to support healing through balancing and alignment of the body's energy biofield. Focuses on therapeutic touch and healing touch, where the practitioner acts as a conduit for the movement of energy and uses their hands to direct or transfer energy according to the area's needs for energy (National Center for Complementary and Integrative Health [NCCIH], 2018b).
- Practitioners require specific training to detect and correct energy imbalances in the body using their hands.
- It is the energy, not the healer, that influences healing. In this way, Reiki differs from other healing systems: Energy travels *through* the healer, not *from* the healer.
- Reiki is said to alleviate physical, emotional, and spiritual blockages. The practitioner gently places his or her hands on or over the client in a particular series of positions. About 5 minutes are spent on each of the 12 positions, although this may vary based on the needs of the client. The client is fully clothed at all times, and there is no direct pressure, massage, or manipulation applied to the client. The environment is kept quiet and soothing.

Level of Evidence

- Two systematic reviews suggested the use of healing touch, touch therapy, and Reiki could be beneficial as adjuvant therapies for cancer pain (Eaton & Hulett, 2019)
- More than 20 RCTs are reported in Medline for Reiki, showing that it may be helpful in the treatment of pain, mood change, and fatigue. One study tested a standardized procedure for placebo Reiki in an effort to provide a foundation for subsequent randomized and placebo-controlled Reiki efficacy studies (Eaton & Hulett, 2019).

Contraindications

Contraindications for Reiki therapy are inability to let go of one's fear and need for control.

Practitioners

Typically, Reiki is taught in three parts:

- Reiki I includes history of Reiki, Reiki hand positions, Reiki symbols and their names, and meditation manifestation.
- Reiki II involves intense training focusing on advanced techniques and includes a review of Reiki I. The training for Reiki II brings knowledge of long-distance healing, scanning techniques, and the long-distance Reiki symbols and their names. Two Usui-REIKI-Tibetan attunements, named after the Japanese Buddhist Mikao Usui, are performed at intervals throughout the course. These are powerful spiritual experiences during which the attunement energies are channeled into the student by the Reiki Master.
- Reiki III (Master) includes a review of previous training and practice and brings to the student knowledge for long-distance healing, scanning techniques, more meditation techniques, and an additional Reiki symbol. There is a Reiki attunement at the end of the course. There is no national curriculum or certifying body, although the Usui approach is the most prevalent. There are no states that license Reiki practitioners.

Mind-Body Interventions

Mind-body interventions, a type of CAM and integrative health, involve techniques designed to enhance the mind's capacity to affect body functions and symptoms. Furthermore, these interventions are not considered part of conventional therapies and focus on the connection between mind, body, and behavior. Examples include meditation, hypnosis, biofeedback, guided imagery, support groups, music therapy, cognitive-behavioral therapy, and aromatherapy. Conventional therapies are the primary treatment modalities for chronic cancer pain; scientific evidence is limited for the effectiveness of mind-body interventions in cancer patients in reducing pain intensity. The use of mind-body interventions is inexpensive and has minimal adverse events.

Mindfulness Meditation

- Mindfulness meditation, when it is practiced in mindfulness-based stress reduction (MBSR), is a self-regulatory approach to stress reduction and management of emotions. Mindfulness is a state in which an individual is highly aware and focused on the reality of the present moment, including acceptance and acknowledgment. The growing interest in the use of MBSR in cancer care reflects a desire for a more holistic approach to cancer treatment and acknowledges the links between social, psychological, and physiologic health determinants.
- MBSR programs are usually 6 to 8 weeks in length, involving daily individual activities and group activities up to several days per week. It is anticipated that individuals will continue to practice the activities for an extended period after completion of the structured program to receive the full benefit of the intervention.
- MBSR focuses on three meditation techniques: breath awareness, body awareness, and mindful movement.
- Recommendations for a daily dose range from 10 to 60 minutes per day, and regular daily practice increases the effects of mindfulness.
- Mindfulness interventions such as 5 to 10 minutes of guided mindfulness induction with three to four sessions of mindfulness meditation strongly supported the reduction of pain symptoms; moreover, they also showed improvement in managing agitation, anxiety, discomfort, and confusion.

Level of Evidence

- MBSR interventions appear to be effective.
- ASCO guidelines give a moderate recommendation for the use of mindfulness-based therapies for managing chronic pain in adult cancer survivors (Eaton & Hulett, 2019).

Contraindications

No contraindications have been reported.

Practitioners

Trained individuals may administer MBSR interventions either separately or in a group situation. It has been recommended that this therapy is best practiced by those licensed in counseling, psychology, or social work.

Aromatherapy

- Aromatherapy is the controlled use of essential oils extracted from plants for therapeutic benefit.
- *Essential oil* is the aromatic essence of a plant in the form of an oil or resin derived from the plant's leaf, stalk, bark, root, flower, fruit, or seed. The diluent, as the *carrier*, is used with a concentrated essential oil for application.
- Types of aromatherapy (e.g., massage, medical, olfactory, and psycho-aromatherapy).
- Currently, there are about 150 recognized essential oils.
- The term *neat* refers to direct application of the essential oil compound (essential oil plus carrier) to the skin.
- The term *note* refers to the unique aromatic variable of the essential oil, which is important when blending combinations of essential oil compounds.
- Essential oils can be applied directly to the skin through a compressor massage, inhaled via a diffuser or steaming water, or added directly to bath water.
- The mechanism of action in the use of essential oils begins after the smell is sensed. The limbic system is activated in retrieving learned memories. Essential oils are also absorbed into the bloodstream via the skin and subcutaneous fat. Entry via the oral route into the digestive system is not recommended.
- Aromatherapy can be practiced with a massage. An aromatherapy massage is used to alleviate symptoms such as anxiety, depression, stress, and insomnia; furthermore, it is used in palliative care settings to improve the quality of life for patients with cancer.

Level of Evidence

- To date, there are no certain guidelines regarding the use of aromatherapy.
- Published data on dosing, comparative methods of administration, and therapeutic outcomes in the use of essential oils in aromatherapy are limited.
- The national guidelines examined for our review (i.e., SIO, ASCO, and NCCN) do not provide recommendations for aromatherapy for cancer pain.
- Massage and aromatherapy massage seem to offer short-term benefits for psychological well-being, but there is limited evidence supporting the effect on anxiety. Mixed evidence exists as to whether aromatherapy enhances the effects of massage. Replication, longer follow-up, and larger trials are needed to accrue the necessary evidence (Eaton & Hulett, 2019).

Contraindications

- Contraindications include allergy, pregnancy, contagious disease, epilepsy, venous thrombosis, varicose veins, open wounds on skin sites, and recent surgery of any type.
- Aromatherapy should not be administered orally and should not be applied to the skin before dilution.
- Possible adverse events associated with the use of essential oils include photosensitivity, allergic reactions, nausea, and headache. Many essential oils have the potential to either enhance or reduce the effects of prescribed medications, including antibiotics, tranquilizers, antihistamines,

anticonvulsants, barbiturates, morphine, and quinidine. Cases of potentially serious reactions involving the use of essential oils have been reported in two individuals who had no known allergies or sensitivities before exposure.
- Special considerations
  - Check resources for safety precautions for each oil before use:
    - Oils should be diluted with a carrier oil such as grapeseed or apricot.
    - Check the FDA's Generally Regarded as Safe (GRAS) list.
    - Check for skin sensitivities and for oils that can increase skin sensitivity to sun exposure.
    - Check for oils that can be hepatotoxic and/or nephrotoxic with prolonged use.
    - Check for estrogenic effects that would make the oil contraindicated in patients with estrogen-sensitive tumors.
- Some essential oils, such as oil of clove, may compete for receptor sites with chemotherapy drugs, so keep the oil dose low (1 to 2 drops/ounce of carrier oil) and do not use oils for 9 to 10 days before or after chemotherapy.

Practitioners
- Certification is available through the National Association for Holistic Aromatherapy (www.naha.org). Schools must provide practice in the fields of aromatherapy, essential oil studies, anatomy, and physiology. Holistic nursing certification is available through the American Holistic Nurses' Certification Corporation (www.ahncc.org). Requirements include a Bachelor of Science in Nursing (BSN) degree, continuing education, 1 year of practice, and a passing score on a written examination.
- Certification in aromatherapy or holistic nursing does not qualify a nurse to work independently, nor does it necessarily meet institutional requirements for practice.

Movement Therapies

Movement therapies are used to improve patterns of body movement. Examples include Qi gong and Tai chi, hatha yoga, dance therapy, qi gong, Rolfing, and the Feldenkrais method. A few of the more common movement therapies are addressed here.

Qi Gong and Tai Chi
- Qi gong and Tai chi are traditional Chinese medicine, related to mind and body practices that involve certain postures and gentle movements with mental connection, breathing, and relaxation. They are believed to enhance energy, improve health, longevity, and harmony within oneself and the world. In contrast to qi gong, traditional Tai chi movements are more lengthy, complicated, and planned out.
- Qi gong is based on four common principles, sometimes referred to as the "secrets" of qi gong:
  - Mind (the presence of intention)
  - Eyes (the focus of intention)
  - Movement (the action of intention)
  - Breath (the flow of intention)

Level of Evidence
- Research suggests that practicing Tai chi may improve balance and stability in people with knee osteoarthritis, help people with knee pain, and promote quality of life and mood in people with heart failure and cancer.
- Less evidence has been found in the effects of qi gong.
- Qi gong may also improve the quality of life, fatigue, and mood.
- Tai chi and qi gong appear to be safe practices (Kamieniarz et al., 2021).

Contraindications
Psychosis has been reported, but it is not known whether there was a latent or undiagnosed psychiatric condition.

Practitioners
Because it is considered a form of Chinese medicine, patients should seek an acupuncturist and those appropriately credentialed in acupuncture and/or Oriental medicine.

Yoga
- Yoga is a popular exercise of mind and body practice with origins in ancient Indian philosophy.
- The various styles of yoga typically combine physical postures, breathing techniques, and meditation or relaxation.
- The popular yoga styles, such as Iyengar, Ashtanga, Vini, Kundalini, Bikram, and Hatha. Hatha yoga is the most commonly practiced method in the United States and Europe.
- NCCIH's website, highlighted the following results of 2017 from the questionnaire that was developed by NCCIH and the NCHS regarding the use of yoga (National Center for Complementary and Integrative Health [NCCIH], 2018a).
- Yoga was the most commonly used complementary health approach among US adults in 2012 (9.5%) and 2017 (14.3%). It has been used in the treatment of numerous medical conditions (National Center for Complementary and Integrative Health [NCCIH], 2018a).
- The use of meditation increased more than threefold, from 4.1% in 2012 to 14.2% in 2017. In 2012, chiropractic care was as popular as yoga, followed by meditation; however, the popularity of meditation surpassed that of chiropractic care to become the second most used approach among those surveyed in 2017.
- The use of chiropractors increased from 9.1% in 2012 to 10.3% in 2017.
- In 2017, women were more than twice as likely to use yoga compared with men (19.8% vs. 8.6%). Women were also more likely than men to use meditation (16.3% vs. 11.8%) and see a chiropractor (11.1% vs. 9.4%).
- Non-Hispanic White adults were more likely to use yoga, meditation, and chiropractors compared with Hispanic and non-Hispanic Black adults.

- The use of yoga was highest among adults aged 18 to 44 compared to older adults, while the use of meditation and chiropractic care was higher among adults aged 45 to 64 years compared with younger and older age groups.

Levels of Evidence
- Studies suggest that yoga may be beneficial for several conditions, including pain and fatigue. Recent studies in people with chronic low-back pain suggest that a carefully adapted set of yoga poses can help reduce pain and improve function.
- Other studies suggest that practicing yoga may have other health benefits, such as reducing heart rate and blood pressure, and may also help relieve anxiety and depression.

Contraindications
- Serious adverse events affecting the musculoskeletal, neurologic, and ocular systems have occurred in people using the "pranayam" or "Kapalabhati pranayama" technique.
- Yoga is contraindicated after abdominal surgery if the Valsalva maneuver is included.
- Research suggests that yoga is not helpful for asthma.
- Aggressive forms of yoga may raise blood pressure.
- Studies looking at yoga and arthritis have had mixed results.
- Those patients with hypertension, glaucoma, or sciatica, and women who are pregnant, should modify or avoid certain yoga poses.

Practitioners
- Certification is available through the Yoga Alliance (www.yogaalliance.org). There is no formal licensure process.
- Choice of instructor is important. The instructor must be able to adapt poses to individual needs.

Nutritional Therapeutics

Nutritional therapies include a variety of nutrients and non-nutrient bioactive food components used as chemopreventive agents, as well as specific foods or diets used as cancer prevention or treatment strategies. Examples include the macrobiotic diet, vegetarianism, Gerson therapy, vitamins, soy phytoestrogens, antioxidants, selenium, and coenzyme Q10. Some of the most notable types are highlighted here.

Antioxidants

Antioxidant vitamins—such as vitamin A (retinol, retinoic acid), vitamin C (L-ascorbic acid, ascorbic acid, ascorbate), vitamin E (α-tocopherol), selenium, lutein, lycopene, and beta-carotene—are natural substances found in food, including fruits and vegetables, that are believed to have health-promoting properties in preventing and delaying some type of cell damage, and each one has a different effect on body cells.

Levels of Evidence
- The belief that antioxidants may interfere with the efficacy of cancer therapy is not new. Limited research supports the belief that chemotherapy diminishes total antioxidant status, but inconsistencies based on cancer site, cancer therapy, research methodologies, patient populations, variability in doses, duration of supplementation, and timing of interventions have prevented the formulation of conclusions or consensus.
- Antioxidants may have a role in primary and secondary cancer prevention. Early studies suggest that high vitamin C intake prior to a diagnosis of breast cancer may positively affect survival.
- There is good evidence that eating a diet rich in vegetables and fruits is healthy.
- Evidence has shown that people who eat more vegetables and fruits have lower risks of several diseases; however, more research is required to prove the relation of antioxidant amounts in vegetables and fruits to other components of these foods, to other factors in people's diets, or to other lifestyle choices.
- Scientific studies with more than 100,000 people combined have tested whether antioxidant supplements can help prevent chronic diseases, such as cardiovascular diseases, cancer, and cataracts. In most instances, antioxidants did not reduce the risk of developing these diseases.
- Antioxidant supplements may interact with medication or conventional therapies.
- Beta-carotene increases the risks of lung cancer and stomach cancer.
- Beta-carotene did not protect against cardiovascular disease.
- *Vitamin E* increases the risks of prostate cancer and colorectal adenoma (National Institutes of Health [NIH], 2022).
- Special Consideration: The use of antioxidants should be discussed with health care providers due to possible food and drug interactions.

Practitioners
- Registered dieticians have a minimum of a bachelor's degree in dietetics.
- Certified nutritional consultants have education and training in clinical nutrition and may be nurses or other health care professionals.
- Caution should be used when choosing a nutrition practitioner to be certain that he or she has expertise in cancer care as well as in supplements and nutrition.

Pharmacologic and Biologic Therapies

The pharmacologic and biologic group of therapies includes drugs, vaccines, off-label use of prescription drugs, and other biologic interventions not yet accepted in conventional medicine. Some of the most common types are highlighted here.

Laetrile/Amygdalin
- Laetrile, also known as amygdalin, is found in pits of many fruits and plants (apricot almonds, apricot kernel oil, apricot seed, laetrile, prunus kernel, vitamin B_{17}, etc.).

- Laetrile is commonly administered intravenously and then orally as a maintenance therapy for cancer.
- Laetrile is also called vitamin B_{17}; it is not approved as a vitamin by the American Institute of Nutrition Vitamins.
- Laetrile treatments are given in some US clinics.
- Sometimes laetrile is given in combination with a metabolic therapy program (special diet, high-dose vitamins, and pancreatic enzymes).

Level of Evidence

- Laetrile is considered unsafe when taken either orally or intravenously.
- Apricot kernels are a source of cyanide. Orally, apricot kernels can cause acute poisoning, with symptoms including dizziness, headache, nausea, vomiting, drowsiness, dyspnea, palpitations, marked hypotension, convulsions, paralysis, coma, and death within 15 minutes. The lethal dose is 50 to 60 kernels, but the amount may vary. It can also cause chronic poisoning, with symptoms of increased blood thiocyanate, goiter, thyroid cancer, optic nerve lesions, blindness, ataxia, hypertonia, cretinism, and mental retardation.
- Demyelinating lesions and neuromyopathies reportedly have occurred secondary to chronic exposure, including long-term therapy.
- Two clinical trials conducted by the National Cancer Institute reported the following:
  - A Phase I study tested doses, schedules, and ways to give amygdalin to six cancer patients. Researchers found that amygdalin caused very few side effects at the prescribed doses when given by mouth or intravenously. Two patients who ate raw almonds while taking amygdalin had side effects.
  - A Phase II study with 175 patients looked at what types of cancer might benefit from treatment with amygdalin. Most of the patients in this study had breast, colon, or lung cancer. In about half of the patients, cancer had grown by the end of the treatment. Cancer had grown in all patients 7 months after treatment ended. Patients reported improved symptoms, such as the ability to work or do other activities. These improvements did not last after treatment ended.
  - The US FDA has not approved laetrile as a treatment for cancer or any other medical condition.
  - Laetrile is made in Mexico. The way that laetrile is made is not regulated by the FDA, so batches of laetrile may vary in purity and contents (National Cancer Institute [NCI], 2021).

714-X

- The main ingredient of 714-X is camphor, which is derived from the wood and bark of the camphor tree. Nitrogen, water, and salts are added to the camphor. It is believed that 714-X helps the immune system fight cancer. No studies of 714-X have been published in a peer-reviewed scientific journal that demonstrates safe and/or effectiveness in treating cancer.
- The development of 714-X was based on the theory that there are tiny living things in the blood called *somatids*. Some types of somatids are found only in the blood of people who have cancer or other serious diseases. These types of somatids are said to make growth hormones that initiate uncontrolled cell growth. The makers of 714-X state that by looking at the numbers and types of somatids in the blood, doctors can see if cancer is starting to form or can diagnose cancer and predict where it will spread. The theory states that cancer cells trap nitrogen needed by normal cells and make a toxic substance that weakens the immune system.
- 714-X is reported to help the body fight cancer by preventing cancer cells from taking nitrogen from the body's normal cells. It is also said to help the immune system by increasing the flow of lymphatic fluid through the body, which carries white blood cells that help fight infection and disease.
- 714-X is usually given by injection near the lymph nodes in the groin but can be sprayed into the nose using a nebulizer in specific cases.
- 714-X should not be injected into a vein (intravenously) or taken by mouth.
- 714-X can be used along with conventional treatments.
- Vitamin B_{12} supplements, vitamin E supplements, shark cartilage, and alcohol should not be used during treatment with 714-X.

Practitioners

- Patients in Canada can get 714-X only from a doctor for compassionate use.
- It is used in Mexico and some western European countries.
- The FDA has not approved 714-X for use in the United States (National Cancer Institute [NCI], 2017).

Complex Natural Products

Complex natural products are a subcategory of pharmacologic and biologic therapies and include many botanicals and extracts of natural substances, including marine organisms. The table on the next page provides information on several herbs and herbal extracts in this category.

- Herbal products are rated by the American Herbal Products Association in their *Botanical Safety Handbook* (American Herbal Products Association [AHPA], 2020).
  - Class 1 herbs can be consumed safely when used appropriately.
  - Class 2 herbs have some restrictions unless otherwise directed by a qualified expert:
    - Class 2a herbs are for external use only.
    - Class 2b herbs are not to be used during pregnancy.
    - Class 2c herbs are not to be used by lactating women.
    - Class 2d herbs may have other restrictions.

Herbs and Spices in the Prevention and Treatment of Cancer

Herb/Spice	Role in Cancer Care	Comments
Allspice	Antimicrobial Antioxidant Anti-Inflammatory Analgesic Antipyretic Anticancer Antitumorigenic	
Basil	Antimicrobial Antimutagenic	• Excess basil exposure may be harmful • Estragole, found in basil, is a potential procarcinogen, although benefits of basil use are thought to outweigh risk
Caraway	Antioxidant in vitro	• Human trials are lacking • May promote carcinogen deactivation
Cardamom	Inhibit carcinogenesis Enhance cytotoxic activity	• May be synergistic with black pepper to enhance splenocyte proliferation
Cinnamon	Inhibits *H. pylori* in vitro Inhibition of VEGF	• Positive results limited to animal studies
Clove	Potential antimutagen	• Contains high amounts of eugenol, which may be carcinogenic at higher doses
Coriander	Promote hepatic antioxidant system	• Human studies lacking
Cumin	Antioxidant Antimicrobial Anti-Inflammatory Chemo-preventive	• Properties are positive for further research in health promotion
Dill	Promotes detoxification	• Human trials are lacking
Garlic	Anti-carcinogenic	• Positive trials in animals but human trials less compelling
Ginger	Antioxidant Anti-inflammatory Antitumorigenic Anti-nausea	• Additional studies needed to demonstrate benefits in humans
Peppermint	Bronchodilator Muscle relaxant	• Some human studies exist but more are needed
Rosemary	Antioxidant Antitumorigenic	• Human trials are lacking
Saffron	Inhibit carcinogenesis Antitumorigenic	• Significant potential to inhibit cancer but human studies are lacking

Data from Kaefer, C. M., & Milner, J. A. (2011). Herbs and Spices in Cancer Prevention and Treatment. In I. F. F. Benzie & S. Wachtel-Galor, (Eds), *Herbal Medicine: Biomolecular and Clinical Aspects* (2nd ed.). Boca Raton (FL): CRC Press/Taylor & Francis. Available at https://www.ncbi.nlm.nih.gov/books/NBK92774/.

- Class 3 herbs are those for which significant data exist to recommend the following labeling: "to be used only under the supervision of an expert qualified in the appropriate use of this substance." Labeling must include the following:
  - Dosage
  - Contraindications
  - Potential adverse events and drug interactions
  - Any other relevant information related to the safe use of the substance
- Class 4 herbs are those for which insufficient data are available for classification.

The Role of Oncology Nurse

Nurses' skill, knowledge, and attitudes, as well as therapeutic communication skills toward CAM, are essential to promote an effective, trust-rapport relationship with the patient. Nurses at the leadership level are taking an active part in supporting and providing the oncology nurses' training needs to ensure integrated care is implemented. Evidence-based practice and research are needed to measure the effectiveness of CAM education and implementation and, finally, to evaluate how nurses can incorporate CAM into practice.

Conclusion

There is an increasing and growing number of leading cancer centers that provide information about CAM and supportive oncology information. Through their websites and published reports, the quality remains highly variable. However, the resources that are available can empower patients and families seeking CAM and supportive therapies to improve their quality of life. CAM therapies are now common mainstream in oncology practice. Nurses should understand the basic foundations of CAM therapies to provide patient education and safely incorporate these therapies into daily practice.

References

American Herbal Products Association (AHPA). (2020). *Botanical safety handbook* (2nd ed.). Available at https://www.ahpa.org/News/Alerts/TabId/100/ArtMID/1052/ArticleID/1508/AHPA-updates-online-Botanical-Safety-Handbook.aspx (accessed March 14, 2022).

Bao, T., Zhi, W. I., Vertosick, E. A., Li, Q. S., DeRito, J., Vickers, A., … Van Zee, K. J. (2018). Acupuncture for breast cancer-related lymphedema: A randomized controlled trial. *Breast Cancer Research and Treatment, 170*(1), 77–87. https://doi.org/10.3747/co.25.3884.

Buckner, C. A., Lafrenie, R. M., Dénommée, J. A., Caswell, J. M., & Want, D. A. (2018). Complementary and alternative medicine use in patients before and after a cancer diagnosis. *Current Oncology (Toronto, Ont.)*, 25(4), e275–e281.

Centers for Disease Control and Prevention (CDC). (2022). *Complementary and alternative medicine.* Available at https://www.cdc.gov/cancer/survivors/patients/complementary-alternative-medicine.htm (accessed March 9, 2023).

Centre for Evidence-Based Medicine, University of Oxford. (2009). *Levels of evidence.* Available at http://www.cebm.net/oxford-centre-evidence-based-medicine-levels-evidence-march-2009/ (accessed February 12, 2016).

Clarke, T. C., Barnes, P. M., Black, L. I., Stussman, B. J., & Nahin, R. L. (2018). Use of yoga, meditation, and chiropractors among U.S. adults aged 18 and over. *NCHS Data Brief*, 325, 1–8.

Deng, G., Bao, T., & Mao, J. J. (2018). Understanding the benefits of acupuncture treatment for cancer pain management. *Oncology (Williston Park)*, 32(6), 310–316.

Donelli, D., & Antonelli, M. (2021). Homeopathy and psychological therapies. *Encyclopedia*, 1(1), 57–64. Available at https://www.mdpi.com/2673-8392/1/1/8.

Eaton, L. H., & Hulett, J. M. (2019). Mind-body interventions in the management of chronic cancer pain. *Seminars in Oncology Nursing*, 35(3), 241–252.

Eisenberg, D. M., Kessler, R. C., Foster, C., Norlock, F. E., Calkins, D. R., & Delbanco, T. L. (1993). Unconventional medicine in the United States. Prevalence, costs, and patterns of use. *New England Journal of Medicine*, 328(4), 246–252.

Food and Drug Administration. (2018). *FDA history.* Available at https://www.fda.gov/about-fda/fda-history (accessed January 18, 2022).

Gentile, D., Boselli, D., O'Neill, G., Yaguda, S., Bailey-Dorton, C., & Eaton, T. A. (2018). Cancer pain relief after healing touch and massage. *Journal of Alternative and Complementary Medicine (New York, NY)*, 24(9–10), 968–973.

Grams, N. (2019). Homeopathy-where is the science? A current inventory on a pre-scientific artifact. *EMBO Reports*, 20(3), e47761.

Greenlee, H., DuPont-Reyes, M. J., Balneaves, L. G., Carlson, L. E., Cohen, M. R., Deng, G., … Tripathy, D. (2017). Clinical practice guidelines on the evidence-based use of integrative therapies during and after breast cancer treatment. *CA: A Cancer Journal for Clinicians*, 67(3), 194–232.

Greenlee, H., Neugut, A. I., Falci, L., Hillyer, G. C., Buono, D., Mandelblatt, J. S., … Hershman, D. L. (2016). Association between complementary and alternative medicine use and breast cancer chemotherapy initiation: The breast cancer quality of care (BQUAL) study. *JAMA Oncology*, 2(9), 1170–1176.

Hook, J. N., Davis, D. E., Owen, J., Worthington, E. L., & Utsey, S. O. (2013). Cultural humility: Measuring openness to culturally diverse clients. *Journal of Counseling Psychology*, 60(3), 353–366.

Institute of Medicine (IOM) (U.S.) and Committee on the Use of Complementary and Alternative Medicine by the American Public. (2005). *Complementary and alternative medicine in the United States.* Washington, DC: National Academies Press.

Judson, P. L., Abdallah, R., Xiong, Y., Ebbert, J., & Lancaster, J. M. (2017). Complementary and alternative medicine use in individuals presenting for care at a comprehensive cancer center. *Integrative Cancer Therapies*, 16(1), 96–103.

Kamieniarz, A., Milert, A., Grzybowska-Ganszczyk, D., Opara, J., & Juras, G. (2021). Tai Chi and Qi Gong therapies as a complementary treatment in Parkinson's disease—a systematic review. *Complementary Therapies in Medicine*, 56, 102589.

Keene, M. R., Heslop, I. M., Sabesan, S. S., & Glass, B. D. (2019). Complementary and alternative medicine use in cancer: A systematic review. *Complementary Therapies in Clinical Practice*, 35, 33–47.

Kwon, S., Jung, W. S., Yang, S., Jin, C., Cho, S. Y., Park, S. U., … Park, M. J. (2018). Safety of acupuncture in patients taking newer oral anticoagulants: A retrospective chart review study. *Evidence-Based Complementary and Alternative Medicine*, 2018, 8042198.

Latte-Naor, S., & Mao, J. J. (2019). Putting integrative oncology into practice: Concepts and approaches. *Journal of Oncology Practice*, 15(1), 7–14.

Li, Q.-W., Yu, M.-W., Wang, X.-M., Yang, G. W., Wang, H., Zhang, C. X., & Yang, Z. (2020). Efficacy of acupuncture in the prevention and treatment of chemotherapy-induced nausea and vomiting in patients with advanced cancer: A multi-center, single-blind, randomized, sham-controlled clinical research. *Chinese Medicine*, 15(1), 57.

National Cancer Institute (NCI). (2017). *714-X (PDQ) overview.* Available at https://www.cancer.gov/about-cancer/treatment/cam/patient/714-x-pdq (accessed March 12, 2022).

National Cancer Institute (NCI). (2019). *NCI-Designated Cancer Centers.* Available at https://www.cancer.gov/research/infrastructure/cancer-centers (accessed 17 March, 2023).

National Cancer Institute (NCI). (2021). *Laetrile/Amygdalin (PDQ).* Available at https://www.cancer.gov/about-cancer/treatment/cam/patient/laetrile-pdq (accessed 17 March, 2023).

National Cancer Institute (NCI). (2022). *About CAM.* Available at https://cam.cancer.gov (accessed 17 March, 2023).

National Center for Complementary and Integrative Health (NCCIH). (2018a). *National survey reveals increased use of yoga, meditation, and chiropractic care among U.S. adults.* Available at https://www.nccih.nih.gov/research/research-results/national-survey-reveals-increased-use-of-yoga-meditation-and-chiropractic-care-among-us-adults (accessed 17 March, 2023).

National Center for Complementary and Integrative Health (NCCIH). (2018b). *Reiki information.* Available at https://nccih.nih.gov/health/reiki (accessed 17 March, 2023).

National Center for Complementary and Integrative Health (NCCIH). (2021a). *Complementary, alternative, or integrative health.* Available at https://nccih.nih.gov/health/integrative-health#types (accessed 17 March, 2023).

National Center for Complementary and Integrative Health (NCCIH). (2021b). *NIH Complementary and Integrative Health Agency gets new name.* Available at https://nccih.nih.gov/news/press/12172014 (accessed 17 March, 2023).

National Institutes of Health (NIH). (2017). National Health Interview Survey 2017. Available from https://www.nccih.nih.gov/research/statistics/nhis/2017 (accessed March 9, 2023).

National Institutes of Health (NIH). (2022). *Antioxidants: In depth.* National Center for Complementary and Integrative Health (NCCIH). Available at https://www.nccih.nih.gov/health/antioxidants-in-depth (accessed 17 March, 2023).

National Library of Medicine. (2023). *Levels of evidence for human studies of cancer complementary and alternative medicine (PDQ).* Available at http://www.ncbi.nlm.nih.gov/pubmedhealth/PMH0032708/ (accessed March 9, 2023).

Natural Medicines. (2023). Available at https://naturalmedicines.therapeuticresearch.com/search.aspx?q=levels+of+evidence&go.x=0&go.y=0 (accessed March 9, 2023).

Oncology Nursing Society. (2014). *Putting Evidence into Practice (PEP) rating system overview.* Available at https://www.ons.org/practice-resources/pep (accessed February 12, 2016).

Xiang, Y., Guo, Z., Zhu, P., Chen, J., & Huang, Y. (2019). Traditional Chinese medicine as a cancer treatment: Modern perspectives of ancient but advanced science. *Cancer Medicine*, 8(5), 1958–1975.

Clinical Trials

Marlon Garzo Saria

Introduction

"Today's standard cancer treatments were yesterday's clinical trials" (National Cancer Institute [NCI], 2002). Cancer research has significantly expanded understanding of the biologic mechanisms that contribute to cancer development, progression, and metastasis. A solid basic science research provides the structural foundation for impactful clinical research (Halushka et al., 2020). Clinical trials make up the significant final steps in an arduous research process that translates basic research findings into clinical interventions for cancer risk reduction, detection, and treatment, allowing many individuals to survive diseases that in the past were almost universally fatal.

The contribution of clinical trials to modern medicine can readily be seen in the advances made in the treatment of pediatric cancers. It has been consistently estimated that less than 5% of adult patients with cancer participate in cancer clinical trials despite estimates that 70% of Americans are interested and willing to participate. In comparison, participation of children less than 15 years old in clinical trials has historically been higher at greater than 50%, resulting to a 2.6% average reduction in mortality per year from 1975 to 1995 for those less than 20 years old (Unger et al., 2016).

Drug Development Process

It takes about 10 to 15 years at a cost of $2.6 billion to develop a new drug, including the cost of the many failures. It is interesting to note that investments in new technologies and research that have spanned decades contributed to the swift response in designing safe and effective treatments to COVID-19 (Congressional Budget Office, 2021; Pharmaceutical Research and Manufacturers of America, 2021).

Development begins with the discovery of a potentially effective agent and includes a series of steps that takes 3 to 6 years.
- Prediscovery: understanding the disease
- Target identification: choosing a molecule to target with a drug
- Target validation: testing the target and confirming its role in the disease
- Drug discovery: finding a promising molecule that could become a drug
- Early safety tests: performing initial tests on promising compounds
- Lead optimization: altering the molecule to improve drug properties
- Preclinical testing: laboratory and animal testing to determine whether the drug is safe enough for human testing

Candidate drugs are extensively studied in humans before they are approved by the US. Food and Drug Administration (FDA). This process involves a series of steps designed with specific goals and requirements, taking an average of 6 to 7 years to complete.

Types of Clinical Trials

Several types of cancer clinical trials exist; each is designed to answer different research questions (NCI, 2020b; NIH, 2021).
- *Prevention trials:* Involve otherwise healthy individuals who may have higher risk characteristics for developing cancer. This type of trial evaluates the safety and efficacy of various risk reduction strategies that may include "action" interventions (e.g., being more active, quitting smoking, eating more fruits and vegetables) or "agent" interventions (e.g., taking certain medications, vitamins, and supplements). Agent trials are also referred to as chemoprevention trials.
- *Screening trials:* Evaluate the effectiveness of new techniques for early detection of cancer in the general population. Screening effectiveness is measured by the reduction in the number of deaths from the cancer being screened.
- *Quality-of-life/supportive care/palliative care trials:* Evaluate interventions designed to improve the comfort and quality of life of individuals diagnosed with cancer and their families. Supportive care trials explore pharmacologic or nonpharmacologic therapies suggested to minimize cancer-related and cancer treatment–related toxicities.
- *Treatment (therapeutic) trials:* Evaluate the safety and efficacy of new drugs, vaccines, biologic agents, approaches to surgery or radiation therapy, treatment combinations, or other interventions in people diagnosed with cancer.
- *Natural history studies:* Collect longitudinal data from people with cancer or people who are at high risk for developing cancer to understand how the medical condition or disease develops and how to treat it.

Phases of Clinical Trials

Cancer therapeutic trials evaluate the safety and efficacy of new pharmaceutical agents, biologic therapies, procedures, or other interventions in people with cancer. Cancer clinical trials include a series of steps, called phases (American Cancer Society, 2020; Congressional Budget Office, 2021; NCI, 2020c). Each phase is designed to answer a distinct research question (see figure on the next page).

Phase I

- Sample: Patients with advanced disease that is resistant to standard therapy
- Sample size: 15-30 patients
- Objective: Determine a dose that will be appropriate for use in phase II studies
- End point: Safety
- Specific end points: Toxicities, dose-limiting toxicity, pharmacokinetics, metabolism, maximum tolerated dose, schedule, pharmacodynamics/biomarkers, early evidence of effectiveness
- Time to complete: 1-6 months

Phase II

- Sample: Patients with maximum performance status and minimum exposure to prior chemotherapy
- Sample size: <100 patients
- Objectives: Determine antitumor activity against specific tumor type; determine short-term side effects and risks
- End point: Efficacy
- Specific end point: Tumor response, toxicity
- Time to complete: 6 months to 2 years

Phase III

- Sample: Patients with specific types of cancer
- Sample size: 100s to 1000s, multiple sites
- Objectives: Determine whether new therapy is more effective or has better toxicity profile than standard treatment
- End point: Efficacy
- Specific end point: Survival time, symptom control, quality of life, long-tern side effects and risks, progression-free survival, disease-free survival, cost-benefit analysis
- Time to complete: 1-10 years

Phase IV

- Objectives: Monitor ongoing safety of marketed drugs and identify additional potential uses of the drug
- End point: Safety and efficacy
- Specific end point: Long-term side effects
- Time to complete: 6 months to 5 years

Phases of Cancer Clinical Trials. (From National Cancer Institute. [2020b]. Phases of clinical trials. Available at https://www.cancer.gov/about-cancer/treatment/clinical-trials/what-are-trials/phases [accessed January 9, 2022]; U.S. Food and Drug Administration. [2018]. *Guidance for industry: Clinical trial endpoints for the approval of cancer drugs and biologic.* Rockville, MD: Author.)

Phase I: Initial Testing in a Small Group of Volunteers

- *Goal:* Evaluate safety, determine a safe dosage range, and identify side effects of a new drug or treatment in a small group of people.
- *Benefits:* If the new drug or treatment under study demonstrates anticancer activity, participants will be among the first to benefit; the intervention may benefit future patients.
- *Risks:* Unpredictable side effects can occur because phase I trials are often the first study of the drug or treatment that involves human subjects.

Phase II: Testing in a Small Group of Patients

- *Goal:* Evaluate the efficacy and further determine the safety of a drug or treatment in a larger group of people.

- *Benefits:* Participants may be among the first to benefit from the treatment.
- *Risks:* Unpredictable side effects may occur.

Phase III: Testing in a Large Group of Patients to Show Safety and Efficacy

- *Goal:* Evaluate the effectiveness, monitor side effects, and compare the drug or treatment with other, commonly used treatments (also known as standard of care).
- *Benefits:* Regardless of randomization, participants will receive the best widely accepted standard treatment.
- *Risks:* New drugs or treatments are not always better than, or even as good as, standard treatment; new treatments may have toxicities that are worse than those of the standard treatment; despite phase I and II testing, unexpected side effects may still occur; participants who are randomized

to standard treatment may not benefit as much as those receiving the experimental drug or treatment.

Phase IV: Ongoing Studies, Sometimes Called Postmarketing Surveillance Studies
- *Goal:* Evaluate the drug's effect in various populations and any side effects associated with long-term use after the treatment has been marketed.

Components of a Clinical Trial

Clinical trials adhere to strict scientific and ethical guidelines to protect participants. Multiple regulatory groups and independent review and advisory boards oversee participation of human subjects in research, monitor progress of clinical trials, and guarantee that the studies are conducted, recorded, and reported according to the protocol, standard operating procedures, good clinical practices, and regulatory requirements (NIH, 2021).

Clinical Research Team

The design and implementation of a clinical trial require the talents and expertise of a multidisciplinary research team (National Cancer Institute, 2020a). There is a wide variation in the composition of research teams that may include but are not limited to any of the following roles: investigators, clinical research associates, research nurses, data managers, and study coordinators who have varying responsibilities, including screening for potential study candidates, determining eligibility, coordinating the patient calendar, preparing documents for submission to institutional review boards (IRBs), filing amendments, submitting safety data, conducting patient education, obtaining informed consent, and assessing potential adverse events.
- *Principal investigator (PI) or clinical investigator:* oversees all aspects of a clinical trial; conducts research that contributes to generalizable knowledge; ultimately responsible for the ethical conduct of the research study (NCI, 2020a).

- *Research nurse:* coordinates and manages the collection of data throughout the clinical trial; responsible for education of staff, patients, and referring health care providers about the trial; assists the PI with toxicity and response monitoring, quality assurance, audits, data management, and analysis (NCI, 2020a).
- *Data manager:* supervises clinical trial data, including electronic data entry; provides data to monitoring agencies; prepares summaries for data analysis (NCI, 2020a).
- *Staff physicians and nurses:* administers treatments to participants as dictated by the protocol; assess and document toxicities, drug tolerance, and adverse events; collaborate with the PI and research nurse in monitoring clinical trends; provide direct care and patient and family education (NCI, 2020a).
- *Clinical research coordinator:* involved in the daily tasks of enrollment, data entry, and all other aspects of clinical trials at the site level (Certified Clinical Research Professionals Society [CCRPS], 2021).
- *Clinical research associate (also known as clinical monitor):* review and verify documents from multiple sites conducting the same trial and do multiple visits to ensure quality and ethical conduct of the clinical trial (CCRPS, 2021).

Clinical Trial Protocol

A clinical trial protocol is a clear, detailed, and transparent action plan that guides the conduct of a clinical trial. Protocols provide investigators with a written plan to carry out the clinical trial; provide trial participants with a precise description of the methodology; provide ethics committees and IRBs with information on the safety plan and assurances to protect participants' welfare and rights; provide funding agencies with a mechanism to evaluate proposed methodologies; and provide systematic reviewers with a description of *a priori* methods to address potential biases. The table below outlines the sections to be included in a clinical trial protocol as reported by an expert consensus panel (Tetzlaff, Chan, et al., 2012; Tetzlaff, Moher, et al., 2012).

Minimum Clinical Trial Protocol Content

Section and Topic	Brief Description
General Information	
Title	Descriptive title identifying study design
Trial identifier	Unique number/name and registration information
Protocol version	Version or amendment number and date
Protocol summary	Short summary of proposed research
Names and addresses	Contact information for primary investigators and sponsor
Table of contents	List of contents and page numbers
Introduction	
Rationale	Outlines topic and provides justification for the study
Background of the study	Summary of all previous studies
Preliminary data	Describe preliminary studies
Objectives	Specific objectives and hypotheses for the study
Study locations	Description of intended site or sites
Methods: Participant	
Population	Target and study population and source of the latter
Eligibility criteria	Description of inclusion and exclusion criteria
Sample size	Estimated number; calculations and assumptions
Recruitment	Process of recruitment and enrollment (e.g., advertisements)

Continued

Minimum Clinical Trial Protocol Content—cont'd

Section and Topic	Brief Description
Methods: Design	
Type of study	Description of type/design and trial framework
Study timeline	Diagram of procedures/visits through trial stages
Sequence generation	Random sequence method; details of any restriction
Allocation concealment	Random sequence implementation and whether concealed
Random implementation	How participants will be assigned to groups
Blinding	Who (e.g., participants, investigators, outcome assessors)
Methods: Interventions	
Interventions A	Precise details; how administered (e.g., dosage, form)
Interventions B	Justification of control
Schedule of interventions	Number and duration of treatment periods (run-in, washout)
Concomitant interventions	Treatments permitted or not before or during trial
Risks or harms	Known or potential risks for each intervention
Methods: Data Collection and Management	
Outcomes	Describes and defines primary and secondary outcomes
Data collection	Instruments and timing of data collection and recording
Biologic specimens	Laboratory evaluation, specimen collection and handling
Validation of instruments	Instrument reliability/validity or plans to validate
Follow-up	Description and schedule of visits and logistics
Data management	Plans for data entry, editing, coding, and storage
Quality control	Quality of outcome assessment and data records
Compliance	Monitoring of participant compliance
Methods: Statistical Methods	
Statistical methods	Methods for primary/secondary outcomes and additional analyses
Withdrawals A	Criteria to withdraw or exclude participants from the intervention
Withdrawals B	Data collected and follow-up, withdrawn participants
Missing data	Methods to account for missing or erroneous data
Interim trial monitoring	Process and timing of any planned interim analyses
Stopping guidelines A	Predefined statistical stopping boundaries
Stopping guidelines B	Nonstatistical criteria for the early trial termination
Methods: Safety and Monitoring	
Safety evaluations	Monitoring of safety plans including methods, timing
Data and Safety Monitoring Board (DSMB)	If relevant, composition and role of DSMB
Adverse event reporting	Recording and reporting events; methods to handle
Emergency code breaking	Establishment and storage of code; when and by whom it can be broken
Trial monitoring	Plans and frequency, whether independent
Trial Organization and Administration	
Monetary and material support	Sources of financial and material support
Data ownership	Who has ownership; contractual limits for principal investigators
Ethical Considerations	
Potential benefits and risks	Potential benefits and risks to participants, society
Agreement and consent	Materials for potential participants
Surrogate consent/assent	Method of obtaining surrogate consent or assent
Confidentiality/anonymity	Provisions for protecting personal data and privacy
Ethics approval	Whether obtained, names of committees
Role of sponsor	Role of sponsor in design, data collection, analysis, dissemination
Conflict of interest	Real or perceived conflicts of interest
Posttrial care	Posttrial follow-up, access to treatment, duration; defines who is responsible
Reporting and Dissemination	
Protocol amendments	Methods of communicating to investigators and institutional review boards, documentation
Dissemination	How results will be disseminated to participants, practitioners, public
Publication policy	Publication rights, restrictions, authorship guidelines
Reporting of early stopping	Dissemination of results if trial is stopped early
Other	
Limitations	Limitations of study, including risk of bias
References	List of references cited in protocol
Data collection forms	Summary of data collection forms and times

From Tetzlaff, J. M., Moher, D., & Chan, A. W. (2012). Developing a guideline for clinical trial protocol content. Delphi consensus survey. *Trials, 13,* 176

Eligibility Criteria

Eligibility criteria define the population under study. They may specify attributes required for patients to be considered for enrollment or identify characteristics that would make them ineligible for enrollment, with the primary purpose of protecting the safety of trial participants (Kim et al., 2017).

Common inclusion and exclusion criteria derived from cumulative experience with agents with narrow therapeutic indices have evolved over time; they include cancer status, performance status, measurable disease, biomarker status. In 2017, the American Society of Clinical Oncology and Friends of Cancer Research issued a joint statement to broaden eligibility criteria and recommended changes to criteria that commonly lead to exclusion of patients from clinical trials: brain metastases, minimum age for enrollment, HIV infection, and organ dysfunction and prior and concurrent malignancies (Kim et al., 2017).

End Points

Clinical end points guide clinical decision making and are essential in evaluating the safety and efficacy of investigational therapeutics. They are objective tools that measure the outcomes of interventions, including survival, symptoms, functional capacity, and the chances of developing a chronic condition (see table below) (Delgado & Guddati, 2021).

Comparison of Important Cancer Approval End Points

End Point	Regulatory Evidence	Study Design	Advantages	Disadvantages
Overall survival	Clinical benefit for regular approval	Randomized studies essential Blinding not essential	Universally accepted direct measure of benefit Easily measured Precisely measured	May involve larger studies May be affected by crossover therapy and sequential therapy Includes noncancer deaths
Symptom end points (patient-reported outcomes)	Clinical benefit for regular approval	Randomized blinded studies	Patient perspective of direct clinical benefit	Blinding is often difficult Data frequently missing or incomplete Clinical significance of small changes unknown Multiple analyses Lack of validated instruments
Disease-free survival	Surrogate for accelerated approval or regular approval*	Randomized studies essential Blinding preferred Blinded review recommended	Smaller sample size and shorter follow-up necessary compared with survival studies	Not validated as surrogate for survival in all settings Not precisely measured; subject to assessment bias, particularly in open-label studies Definitions vary
Objective response rate	Surrogate for accelerated approval or regular approval*	Single-arm or randomized studies may be used Blinding preferred in comparative studies Blinded review recommended	Can be assessed in single-arm studies Assessed earlier and in smaller studies compared with survival studies Effect attributable to drug, not natural history	Not a direct measure of benefit Not a comprehensive measure of drug activity Only a subset of patients benefit
Complete response	Surrogate for accelerated approval or regular approval*	Single-arm or randomized studies may be used Blinding preferred in comparative studies Blinded review recommended	Can be assessed in single-arm studies Durable complete responses can represent clinical benefit Assessed earlier and in smaller studies compared with survival studies	Not a direct measure of benefit in all cases Not a comprehensive measure of drug activity Small subset of patients with benefit
Progression-free survival	Surrogate for accelerated approval or regular approval*	Randomized studies essential Blinding preferred Blinded review recommended	Smaller sample size and shorter follow-up necessary compared with survival studies Measurement of stable disease included Not affected by crossover or subsequent therapies Generally based on objective and quantitative assessment	Not validated as surrogate for survival in all settings Not precisely measured; subject to assessment bias particularly in open-label studies Definitions vary Frequent radiologic or other assessments Involves balanced timing of assessments of treatment arms

* Adequacy as a surrogate end point for accelerated approval or regular approval is highly dependent on other factors such as effect size, effect duration, and benefits of other available therapies.

From Wilson, M. K., Karakasis, K., & Oza, A. M. (2015). Outcomes and endpoints in trials of cancer treatment: The past, present, and future. *Lancet Oncology, 16*(1), e32–e42.

Randomization

Randomization is indispensable in any clinical trial involving treatment comparison. It prevents selection bias, allows comparability between or among groups with respect to known and unknown confounders, and contributes to the rigor of statistical analysis (Berger et al., 2021).

Blinding

Blinding is defined as withholding information that has the potential to influence study results from one or more parties involved in a research study that may include study participants, research team, and clinical team. Blinding mitigates several sources of bias, including participants' expectations, adherence to protocol, treatment-seeking behavior outside of the trial, and assessment of efficacy and safety of the intervention; mitigates research or clinical team's differential treatment, attention, or attitudes toward subjects (Monaghan et al., 2021).

Considerations for Nursing Care

Oncology nurses have contributed to the body of evidence defining, validating, and advancing the role of clinical research nursing (see table below). Nurses work directly or indirectly in multiple roles that include direct care provider, research coordinator, advanced clinician, manager, educator, scientist, monitor, regulatory specialist, and IRB administrator (Ness, 2020). Clinical trials nurses are essential members of the research team and are crucial to the successful completion of clinical trials. In addition to their research-related responsibilities, oncology nurses are known to harness the therapeutic relationship they establish with research participants. One cannot overemphasize the contributions of oncology nurses in the scientific advancement of new cancer therapies that allow patients to live longer and with greater quality of life.

Oncology Clinical Trials Nurse Competencies

Category	Competency
Adherence to ethical standards	Demonstrates leadership in ensuring adherence to ethical practices during the conduct of clinical trials to protect the rights and well-being of patients and the collection of quality data.
Protocol compliance	Facilitates compliance with the requirements of the research protocol and good clinical research practice while remaining cognizant of the needs of diverse patient populations.
Informed consent	Demonstrates leadership in ensuring patient comprehension and safety during initial and ongoing clinical trial informed consent discussions.
Patient recruitment and retention	Utilizes a variety of strategies to enhance recruitment and retention while being aware of and respectful of the needs of diverse patient populations.
Management of clinical trial patients	Uses a variety of resources and strategies to manage the care of patients participating in clinical trials, ensuring compliance with protocol procedures, assessments, and reporting requirements as well as management of symptoms.
Documentation and document management	Provides leadership to the research team in ensuring accurate source documentation and maintaining essential documents that validate integrity in the conduct of the clinical trial.
Data management and information technology	Provides leadership in the collection of data and demonstrates basic information technology and computer skills to ensure data quality and patient confidentiality.
Financial stewardship	Identifies the financial variables that affect research and supports good financial stewardship in clinical trials.
Leadership and professional development	Utilizes leadership skills to inspire and motivate the clinical research team toward the common goal of conducting quality clinical research to enhance cancer care across the continuum and takes responsibility for his or her ongoing professional development.

Data from Oncology Nursing Society. (2016). *Oncology clinical trials nurse competencies*. Pittsburgh, PA: Author.

References

American Cancer Society. (2020). *Types and phases of clinical trials*. Available at https://www.cancer.org/treatment/treatments-and-side-effects/clinical-trials/what-you-need-to-know/phases-of-clinical-trials.html (accessed January 9, 2022).

Berger, V. W., Bour, L. J., Carter, K., Chipman, J. J., Everett, C. C., Heussen, N., … Randomization Innovative Design Scientific Working Group. (2021). A roadmap to using randomization in clinical trials. *BMC Medical Research Methodology, 21*(1), 168.

Congressional Budget Office. (2021). *Research and development in the pharmaceutical industry*. Available at https://www.cbo.gov/publication/57126 (accessed January 9, 2022).

Certified Clinical Research Professionals Society (CCRPS). (2021). *Clinical research certification*. Available at https://ccrps.org/ (accessed January 9, 2022).

Delgado, A., & Guddati, A. K. (2021). Clinical endpoints in oncology—a primer. *American Journal of Cancer Research, 11*(4), 1121–1131.

Halushka, P., Loucks, T. L., Paranal, R., Harvey, J., Briggman, K., Lee-Chavarria, D., & Feghali-Bostwick, C. (2020). The translational sciences clinic: From bench to bedside. *Journal of Clinical and Translational Science, 5*(1), e36.

Kim, E. S., Bruinooge, S. S., Roberts, S., Ison, G., Lin, N. U., Gore, L., … Schilsky, R. L. (2017). Broadening eligibility criteria to make clinical trials more representative: American Society of Clinical Oncology and friends of cancer research joint research statement. *Journal of Clinical Oncology, 35*(33), 3737–3744.

Monaghan, T. F., Agudelo, C. W., Rahman, S. N., Wein, A. J., Lazar, J. M., Everaert, K., & Dmochowski, R. R. (2021). Blinding in clinical trials: Seeing the big picture. *Medicina (Kaunas, Lithuania), 57*(7), 647.

National Cancer Institute. (2002). *Cancer clinical trials: The in-depth program*. Bethesda, MD: NCI.

National Cancer Institute. (2020a). *Research team members*. Available at https://www.cancer.gov/about-cancer/treatment/clinical-trials/what-are-trials/team (accessed January 9, 2022).

National Cancer Institute. (2020b). *Types of clinical trials*. Available at https://www.cancer.gov/about-cancer/treatment/clinical-trials/what-are-trials/types (accessed January 9, 2022).

National Cancer Institute. (2020c). *Phases of clinical trials*. Available at https://www.cancer.gov/about-cancer/treatment/clinical-trials/what-are-trials/phases (accessed March 4, 2023).

National Institutes of Health. (2021). *NIH clinical research trials and you: The basics*. Available at https://www.nih.gov/health-information/nih-clinical-research-trials-you/basics (accessed January 9, 2022).

Ness, E. (2020). The oncology clinical research nurse study Co-Ordinator: Past, present, and future. *Asia-Pacific Journal of Oncology Nursing, 7*(3), 237–242.

Oncology Nursing Society. (2016). *Oncology clinical trials nurse competencies*. Pittsburgh, PA: Author.

Pharmaceutical Research and Manufacturers of America. (2021). *Research & development policy framework*. Washington, DC: Author. Available at https://www.phrma.org/policy-issues/research-and-development-policy-framework (accessed January 9, 2022).

Tetzlaff, J. M., Chan, A. W., Kitchen, J., Sampson, M., Tricco, A. C., & Moher, D. (2012). Guidelines for randomized clinical trial protocol content: A systematic review. *Systematic Reviews, 1*, 43.

Tetzlaff, J. M., Moher, D., & Chan, A. W. (2012). Developing a guideline for clinical trial protocol content: Delphi consensus survey. *Trials, 13*, 176.

Unger, J. M., Cook, E., Tai, E., & Bleyer, A. (2016). The role of clinical trial participation in cancer research: Barriers, evidence, and strategies. American Society of Clinical Oncology educational book. *American Society of Clinical Oncology. Annual Meeting, 35*, 185–198.

Oncology Symptoms

Alopecia

Wendy H. Vogel

Definition

- Alopecia is the absence or loss of hair.
- It can result from genetic factors, aging, a local or systemic disease, or it can be therapy induced.
- Loss of less than 25% of the hair is considered minimal, 25% to 50% is considered moderate hair loss, and more than 50% is severe hair loss.
- At least 50% of the hair must be lost for it to be noticeable.
- In oncology settings, toxic alopecia typically occurs because of chemotherapeutic agents or radiation therapy; the estimated incidence is 65% (see table below). Some targeted therapies, such as kinase inhibitors, may cause varying degrees of alopecia.
- Toxic alopecia is usually temporary and can include body hair as well as the hair of the head.
- The average daily hair loss (under normal conditions) is approximately 100 hairs.
- Because hair follicles are mitotically active structures, they are at risk for damage from radiation therapy and chemotherapy.
- The scalp is the area most sensitive to hair damage, followed by the male beard, the eyebrows, axillary hair, pubic hair, and fine hair.
- The degree of alopecia depends on the treatment given, the dose, the schedule, and the route of administration.
- Bolus-dosing schedules of chemotherapy cause more alopecia than cumulative doses given over an extended period.
- Radiation doses of 2500 to 3000 cGy fractionated over 2 or 3 weeks will cause hair loss. A single dose as small as 500 cGy may cause hair loss.
- Radiation doses greater than 4500 cGy can cause permanent alopecia.
- Radiation doses greater than 6000 cGy may cause sebaceous and sweat glands to stop functioning.

Oncology Agents That Cause Hair Loss (Listed in Order of Toxicity)

Class	Drug Examples	Incidence of Hair Loss (%)*
Antimicrotubule agents	Docetaxel, paclitaxel, vincristine	>80
Topoisomerase	Doxorubicin, epirubicin, etoposide	60–100
Alkylators	Bendamustine, cisplatin, cyclophosphamide	>60
Antimetabolites	5-Fluorouracil, capecitabine, pemetrexed	10–50
Kinase Inhibitors	Sunitinib, sorafenib	14

*Incidence and severity vary by selected agent and dose density. The combination of agents may increase toxicity.

Pathophysiology and Contributing Factors

- When cells in the hair bulb absorb the chemotherapeutic agent or are damaged by radiation therapy, cellular division and protein synthesis may be suppressed or halted.
- Cells can enter the telogen phase early, enabling the hair to be shed, either in clumps or gradually, depending on the mitotic activity of the hair follicle at the time of the exposure.
- Hair loss usually occurs within 2 to 3 weeks after the first exposure to the toxin.
- Continued loss can occur over the next 3 to 4 weeks, although this varies according to the chemotherapeutic agent.
- In general, hair loss begins on the crown and on the sides of the head above the ear.
- Regrowth occurs within 3 to 5 months. New hair growth may be of a different texture, color, or consistency.
- Regrowth may occur before the end of therapy because of the tricyclic nature of hair growth phases.
- Permanent alopecia is rare after cancer treatment, although it has been reported after bone marrow transplantation, and it is associated with chronic graft-versus-host reaction, previous exposure to radiation, and advanced age.

Signs and Symptoms

- Loss of hair usually begins 2 to 3 weeks after exposure. The scalp may become sensitive before hair is lost.

Assessment Tools

- Thorough history
  - Comorbid diseases
  - Nutrition
  - Drug history
  - Psychiatric history
- Physical examination
  - Inspection for a pattern of hair loss
  - Density of remaining hair
  - Color (dull or bright)
  - Condition of scalp
  - Length and texture of hair
- A hair pull test involves gentle traction on about 50 hairs. If two to three or more hairs are dislodged, then accelerated hair loss is likely.
- Common Terminology Criteria for Adverse Events (version 4.03)
  - Grade 1 indicates thinning or patchy hair.
  - Grade 2 is complete hair loss.
- Eastern Cooperative Oncology Group grading scale
- World Health Organization toxicity grading criteria

313

Laboratory and Diagnostic Tests

- None

Differential Diagnoses

- Malnutrition
- Hypothyroidism
- Noncytotoxic drugs such as allopurinol, amphetamines, anticoagulants, antithyroid drugs, heavy metals, hypocholesterolemic drugs, levodopa, oral contraceptives, propranolol, and retinoids
- Chronic stress
- Postpartum state
- Lupus erythematosus
- Alopecia of other causes, such as congenital alopecia, alopecia areata, androgenetic alopecia, alopecia associated with trauma, tinea capitis, folliculitis decalvans, and alopecia neoplastica

Interventions

- Prevention has been a subject of debate since the 1960s.
- Various preventive methods have been used, including scalp tourniquets and scalp hypothermia. Discomfort and the risk of creating a "drug-free area" that could be a site for recurrence (e.g., skin metastases) have discouraged these practices.

Pharmacologic Interventions

- None is used as the standard of care.
- Several agents for prevention and treatment of alopecia have been studied with varying results, although none has been approved by the US Food and Drug Administration (FDA):
  - Tocopherol (vitamin E)
  - ImuVert, a biologic response modifier
  - Minoxidil (topical) may shorten duration or severity but does not prevent hair loss

Nonpharmacologic Interventions

- Alopecia can cause the skin to be sensitive or tender. Warmth, lotions, massage, or other symptomatic treatments may be used, although there are no guidelines in the medical literature to advise these.
- Scalp tourniquets—limited use due to patient discomfort.
- Scalp cooling is the only FDA-approved technique with an evidence base. Concerns regarding higher incidence of scalp metastasis have no supporting evidence. Side effects of scalp cooling include headaches and feelings of cold throughout the body.
- Patients should be reassured that hair regrowth will occur.
- Psychosocial adjustment (in both men and women) should be continually assessed throughout the treatment period until regrowth occurs.

Patient Teaching

- Instruct the patient as to when hair loss will occur.
- Advise the patient to obtain a wig or head covering, if desired, before hair loss occurs, while a good color and style match can be made.

- Encourage use of sunscreen and sun hats.
- Care should be taken to avoid cuts or nicks to the scalp if the head is shaved.

Follow-Up

- Hair should begin to regrow within 3 to 5 months after therapy ends. The rate of growth depends on the individual's growth rate. If hair has not begun to regrow within 6 months, alopecia may be permanent.

Resources

- American Academy of Dermatology: www.aad.org/default.htm
- Cancer Care.org: www.cancercare.org
- Oncolink: www.oncolink.com

Bibliography

Callaghan, M., & Cooper, A. (2014). Alopecia. In C. Yarbro, D. Wujcik, & B. Gobel (Eds.), *Cancer symptom management* (4th ed.). Burlington, MA: Jones & Bartlett.

Camp-Sorrell, D. (2018). Chemotherapy toxicities and management. In C. Yarbro, D. Wujcik, & B. Gobel (Eds.), *Cancer nursing principles and practice* (8th ed.). Sudbury, MA: Jones & Bartlett.

Dest, V. (2018). Radiation therapy: Toxicities and management. In C. Yarbro, D. Wujcik, & B. Gobel (Eds.), *Cancer nursing principles and practice* (8th ed.). Sudbury, MA: Jones & Bartlett.

Dunnill, C. J., Al-Tameemi, W., Collett, A., Haslam, I. S., & Georgopoulos, N. T. (2018). A clinical and biological guide for understanding chemotherapy-induced alopecia and its prevention. *Oncologist, 23*(1), 84–96.

Nail, L., & Lee-Lin, F. (2015). Alopecia. In C. Brown (Ed.), *Guide to oncology symptom management* (2nd ed.). Pittsburg, PA: Oncology Nursing Society.

National Cancer Institute, National Institutes of Health. (2017). Common terminology criteria for adverse events, version 5.0. Available at https://ctep.cancer.gov/protocoldevelopment/electronic_applications/docs/CTCAE_v5_Quick_Reference_8.5x11.pdf (accessed December 30, 2021).

Polovich, M., Olsen, M., & LeFebvre, K. (2014). *Chemotherapy and biotherapy guidelines and recommendations for practice* (4th ed.). Pittsburgh, PA: Oncology Nursing Society.

Renehan, S., Tencic, M., Jackson, K., & Krishnasamy, M. (2021). Improving preparation for scalp cooling: Learning from women undergoing chemotherapy for early-stage breast cancer—the COOL study. *Journal of Clinical Nursing, 31*(21-22), 3222–3234.

Trusson, D., & Quincey, K. (2021). Breast cancer and hair loss: Experiential similarities and differences in men's and women's narratives. *Cancer Nursing, 44*(1), 62–70.

Anorexia

Mary Steinbach

Definition

- Anorexia is an abnormal loss of appetite or aversion to food, with or without weight loss.
- Anorexia is often associated with cachexia (lean tissue wasting), although it can occur without it.
- Cancer anorexia-cachexia syndrome comprises appetite loss and weight loss plus muscle wasting, which affects physical functioning and nutritional well-being.
- It occurs in more than half of newly diagnosed cancer patients and in 30% to 80% of those with advanced cancer.
- The highest incidences are in patients with gastrointestinal cancers.
- Weight loss is a major cause of morbidity and mortality in patients with advanced cancer.

- Anorexia is associated with a lower quality of life, a poor response to chemotherapy, reduced performance status, and a reduction in survival.

Pathophysiology and Contributing Factors

- End result of altered central and peripheral neurohormonal signals that govern appetite
- Involuntary systemic effect of underlying disease
- Inflammation can drive symptoms but also contribute
- Predisposed by disease progression
- Direct result of supportive treatment modalities, including surgery, radiation therapy, and chemotherapy
- Secondary effect of
  - Taste alterations
  - Pain
  - Nausea
  - Lowered immune competence
- Humoral and inflammatory responses
  - Production of inflammatory cytokines
- Local effects of tumor
  - Dysphagia
  - Gastric obstruction and permeability changes
- Psychological factors, including depression/anxiety
- Metabolic disturbances

Signs and Symptoms

- Lack of appetite
- Weight loss
- Dry mouth
- Muscle wasting (sarcopenia)
- Early satiety
- Fatigue
- Nausea
- Vomiting
- Weakness
- Sleep disturbances
- Depression/anxiety
- Eating-related anxiety

Assessment Tools

- Patient history and physical examination
- The Functional Assessment of Anorexia/Cachexia Therapy Questionnaire
- Simplified Nutrition Assessment Questionnaire
- Rotterdam Symptom Checklist

Laboratory and Diagnostic Tests

- Complete blood cell count
- Creatinine clearance
- Albumin, prealbumin, transferrin, and retinol-binding protein levels

Differential Diagnoses

- Dysphagia
- Malnutrition
- Cachexia
- Nausea and vomiting

- Dehydration
- Fatigue
- Depression
- Hypercalcemia

Interventions

- Treat underlying cause and symptoms.
- Provide nutritional counseling.

Pharmacologic Interventions

- Progestational agents (appetite stimulants)
  - Megestrol acetate (Megace)
  - Medroxyprogesterone
- Corticosteroids
  - Dexamethasone
  - Prednisone
- Cannabinoids
  - Tetrahydrocannabinol (THC)/Dronabinol
  - Other drugs
    - Mirtazapine
    - Olanzapine

Nonpharmacologic Interventions

- Increased food intake
- Screening at diagnosis and at regular intervals
  - Weight change
  - Dietary intake
  - Physical examination findings
  - Laboratory findings
- Management of underlying causes
  - Nausea
  - Constipation
  - Mucositis
- Nutritional counseling
- Enteral or parenteral nutrition
- Minimizing factors that decrease food intake

Patient Teaching

- Eat small, frequent meals.
- Decrease energy expenditure when possible.
- Minimize factors that decrease food intake.
- Avoid offensive odors.
- Eat energy-dense foods.
- Limit fat intake.
- Avoid extremes in taste and smell of food.
- Enhance presentation of food.

Follow-Up

- Consultation with nutritionist or dietician
- Reassessment of patient status
- Assessment of new-onset or continued weight loss

Resources

- Oncology Nursing Society: https://www.ons.org/practice-resources/pep/anorexia
- FAACT Version 4: obtained from FACIT.org

Bibliography

Berry, D. L., Blonquist, T., Nayak, M. M., Roper, K., Hilton, N., Lombard, H., & McManus, K. (2018). Cancer anorexia and cachexia: Screening in an ambulatory infusion service and nutrition consultation. *Clinical Journal of Oncology Nursing, 22*(1), 63–68.

Blauwhoff-Buskermolen, S., Ruijgrok, C., Ostelo, R. W., de Vet, H. C., Verheul, H. M., de van der Schueren, M. A., & Langius, J. A. (2016). The assessment of anorexia in patients with cancer: cut-off values for the FAACT–A/CS and the VAS for appetite. *Supportive Care in Cancer, 24*(2), 661–666.

Childs, D. S., & Jatoi, A. (2019). A hunger for hunger: A review of palliative therapies for cancer-associated anorexia. *Annals of Palliative Medicine, 8*(1), 50–58.

Peixoto da Silva, S., Santos, J. M., Costa e Silva, M. P., Gil da Costa, R. M., & Medeiros, R. (2020). Cancer cachexia and its pathophysiology: Links with sarcopenia, anorexia and asthenia. *Journal of Cachexia, Sarcopenia and Muscle, 11*(3), 619–635.

Zhang, F., Shen, A., Jin, Y., & Qiang, W. (2018). The management strategies of cancer-associated anorexia: A critical appraisal of systematic reviews. *BMC Complementary & Alternative Medicine, 18*(1), 1–9.

Anxiety

Darcy Burbage

Definition

- Anxiety is a subjective feeling of distress, apprehension, tension, insecurity, or uneasiness, usually without a known stimulus or cause, and a fear of real or perceived threat to oneself.
- It is most often rated as mild, moderate, or severe.
- Anxiety related to cancer is considered a normal reaction to a potentially life-threatening illness.

Pathophysiology and Contributing Factors

- Anxiety is thought to result from an inappropriate activation of the sympathetic nervous system.
- Increased levels of norepinephrine and decreased levels of serotonin and γ-aminobutyric acid are present.
- Hormonal inputs, such as from the hypothalamus, pituitary, and adrenal glands, interfere with normal processes, leading to feelings of panic or a sense of dread.
- Cardiovascular abnormalities contribute to anxiety because of altered regulation of the autonomic nervous system.
- Anxiety can be medication induced (see list under "Assessment Tools").
- It can be caused by withdrawal from alcohol or nicotine.
- It can be related to disease stage: Anxiety increases as disease advances or physical status declines.
- It can be related to difficulty with treatment regimens or lifestyle changes and financial concerns.
- It can be related to transitions in care, such as a change in treatment modality, transition to survivorship, or transition to end-of-life care.
- It can be related to dealing with family issues or conflicts and facing death.
- Family and staff anxiety can contribute to the patient's level of anxiety, and vice versa.

Signs and Symptoms

- Restlessness, panic, tachycardia, difficulty concentrating, palpitations, sweating, dizziness, urinary frequency, abdominal discomfort, and sleep disturbances.
- Chest pain, irritability, headache, apprehension, and anorexia.
- Repetitive behaviors to prevent discomfort (e.g., pacing, rubbing hands, scratching).
- Changes in vital signs: elevated heart rate, blood pressure, or respiratory rate and temperature.
- Endocrine-associated changes to the skin that contribute to anxiety (e.g., dry skin in thyroid disorder, Addison disease symptoms), facial puffiness, and increased skin pigmentation.
  - Skin turgor may predict poor appetite, dehydration, or hypernatremia.

Assessment Tools

- Depression and anxiety screening tools to help evaluate subjective feelings of anxiety and the level of anxiety the patient is experiencing. Anxiety can be rated on a visual analog scale or on a verbal rating scale from 1 to 10 (similar to pain ratings).
  - Screening tools include:
    - GAD-7 (General Anxiety Disorder-7) scale, which is used to measure the level of anxiety.
    - National Comprehensive Cancer Network Distress Thermometer, which measures physical, emotional, social, and practical concerns.
    - Patient health questionnaire-4, which measures anxiety and depression.
  - Ask questions such as, "Do you feel nervous?" and "Do you worry about your diagnosis or treatment?" The goal is to understand what may be contributing to the anxiety.
- The history should include any history of psychosocial disorders, adjustment disorders, or panic attacks.
- Any history of generalized anxiety disorders or phobias or a history of agitated depression.
- What are the presenting symptoms, including precipitating factors, onset, and duration?
- What makes the symptoms better or worse?
- How does the patient cope with anxiety? What methods does the patient use to manage anxiety?
- Medication history, including over-the-counter medications. Medications associated with anxiety include stimulants, thyroid replacement medications, corticosteroids, bronchodilators and decongestants, epinephrine, antihypertensives, antihistamines, anticholinergics, anesthetics, and analgesics.
- Uncontrolled pain, hypoxia, sepsis, adverse drug effects, and withdrawal effects.
- Cardiac examination to identify irregular heart rate or abnormal heart sounds.
- Pulmonary examination to rule out hypoxia related to pneumonia, pleural effusions, or embolus.
- Neurologic examination to identify cranial nerve palsies, neuropathies, and cognitive disruptions.

Laboratory and Diagnostic Tests

- Complete blood cell count and comprehensive metabolic panel to identify infections and any metabolic imbalances

- Thyroid-stimulating hormone to detect thyroid abnormalities
- Oxygen saturation measurement to identify respiratory conditions
- Electrocardiography to evaluate cardiac functioning
- Chest radiography to rule out pneumonia, pleural effusion, and embolus

Differential Diagnoses

- Phobic disorders
- Panic attack
- Obsessive-compulsive disorder
- Posttraumatic stress disorder
- Delirium (may be misdiagnosed as anxiety or depression)
- Medications that contribute to anxiety
  - Stimulants: caffeine, amphetamines, cocaine
  - Psychotropics: antipsychotics, buspirone
  - Central nervous system depressant withdrawal: barbiturates, benzodiazepines
  - Antihistamines
  - Anticholinergics
  - Other medications: steroids, theophylline, thyroid replacement hormones, cannabis

Interventions

- Treatment of anxiety is related to the patient's subjective level of distress.
- Moderate to severe anxiety can interfere significantly with a patient's ability to comply with treatments.
- The goal of treatment is to diagnose the presence and level of anxiety and to modify potential contributing factors.

Pharmacologic Interventions

- Benzodiazepines: diazepam, alprazolam, temazepam
- Azapirones: buspirone
- Antidepressants: amitriptyline, imipramine, nortriptyline, doxepin, fluoxetine, sertraline, paroxetine, venlafaxine
- Other medications used for anxiety: propranolol, haloperidol
- Atypical neuroleptics: olanzapine, risperidone

Nonpharmacologic Interventions

- Provide a safe, supportive environment.
- Cognitive-behavioral interventions provide the greatest evidence-based benefit.
- Initiate a discussion of concerns that may be contributing to the feeling of anxiety, such as pain, fear, or dependence issues. Use open-ended questions and clarification remarks.
- Help the patient identify what has helped him or her get through times like this before; "How can we help you use those strategies now?"
- Encourage the patient to identify people who can support him or her through this anxiety.
- Recognize that as patients move from mild to severe anxiety, the cause may be lost as the anxiety takes over. Preventive strategies can be useful to minimize anxiety or stabilize the escalation.

- Increase opportunities for control.
- Refer patients to individual counseling or group support programs.
- Evaluate dietary intake to reduce caffeine and alcohol intake to promote sleep.
- Relieve pain.

Patient Teaching

- Provide patient and family education to support reduction of fear and anticipatory reactions. Give instructions on medications and management of side effects. The goal of education is to reduce stress and anxiety.
- Increase patient and family participation in activities.
- Encourage hope.
- Use a family member or friend as the support person to stay present and help the patient.
- Provide accurate information to help restructure unrealistic fearful beliefs.
- Teach anxiety-reducing interventions such as relaxation, visualization, deep breathing, massage, touch, and physical exercise.
- Stress management may include journaling, music and art therapy, yoga, and meditation.
- Suggest web-based and mobile apps as a resource for meditation.

Follow-Up

- Refer patients to supportive psychiatric care when necessary.
- Multidisciplinary management can be the most effective way to achieve relief of anxiety. Psychologists, social workers, and chaplains should be part of the team to help support patients experiencing anxiety.

Resources

- American Cancer Society: https://www.cancer.org/treatment/treatments-and-side-effects/physical-side-effects/emotional-mood-changes/anxiety.html
- Cancer.Net: Coping with cancer: Anxiety. http://www.cancer.net/coping-and-emotions/managing-emotions/anxiety
- National Cancer Institute: Adjustment to cancer: Anxiety and distress. www.cancer.gov/cancertopics/pdq/SupportiveCare/Adjustment//Patient/page1

Bibliography

Bush, N. J. (2018). Anxiety. In N. J. Bush & L. M. Gorman (Eds.), *Psychosocial nursing care along the cancer continuum* (3rd ed.). Pittsburgh, PA: Oncology Nursing Society.

Hammelef, K. J. (2015). Anxiety. In C. G. Brown (Ed.), *A guide to oncology symptom management* (2nd ed.). Pittsburgh, PA: Oncology Nursing Society.

Löwe, B., Wahl, I., Rose, M., Spitzer, C., Glaesmer, H., Wingenfeld, K., … Brähler, E. (2010). A 4-item measure of depression and anxiety: Validation and standardization of the patient health questionnaire-4 (PHQ-4) in the general population. *Journal of Affective Disorders, 122*(1), 86–95.

Mahon, S. M., & Carr, E. (2021). Distress: Common side effect. *Clinical Journal of Oncology Nursing, 25*(6), 24.

National Comprehensive Cancer Network. (2022). NCCN clinical practice guidelines in oncology (NCCN guidelines). Distress Management. (version 2.2022). Available at https://www.nccn.org/professionals/physician_gls/pdf/distress.pdf.

Pasacreta, J., Minarik, P. A., Nield-Anderson, L., & Paice, J. (2015). Anxiety and depression. In B. Ferrell, N. Coyle, & J. Paice (Eds.), *Textbook of palliative nursing* (4th ed.). New York: Oxford University Press. https://doi.org/10.1093/med/9780199332342.003.0021.

Rucker, Y., & Gobel, B. C. (2014). Anxiety. In C. Yarbro, D. Wujcik, & B. H. Gobel (Eds.), *Cancer symptom management* (4th ed.). Burlington, MA: Jones & Bartlett Learning.

Spitzer, R. L., Kroenke, K., Williams, J. B., & Löwe, B. (2006). A brief measure for assessing generalized anxiety distress: The GAD-7. *Archives of Internal Medicine, 166,* 1092–1097.

Zigmond, A. S., & Snaith, R. P. (1983). The hospital anxiety and depression scale. *Acta Psychiatrica Scandinavica, 67*(6), 361–370.

Arthralgias and Myalgias

Carol Stein Blecher

Definition

- Arthralgias are pains in the joints.
- Myalgias are diffuse, generalized muscle pains.
- Both symptoms may be accompanied by a general feeling of malaise.

Pathophysiology and Contributing Factors

- The pathophysiology of arthralgias and myalgias in the oncology context is unclear.
- Proposed theories include the following:
  - They occur in response to a noxious stimulus or trauma that damages the muscle tissue, leading to release of bradykinin and stimulation of muscle nociceptors.
  - They may be related to the taxanes and vinca alkaloids and possibly to microtubule stabilization or an inflammatory reaction to the drug.
  - They may also be related to aromatase inhibitors, hormonal therapies, targeted therapies, and immunotherapy.
  - Other causes include white blood cell growth factors and bisphosphonates.
- Risk factors include the following:
  - History of peripheral neuropathy
  - History of diabetes
  - Alcohol use
  - Chemotherapy agents, including 13-*cis*-retinoic acid, alemtuzumab, altretamine, aromatase inhibitors as a class, azacytidine, bacille Calmette-Guérin (BCG), bevacizumab, bleomycin, cetuximab, cladribine, cytarabine, dacarbazine, docetaxel, etoposide, filgrastim, fludarabine, 5-fluorouracil, gemcitabine, immunotherapy as a class, interferon, interleukin-2, isotretinoin, L-asparaginase, olaparib, paclitaxel (especially in combination with cisplatin), procarbazine, rituximab, sargramostim, topotecan, trastuzumab, other targeted therapies, trimetrexate, vincristine, vinblastine, and vinorelbine
  - Age
  - Prior neurotoxic chemotherapy
  - History of arthritis
  - History of neuromuscular disease

Signs and Symptoms

Myalgias

- Generalized or localized muscle aches

- Edema
- Induration
- Fever
- Warm, flushed skin
- Tachycardia
- Shortness of breath
- Headache
- Thirst

Arthralgias

- Painful joints
- Swelling and redness of joints
- Limited range of motion
- Fever and chills
- Fatigue
- Depression

Assessment Tools

Assessment of the patient with arthralgias or myalgias should include the following:

- History, including diagnosis and cancer treatment, current medications, presenting symptoms, precipitating factors, location, and duration
- Vital signs
  - Elevated temperature
  - Tachycardia
  - Tachypnea
- Musculoskeletal system
  - Edema
  - Spasm
  - Erythema
  - Warmth and tenderness
  - Strength and range of motion
- Complete pain assessment
  - Character of the pain
  - Location
  - Quality
  - Onset
  - Factors that cause pain to worsen
  - Factors that alleviate pain
    - Current medication
    - Severity of the pain—current pain score, worst pain score, best pain score, and pain goal
    - Effects of pain on activities of daily living (ADLs) and quality of life
- National Cancer Institute, Common Terminology Criteria for Adverse Events
  - Grade 1: Mild pain not interfering with function
  - Grade 2: Moderate pain, limiting instrumental ADLs
  - Grade 3: Severe pain, limiting self-care ADLs

Laboratory and Diagnostic Tests

- Complete blood cell count with differential to evaluate neutropenia and rule out infection
- Chemistry studies to rule out hypokalemia, hyperkalemia, hypomagnesemia, hypocalcemia, hyponatremia, hypernatremia, and hypophosphatemia

- Creatine phosphokinase levels to rule out muscle inflammation or damage
- Urinalysis focusing on red blood cells
- Thyroid-stimulating hormone level
- Blood cultures if neutropenia is suspected
- Electromyelography to differentiate myelopathy from neuropathy
- Muscle biopsy to identify specific myopathies

Differential Diagnoses

- Cancer or metastatic disease
- Hematoma
- Ruptured tendon
- Thrombophlebitis
- Pyomyositis
  - Bacterial infection of the skeletal muscles that results in a pus-filled abscess
  - Most often caused by *Staphylococcus aureus*
- Fasciitis
- Sarcoidosis
- Ischemia or infarction
- Alcoholic myopathy
- Exertional muscle damage
- Fibromyalgia
- Inflammation
- Infections such as toxoplasmosis, trichinosis, influenza, herpes
- Electrolyte imbalance such as hypokalemia, hyperkalemia, hypomagnesemia, hypocalcemia, hyponatremia, hypernatremia, or hypophosphatemia
- Hypothyroidism
- Drugs: steroid withdrawal, paclitaxel (especially in combination with cisplatin), docetaxel, vincristine, vinblastine, vinorelbine, rituximab, etoposide, BCG, filgrastim, sargramostim, interferon, interleukin-2, dacarbazine, altretamine, topotecan, gemcitabine, procarbazine, fludarabine, letrozole (aromatase inhibitors as a class), azacytidine, cladribine, L-asparaginase, olaparib
- Amyloidosis
- Osteomalacia
  - The adult equivalent of the disease rickets
  - Defective mineralization of newly formed bone matrix
- Guillain-Barré syndrome
- Polymyalgia rheumatica
- Fabry disease
  - An X-linked recessive inherited lysosomal storage disease
- Parkinson disease

Interventions

- Treatment of the underlying disease
- Frequent rests interspersed with activity
- Maintain adequate nutrition and hydration

Pharmacologic Interventions

- Add medications as needed, using the World Health Organization analgesic ladder as a reference

- Acetaminophen (Tylenol), 650 mg orally every 4 hours as needed, not to exceed 4 g/day
- Ibuprofen (Motrin, Advil, Nuprin), 200 to 400 mg every 6 hours
- Indomethacin (Indocin), 25 to 50 mg orally twice or three times a day, not to exceed 200 mg/day
- Prednisone, 10 mg orally twice a day for 5 days after chemotherapy
- Amitriptyline, 25 mg orally at night
- Terfenadine (Seldane), 60 mg twice daily
- Glutamine, 10 g orally, three times daily

Nonpharmacologic Interventions

- Heating pad or hot water bottle on the painful area
- Ice pack on the painful area
- Warm baths
- Physical therapy
- Exercise
- Complementary therapies such as massage, relaxation techniques, whirlpool, magnets

Patient Teaching

- Keep a diary of your pain
- If you are having pain for any reason, your health care provider will ask certain questions to determine the cause of your pain. Things to include are:
  - Onset: When did the pain start? What was I doing when I had pain?
  - Quality: What does the pain feel like? Is it knifelike and stabbing, or dull and constant?
  - Location: Where is the pain? Can I point to it with my finger, or is it spread all over?
  - Intensity: How bad is your pain all the time? How bad is it with certain activities that cause you to feel pain, on a 1 to 10 scale, with the number "10" being the worst pain imaginable?
  - Duration: How long did the pain last?
  - Character: Does the pain come and go whenever I perform a certain activity, or is it unpredictable?
  - Relieving factors: What can I do to make the pain go away? Does anything help? What have I used in the past that has worked, and does this work now?
  - Your mood: Are you depressed or anxious? Does this make the pain worse?

Follow-Up

- Pain service referral
- Physical therapy
- Occupational therapy
- Instruct patients to call the health care provider if they experience
  - New and increasingly severe back pain
  - A new symptom of numbness and tingling down the legs
  - Weakness or decreased sensation in the lower extremities
  - Loss of bowel function or bladder control

Resources

- Arthritis Foundation: Arthritis pain management. Available at https://www.arthritis.org/health-wellness/detail?content=healthyliving (accessed March 6, 2022).
- Chemocare: Muscle pain (myalgias). Available at http://chemocare.com/chemotherapy/side-effects/muscle-pain-myalgias.aspx (accessed March 6, 2022).

Bibliography

Brant, J. M. (2014). Bone pain. In D. Camp-Sorrell & R. A. Hawkins (Eds.), *Clinical manual for the oncology advanced practice nurse* (3rd ed.). Pittsburgh, PA: Oncology Nursing Press.

Chemocare. Pain & chemotherapy. Available at http://chemocare.com/chemotherapy/side-effects/pain-and-chemotherapy.aspx (accessed March 6, 2022).

Chiu, N., Chiu, L., Chow, R., Lam, H., Verma, S., Pasetka, M., … DeAngelis, C. (2017). Taxane-induced arthralgia and myalgia: A literature review. *Journal of Oncology Pharmacy Practice, 23*(1), 56–67.

Gupta, A., Henry, N. L., & Loprinzi, C. L. (2020). Management of aromatase inhibitor-induced musculoskeletal symptoms. *Journal of Clinical Oncology, 16*(11), 733–741.

Mahon, S. M., & Carr, E. (2021). Pain: Common side effect. *Clinical Journal of Oncology Nursing, 25*(6), 31.

Martin, V. R. (2014). Arthralgias and myalgias. In C. H. Yarbro, M. H. Frogge, & M. Goodman (Eds.), *Cancer symptom management*. Jones & Bartlett: Sudbury, MA.

MedlinePlus Medical Encyclopedia. (2016). Joint pain. Available at http://www.nlm.nih.gov/medlineplus/ency/article/003261.htm (accessed March 6, 2022).

MedlinePlus Medical Encyclopedia. (2016). Muscle aches. Available at http://www.nlm.nih.gov/medlineplus/ency/article/003178.htm (accessed March 6, 2022).

National Cancer Institute. (2017). Common terminology criteria for adverse events, version 4.03. Available at https://ctep.cancer.gov/protocoldevelopment/electronic_applications/docs/ctcae_v5_quick_reference_8.5x11.pdf (accessed March 6, 2022).

Noonan, K. A. (2014). Arthralgia. In D. Camp-Sorrell & R. A. Hawkins (Eds.), *Clinical manual for the oncology advanced practice nurse* (3rd ed.). Pittsburgh, PA: Oncology Nursing Press.

Noonan, K. A. (2014). Myalgia. In D. Camp-Sorrell & R. A. Hawkins (Eds.), *Clinical manual for the oncology advanced practice nurse* (3rd ed.). Pittsburgh, PA: Oncology Nursing Press.

Cardiac Symptom: Hypertension

Deborah Lynn Kirk

Definition

- Blood pressure is the force of blood on arterial walls.
  - Systolic blood pressure is the pressure measured when the heart beats.
  - Diastolic blood pressure is the pressure measured when the heart is at rest.
- Blood pressure classifications have been established (see table below).
- Diagnosis is made after reviewing the average readings taken on ≥2 occasions.

Blood Pressure Goals

Classification	Systolic (mm Hg)	Diastolic (mm Hg)
Normal	<120	<80
Elevated	120–129	<80
Stage 1	130–139	80–89
Stage 2	≥140	≥90

- In primary (essential) hypertension, the cause is unknown; it develops gradually over years.
- Secondary hypertension is caused by an underlying condition or stimulus; it is often sudden in onset.

Pathophysiology and Contributing Factors

- Increased vascular stiffness, systemic resistance, and responsiveness contribute to hypertension.
- Contributing factors:
  - Age: men, above 55 years; women, above 65 years
  - Gender: men > women
  - Race: African Americans are at greatest risk and can develop hypertension early in life.
  - Genetic predisposition
  - Diabetes
  - Diets high in sodium (often found in processed foods) or table salt
  - Diets low in potassium, calcium, magnesium, protein, fiber, and fish fats
  - Physical inactivity causing weight gain
  - Overweight or obesity
  - Alcohol in excess (women, >1 drink per day; men, >2 drinks per day)
  - Smoking
  - Stressful situations
  - Pain
  - Drugs: vascular endothelial growth factor inhibitors, angiogenesis inhibitors, oral contraceptives, over-the-counter cold medications, illegal drugs, herbals, antidepressants, caffeine, decongestants, immunosuppressants, nonsteroidal antiinflammatory drugs, systemic corticosteroids
  - Kidney problems
  - Adrenal gland problems

Signs and Symptoms

- Some patients experience no signs or symptoms.
- Some patients have headaches, dizziness, nosebleeds, or flushing.
- Peripheral edema, blurred vision, and dyspnea may be seen with uncontrolled blood pressure.

Assessment Tools

- Medical and family history for evaluation of any conditions that may contribute to development of high blood pressure
- Review of current medications
- Social history, including alcohol, tobacco, and illegal drugs; diet history; and job-related stress
- Physical examination:
  - Vital signs including several blood pressure readings at different times and in different positions
  - Height and weight
  - Eye examination, noting any narrowing of blood vessels, retinopathy, papilledema, or exudate
  - Neck examination, evaluating carotid arteries, jugular veins, and thyroid
  - Cardiovascular examination

- Pulmonary examination, noting any adventitious breath sounds
- Abdominal evaluation for enlarged kidneys, aneurysms, and hepatomegaly
- Peripheral vascular system, evaluating pulses, edema, and muscle weakness or atrophy
- Neurologic evaluation, including reflexes

Laboratory and Diagnostic Tests

- Chest radiograph for evaluation of heart size, lung disease, or other heart abnormalities
- Electrocardiograph to evaluate for any damage to the heart
- Complete blood cell count (CBC) looking for anemia or polycythemia
- Urine analysis to evaluate for proteinuria
- Thyroid-stimulating hormone to check for abnormalities
- Lipid profile
- Complete metabolic panel
  - Evaluation of electrolytes before any treatment with diuretics is started
  - Fasting glucose level for diabetes
  - Serum creatinine with estimated glomerular filtration rate and blood urea nitrogen (BUN) for kidney disease

Differential Diagnoses

- Renal artery stenosis
- Kidney disease
- Cushing syndrome
- Tumors of the pituitary
- Tumors of the adrenal glands
- Blood vessel diseases
- Thyroid disorders
- Alcoholism
- Arteriosclerosis
- Drug-induced hypertension
  - Steroids, erythropoietin, and certain chemotherapy agents (i.e., antiangiogenesis agents)
  - Over-the-counter cold preparations

Interventions

- Individualized treatment plans to help lower blood pressure (see table below)

Pharmacologic Interventions

First-line treatment should consist of a thiazide-type diuretic, calcium channel blocker, angiotensin-converting enzyme inhibitor (ACEI), or angiotensin receptor blocker (ARB), as follows:

- For Blacks: initial treatment with a thiazide-type diuretic, calcium channel blocker, or both
- For races other than Black: initial treatment with a thiazide-type diuretic, an ACEI, an ARB, or a calcium channel blocker
- For patients with chronic kidney disease: initial treatment with an ACEI, ARB, or both
- Thiazide diuretics are the preferred agents; monitor electrolytes and blood sugar
- ACEIs may be less tolerated in African Americans; monitor electrolytes and creatinine; may cause coughing
- Co-morbidities should be considered when prescribing medications
- Alternative classes of drugs to consider as additional therapy in late management of hypertension or include the following:
  - β-Blockers
  - α-Blockers (given at bedtime)
  - α/β-Blockers (more effective in African Americans)
  - Vasodilators (used in combination with other agents)
  - Peripherally acting adrenergic antagonists
  - Loop diuretics
  - Aldosterone antagonists
  - Central α_2-adrenergic agonists

Nonpharmacologic Interventions

- Lifestyle changes
  - Low-sodium, low-fat diet
  - Weight loss
  - Regular exercise
  - Smoking cessation
  - Reduced alcohol consumption
  - Stress management

Patient Teaching

- Monitor blood pressure at home.
- Control of high blood pressure is important to avoid complications such as damage to heart or other organs.
- Maintain regular medication administration to control blood pressure.
- Avoid or eliminate known modifiable risk factors.
- Reduce salt and fat in the diet.
- Lose or control weight.
- Exercise regularly.
- Cease smoking.
- Limit alcohol consumption.

Follow-Up

- One month after initiation of treatment to monitor progress
- Monthly until desired blood pressure is met
- Every 3 to 6 months for maintenance follow-up
- If goal is not met, medication dose should be increased or a second agent added.
- Consider referral to cardiology, if needed.

Stages of BP and Recommendations

Classification	Interventions	Follow-Up
Normal BP		Every year
Elevated BP or stage 1 with low risk factors	Nonpharmacologic	Every 3–6 months
Stage 1 with increased risk	Nonpharmacologic and pharmacologic	Every 3–6 months
Stage 2	Nonpharmacologic and pharmacologic	1 month
Very high systolic BP ≥180 mm Hg and diastolic BP ≥110 mm Hg	Prompt pharmacologic treatment	

Resources

- http://www.nlm.nih.gov/medlineplus/highbloodpressure.html
- http://www.heart.org/HEARTORG/Conditions/HighBloodPressure/High-Blood-Pressure_UCM_002020_SubHomePage.jsp
- http://www.nhlbi.nih.gov/health/health-topics/topics/hbp/
- http://www.fda.gov/Drugs/ResourcesForYou/SpecialFeatures/ucm358442.htm
- http://www.cdc.gov/bloodpressure/hypertension_iom.htm
- http://smokefree.gov/
- http://www.cdc.gov/bloodpressure/

Cardiac Symptom: Tachycardia

Deborah Lynn Kirk

Definition

- A faster than normal resting heart rate, generally more than 100 beats/min

Pathophysiology and Contributing Factors

- Electrical signals in the heart may cause the ventricles, atria, or both to beat faster than normal
- Contributing factors:
  - Anemia
  - Medications
  - Thyroid problems
  - High levels of caffeine
  - Alcohol use or withdrawal
  - High or low blood pressure
  - Smoking
  - Drug misuse
  - Myocarditis
  - Family history of heart arrhythmias
  - Electrolyte abnormalities

Signs and Symptoms

- From no symptoms to severe
- Dizziness, lightheadedness
- Palpitations
- Shortness of breath
- Chest pain

Assessment Tools

- Medical and family history for evaluation of any conditions that may contribute to development of tachycardia
- Review of current medications
- Social history, including alcohol, tobacco, and illegal drugs; diet history; and job-related stress
- Physical examination:
  - Vital signs
  - Neck examination, evaluating carotid arteries, jugular veins, and thyroid
  - Cardiovascular detailed examination
  - Pulmonary examination, noting any adventitious breath sounds
  - Abdominal evaluation for enlarged kidneys, aneurysms, and hepatomegaly
  - Peripheral vascular system, evaluating pulses, edema, and muscle weakness or atrophy

Laboratory and Diagnostic Tests

- Electrocardiogram (ECG) to evaluate for any damage to the heart
- Exercise stress test to evaluate heart's response to stress
- Holter monitor monitoring rhythm over time
- Echocardiogram to look at structure
- Chest radiograph for evaluation of heart size, lung disease, or other heart abnormalities
- CBC looking for anemia or polycythemia
- Complete metabolic panel
  - Evaluation of electrolytes
  - Creatinine and BUN for kidney disease
- Thyroid function study
- Cardiac markers
- Drugs levels if suspected misuse or toxicity

Differential Diagnoses

- Sinus tachycardia
- Acute atrial fibrillation
- Chronic atrial fibrillation
- Atrial flutter
- Atrial tachycardia

Interventions

- Correct underlying issue
- Radioablation or defibrillator if severe

Pharmacologic Interventions

- Medications to slow rate or prevent abnormal rhythm
- Treatment of underlying medical condition

Nonpharmacologic Interventions

- Healthy lifestyle with diet and exercise
- Healthy weight
- Manage stress
- Drink less caffeine or alcohol
- Smoking cessation
- Adequate sleep
- Vagal maneuvers
- Maintain good blood pressure and cholesterol levels

Patient Teaching

- Lifestyle modifications—healthy diet, regular exercise, healthy weight
- Smoking cessation
- Drink in moderation, avoid illegal substances
- Manage stress
- Limit caffeine
- If underlying causes, adherence to treatment
- How to monitor heart rate and blood pressure if started on medication

Follow-Up

- Will depend on symptoms, testing required, and results
- Refer to cardiology for further workup
- If medications started, follow up 2 to 3 months

Resources

- https://www.heart.org/en/health-topics/arrhythmia/about-arrhythmia/tachycardia--fast-heart-rate
- https://cpr.heart.org/-/media/cpr-files/cpr-guidelines-files/algorithms/algorithmacls_tachycardia_200612.pdf

Cardiac Symptom: Electrocardiography Changes

Deborah Lynn Kirk

Definition

- Changes to the electrical impulses of each heartbeat that are recorded with a machine

Pathophysiology and Contributing Factors

- Changes that may occur with cancer treatment when there is direct damage to the myocardial cell, induction of myocardial ischemia, impairment at the level of the ion channels, or effects on the conduction system.
- Contributing factors:
  - Cancer diagnosis
  - Cancer therapies such as radiation and/or chemotherapy may cause disruption or damage to the muscles of the heart
  - Chronic inflammation
  - Metabolic changes
  - Obesity
  - Alcohol use
  - Co-morbid conditions
  - Damage to heart muscle

Signs and Symptoms

- Symptoms depend on type of abnormality identified
- QTc prolongation, abnormal atrial or ventricular beats, increased heart rate, decreased heart rate, QRS complex abnormalities, ST segment and T wave changes
- Atrioventricular conduction system effects

Assessment Tools and Laboratory and Diagnostic Tests

- ECG to evaluate for any damage to the heart
- Cardiac markers
- Echocardiography to assess left ventricular function
- Troponin I

Differential Diagnoses

- Arrhythmias
- Metabolic disorders
- Drug abnormality
- Myocardial infarction
- Pericarditis
- Pulmonary embolism

- Acute or chronic lung disease
- Congenital syndromes
- Severe obesity
- Pacemaker

Interventions

- Depend on the underlying cause

Patient Teaching

- ECG procedure
- On risk factors associated with results
- Interpretation of the results

Follow-Up

- Based on outcome of test

Resources

- https://www.heart.org/en/health-topics/heart-attack/diagnosing-a-heart-attack/electrocardiogram-ecg-or-ekg
- https://oxfordmedicaleducation.com/ecgs/ecg-interpretation/
- https://www.cancer.net/navigating-cancer-care/diagnosing-cancer/tests-and-procedures/electrocardiogram-ekg-and-echocardiogram#:~:text=%20You%20may%20need%20an%20echo%20before%2C%20during%2C,How%20well%20the%20heart%20pumps%20blood%20More%20

Bibliography

American Heart Association (AHA). (2022). *Tachycardia: Fast heart rate.* Available at https://www.heart.org/en/health-topics/arrhythmia/about-arrhythmia/tachycardiaSPI_Doublefast-heart-rate.

American Heart Association (AHA). (2022). *Understanding blood pressure readings.* Available at https://www.heart.org/en/health-topics/high-blood-pressure/understanding-blood-pressure-readings#:~:text=You%20could%20be%20experiencing%20a%20hypertensive%20crisis.%20If,pressure%20comes%20down%20on%20its%20own.%20Call%20911.

Bohdan, M., Kowalczys, A., Mickiewicz, A., Gruchała, M., & Lewicka, E. (2021). Cancer therapy-related cardiovascular complications in clinical practice: Current perspectives. *Journal of Clinical Medicine, 10,* 1647.

Buza, V., Rajagopalan, B., & Curtis, A. B. (2017). Cancer treatment-induced arrhythmias. *Circulation: Arrhythmia and Electrophysiology, 10*(8), e005443.

Cohen, J. B., Geara, A. S., Hogan, J. J., & Townsend, R. R. (2019). Hypertension in cancer patients and Survivors: Epidemiology, diagnosis, and management. *JACC: CardioOncology, 1*(2), 238–251.

Glenn, K. (2019). *Tachycardia in cancer patients may signal increased mortality risk. American College of Cardiology.* Available at https://www.acc.org/about-acc/press-releases/2019/01/25/14/19/tachycardia-in-cancer-patients-may-signal-increased-mortality-risk.

Okwuosa, T., Hemu, M., Chiang, C., Ahmed, A., Hein, K. Z., Mourad, T., … Fogg, L. (2021). Associations between sinus tachycardia and adverse cardiovascular outcomes and mortality in cancer patients. *Research Square.*

Shadman, R., & Rho, R. W. (2021). Assessment of tachycardia: Differentials. In *BMJ Best Practice.* Available at https://bestpractice.bmj.com/topics/en-gb/830/differentials#diffCommon.

Spînu, Ş., Cismaru, G., Boarescu, P. M., Istratoaie, S., Negru, A. G., Lazea, C., … Burz, C. (2021). ECG markers of cardiovascular toxicity in adult and pediatric cancer treatment. *Disease Markers, 6653971,* 10. https://www.heart.org/en/health-topics/heart-attack/diagnosing-a-heart-attack/electrocardiogram-ecg-or-ekg.

Whelton, P. K., Carey, R. M., Aronow, W. S., Casey, D. E., Collins, K. J., Dennison Himmelfarb, C., … MacLaughlin, E. J. (2018). 2017 ACC/AHA/AAPA/ABC/ACPM/AGS/APhA/ASH/ASPC/NMA/PCNA guideline for the prevention, detection, evaluation, and management of high blood pressure in adults: A report of the American College of Cardiology/American Heart Association Task Force on Clinical Practice Guidelines. *Journal of the American College of Cardiology, 71*(19), e127–e248.

Yano, Y., & Lloyd-Jones, D. M. (2021). USPSTF recommendations for screening for hypertension in adults: It is time to unmask hypertensive risk. *JAMA Cardiology, 6*(8), 869–871.

Confusion/Cognitive Dysfunction

Carol Stein Blecher

Definition

- Decline in function in attention, concentration, executive function, information processing, language, and the ability to identify visual and special relationships among objects.
- It has variable subjective symptoms and objective behaviors.
- It may be operationally defined as behaviors that fall into the following four categories:
  - Disorientation to time, place, or person
  - Inappropriate communication
  - Inappropriate behavior
  - Illusions, misinterpretation of real stimuli, or hallucinations, which are subjective sensory perceptions without real stimuli.
- End-of-life confusion refers to cognitive failure caused by metastatic cancer and multiorgan system failure.

Pathophysiology and Contributing Factors

- The pathogenesis is not well understood.
- Contributing factors may include:
  - Reduced cerebral oxygen metabolism
  - Damaged neuronal enzyme synthesis
  - Neurotransmitter imbalance
  - Neuronal loss
  - Metabolic abnormality

Signs and Symptoms

- Hypoactive behavior, such as mental slowness, a generalized slowing down, or somnolence
- Hyperactive behavior, such as restlessness, pacing, searching, or picking
- Delusions
- Paranoia
- Poor memory or forgetfulness
- Inability to concentrate
- Changes in personality
- Changes in habits or ability to care for self

Assessment Tools

- There are no evidence-based screening tools for cognitive dysfunction, but the following have been used to assess confusion:
- Brief Cognitive Assessment/Mini Mental Status Examination, which includes
  - Orientation to time and place
  - Memory test through repetition of the names of three unrelated objects
  - Attention and calculation with serial numbers testing
  - Language testing through identification of two items and repetition of a sentence

- Following a multistep command, writing a sentence, and then copying a sentence
- Confusion assessment measurement: 10-item scale administered by the clinician to assess nine domains of cognitive function
- Common terminology criteria for adverse events: grading for cognitive disturbance
  - Cognitive disturbance
    - Grade 1: Mild cognitive disability; not interfering with work/school/life performance; specialized educational services/devices not indicated.
    - Grade 2: Moderate cognitive disability; interfering with work/school/life performance but capable of independent living; specialized resources on part-time basis indicated.
    - Grade 3: Severe cognitive disability; significant impairment of work/school/life performance.
  - Concentration impairment
    - Grade 1: Mild inattention or decreased level of concentration
    - Grade 2: Moderate impairment in attention or decreased level of concentration, limiting instrumental activities of daily living (ADLs)
    - Grade 3: Severe impairment in attention or decreased level of concentration, limiting self-care ADLs
- Physical examination to rule out neurologic problems
- Cardiovascular examination to rule out cardiac abnormalities
- Pulmonary examination to rule out adventitious breath sounds

Laboratory and Diagnostic Tests

- Chemistry panel to evaluate for metabolic abnormalities:
  - Hypernatremia
  - Hyponatremia
  - Hypercalcemia
  - Hypomagnesemia
  - Hyperglycemia
  - Hypoglycemia
  - Liver function
- Complete blood cell count to evaluate for
  - Leukocytosis
  - Anemia
- Serum therapeutic drug levels of
  - Digoxin
  - Lithium
  - Alcohol
  - Phenytoin
  - Gabapentin
- Ammonia level
- Magnetic resonance imaging of the head to rule out brain metastases or hemorrhage
- Pulse oximetry or arterial blood gas analysis to rule out hypoxia
- Lumbar puncture to assess for carcinomatous meningitis
- Electroencephalography

Differential Diagnoses

- Electrolyte abnormalities
- Dehydration
- Renal failure
- Cirrhosis
- Sepsis
- Hypothermia
- Hyperthermia
- Meningitis
- Airway obstruction
- Syndrome of inappropriate antidiuretic hormone secretion
- Tumor lysis syndrome
- Constipation
- Drug-induced confusion related to
  - Cardiac drugs such as procainamide, propranolol, quinidine, lidocaine, clonidine, methyldopa, reserpine, digitalis
  - Gastrointestinal drugs such as atropine, belladonna, phenothiazine, scopolamine, cimetidine, ranitidine, metoclopramide
  - Musculoskeletal drugs such as corticosteroids, indomethacin, salicylate, diazepam
  - Neurologic/psychiatric drugs such as barbiturates, phenytoin, levodopa, amantadine, chloral hydrate, glutethimide, benzodiazepines, lithium salts, antidepressants
  - Respiratory/allergy drugs such as chlorpheniramine, cyproheptadine, diphenhydramine, theophylline
  - Analgesics such as opioids
  - Antidiabetic drugs such as insulin, oral hypoglycemics
  - Antineoplastic agents such as methotrexate, mitomycin, procarbazine, ifosfamide, interferon, L-asparaginase, cytarabine

Interventions

Pharmacologic Interventions

- Donepezil (Aricept) 25 mg orally (PO) at night.
- Haloperidol (Haldol)
  - Mild confusion: 0.5 to 1.0 mg PO, intramuscularly (IM), or intravenously (IV) twice a day
  - Agitated confusion: 1 to 2 mg every 30 to 60 minutes; after agitation is controlled, assess the 24-hour dose and adjust to a twice-daily dose
  - Terminal confusion: treat per protocol for mild confusion.
- Lorazepam (Ativan) for use in confusion associated with alcohol withdrawal and hepatic encephalopathy; dose is 0.5 to 2.0 mg every 1 to 4 hours PO, IM, or IV.
- Phenothiazine (Thorazine) for severe symptoms when sedation is required. Usual dose is 12.5 to 50 mg every 12 hours PO, IM, or IV.
- Diazepam (Valium) may be used, but with caution because the active metabolites can cause prolonged sedation; dose is 2 to 10 mg PO or IV two to four times a day.
- Midazolam (Versed) used only if all other methods fail to control symptoms; short half-life, so titration is easy; dose is 1 to 4 mg continuous IV or subcutaneous infusion.

Nonpharmacologic Interventions

Cognitive Dysfunction

- Prevention—exercise, yoga, mind/body practices, and relaxation therapy
- Interventions—cognitive training, memory aids, reminders, technology, exercise, yoga, mind/body practices, and relaxation therapy
- Correct or manage causative factors
- Orient patient frequently with calendars, clocks, and reorientation to place
- Ensure safety:
  - Keep bed in low position; if patient is hospitalized, keep call bell within reach.
  - Assist with toileting, ambulation, and positioning.
  - Check often for thirst, dry mouth, indigestion, hunger, pain, and hypothermia or hyperthermia.
  - Have support people stay with the patient and avoid restraints.
  - Encourage the patient to use hearing aids and glasses if necessary.
  - Patient is not to drive.
  - Reassure patient frequently.

Patient Teaching

- If the patient has early-stage confusion, aim patient teaching toward offering reassurance, frequent orientation, and encouraging the safety mechanisms listed above while correcting or managing the causative factors.
- If the patient has late-stage confusion, direct education efforts toward the caregiver or family, offering reassurance and teaching them how to assist the patient according to the nonpharmacologic interventions listed above.

Follow-Up

- Short term:
  - Monitor the effectiveness of the drug regimen over the first 24 to 48 hours.
  - Correct the underlying cause of confusion and monitor for clearing of confusion.
  - Continue safety measures to reduce the risk for falls or self-injury.
  - In terminal-stage confusion, balance sedation with wakefulness to facilitate patient/caregiver/family communication.
- Long term
  - Follow at-risk patients closely (e.g., elopement, self-injury).
  - Refer patient to psychiatrist or psychologist.
  - Refer patient for home care.
  - Refer patient to hospice if appropriate.

Resources

- Common terminology criteria for adverse events: https://evs.nci.nih.gov/ftp1/CTCAE/CTCAE_4.03/CTCAE_4.03_2010-06-14_QuickReference_8.5x11.pdf

- MedlinePlus Medical Encyclopedia. Confusion: http://www.nlm.nih.gov/medlineplus/ency/article/003205.htm
- National Comprehensive Cancer Network palliative care guidelines addressing distress: http://www.nccn.org/professionals/physician_gls/pdf/distress.pdf
- NCCN Guidelines for Patients Survivorship Care for Cancer-Related Late and Long-Term Effects: https://www.nccn.org/patients/guidelines/content/PDF/survivorship-crl-patient.pdf

Bibliography

Dahlin, C. (2014). Confusion/delirium. In D. Camp-Sorrell, & R. A. Hawkins (Eds.), *Clinical manual for the oncology advanced practice nurse* (3rd ed.). Pittsburgh, PA: Oncology Nursing Society.

Mahon, S. M., & Carr, E. (2021). Cognitive dysfunction: Common side effect. *Clinical Journal of Oncology Nursing, 25*(6), 23.

National Cancer Institute. (2017). Common terminology criteria adverse events, version 4.03. Available at https://ctep.cancer.gov/protocoldevelopment/electronic_applications/docs/ctcae_v5_quick_reference_8.5x11.pdf (accessed March 6, 2022).

NCCN Clinical Practice Guidelines in Oncology Survivorship (v.3.2021). Available at: www.nccn.org/professionals/physician_gls/pdf/survivorship.pdf (accessed March 6, 2022).

NCCN Guidelines for Patients Survivorship Care for Cancer-Related Late and Long-Term Effects. Available at: https://www.nccn.org/patients/guidelines/content/PDF/survivorship-crl-patient.pdf (accessed March 6, 2022).

National Institutes of Health, U.S. Library of Medicine. (2014). Confusion. Available at http://www.nlm.nih.gov/medlineplus/ency/article/003205.htm (accessed March 6, 2022).

Oncology Nursing Society Putting Evidence into Practice: Cognitive Impairment. Available at: https://www.ons.org/pep/cognitive-impairment?display=pepnavigator&sort_by=created&items_per_page=50 (accessed March 6, 2022).

Constipation

Jill Reese

Definition

- Passage of hard, dry stools with difficulty or discomfort
- Feeling of incomplete evacuation
- Decrease in frequency of defecation
- Obstipation
  - A more severe form of constipation
  - Absence of bowel movement despite large volumes of stool in the bowel
- Occurs in approximately 50% of cancer patients and in as many as 75% of terminally ill patients
- More common in women and the elderly

Pathophysiology and Contributing Factors

- Bowel function is determined by the state of intestinal motility and management of fluid in terms of absorption and secretion.
- Primary causes are related to extrinsic and lifestyle factors, including the following:
  - Age
  - Low-fiber diet
  - Dehydration
  - Decreased activity
  - Weakness/poor muscle tone
  - Extreme fatigue

- Secondary causes are related to medical conditions or disease processes that may cause hypomotility or obstruction.
- Iatrogenic causes result from medical interventions or from pharmacologic agents, including the following drug classes:
  - Opioids
  - Anticonvulsants
  - Anesthetics
  - Anticholinergics
  - Tricyclic antidepressants
  - Diuretics
  - Iron supplements
  - Serotonin antagonists
  - Vinca alkaloids
- Surgical anastomosis may lead to narrowing of the colon lumen from scar tissue.

Signs and Symptoms

- Abdominal fullness
- Bloating
- Nausea
- Vomiting
- Excessive gas
- Cramping
- Change in bowel elimination pattern (size and consistency of stools)

Assessment Tools

- Comprehensive history:
  - Extent of cancer, past and current treatments
  - Dietary habits including fluid intake
  - Alcohol use
  - Medication list of prescribed and over-the-counter drugs with doses and frequency
  - Previous laxative or enema use and its effect
- Baseline frequency pattern of bowel elimination
- Description of last bowel movement:
  - Frequency
  - Amount
  - Consistency and color of stool
  - Presence of blood
  - Distinct odor change
- Comprehensive physical examination:
  - Abdominal examination, including auscultation for bowel sounds, percussion of all four quadrants, palpation for masses or hepatomegaly
  - Examination of anus for fissures, external hemorrhoids, inflammation
  - Rectal or stoma examination for masses, fecal impaction, stricture
  - Examination of stool for occult blood
- Accurate assessment tools are lacking in making the diagnosis of constipation. Given the subjective nature of constipation, the Rome criteria were developed to assist in diagnosing this symptom. Criteria to establish a diagnosis of constipation require that a patient has experienced the following within the past 3 months:

- Straining with defecation
- Hard stools
- Incomplete evacuation
- Anorectal blockage
- Disimpaction
- Fewer than three bowel movements in a week
- The patient should not have loose stools or symptoms of irritable bowel syndrome.
- The National Cancer Institute has outlined the common terminology criteria for adverse events grading system to assist in categorizing the severity of the event. Grading for constipation is as follows:
  - Grade 1: occasional or intermittent symptoms; occasional use of stool softeners, laxatives, dietary modification, or enema
  - Grade 2: persistent symptoms with regular use of laxatives or enemas indicated; limiting instrumental activities of daily living (ADL)
  - Grade 3: symptoms interfering with activities of daily living, obstipation with manual evacuation indicated
  - Grade 4: life-threatening consequences (e.g., obstruction, toxic megacolon); intervention urgently indicated
  - Grade 5: death

Laboratory and Diagnostic Tests

- Complete blood cell count, electrolyte panel including calcium and potassium, renal and liver function tests, thyroid function tests
- Supine and upright radiographic films to differentiate between mechanical obstruction and ileus
- Computed tomography of abdomen and pelvis if an extraluminal site is suspected
- Barium enema
- Sigmoidoscopy or colonoscopy

Differential Diagnosis

- Cancer
  - Mass obstruction
  - Spinal cord tumor compression at T8 to L3
  - Ascites
- Metabolic causes
  - Hypercalcemia
  - Hypokalemia
  - Uremia
  - Hypothyroidism
  - Hyponatremia
- Diseases and other conditions
  - Anorectal abscess
  - Anal fissure
  - Cirrhosis
  - Depression
  - Diabetes
  - Diverticulosis
  - Hepatic porphyria
  - Intestinal obstruction
  - Irritable bowel syndrome

- Mesenteric artery ischemia
- Other
  - Dehydration
  - Nutritional compromise
  - Extreme fatigue/weakness
  - Poor muscle tone

Interventions

Pharmacologic Interventions

- Laxatives and cathartics are divided into categories on the basis of the mechanism of action.
- Bulk formers: onset of effect in 12 hours to 3 days
  - Psyllium (Metamucil)
  - Methylcellulose (Cologel, Citrucel)
- Bowel stimulants: onset of effect in 6 to 10 hours, rectally in 15 to 60 minutes
  - Phenolphthalein (Feen-A-Mint, Correctol)
  - Bisacodyl (Dulcolax), 5 mg tablet, one to three times a day; suppository 10 mg as needed
  - Senna (Senokot), 187 mg tablet, maximum eight per day
  - Cascara sagrada, 5 mL or one tablet as needed at bedtime
  - Casanthranol, 30 mg usually in combination with docusate
- Osmotic laxatives
  - MiraLAX: onset of effect in 2 to 4 days; 1 tablespoon (17 g) in 4 to 8 ounces of water, juice, soda, coffee, or tea daily
  - Lactulose: onset of effect in 24 to 48 hours
    - Cephulac, 30 to 45 mL three or four times daily, or hourly to induce rapid effect
    - Chronulac, 15 to 30 mL/day, maximum 60 mL/day
    - Sorbitol, 3 to 150 mL/day
  - Polyethylene glycol electrolyte solution: onset of effect within 1 hour
    - GoLYTELY, 8 ounces orally every 15 minutes as tolerated over 3 to 4 hours until 1 L has been taken or diarrhea results
  - Glycerin suppositories: onset of effect within 30 minutes; one or two per day, as needed or 5 to 15 mL as enema
- Lubricants: onset of effect within 8 hours
  - Mineral oil, 15 to 40 mL/day, once or in divided doses; as a retention enema, 60 to 150 mL/day
- Detergent laxatives: onset of effect in 24 to 72 hours
  - Docusate, 50 to 500 mg/day, once or in divided doses
    - Docusate sodium (Colace)
    - Docusate calcium (Surfak)
- Saline laxatives
  - Magnesium salts:
    - Magnesium citrate, ½ to 1 full bottle orally as needed, onset of effect in 30 minutes to 6 hours depending on dose
    - Magnesium hydroxide (milk of magnesia), 30 to 60 mL/day orally in single or divided doses, onset of effect in 4 to 8 hours
  - Sodium salts:

- Sodium phosphate (Fleet Phospho-soda), 20 to 30 mL as a single dose, onset of effect in 3 to 6 hours
- Fleet enema, onset of effect in 3 to 5 minutes
- Use of these agents can be initiated with a four-step approach. Advancement to the next step is indicated if the prior step at maximal doses was ineffective. Allow at least 48 hours to evaluate effectiveness of an intervention:
  - Step 1: bulk laxatives or milk of magnesia
  - Step 2: docusate sodium, senna, or milk of magnesia
  - Step 3: sorbitol or lactulose
  - Step 4: magnesium citrate or GoLYTELY
- Drug and dosage should be determined by patient condition, response, and tolerance of side effects. For patients receiving opioids for chronic pain or who have vinca alkaloid–containing chemotherapy regimens, prophylaxis for constipation with a stool softener and a stimulant laxative should be used.

Nonpharmacologic Interventions

- Increase daily intake of dietary fiber; gradually titrate from 3 to 4 g/day to total of 10 to 20 g/day. For patients with structural blockage, this method should be avoided because it may increase the obstruction. Sources of fiber include the following:
  - Wheat bran
  - Whole grain breads
  - Peanuts
  - Peanut butter
  - Peas
  - Raw, unpeeled vegetables and fruits, and salads
  - Dried apricots, prunes, raisins
  - Beans
  - Oatmeal
  - Coconut
- Increase fluid intake to eight to ten 8-ounce glasses of water daily; avoid coffee, tea, and grapefruit juice because they can have a diuretic effect.
- Establish a toileting routine after breakfast when contractions within the intestines are strongest.
- Increase exercise to improve gastrointestinal motility.

Patient Teaching

- Prevention of constipation is the goal.
- Recommend that patients consistently carry a water bottle to sip on throughout the day. Strive for 2 L of noncaffeinated fluids per day. Eating foods that contain water may help stool remain soft.
- Develop a routine for toileting, at the same time each day.
- Establish an exercise routine of at least 20 to 30 minutes/day.
- Incorporate at least 10 g of dietary fiber per day into the meal plan.
- Initiate bowel regimen as specified by physician or nurse, concurrently with chronic opioid use for pain management.
- Initiate prophylactic bowel regimen as specified by a physician or nurse with chemotherapy regimens containing vincristine or vinblastine.

- Avoid drinks with alcohol, caffeine, or milk products that may make constipation worse. Avoid fried and greasy foods.

Follow-Up

- Contact the nurse or physician for persistent constipation or if pain or bleeding ensues.

Resources

- Chemocare: Constipation and chemotherapy. Available at https://chemocare.com/chemotherapy/side-effects/constipation-and-chemotherapy.aspx (accessed December 16, 2021)

Bibliography

Brown, C. (2015). *A guide to oncology symptom management*. Pittsburgh, PA: Oncology Nursing Society.

Ginex, P. K., Hanson, B. J., LeFebvre, K. B., Lin, Y., Moriarty, K. A., Maloney, C., … Morgan, R. L. (2020). Management of opioid-induced and non-opioid-related constipation in patients with cancer: Systematic review and meta-analysis. *Oncology Nursing Forum, 47*(6), E211–E224.

Mahon, S. M., & Carr, E. (2021). Constipation: Common side effect. *Clinical Journal of Oncology Nursing, 25*, 26.

McQuade, R. M., Stojanovska, V., Abalo, R., Bornstein, J. C., & Nurgali, K. (2016). Chemotherapy-induced constipation and diarrhea: Pathophysiology, current and emerging treatments. *Frontiers in Pharmacology, 7*, 414.

National Cancer Institute, National Institutes of Health. (2017). Common terminology criteria for adverse events (CTCAE) v5.0. Available at https://ctep.cancer.gov/protocolDevelopment/electronic_applications/ctc.htm (accessed December 16, 2021).

Depressed Mood

Darcy Burbage

Definition

- Major depressive disorder is diagnosed according to the *Diagnostic and Statistical Manual of Mental Disorders, Fifth Edition* (DSM-V).
- Patients report a depressed mood or state that they have experienced a loss of interest or pleasure, lasting most of the day, in almost all their activities for at least 2 weeks.
- Four of the following additional conditions must exist:
  - Decreased energy
  - Feelings of guilt or lack of worth
  - Difficulty concentrating or making decisions
  - Recurrent thoughts of death or suicidal thoughts or plans
  - Changes in appetite or weight
  - Changes in sleep patterns
- Many of the physical symptoms that relate to appetite, concentration, and lack of energy can also result from a cancer patient's treatment regimen. For this reason, depression in oncology patients is often missed or undertreated.
- Depression affects treatment adherence due to lack of motivation, withdrawal, and isolation.

Pathophysiology and Contributing Factors

- Both biologic and psychosocial factors influence mood disturbances in patients.
- Genetic factors may make some patients more susceptible to the development of depression.

- A current or history of alcohol or substance abuse.
- Physiologic stressors, including medications, endocrine or nutritional disturbances, poorly controlled pain, and infections, can induce biochemical changes that precipitate depression.
- Developmental events or multiple losses may sensitize a patient, causing the patient to lose the ability to cope with their illness.
- These factors contribute to changes in neurotransmission, affecting mood, motivation, and psychomotor function. Norepinephrine and serotonin are the neurotransmitters most often associated with depression. Medications used to manage depression are related to regulation of these transmitters.
- Medication classes associated with depressive side effects include analgesics, anticonvulsants, antihypertensives, antiinflammatory agents, antimicrobials, antineoplastics, cytotoxics, hormones, immunosuppressive agents, sedatives, steroids, stimulants, tranquilizers, and benzodiazepines.
- Cancer diagnosis causes fear of pain, dependence, and altered body image; distress; and fear of death.
- Psychological factors contribute to feelings of depression (i.e., coping ability, emotional maturity, disruption of life's plans).
- Social factors associated with depressed mood include financial stability, emotional support from family or friends, and occupational successes or failures.
- The mood state of depression includes feelings of gloom, despair, numbness, emptiness, lack of worth, hopelessness, and helplessness.

Signs and Symptoms

- Mood that seems depressed for at least 2 weeks
- Unable to find pleasure in activities that used to be enjoyable
- Feelings of worthlessness
- Sadness, crying
- Difficulty concentrating
- Difficulty sleeping or sleeping too much
- Fatigue
- Verbalizes thoughts of dying or committing suicide

Assessment Tools

- All patients should be screened for depression at their initial visit and as appropriate thereafter.
- One of the most accurate screening measurements is a single question: "Are you depressed most of the day nearly every day?" A positive response necessitates further evaluation. A study of 197 patients with advanced cancer found that this question showed 100% sensitivity and 100% specificity for depression.
- The Beck Depression Inventory (BDI) is a 21-item questionnaire that takes about 2 to 5 minutes to complete and has an average specificity of 90%.
- Hospital Anxiety and Depression Scale (HADS)
- National Comprehensive Cancer Network (NCCN) Distress Thermometer Scale

- Two items from the nine-item Personal Health Questionnaire, based on American Society of Clinical Oncology guideline for screening and assessment of depression in adults with cancer, to guide further assessment:
  - Little interest or pleasure in doing things
  - Feeling down, depressed, or helpless (depressed mood)
- Assessment should include the following:
  - Report of depression
  - Signs and symptoms (four or more of those listed in the "Definition" section)
  - History of depression or substance abuse (drugs or alcohol)
  - Medications associated with depression
  - Patient with head and neck, pancreatic, or lung cancer (higher risk for suicide)
  - Unrelieved pain
- Social worker assessment can be beneficial to assist with evaluation and management of appropriate problems.
- Predictors of risk include a history of poor coping or psychological adjustment skills. Patients with a history of clinically significant anxiety or depression or major psychiatric syndromes should be monitored closely throughout treatment.
- Social support: Patients who can maintain close connections with family and friends cope more effectively with their illness and their outlook for the future.
- Cultural considerations: What is the language used to describe feelings of depression? Latin and Mediterranean cultures may complain of nerves or headaches. Asian or Chinese cultures may use words related to weakness, tiredness, or imbalance. Middle Eastern cultures may refer to problems of the heart or feeling heartbroken.

Laboratory and Diagnostic Tests

- There are no laboratory or diagnostic tests to screen for depressed mood (refer to "Assessment Tools").

Differential Diagnoses

- Fatigue
- Hypothyroidism
- Bipolar disorder
- Anxiety

Interventions

Pharmacologic Interventions

- Antidepressant medications used in the cancer setting include selective serotonin reuptake inhibitors (SSRIs) and serotonin-norepinephrine reuptake inhibitors (SNRIs) aimed at symptomatic benefit. Antidepressants are especially effective when used in conjunction with behavioral interventions and follow-up.
  - SSRIs: fluoxetine, mirtazapine, paroxetine, sertraline (helpful as a sleep aid, appetite stimulant, less gastrointestinal effects, few P450 interactions)
  - SNRIs: duloxetine, venlafaxine (helpful for hot flashes and neuropathic pain; least interaction with tamoxifen)

- Atypical antidepressants: trazodone (helpful as a sleep aid)
- Psychostimulants: bupropion (may be helpful for low energy or concentration issues)
- When prescribing, consider the short- and long-term side effects, possible interactions with other medications and other illnesses, and prior response to antidepressants.
- Monitor patients who are taking psychotropic medications for dosing accuracy, especially when therapies change or invasive procedures (e.g., surgery, chemotherapy), or disease progression occurs.
- Common side effects of antidepressants include sedation, anticholinergic effects, orthostatic hypotension, and weight gain.

Nonpharmacologic Interventions
- Cognitive behavioral therapy.
- Mindfulness-based stress reduction techniques such as meditation, yoga.
- Psychoeducational interventions to increase knowledge and lessen uncertainty surrounding cancer diagnosis and treatment.
- Referral to social work or a chaplain.
- If a patient verbalizes thoughts or plans for committing suicide, immediate evaluation is necessary. If a patient verbalizes thoughts of jumping out a window, shooting himself or herself, or self-harm in other ways, the nurse must assess whether the patient has access to complete these threats and must remove the patient from harm. It is vital for oncology nurses to respond to expressions of suicidal thoughts directly:
- Ask the patient, "Are you planning to end your life?" "What are you going to do?"
- If the patient answers yes or has a specific plan:
  - If in person, stay with patient and contact mental health professional/team member
  - If on telehealth visit, remain on phone with patient, ask if anyone is in the home with them, and have a colleague contact 9-1-1. Remain on phone until help arrives.
  - Follow-up with patients' primary oncology team.
- Statements such as "I should just kill myself" or "I have no reason to go on living" require further evaluation. Always ask, "Do you have a plan?" and "Can you tell me what it is?"
- Statements of feeling hopeless or helpless must be evaluated because these patients are at high risk for suicide.
- Help patients identify and build adaptive coping mechanisms.
- Help patients regain a sense of control over their lives; provide options when possible.
- Be available to your patient. Help to normalize the patient's feelings and maintain realistic hope.
- Any reference to suicide must be referred for further evaluation beyond the nurse who is taking care of the patient.
- Counseling

Patient Teaching
- Patients with depressed mood are at higher risk for non-compliance with their treatments; monitor and encourage adherence.
- Reinforce hope and educate family and caregivers on the patient's needs as appropriate.
- If suicidal thoughts have been identified, caregivers must be aware of these feelings and take preventive actions in the home to remove items that may be used to complete these threats (e.g., guns, knives, ropes). A suicide hotline phone number should be accessible.
- Discuss plans with the patient so that suicide is not thought of as an automatic solution to problems. Interventions should be provided to relieve extreme symptoms and improve quality of life.
- Feelings of hopelessness, helplessness, and worthlessness need to be discussed, and the patient's ability to mobilize personal support systems needs to be established.
- Caregiver support is essential.

Follow-Up
- If the patient screens positively for depression, notify the physician for referral to a mental health professional for further assessment.
- If the patient reports a desire to commit suicide, discuss the plan with the patient and notify the physician immediately. Take necessary steps to protect the patient from self-harm and arrange for immediate follow-up.
- Ask specific questions regarding mood. Be aware of statements that refer to feelings of hopelessness, being a burden to one's family, financial concerns, or unrelieved symptoms.
- Assess distress levels related to fatigue, pain, mood, or family and financial concerns.
- Continue to provide hope and support.

Resources
- American Cancer Society: https://www.cancer.org/treatment/treatments-and-side-effects/physical-side-effects/emotional-mood-changes/depression.html
- Cancer Net: https://www.cancer.net/coping-and-emotions/managing-emotions/depression
- National Cancer Institute: https://www.cancer.gov/about-cancer/coping/feelings/depression-hp-pdq
- National Suicide Prevention Lifeline 1-800-273-TALK [8255]

Bibliography

Albright, A. V., & Valente, S. (2018). Depression and suicide. In N. J. Bush & L. M. Gorman (Eds.), *Psychosocial nursing care along the cancer continuum* (3rd ed.). Pittsburgh, PA: Oncology Nursing Society.

Andersen, B. L., DeRubeis, R. J., Berman, B. S., Gruman, J., Champion, V. L., Massie, M. J., … American Society of Clinical Oncology. (2014). Screening, assessment, and care of anxiety and depressive symptoms in adults with cancer: An American Society of Clinical Oncology guideline adaptation. *Journal of Clinical Oncology, 32*(15), 1605–1620.

Badger, T. A., & Lazenby, M. (2015). Depression. In C. G. Brown (Ed.), *A guide to oncology symptom management* (2nd ed.). Pittsburgh, PA: Oncology Nursing Society.

Decker, V. B., & Tofthagen, C. (2021). Depression: Screening, assessment, and interventions in oncology nursing. *Clinical Journal of Oncology Nursing, 25*(4), 413–421.

Pasacreta, J., Minarik, P. A., Nield-Anderson, L., & Paice, J. (2015). Anxiety and depression. In B. Ferrell, N. Coyle, & J. Paice (Eds.), *Textbook of palliative nursing* (4th ed.). New York: Oxford University Press. https://doi.org/10.1093/med/9780199332342.003.0021.

Diarrhea

Jill Reese

Definition

- Increase in frequency, volume, and consistency of stool
- Passage of ≥200 g of stool/day
- Can be acute or chronic
- Experienced by 10% of advanced cancer patients and 43% of bone marrow transplantation patients
- Diarrhea classifications:
  - *Osmotic diarrhea* is related to mechanical disturbances resulting from ingestion of hyperosmolar substances such as sorbitol or enteral feeding solutions (J-tubes, G-tubes). The diarrhea is watery and voluminous, resolving when the causative agent is withdrawn.
  - *Secretory diarrhea* is related to biochemical disturbances causing a mechanical response. The origins of these disturbances are enterotoxin-producing pathogens such as *Clostridium difficile* and *Escherichia coli* or endocrine tumors. The diarrhea is watery and voluminous.
  - *Exudative diarrhea* is often the toxic effect of radiation therapy (RT) to the bowel mucosa. This diarrhea is characterized by high frequency (>6 stools/day) with variable volume, although less than 1000 mL/day. Stools are characterized by mucus and blood.
  - *Malabsorptive diarrhea* is related to both mechanical and biochemical disturbances. These disturbances can result from enzyme deficiencies. Stools are voluminous, foul smelling, and steatorrhea type.
  - *Dysmotility associated diarrhea* is related to a mechanical disturbance or peristaltic dysfunction that results in rapid transit time of stool through the small and large intestine. Stools are small, semisolid to liquid in consistency, with variable volume and frequency.
  - *Chemotherapy-induced diarrhea* results from mechanical and biochemical disturbances caused by the effects of chemotherapy on the bowel mucosa. Stools are watery or semisolid.

Pathophysiology and Contributing Factors

- Gastrointestinal (GI) motility involves processes that promote the absorption of nutrients. Movement through the GI tract requires coordination of intraluminal pressures and smooth muscle contractions controlled by the enteric nervous system and peptide hormonal release. Diarrhea is caused by an imbalance in the physiologic mechanisms of the GI tract. It is the result of impaired absorption and excessive secretion.

- Decreased absorption of fluid and electrolyte can result from:
  - Presence of osmotically active substances in the lumen
  - Increased intestinal motility
- Increased secretion of fluid and electrolytes can result from:
  - Endogenous secretions
  - Exogenous toxins
- With RT that involves the abdomen or pelvis and in chemotherapy-induced diarrhea, acute damage to the epithelial crypt cells results in necrosis, inflammation, and ulceration of the intestinal mucosa. Atrophy and fibrosis of the lining can occur over time, resulting in decreased absorption of water and electrolytes and producing diarrhea.
- Risk factors for diarrhea:
  - Chemotherapy
    - Diarrhea from previous chemotherapy cycles
    - Types of chemotherapeutic agents, including fluoropyrimidines, topoisomerase I inhibitors (irinotecan, topotecan), antitumor antibiotic (actinomycin D), and toxoid (paclitaxel)
  - Other factors, such as the presence of primary tumor
  - RT—diarrhea is dependent on:
    - Total RT dose
    - Size of the RT field
    - Site being irradiated
    - Dose per fraction

Signs and Symptoms

- Increased number of stools/day
- Nocturnal stool
- Incontinence
- Cramping
- Patient may have other symptoms:
  - Nausea/vomiting
  - Hypotension
  - Dizziness
  - Decreased skin turgor
  - Dry mouth
  - Perianal irritation
  - Flushing
  - Diaphoresis

Assessment Tools

- Comprehensive history:
  - Cancer diagnosis, past and current treatments
  - Sites of metastasis
  - Complete medication list:
    - Laxatives
    - Opioids or recent opioid withdrawal
    - Recent antibiotic therapy
    - Regular and as-needed prescription medications
    - Over-the-counter medications
    - Herbal and vitamin supplements
    - Chemotherapy/biotherapy agents

- The hallmark assessment tool is the patient report.
  - Description of baseline bowel movements and current bowel movement history:
    - Frequency
    - Amount
    - Consistency and color of stool
    - Incontinence
    - Presence of blood
    - Distinct odor change
  - Assess for signs and symptoms of dehydration:
    - Orthostatic hypotension
    - Dry mouth
    - Excessive thirst
    - Dizziness
    - Feelings of weakness
    - Decreased urination
    - Weight loss
  - Comprehensive physical examination
    - Abdomen
      - Palpate for tenderness, distention
      - Percuss—dullness may indicate obstruction, fecal impaction
      - Auscultate for bowel sounds
- The National Cancer Institute has outlined the common terminology criteria for adverse events (CTCAE) grading system to assist in categorizing the severity of the event (see table below).
- Diarrhea can originate in the small bowel or in the colon, or it can occur in an ostomy.

Laboratory and Diagnostic Tests

- Complete blood cell count
- Stool test for occult blood
- Metabolic panel to assess electrolyte levels, blood urea nitrogen (BUN)/creatinine, albumin
- Stool cultures for enteric pathogens, *C. difficile*, and ova and parasites
- Radiography: flat plate of the abdomen or obstruction series (as indicated by history and physical examination)

Differential Diagnoses

- Carcinoid syndrome
- Chemotherapy-induced or targeted therapy–induced diarrhea
- RT–induced diarrhea
- *C. difficile* infection
- Enzyme deficiency
- Crohn disease
- Acute viral, bacterial, or protozoal infections
- Intestinal obstruction
  - Tumor
  - Stool
  - Scar tissue
- Irritable bowel disease
- Ischemic bowel disease
- Lactose intolerance
- Pseudomembranous enterocolitis
- Rotavirus gastroenteritis
- Thyrotoxicosis
- Ulcerative colitis
- Laxative overuse
- Opioid withdrawal

Interventions

Pharmacologic Interventions

The intervention selected should be correlated with the root cause of the diarrhea. Maximizing the use of a particular intervention, while monitoring patient adherence to the prescribed regimen, is critical in determining efficacy. Antidiarrheal agents are divided into categories based on the mechanism of action:

- Opioids
  - Lomotil: 2.5 mg diphenoxylate with 0.025 mg atropine sulfate/tablet. May give a loading dose with two tablets, then one to two tablets four times daily every 6 hours, not to exceed eight tablets per day
  - Codeine: 30 to 60 mg orally every 4 to 6 hours as needed

Common Terminology Criteria for Adverse Events (CTCAE) Reporting: Diarrhea*

Adverse Event	Grade 1	Grade 2	Grade 3	Grade 4	Grade 5
Diarrhea	Increase of <4 stools/day over baseline; mild increase in ostomy output compared with baseline	Increase of 4-6 stools/day over baseline; moderate ostomy output compared with baseline	Increase of ≥7 stools/day; incontinence; hospitalization indicated; severe increase in ostomy output compared with baseline; limiting self-care activities of daily living (ADLs)	Life-threatening consequence; urgent intervention needed	Death

*A semicolon indicates "or" in the grade description.
From National Cancer Institute, National Institutes of Health. (2017). Common terminology criteria for adverse events (CTCAE), version 5.0. Available at https://ctep.cancer.gov/protocolDevelopment/electronic_applications/ctc.htm#ctc_60 (accessed December 13, 2021).

- Opium tincture: 10% opium liquid (10 mg morphine/mL with 19% alcohol); 0.3 to 1 mL orally every 2 to 6 hours until controlled, not to exceed 6 mL/24 h.
- Paregoric: 0.4 mg morphine/mL orally one to four times daily or 4 mL every 4 hours
- Absorbents
  - Bismuth subsalicylate (Pepto-Bismol): chewable tablets 262 mg or suspensions 262 mg/15 mL or 524 mg/15 mL. Dosing is 524 mg every 30 minutes, not to exceed 5 g/day
  - Kaopectate (5.85 g kaolin and 130 mg pectin/30 mL): 2 to 6 g every 4 hours as needed
- Somatostatin analogs
  - Octreotide
  - Lanreotide
  - Pasireotide

Nonpharmacologic Interventions

- Nonopioids
  - Imodium (loperamide): 2-mg capsules or liquid 1 mg/mL or 1 mg/5 mL; may give a loading dose of 4 mg orally, then 2 mg after each loose stool, not to exceed 16 mg/day
- Diet modifications, including
  - Foods that build stool consistency (i.e., low in fiber, pectin containing)
  - Foods high in potassium
  - Foods at room temperature to minimize peristalsis
  - Lactose-free diet if indicated
  - Fluid intake at least 3 to 4 L/day

Patient Teaching

- Encourage foods that are low in fiber and that contain pectin (∗ = high in potassium):
  - Beets
  - Applesauce (without spice)
  - Peeled apple
  - White rice
  - Banana∗
  - Baked potato without skin
  - White bread
  - Plain pasta
  - Avocados∗
  - Asparagus tips∗
- Encourage foods high in potassium:
  - Peach and apricot nectar
  - Boiled or mashed potatoes, without skin
  - Lactose-free milk
  - Fish, turkey, skinned chicken
  - Bananas
- Avoid high-fiber, high-fat, greasy, spicy, or caffeine- containing foods:
  - Whole grain breads or cereals
  - Raw vegetables
  - Nuts
  - Seeds
  - Popcorn
  - Relishes or pickles
  - High-fat spreads or dressings
  - Chocolate
  - Coffee/tea
- Increase fluids to at least 3 L/day:
  - Bouillon
  - Fruitades
  - Gatorade, Propel, or other sports drinks
  - Pedialyte or Pedialyte ice pops
  - Ice pops
  - Gelatin
- Avoid alcohol and carbonated beverages.
- Maintain a lactose-free diet when indicated.
  - Avoid milk and dairy products.
  - May use lactose-free dairy products or soymilk products.
- Maintain skin integrity.
  - Cleanse rectal area after each bowel movement with soft wipes; pat rather than rub perianal area when cleansing.
  - Apply a topical skin barrier ointment such as Desitin or A&D ointment.
  - Take sitz baths as needed.
- Take antidiarrheal medication as prescribed.

Follow-Up

- Have patient or caregiver record number and consistency of stools.
- Call physician or nurse if diarrhea persists in frequency and volume greater than 24 hours after following outlined plan of care.

Resources

- Chemocare: Diarrhea and chemotherapy. Available at https://chemocare.com/chemotherapy/side-effects/diarrhea-and-chemotherapy.aspx (accessed December 13, 2021)

Bibliography

Brown, C. (2015). *A guide to oncology symptom management*. Pittsburgh, PA: Oncology Nursing Society.

McQuade, R. M., Stojanovska, V., Abalo, R., Bornstein, J. C., & Nurgali, K. (2016). Chemotherapy-induced constipation and diarrhea: Pathophysiology, current and emerging treatments. *Frontiers in Pharmacology, 7*, 414.

National Cancer Institute, National Institutes of Health. (2017). Common terminology criteria for adverse events (CTCAE), version 5.0. Available at https://ctep.cancer.gov/protocolDevelopment/electronic_applications/ctc.htm#ctc_60 (accessed December 13, 2021).

Oncology Nursing Society. (2017). Chemotherapy induced diarrhea. Available at https://www.ons.org/pep/chemotherapy-induced-diarrhea (accessed February 6, 2022).

Dizziness and Vertigo

Joshua Carter

Definition

- Described in terms of sensations
- Lightheadedness, fainting, spinning, confusion, blurred vision, tingling
- Nonspecific symptoms
- Clustered with vertigo, dizziness, disequilibrium, and presyncope (prodromal symptom for fainting or near fainting)
- Unsteadiness

- Must fit patient into category of dizziness, vertigo, or presyncope
- May include nausea and/or vomiting

Pathophysiology and Contributing Factors

- Vertigo (a symptom of dizziness) is caused by a disturbance in the vestibular system: sensory, visual, or somatosensory. The vestibular system includes apparatus in inner ear, the vestibular nerve and nucleus in the medulla, and connections from the cerebellum.
- Contributing factors may be specific or nonspecific.
- Symptoms are never continuous.
- It may be made worse by movement of the head or cervical spine.
- There is a disruption between vestibular apparatus and the brain.
- A prior psychological disorder may be a factor.

Signs and Symptoms

- Lightheadedness
- Feeling of spinning (similar to coming off a roller coaster or when spun multiple times)
- Imbalance, tipping to one side
- Nausea and vomiting with the spinning
- Visual changes
- Auditory changes
- May be episodic or regular, in short or long duration
- Out-of-body feeling
- Additional paresthesias of face or limbs possible

Assessment Tools

- Patient history, including head injury, comorbid conditions
- Identify what dizziness means to patient, full sensations, duration, and aggravating, triggering, and alleviating factors
- Neurologic examination
- Orthostatic assessment
- Ear, nose, and throat (ENT) examination (dizziness with vertigo involves the peripheral vestibular system)
- Medication review
- Assessment for nystagmus, hearing loss, ataxic gait, nausea, vomiting, visual changes, numbness, incoordination
- Social history, including any history of substance abuse
- Psychological assessment
- Fall risk assessment

Laboratory and Diagnostic Tests

- Complete blood count (CBC), blood glucose level, thyroid-stimulating hormone (TSH) level
- Range of motion with emphasis on cervical spine
- Cervical spine radiographic film
- Vestibular function tests
- Stimulate to hyperventilate
- Magnetic resonance imaging (MRI) if focal neurologic symptoms are present

Differential Diagnoses

- Ménière disease

- Benign paroxysmal positional vertigo
- Diseases of the central nervous system (CNS)
- Cerebrovascular disease
- Orthostasis
- Neurologic deficit
- Dehydration
- Hyperventilation
- Parkinson disease
- Medication side effect
- Labyrinthitis
- Malignancy
- Cervical spine disorders

Interventions

Pharmacologic Interventions

- Antihistamines: meclizine
- Anticholinergics: scopolamine
- Benzodiazepines
- Antiemetics as needed

Nonpharmacologic Interventions

- Hydration
- Repositioning
- Vestibular rehabilitation
- Bed rest if needed
- Treat the cause
- Physical and occupational therapy
- Sodium-restricted diet

Patient Teaching

- Avoid sudden changes in position.
- Chief concern is patient safety.
- Sit or lie down if feeling dizzy.
- Increase fluids; drink 3 L/day.
- Ensure good lighting to prevent falls.
- Use assistive devices as needed for support.
- Do not drive or use machinery if dizzy.
- Do not use alcohol, tobacco, or caffeine if symptomatic.
- Use energy conservation techniques.

Follow-Up

- Seek immediate medical assistance if there is a change in level of consciousness, respiratory difficulty, or sudden loss of vision or hearing.
- Alert health care provider if there is sudden, severe ear pain or a temperature greater than 100.5°F (38.3°C).
- Report all ear infections, sinus congestion, and respiratory complaints.
- Ensure that the patient's environment remains safe.

Resources

- Mayo Clinic (Mayo Foundation for Medical Education and Research): www.mayoclinic.com
- WebMD: www.webmd.com
- Chemo Care (Cleveland Clinic): http://www.chemocare.com/

Bibliography

ADAM Medical Encyclopedia [Internet]. (2015). *Light-headedness, dizzy, loss of balance, vertigo*. Available at https://www.nlm.nih.gov/medlineplus/ency/article/003093.htm (accessed February 18, 2016).

Alyono, J. C. (2018). Vertigo and dizziness: Understanding and managing fall risk. *Otolaryngologic Clinics of North America*, 51(4), 725–740.

Branch, W., & Barton, J. (2015). *Approach to the patient with dizziness*. Available at http://www.uptodate.com/contents/approach-to-the-patient-with-dizziness?source=search_result&search=dizziness&selectedTitle=1%7E150 (accessed February 18, 2016).

Tucci, D. L. (2013). *Dizziness and vertigo*. Available at http://www.merck-manuals.com/professional/ear,-nose,-and-throat-disorders/approach-to-the-patient-with-ear-problems/dizziness-and-vertigo (accessed February 18, 2016).

Zwergal, A., & Dieterich, M. (2020). Vertigo and dizziness in the emergency room. *Current Opinion in Neurology*, 33(1), 117–125.

Dysphagia

Mary Steinbach and Jennifer S. Webster

Definition

- Dysphagia is the sensation of difficulty swallowing. It can occur at the initiation of swallow (oropharyngeal dysphagia) or afterwards with the sensation of food getting stuck (esophageal dysphagia).
- Malignant dysphagia is directly related to the disease itself.
- Treatment-related dysphagia is a result of injury to the tissues from radiation or chemotherapy.
- It is a common sequela of head and neck cancer and its treatment, occurring in 96% of those patients. Approximately 60% of these patients experience dysphagia prior to treatment, as a result of the tumor itself.
- Classifications:
  - Oropharyngeal dysphagia—difficulty initiating the swallowing process and propelling food through the esophagus
  - Esophageal dysphagia—ability to swallow food, yet having the sensation that food is not able to pass from esophagus into the stomach (often associated with pain)
- Chemotherapy and radiation therapy may reduce symptoms of dysphagia when it is related to tumor size, thus prolonging life, but may also exacerbate dysphagia, especially in the acute phase post-treatment.
- Dysphagia is strongly associated with lower quality of life for patients.

Pathophysiology and Contributing Factors

- Swallowing is a complex process requiring more than 30 pairs of muscles and 6 cranial nerves in a coordinated action. Patients with head and neck cancer or lung cancer requiring radiation therapy are at greatest risk for disruption of this finely tuned bodily function. Patients with esophageal cancer requiring radiation may experience esophageal dysphagia.
- Multiple other tumor types such as breast, colorectal, gastric, and bone and soft tissue put patients at risk for dysphagia depending on tumor location or treatment.
- Radiation therapy initially may negatively affect dysphagia due to tissue inflammation, edema, xerostomia, mucositis, and pain.

- Chronic dysphagia may result if tissues become permanently damaged or weakened.
- Approximately 20% of patients with head and neck cancer receiving concurrent chemoradiation will require a gastrostomy tube permanently due to persistent dysphagia.
- Results from any condition that weakens or damages the muscles and nerves involved in swallowing:
  - Obstructive lesions
  - Tumors
  - Inflammatory changes in the esophagus, such as a stricture, narrowing of the lower part of the esophagus
    - Trauma/surgical resection
    - Esophageal webs
    - Extrinsic structural lesions
    - Anterior mediastinal masses
    - Esophageal spasms
    - Mucositis
    - Xerostomia
    - Post radiation sequelae
    - Laryngeal penetration
    - Zenker diverticulum (a pharyngeal pouch just above the upper sphincter of the esophagus)
  - Nerve paralysis
  - Age-related factors
- Gastroesophageal reflux disease (GERD) may exacerbate painful swallowing

Signs and Symptoms

- Difficulty swallowing, manifested as choking, coughing, drooling, or regurgitating when swallowing
- Pain with swallowing
- Hoarse voice
- Dry mouth
- Weight loss
- Dehydration
- Taste alterations
- Atrophy of neck muscles
- Aspiration
- Infection

Assessment Tools

- History and physical examination, including history of GERD, hiatal hernia, aspiration, or pneumonia. Physical exam should include oral cavity, head and neck, supraclavicular lymph nodes
- Character and quality of pain
- Precipitating factors and relieving factors

Laboratory and Diagnostic Tests

- Comprehensive metabolic panel (creatinine)
- Albumin, prealbumin, transferrin, and retinol-binding protein
- Clinical swallowing evaluation (CSE)
- Water swallow test (WST)
- Barium study (esophagram)/barium swallow
- Videofluoroscopic swallowing study (VFSS)
- Fiberoptic endoscopic evaluation of swallowing (FEES)

- Nasopharyngeal laryngoscopy
- Endoscopy
- Manometry—measures pressure within the esophagus
- Chest radiographic film

Differential Diagnoses

- Xerostomia
- Anorexia
- Aspiration
- Malnutrition
- Dehydration
- Pain
- Cough
- Mucositis
- Gastroesophageal reflux
- Tissue fibrosis
- Aspiration pneumonia
- Anxiety
- Infection
- Depression
- Isolation (may avoid social gatherings where food is involved)

Interventions

- Treat the underlying causes. An expert swallowing evaluation prior to any head and neck cancer therapy, along with continued monitoring during and after treatment, is extremely valuable in ameliorating the effects of therapy on dysphagia.

Pharmacologic Interventions

- Histamine receptor 2 antagonists (blockers)
- Proton pump inhibitors
- Prokinetic agents
- Antacids
- Hydration
- Pain management

Nonpharmacologic Interventions

- Aggressive nutritional and supportive care may be required for patients experiencing dysphagia as an acute side effect of therapy
  - Feeding tube insertion and enteral feedings
  - Parenteral nutrition
  - Hydration therapy
  - For chronic dysphagia: esophageal dilation and/or stenting

Patient Teaching

- Swallowing techniques:
  - Chin tuck and or modified head maneuver based on area of weakness.
  - Head rotation to modify pharyngeal pressure.
  - Eat sitting upright at a 90-degree angle.
- Diet modification:
  - Avoid solid, abrasive foods; incorporate a pureed, liquid diet.
  - Maintain adherence with medications.
- Avoidance of aspiration:
- Avoid lying down after meals for 30 minutes.
- Keep head of bed elevated while sleeping.

Follow-Up

- Nutritional counseling/referral to dietician
- Speech and language pathologist referral
- ENT or GI referral
- Call health care provider if experiencing the following:
  - Difficulty or pain when swallowing continues
  - Pain is unrelieved
  - Continued weight loss

Resources

- Dysphagia Resource Center: www.dysphagiaonline.com
- Cancer.net—Difficulty swallowing or dysphagia: http://www.cancer.net/navigating-cancer-care/side-effects/difficulty-swallowing-or-dysphagia
- The Oral Cancer Foundation—Dysphagia: http://oralcancerfoundation.org/complications/dysphagia.php
- Oncology Nursing Society: www.ons.org
- National Cancer Institute: Oral complications of chemotherapy and head/neck radiation (PDQ): https://www.cancer.gov/about-cancer/treatment/side-effects/mouth-throat/oral-complications-hp-pdq#_592_toc (accessed June 1, 2022).

Bibliography

Ashman, J. B., Hallemeier, C. L., Wu, Z., Bass, A., Beamer, S., & Tepper, J. E. (2021). Esophagus-gastric cancer. In L. L. Gunderson & J. E. Tepper (Eds.), *Clinical radiation oncology* (5th ed.). Philadelphia: Elsevier.

Cannon, G. M., Saba, N. F., & Harari, P. M. (2021). Oropharyngeal cancer. In L. L. Gunderson, & J. E. Tepper (Eds.), *Clinical radiation oncology* (5th ed.). Philadelphia: Elsevier.

Eastburn, K., Lyu, L., Harrison, C., Atchison, K., Moore, K., Pomfret, S., … Nilsen, M. (2022). Association between patient-reported symptoms of dysphagia and psychological distress in head and neck cancer survivors. *Oncology Nursing Forum, 49*(1), 81–89.

Espitalier, F., Fanous, A., Aviv, J., Bassiouny, S., Deshter, G., Nerurkar, N., … Crevier-Buchman, L. (2018). International consensus (ICON) on assessment of oropharyngeal dysphagia. *European Annals of Otorhinolaryngology, Head and Neck Diseases, 135*(1), S17–S21.

Frowen, J., Hughes, R., & Skeat, J. (2020). The prevalence of patient-reported dysphagia and oral complications in cancer patients. *Support Care Cancer, 28*, 1141–1150.

Laursen, A. (2020). Nutritional screening: Development and implementation of a protocol in patients with head and neck cancer. *Clinical Journal of Oncology Nursing, 24*(4), 415–420.

Mathey, K. (2022). Dysphagia. In D. Camp-Sorrell, R. A. Hawkins, & D. G. Cope (Eds.), *Clinical manual for the advanced practice nurse* (4th ed.). Pittsburgh: Oncology Nursing Society.

Munoz-Schuffenegger, P., Chu, R. W. K., & Wong, R. K. S. (2018). Dysphagia, reflux, and hiccups. In I. Olver (Ed.), *The MASCC textbook of cancer supportive care and survivorship* (2nd ed.). Cham: Springer.

Valdez, J. A., & Brennan, M. T. (2018). Impact of oral cancer on quality of life. *Dental Clinics of North America, 62*(1), 143–154.

Epistaxis

Joshua Carter

Definition

- Epistaxis is defined as nasal bleeding.
- Severity can range from minor to intractable.

- Approximately 10% of epistaxis cases require medical treatment; 1% to 2% require surgery.
- Epistaxis can be spontaneous with hematologic disorders, malignancies, or thrombocytopenia.
- Epistaxis has been estimated to account for 0.5% of all emergency department visits and up to one-third of all otolaryngology-related emergency department encounters. Inpatient hospitalization for aggressive treatment of severe nosebleeds has been reported in 0.2% of patients with nosebleeds.

Pathophysiology and Contributing Factors

- Epistaxis is described as either anterior or posterior, depending on origin site.
- Epistaxis from the anterior region accounts for 80% of cases.
- Local causes of epistaxis include trauma to the nasal cavity, facial injury, or a foreign body in the nasal cavity.
- Systemic causes of epistaxis include environmental factors (e.g., temperature, humidity, being at a high altitude) and other systemic causes (e.g., inflammation, neoplastic conditions, organ failure).
- Antiplatelet or anticoagulant therapy is a common cause of epistaxis. In these cases, epistaxis usually is caused by nasal dryness, trauma, and the effects of therapy.
- For nasopharyngeal carcinoma patients treated with radiation therapy, epistaxis can be a treatment-related toxicity.
- Immune thrombocytopenia can cause a sudden onset of epistaxis.

Signs and Symptoms

- Bleeding from the nose
- Blood running into throat from nose
- Difficulty breathing
- Fatigue
- Disorientation (from uncontrolled epistaxis)

Assessment Tools

- History, including all past medical history; medications and supplements that the patient is currently taking.
- Nasal examination by primary care physician; ear, nose, and throat (ENT) doctor; and/or head and neck surgeon.
- From patient's report, suspected cause for epistaxis (if from trauma or other preceding known cause).
- To establish the cause of uncontrolled epistaxis, the head and neck surgeon may evaluate the patient under anesthesia, examining the patient's nose and nasopharynx; biopsy procedures may be warranted.
- Establish whether the patient has any hematologic disorders or malignancies.

Laboratory and Diagnostic Tests

- Complete blood count
- Platelet studies
- Coagulation studies
- Angiography
- Computed tomography, magnetic resonance imaging

Differential Diagnoses

- Trauma
- Head and neck malignancy
- Medication-related
- Treatment-related
- Environment-related
- Immune-related thrombocytopenia
- Hematologic disorders and malignancies

Interventions

Invasive Interventions

- Cauterization of the bleeding site
- Angiography with embolization
- Surgical biopsy if the lesion is in the nasal passage
- Transnasal endoscopic sphenopalatine artery ligation

Noninvasive Interventions

- Patient sits upright with head tilted forward and applies direct external pressure to the nares with index finger and thumb
- Anterior nasal packing
- Posterior nasal packing

Patient Teaching

- Avoid nonsteroidal antiinflammatory drugs (NSAIDs), alcoholic beverages, and smoking.
- Do not blow, pick, or clean the inside of the nose.
- Inform patient that there may be a dark red or brown discharge from the nose.
- Use a cool-mist room humidifier.
- Use strategies to prevent constipation and straining.
- Avoid forceful blowing of the nose.
- If packing is in place, moisturize lips and nostrils with water-soluble ointment.
- For 24 hours after epistaxis episode, avoid bending over.
- Before starting any supplements, discuss with physician.
- If epistaxis remains uncontrolled, present to emergency department for a full workup and evaluation.

Follow-Up

- Reinforce need for prompt communication with health care providers when future epistaxis episodes occur.

Resources

- Chemo Care (The Cleveland Clinic Foundation): www.chemocare.com
- Uptodate.com: Patient Information, beyond the basics: www.uptodate.com; http://www.uptodate.com/contents/search?search=epistaxis&x=0&y=0

Bibliography

Heining, C. J., Amlani, A., & Doshi, J. (2021). Ambulatory management of common ENT emergencies—What's the evidence? *The Journal of Laryngology and Otology, 135*(3), 191–195.

Kasle, D. A., Fujita, K., & Manes, R. P. (2021). Review of clinical practice guideline: Nosebleed (epistaxis). *JAMA Surgery, 156*(10), 974–975.

Krulewitz, N. A., & Fix, M. L. (2019). Epistaxis. *Emergency Medicine Clinics of North America, 37*(1), 29–39.

Mcleod, R. W. J., Price, A., Williams, R. J., Smith, M. E., Smith, M., & Owens, D. (2017). Intranasal cautery for the management of adult epistaxis: Systematic review. *The Journal of Laryngology and Otology, 131*(12), 1056–1064.

Randall, D. A. (2021). Simplified management of epistaxis. *Journal of the American Association of Nurse Practitioners, 33*(11), 1024–1029.

Seikaly, H. (2021). Epistaxis. *The New England Journal of Medicine, 384*(10), 944–951.

Sowerby, L., Rajakumar, C., Davis, M., & Rotenberg, B. (2021). Epistaxis first-aid management: a needs assessment among healthcare providers. *Journal of Otolaryngology—Head & Neck Surgery, 50*(1), 7.

Tunkel, D. E., Holdsworth, S. M., Alikhaani, J. D., Monjur, T. M., & Satterfield, L. (2020). Plain language summary: Nosebleed (epistaxis). *Otolaryngology—Head and Neck Surgery, 162*(1), 26–32.

Womack, J. P., Kropa, J., & Jimenez Stabile, M. (2018). Epistaxis: Outpatient management. *American Family Physician, 98*(4), 240–245.

Zhou, A. H., Chung, S. Y., Sylvester, M. J., Zaki, M., Svider, P. S., Hsueh, W. D., … Eloy, J. A. (2018). To pack or not to pack: Inpatient management of epistaxis in the elderly. *American Journal of Rhinology & Allergy, 32*(6), 539–545.

Esophagitis

Jennifer S. Webster

Definition

- Damage to the basal epithelial cell layer of the esophagus, resulting in reduced cell proliferation, mucosal thinning, inflammation and eventual ulceration, and/or edema.
- A common complication, often acute, associated with patients receiving radiation therapy to the thoracic cavity. Concurrent chemotherapy worsens the toxicity.
- May cause significant pain and interfere with normal swallowing, leading to a profound effect on nutrition and hydration status, energy and activity level, and quality of life.
- Affects the course of treatment, causing delays or dose reductions in therapy.
- Usually begins in the first 2 to 3 weeks after initiation of radiation therapy. Is frequently self-limiting.
- Late esophageal toxicities include strictures, esophageal erosion and, rarely, fistulas.
- Although rare, Barrett esophagus (a thickening and chronic inflammation of the lining of the esophagus) may develop, which is a risk factor for cancer of the esophagus.

Pathophysiology and Contributing Factors

- Breakdown of rapidly dividing epithelial cells caused by radiation treatment and chemotherapy, primarily in the gastrointestinal (GI) tract.
- Any cancer requiring radiation to the chest such as lung, breast, esophageal, or gastric cancer, or due to mediastinal lymph node involvement (e.g., the lymphomas). The addition of systemic chemotherapy increases patient susceptibility to esophagitis. The effect is not only additive but synergistic due to radiation-sensitizing of the tissues.
- Treatment regimen, dose, and frequency:
  - It is estimated that patients with advanced lung cancer undergoing chemoradiotherapy may have up to a 50% risk of developing esophagitis and dysphagia, depending on treatment regimen.
  - Gynecologic cancers are commonly treated with highly emetic chemotherapy regimens that may result in GI disturbances such as esophagitis and gastroenteritis.

- The advent of immune-checkpoint inhibitors such as nivolumab or pembrolizumab in the treatment of advanced malignancies can contribute to esophagitis, although it is not a common side effect of these agents.
- Cancer of the stomach or esophagus requiring surgery
- History of esophagitis or mucositis
- History of gastroesophageal reflux disease (GERD)
- Presence of *Helicobacter pylori* infection/history of stomach ulcers
- History of irritable bowel syndrome
- Age
- Poor oral hygiene, prior dental disease
- Alcohol and tobacco use are risk factors
- Medications such as dexamethasone, aspirin, or nonsteroidal antiinflammatories can cause or exacerbate GI disturbances.

Signs and Symptoms

- Difficult swallowing (dysphagia) or painful swallowing (odynophagia)
- A feeling of something being stuck in the throat or sternal area of the chest
- Dull, substernal discomfort or ache
- Retrosternal burning that radiates upward
- Heartburn or acid reflux
- Mouth sores (an indication of GI tract erosion)
- Bleeding
- Infection
- Nausea
- Vomiting

Assessment Tools

- History, physical examination, and a thorough oral examination
- Common terminology criteria for adverse events (CTCAE), version 5.0, "Esophagitis" and "Esophageal Pain"
- Are there factors that contribute to or alleviate the pain (e.g., certain food, times of day, body position)?
- Assess ability to swallow
- Nutritional status

Laboratory and Diagnostic Tests

- Complete blood cell count (CBC) (The presence of neutropenia can compound the esophagitis risk)
- Blood, urine, and sputum culture to identify possible infection
- Upper endoscopy and pH studies (not always necessary)
- Upper GI series (or barium swallow)
- Biopsy of esophageal tissue sample

Differential Diagnoses

- Infection, such as esophageal candidiasis
- GERD
- Esophageal stricture
- Dysphagia
- Pain
- Dehydration
- Anorexia

Interventions

- If possible, treat the underlying cause (e.g., infection) to promote more rapid healing.
- Most interventions are aimed at providing symptom relief.

Pharmacologic Interventions

- Antibiotics, antifungals, or antivirals to treat infection
- Topical anesthetics: viscous lidocaine, analgesics that can be gargled or swallowed
- Systemic analgesics, if necessary
- Corticosteroid medication to reduce inflammation
- Antacid therapy, such as proton pump inhibitors (preferred) or H_2 receptor antagonists
- Promotility/prokinetic agents to promote gastric emptying (e.g., metoclopramide)
- Amifostine (Ethyol); a radioprotective agent used as prophylaxis; however, contradictory results, side effects, and cost have prevented widespread routine adoption
- Enteral/Parenteral nutrition and intravenous hydration to allow the esophagus to heal and to reduce the likelihood of malnourishment or dehydration

Nonpharmacologic Interventions

- Dietary modifications, such as small frequent low-fat meals, pureed or liquid diets, nutritional supplements, and avoidance of spicy foods
- Good oral hygiene as listed below
- In small clinical trials, oral glutamine shows promise in reducing the severity of esophagitis but due to lack of randomized trials and inconsistent results it has not been widely adopted
- Avoidance or reduction of alcohol intake and smoking

Patient Teaching

- Good oral health reduces risk of infection along the entire GI tract. A dental evaluation to establish an oral care plan before treatment is highly recommended.
- Dental cleaning:
  - Brush with soft toothbrush two to four times a day.
  - Continue despite thrombocytopenia or neutropenia unless uncontrolled bleeding develops.
  - Use fluoride toothpaste.
  - Brush tongue gently at least once a day with a toothbrush or tongue scraper.
- Floss daily with unwaxed dental floss or alternative interproximal plaque removing device.
- Rinsing:
  - Normal saline solution (NS), sodium bicarbonate ($NaHCO_3$), $NS/NaHCO_3$, and water are all acceptable agents to keep the mouth clean
  - Nonalcoholic unsweetened mouthwash
- Dental appliances should be left out as much as possible if mucous membranes become irritated.
- Report any pain that is unrelieved with pain medication.
- Dietary modifications:
  - Patient may benefit from a consult with a nutritionist.

- Follow a low-acid and bland diet. Eat soft foods such as scrambled eggs, mashed potatoes, milkshakes, and ice cream.
- Food served at room temperature or cold may be easier to tolerate. Cool liquids, jello, and popsicles can help to maintain hydration.
- Avoid coffee, hot beverages, spicy foods, citrus fruits and juices, alcohol, and tobacco.
- Sit upright while eating and drinking. If gastric reflux is a problem, maintain an upright position for at least 30 minutes after eating or drinking. Elevate head of bed while sleeping.
- Report any fever of 100.5°F (38°C) or greater.
- Report changes in oral mucosa or tongue (e.g., erythema, bleeding, white patches, or ulcerations).

Follow-Up

- Assess for increased risk of esophagitis with continuing treatments.
- Assess for pain unrelieved with pain medication.
- Monitor nutritional status and weight closely.
- Reinforce the importance of communication of any changes to the patient's care team.

Resources

- National Cancer Institute: Oral complications of chemotherapy and head/neck radiation (PDQ). Available at https://www.cancer.gov/about-cancer/treatment/side-effects/mouth-throat/oral-complications-hp-pdq#_592_toc (accessed June 1, 2022)
- Metz, J., & Millar, L. B. (2022). Esophagitis. *Oncolink*. Available at https://www.oncolink.org/cancer-treatment/radiation/side-effects-of-radiation-therapy/esophagitis#:~:text=Esophagitis%20is%20a%20common%20side%20effect%20of%20cancer,receiving%20treatment%20to%20the%20chest%20and%20neck%20area (accessed June 8, 2022)
- Oncolink. (2022). Nutrition for patients with esophageal cancer. Available at https://www.oncolink.org/cancers/gastrointestinal/esophageal-cancer/support-resources-for-people-with-esophageal-cancer/nutrition-for-patients-with-esophageal-cancer (accessed June 8, 2022)
- Oncology Nursing Society. (2019). Mucositis. Putting evidence into practice. Available at https://www.ons.org/pep/mucositis?display=pepnavigator&sort_by=created&items_per_page=50 (accessed June 11, 2022)

Bibliography

Ashman, J. B., Hallemeier, C. L., Wu, Z., Bass, A., Beamer, S., & Tepper, J. E. (2021). Esophagus-gastric cancer. In L. L. Gunderson & J. E. Tepper (Eds.), *Clinical radiation oncology* (5th ed.). Philadelphia: Elsevier.

Bowen, J. M., Gibson, R. J., Coller, J. K., Blijlevens, N., Bossi, P., Al-Dasooqi, N., … Mucositis Study Group of the Multinational Association of Supportive Care in Cancer/International Society of Oral Oncology (MASCC/ISOO). (2019). Systematic review of agents for the management of cancer treatment-related gastrointestinal mucositis and clinical practice guidelines. *Support Care Cancer, 27,* 4011–4022.

Chang, S. C., Lai, Y. C., Hung, J. C., & Chang, C. Y. (2019). Oral glutamine supplements reduce concurrent chemoradiotherapy-induced esophagitis in patients with advanced non-small cell lung cancer. *Medicine, 98*(8), e14463.

Hydzik, C., & Perialis, K. M. (2018). Gynecologic cancers. In L. Parks & M. Routt (Eds.), *Critical care nursing of the oncology patient*. Pittsburgh: Oncology Nursing Society.

Mathey, K. (2022). Heartburn/indigestion/dyspepsia. In D. Camp-Sorrell, R. A. Hawkins, & D. G. Cope (Eds.), *Clinical manual for the advanced practice nurse* (4th ed.). Pittsburgh: Oncology Nursing Society.

Milano, M. T., Marks, L. B., & Constine, L. S. (2021). Late effects after radiation. In L. L. Gunderson & J. E. Tepper (Eds.), *Clinical radiation oncology* (5th ed.). Philadelphia: Elsevier.

Munoz-Schuffenegger, P., Chu, R. W. K., & Wong, R. K. S. (2018). Dysphagia, reflux, and hiccups. In I. Olver (Ed.), *The MASCC textbook of cancer supportive care and survivorship* (2nd ed.). Cham: Springer.

Patil, P. A., & Zhang, Xuchen. (2021). Pathologic manifestations of gastrointestinal and hepatobiliary injury in immune checkpoint inhibitor therapy. *Archives of Pathology & Laboratory Medicine, 145*(5), 571–582.

Valdez, J. A., & Brennan, M. T. (2018). Impact of oral cancer on quality of life. *Dental Clinics of North America, 62*(1), 143–154.

Fatigue

Susie Maloney-Newton

Definition

- Fatigue is a distressing, persistent, and subjective sense of physical, emotional, and/or cognitive tiredness or exhaustion that is not proportional to activity and interferes with usual function.
- Cancer-related fatigue is a subjective feeling of weariness or tiredness that is different from any other fatigue that the person has experienced.
- It is typically not relieved by sleep or rest.
- It has a serious detrimental effect on the cancer patient's quality of life.
- It affects as many as 80% to 100% of cancer patients.

Pathophysiology and Contributing Factors

- Exact pathophysiologic mechanism unknown
- Many contributing factors:
  - Underlying disease
  - Treatment-related toxicity:
    - Chemotherapy
    - Radiation therapy
    - Surgery
    - Biotherapy
  - Cytokines
  - Performance status/excessive inactivity
  - Pain
  - Depression
  - Anemia
  - Dyspnea
  - Infection
  - Anorexia/cachexia and other nutritional deficiencies
  - Dehydration
  - Metabolic disturbances
  - Hormone imbalance
  - Sleep disorders
  - Polypharmacy or other medications
  - Other health issues
  - Psychological distress

Signs and Symptoms

- Fatigue is reported as the most distressing symptom associated with cancer treatments, including chemotherapy, radiation therapy, bone marrow transplant, and selected biologic response modifiers.
- It is rated as more distressing than pain, nausea, and vomiting, which can frequently be treated with medications.
- Patients report whole-body tiredness and inability to perform basic tasks.
- Other reported physical symptoms include the following:
  - Dyspnea
  - Heart palpitations
  - Depressed mood
  - General lack of energy
- Fatigue often manifests with other symptoms:
  - Pain
  - Insomnia
  - Depression or anxiety

Assessment Tools

- The key assessment finding is the patient's self-report.
  - Fatigue is whatever the patient says it is.
  - Neither clinicians, family members, nor anyone else can judge fatigue level.
- Other assessment information includes the following:
  - Physical examination
  - Related laboratory data
  - Caregiver information
- Methods and tools for measuring fatigue include the following:
  - Functional Assessment of Cancer Therapy: Fatigue (FACT-F)
  - Brief Fatigue Inventory (BFI)
  - Linear Analog Scale Assessment (LASA)
  - Visual Analog Scale (VAS)
  - Fatigue Intensity Scale (FIS)

Laboratory and Diagnostic Tests

- Laboratory tests to assess for the cause of fatigue include the following:
  - Complete blood cell count
  - Serum iron testing, including transferrin, total iron-binding capacity, ferritin, and iron levels
  - Folic acid and vitamin B_{12}
  - Thyroid function, including thyroxine (T_4) total, triiodothyronine (T_3) uptake, thyroid-stimulating hormone (TSH)
- There are no diagnostic tests to screen for fatigue.

Differential Diagnoses

- Anemia
- Depression
- Infection
- Sleep disturbances
- Anorexia
- Hypothyroidism

- Dehydration
- Medications that cause fatigue

Interventions
Pharmacologic Interventions
- Psychostimulants
  - Psychostimulants are not approved by the U.S. Food and Drug Administration (FDA) for the treatment of cancer-related fatigue (CRF). However, preliminary evidence from randomized controlled studies suggests that these medications might be helpful in a subpopulation of patients experiencing moderate to severe fatigue. Of the psychostimulants, methylphenidate is the most studied pharmacological agent for fatigue, yet the evidence for its efficacy is mixed.
- Ginseng
  - There are two types of ginseng: Asian and American. Ginseng is reported to have many effects, including boosting of the immune system, antidepressive properties, and increased energy, concentration, and libido.
- Erythropoiesis-stimulating factors (ESAs) if fatigue is related to anemia
  - ESAs such as erythropoietin, darbepoetin, and erythropoietin alfa are agents that control red blood cell (RBC) production.

  ESAs (including biosimilars) may be offered to patients with chemotherapy-associated anemia whose cancer treatment is not curative in intent and whose hemoglobin levels have declined to lower than 10 g/dL. RBC transfusion is also an option.
  - The effects of erythropoietin on fatigue and cognitive impairment have been studied in patients with chemotherapy-related anemia. The U.S. Food and Drug Administration has issued several warnings related to the use of ESAs. Related concerns include risk of increased tumor growth, decreased survival time, and thromboembolism.
- Antidepressants, if depression is suspected
  - The prevalence and incidence of depression in patients with cancer vary widely depending on the diagnostic criteria and the instruments used; however, a significant number of patients with cancer have depression.
  - Patients who are at greatest risk of depression are those with advanced disease, those who have uncontrolled physical symptoms, and those who have had previous psychiatric disorders.
  - Oncology professionals should seek the expertise of mental health providers if they have questions regarding the prescribing of antidepressants or for referral to cognitive/psychological counseling.
- Corticosteroids such as methylprednisolone (prednisone) have been shown to reduce the significance of fatigue in some patient populations (e.g., those with chronic fatigue syndrome). However, because of the side effects associated with long-term use of these drugs (e.g., alterations in bone metabolism, adrenal suppression), they are not good options for the cancer population.

Nonpharmacologic Interventions
- As outlined in the National Comprehensive Cancer Network (NCCN) guidelines on fatigue. NCCN category 1 interventions for CRF include the following:
  - Physical activities (yoga)
  - Physically based therapies (massage)
  - Psychosocial interventions (cognitive behavioral therapy/ behavioral therapy and psychoeducational therapies)
- Other nonpharmacologic interventions in the literature include:
  - Exercise, such as walking on a regular basis
  - Delegating tasks
  - Energy conservation principles
  - Frequent rest periods that do not interfere with nighttime sleep
  - Stress reduction techniques, such as progressive muscle relaxation or relaxation breathing

Patient Teaching
- Instruct patient regarding factors that contribute to fatigue:
  - Cancer itself
  - Cancer treatments
  - Anemia
  - Nutritional problems
  - Sleep problems
- Teach patient to recognize the signs of fatigue:
  - Feeling weary or exhausted (may be physical, emotional, or mental exhaustion)
  - A feeling of heaviness in the body, especially arms and legs
  - Less desire to do normal activities such as eating or shopping
  - Difficulty concentrating or thinking clearly
- Instruct patient regarding ways to manage fatigue:
  - Take time to rest but be aware that too much rest can decrease energy levels.
  - Stay as active as possible; take part in enjoyable physical activities at least three times a week.
  - Practice yoga.
  - Eat nutritious foods and drink plenty of liquids.
  - Conserve energy when possible.
  - Perform stress-relieving activities.

Follow-Up

Fatigue is one of the most common side effects experienced by patients with cancer. Patients will need education before beginning therapy for their cancer, as well as continuing evaluation and support to help them through the effects of this symptom.

After consulting with a health care provider, patients may begin an exercise program with activities such as walking, stretching, or riding a bicycle. Begin slowly with exercise for 5 to 10 minutes twice a day. Increase the exercise by 1 minute per day. Strive for consistency in the exercise without overdoing it.

Resources

- Abramson Cancer Center of the University of Pennsylvania: www.oncolink.com
- American Society of Clinical Oncology (ASCO): Cancer.net
- CancerCare, Inc.: www.cancercare.org
- Oncology Nursing Society: www.ons.org

Bibliography

Bohlius, J., Bohlke, K., Castelli, R., Djulbegovic, B., Lustberg, M. B., Martino, M., … Lazo-Langner, A. (2019). Management of cancer-associated anemia with erythropoiesis-stimulating agents: ASCO/ASH clinical practice guideline update. *Journal of Clinical Oncology, 37*(15), 1336–1351.

Fabi, A., Bhargava, R., Fatigoni, S., Guglielmo, M., Horneber, M., Roila, F., … ESMO Guidelines Committee. (2020). Cancer-related fatigue: ESMO Clinical Practice Guidelines for diagnosis and treatment. *Annals of Oncology, 31*(6), 713–723.

Juvet, L. K., Thune, I., Elvsaas, I. K.Ø., Fors, E. A., Lundgren, S., Bertheussen, G., … Oldervoll, L. M. (2017). The effect of exercise on fatigue and physical functioning in breast cancer patients during and after treatment and at 6 months follow-up: A meta-analysis. *Breast, 33*, 166–177.

Lemke, E. A. (2021). Ginseng for the management of cancer related fatigue: An integrative review. *Journal of the Advanced Practitioner in Oncology, 12*(4), 406–414.

Lin, P. J., Kleckner, I. R., Loh, K. P., Inglis, J. E., Peppone, L. J., Janelsins, M. C., … Mustian, K. M. (2019). Influence of yoga on cancer-related fatigue and on mediational relationships between changes in sleep and cancer-related fatigue: A nationwide, multicenter randomized controlled trial of yoga in cancer survivors. *Integrative Cancer Therapies, 18*, 1534735419855134.

Mitchell, S. A., Hoffman, A. J., Clark, J. C., DeGennaro, R. M., Poirier, P., Robinson, C. B., & Weisbrod, B. L. (2014). An update of evidence based interventions for cancer related fatigue during and following treatment. *Clinical Journal of Oncology Nursing, 18*(6), 38–58.

National Comprehensive Cancer Network. (2020). *NCCN clinical practice guidelines in oncology: Cancer-related fatigue version 1.2021.* Plymouth Meeting, PA: National Comprehensive Cancer Network.

Williams, A. M., Khan, C. P., Heckler, C. E., Barton, D. L., Ontko, M., Geer, J., & Janelsins, M. C. (2021). Fatigue, anxiety, and quality of life in breast cancer patients compared to non-cancer controls: A nationwide longitudinal analysis. *Breast Cancer Research and Treatment, 187*(1), 275–285.

Fever

Becky Collins

Definition

- Fever, or pyrexia, is elevation of core body temperature.
- The mean oral temperature is 98.6° ± 7° F or 37° ± 0.4° C.
- A fever, or high temperature, is considered when a person's temperature is above 100.3° F (38.5° C).
- Fever is an emergency medical condition in a person who has neutropenia or is on immunosuppressive therapy.

Pathophysiology and Contributing Factors

- Pathophysiology of fever in general:
  - The hypothalamus regulates and controls body temperature in the thermoregulatory center.
  - The thermoregulatory center balances heat production with heat dissipation.
  - When the balance is disrupted (i.e., elevation of the hypothalamic set point), vasoconstriction and heat production occur.
  - Fever has three phases: chill, fever, and flush.

- Pathophysiology in neoplastic fever:
  - Neoplastic fever is a unique feature of malignancies such as colon cancer, renal cell carcinoma, liver cancer, and hematologic malignancies.
  - Fever can be induced when a tumor produces pyrogens.
  - Pyrogens interfere with the normal functioning of the hypothalamus.
  - Exogenous pyrogens originate from outside the body; they are primarily infectious agents and toxins. Endogenous pyrogens originate from inside the body; normal flora are altered by neutropenia, toxins, and tumors.
  - Pyrogenic cytokines cause fever when activated; they include interleukins, interferons, and tumor necrosis factor.
- Contributing factors:
  - Elderly persons are more susceptible to temperature change; they may present apyrexia or manifest a lower fever than others.
  - Persons with cancer may mount a febrile response to infection, drugs, tumor, thrombosis, graft-versus-host disease, or a blood transfusion.
  - Persons receiving biologic therapy may experience a fever as a likely side effect of the treatment.

Signs and Symptoms

- Vasoconstriction of hands and feet
- Shivering, followed by need for warmth
- Chills, rigors
- Flush
- Dry skin
- Diaphoresis
- Generalized body aches and fatigue

Assessment Tools

- Determine whether the patient is at high or low risk for febrile neutropenia, is undergoing chemotherapy or biotherapy, and/or has hematologic malignancy.
- High-risk assessment of fever:
  - Multinational Association for Supportive Care in Cancer (MASCC) score of greater than 21 and/or Talcott's Risk Assessment in Group I to III
  - Inpatient at time of fever onset
  - Comorbidities leading to hospitalization
  - Neutropenia
  - Elevated serum creatinine level
  - Elevated liver function tests
- Low-risk assessment of fever:
  - MASCC score of less than 21 and/or Talcott Risk Assessment in Group IV
  - Outpatient at time of fever onset
  - No comorbidities
  - Short duration of neutropenia
  - Good performance status
- Risk assessment tools:
  - MASCC risk score
  - Talcott Risk Assessment
  - History and physical examination

- Areas to examine:
  - Skin assessment for areas of pressure, ulcerations, or wounds
  - Vascular access devices as sources of infection
  - Lungs and sinuses
  - Alimentary canal: mouth, pharynx, esophagus, rectum, bowel
  - Perineal, vaginal, perirectal areas
  - Lymph nodes
- Assessment for nausea, vomiting, diarrhea
- Review of the medical history
- Medications, previous or current use of antibiotics
- Review of potential exposures: family, friends, pets, travel, recent blood transfusion, exposure to tuberculosis
- Time from last treatment and agents received
- Neurologic assessment (confusion and cognitive impairment can occur with high fevers)
- Vital signs: evaluate for any signs of sepsis; check temperature at regular intervals
- In persons with cancer, consider infection as the cause of fever unless proven otherwise
- Skin ulcerations or decubitus formation

Laboratory and Diagnostic Tests

- Complete blood cell count (CBC) with differential, sedimentation rate
- Renal panel, liver function tests
- Chest radiographic film
- Cultures: urine, sputum, blood, stool, central and peripheral devices

Differential Diagnoses

- Neoplastic fever
- Blood product transfusion-associated fever
- Biologic treatment-associated fever
- Infection: neutropenic fever (bacterial, viral, fungal, or opportunistic)
- Fever of unknown origin (FUO)
- Deep vein thrombosis

Interventions

- Determined by cause of fever
- Treatment based on the cause of fever

Pharmacologic Interventions

- Antipyretics to reduce temperature, myalgias, rigors
- Empirical broad-spectrum antibiotics based on institutional isolates
- Anaerobic therapy as needed
- Specific therapy for documented infection sites or pathogens
- Prophylaxis as required

Nonpharmacologic Interventions

- Hydration
- Nutritional support
- Comfort care, oral care, keep mucous membranes moist, sponge bathing with cool or cold cloth, changing bed linen and clothes, use of a fan for cooling

Patient Teaching

- Prevention includes good handwashing and hygiene.
- Neutropenic precautions should be reviewed and stressed during chemotherapy treatment.
- Report fevers (>38.3° C or 100.4° F) or chills to health care provider as soon as possible.
- Take the complete course of antibiotics or other medications as prescribed.
- Monitor temperature at least two times daily at home throughout duration of chemotherapy.
- Assure patient has access to a thermometer and review with return demonstration the use of thermometer.
- Future treatments may include a colony-stimulating factor.
- Teach when to contact a health care provider (e.g., presenting with unusual symptoms, signs of infection or bleeding).
- A neutropenic person will not experience the usual signs of infection (i.e., redness, swelling, pus); fever may be the first sign of infection.
- Instruct the patient and family to not take any rectal medications or treatments.
- Educate the patient and family to avoid contact with anyone who is ill.
- Instruct patient to avoid dental work unless approved by the health care provider.
- Oral care hygiene should be performed at least four times a day.

Follow-Up

- Daily follow-up when hospitalized.
- Outpatient daily follow-up for the first 72 hours at home or in the clinic, and then as needed for signs and symptoms of persistent or recurrent fever.

Resources

- Centers for Disease Control and Prevention: www.cdc.gov
- National Comprehensive Cancer Network: www.NCCN.org
- Oncology Nursing Society: www.ons.org
- National Cancer Institute: www.cancer.gov
- American Cancer Society: www.cancer.org

Bibliography

Goldsmith, C., Kalis, J., & Jeffers, K. D. (2018). Assessment of initial febrile neutropenia management in hospitalized cancer patients at a community cancer center. *Journal of the Advanced Practitioner in Oncology, 9*(6), 659–664.

NCCN Guidelines for Patients. (2021). *Anemia and neutropenia*. https://www.nccn.org/patients/guidelines/content/PDF/anemia-patient-guideline.pdf (accessed November 10, 2021).

Talcott, J. A. (2018). Decision rules in a guideline: Allow the science to speak. *Journal of Clinical Oncology, 36*(31). JCO2018788430. Published online ahead of print, September 4, 2018. Published correction appears in *J Clin Oncol.* 2020 May 1;38(13):1500.

Taplitz, R. A., Kennedy, E. B., Bow, E. J., Crews, J., Gleason, C., Hawley, D. K., … Flowers, C. R. (2018). Outpatient management of fever and neutropenia in adults treated for malignancy: American Society of Clinical Oncology and Infectious Diseases Society of America Clinical Practice Guideline Update. *Journal of Clinical Oncology, 36*(14), 1443–1453.

Flu-Like Symptoms

Becky Collins

Definition

- Consists of a group of symptoms similar to influenza
- Characterized by fever, chills, rigors, myalgias/arthralgias, malaise, headache, cough, and nasal congestion
- Is a side effect after administration of certain oncologic therapies
- Symptoms resolve within a specific time frame

Pathophysiology and Contributing Factors

- Flu-like symptoms occur as a result of pyrogens causing an increase in the thermoregulatory set point.
- Pyrogens may be exogenous (virus, bacteria, neoplastic cells, or drugs) or endogenous (cytokines).
- Flu-like symptoms occur with the following agents (a representative but not inclusive list):
  - Chimeric antigen receptor (CAR) T-cell therapy (CAR-T)
  - Interferons
  - Interleukins
  - Granulocyte colony-stimulating factor (G-CSF)
  - Granulocyte-macrophage colony-stimulating factor (GM-CSF)
  - Monoclonal antibodies
  - Bleomycin
  - Cladribine
  - Cytarabine
  - Dacarbazine
  - Fluorouracil
  - L-Asparaginase
  - Procarbazine
  - Trimetrexate

Signs and Symptoms

- Chills or rigors that occur 3 to 6 hours after biotherapy treatment
- Fever of 100.4° F or above
- Myalgia or arthralgia
- Headache
- Fatigue
- Nausea or vomiting
- Anorexia
- Diarrhea
- Nasal congestion (runny nose, clear)
- Cough without increased sputum

Assessment Tools

- Physical examination with review of systems: cardiopulmonary, abdomen, lymph nodes, musculoskeletal, and skin
- Vital signs: blood pressure, temperature, pulse, respirations, and pulse oximetry
- Neurologic assessment

Laboratory and Diagnostic Tests

- Complete blood cell count (CBC) to determine whether the symptoms are related to neutropenia
- If patient is neutropenic, need to pan culture and rule out infection
- Chest x-ray film if neutropenic
- COVID-19 polymerase chain reaction (PCR) test as directed

Differential Diagnosis

- Infection or sepsis
- Influenza
- COVID-19 infection
- Oncology treatment-related side effects

Interventions

Pharmacologic Interventions

- Antipyretics such as nonsteroidal antiinflammatory drugs (NSAIDs), if patient is not thrombocytopenic or acetaminophen
- Antihistamines
- Opiates to relieve rigors (e.g., meperidine, morphine, hydromorphone)
- Monitor temperature patterns; if there is no response to antipyretics, an infectious process may be present.
- Analgesics for headache, myalgias, arthralgias

Nonpharmacologic Interventions

- Provide warm blankets, heating pads, warm bath.
- Provide a quiet, dark room for patients with headache.
- Increase fluids.
- Encourage relaxation techniques.
- Provide emotional support and reassurance.
- Provide for rest.

Patient Teaching

- Teach patient that this is a possible side effect of therapy.
- Use antipyretics for fever.
- Use warm blankets to relieve chills.
- Use an NSAID (if no thrombocytopenia) or acetaminophen for myalgias or arthralgias.
- Instruct patient that this side effect is short lived and usually reduces with future drug administration.
- Encourage monitoring of side effects and temperature.

Follow-Up

- Report fevers or chills not controlled with above interventions.
- Obtain emergency care if vomiting, seizures, mental status change, increased shortness of breath, or uncontrolled fever occurs.
- Patients have 24-hour emergency numbers for access to providers.

Resources

- Oncology Nursing Society: www.ons.org/patientEd
- Chemocare.com
- National Cancer Institute: www.cancer.gov

Bibliography

Cavalieri, S., Colombo, E., Bottiglieri, A., Massa, G., Platini, F., Ottini, A., … Licitra, L. (2022). Monitoring patients with head and neck cancer for flu-like symptoms during the COVID-19 pandemic. *Tumori Journal, 108*(3), 240–249.

Long, B., Brém, E., & Koyfman, A. (2020). Oncologic emergencies: Immune-based cancer therapies and complications. *The Western Journal of Emergency Medicine.*, 21(3), 566–580.

Schirrmacher, V. (2019). From chemotherapy to biological therapy: A review of novel concepts to reduce the side effects of systemic cancer treatment (Review). *International Journal of Oncology*, 54, 407–419. Science Direct. *Flu like syndrome*. Available at https://www.sciencedirect.com/topics/pharmacology-toxicology-and-pharmaceutical-science/flu-like-syndrome (accessed December 2021).

Hand-Foot Syndrome

Laura S. Wood

Definition

- Dermatologic reaction associated with certain anticancer therapies.
- Presentation varies depending on agent, dose, and patient characteristics.
- Involvement of hands and feet is most common but can involve other skin surfaces.
- Hand-foot syndrome (HFS) is also known as
  - Palmar-plantar erythrodysesthesia (PPE)
  - Acral erythema
  - Hyperkeratosis
  - Hand-foot skin reaction

Pathophysiology and Contributing Factors

- HFS is a cutaneous eruption of the integument of the hands and feet.
- Chemotherapy drugs with sustained serum levels (e.g., liposomal doxorubicin, capecitabine, pyrimidine analogs, and fluoropyrimidines) are most likely to cause HFS.
- Multikinase inhibitors, including sorafenib, sunitinib, axitinib, regorafenib, lenvatinib, and cabozantinib, are associated with HFS.
- HFS may result from prolonged drug exposure via superficial capillaries, keratinocyte damage, or keratinocyte necrosis. Investigations to identify other etiologies are ongoing.
- It is dependent on both peak drug concentration and total cumulative dose.
- It may occur earlier and more severely with bolus or short-term dose-intensive therapy.
- It may result from friction and pressure (weight bearing) on hands, feet, or other areas.
- Patients with diabetes or peripheral vascular disorders are at increased risk.
- Cytochrome P450 subsystem inhibitors must be considered as potential contributing factors.

Signs and Symptoms

- Often characterized by initial paresthesias (tingling sensations, numbness, or sensitivity to warmth), followed by erythema.
- May occur concurrently with dry skin.
- May include hyperkeratosis and callus formation.
- May include blisters, bullae, or fissures.
- Acral erythema consists of painful, symmetric erythematous and edematous areas.
- Dry or moist desquamation may occur.
- May include swelling or edema.
- May become painful and/or interfere with both function and activities of daily living (ADLs).
- May have a negative impact on quality of life.

Assessment Tools

- Patient history
- Medication review during each interaction
- Physical examination of hands and feet before initiation of therapy and at every clinic visit
- Common Toxicity Criteria (CTC, version 5.0) grading scale:
  - Grade 1 (mild): minimal skin changes or dermatitis (e.g., erythema, edema, hyperkeratosis without pain)
  - Grade 2 (moderate): skin changes (e.g., peeling, blisters, bleeding, fissures, edema, or hyperkeratosis) with pain; limiting instrumental ADLs
  - Grade 3 (severe): severe skin changes (e.g., peeling, blisters, bleeding, fissures, edema, or hyperkeratosis) with pain; limiting self-care ADLs

Laboratory and Diagnostic Tests

- There are no specific laboratory tests.
- Physical examination and patient-reported symptoms facilitate accurate diagnosis.
- Patients with diabetes, peripheral vascular disease, or peripheral neuropathy should have more frequent examinations of the hands and feet.

Differential Diagnoses

- Cellulitis
- Rash
- Contact dermatitis
- Allergic reaction

Interventions

Pharmacologic Interventions

- Topical high-potency steroids twice daily for erythema and burning sensation associated with HFS
- Dexamethasone for severe HFS not responsive to other interventions
- Pain control: nonsteroidal antiinflammatory agents (NSAIDs, as long as thrombocytopenia is not present), γ-aminobutyric acid (GABA) agonist
- Urea 10% cream
- Topical clobetasol 0.05% cream BID at initiation of therapy
- Celecoxib 200 mg/m^2 twice daily plus topical high-potency steroid twice daily for capecitabine-induced HFS
- Treatment interruption and/or dose reduction for severe HFS

Nonpharmacologic Interventions

- Prevention is not possible. Patient education regarding frequent self assessment and compliance with skin care regimen is critical to minimize risk of severe or treatment-limiting HFS.
- Initiation of skin care regimen with first dose of therapy:
  - Frequent application of moisturizing lotion (e.g., Bag Balm, Udderly Smooth cream, Eucerin cream, Aquaphor)

- Urea 10% cream
- Clobetasol 0.05% cream BID
- Avoidance of activities resulting in excessive friction or pressure to hands or feet
- Minimize duration of exposure to heat (i.e., bathing, dishwashing)
- Well-fitting, cushioned, comfortable shoes
- Gel insole liners
- Early notification of provider for development of symptoms associated with HFS
- Exfoliating agents for hyperkeratotic areas
- Referral to podiatrist for evaluation and management

Patient Teaching

- Emphasize compliance with skin care regimen.
- Emphasize early notification for development of symptoms associated with HFS.
- If skin blisters are noted, soak the area with cool water for 10 minutes, and then apply petroleum jelly to the wet skin to trap the moisture.

Follow-up

- If the patient reports any changes to the palms or soles, a physical assessment with diagnosis and a treatment plan must occur.

Resources

- https://www.ons.org
- https://www.asco.org
- https://www.sitcancer.org
- https://nccn.org
- https://mascc.org
- https://chemocare.com
- https://ascc.org
- https://ctep.cancer.gov/protocoldevelopment/electronic_applications/docs/CTCAE_v5_Quick_Reference_5x7.pdf

Bibliography

Anderson, R., Jatoi, A., Robert, C., Wood, L. S., Keating, K. N., & Lacouture, M. E. (2009). Search for evidence-based approaches for the prevention and palliation of hand-foot skin reaction (HFSR) caused by multikinase inhibitors (MKIs). *The Oncologist, 14,* 291–302.

Anoop, T. M., Rona Joseph, P., Mini, P. N., Pranab, K. P., Gopan, G., & Chacko, S. (2021). Cutaneous toxicities in breast cancer patients receiving chemotherapy and targeted agents—An observational clinical study. *Clinical Breast Cancer, 21,* e434–e447.

Ding, F., Liu, B., & Wang, Y. (2019). Risk of hand-foot skin reaction associated with vascular endothelial growth factor-tyrosine kinase inhibitors: A meta-analysis of 57 randomized controlled trials involving 24,956 patients. *American Academy of Dermatology, 83,* 788–796.

Ding, J., Farah, M. H., Nayfeh, T., Malandris, K., Manolopoulos, A., Ginex, P. K., … Murad, M. H. (2020). Targeted therapy- and chemotherapy-associated skin toxicities: Systematic review and meta-analysis. *Oncology Nursing Forum, 47,* E149–E160.

Jatoi, A., Ou, F. S., Ahn, D. H., Zemla, T. J., Le-Rademacher, J. G., Boland, P., … Bekaii-Saab, T. (2021). Preemptive versus reactive topical clobetasol for regorafenib-induced hand foot reactions: A preplanned analysis of the ReDOS trial. *The Oncologist, 26,* 610–618.

Kwakman, J. J. M., Elshot, Y. S., Punt, C. J. A., & Koopman, M. (2020). Management of cytotoxic chemotherapy-induced hand-foot syndrome. *Oncology Reviews, 14*(442), 57–63.

Lan, T. C., Tsou, P. H., Tam, K. W., & Huang, T. W. (2021). Effect of urea cream on hand-foot syndrome in patients receiving chemotherapy: A meta-analysis. *Cancer Nursing, 45*(5), 378–386.

Lian, S., Zhang, X., Zhang, Y., & Zhao, Q. (2021). Pyroxidine for prevention of hand-foot syndrome caused by chemotherapy agents: A meta-analysis. *Clinical and Experimental Dermatology, 46,* 629–635.

Mahon, S. M., & Carr, E. (2021). Skin toxicities: Common side effects. *Clinical Journal of Oncology Nursing, 25*(6), 32.

Manchen, E., Robert, C., & Porta, C. (2011). Management of tyrosine kinase inhibitor-induced hand-foot skin reaction: Viewpoints from the medical oncologist, dermatologist, and oncology nurse. *Journal of Supportive Oncology, 9*(1), 13–23.

National Cancer Institute. (2017). *Common Terminology Criteria for Adverse Events (CTCAE), version 4.03.* Available at https://ctep.cancer.gov/protocoldevelopment/electronic_applications/docs/ctcae_v5_quick_reference_5x7.pdf (accessed February 11, 2022).

Pereira, P. P., Nunes Filho, M., Moreira, T. A., Duarte Silva Malvino, L., de Araújo, L. B., Dos Santos Pedroso, R., & Ângela Ribeiro, M. (2022). Hand-foot syndrome and nail disorders secondary to treatment with paclitaxel: Is there a relationship with the presence of fungi? *Journal of Oncology Pharmacy Practice, 28*(8), 1798–1806.

Richards, R. M., Keathing, E. A., & Boucher, J. E. (2019). Targeted therapies: Treatment options for patients with metastatic breast cancer. *Clinical Journal of Oncology Nursing, 23,* 434–438.

Rosen, A., Amitay-Laish, I., & Lacouture, M. E. (2014). Management algorithms for dermatologic adverse events. In M. E. Lacouture (Ed.), *Dermatologic principles and practice in oncology: Conditions of the skin.* Hoboken, NJ: Wiley-Blackwell.

Rubin, K. M. (2017). MAPK pathway-targeted therapies: Care and management of unique toxicities in patients with advanced melanoma. *Clinical Journal of Oncology Nursing, 21,* 699–709.

Wiley, K., Ebanks, G. L., Jr., Shelton, G., Strelo, J., & Ciccolini, K. (2020). Skin toxicity: Clinical summary of the ONS guidelines for cancer treatment-related skin toxicity. *Clinical Journal of Oncology Nursing, 24,* 561–565.

Williams, L. A., Ginex, P. K., Ebanks, G. L., Jr., Ganstwig, K., Ciccolini, K., Kwong, B. K., … Morgan, R. L. (2020). ONS guidelines for cancer treatment-related skin toxicity. *Oncology Nursing Forum, 47,* 539–556.

Wood, L. S., Gornell, S., & Rini, B. I. (2012). Maximizing clinical outcomes with axitinib therapy in advanced renal cell carcinoma through proactive side effect management. *Community Oncology, 9,* 46–55.

Wood, L. S., Lemont, H., Jatoi, A., Lacouture, M. E., Robert, C., Keating, K., & Anderson, R. (2010). Practical considerations in the management of hand-foot skin reaction caused by multikinase inhibitors. *Community Oncology, 7*(1), 23–29.

Zhang, R. X., Wu, X. J., Wan, D. S., Lu, Z. H., Kong, L. H., Pan, Z. Z., & Chen, G. (2012). Celecoxib can prevent capecitabine-related hand-foot syndrome in stage II and III colorectal cancer patients: Result of a single-center, prospective randomized phase III trial. *Annals of Oncology, 23,* 1348–1353.

Headache

Carol Stein Blecher

Definition

- Headache is defined as pain that is referred to the surface of the head from deep structures.
- Headache can be caused by some other physical disorder, or it can be an independent disorder.
- When there is damage to the venous sinuses or to the membranes that cover the brain, intense pain may occur, although the brain itself is almost completely insensitive to pain.

Pathophysiology and Contributing Factors

- There are three major types of headaches:
  - Tension (or stress) headache: caused by the tightening of muscles in the head and neck
  - Migraine headache: caused by vasodilation of the blood vessels in the brain
  - Cluster headache: a form of chronic, recurrent headaches characterized by sudden onset with no specific cause, although it appears to be related to a sudden release of histamine or serotonin

- Contributing factors vary with the type of headache; in cancer patients, headaches are most frequently related to
  - Primary brain tumors or brain metastases
  - An increase in intracranial pressure (ICP) from mass effect or edema
  - Radiation therapy treatments that initially increase edema and cause headaches
  - Intrathecal chemotherapy causing headaches and the procedure of administering chemotherapy by Ommaya reservoir or lumbar puncture
  - Chemotherapy and biotherapy agents, including but not limited to the following:
    - Antithymocyte globulin (ATG)
    - Erythropoietin
    - Granulocyte colony-stimulating factor (G-CSF)
    - Granulocyte-macrophage colony-stimulating factor (GM-CSF)
    - Oprelvekin (Neumega)
    - Hormonal therapies as a class
    - Immunoglobulin G (IgG)
    - Immunotherapy in general
    - Interferon
    - Interleukin
    - Levamisole
    - All-*trans* retinoic acid (ATRA)
    - Monoclonal antibodies in general
    - Tumor necrosis factor
    - Dacarbazine
    - Gemcitabine
    - Paclitaxel
    - Targretin
    - Temozolomide

Signs and Symptoms

- Patients with brain tumors may have headaches that are worse in the morning.
- Initially, these headaches ease during the day, but ultimately they become persistent.
- Pain is usually described as dull, but if it occurs during sleep, it awakens the patient.
- The pain may be associated with morning nausea and vomiting, papilledema, and seizures.

Assessment Tools

- History, including diagnosis and cancer treatment, current medications, presenting symptoms, precipitating factors, location, and duration (assess for any associated symptoms).
- Neurologic examination, evaluating for confusion, decrease in attention span, memory loss, drowsiness, weakness, or ataxia
- Vital signs: changes in vital signs may indicate an increase in ICP. Blood pressure should be monitored for a widening pulse pressure and for hypertension. Heart rate should be monitored for bradycardia and for irregular or thready pulse.
- Examine the head for signs of trauma: skull tenderness (subdural hematoma), poor dentition or grinding of the teeth, bogginess of the sinuses, papilledema, otitis media, and mastoiditis.

- Examine the neck for nuchal rigidity, tenderness of the shoulders or neck, and decreased range of motion.
- National Cancer Institute (NCI) common terminology criteria adverse events (CTCAE) grading system for pain:
  - Grade 1: mild pain not interfering with function
  - Grade 2: moderate pain; pain or analgesics interfering with function but not interfering with activities of daily living (ADLs)
  - Grade 3: severe pain; pain or analgesics severely interfering with ADLs
  - Grade 4: disabling pain

Laboratory and Diagnostic Tests

- Complete blood cell count (CBC) with differential to rule out infection or anemia
- Chemistry studies to rule out renal failure and other underlying systemic diseases
- Platelet count, prothrombin time (PT), and international normalized ratio (INR)/partial thromboplastin time (PTT) to identify a risk for intracranial bleeding
- Arterial blood gas analysis (ABGs) to assess for hypoxia
- Drug screening for cocaine and amphetamines
- Computed tomography (CT) scan of the head to identify a tumor, metastases, or edema
- Magnetic resonance imaging (MRI) of the head to identify a tumor, metastases, or edema
- Lumbar puncture to assess infection (meningitis or encephalitis) or meningeal carcinomatosis

Differential Diagnoses

- Acute glaucoma
- Anemia
- Arteriovenous malformation
- Brain metastases
- Dental abscess
- Hypertension
- Meningeal carcinoma
- Meningitis
- Migraine
- Primary brain tumor
- Sinusitis
- Stroke
- Subarachnoid hemorrhage
- Subdural hematoma
- Systemic lupus erythematosus
- Trigeminal neuralgia
- Drug-related headaches from chemotherapy and biotherapy agents, including but not limited to the following:
  - ATRA
  - Dacarbazine
  - Erythropoietin
  - 5-Fluorouracil (5FU)
  - G-CSF
  - GM-CSF
  - Gemcitabine
  - Oprelvekin (Neumega)
  - IgG

Principles of Symptom Management

4

- Interferon
- Interleukin
- Intrathecal chemotherapy
- Levamisole
- Monoclonal antibodies in general
- Paclitaxel
- Procarbazine
- Tumor necrosis factor
- Drug-related headaches from analgesics, including but not limited to the following:
  - Acetaminophen (Tylenol)
  - Caffeine
  - Ergot preparations
  - Opioids
  - Tranquilizers/muscle relaxers
- Drug-related headaches from other agents, including but not limited to the following:
  - Amphotericin B
  - Azathioprine
  - Aztreonam
  - Cyclosporine
  - Foscarnet
  - Ganciclovir
  - Pamidronate
  - Rifampicin
  - Voriconazole

Interventions

Treatment of the Underlying Disease

- Surgery for primary brain tumor, radiation therapy, chemotherapy, targeted therapy
- Radiation therapy for metastatic disease
- Steroids for cerebral edema due to increased ICP

Pharmacologic Interventions

- Acetaminophen (Tylenol)
- Aspirin
- Aspirin or acetaminophen/caffeine
- Beta-blockers: propranolol (Inderal), nadolol (Corgard), metoprolol (Lopressor)
- Calcium channel blockers: verapamil (Calan) for prevention of migraines
- Ergotamine tartrate/caffeine (Cafergot, Wigraine, Ergomar)
- Naproxen (Naprosyn, Anaprox, Aleve)
- Ibuprofen (Motrin, Advil, Nuprin)
- Indomethacin (Indocin)
- Ketorolac (Toradol)
- Sumatriptan (Imitrex)
- Tricyclic antidepressants: amitriptyline (Elavil, Endep), nortriptyline (Pamelor)

Nonpharmacologic Interventions

- Complementary therapies, such as biofeedback, acupuncture, acupressure, massage, relaxation, and transcutaneous electrical nerve stimulation (TENS)
- Dietary modifications: avoid dairy products, caffeinated drinks, chocolate, salted or preserved meats, and foods containing monosodium glutamate (MSG)

- Herbal and nutrient therapies suggested for relief of headaches include skullcap, rosemary, thyme, chamomile, feverfew, valerian, white willow, vitamin B complex, vitamin E, calcium, and magnesium

Patient Teaching

- Treatment for headache is determined on the basis of the following:
  - Age, health status, and medical history
  - Severity of symptoms
  - Individual tolerance of specific medications, procedures, or therapies
  - Expectations for the course of the condition
  - Personal opinions and preferences
- Treatment may include the following:
  - Biofeedback training
  - Complementary medicine
  - Dietary evaluation to eliminate foods that might contribute to headaches
  - Drug therapy (medication)
  - Regular exercise, such as swimming or vigorous walking
  - Stress reduction
  - Use of cold packs

Follow-Up

- Call health care provider if any of the following occurs:
  - This is the first time the person has had a headache.
  - The headache occurs rapidly or is persistent.
  - The headache is associated with fever, stiff neck, or projectile or uncontrollable vomiting.
  - The headache is associated with confusion, seizures, or loss of consciousness.
  - There is numbness, weakness, or vision loss with the headache.
  - The headache interferes with the ability to function normally.
  - Medication for the headache is taken on more than 2 days/week.
- Also consider the following:
  - Pain service referral
  - Headache center referral
  - Physical therapy
  - Occupational therapy

Resources

- American Council for Headache Education: www.achenet.org
- Breastcancer.org: Breast Cancer Information and Support: https://www.breastcancer.org
- Cancer.Net: Headaches: https://www.cancer.net/coping-with-cancer/physical-emotional-and-social-effects-cancer/managing-physical-side-effects/headaches
- Chemocare: Headache: https://chemocare.com/chemotherapy/side-effects/headache.aspx
- National Headache Foundation: www.headaches.org

Bibliography

Cancer.Net. (2018). *Headaches*. Available at http://www.cancer.net/navigating-cancer-care/side-effects/headaches (accessed March 6, 2022).

MedlinePlus Medical Encyclopedia. (2013). *Headache*. Available at http://www.nlm.nih.gov/medlineplus/ency/article/003024.htm (accessed March 6, 2022).

National Cancer Institute. (2017). *Common terminology criteria for adverse events, version 5*. Available at http://evs.nci.nih.gov/ftp1/CTCAE/About.html (accessed March 6, 2022).

Rice, L. (2014). Headache. In D. Camp-Sorrell & R. A. Hawkins (Eds.), *Clinical manual for the oncology advanced practice nurse*. Pittsburgh, PA: Oncology Nursing Press.

Hiccups

Darcy Burbage

Definition

- Sudden, involuntary diaphragmatic spasm causing a sudden inhalation and interrupted by a spasmodic closure of the glottis, resulting in the "hic" sound.
- Three types of hiccups:
  - Benign: lasting as long as 48 hours
  - Persistent or chronic: lasting longer than 48 hours but less than 1 month
  - Intractable: lasting longer than 1 month

Pathophysiology and Contributing Factors

- A reflex arc in the cervical spine (C3 to C5) travels afferent pathways over fibers of the phrenic and vagus nerves and thoracic segments T6 to T12.
- Hiccups are a response to vagus and phrenic nerve irritation.
- Causes of hiccups are organized into four conditions:
  - Structural
  - Metabolic
  - Inflammatory
  - Infectious
- Hiccups can contribute to fatigue and exhaustion, especially if sleep and eating are interrupted.
- Unrelieved hiccups can also lead to feelings of depression, anxiety, and frustration over the long term.
- Common causes of hiccups in terminal illness include stroke, brain tumor, sepsis, and nerve irritation such as gastric distention, gastritis, gastroesophageal reflux disease (GERD), pancreatitis, *Helicobacter pylori* infection, hepatitis, and myocardial infarction.
- Cancers associated with hiccups include esophageal, gastric, colon, lung, pancreatic, and renal cancers; primary or metastatic brain tumors; leukemia; and lymphoma.
- Excessive drinking or smoking can be a factor.
- Medications that may contribute to hiccups include the following:
  - Steroids
  - Chemotherapy agents
  - Nicotine
  - Opioids
  - Muscle relaxants

Signs and Symptoms

- Brief, irritable spasms of the diaphragm.

Assessment Tools

- Obtain a history of presenting symptoms.
- Identify precipitating factors or triggers (e.g., eating, drinking, positioning).
- Obtain medical history regarding abdominal, thoracic, or neurologic surgery and social history of alcohol use.
- Determine the level of distress hiccups are causing.
- Determine interference with activities of daily living (ADLs), including eating and sleeping.
- Observe patient for other causes of hiccups.
- Evaluate for other causes such as temporal artery tenderness and hair or foreign body in the ear.
- Perform an oral examination to identify any swelling or obstruction that may be contributing to hiccups.
- Evaluate for infection or a septic process.
- Assess for pneumonia, pericarditis, abdominal distention, or ascites.
- Identify peritumor edema in the abdominal area.

Laboratory and Diagnostic Tests

- Complete blood count (CBC) and electrolytes to rule out infection or renal failure.
- Chest radiographic film to rule out pulmonary processes.
- Fluoroscopy to determine whether one hemidiaphragm is dominant.
- The extent of the workup is proportional to the duration of hiccups and the impact on the patient's quality of life.

Differential Diagnoses

- Diaphragmatic or phrenic nerve irritation
- Gastric dilation
- Hiatal hernia
- Pancreatitis
- Alcohol abuse
- Central nervous system (CNS) dysfunction
- Psychogenic cause

Interventions

Pharmacologic Interventions

- Attempt to decrease gastric distention with medications such as simethicone and metoclopramide. A nasogastric (NG) tube or fasting may be necessary to help relieve this symptom.
- Anecdotal results have been seen with baclofen, chlorpromazine (Thorazine), or haloperidol.
- Additional medications may include muscle relaxants, anticonvulsants, antidepressants, and dopamine agonists.

Nonpharmacologic Interventions

- Respiratory measures may help. Consider having the patient perform breath-holds. Try rebreathing in a paper bag or causing sneeze or cough with spices. Try an ice-cold, wet cotton tip applied between the hard and soft palates for 1 minute.
- Drinking large gulps of water, swallowing sugar, or sucking on a lemon wedge may interfere with hiccups.
- Psychological interventions include distraction techniques and breathing exercises.
- Intractable hiccups may require anesthetic block of the phrenic and cervical nerves, acupressure, or acupuncture.
- Peppermint water helps to relax the lower esophagus.

Patient Teaching

- Provide education and information regarding different classes of medications used for relief, along with nonpharmacologic management approaches.

Follow-Up

- Gastrointestinal (GI) consultation if the cause is GI related.
- Anesthesia consultation if nerve block is necessary.
- Provide support to the patient and continual assessment of interventions until hiccups are relieved.

Resources

- American Cancer Society: https://www.cancer.org/treatment/treatments-and-side-effects/physical-side-effects/hiccups.html
- Mayo Clinic: http://www.mayoclinic.com/health/hiccups/DS00975

Bibliography

Calsina-Berna, A., Garcia-Gomez, G., Gonzalez-Barboteo, J., & Porta-Sales, J. (2012). Treatment of chronic hiccups in cancer patients: A systematic review. *Journal of Palliative Medicine, 15*(10), 1142–1150.

Dahlin, C., & Cohen, A. (2015). Dysphagia, xerostomia, and hiccups. In B. R. Ferrell, N. Coyle, & J. Paice (Eds.), *Textbook of palliative nursing* (4th ed.). New York: Oxford University Press.

Jeon, Y. S., Kearney, A. M., & Baker, P. G. (2018). Management of hiccups in palliative care patients. *BMJ Supportive and Palliative Care, 8*, 1–6.

Moretto, E. N., Wee, B., Wiffen, P. J., & Murchison, A. G. (2013). Interventions for treating persistent and intractable hiccups in adults [review]. *Cochrane Database of Systematic Reviews*, (1), CD008768.

Wickham, R. (2019). Hiccups (singultus). In M. Hickey & S. Newton (Eds.), *Telephone triage for oncology nurses* (3rd ed.). Pittsburgh: Oncology Nursing Society.

Hyperglycemia

Deborah Lynn Kirk

Definition

- Increased amount of glucose in the blood
- Type 1: destruction of pancreatic β-cells due to a cellular-mediated autoimmune response
  - Rate of destruction is variable
- Type 2: combination of insulin resistance and insulin deficiency
  - Usually develops gradually

Pathophysiology and Contributing Factors

Prolonged elevated insulin levels may stimulate cancer cell proliferation in certain cancers. Diabetes increases risk for pancreatic, liver, breast, colorectal, urinary tract, gastric, and female reproductive cancers. Diabetes increases mortality rates in the cancer population. Glucose control is important for survivors to protect the health of their organs (e.g., eyes, heart, kidneys). Cancer survivors are often at increased risk for comorbidities such as diabetes, with variations seen based on risk factors and type of treatment.

- Type 1: Insulin deficiency is usually related to β-cell destruction.
  - Family history: A first-degree relative with diabetes greatly increases a person's risk.
  - Autoimmune disorders increase risk, including Addison disease, myasthenia gravis, celiac sprue, pernicious anemia, and Graves disease, among others.
  - The presence of certain genes may increase risk.
  - There is an increased risk for those farthest away from the equator.
  - Age: There are two peak periods: between 4 and 7 years, and between 10 and 14 years.
- Type 2: Defective insulin secretion with insulin resistance (typically obese).
  - Women with polycystic ovary syndrome, who delivered a baby weighing more than 9 lb, or who had a diagnosis of gestational diabetes mellitus.
  - Physical inactivity
  - Age 45 years or older
  - Overweight and obesity
  - Dietary factors:
    - High-fat foods
    - Processed foods
    - Red meats
    - Excessive alcohol intake
  - Hypertension
  - Hyperlipidemia
    - Fasting triglyceride level of 250 mg/dL or greater
    - High-density lipoprotein cholesterol level of 35 mg/dL or lower
  - Smoking
  - Family history: First-degree relative with diabetes greatly increases risk
  - Race/ethnicity:
    - African American
    - Latino
    - Native American
    - Asian American
    - Pacific Islander
  - History of cardiovascular disease
  - Infections
  - Kidney, liver, and pancreatic disease
  - Glycated hemoglobin (A_{1C}) of 5.7% or higher, impaired glucose tolerance (IGT), or impaired fasting glucose (IFG) on previous testing
  - Drugs (may alter glucose homeostasis)
    - Mammalian target of rapamycin (mTor): hyperglycemia
    - Tyrosine kinase inhibitor (TKI): hyperglycemia or hypoglycemia
    - Immune checkpoint inhibitors
    - Protease inhibitors
    - Corticosteroids
    - Octreotide
    - L-Asparaginase
    - Thiazides
    - Thyroid hormone
    - Atypical antipsychotics
    - Nonselective B-adrenergic antagonist
    - B-receptor agonist

Signs and Symptoms

- Symptoms vary from none to severe and life-threatening (e.g., diabetic ketoacidosis [DKA])
  - DKA: frequent urination, extreme thirst, nausea, vomiting, abdominal pain, confusion, breath that smells fruity, a flushed face, fatigue, weakness, and increased ketones in urine.
- Type 1 diabetics are more likely to present with elevated glucose levels and to have acute symptoms.
- Elevated glucose
- Frequent infections
- Slow wound healing
- Weight loss that is not intentional
- Visual changes
- Polyuria, polydipsia, polyphagia
- Tremors
- Tingling in hands and feet (early)
- Neuropathy in hands and feet (late)
- Fatigue
- Mood changes

Assessment Tools

- A complete past medical history, social history, and family history
- Vital signs, including body mass index (BMI), orthostatic blood pressure measures when indicated
- Physical examination
  - Eye examination to evaluate for retinopathy
  - Thyroid palpation
  - Skin evaluation to evaluate for integrity and any infections
  - Cardiac examination to look for any evidence of cardiac disease caused by elevated blood sugar levels
  - Peripheral vascular examination (pulses may be decreased with vascular disease)
  - Abdominal examination for hepatomegaly and assessment of injection sites if injecting insulin
  - Neurologic examination including reflexes and evaluation of proprioception
  - Comprehensive foot examination that includes evaluation for any fungal infection or breaks in skin
  - Psychiatric examination

Laboratory and Diagnostic Tests

- Consider testing overweight adults (BMI ≥ 25 kg/m^2, or 23 kg/m^2 in Asian Americans).
- Hemoglobin A_{1C}
  - Fasting is not required.
  - Stress and illness do not affect results as much as they do for random glucose levels.
  - Hemoglobinopathies and anemia may alter results.
  - Levels of hemoglobin A_{1C}: recommend individualizing goals; normal less than 5.7% for many nonpregnant adults with diabetes; prediabetes 5.7% to 6.4%; diabetes 6.5% or higher.
- Plasma glucose levels

- Fasting plasma glucose (FPG): normal is less than 100 mg/dL; prediabetes is 100 to 125 mg/dL; diabetes is 126 mg/dL or higher
- Two-hour plasma glucose (on the 75-g oral glucose tolerance test [OGTT]): normal is less than 140 mg/dL; prediabetes is 140 to 199 mg/dL; diabetes is 200 mg/dL or higher
- Other
  - Fasting lipid profile
  - Liver function studies
  - Serum creatinine and calculated glomerular filtration rate (GFR)
  - Thyroid-stimulating hormone level in type 1
  - Screen for increased urinary albumin excretion yearly
  - Serum creatinine level yearly
  - Vitamin B_{12} if on metformin
  - Spot urinary albumin-to-creatinine ratio

Differential Diagnoses

- Secondary diabetes mellitus
  - Drugs
  - Chemicals
- Pancreatitis
- Infection
- Paraneoplastic syndrome
- Cushing disease
- Diabetes insipidus

Interventions

- Individualized: weight loss through healthy diet and exercise if obese
- Prevention
- Treatment of disease
- Prevention and treatment of secondary effects and complications

Pharmacologic Interventions

- Type 1
  - Insulin
- Type 2
  - Metformin initially
  - May add a second oral agent (or basal insulin) if monotherapy is ineffective:
    - Orlistat
    - Thiazolidinediones
    - Gamma-glucosidase inhibitors
- For those with hypertension with low risk, the goal is less than 140/90 mm Hg; for those with high-risk less than 130/80 mm Hg
  - Angiotensin-converting enzyme inhibitor (ACEI), angiotensin receptor blocker (ARB), thiazide diuretics, or dihydropyridine calcium channel blockers
- Cholesterol management and control
  - Statin therapy should be initiated for those with cardiovascular disease

Nonpharmacologic Interventions

- Psychosocial assessment for depression, distress, anxiety, eating disorders, and cognitive impairment

- Lifestyle modifications
  - Weight loss
  - Moderate-intensity physical activity for 150 minutes per week
  - Nutrition

Patient Teaching

- Individualize the use of technology in the management of diabetes.
- Emphasis on self-management, helping the patient understand the following:
  - Diabetes as a disease
  - Healthy eating
  - Physical activity
  - Medications
  - Blood glucose monitoring
  - Blood pressure monitoring
  - Increased needs during illness
  - Long-term complications of diabetes
  - Health promotion
  - Behavior change
- Lifestyle
  - Nutrition
    - Healthy eating patterns that are personalized and culturally appropriate
    - Carbohydrate management with portion control and healthy food choices
    - Weight loss
    - Limited alcohol
    - Individualized sodium reduction
    - Limited calories from fat
    - Low-fat protein sources
    - Encouragement to record food intake
    - Importance of a healthy breakfast
    - Small portions when eating out
    - Self-weighing once per week
    - Choosing water to drink
    - Avoiding television watching while eating
  - Exercise
    - 150 minutes per week of moderate-intensity aerobic physical activity
    - No more than 2 days in a row without exercise
    - Resistance training twice a week
    - Exercise record keeping
    - Setting goals
  - Home blood pressure monitoring and blood pressure control (<140/90 mm Hg)
  - Routine cholesterol screening and control
  - Smoking cessation
    - Because of the increased risk of cardiovascular disease in those with diabetes, smoking cessation is recommended.
    - Refer to counseling if needed.
  - Self-monitoring of blood glucose
    - Frequency is individualized based on severity of hyperglycemia and agents used for treatment.
  - Foot care

- Risk of diabetic kidney disease
  - Importance of blood pressure control

Follow-Up

A multidisciplinary, comprehensive approach is needed and is individualized based on severity of symptoms. Follow-up and referrals should be made for the following:

- Eye care: annual eye examination for evaluation of retinal disease
- Foot examination at least annually, including pulse check
- Dietitian or diabetes educator
- Diabetes self-management support
- Dentist
- Mental health
- Immunizations (influenza, pneumococcus, hepatitis A)
- Hemoglobin A_{IC} measured at least twice a year, more often with changes in management or if not well controlled
- Endocrinology referral
- Cardiovascular workup including blood pressure control and monitoring
- Nephrologist if renal disease is apparent
- Neurologist for neuropathy

Resources

- List of interferences with A_{1C} measurement: https://ngsp.org/interf.asp
- Evidence-based lifestyle change programs: www.cdc.gov/diabetes/prevention/index.html
- Information for patients from National Institute of Diabetes and Digestive and Kidney Diseases: http://go.usa.gov/8n7F
- Diabetes and diet: https://www.heart.org/en/health-topics/diabetes/prevention--treatment-of-diabetes/the-diabetic-diet
- ChooseMyPlate: https://www.myplate.gov/
- 2018 Physical Activity Guidelines for Americans: https://health.gov/sites/default/files/2019-09/Physical_Activity_Guidelines_2nd_edition.pdf
- Resources for smoking cessation:
  - www.smokefree.gov
  - 1-800-QUIT-NOW
- American Association of Diabetes Educators: https://www.adcesconnect.org/home
- American Diabetes Association: https://diabetes.org/

Bibliography

American Diabetes Association. (2021). 2. Classification and diagnosis of diabetes: Standards of Medical Care in Diabetes—2021. *Diabetes Care, 44*(Suppl. 1). S15–S33.

American Diabetes Association. (2021). 3. Prevention or delay of type 2 diabetes: Standards of Medical Care in Diabetes—2021. *Diabetes Care, 44*(Suppl. 1), S34–S39.

American Diabetes Association. (2021). 4. Comprehensive medical evaluation and assessment of comorbidities: Standards of Medical Care in Diabetes—2021. *Diabetes Care, 44*(Suppl. 1), S40–S52.

American Diabetes Association. (2021). 5. Facilitating behavior change and wellbeing to improve health outcomes: Standards of Medical Care in Diabetes—2021. *Diabetes Care, 44*(Suppl. 1), S53–S72.

American Diabetes Association. (2021). 6. Glycemic targets: Standards of Medical Care in Diabetes—2021. *Diabetes Care, 44*(Suppl. 1), S73–S84.

American Diabetes Association. (2021). 7. Diabetes technology: Standards of Medical Care in Diabetes—2021. *Diabetes Care, 44*(Suppl. 1), S85–S99.

American Diabetes Association. (2021). 8. Obesity management for the treatment of type 2 diabetes: Standards of Medical Care in Diabetes—2021. *Diabetes Care*, 44(Suppl), S100–S110.

American Diabetes Association. (2021). 9. Pharmacologic approaches to glycemic treatment: Standards of Medical Care in Diabetes—2021. *Diabetes Care*, 44(Suppl. 1), S111–S124.

American Diabetes Association. (2021). 10. Cardiovascular disease and risk management: Standards of Medical Care in Diabetes—2021. *Diabetes Care*, 44(Suppl. 1), S125–S150.

American Diabetes Association. (2021). 11. Microvascular complications and foot care: Standards of Medical Care in Diabetes—2021. *Diabetes Care*, 44(Suppl. 1), S151–S167.

American Diabetes Association. (2021). *Understanding A1C diagnosis*. Available at https://www.diabetes.org/a1c/diagnosis.

Banday, M. Z., Sameer, A. S., & Nissar, S. (2020). Pathophysiology of diabetes: An overview. *Avicenna Journal of Medicine*, 10(4), 174–188.

Lega, I. C., & Lipscombe, L. L. (2020). Review: Diabetes, obesity, and cancer—pathophysiology and clinical implications. *Endocrine Reviews*, 41(1), 33–52.

McCoy, R. G., Galindo, R. J., Swarna, K. S., Van Houten, H. K., O'Connor, P. J., Guillermo, E., … Shah, N. D. (2021). Sociodemographic, clinical and treatment-related factors associated with hyperglycemic crises among adults with type 1 or type 2 diabetes in the US from 2014 to 2020. *JAMA Network Open*, 4(9), e2123471.

Srivastava, S. P., & Goodwin, J. E. (2020). Cancer biology and prevention of diabetes. *Cells*, 9, 1380.

Hypersensitivity Reactions

Colleen O'Leary

Definition

- Terms such as *drug reaction*, *drug allergy*, and *drug hypersensitivity* are often used interchangeably.
- Drug reaction includes all unwanted, uncomfortable, or dangerous adverse events from a drug regardless of cause.
- Drug allergies are specifically mediated by the immune system, causing an abnormal reaction.
- Drug hypersensitivity is an immune-mediated response to a drug in a patient who has been sensitized to the drug.
- Hypersensitivity reactions (HSRs) to chemotherapy and/or biotherapy are unexpected reactions with symptoms that are different from the normal side effects of the agent.
- Severity ranges from mild to anaphylaxis.
- Four categories have been identified:
  - Type I: immediate immunoglobulin E (IgE) mediated (most common type with chemotherapy)
  - Type II: antibody mediated
  - Type III: immune complex mediated
  - Type IV: delayed or cell mediated

Pathophysiology and Contributing Factors

- Type I reactions
  - Occur after exposure to a foreign substance or antigen.
  - Exposure causes IgE antibodies to form; they bind to receptors on mast cells in tissues or basophils in the peripheral blood.
  - With subsequent exposure to the antigen, the antigen attaches to the IgE antibody, causing mast cells to degranulate and release chemical mediators of this type of reaction into the peripheral blood.
  - Early-phase reactions occur within 15 minutes.
  - Late-phase reactions occur within 4 to 8 hours when cytokines, tumor necrosis factors, or granulocyte monocyte colony-stimulating factor (GM-CSF) are produced by the mast cells.
  - Histamines, leukotrienes, prostaglandins, and chemotactic are the chemical mediators.
  - Some drugs, such as paclitaxel and docetaxel, require mixture with synthetic solvents such as chremophor so they can be given parenterally. These solvents have been connected with severe to life-threatening reactions.
  - Nanoparticle albumin-bound paclitaxel (nabP) is solvent free, and there are few to no reactions associated with its administration.
- Type II reactions
  - They are caused by immunoglobulin G (IgG) or immunoglobulin M (IgM).
  - The immunoglobulin is released and forms an antibody-antigen complex, resulting in the signs and symptoms of this type of reaction.
- Type III reactions
  - IgG and IgM antibodies bind to antigens, causing immune complexes to be formed in the circulation and deposited in various tissues.
- Type IV reactions
  - These are cell-mediated or delayed-type reactions that involve the interaction of sensitized T lymphocytes with the antigen.
- Factors that influence the development and severity of reactions include the amount of antigen introduced, the route of entry (i.e., oral [PO], intravenous [IV]), and the rate of absorption (length of infusion).
- Cytokine release syndrome
  - It is a drug reaction common to biologic agents.
  - It results from a massive release of pro-inflammatory cytokines along with an imbalance in normal immune system.
  - It is associated with drugs that are directed to specific immune system targets, such as anti-CD19 and anti-CD20 antibodies.
  - The drug reacts with the antibody and releases cytokines such as tumor necrosis factor-α (TNF-α), interleukin-6 (IL-6), and interferons.
  - It can be exhibited by high fever, delirium, nausea, vomiting, abdominal pain, and/or diarrhea.
  - If left untreated, it can progress to hypotension and multiorgan failure.
- Risk factors for HSRs include type of drug administered, high doses, female gender, and history of prior allergic reactions to any type of medications.
  - Chemotherapy drugs with the highest potential for HSRs include L-asparaginase, taxanes, platinum compounds, epipodophyllotoxins, and procarbazine.
  - Chemotherapy drugs that occasionally cause HSRs include anthracyclines, dacarbazine, and 6-mercaptopurine.
  - Biotherapy drugs associated with HSRs and cytokine release syndrome include interferons, interleukins, and monoclonal antibodies.

Principles of Symptom Management

- Patients with a history of prior allergic reactions to food, insulin, opiates, penicillins, bee stings, blood products, or contrast media are at a higher risk for HSRs.

Signs and Symptoms

- Type I HSR: fever, rash, nausea, vomiting, flushing, urticaria, bronchospasm, hypotension, angioedema, feeling of impending doom, respiratory and cardiovascular collapse
- Type II HSR: hemolysis
- Type III HSR: tissue injury including vasculitis, nephritis, and arthritis
- Type IV HSR: contact dermatitis, graft rejection, formation of granulomas

Assessment Tools

- Baseline vital signs and assessment: frequent measurement of vital signs and assessment of symptoms throughout administration.

Laboratory and Diagnostic Tests

- There are no specific laboratory or diagnostic tests for HSRs; diagnosis is based on symptom assessment.

Differential Diagnoses vs. Diagnosis

- Drug allergy
- Drug reaction

Interventions

Pharmacologic Interventions

- Prevention is the mainstay of interventions. Premedication with corticosteroids such as dexamethasone; histamine receptor 1 (H_1) antagonists such as diphenhydramine; histamine receptor 2 (H_2) antagonists such as cimetidine, famotidine, and ranitidine; and antipyretics such as acetaminophen are commonly used.
- Desensitization protocols have been shown to be effective in type 1 and type 4 reactions.
- Medications for severe HSRs include adrenaline, crystalloid solutions, and oxygen.
- Rechallenge with premedications is often accomplished.

Nonpharmacologic Interventions

- At the first suspicion of HSRs, administration of the drug should be stopped.
- Place patient in supine position to promote organ profusion.
- Maintain airway, breathing, and circulation as indicated.
- Vital signs should be taken every 2 to 5 minutes until stable, and then every 15 minutes.

Patient Teaching

- Patients should be taught to tell the nurse of any changes experienced during their treatment, including itching, hives, shortness of breath, and cough.
- Often, patients cannot verbalize exactly what is wrong, but they know they just do not feel right. This is often the first indication of HSRs and should be taken seriously.

Follow-Up

- As needed to assess resolution of symptoms.

Resources

- American Cancer Society: www.cancer.org
- Chemocare.com: www.chemocare.com
- Canadian Cancer Society: www.cancer.ca
- National Cancer Institute: www.cancer.gov
- Oncology Nursing Society: www.ons.org

Bibliography

Buelow, B. (2020). Immediate hypersensitivity reaction clinical presentation. *Medscape*. Available at https://emedicine.medscape.com/article/136217-clinical.

Capelle, H., Tummino, C., Greillier, L., Gouitaa, M., Birnbaum, J., Ausias, N., … Montana, M. (2018). Retrospective study of hypersensitivity reactions to chemotherapeutic agents in a thoracic oncology service. *Journal of Clinical Pharmacy and Therapeutics, 43*(3), 320–326.

Dispenza, M. C. (2019). Classification of hypersensitivity reactions. *Allergy and Asthma Proceedings, 40*(6), 470–473.

Kang, Y., Kwon, O. Y., Jung, H., Kang, M., An, J., Lee, J. H., … Kim, T.-B. (2019). Breakthrough reactions during rapid drug desensitization: Clinical outcome and risk factors. *Annals of Allergy, Asthma & Immunology, 123*(1), 48–56.e1.

O'Leary, C., & DeVilliers, A. (2018). Hypersensitivity reactions to antineoplastic drugs. In C. H. Yarbro, D. Wujcik, & B. H. Gobel (Eds.), *Cancer nursing: Principles and practice* (8th ed.). Burlington, MA: Jones & Bartlett.

Pagani, M., Bavbek, S., Alvarez-Cuesta, E., Berna Dursun, A., Bonadonna, P., Castells, M., … Sanchez, S. S. (2022). Hypersensitivity reactions to chemotherapy: An EAACI position paper. *Allergy, 77*(2), 388–403.

Rosello, S., Blasco, I., Fabregat, L. G., Cervantes, A., Jordan, K., & ESMO Guidelines Committee. (2017). Management of infusion reactions to systemic anticancer therapy: ESMO clinical practice guidelines. *Annals of Oncology, 28*(Suppl. 4), 100–118.

Rounds, I. V. (2008). Handling a Type I hypersensitivity reaction. *Nursing, 38*(4), 60.

Tsao, L. R., Young, F. D., Otani, I. M., & Castells, M. C. (2021). Hypersensitivity reactions to platinum agents and taxanes. *Clinical Reviews in Allergy & Immunology, 62*(3), 432–448.

Vetter, M. H., Khan, A., Backes, F. J., Bixel, K., Cohn, D. E., Copeland, L. J., … O'Malley, D. M. (2019). Outpatient desensitization of patients with moderate (high-risk) to severe platinum hypersensitivity reactions. *Gynecologic Oncology, 152*(2), 316–321.

Yang, B. C., & Castells, M. C. (2022). The who, what, where, when, why, and how of drug desensitization. *Immunology and Allergy Clinics of North America, 42*(2), 403–420.

Lymphedema

Wendy H. Vogel

Definition

- Lymphedema is swelling from abnormal production of lymph fluid or because of an obstruction in the lymph circulation, usually in the upper or lower extremities.
- It occurs in approximately 20% of patients after a radical mastectomy and in 6% to 7% after modified radical mastectomy (worldwide statistics report incidences of up to 40%).
- Lower extremity lymphedema after pelvic or inguinal lymphadenectomy occurs in about 20% of patients.

Pathophysiology and Contributing Factors

- Primary lymphedema is rare, most often occurring as a birth defect.

- Secondary lymphedema usually develops as the result of obstruction or disruption of the lymphatic system by a tumor or trauma such as infection, surgery, or radiation therapy.
  - It may occur acutely or chronically, years after treatment.
  - Acute lymphedema subsides within a few weeks after surgery, when collateral circulation has developed.
  - The most common sites of lymph obstruction are the axillary, pelvic, and inguinal nodes.
- After surgery, if lymph fluid does not get rerouted or collateral circulation does not develop, the lymphatic system may not be able to accommodate the demand for drainage, and fluid may accumulate in the interstitial spaces, resulting in edema.
- If edema persists, the high protein concentration causes fibrosis of the subcutaneous tissue, leading to irreversible damage to the lymphatic system. Chronic lymphedema increases the risk of cellulitis, infections, and lymphangitis and decreases the quality of life.
- Lymphedema is more common in women who have undergone axillary dissection and radiation therapy with a dose greater than 46 Gy.
- Most patients develop lymphedema within 3 years after cancer treatment.
- Chronic lymphedema is lymphedema that persists for longer than 3 months.
- Risk factors include the following:
  - Lymph node dissection (usually, the greater the number of lymph nodes removed, the greater the risk of lymphedema)
  - Radiation therapy
  - Infection
  - Obesity
  - Trauma
  - Age
  - Breast cancer, ovarian cancer, lymphoma, or prostate cancer
  - Comorbidities such as congestive heart failure and neurologic, kidney, or liver disease
- Lymphedema is considered incurable; treatment is palliative, to prevent disease progression and alleviate symptoms.

Signs and Symptoms

- Swollen limb
- Swollen axilla or groin area
- May extend to face, neck, or genitalia.
- Signs of infection or inflammation may be present.
- Patients may report edema, heaviness, tightness, firmness, pain, aching, numbness, tingling, stiffness, limb fatigue, or impaired limb mobility even in early stages before lymphedema is visually noticeable.

Assessment Tools

- Obtain a thorough history:
  - Possible sources, signs, and symptoms of infection
  - Any unusual or heavy lifting or activity
  - Repetitive-type movements

- Time frame with regard to surgery or trauma
- Activity level
- Nutrition
- Comorbid conditions
- Evaluate psychosocial factors:
  - Assess impact on body image, sexuality, social activities, work.
  - Assess for anger, social avoidance, sexual dysfunction, poor adjustment.
- Assess for pain.
- Perform a physical examination:
  - Measure the affected limb, using anatomic landmarks for accuracy in follow-up assessments. Compare with unaffected limb. Serial measurements allow assessment of changes over time.
  - Assess for signs and symptoms of infection.
  - Measure pulses and range of motion.
  - Assess the strength of the affected limb.
  - Check affected areas for the presence of suspicious masses or tumor recurrence.
  - Grade the severity (International Society of Lymphology):
    - *Stage 0:* Subclinical lymphedema—no visible edema, but symptoms of heaviness (may be present for months or years before progressing).
    - *Stage I:* Mild—2- to 3-cm difference between limbs; feelings of heaviness, throbbing, or soreness. May subside with elevation.
    - *Stage II:* Moderate—3- to 5-cm difference between limbs, visibly noticeable; skin may be stretched and shiny; pitting edema may be present; tissue is soft. Elevation rarely reduces edema.
    - *Stage III:* Severe—greater than 5-cm difference between limbs; skin stretched and discolored to purple or brown; skin tough, brawny, with peau d'orange appearance; tissue may be firm, nonpitting.

Laboratory and Diagnostic Tests

- Rule out venous swelling (e.g., venous obstruction or thrombus) with color flow Doppler ultrasonography or venography.
- Perform computed tomography (CT) or magnetic resonance imaging (MRI) of the axilla or groin to rule out tumor recurrence.
- Bioelectric impedance analysis measures impedance and resistance of extracellular fluid.
- Perform lymphoscintigraphy as indicated.
- Perform blood urea nitrogen (BUN), creatinine, liver function tests, albumin, urinalysis, and liver function tests to rule out possible systemic causes.

Differential Diagnoses

- Thrombus
- Infection
- Cirrhosis
- Nephrosis

- Congestive heart failure
- Myxedema (severe hypothyroidism)
- Hypoalbuminemia
- Chronic venous stasis
- Obstruction from pelvic or abdominal malignancy

Interventions

Pharmacologic Interventions

- Gold standard: complete decongestive physiotherapy (CDP) after recurrent malignancy is ruled out:
  - Phase I: Therapist administers manual lymphatic massage, compression bandaging, exercises, and skin care.
  - Phase II: Patient self-care activities, including use of compression garments, night wrappings, skin care, self-massage (manual lymph drainage), and continued exercises.
  - Maintenance activities are time-consuming and are required lifelong; cost may be problematic for some patients. Adherence can be difficult but is necessary to prevent progression.
- Intermittent pneumatic gradient sequential pump therapy
- Compression garments that are properly fitted
- Elevation of edematous extremity
- Referral to physical therapy or surgery as indicated; specific exercises and surgical interventions may improve mobility but must be balanced with potential harms
- Pain management
- Referral to support group or support resources as appropriate
- Diuretics, used only temporarily if at all; effects are generally minimal. Little evidence exists for pharmacologic therapy of cancer-related lymphedema.

Nonpharmacologic Interventions

- Prevention is key:
  - Encourage exercise, particularly strengthening exercises and aerobic activities.
  - Perform no heavy, dependent lifting of more than 15 lb.
  - Avoid breaks in the skin (e.g., wear gloves when gardening).
  - Prevent infection or treat promptly if it occurs.
  - Encourage good hygiene and precautions against trauma.
  - Encourage a well-balanced, low-sodium, high-fiber diet.
  - Maintain ideal body weight.
  - Consider wearing a well-fitted compression garment on long flights (National Lymphedema Network, Position Statement on Air Travel, May 2011. Available at https://issuu.com/lymphnet/docs/air.travel [accessed December 31, 2021]).

Patient Teaching

- Prevention education is the best risk reduction tool.
- Avoid trauma and breaks in the skin in the affected extremity.
- Practice good hygiene to avoid introduction of bacteria to potential open areas of the affected extremity.
- Avoid heavy, dependent lifting or vigorous, repetitive motions against resistance.
- Avoid venipuncture, chemotherapy, blood product administration, injection, and assessment of blood pressure in the affected extremity unless need outweighs the potential consequences.
- Be aware of and report signs and symptoms of infection.
- Avoid having the limb in a dependent position for long periods, as with travel.
- Refer to patient teaching sheet in "Section Seven."

Follow-Up

- Periodically assess for intervention success with visual inspection and serial measurements of anatomic landmarks.
- Provide referrals as appropriate, especially for CDP if necessary.

Resources

- American Cancer Society: www.cancer.org
- Breast cancer.org: www.breastcancer.org
- National Cancer Institute: www.cancer.gov
- The National Lymphedema Network: www.lymphnet.org

Bibliography

Armer, J. M., Ostby, P. L., Ginex, P. K., Beck, M., Deng, J., Fu, M. R., … Morgan, R. L. (2020). ONS Guidelines™ for cancer treatment–related lymphedema. *Oncology Nursing Forum*, 47(5), 518–538.

Ding, J., Hasan, B., Malandris, K., Farah, M. H., Manolopoulos, A., Ginex, P. K., … Murad, M. H. (2020). Prospective surveillance and risk reduction of cancer treatment–related lymphedema: Systematic review and meta-analysis. *Oncology Nursing Forum*, 47(5), E161–E170.

Eidenberger, M. (2021). Patient-reported outcome measures with secondary lower limb lymphedemas: A systematic review. *Journal of the Advanced Practitioner in Oncology*, 12(2), 174–187.

Lytvyn, L., Zeraatkar, D., Anbari, A. B., Ginex, P. K., Zoratti, M., Niburski, K., … Morgan, R. L. (2020). Conservative intervention strategies for adult cancer-related lymphedema: A systematic review and network meta-analysis. *Oncology Nursing Forum*, 47(5), E171–E189.

McLaughlin, S., Brunelle, C., & Taghian, A. (2020). Breast cancer–related lymphedema: Risk factors, screening, management, and the impact of locoregional treatment. *Journal of Clinical Oncology*, 38(20), 2341–2350.

National Lymphedema Network. (2011a). *Position statement of the National Lymphedema Network: Air travel.* Available at https://issuu.com/lymphnet/docs/air.travel (accessed December 31, 2021).

National Lymphedema Network. (2011b). *Position statement of the National Lymphedema Network: Exercise.* Available at https://issuu.com/lymphnet/docs/exercise (accessed December 31, 2021).

National Lymphedema Network. (2012). *Position statement of the National Lymphedema Network: Lymphedema risk reduction practices.* Available at https://issuu.com/lymphnet/docs/risk_reduction (accessed December 31, 2021).

Menopausal Symptoms

Wendy H. Vogel

Definition

- Menopause is a hormonal change that occurs when estrogen and progesterone levels begin to drop.
- It usually occurs between the ages of 45 and 55 years; however, it can also be surgically or chemically induced.
- The average age at menopause in the United States is 51 years.

- There are increasing numbers of women who have menopausal symptoms after treatment for cancer.
- Early menopause can have long-lasting effects on a woman's quality of life.

Pathophysiology and Contributing Factors

- Physiologic menopause is caused by exhaustion of the ovarian follicles, which contain the germ cells that produce the steroid hormones estrogen and progesterone.
- Premature ovarian failure is cessation of ovarian function before the age of 40 years.
- Ovarian failure may be induced by radiation therapy, chemotherapy, surgery, or infection.
- When a decreased level of hormone is detected by the hypothalamus, the pituitary gland secretes follicle-stimulating hormone (FSH) and luteinizing hormone (LH). In menopause, the ovaries are unable to respond to the FSH and LH; therefore, estrogen deficiency occurs, ovulation does not occur, and the woman becomes amenorrheic.
- Vasomotor instability (a hot flash) is caused by dysfunction of the thermoregulatory center in the hypothalamus.
  - There is a sharp rise in epinephrine, which stimulates heart function, a rise in blood pressure, and an intense feeling of warmth throughout the upper body with flushing and perspiration that may last as little as a few seconds or as long as 20 minutes.
  - Estrogen influences the firing rate of the thermosensitive neurons in the preoptic area of the hypothalamus and affects how responsive vascular smooth muscle is to vasoactive substances such as epinephrine and norepinephrine.
  - Symptoms may resolve spontaneously over time without treatment.
- Cancer survivors, especially those who have had breast cancer (65% to 80% of breast cancer survivors), may experience more vasomotor symptoms and at an earlier age.
- A few years after estrogen deprivation, women begin to experience genitourinary symptoms, primarily as a result of decreased arterial blood flow to vagina and vulva. This occurs in an estimated 50% to 75% of breast cancer survivors. The following symptoms may increase over time and may persist indefinitely:
  - Atrophy of the vaginal wall
  - Vaginal dryness, infections, bleeding, and burning sensations
  - Dyspareunia
  - Urinary symptoms occurring as a result of urogenital atrophy
  - Decreased libido, which may occur because of loss of ovarian function, also decreases serum androgen levels.
- Psychological changes:
  - Estrogen increases the degradation rate of monoamine oxidase, the enzyme that catabolizes serotonin.
  - Serotonin deficiency is believed to contribute to depression.
  - Decreased bone density occurs because of the imbalance between bone resorption and formation. Early estrogen deprivation can lead to osteoporosis and potential fractures.
- The risk for heart disease is increased because risk is relative to the age at which estrogen deprivation occurs.

Signs and Symptoms

- Can be mild or severe
- Change in or cessation of menses
- Vasomotor symptoms such as hot flashes and night sweats
- Vaginal atrophy, thinning of the vaginal wall, dryness, dyspareunia, postcoital bleeding
- Urinary symptoms such as urgency, stress incontinence, and frequent urinary tract infections
- Emotional lability, mood changes, irritability
- Cognitive changes such as forgetfulness or decreased ability to concentrate or make decisions; depression
- Weight gain in hips and thighs
- Sleep disturbances
- Decreased skin elasticity

Assessment Tools

- Thorough history and physical examination to determine the cause of menopausal symptoms.
- Pelvic examination, observing for vaginal atrophy and associated difficulties
- Assessment of the characteristics, frequency, and severity of symptoms

Laboratory and Diagnostic Tests

- FSH
- LH
- Serum estradiol
- Mean estrone level
- Urinalysis, presence of urinary tract symptoms
- Bone density testing
- Lipid panel

Differential Diagnoses

- Ovarian abnormalities
- Polycystic ovarian syndrome
- Pregnancy
- Hypothalamic dysfunction
- Hypothyroidism
- Pituitary tumors
- Adrenal abnormalities
- Ovarian neoplasm
- Tuberculosis
- Bone loss
- Lipid profile elevations

Interventions

Pharmacologic Interventions

- Hormone replacement therapy (HRT) is a controversial subject in postmenopausal women because of various health risks, including breast cancer. However, it is not always contraindicated.

- HRT options involve different doses of estrogen or combinations of estrogen and progesterone or testosterone and different levels of systemic absorption depending on the route of administration.
- HRT is contraindicated in patients who have experienced a stroke or thromboembolic event, recent myocardial infarction, acute liver or pancreatic disease, or undiagnosed vaginal bleeding.
- For menopausal symptoms, HRT may be considered but should be given for the shortest period possible (ideally, <5 years).
- HRT should be chosen to match the specific menopausal complaints and to provide maximum safety.
- HRT options include oral estrogens, vaginal estrogens, and transdermal estrogens, each of which can involve various hormone combinations. A full discussion of benefits and risks of HRT should ensue between the patient and the health care provider.
- In the oncology patient, careful consideration should be given to hormone-related cancer, and the risks of cancer stimulation should be evaluated.
- The lowest possible dose of estrogen should be chosen. Oral doses and vaginal doses as low as 0.3 mg may provide relief from hot flashes and vaginal discomfort, although the lower doses may have a somewhat delayed response. Consider adding a progestin if a patient remains symptomatic.
- Local estrogen products may be used for vaginal and urinary complaints and have less systemic absorption.
- Minimizing progestin exposure decreases the rate of endometrial hyperplasia. Progestins may be given less frequently, such as quarterly or biannually, to women taking lower dose estrogens.
- Topical estrogens may be useful for vaginal and urinary symptoms, but the potential risks should be reviewed with the patient.
- Zoledronic acid is in clinical trials for the prevention of bone loss in postmenopausal women with breast cancer who are taking an aromatase inhibitor.
- Nonhormonal pharmacologic options for vasomotor symptoms include the following:
  - Clonidine, oral or transdermal
- Venlafaxine, fluoxetine, citalopram, or paroxetine (caution is advised because of possible interactions between selective serotonin reuptake inhibitors or serotonin-norepinephrine reuptake inhibitors and tamoxifen)
- Bellergal or Bellergal-S (ergotamine, belladonna, and phenobarbital)
- Propranolol
- Lofexidine
- Vitamin E 400 IU twice daily; also vitamins B and C
- Ginseng
- Megace acetate and medroxyprogesterone have been used; however, their safety in patients with a hormonally sensitive tumor is not fully known. Progestins can stimulate proliferation of the endometrium when given alone. Potential risks and benefits of treatment must be considered carefully and discussed with the patient.

- Phytoestrogens and black cohosh have been used, but the safety of these interventions is not known, and the results in many studies show effects similar to those of placebo.
- Gabapentin is being evaluated in clinical trials for the treatment of hot flashes, but side effects may limit its use.

Nonpharmacologic Interventions

- For hot flashes (effectiveness not established):
  - Yoga
  - Acupuncture
  - Paced respirations
  - Trained relaxation techniques
  - Cognitive behavioral therapy
  - Avoidance of hot flash triggers such as alcohol, hot drinks, or spicy foods
- Follow a low-fat diet, cease smoking, allow low to moderate alcohol intake, maintain a healthy weight, and avoid a sedentary lifestyle.
- Weight reduction and moderate exercise of 30 minutes or more on most days of the week should be recommended.
- Vaginal lubricants, such as Replens (Auspharm, Australia), may be helpful for vaginal dryness.
- Insomnia may be treated both pharmacologically and nonpharmacologically.
- Osteoporosis prevention and treatment:
  - Bisphosphonates may be prescribed for patients with osteopenia or osteoporosis.
  - Raloxifene, a selective receptor modulator, is also approved for the prevention and treatment of osteoporosis. It should not be given with an aromatase inhibitor or with tamoxifen. Raloxifene may increase hot flashes.
  - Patients should be advised to take calcium and vitamin D, to perform weight-bearing exercise, and to avoid smoking and excessive alcohol intake.

Patient Teaching

- Patients should understand the fertility risks and the potential for early menopause before undergoing cancer treatment.
- If HRT is considered, the risks and benefits must be fully explored with the patient.
- Prevention and screening for osteoporosis and maintenance of bone health are important.

Follow-Up

- Follow up as needed to assess symptom management
- Sleep hygiene or bladder training as appropriate

Resources

- American Cancer Society: www.cancer.org
- Breastcancer.org: www.breastcancer.org
- Chemocare.org: www.chemocare.org
- National Cancer Institute: www.cancer.gov

Bibliography

Crean-Tate, K. K., Faubion, S. S., Pederson, H. J., Vencill, J. A., & Batur, P. (2020). Management of genitourinary syndrome of menopause in female cancer patients: A focus on vaginal hormonal therapy. *American Journal of Obstetrics and Gynecology, 222*(2), 103–113.

Frazier, S., & Egger, M. (2014). Menopausal symptoms. In C. Yarbro, D. Wujcik, & B. Gobel (Eds.), *Cancer symptom management* (4th ed.). Burlington, MA: Jones & Bartlett.

Kaplan, M., Mahon, S. M., Lubejko, B. G., & Ginex, P. K. (2020). Hot flashes: Clinical summary of the ONS Guidelines™ for cancer treatment-related hot flashes in women with breast cancer and men with prostate cancer. *Clinical Journal of Oncology Nursing, 24*(4), 430–433.

Lupo, M., Dains, J. E., & Madsen, L. T. (2015). Hormone replacement therapy: An increased risk of recurrence and mortality for breast cancer patients? *Journal of the Advanced Practitioner in Oncology, 6*(4), 322–330.

Mahon, S. M., & Carr, E. (2021). Hot flashes: Common side effect. *Clinical Journal of Oncology Nursing, 25*(6), 28.

Matthews, E. (2018). Sleep disturbances. In C. Yarbro, D. Wujcik, & B. Gobel (Eds.), *Cancer symptom management* (8th ed.). Burlington, MA: Jones & Bartlett.

Potter, B., Schrager, S., Dalby, J., Torell, E., & Hampton, A. (2018). Menopause. *Primary Care, 45*(4), 625–641.

Rees, M., Angioli, R., Coleman, R. L., Glasspool, R., Plotti, F., Simoncini, T., & Terranova, C. (2020). European Menopause and Andropause Society (EMAS) and International Gynecologic Cancer Society (IGCS) position statement on managing the menopause after gynecological cancer: Focus on menopausal symptoms and osteoporosis. *Maturitas, 134,* 56–61.

Santen, R. J., Stuenkel, C. A., Davis, S. R., Pinkerton, J. V., Gompel, A., & Lumsden, M. A. (2017). Managing menopausal symptoms and associated clinical issues in breast cancer survivors. *The Journal of Clinical Endocrinology and Metabolism, 102*(10), 3647–3661.

Sheng, Y., Carpenter, J. S., Cohee, A. A., Storey, S., Stump, T. E., Monahan, P. O., & Champion, V. L. (2021). Genitourinary symptoms in breast cancer survivors: Prevalence, correlates, and relationship with sexual functioning. *Oncology Nursing Forum, 48*(2), 229–241.

Szabo, R., Marino, J., & Hickey, M. (2019). Managing menopausal symptoms after cancer. *Climacteric, 22*(6), 572–578.

Mucositis

Annette Brant Isozaki

Definition

- Mucositis is an inflammatory process that affects the mucous membranes of the oral cavity and gastrointestinal tract.
- It is commonly associated with chemotherapy, radiation therapy, and hematopoietic stem cell and bone marrow transplantation.
- It can occur anywhere along the digestive tract, from the mouth to the anus; in the mouth or oropharynx, it is referred to as oral mucositis.
- It occurs in 30% to 40% of patients treated with chemotherapy.
- Approximately 90% of patients receiving chemotherapy and radiation therapy for head and neck cancer and as many as 60% to 85% of patients undergoing hematopoietic stem cell transplantation (HSCT) experience mucositis.
- It is the most significant adverse symptom of cancer treatment reported by patients.
- Mucositis adds substantial health care costs and prolongs hospitalization.

Pathophysiology and Contributing Factors

- Breakdown of rapidly dividing epithelial cells caused by chemotherapy and radiation treatment, primarily in the gastrointestinal tract
- Previous history of mucositis
- Poor oral hygiene, prior dental disease
- Ill-fitting dentures
- Type of treatment and dose regimen

- Size and location of tumor
- History of kidney disease, diabetes, or human immunodeficiency virus (HIV) infection
- Age younger than 20 years or older than 50 years
- History of alcohol use and smoking
- Poor performance status
- Inflammatory bowel disease increases risk of gastrointestinal mucositis
- Genetic factors that can alter the metabolism of the chemotherapy

Signs and Symptoms

- Dry, cracked lips
- Pain and difficulty swallowing
- Soreness or pain in the mouth or throat; usually begins as asymptomatic erythema of the oral mucosa that may feel like burning or tingling in the mouth
- Red, shiny, or swollen mouth and gums
- Ulcers or sores in the mouth, on gums, and on the tongue; the sores may be reddish and may have white centers
- Mucosal bleeding
- Sensitivity to hot and cold foods
- Feeling of dryness (xerostomia), mild burning, or pain
- Infection
- Weight loss
- Dehydration
- Diarrhea
- Epigastric pain, dysphagia

Assessment Tools

- Oral Assessment Guide (OAG)
- Oral Mucositis Index (OMI)
- Oral Mucositis Assessment Scale (OMAS)
- Common terminology criteria for adverse events (CTCAE) v4.0
- World Health Organization (WHO) scale for oral mucositis
- Head and Neck Radiotherapy Questionnaire
- Inflammatory Bowel Disease Questionnaire
- Eastern Cooperative Oncology Group (EGOG) common toxicity criteria
- Important to include patient's subjective report as there is relatively low inter-rater reliability between tools
- History and physical examination; clinical examination based on inspection of oral cavity
- Risk for mucositis
- Current oral hygiene and dental care
- Nutritional status
- Symptomatic functional assessment based on ability to swallow
- Pain, using a scale of 0 to 10 or a categorical scale (none, mild, moderate, or severe)

Laboratory and Diagnostic Tests

- Complete blood count (CBC)
- Blood, urine, and sputum cultures
- Stool specimen
- Endoscopy and flexible sigmoidoscopy

Differential Diagnoses

- Infection—oral or gastrointestinal
- Dysphagia
- Heartburn
- Bleeding—oral
- Xerostomia
- Peptic ulcer disease
- Gastritis
- Chemotherapy-induced diarrhea

Interventions

- Prevent mucositis
- Adequate nursing assessment and early identification
- Treat the underlying cause
- Provide pain and symptom management

Pharmacologic Interventions

- Palifermin (Kepivance)
- Benzydamine mouthwash
- Viscous lidocaine
- Opioids
- Total parenteral nutrition (TPN), if mucositis is severe
- Hyperbaric oxygen therapy
- Probiotics containing *Lactobacillus*
- Oral glutamine
- Zinc

Nonpharmacologic Interventions

- Basic oral care/hygiene
- Monitor nutritional intake and weight; consult a dietician
- Cryotherapy
- Low-level laser therapy (LLLT) for patients undergoing HSCT
- Saline and sodium bicarbonate rinses
- Intraoral photobiomodulation

Patient Teaching

- Dental evaluation before initiation of treatment and biannually.
- Dietary counseling
  - A soft, bland diet may be more tolerable.
  - High-protein diet
  - Limit salty, acidic, spicy, or rough foods.
- Cleaning:
  - Brush with a soft toothbrush.
  - Continue despite thrombocytopenia or neutropenia unless uncontrolled bleeding develops.
  - Use fluoride toothpaste.
- Floss daily
  - Patients who floss regularly should continue unless there is uncontrolled bleeding, the platelet level falls to less than 20,000 per microliter, or the absolute neutrophil count (ANC) is less than 1 per microliter.
- Rinsing:
  - Normal saline solution (NS), sodium bicarbonate (NaHCO$_3$), NS/NaHCO$_3$, water
  - Nonalcoholic, nonmedicated, unsweetened mouthwash

- Before meals, and increasing to every 2 hours as needed for comfort (swish/gargle for 15 to 30 seconds).
- Dental appliances should be left out as much as possible once mucous membranes become irritated.
- Maintain adequate hydration.
- Avoid tobacco and alcohol
- Report any fever of 100.5°F (38°C) or greater.
- Report any pain that is unrelieved with pain medication.

Follow-Up

- Assess for increased risk of mucositis with continuing treatments.
- Assess for pain that is unrelieved with pain medication.
- Reinforce the importance of communication with physician and nurse.

Resources

- American Cancer Society. Caring for the patient with cancer at home: Mouth sores: http://www.cancer.org/treatment/treatmentsandsideeffects/physicalsideeffects/dealingwithsymptomsathome/caring-for-the-patient-with-cancer-at-home-mouth-sores
- National Cancer Institute. Oral complications of chemotherapy and head/neck radiation (PDQ): http://www.cancer.gov/about-cancer/treatment/side-effects/mouth-throat/oral-complications-pdq
- National Institute of Dental and Craniofacial Research. Oral complications of cancer treatment: What the oncology team can do: http://www.nidcr.nih.gov/oralhealth/Topics/CancerTreatment/OralComplicationsCancerOncology.htm
- Oncolink: Cancer resources for patients and health care professionals. Mucositis: The basics: http://www.oncolink.org/coping/article.cfm?id=965
- Oncology Nursing Society. Putting evidence into practice: Mucositis: https://www.ons.org/practice-resources/pep/mucositis

Bibliography

Abreu, A. M., Fraga, D. R. D. S., Giergowicz, B. B., Figueiró, R. B., & Waterkemper, R. (2021). Effectiveness of nursing interventions in preventing and treating radiotherapy side effects in cancer patients: A systematic review. *Revista da Escola de Enfermagem da U S P, 55*, e03697.

Ariyawardana, A., Cheng, K. K. F., Kandwal, A., Tilly, V., Al-Azri, A. R., Galiti, D., ... Mucositis Study Group of the Multinational Association of Supportive Care in Cancer/International Society for Oral Oncology (MASCC/ISOO). (2019). Systematic review of anti-inflammatory agents for the management of oral mucositis in cancer patients and clinical practice guidelines. *Support Care Cancer, 27*(10), 3985–3995.

Bowen, J., Al-Dasooqi, N., Bossi, P., Wardill, H., Van Sebille, Y., Al-Azri, A., ... Mucositis Study Group of the Multinational Association of Supportive Care in Cancer/International Society for Oral Oncology (MASCC/ISOO). (2019). The pathogenesis of mucositis: Updated perspectives and emerging targets. *Support Care Cancer, 27*(10), 4023–4033.

Bowen, J. M., Gibson, R. J., Coller, J. K., Blijlevens, N., Bossi, P., Al-Dasooqi, N., ... Mucositis Study Group of the Multinational Association of Supportive Care in Cancer/International Society for Oral Oncology (MASCC/ISOO). (2019). Systematic review of agents for the management of cancer treatment-related gastrointestinal mucositis and clinical practice guidelines. *Support Care Cancer, 27*(10), 4011–4022.

Hong, C. H. L., Gueiros, L. A., Fulton, J. S., Cheng, K. K. F., Kandwal, A., Galiti, D., ... Mucositis Study Group of the Multinational Association of Supportive Care in Cancer/International Society for Oral Oncology (MASCC/ISOO). (2019). Systematic review of basic oral care for the management of oral mucositis in cancer patients and clinical practice guidelines. *Support Care Cancer, 27*(10), 3949–3967.

Pulito, C., Cristaudo, A., Porta, C. L., Zapperi, S., Blandino, G., Morrone, A., & Strano, S. (2020). Oral mucositis: the hidden side of cancer therapy. *Journal of Experimental & Clinical Cancer Research, 39*(1), 210.

Steinmann, D., Babadağ Savaş, B., Felber, S., Joy, S., Mertens, I., Cramer, H., & Voiss, P. (2021). Nursing procedures for the prevention and treatment of mucositis induced by cancer therapies: Clinical practice guideline based on an interdisciplinary consensus process and a systematic literature search. *Integrative Cancer Therapies, 20.* 1534735420940412.

Wardill, H. R., Sonis, S. T., Blijlevens, N. M. A., Van Sebille, Y. Z. A., Ciorba, M. A., Loeffen, E. A. H., ... Mucositis Study Group of the Multinational Association of Supportive Care in Cancer/International Society of Oral Oncology (MASCC/ISOO). (2020). Prediction of mucositis risk secondary to cancer therapy: A systematic review of current evidence and call to action. *Support Care Cancer, 28*(11), 5059–5073.

Yarom, N., Hovan, A., Bossi, P., Ariyawardana, A., Jensen, S. B., Gobbo, M., ... Mucositis Study Group of the Multinational Association of Supportive Care in Cancer/International Society of Oral Oncology (MASCC/ISOO). (2019). Systematic review of natural and miscellaneous agents for the management of oral mucositis in cancer patients and clinical practice guidelines—Part 1: Vitamins, minerals, and nutritional supplements. *Support Care Cancer, 27*(10), 3997–4010.

Nail Changes

Colleen O'Leary

Definition

- The types and severity of nail changes depend on the drug, dose, duration, and frequency of treatment.
- Nail changes include the following:
  - Changes in nail color
  - Growth reduction
  - Beau lines—deep horizontal grooves across the nails
  - Mees' lines—horizontal lines of white/opaque discoloration across nails reflecting damage to the distal nail matrix and moving distally with nail growth
  - Onycholysis—lifting of the nail from nail bed
  - Paronychia—inflammation of skin folds around nail
  - Onychomycosis—fungal nail infection
  - Ingrown toenails
  - Pincer nails—type of ingrown nail in which an overcurvature causes the nail to penetrate into the soft tissue
- Nail changes occur frequently, especially with the use of taxanes, epidermal growth factor receptor (EGFR) inhibitors, mammalian target of rapamycin (mTOR) inhibitors, and monoclonal antibodies.
- Nail changes seen with chronic graft-versus-host disease (GVHD) can range from mild nail dystrophy to anonychia and include the following:
  - Nail loss
  - Dystrophy
  - Longitudinal ridging
  - Splitting or brittle nails
  - Onycholysis
  - Pterygium—abnormal adherence of the nail plate to the proximal nail fold
- It is important to distinguish between GVHD nail changes and infectious processes.
- The most common nail infections are paronychial infections and onychomycosis.

Pathophysiology and Contributing Factors

- There are multiple mechanisms of adverse nail changes, including changes to the nail bed and surrounding tissue and sensitivity to environmental factors such as exposure to chemicals, polishes, or harsh detergents and prolonged water or ultraviolet exposure.
- Often more than one process is involved.
- Changes to the nail bed and nail can be caused by defective nail matrix production, resulting from effects of cancer treatments (chemotherapy and molecularly targeted agents) on maturation of cells, and by direct toxicity to structures surrounding the nail.
- Nail color changes result from toxins related to chemotherapy that alter melanocytes in the epithelium of the nail matrix.
- Toxins from the chemotherapy can cause damage to the nail bed and edema under the nail bed, resulting in onycholysis.
- Toxin-related damage to soft tissue surrounding the nails can lead to paronychia and possible secondary infection.
- Changes such as splinter hemorrhage and subungual hemorrhage may result when patients are thrombocytopenic.
- Frequency and duration of treatment contribute to nail changes; patients receiving taxanes for longer than 6 weeks are predisposed to nail changes.
- More adverse nail changes are seen in patients receiving treatments every week rather than every 3 weeks.
- Some research indicates that chemotherapy makes nails more sensitive to ultraviolet light, which can cause further damage.
- Certain types of chemotherapy, such as taxanes, EGFR inhibitors, and mTOR inhibitors, confer a greater risk for nail changes.

Signs and Symptoms

- The National Cancer Institute's common terminology criteria for adverse effects (CTCAE) are used to grade nail changes based on symptoms such as nail discoloration, nail loss, and nail ridging.
  - Nail discoloration:
    - Grade 1: Asymptomatic; clinical or diagnostic observations only
  - Nail loss:
    - Grade 1: Asymptomatic separation of the nail bed from the nail plate or nail loss
    - Grade 2: Symptomatic separation of the nail bed from the nail plate or nail loss; limiting instrumental activities of daily living
  - Nail ridging:
    - Asymptomatic; clinical or diagnostic observations only
    - Intervention not indicated.
- Painful paronychias are most common and can involve multiple nails, especially the thumbs and great toes.
- Paronychial lesions may bleed easily.

Assessment Tools

- Observation of nails and surrounding skin is the most effective means of assessing for nail changes.

Laboratory and Diagnostic Tests

- There are no specific tests for nail changes other than observation. However, if infection is suspected, consideration should be given to obtaining cultures to tailor treatment.

Differential Diagnoses

- Infection
- Trauma

Interventions

Pharmacologic Interventions

- Oral or intravenous antibiotics for culture-proven paronychia.
- Empiric antibiotics initiated in immunocompromised patients.
- Soaks with Burow solution (4% thymol in alcohol with aluminum acetate).
- Silver nitrate and ferric subsulfate to act as chemical cautery.
- Topical corticosteroids to reduce inflammation.

Nonpharmacologic Interventions

- Soaking nails in warm water two or three times a day can help reduce swelling and pain.
- Soaking with white vinegar (1:10) or bleach (0.25 cup bleach to 3 gallons water) for 10 minutes a day can provide relief from pain, decrease the microbe count, and prevent superinfections.
- Hydrating nail solutions consisting of purified thermal spring water, polyacrylate-16, chlorphenesin, xanthan gum, phenoxyethanol, caprylyl glycol, and piroctone olamine painted on docetaxel-induced onycholytic nails can reduce the grading of nail changes.
- Frozen glove cryotherapy reduces nail toxicity associated with taxane therapy.

Patient Teaching

- Keep nails trimmed and clean.
- Wear gloves when gardening or house cleaning.
- Paint nails to hide blemishes and increase nail strength.
- Remove nail polish with nonacetone remover only.
- Do not bite or tear nails.
- Do not pick at cuticles.
- Use cuticle removal cream or gel.
- Massage cuticle cream into nail area daily to avoid dryness and hangnails.
- Limit the time your hands are in water.
- Avoid professional manicures unless you bring all of your own equipment.
- Do not use artificial nails.
- If ingrown nails occur, soak them in warm water and apply antibiotic cream. If area is painful, is swollen, or has discharge, contact your health care provider.
- Tell your health care provider about any signs of inflammation or infection.
- If you need to bandage an area, use paper tape.
- Soak nails in vegetable or olive oil daily and gently massage.
- Wear comfortable shoes that do not rub.
- If an infectious organism is identified, discard or wash in hot, soapy water with bleach any slippers, socks, or gloves that might have become contaminated.

Follow-Up

- As needed to assess signs and symptoms.
- Refer patient to podiatry and/or dermatology specialists for assistance in management of nail disorders.
- Consult with an infectious disease specialist if infection is suspected.

Resources

- American Cancer Society: www.cancer.org
- Patient Resource: www.patientresource.com
- Breastcancer.org: www.breastcancer.org
- Chemocare.org: www.chemocare.org
- American Podiatric Medical Association: www.apma.org
- American Academy of Dermatology: www.aad.org
- Podiatry Today: http://www.podiatrytoday.com/diagnosing-and-treating-chemotherapy-induced-nail-changes
- National Cancer Institute: http://evs.nci.nih.gov/ftp1/CTCAE/CTCAE_4.03_2010-06-14_QuickReference_5x7.pdf

Bibliography

American Cancer Society. (2020, February 1). *Nail changes.* Available at https://www.cancer.org/treatment/treatments-and-side-effects/physical-side-effects/nail-changes.html.

Barton-Burke, M., Ciccolini, K., Mekas, M., & Burke, S. (2017). Dermatologic reactions to targeted therapy: A focus on epidermal growth factor receptor inhibitors and nursing care. *The Nursing Clinics of North America, 52*(1), 83–113.

Cury-Martins, J., Eris, A. P. M., Abdalla, C. M. Z., Silva, G. B., Moura, V. P. T., & Sanches, J. A. (2020). Management of dermatologic adverse events from cancer therapies: Recommendations of an expert panel. *Anais brasileiros de dermatologia, 95*(2), 221–237.

Ferreira, M. N., Ramseier, J. Y., & Leventhal, J. S. (2019). Dermatologic conditions in women receiving systemic cancer therapy. *International Journal of Women's Dermatology, 5*(5), 285–307.

Gupta, M. K., & Lipner, S. R. (2022). Review of chemotherapy-associated paronychia. *International Journal of Dermatology, 61*(4), 410–415.

Kim, J. Y., Ok, O. M., Seo, J. J., Lee, S. H., Ahn, J. S., Im, Y. H., & Park, Y. H. (2017). A prospective randomized controlled trial of hydrating nail solution for prevention or treatment of onycholysis in breast cancer patients who received neoadjuvant/adjuvant docetaxel chemotherapy. *Breast Cancer Research and Treatment, 164,* 617–625.

LaCouture, M., & Sibaud, V. (2018). Toxic side effects of targeted therapies and immunotherapies. *American Journal of Clinical Dermatology, 19*(Suppl. 1), S31–S39.

Mittal, S., Khunger, N., & Kataria, S. P. (2022). Nail changes with chemotherapeutic agents and targeted therapies. *Indian Dermatology Online Journal, 13,* 13–22.

National Cancer Institute. (2017, November 27). *Common Terminology Criteria for Adverse Events, v5.0. National Cancer Institute, National Institutes of Health, Department of Health and Human Services.* Available at https://ctep.cancer.gov/protocolDevelopment/electronic_applications/docs/CTCAE_v5_Quick_Reference_5x7.pdf

National Cancer Institute. (2019, June 14). *Skin and nail changes during cancer treatment.* Available at https://www.cancer.gov/about-cancer/treatment/side-effects/skin-nail-changes.

National Institutes of Health. (2021, April 14). *Medline plus medical encyclopedia.* Paronychia. U.S. Library of Medicine. Available at https://medlineplus.gov/ency/article/001444.htm.

Peyton, L., & Fischer-Cartlidge, E. (2019). Extremity cooling: A synthesis of cryotherapy interventions to reduce peripheral neuropathy and nail changes from taxane-based chemotherapy. *Clinical Journal of Oncology Nursing, 23*(5), 522–528.

Ramachadran, V., Kolli, S. S., & Strowd, C. (2019). Review of graft-versus-host disease. *Dermatologic Clinics, 37*(4), 569–582.

Russo, I., Zorzetto, L., Frigo, A. C., Chiarion Sileni, V., & Alaibac, M. (2017). A comparative study of the cutaneous side effects between BRAF monotherapy and BRAF/MEK inhibitor combination therapy in patients with advanced melanoma: A single-centre experience. *European Journal of Dermatology, 27*(5), 482–486.

Nausea and Vomiting

Jill Reese

Definition

Nausea

- Nausea is an unpleasant subjective sensation of sickness in stomach that may come and go. It may be accompanied by an involuntary impulse to vomit or queasiness in the stomach.
- It can be classified as anticipatory, acute, delayed, breakthrough, or refractory.
- Severity can lead to poor compliance with treatment regimen and decreased quality of life.

Vomiting

- Vomiting is an uncontrollable, forceful expulsion of gastric contents from the stomach through the mouth.
- Matter is ejected from the stomach through the mouth.

Patterns of Nausea and Vomiting

- *Anticipatory*: A conditioned response that occurs before chemotherapy. It typically occurs after a negative experience with chemotherapy when nausea and vomiting were not controlled. Typically, it begins after the third or fourth treatment.
- *Acute*: Onset within a few minutes to several hours after drug administration; usually resolves within 24 hours.
- *Delayed*: Onset more than 24 hours after chemotherapy; achieves maximum intensity 48 to 72 hours after chemotherapy and can last 6 to 7 days.
- *Breakthrough*: Occurs if prophylactic medications fail; requires rescue medications to be used.
- *Refractory*: Occurs in subsequent chemotherapy cycles when prior antiemetic prophylactic and breakthrough medications have failed.

Pathophysiology and Contributing Factors

- Mechanisms include activation of efferent impulses to the vomiting center (medulla) in the brain from the chemotherapy trigger zone (CTZ); peripheral mechanisms in the gastrointestinal (GI) tract; vestibular mechanisms; cortical mechanisms; and alterations of taste and smell.
- Efferent impulses sent from the medulla (vomiting center) initiate a series of events leading to vomiting. Several neuroreceptors are involved in emesis, most notably serotonin (5-hydroxytryptamine [5-HT3]) and neurokinin-1 (NK-1).

Anticipatory nausea and vomiting involve a psychological mechanism because the experience is not related to the administration of chemotherapy or radiation therapy.

- The exact mechanism of radiation-induced vomiting is not clear; however, it is believed that a peripheral mechanism in the GI tract or central mechanisms in the CTZ may contribute.
- Contributing factors include the following:
  - Underlying tumor
  - Medications such as opioids
  - Treatment-related toxicity:
    - Surgery
    - Chemotherapy
    - Radiation therapy
    - Blood and marrow transplantation
- Patient-specific factors:
  - Sex—females are more susceptible
  - Age—younger than 50 years of age
  - Alcohol history—higher consumption over time correlates with lower incidence
  - Performance status—lower performance status correlates with higher incidence
  - History of morning sickness or motion sickness—positive history increases susceptibility
  - Level of chemotherapy emetogenicity: low, moderate, or high (see table below)
  - Tumor burden—greater susceptibility as tumor burden increases
  - Combined-modality therapy—greater susceptibility compared with monotherapy
  - Dehydration—increases incidence
  - Comorbid conditions: anxiety, GI malignancies, intestinal obstruction, impaired liver or renal function, hypercalcemia, hepatitis, pancreatitis, peritonitis, cerebellar metastasis, dehydration, constipation.

Emetic Risk Classifications for Chemotherapy-Induced Nausea and Vomiting

Risk	Emesis Risk Without Use of Antiemetics (%)
High	>90
Moderate	30–90
Low	10–30
Minimal	<10

Modified from Grunberg, S., & Hawkins, R. (2009). Chemotherapy-induced nausea and vomiting: Challenges and opportunities for improved patient outcomes. *Clinical Journal of Oncology Nursing, 13*(1), 54–64; Multinational Association of Supportive Care in Cancer (MASCC). (2014). MASCC/ESMO antiemetic guideline 2016 with updates in 2019. Available at https://www.mascc.org/assets/Guidelines-Tools/mascc_antiemetic_guidelines_english_v.1.5SEPT29.2019.pdf (accessed December 18, 2021); National Comprehensive Cancer Network. (2015). NCCN clinical practice guidelines in oncology (NCCN guidelines): Antiemesis, v.1.2015. Available at https://www.nccn.org/professionals/physician_gls/pdf/antiemesis.pdf (accessed December 18, 2021).

Signs and Symptoms

- Ill feeling of the stomach
- Hypersalivation
- Diaphoresis
- Tachycardia

- Tachypnea
- Urge to vomit

Assessment Tools

- The hallmark assessment tool is patient report.
- Other assessment information:
  - Physical examination, including vital signs and weight
  - Laboratory data
  - Caregiver report

The common terminology criteria for adverse events (CTCAE) provides a grading system ranked from 1 to 5 for assessing severity of side effects associated with cancer therapy. Grade 1 represents the mildest effects and Grade 5 represents the most severe effects (see table below).

Laboratory and Diagnostic Tests

- Laboratory tests to assess for a primary cause or secondary complications from persistent nausea and vomiting.
- Diagnostic tests to rule out differential diagnoses. There are no diagnostic tests for nausea/vomiting.

Common Terminology Criteria for Adverse Events (CTCAE) for Nausea and Vomiting

CTCAE Grade	Nausea	Vomiting
1	Loss of appetite without alteration in eating habits	1–2 episodes (separated by 5 min) in 24 h
2	Oral intake decreased without significant weight loss, dehydration, or malnutrition	3–5 episodes (separated by 5 min) in 24 h
3	Inadequate oral caloric or fluid intake; tube feeding, total parenteral nutrition, or hospitalization indicated	≥6 episodes (separated by 5 min) in 24 h; tube feeding, total parenteral nutrition, or hospitalization indicated
4	—	Life-threatening consequences; urgent intervention indicated
5	—	Death

Adapted from National Cancer Institute. (2017). Common terminology criteria for adverse events (CTCAE), version 5.0. Available at https://ctep.cancer.gov/protocolDevelopment/electronic_applications/ctc.htm (accessed December 13, 2021).

- Complete blood count (CBC), electrolyte panel including sodium, potassium, and chloride; carbon dioxide level; blood urea nitrogen (BUN) and creatinine; liver function tests
- Radiography: flat plate of the abdomen, obstruction series

Differential Diagnoses

- Chemotherapy-induced nausea/vomiting
- Radiation therapy–induced nausea/vomiting
- Underlying disease
- Brain metastases
- Intestinal obstruction
- Cholecystitis
- Cirrhosis
- Diverticulitis
- Gastritis
- Hepatitis
- Migraine headache
- Pancreatitis
- Medication-induced nausea

Interventions

- Prevention of nausea and vomiting is the goal.

Pharmacologic Interventions

Anticipatory Nausea or Vomiting

- Benzodiazepines (select one)
  - Alaprazolam (Xanax) to 0.25 to 0.5 mg orally three times per day, starting the day before treatment, then repeat the next day 1 to 2 hours before chemotherapy OR
  - Lorazepam (Ativan) 0.5 to 2 mg orally the night before treatment and then repeat 1 to 2 hours before chemotherapy

Acute and Delayed Nausea/Vomiting: Highly Emetogenic Chemotherapy

- Olanzapine 5 to 10 mg oral (PO) once and daily on days 2, 3, 4
- NK-1 receptor antagonist-containing regimen (select one)
  - Aprepitant injectable emulsion 130 mgmg intravenous (IV) once OR
  - Netupitant 300 mg/palonosetron 0.5 mg (Akynzeo) orally OR
  - Fosnetupitant 235 mg/palonosetron 0.25 mg IV once OR
  - Rolapitant 180 mg PO once
- Corticosteroid (select one)
  - Dexamethasone (Decadron) 12 mg orally or IV on day 1, 8 mg orally or IV on days 2 to 4 (with aprepitant 125 mg on day 1) OR
  - Dexamethasone 12 mg orally or IV on day 1, 8 mg orally on day 2, then 8 mg orally twice daily on days 3 and 4 (with fosaprepitant 150 mg IV on day 1) AND
- 5-HT3 receptor antagonist (select one)
  - Dolasetron (Anzemet) 100 mg orally on day 1
  - Granisetron (Kytril) dosing options include:
    - Either 2 mg orally or 1 mg orally twice a day (day of chemo)
    - 0.01 mg/kg IV on day 1
    - 10 mg subcutaneous (SQ) once on day one
    - Transdermal patch (Sancuso), 3.1 mg/24-h patch, applied 24 to 48 h before chemotherapy administration, to remain in place no longer than 7 days.
  - Ondansetron (Zofran) 16 to 24 mg orally or 8 to 16 mg IV on day 1
  - Palonosetron (Aloxi) 0.25 mg IV on day 1 OR
- Olanzapine (Zyprexa)-containing regimen
  - Olanzapine 5 or 10 mg orally on days 1 to 4 AND
  - Palonosetron 0.25 mg IV on day 1 AND
  - Dexamethasone 12 mg PO/IV on day 1

Acute and Delayed Nausea/Vomiting: Moderately Emetogenic Chemotherapy

- 5-HT3 receptor antagonist (select one)
  - Dolasetron 100 mg orally on days 1 to 3
  - Granisetron 2 mg orally once or 1 mg orally twice a day; or 0.01 mg/kg IV on days 1 to 3; or 10 mg SQ once.
  - Transdermal patch (Sancuso), 3.1 mg/24-h patch, applied 24 to 48 hours before chemotherapy administration, to remain in place no longer than 7 days
  - Ondansetron 16 to 24 mg orally or 8 to 16 mg IV on day 1; then 8 mg orally twice a day or 16 mg orally daily or 8 to 16 mg IV daily on days 2 and 3
  - Palonosetron 0.25 mg IV on day 1
- Corticosteroid
  - Dexamethasone 12 mg orally or IV once on day 1 and 8 mg orally or IV on days 2 and 3, WITH OR WITHOUT
- NK-1 antagonist (select one)
  - Aprepitant injectable emulsion 130 mg IV once
  - Aprepitant (Emend) 125 mg orally on day 1, 80 mg orally daily on days 2 and 3
  - Fosaprepitant (Emend injectable) 150 mg IV on day 1 only OR
- Netupitant-containing regimen
  - Netupitant 300 mg/palonosetron 0.5 mg (Akynzeo) orally, AND
  - Fosnetupitant 235 mg/palonosetron 0.25 mg IV once OR
  - Rolapitant 180 mg PO once
- Olanzapine (Zyprexa)-containing regimen
  - Olanzapine 5 to 10 mg orally on days 1 to 3 AND
  - Palonosetron 0.25 mg IV on day 1 AND
  - Dexamethasone (Decadron) 12 mg PO/IV once

Acute and Delayed Nausea/Vomiting: Low Emetogenic Chemotherapy

Start before chemotherapy and repeat daily for multiday doses:
- Dexamethasone 8 to 12 mg PO/IV once OR
- Metoclopramide 10 to 20 mg PO/IV once OR
- Prochlorperazine 10 mg PO/IV once OR
- 5-HT3 antagonist (select one)
  - Dolasetron 100 mg orally daily
  - Granisetron 2 mg orally daily or 1 mg twice daily
  - Ondansetron 8 to 16 mg orally daily

Breakthrough Nausea or Vomiting

The general rule is to consider administering an additional agent from a different class not previously given:
- Corticosteroid: Dexamethasone 12 mg orally or IV daily, OR
- 5-HT3 receptor antagonist (select one)
  - Dolasetron 100 mg orally
  - Granisetron either 1 to 2 mg orally daily, 1 mg orally twice daily, 0.01 mg/kg (maximum 1 mg) IV
  - After IV dose 3.1 mg/24-h transdermal patch every 7 days
  - Ondansetron 8 mg PO/IV every 8 to 12 hours (16 to 24 mg total daily dose)

- Phenothiazine
  - Prochlorperazine either 25 mg suppository every 12 hours, 10 mg orally every 12 hours or 15 mg every morning. Can also be given IM or IV.
  - Promethazine 25 mg suppository per rectum every 6 hours, or 12.5 to 25 mg orally or IV (central line only) every 4 to 6 hours
- Substituted benzamide: metoclopramide 10 to 20 mg PO/IV every 4 to 6 hours
- Butyrophenone: haloperidol (Haldol) 0.5 to 2 mg orally every 4 to 6 hours
- Benzodiazepine: lorazepam 0.5 to 2 mg orally, sublingual, or IV every 4 to 6 hours
- Cannabinoid (select one)
  - Dronabinol (Marinol) capsules 5 to 10 mg, or dronabinol PO solution 2.1 to 4.2 mg/m^2, PO 3 to 4 times daily
- Atypical antipsychotic: olanzapine 5 to 10 mg PO daily for 3 days
- Anticholinergic belladonna alkaloid: scopalamine transdermal patch, 1 patch every 72 hours

Nausea and Vomiting Prevention for Oral Anticancer Agents

Acute and Delayed Nausea/Vomiting: High to Moderate Emetic Risk

- Start before therapy and continue daily
- 5HT3 RA (choose one)
  - Dolasetron 100 mg PO daily OR
  - Granisteron 1–2 mg (total dose) PO daily or 3.1 mg/24-h transdermal patch every 7 days OR
  - Ondansetron 8–16 mg (total dose) PO daily OR

See breakthrough treatment for nausea/vomiting.

Acute and Delayed Nausea/Vomiting: Low to Minimal Emetic Risk

- Take as needed is recommended and follow the breakthrough treatment
- If nausea/vomiting is not controlled consider following the high to moderate emetic risk guidelines
- If nausea/vomiting not controlled with above then begin before anticancer therapy and continue daily (choose one)
  - Metocloporamide 10–20 mg PO and then every 6 hours as needed OR
  - Prochlorperazine 10 mg PO and then every 6 hours as needed (do not exceed 40 mg/day) OR
  - 5HT3 RA (choose one)
    - Dolasteron 100 mg PO daily PRN OR
    - Granisteron 1–2 mg (total dose) PO daily PRN OR
    - Ondansetron 8–16 mg (total dose) PO daily PRN

Nonpharmacologic Interventions

- Behavioral management
- Acupuncture, acupressure
- Guided imagery, progressive muscle relaxation
- Music therapy

Patient Teaching

- Take antinausea medication on a timed schedule before nausea begins.
- Eat small, frequent meals. Nausea is more likely to occur on an empty stomach.
- Avoid spicy, greasy, or fatty foods, and overly sweet foods.
- Cold foods, salty foods, dry crackers, and dry toast may be more tolerable.
- Consider diversionary activities (i.e., music therapy, relaxation techniques).
- Reduce food aromas and other strong odors.

Follow-Up

- If vomiting is severe, restrict diet to clear liquids and notify doctor or nurse.
- If emesis is red or brown (coffee-ground appearance), recall foods eaten and notify doctor or nurse.

Resources

- Chemocare: https://chemocare.com/chemotherapy/side-effects/nausea-vomiting-chemotherapy.aspx (accessed 13 December 2021)
- CancerCare.org: https://www.cancercare.org/publications/7-chemotherapy-induced_nausea_and_vomiting (accessed 13 December 2021)

Bibliography

Brown, C. (2015). *A guide to oncology symptom management*. Pittsburgh, PA: Oncology Nursing Society.

Multinational Association of Supportive Care in Cancer (MASCC). (2019). Antiemetic guideline 2016 with updates in 2019. Available at https://www.mascc.org/assets/Guidelines-Tools/mascc_antiemetic_guidelines_english_v.1.5SEPT29.2019.pdf (accessed December 18, 2021).

National Cancer Institute. (2015). Nausea and vomiting—For health professionals (PDQ). Available at https://www.cancer.gov/about-cancer/treatment/side-effects/nausea/nausea-hp-pdq (accessed December 13, 2021).

National Cancer Institute. (2017). Common terminology criteria for adverse events (CTCAE), version 5.0. Available at https://ctep.cancer.gov/protocolDevelopment/electronic_applications/ctc.htm (accessed December 13, 2021).

National Comprehensive Cancer Network. (2023). *Antiemesis (Version 1.2023)*. Available at https://www.nccn.org/professionals/physician_gls/pdf/antiemesis.pdf (accessed March 8, 2023).

National Comprehensive Cancer Network. (2015). *NCCN clinical practice guidelines in oncology (NCCN guidelines): Antiemesis, v.1.2015*. Available at https://www.nccn.org/professionals/physician_gls/pdf/antiemesis.pdf (accessed 13 December 2021).

Oncology Nursing Society. (2019). Chemotherapy induced nausea and vomiting—adult. Available at https://www.ons.org/pep/chemotherapy induced nausea and vomiting (accessed February 6, 2022).

Rapoport, B. L. (2017). Delayed chemotherapy-induced nausea and vomiting: Pathogenesis, incidence, and current management. *Frontiers in Pharmacology, 8*, 19.

Ocular and Visual Changes

Colleen O'Leary

Definitions

- Blepharitis
  - Inflammation of the eyelids that may include reddened eyelids with drainage and crusting around the eyelashes
  - Often accompanied by eye redness
  - Irritation on the inside of the eye is accompanied by dry eye syndrome
  - Often occurs with other conditions such as dry eye syndrome (see figure below)

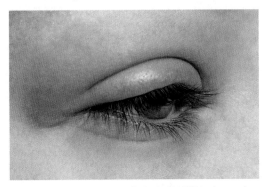

Blepharitis. (Copyright © Andrei310/iStock.com.)

- Epiphora
  - Watery eyes or excessive tearing
  - Excessive painless tearing, not related to crying
- Dry eye syndrome (ocular sicca)
  - It occurs when the eyes do not produce enough tears.
  - Although the eyes may produce excessive tearing, dry eye syndrome may cause a lack of chemicals needed to form tears in order to lubricate eyes, which makes them feel dry.
- Conjunctivitis (see figure below)
  - Commonly called "pink eye"
  - Redness and inflammation around the conjunctiva
  - Can be caused by allergies, bacteria, or viruses

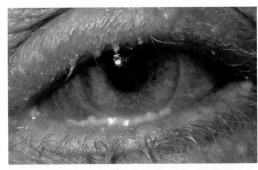

Conjunctivitis. (From Cuppett, M., & Walsh, K. M. [2012]. *General medical conditions in the athlete* [2nd ed.]. St. Louis: Elsevier.)

- Conjunctival injection, commonly referred to as red or bloodshot eyes
- Chemosis: the conjunctiva may have the appearance of a blister or appears filled with fluid.
- Trichomegaly
  - Excessive growth of eyelashes and eyebrows as a result of cancer treatment
- Cataracts (see figure on next page)
  - A cloudy area in the lens of the eye that prevents light from passing through
  - Painless but lead to progressive loss of vision over time
  - Most often develops symmetrically in both eyes

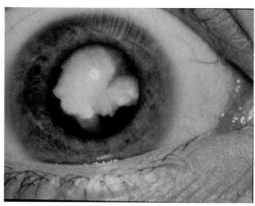

Cataracts. (From National Eye Institute, National Institutes of Health. Cataract. Available at https://medialibrary.nei.nih.gov/search?keywords =cataract&photographer=&orientation=All&type=1.)

- Glaucoma
  - Glaucoma occurs when the optic nerve is damaged, most commonly from an increase in intraocular pressure (IOP) greater than 22 mm Hg.
  - Increased IOP results from a buildup of the aqueous humor fluid, which normally flows through the eye and is subsequently drained.
  - There are several types, with the most common being open-angle glaucoma, which occurs over time.
  - Closed-angle glaucoma occurs suddenly.
  - Because the only symptom is loss of peripheral vision, regular ophthalmic evaluations are critical to early detection.
- Photophobia
  - Photophobia is the avoidance of light due to eye pain.
  - It is a common result of injury to the cornea.
  - Swelling of any eye structure may cause pain when the pupil is constricting.
  - Pain may be noticed when changing from dark to brightly lit environments or when going outside into the bright light.
- Uveitis
  - Inflammation of the middle layer of tissue in the eye wall
  - Most common is inflammation of the iris (iritis)
  - Warning signs often come on suddenly and worsen quickly
- Keratopathy
  - A disease of the outer lens of the eye (cornea)
  - Noninflammatory
  - May be due to environmental or systemic causes

Pathophysiology and Contributing Factors

- Blepharitis
  - Anterior blepharitis is less common and is found mainly around eyelashes and follicles.
  - Posterior blepharitis involves inflammation of the inner portion of the eye around the meibomian gland.
  - Meibomian glands secrete an oily layer of tear film to help prevent tears from evaporating.
  - Posterior blepharitis often occurs with dry eye syndrome, conjunctivitis, and keratitis.
  - Two classes of drugs most commonly associated with blepharitis are epidermal growth factor receptor (EGFR) inhibitors and bortezomib.

- Between 30% and 50% of patients receiving 5-fluorouracil (5-FU) develop blepharitis.
- Eighty percent of patients receiving cetuximab develop blepharitis, and 15% experience severe blepharitis.
- Thirty-five percent of patients receiving aromatase inhibitors experience blepharitis but most are not severe.
- Patients with chronic graft-versus-host disease (cGVHD) are at greater risk for ocular GVHD, which can affect the lids, meibomian glands, and cornea.
- Epiphora
  - Epiphora is divided into four categories: lid-globe growth abnormalities, obstructive lacrimal drainage disorders, ocular surface disorders, and neurogenic lacrimal hypersecretory disorders.
  - Epiphora resulting from cancer treatment is most often caused by ocular surface disorders.
  - Blepharitis, foreign bodies, ptosis, or allergies can contribute to epiphora.
  - Agents known to be associated with epiphora include 5-FU, high-dose cytarabine, doxorubicin, bevacizumab, docetaxel, and imatinib.
  - Epiphora is a typical symptom of ocular GVHD.
- Dry eye syndrome (ocular sicca)
  - In dry eye syndrome, the eyes fail to produce a sufficient amount of tears.
  - Tears provide moisture, oxygen, and nutrients for the eye.
  - A decrease in tear production results in irritation.
  - The decrease in tear formation is usually caused by lacrimal aqueous insufficiency.
  - Ocular sicca is commonly seen with the use of 5-FU and retinoids as well as antihistamines, antidepressants, and antipsychotic medications.
  - The retinoid isotretinoin, used in the treatment of acute promyelocytic leukemia, is often associated with dry eye syndrome.
  - Ocular sicca is commonly seen with ocular GVHD.
- Conjunctivitis
  - Conjunctivitis is usually caused by viral infections, but noninfectious conjunctivitis is seen with the use of certain chemotherapeutic agents, including the BRAF inhibitors vemurafenib and pemetrexed and anthracyclines such as doxorubicin and epirubicin as well as 5-FU, capecitabine, carmustine, methotrexate, and erlotinib.
  - Incidence is 25% with docetaxel and 39% with 5-FU and cyclophosphamide.
  - The conjunctiva, the transparent mucous membrane that lines the inner surface of the eyelid and covers the front part of the orbit, becomes inflamed, causing cellular infiltration, vascular engorgement, and diffuse exudation accompanied by itching and irritation.
  - Conjunctival injection and chemosis are common manifestations.
  - Most cases can be managed conservatively.
- Trichomegaly
  - The EGFR pathway is important to normal development of hair follicles.

- The biotherapy agents cetuximab, gefitinib, and erlotinib block the EGFR signaling pathway.
- The cyclin-dependent kinase inhibitor 1C (P57) pathway is important in the regulation of hair follicle growth. EGFR inhibitors upregulate P57, causing an increase in maturation of hair follicles and leading to trichomegaly.
- Cataracts
  - The lens of the eye, which is normally clear, allows light to pass through the iris to the retina, where it is converted into nerve signals that are sent to the brain.
  - The lens is made mostly of water and crystalline proteins that are arranged in a particular pattern to allow light to pass through the lens.
  - When the crystalline proteins change over time, most often due to aging, they begin to clump together, resulting in the clouding seen with cataracts.
  - Cataracts can occur secondary to treatment with specific anticancer therapies or supportive care medications commonly used in cancer treatment (e.g., corticosteroids).
  - Patients with leukemia or lymphoma who are receiving long-term prednisone or dexamethasone therapy can experience cataracts.
  - Tamoxifen has been associated with the development of cataracts.
  - Patients who receive total body irradiation with bone marrow transplantation are at a greater risk for development of cataracts.
  - Patients with diabetes are at a greater risk for cataract formation.
- Glaucoma
  - The aqueous humor flows through the posterior and anterior chambers of the eye and eventually drains out of the eye through outflow mechanisms.
  - The flow of aqueous humor helps to preserve the integrity and functioning of ocular structures.
  - When the outflow mechanisms do not function correctly, the fluid builds up, causing increased IOP.
  - Increased IOP can cause damage to the optic nerve, resulting in loss of vision.
  - Glaucoma associated with chemotherapy is related to capillary protein leakage.
  - Administration of paclitaxel or docetaxel is associated with increased risk of glaucoma.
  - Corticosteroids, especially in eye drops, increase the risk for glaucoma.
  - Other medications that can increase the risk for development of glaucoma include sulfamethoxazole and trimethoprim, topiramate, ranitidine, epinephrine, and venlafaxine.
- Photophobia
  - When the rapidly dividing cells of the corneal epithelium are exposed to chemotherapeutic agents, small (pinpoint) areas on the outer layer of the epithelium are destroyed, resulting in oversensitivity to light.
  - Agents associated with photophobia include procarbazine, vincristine, vinblastine, and 5-FU.

- Uveitis
  - Usually happens when the immune system is fighting an infection
  - Can occur when the immune system attacks healthy tissue in the eyes
  - Three types depending on what part of the uvea is affected
    - Anterior uveitis occurs in the front of the eye
    - Intermediate uveitis affects the middle of the eye
    - Posterior uveitis affects the back of the eye
  - Some forms are ongoing while others go away and come back
  - Immune checkpoint inhibitors (ICIs) such as ipilimumab, nivolumab, pembrolizumab, atezolizumab, avelumab, durvalumab, and cemiplimab.
  - Incidence between 0.3% and 0.6% when taking ICIs
- Keratopathy
  - Predominately seen with belantamab mafodotin in the treatment of relapsed refractory multiple myeloma (RRMM)
  - Superficial bilateral, microcyst-like lesions seen with exam
  - Can occur in corneal periphery, mid-periphery or center
  - Incidence is frequent with 72% of patients experiencing early in treatment
  - May be asymptomatic

Signs and Symptoms

- Blepharitis
  - Conjunctival injection
  - Foreign body or gritty sensation
  - Burning sensation
  - Excessive tearing
  - Itchy eyelids
  - Red, swollen eyelids
  - Crusting or matting of eyelashes
  - Flaking or scaling of the eyelid
  - Light sensitivity
  - Blurred vision
- Epiphora
  - Watery eyes
  - Excessive tearing when not crying
  - Painless
- Dry eye syndrome
  - Dry or gritty feeling in the eye
  - Sensation of foreign body in eye
  - Excessive watering of eyes
  - Blurred vision that improves with blinking
- Conjunctivitis
  - Redness or swelling of eyelids
  - Chemosis, scleral injection, and conjunctival erythema
  - Scratchy, watery, itchy eyes
  - Purulent discharge from the eye
  - Sensitivity to light
- Trichomegaly
  - Long, wiry eyelashes or eyebrows
- Cataracts
  - Cloudy or blurry vision
  - Difficulty seeing in the dark or at night

- Difficulty driving at night
- Lights appearing bright or with a halo around them
- Frequent changes in eyeglasses prescription
- Diplopia (double vision) that worsens over time
- Glaucoma
  - Loss of side vision over time
- Photophobia
  - Pain in the eye when changing from dark to light areas, especially when going outside in bright light
- Uveitis
  - Blurry vision
  - Floaters
  - Eye pain
  - Red eyes
  - Sensitivity to light
- Keratopathy
  - When on corneal center, associated with changes in vision including blurred vision
  - Only 56% had symptoms such as blurred vision and dry eye
  - Often short lived with return to normal vision

Assessment Tools

- A comprehensive history and assessment are important to help determine the etiology of the ocular signs and symptoms.
  - Symptom initiation, duration, and exacerbation
  - Smoking history
  - Allergies
  - History of light sensitivity
  - History of eye pain
- Physical examination
  - Thorough eye examination:
    - Visual acuity
    - Visual field testing
    - Examination of eye structures for erythema, edema, and crusting of eyelashes or eyelids
    - Examination of eyelashes for
      - Misdirected eyelashes
      - Loss of lashes
      - Loss of pigmentation
      - Abnormal growth
  - If glaucoma is suspected, a complete ophthalmoscopic examination, including examination of the optic disc, should be performed and IOPs should be measured.

Laboratory and Diagnostic Tests

- There are no laboratory or diagnostic tests to confirm most ocular toxicities.
- Tear cultures can be used with epiphora.
- Schirmer test is used with ocular sicca to evaluate millimeters of wetting.
  - Filter paper is placed inside the lower eyelid pouch to measure tear production.

Differential Diagnoses

- Allergy
- Injury to eye

- Foreign body in eye
- Viral, bacterial, or fungal infection

Interventions

Pharmacologic Interventions

- Blepharitis
  - Erythromycin or bacitracin ointment
  - Topical azithromycin ophthalmic solution
  - Doxycycline or tetracycline for prolonged cases
- Epiphora
  - Antibiotic eye drops with bacterial infections
- Dry eye syndrome
  - Preservative-free single-use artificial tears or ointment
  - Topical cyclosporine
  - Topical steroids
  - Punctal plugs or punctal cautery
  - Scleral lenses
- Conjunctivitis
  - Antihistamine (tablets or drops)
  - Antibiotic eye drops for bacterial infections
- Glaucoma
  - Prostaglandin drops
  - β-Blocker drops
  - α_2-Adrenergic agonist drops
  - Carbonic anhydrase inhibitor drops
  - Parasympathomimetic drops
  - Epinephrine drops
  - Hyperosmotic drops
  - Combination drops
- Uveitis
  - Prescription eye drops
  - Oral steroids
  - Surgical implant to release small doses of steroids over time
- Keratopathy
  - Dose reduction of belantamab mafodotin
  - Treatment of dry eye

Nonpharmacologic Interventions

- Blepharitis
  - Warm compresses placed over eyes for 5 to 10 minutes two to four times a day
  - Lid massage after warm compresses, massaging the edge of the eyelid toward the eye with circular motions
  - Lid washing using warm water or warm water and baby shampoo
- Epiphora
  - Warm compresses applied to eyes to help them drain if there is an infection
  - Use of an air cleaner to help eliminate other eye irritants such as dust
  - Wearing dark or colored glasses to help protect eyes from light
- Dry eye syndrome
  - Preservative-free, single-use artificial tears should be used routinely
  - Panoptx eyewear for use in windy conditions

- Conjunctivitis
  - Wash hands often and avoid people with compromised immune systems
  - Gently wash eyelids with a warm, clean, moist towel to remove drainage
- Trichomegaly
  - Carefully trim eyelashes with small scissors
  - Electrolysis, laser or phototherapy, and/or waxing can be used to remove eyelashes in severe cases
- Cataracts
  - Intraocular lens implant to improve vision
- Photophobia
  - Wear dark glasses to decrease the amount of light that reaches the eyes

Patient Teaching

- Patients should be taught how to cleanse around eyes and how to instill eye drops.
- Protecting eyes from light with dark glasses and/or the use of Panoptx eyewear in windy conditions should be encouraged to limit environmental sources of irritation.
- Use of a bright light when reading can be helpful to patients with cataracts.
- Patients with conjunctivitis should be taught to avoid sharing cosmetics, towels, sheets, contacts lenses, and lens cleaning products and to use a separate washcloth for each eye when cleansing.
- Teach patients to call their health care provider in the following situations:
  - Sudden severe eye pain
  - Eyelashes that are growing in toward the eye
  - Sudden loss of vision, floaters
  - Eyes becoming sensitive to light
  - Seeing halos around lights
  - Worsening symptoms or no improvement in symptoms

Follow-Up

- Follow-up with any new or worsening symptoms
- Follow-up as needed to assess prior symptoms

Resources

- American Cancer Society: www.cancer.org
- Chemocare.org: www.chemocare.org
- National Cancer Institute: Chemotherapy and you: www.cancer.gov
- American Academy of Ophthalmology: www.aao.org
- Eye Health: www.myeyes.com
- National Eye Institute: https://nei.nih.gov/health

Bibliography

Amescua, G., Akpek, E. K., Farid, M., Garcia-Ferrer, F. J., Lin, A., Rhee, M. K., ... American Academy of Ophthalmology Preferred Practice Pattern Cornea and External Disease Panel. (2019) Blepharitis: Preferred practice pattern. *Ophthalmology, 26*(1), 56–93.

Azka, A., Shad, A. A., Jeang, L. J., Fallgatter, K. S., George, T. J., & DeRemer, D. L. (2022). Emergence of ocular toxicities associated with novel anticancer therapeutics: What the oncologist needs to know. *Cancer Treatment Reviews, 105*, 102376.

Chiang, J., Zahari, I., Markoulli, M., Krishnan, A. V., Park, S. B., Semmler, A., ... Edwards, K. (2020). The impact of anticancer drugs on the ocular surface. *The Ocular Surface, 18*(3), 403–417.

Criado, P. R., & Lima, A. A. (2010). Blepharitis and trichomegaly induced by cetuximab. *Anais Brasileiros de Dermatologia, 85*(6), 919–920.

Deutsch, A., Leboeuf, N. R., Lacouture, M. E., & McLellan, B. N. (2020). Dermatologic adverse events of systemic anticancer therapies: Cytotoxic chemotherapy, targeted therapy, and immunotherapy. *American Society of Clinical Oncology Educational Book. American Society of Clinical Oncology. Annual Meeting, 40*, 485–500.

Fortes, B. H., Tailor, P. D., & Dalvin, L. A. (2021). Ocular toxicity of targeted anticancer agents. *Drugs, 81*, 771–823.

Fu, C., Gombos, D. S., Lee, J., George, G. C., Hess, K., Whyte, A., ... Hong, D. S. (2017). Ocular toxicities associated with targeted anticancer agents: An analysis of clinical data with management suggestions. *Oncotarget, 8*(35), 58709–58727.

Goyal, A., & Blaes, A. (2020). Trichomegaly associated with panitumumab. *The New England Journal of Medicine, 383*(16), e94.

Lacouture, M. E., Sibaud, V., Gerber, P. A., van den Hurk, C., Fernández-Peñas, P., Santini, D., ... ESMO Guidelines Committee. (2021). Prevention and management of dermatological toxicities related to anticancer agents: ESMO Clinical Practice Guidelines. *Annals of Oncology, 32*(2), 157–170.

Lonial, S., Nooka, A. K., Thulasi, P., Badros, A. Z., Jeng, B. H., Callander, N. S., ... Jakubowiak, A. (2021). Management of belantamab mafodotin-associated corneal events in patients with relapsed or refractory multiple myeloma (RRMM). *Blood Cancer Journal, 11*(5), 103.

Manthri, S., & Chakraborty, K. (2019). Blepharitis: A rare side effect related to cetuximab in patient with colorectal cancer. *BMJ Case Reports, 12*(8), e231774.

O'Leary, C. (2014). Ocular and otic complications. In C. H. Yarbro, D. Wujcik, & B. H. Gobel (Eds.), *Cancer symptom management* (4th ed.). Burlington, MA: Jones & Bartlett.

O'Leary, C. (2014). Optic and otic side effects of molecular targeted therapies. *Seminars in Oncology Nursing, 30*(3), 169–174.

Villegas, V. M., & Murray, T. A. (2021). Alphabet soup: Clinical pearls for the retina Specialist—Ocular toxicity of advanced antineoplastic agents in systemic cancer care. *Ophthalmology Retina, 5*(12), 1181–1186.

Wahab, A., Rafae, A., Mushtaq, K., Masood, A., Ehsan, H., Khakwani, M., ... Khan, A. (2021). Ocular toxicity of belantamab mafodotin, an oncological perspective of management in relapsed and refractory multiple myeloma. *Frontiers in Oncology, 11*, 678634.

Pain

Nezar Ahmed Salim

Definition

- Pain is a pervasive, multifaceted sensation that is one of the most distressing symptoms for cancer patients.
- The International Association of the Study of Pain defines pain as "An unpleasant sensory and emotional experience associated with, or resembling that associated with, actual or potential tissue damage." The definition includes six additional factors: (1) pain is a personal experience—but influenced by biopsychosocial factors, (2) pain is not the sole result of sensory neuron activity, (3) individuals learn the concept of pain through life experiences, (4) individual experience of pain should be respected, (5) pain can have functional, social, and psychological adverse effects, and (6) inability to communicate does not mean the individual cannot experience pain.
- It's the one symptom that cancer patients fear the most, and uncontrolled pain has the biggest effect on a patient's quality of life (QOL).
- Despite numerous research studies involving pain management, cancer pain continues to be undertreated.

Pain Prevalence

- One of the most common symptoms among cancer patients is pain, which can have a significant impact on their functional status and QOL. Increased emotional distress is associated with cancer pain. Both the duration and severity of pain are linked to the risk of developing depression. Cancer patients miss an average of 12 to 20 days each month due to their disease, with 28% to 55% unable to work.
- The incidence of pain in cancer patients varies widely and is impacted by a variety of factors, including the population evaluated, the type and stage of disease, and the therapeutic context.
- Pain affects 20% to 50% of cancer patients. Approximately 80% of patients with advanced-stage cancer have moderate to severe pain. More than half of patients experienced pain, according to a meta-analysis of data from 52 trials.

Pathophysiology and Contributing Factors

- The basic causes of cancer pain are associated with the cancer or its treatment or with unrelated iatrogenic causes.
- Somatosensory primary afferent fibers carry sensory information to the spinal cord; these can be grouped based on transduction properties of the individual nerve fibers.
- Noxious stimuli activate nociceptor A-delta and C-fibers in the peripheral nerve.
- Nociceptors are polymodal and respond to mechanical, thermal, and chemical stimuli; the resulting action potentials are conducted by the axon to the dorsal horn of the spinal cord and the brainstem.
- Transmission of acute pain involves the activation of sensory receptors on peripheral C-fibers (nociceptors).
- Once tissue damage and inflammation occur, prostaglandins, bradykinin, histamine, adenosine triphosphate (ATP), and acetylcholine act on excitatory receptors on the sensory ending and play a major role in sensitization and activation.
- Impaired nerve fibers, either at the site of nerve injury or in the cell body of impaired fibers in the dorsal root ganglia, have ectopic discharges that are characterized as neuropathic pain.
- Multiple factors come together to determine a patient's perception of pain and his or her ability to get relief from the pain. Gender, culture, and social and societal inputs affect a patient's pain response.
- Major barriers to pain management continue to be related to the patient's belief in myths associated with the management of pain, including fear of tolerance, addiction, and dependence.
  - *Tolerance:* the physiologic adaptation of receptors that are continually exposed to opioids in circulation such that the dose of medication needs to be increased to achieve the same level of pain relief. Tolerance is not an issue in cancer patients because studies have shown that the primary reason for oncology patients to need an increase in dose is related to a change in the source of their pain (e.g., metastasis, bone fractures, impingement of nerves from

growing tumors). Oncology patients on stable doses of opioids over time can reduce the dose of their medications and achieve the same level of pain relief.
  - *Addiction:* a neurobehavioral syndrome with genetic and environmental influences that results in psychological dependence on the use of a substance for its psychic effects. Addiction is characterized by compulsive use despite harm. Use of opioids to relieve pain cannot by itself lead to addiction to the medications.
  - *Physiologic dependence:* symptoms of withdrawal are experienced when opioids are discontinued immediately, without tapering of the medication. The experience of dependence does not signify addiction; acute symptoms occur with abrupt withdrawal because the receptors are used to being bathed in the medication. Other drugs that may cause withdrawal symptoms if stopped abruptly include sedative-hypnotics, β-blockers, corticosteroids, and antidepressants.

Pain Mechanisms (Nociceptive Pain, Neuropathic Pain, and Psychogenic Pain)

- The underlying pathophysiologic mechanisms, the duration, or the description of identifiable pain syndromes are used to classify pain. The three mechanisms underlying the pathophysiology of pain are:
  - Nociceptive pain
  - Neuropathic pain
  - Psychogenic pain

Nociceptive Pain

- Nociceptors, which are free nerve endings found in tissues and organs, detect painful impulses. They have high thresholds and only respond to painful stimuli. There are two distinct types of nociceptors:
  - High threshold mechanoreceptors stimulate tiny, myelinated A-fibers and transmit a sharp or stinging sensation that is well-localized and lasts as long as the stimulus.
  - Small unmyelinated slowly conducting "C fibers" are stimulated by polymodal nociceptors. They are triggered by temperature and chemical stimuli, such as hydrogen ions, potassium ions, bradykinin, serotonin, ATP, and prostaglandins, in addition to mechanical stimulation.
- Nociceptive pain, which is either somatic or visceral, is caused by a chemical, mechanical, or thermal injury to tissue, which triggers pain receptors, which send a signal to the central nervous system (CNS), generating pain perception.
- Visceral pain is explained by the commingling of nerve fibers from somatic and visceral nociceptors at the level of the spinal cord.
- The pain is misinterpreted by patients as originating from the innervated somatic tissue. Visceral pain may be accompanied by autonomic symptoms such as sweating, pallor, or bradycardia. While somatic pain is easier to recognize which is localized.

Neuropathic Pain

- Neuropathic pain caused by damage to the peripheral or CNS (spinal cord or brain).
- Chemotherapy (e.g., vinca alkaloids), tumor infiltration of the nerve roots, or injury to nerve roots (radiculopathy) are the most common causes of neuropathic pain.
- Pain can be triggered by stimuli or develop spontaneously (e.g., allodynia).
- Allodynia is defined as "pain due to a stimulus that does not normally provoke pain." For instance, a light touch (that should only produce sensation), causing pain. Although both can and frequently do coexist, allodynia differs from hyperalgesia, which is an excessive response to a normally painful stimulus.

Psychogenic Pain

- Pain that is related to underlying psychological, emotional, or behavioral factors.
- Pain experienced when there is no physical source. Can be acute or chronic.
- The most common types of psychogenic pain are headaches, backaches, stomach pain, and muscle pain.
- A diagnosis is made when all other sources of pain are ruled out.
- Typically treated with psychotherapy, nonnarcotic pain killers, and antidepressants.

Types of Pain (Acute, Chronic, and Breakthrough Cancer Pain)

- Pain is often classified as either acute or chronic or by how it varies over time with terms such as breakthrough, persistent, or incidental.

Acute Pain

- Acute pain is usually caused by tissue injury, and it occurs suddenly after the injury and diminishes over time as the tissue heals.
- There is no set duration for acute pain, although it usually resolves in 3 to 6 months.
- Acute pain is treated by blocking nociceptive pathways until the tissue heals.

Chronic Pain

- Chronic pain can occur suddenly or gradually, and it can range in severity from moderate to severe.
- Unlike acute pain, chronic or persistent pain lasts for long periods.
- Pain that lasts longer than 3 months is typically called chronic. If not treated properly, it can disrupt the patient life and normal activities.
- Chronic pain does not go away until the underlying cause is treated, but it can typically be managed or controlled by taking pain medications on a regular basis.
- Sometimes in chronic pain, patients are required to take pain medicines around the clock.

Breakthrough Pain

- Breakthrough pain is a flare-up of pain that occurs amid well-controlled background pain. It "breaks through" the pain relief provided by traditional pain medications. It involves incident pain related to predictable events such as movement or activity or pain is insidious and unpredictable.
- As a rule, breakthrough pain comes on quickly, lasts as long as an hour, and it can vary in intensity.
- Breakthrough opioid doses should be 10% to 20% of the 24-hour opioid dose requirement.

Cancer Pain Syndromes

- Pain can be associated with all types of antineoplastic therapy, including chemotherapy, hormonal therapy, immunotherapy, and radiation therapy, and postoperative pain.

Treatment-Related Mucositis

- Myeloablative chemotherapy and standard-intensity treatment frequently induce severe mucositis.
- Mucositis is commonly associated with oral pain, which can interfere with oral intake, nutritional status, and QOL.

White Blood Cell Growth Factor–Related Bone Pain

- Filgrastim and pegfilgrastim are recombinant granulocyte colony-stimulating factors (G-CSFs) that stimulate neutrophil precursor proliferation and differentiation.
- Bone pain starts within 2 days of a pegfilgrastim dose and lasts for 2 to 4 days.
- Although the specific process of how G-CSFs cause bone pain is unknown, histamine release, which causes local inflammation and edema, is known to play a role.

Chemotherapy-Related Musculoskeletal Pain

- Some chemotherapies such as paclitaxel or oral agents such as aromatase inhibitors cause a syndrome of diffuse myalgias and arthralgias in 10% to 20% of patients.
- Diffuse pain in joints and muscles appears 1 to 2 days after the infusion and lasts a median of 4 to 5 days.
- The back, hips, shoulders, thighs, legs, and feet are all affected. The pain is exacerbated by weight bearing, walking, or tactile touch.
- Steroids may help to prevent the onset of myalgia and arthralgias.

Dermatologic Complications and Chemotherapy

- Epidermal growth factor receptor cause dermatitis with ensuing pain.
- Acute herpetic neuralgia is more common in cancer patients, particularly those with hematologic malignancies and those on immunosuppressive therapy.
- The pain usually resolves within 2 months but can persist and become postherpetic neuralgia.
- Continuously infused 5-FU, capecitabine, liposomal doxorubicin, and paclitaxel have been associated to palmar-plantar erythrodysesthesia syndrome.

Radiation-Induced Pain

- Radiation is associated with several distinct pain syndromes.
- Patients may experience pain from brachytherapy and from positioning during treatment (i.e., placement on a radiation treatment table).

Principles of Symptom Management

4

Pain Assessment

- Given the high incidence of cancer pain and the potential for serious consequences, all patients with cancer should be screened for pain on a regular basis.
- There is no objective test to establish a patient's experience of pain.
- Verbal report of pain is the single most accurate tool in identifying pain.
- Pain can be associated with many signs and symptoms.

Signs and Symptoms

Signs and Symptoms of Physical Pain

- Frowning
- Grimacing
- Appetite changes
- Poor sleeping
- Fearful expression
- Teeth grinding
- Fidgeting
- Groaning or moaning
- Crying
- Sighing
- Heavy breathing
- Decreasing activity
- Change in gait
- A loss of function

Signs and Symptoms of Emotional Pain

- Forgetfulness
- Poor concentration
- Dull senses
- Lethargy
- Boredom
- Low productivity
- Negative attitude
- Anxiety

Nonverbal Indicators of Pain

- Tense body language
- Restlessness
- Strained facial expressions
- Sad facial expressions
- Tearfulness
- Increased resistance/agitation with movement

- Increased breathing
- Shortness of breath
- Changes in sleeping patterns
- Loss of appetite
- Withdrawing from family/others, as well as activities and pastimes
- Decreased communication
- Decreased activity because of increased pain with activity
- Verbalizations or sounds of distress

Assessment Tools

Various pain assessment tools exist. Be sure to choose a tool that's appropriate for the patient's condition. Self-report of pain is the gold standard and should be used whenever possible.

- Numeric Pain Scale
- Wong-Baker FACES Pain Rating Scale
- Visual Analog Scale (VAS): A straight line with one end meaning no pain and the other end meaning the worst pain imaginable. Usually measured from 0 to 100 mm. 0 to 4 mm can be considered no pain; 5 to 44 mm, mild pain; 45 to 74 mm, moderate pain; and 75 to 100 mm, severe pain.
- FLACC pain scale: For nonverbal or preverbal patients. Assesses face, legs, activity, cry, and consolability

Numeric Pain Scale

- A numeric pain scale is a tool for self-report. To use this scale, the patient must have a basic understanding of numbers and how they relate to each other.
- The scale can be used vertically or horizontally. The numbers range from 0 to 10, where 0 is no pain and 10 is the worst possible pain.
- The nurse should ask the patient to pick which number corresponds to the pain level.
- A scale of mild, moderate, to severe can be used in patients unable to provide a 0 to 10 number.
- For patients who cannot self-report, such as those who are nonverbal, have cognitive issues, or have an intellectual disability, a pain assessment tool that may be helpful is the FLACC (Face, Legs, Activity, Cry, Consolability) Scale.

Wong-Baker FACES Pain Rating Scale

- Patients with mild to moderate dementia or those who cannot interpret a numeric pain scale can, nurse can use the Wong-Baker FACES Pain Rating Scale (see figure below).

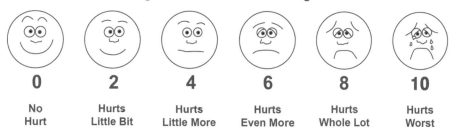

Wong-Baker FACES® Pain Rating Scale

0	2	4	6	8	10
No Hurt	Hurts Little Bit	Hurts Little More	Hurts Even More	Hurts Whole Lot	Hurts Worst

Wong-Baker FACES Pain Rating Scale. (Copyright © Wong-Baker FACES Foundation. www. WongBaker FACES.org. Used with permission. Originally published in *Whaley & Wong's nursing care of infants and children.* © Elsevier Inc.)

- In a self-report tool, the patient points to the face that corresponds to the pain level. It uses a 0 to 10 scale.
- Explain to the patient that each face represents a person who is happy because they have no pain or sad because they have some or a lot of pain while using the FACES scale.

Pain Assessment

- Each facility should have defined criteria to screen for, assess, and reassess a patient's pain. For example, a facility may designate a specific pain assessment tool as appropriate for use with cognitively impaired adults or for those who have an intellectual disability.
- Nurses should use another tool if one does not work. Unless the patient's condition changes, nurses should use a tool that works for the patient on a regular basis (such as if the patient becomes comatose).
- Pain is subjective and pain assessment criteria should be used to compare the patient's pain intensity at different times, evaluate response to the intervention, and help evaluate progress toward pain management goals.
- For cancer patients, determining the source of pain is important to determine how to manage it, as the pain might be caused by the tumor itself, a medication, or painful procedures.
- Depending on the type of pain management, reassess the cancer pain at scheduled times following the intervention (oral, IV, or transdermal route, for example) to evaluate progress toward pain management goals.
- The pain assessment includes the following:
  - Location: Where does the patient report pain? There may be more than one site of pain.
  - Intensity: How does the patient rate the level of pain? The most common tool is the numerical rating scale that asks the patient to rate the pain on a scale of 0 to 10. Children older than 3 years of age and adults who have difficulty using the 0 to 10 scale may use one of the faces scales. Nonverbal scales are also available.
  - Description/quality: What words does the patient use to describe the pain: sharp, shooting, dull, aching? These are indicators of the potential source of pain, that is, somatic, visceral, or neuropathic.
  - Temporality: How does the pain occur over time? Is it constant? Intermittent? Have breakthrough episodes? Determine what makes the pain exacerbates and what makes it relieved.
- Discuss the impact of pain on the patient's mood and activities; determine the level of interference on general activities, mood, walking ability, work, relationships, sleep, and enjoyment of life.

Physical Examination

- Examine the site of pain and any patterns of referred pain.
- Perform a neurologic examination as appropriate to the site of pain.
- Head and neck pain: cranial nerve and funduscopic evaluation

- Back and neck pain: examine patient for motor and sensory function in limbs, gross motor weakness, or sensory deficit. Report deficits to physician immediately.

Pain History

- Find out whether the patient is taking any drugs that might alter their pain perception or ability to communicate pain.
- Past experience with pain or pain medications. Include the family or caregiver when assessing pain; the patient may be stoic and may underreport the pain, or the family may overrate their loved one's pain. What do they call the pain (e.g., discomfort, hurt)? Is this pain acute (i.e., lasting <1 to 3 months) or chronic (i.e., lasting longer than 1 to 3 months)?
- Diagnostic evaluation: evaluate disease status as appropriate to cancer diagnosis and treatment, including tumor markers and radiologic examinations (e.g., computed tomographic [CT] scan, bone scan, magnetic resonance imaging [MRI] scan).

Pain in the Older Adult Population

- A majority of older adults suffer from chronic pain that significantly alters their daily activities and imposes an enormous burden on health care.
- Chronic pain is one of the most common conditions encountered by health care professionals, particularly among older (≥65 years) patients; this often accompanies cancer-related pain.
- A comprehensive assessment can guide selection of treatments most likely to benefit the patient and identify targets for intervention besides pain relief.
- A multimodal approach that includes both drug and nondrug modalities for pain is recommended.
- Given the limited reach of cognitive behavioral and exercise approaches to manage pain in later life, patients should be encouraged to engage in and adopt these techniques.
- Involve and engage family members and paid caregivers and seek out other resources that can help to reinforce adherence to treatment and maintain gains from treatment.
- Recognize the potential for drug-drug interactions due to polypharmacy in older adults.
- Start low and go slow with medications as older adults metabolize drugs more slowly or have organ compromise that can lead to drug toxicity.
- Use caution with metabolite-forming drugs such as morphine in older adults with renal insufficiency.

Pain Assessment in Cognitively Impaired Patients (Hierarchy of Pain Assessment)

- Do not assume that patients who cannot self-report their pain are not experiencing pain.
- Identify procedures or pathologic conditions that may cause pain.
- Observe for behavior associated with painful conditions Use a behavioral assessment tool.
- Gather information from family members or caregivers familiar with the patient.

- If pain is expected, medicate for pain and observe for changes in pain-related behaviors.

Laboratory and Diagnostic Tests

- No blood test can detect the existence of pain. Laboratory testing such as carcinoembryonic antigen (CEA) or cancer antigen (CA 125) levels could detect disease recurrence or metastasis which could be a source of pain.
- Diagnostic testing is related to the location of pain or to known disease locations or both and may include CT scans, positron emission tomographic (PET) scans, and radiology examinations.

Differential Diagnoses

- Rule out a history of nonmalignant chronic pain.
- Arthritis
- Neuralgia
- Chronic abdominal pain
- Fibromyalgia
- Headaches
- Low back pain
- Peripheral neuropathy related to diabetes
- AIDS
- Phantom limb pain
- Reflex sympathetic dystrophy
- Sickle cell disease

Barriers to Pain Assessment and Management

- Patients may downplay or report pain for fear that increased symptoms indicate disease progression and that the oncologist may stop treatment.
- Underreporting may also occur if a patient feels that pain is an inevitable consequence of the disease, its treatment, or dying.
- Patients may avoid speaking about concern connected to a specific complaint if they do not receive attention to frequently reported problems.
- Patients and/or their families may have been harmed by the health care system and have lost faith in it and/or its providers. As a result, they may be hesitant to discuss psychological symptoms.
- Cultural factors play an important role in pain assessment and management. For example, if a female Muslim patient feels shy about discussing pain in a specific area like the breast or pain in a gynecologic area. However, at least one study suggests that for most symptoms, culture may have a limited impact on how patient-reported symptoms are ultimately interpreted.
- Language can pose barriers.
- Patients may become depressed, tired of being sick, and hopeless, to the point that they stop reporting symptoms.
- Lacking knowledge and attitude toward pain assessment and management are the most challenge in delivering successful pain management. A recent study found that nurses had inadequate knowledge and nonstandard attitude toward pain management.

Pain Management Plan of Care

- Involve the patient in the pain management planning process in collaboration with the multidisciplinary team. When opioid and nonopioid drugs are provided, provide information on pain management, treatment options, and the safe use of both.
- Develop realistic expectations and measurable goals that the patient understands for the degree, duration, and reduction of pain.
- The nurse should monitor for potential high-risk adverse events such as respiratory depression and sedation.
- Assess for side effects that may occur because of treatment such as constipation, nausea, dizziness, and urinary retention.
- Treatment of persistent pain should include around-the-clock analgesia for continuous pain relief.
- The practitioner may prescribe a PRN dose if the patient has acute or breakthrough pain (pain that is not relieved by the around-the-clock dose).
- In the 1980s, the World Health Organization described an "analgesic ladder" approach to the use of drugs for cancer pain (see figure below).
- This influential model included references to adjuvant drugs that may be used to provide additional analgesia, treat side effects, or manage a coexisting symptom.

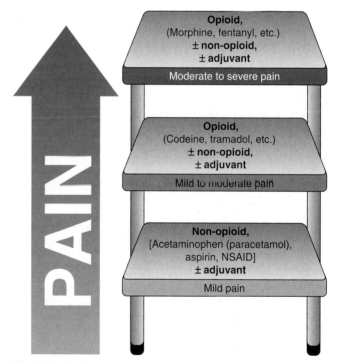

World Health Organization's Analgesic Ladder. (From World Health Organization. [1987]. *Traitement de la douleur cancéreuse.* World Health Organization.)

Interventions

Pharmacologic Interventions

- Combined opioid/nonopioid medications: acetaminophen with codeine (Tylenol 3), hydrocodone with acetaminophen

(Vicodin), hydrocodone with acetaminophen (Norco, Lortab), oxycodone with acetaminophen (Percocet, Tylox), and hydrocodone with ibuprofen (Vicoprofen)

- Compounded opioids are dose limited by the amount (milligrams) of acetaminophen and nonsteroidal antiinflammatory drug (NSAIDs). The recommended daily dose of acetaminophen should not exceed 4000 mg, however taking the maximum dose for extended periods can severely damage the liver. It is best to take the lowest dose necessary and stay closer to 3000 mg per day as the maximum dose.
- Pain medication must be titrated for effectiveness. Increasing or decreasing the dose for comfort is essential to achieve effective management of a patient's pain.
- If patients are not receiving effective management of their pain and are experiencing multiple side effects related to their medication, opioid rotation may be necessary. Another opioid may provide more effective pain management with fewer side effects (see table below).
- If a patient becomes overly sedated from the medication and is experiencing respiratory distress, reversal of the opioid dose may be necessary. Dilute naloxone in 10 mL of normal saline solution and titrate until alertness and respirations are improved.
- Consult with an anesthetist for management with appropriate pain blocks.
- Radiopharmaceuticals may be used for bone pain if appropriate.
- Spinal infusion of medications (epidural/intrathecal) may be necessary if large doses of opioids, orally or peripherally, are required to achieve pain relief.

Types of Pharmacologic Interventions

OPIOIDS

Pain Level	Pain Management
Mild pain (1–3)	• Begin a regular dosing schedule with an opioid for persistent pain, including a rescue dose, as prescribed. • Continue a bowel regimen, as prescribed to prevent constipation. • Reassess and modify pain management interventions to decrease possible adverse effects.
Moderate pain (4–6)	• Provide opioid analgesia and titrate, as prescribed. • Assess the patient for specific pain syndrome problems. • Evaluate the need for consultation with a pain specialist and discuss concerns with the health care team. • Titrate adjuvant analgesia, as prescribed.
Severe pain (7–10)	• Reevaluate opioid titration and adjuvant analgesia, as prescribed. • Perform a comprehensive pain reassessment. • Assess the patient for specific pain syndrome problems. • Evaluate the need for consultation with a pain specialist and discuss concerns with the health care team.

Example of opioids:
- Morphine
- Hydromorphone
- Oxycodone
- Hydrocodone
- Methadone
- Fentanyl (transdermal and transmucosal)
- Tramadol

Adjuvant Analgesia

- Use of anticonvulsants is common for neuropathic pain.
- Use of antidepressants is effective (e.g., amitriptyline, imipramine) with well-established analgesic benefits for many neuropathic pain syndromes.
- Use of corticosteroids (e.g., acetaminophen (paracetamol) or an NSAID is common as adjuvant analgesia for bone cancer pain and pain of visceral or neuropathic origin.
- Use of bisphosphonates (e.g., oral clodronate, intravenous pamidronate, and intravenous zoledronic acid) is common in managing bone pain as well as preventing skeletal complications of metastatic bone disease.
- Use of topical anesthetics (e.g., benzocaine, butamben, dibucaine, lidocaine) in combination with opioids, antidepressants, and anticonvulsants can serve as adjuvant analgesia for neuropathic pain associated with cancer or cancer-related treatments.
- Adjuvant medicines can improve the effectiveness of prescription analgesia and alleviate side effects at any stage of pain management.
- Adjuvant analgesia medicines can also be used to treat particular pain syndromes. Below is a list of some common pain medications and their uses.

Adjuvant Examples
- Corticosteroids
- Antidepressants
- Anticonvulsants
- Bisphosphonates
- Benzodiazepines

Nonopioids
- Aspirin
- Acetaminophen
- NSAIDs

Nonpharmacologic Interventions

- Use distraction, guided imagery, deep breathing, music therapy, muscular relaxation, visual concentration, and rhythmic massage to help the patient enhance the effect of analgesics
- Radiation therapy for pain related to bone metastases
- Heat or cold compresses for musculoskeletal pain (somatic)
- Surgical interventions to relieve compression
- Physical activity to maintain mobility and prevent secondary pain sources
- Cutaneous stimulation (transcutaneous electrical nerve stimulation—TENS), massage, pressure, or vibration for pain associated with muscle tension or muscle spasm
- Relaxation or visualization techniques for distraction
- Acupuncture
- Community resources such as pastoral care and psychosocial care based on patient assessment

Patient Teaching

- During discharge planning, teach the patient and family (if applicable) about pain assessment and management options. Include information regarding the patient's pain management plan as well as the treatment's side effects.

- Discuss daily activities things that may aggravate pain or reduce the effectiveness of the pain management strategy, as well as options for dealing with these difficulties.
- Inform the patient that managing cancer pain is an important part of their treatment, and that the best approach to manage pain is to prevent it from starting or worsening. The pain may worsen, and the pain medication may not function as well if the patient does not address the pain early and waits extended periods of time between doses.
- Explain that the patient has a right to have the pain treated and that pain is not a sign of weakness.
- Encourage the patient to keep a record of pain in a diary or journal to track details.
- Instruct the patient to describe the pain and activities that increase or decrease it; medication information, such as names, dosages, and frequency; complementary pain-relieving methods, such as rest, massage, and distraction; pain ratings before and after pain-relief measures; ways in which pain interferes with daily activities; and pain level changes throughout the day.
- Inform the patient about the drugs he or she is taking, including any potential side effects. The patient should be able to explain the doses and frequency of all drugs used around the clock, as well as how to handle breakthrough pain with PRN doses.
- Describe how pain drugs can cause side effects such as gastrointestinal irritation and bleeding with ibuprofen and constipation with opioids. If opioids are given, teach the patient and family how to use, store, and dispose of them safely.
- Counsel the patient not to discontinue opioids without first discussing the need for a gradual tapering regimen with the health care provider.
- Teach the patient and the family (if applicable) how to use an appropriate pain assessment tool and to use it as soon as possible before a painful event to establish a baseline for comparison. The tool should be selected based on the patient's cognitive level, the type of pain or medical condition that the patient is experiencing, and the patient's ability to self-report. Make sure that the patient understands the assessment tool; if not, introduce a different tool.
- Explain to the patient and family the pain assessment guidelines, including the frequency of reassessment. Assess that the patient and family are aware that if pain does not maintain at or below the desired pain level, they should contact the practitioner.

Follow-Up

- Reassess the patient's pain ratings daily (or every shift if inpatient and no pain is reported).
- Reassess the patient's comfort level 30 minutes after an intravenous or subcutaneous injection and 1 hour after oral medications. If pain is not improved, the physician or advanced practice nurse must be notified to increase or change the pain management plan as necessary.
- Documentation is the most important follow-up intervention. Communicating the patients' medication regimen and response can prevent needless suffering.

Resources

- Pain Medicine and Palliative Care at Beth Israel NY: www.stoppain.org
- Pain Resource Center at City of Hope: http://prc.coh.org
- National Comprehensive Cancer Network (NCCN): Cancer pain guidelines: https://www.nccn.org/store/login/login.aspx?ReturnURL=http://www.nccn.org/professionals/physician_gls/pdf/pain.pdf

Bibliography

Ali, A., Arif, A. W., Bhan, C., Kumar, D., Malik, M. B., Sayyed, Z., … Ahmad, M. Q. (2018). Managing chronic pain in the elderly: An overview of the recent therapeutic advancements. *Cureus, 10*(9), e3293.

American Cancer Society. (2018). *Type of pain.* Available at https://www.cancer.org/treatment/treatments-and-side-effects/physical-side-effects/pain/other-types.html#references.

American Cancer Society. (2019). *Non-medical treatments for pain.* Available at https://www.cancer.org/treatment/treatments-and-side-effects/physical-side-effects/pain/non-medical-treatments-for-cancer-pain.html (accessed October 2021).

American Cancer Society. (2019). *Facts about cancer pain.* Available at https://www.cancer.org/treatment/treatments-and-side-effects/physical-side-effects/pain/facts-about-cancer-pain.html (accessed October 2021).

Bannister, K. (2015). Opioid-induced hyperalgesia: Where are we now? *Current Opinion in Supportive and Palliative Care, 9*(2), 116–121.

Bennett, M. I., Kaasa, S., Barke, A., Korwisi, B., Rief, W., & Treede, R. D. (2019). The IASP classification of chronic pain for ICD-11: Chronic cancer-related pain. *Pain, 160*(1), 38–44.

Bluethmann, S. M., Mariotto, A. B., & Rowland, J. H. (2016). Anticipating the "silver tsunami": Prevalence trajectories and comorbidity burden among older cancer survivors in the United States. *Cancer Epidemiology, Biomarkers & Prevention: A Publication of the American Association for Cancer Research, Cosponsored by the American Society of Preventive Oncology, 25*(7), 1029–1036.

Brant, J. M. (2022). The assessment and management of acute and chronic cancer pain syndromes. *Seminars in Oncology Nursing, 38,* 151248.

Brant, J. M., & Stringer, L. H. (2018). Cancer pain. In C. H. Yarbro, D. Wujcik, & B. H. Gobel (Eds.), *Cancer nursing: Principles and practice* (8th ed., pp. 781–816). Jones and Bartlett.

Eaton, L. H., & Hulett, J. M. (2019). Mind-body interventions in the management of chronic cancer pain. *Seminars in Oncology Nursing, 35*(3), 241–252.

Gallagher, E., Rogers, B. B., & Brant, J. M. (2017). Cancer-related pain assessment: Monitoring the effectiveness of interventions. *Clinical Journal of Oncology Nursing, 21*(3), 8–12.

He, Y., & Kim, P. Y. (2021, September 9). Allodynia. In *StatPearls [Internet]* (p. 2021). StatPearls Publishing. Available at https://www.ncbi.nlm.nih.gov/books/NBK537129/.

HealthCareAssociationofNewJersey.(2017).Painmanagementguidelines.Available at https://www.hcanj.org/files/2013/09/Pain-Management-Guidelines-_HCANJ-May-12-final.pdf (accessed October 2021) (Level VII).

Howard, A., & Brant, J. M. (2019). Pharmacologic management of cancer pain. *Seminars in Oncology Nursing, 35*(3), 235–240.

International Association for the Study of Pain. (2017). *IASP terminology [Online].* Available at https://www.iasp-pain.org/Education/Content.aspx?ItemNumber=1698 (accessed January 2022).

Jiang, C., Wang, H., Wang, Q., Luo, Y., Sidlow, R., & Han, X. (2019). Prevalence of chronic pain and high-impact chronic pain in cancer survivors in the United States. *JAMA Oncology, 5*(8), 1224–1226.

Kindler, C. H., Evgenov, O. V., Crawford, L. C., Vazquez, R., Lewis, J. M., & Nozari, A. (2020). *64 Anesthesia for orthopedic surgery (post operative pain). Miller's anesthesia.* Elsevier.

Leblanc, T. W., & Kamal, A. H. (2018). Management of cancer pain. In V. T. DeVita, T. S. Lawrence, & S. A. Rosenberg (Eds.). *DeVita, Hellman, and Rosenberg's (2019). Cancer: Principles and practice of oncology* (11th ed., pp. 2190–2390). Lippincott Williams & Wilkins.

Li, X. M., Xiao, W. H., Yang, P., & Zhao, H. X. (2017). Psychological distress and cancer pain: Results from a controlled cross-sectional survey in China. *Scientific Reports, 7,* 39397.

Moore, D. C., & Pellegrino, A. E. (2017). Pegfilgrastim-induced bone pain: A review on incidence, risk factors, and evidence-based management. *The Annals of Pharmacotherapy, 51*(9), 797–803.

Moukharskaya, J., Abrams, D. M., Ashikaga, T., Khan, F., Schwartz, J., Wilson, K., ... Ades, S. (2016). Randomized phase II study of loratadine for the prevention of bone pain caused by pegfilgrastim. *Supportive Care in Cancer: Official Journal of the Multinational Association of Supportive Care in Cancer, 24*(7), 3085–3093.

National Cancer Institute. (2021). *Cancer pain (PDQ®): Health professional version.* Available at https://www.cancer.gov/about-cancer/treatment/side-effects/pain/pain-hp-pdq/#_41 (accessed January 2022).

National Comprehensive Cancer Network (NCCN). (2020). NCCN guidelines version 2.2021: Adult cancer pain. Available at https://www.nccn.org/guidelines/guidelines-detail?category=3&id=1413. (Level VII) (accessed October 2021).

National Comprehensive Cancer Network (NCCN). (2021). NCCN guidelines version 2.2021: Adult cancer pain. Available at https://www.nccn.org/guidelines/guidelines-detail?category=3&id=1413. (Level VII) (accessed October 2021).

Portenoy, R. K., Ahmed, E., & Keilson, Y. Y. (2021). Cancer pain management: Adjuvant analgesics (coanalgesics). In J. Abrahm (Ed.), *UpToDate.*

Portenoy, R. K., & Dhingra, L. K. (2020). Assessment of cancer pain. In J. Abrahm (Ed.), *UpToDate.*

Raja, S. N., Carr, D. B., Cohen, M., Finnerup, N. B., Flor, H., Gibson, S., ... Vader, K. (2020). The revised International Association for the Study of Pain definition of pain: Concepts, challenges, and compromises. *Pain, 161*(9), 1976–1982. Available at https://journals.lww.com/pain/Fulltext/2020/09000/The_revised_International_Association_for_the.6.aspx.

Reid, M. C., Eccleston, C., & Pillemer, K. (2015). Management of chronic pain in older adults. *BMJ (Clinical Research ed.), 350*, h532.

Robinson, S., Kissane, D. W., Brooker, J., & Burney, S. (2016). A review of the construct of demoralization: History, definitions, and future directions for palliative care. *American Journal of Hospice and Palliative Medicine, 33*, 93.

Tauben, D., & Stacey, B. R. (2020). Evaluation of chronic non-cancer pain in adults. In S. Fishman (Ed.), *UpToDate.*

The Joint Commission. (2021). *Standard PC.01.02.07. Comprehensive accreditation manual for hospitals.* (Level VII). Available at https://www.joint-commission.org/standards/standard-faqs/hospital-and-hospital-clinics/leadership-ld/000002161/.

U.S. Food and Drug Administration, Drug. (2019). *Drug safety communications: FDA identifies harm reported from sudden discontinuation of opioid pain medicines and requires label changes to guide prescribers on gradual, individualized tapering.* Available at https://www.fda.gov/media/122935/download (accessed October 2021).

van den Beuken-van Everdingen, M. H., de Rijke, J. M., Kessels, A. G., Schouten, H. C., Van Kleef, M., & Patijn, J. (2016). Prevalence of pain in patients with cancer: A systematic review of the past 40 years. *Annals of Oncology: Official Journal of the European Society for Medical Oncology, 18*(9), 1437–1449.

WHO Pain Management Ladder. (2022). Comprehensive cancer pain management. In *Cancer pain relief* World Health Organization. Available at https://www.uptodate.com/contents/image?imageKey=ONC%2F63298.

World Health Organization. (n.d.). WHO's cancer pain ladder for adults. Available at https://www.who.int/cancer/palliative/painladder/en/ (Level I) (accessed October 2021).

Peripheral Neuropathy

Carol Stein Blecher

Definition

- A functional or structural disorder of the motor, sensory, and autonomic neurons that lead from the skin, joints, and muscles of the face, arms, legs, and torso to the central nervous system
- Causes a lack of communication between the brain and the periphery
- Characterized by symptoms of pain and numbness

Pathophysiology and Contributing Factors

- Direct damage to the neurons

- Chemotherapy-induced peripheral neuropathy: damage to the nerve fibers caused by demyelination of the large-fiber sensory nerves (cisplatinum), microtubule inhibition resulting in axonal degeneration (vinca alkaloids), or axonal degeneration and demyelination (taxanes).
- Tumor pressing on the nerves
- Many contributing factors, including the following:
  - Alcohol abuse
  - Arthrosclerosis/ischemic disease
  - Concurrent neuropathic medication (isoniazid, gentamicin, ciprofloxacin hydrochloride, phenytoin)
  - Infections: human immunodeficiency virus (HIV) infection, syphilis, Epstein-Barr virus, shingles, sarcoidosis
  - Metabolic disorders: diabetes mellitus, hypothyroidism, acromegaly
  - Nutritional imbalance: vitamin B_{12} deficiency
  - Treatment-related toxicity
    - Radiation
    - Phantom limb pain
    - Postherpetic neuralgia

Signs and Symptoms

- A perception of wearing a sock or glove when there is none
- Extreme sensitivity to touch
- Muscle weakness, tremor, cramps or spasms, loss of dexterity or coordination
- Numbness or tingling and loss of feeling
- Pain, which may be described as burning, pins-and-needles, sharp, stabbing, or an electric or shooting type of pain

Assessment Tools

- Clinical evaluation of sensory, motor, autonomic, and cranial nerve functions
- History, including risk factors for the development of neuropathy (e.g., diabetes, alcoholism)
- Any concomitant medications that cause neuropathy
- Symptom assessment: onset, intensity, location, quality, intermittent or constant, alleviating and aggravating factors, accompanying symptoms, and impact on ability to perform activities of daily living (ADLs) and quality of life
- Physical examination: monitoring for orthostatic hypotension, cranial nerve examination, assessment of motor function, reflexes, and sensory function
- Common terminology criteria for adverse events (CTCAE):
  - Neuropathy, motor
    - Grade 1—asymptomatic; clinical or diagnostic observations only
    - Grade 2—moderate symptoms; limiting instrumental ADLs
    - Grade 3—severe symptoms; limiting self-care ADLs; assistive device indicated
    - Grade 4—life-threatening consequences; urgent intervention indicated
    - Grade 5—death

- Neuropathy, sensory
  - Grade 1—asymptomatic
  - Grade 2—moderate symptoms; limiting instrumental ADLs
  - Grade 3—severe symptoms; limiting self-care ADLs
  - Grade 4—life-threatening consequences; urgent intervention indicated
- Toxicity grading scales
  - World Health Organization (WHO) toxicity criteria
  - Eastern Cooperative Oncology Group (ECOG)
  - National Cancer Institute of Canada (NCIC) common toxicity criteria:
    - Sensory neuropathy
    - Motor neuropathy
  - Ajani Motor Neuropathy tool for assessing chemotherapy-induced neuropathy in patients with cancer
    - Sensory neuropathy
    - Motor neuropathy
  - Total neuropathy scale
    - Sensory symptoms
    - Motor symptoms
    - Pin sensibility
    - Vibration sensibility
    - Reflex
    - Autonomic symptoms
    - Vibration sensation
    - Sural amplitude: The sural nerve is the nerve leading from the tibial nerve that enervates the gastrocnemius and lateral portion of the leg. The conduction amplitude may be decreased in chemotherapy-induced peripheral neuropathies.
    - Peroneal amplitude: The peroneal nerve is the nerve leading from the sciatic nerve to the biceps femoris and gastrocnemius muscles. The conduction amplitude may be decreased in chemotherapy induced peripheral neuropathies.
  - Functional Assessment of Cancer Therapy/Gynecologic Oncology Group—Neurotoxicity (FACT/GOG-Ntx)
  - Functional Assessment of Cancer Therapy—Taxane
  - Peripheral Neuropathy Scale

Laboratory and Diagnostic Tests

- Audiometry to assess hearing
- Electromyelography (EMG) to evaluate axonal neuropathy and muscle atrophy related to the neuropathy
- Nerve biopsy to assess for abnormalities
- Nerve conduction studies to identify the severity and location of the peripheral neuropathy
- Blood screening for
  - Anemia
  - Diabetes
  - Electrolyte imbalance
  - Hepatitis
  - Homocysteine/methylmalonic acid levels
  - Lupus erythematosus
  - Lyme disease

- Thyroid-stimulating hormone (TSH) deficiency
- Vitamin deficiency

Differential Diagnoses

- Alcoholism/Malnutrition
- Diabetes mellitus
- Motor neuron disease
- Disorders of the neuromuscular junction
- Myopathy
- Myelopathy
- Syringomyelia
- Dorsal column disorders
  - Tabes dorsalis
- Hysterical disorders

Interventions

Pharmacologic Interventions

- Anticonvulsants
  - Phenytoin
  - Carbamazepine
  - Gabapentin
  - Pregabalin (Lyrica)
- Lidocaine patches
- Opioid analgesics
- Over-the-counter pain relievers
  - Acetaminophen
  - Nonsteroidal antiinflammatory drugs (NSAIDs)
- Tricyclic antidepressants
  - Amitriptyline (Elavil)
  - Nortriptyline (Pamelor)
  - Desipramine (Norpramin)
  - Imipramine (Tofranil)
- Vitamin B_{12} supplements

Nonpharmacologic Interventions

- Treatment of the underlying disease
- Physical therapy
- Massage
- Exercise
- Occupational therapy
- Transcutaneous electrical nerve stimulation (TENS)
- Biofeedback
- Acupuncture
- Hypnosis
- Relaxation techniques
- Support groups
- Safety measures
  - Orthotics
  - Ergonomic chairs
  - Braces
  - Splints
  - Positioning
  - Adequate lighting
  - Rails or other appliances to promote safety
  - Removal of obstacles such as loose rugs
  - Bed frames to keep sheets off tender body parts

Patient Teaching

- Help patients to describe their symptoms
  - Pain
  - Numbness or tingling and loss of feeling
  - Feeling as if one is wearing a sock or glove
  - Muscle weakness, loss of dexterity or coordination
  - Burning pain
  - Sharp stabbing or electric type of pain
  - Extreme sensitivity to touch
- Prevention
  - Avoid alcohol.
  - Increase intake of B vitamins.
  - Avoid repetitive activities that may place stress on a nerve (such as golf, tennis, playing a musical instrument, or typing at a computer keyboard).
- Management
  - Controlling diabetes
  - Correction of vitamin deficiency
  - Relieving nerve pressure by eliminating the source of the pressure, if possible, or through surgical repair of the problem
  - Medications: pain relief medication following the WHO ladder, antiseizure medication, lidocaine patches, tricyclic antidepressants
  - Therapies: TENS, biofeedback, acupuncture, hypnosis, relaxation techniques
- Safety
  - Orthotics
  - Ergonomic chairs
  - Braces
  - Splints
  - Positioning
  - Adequate lighting
  - Rails or other appliances to promote safety
  - Removal of obstacles such as loose rugs
  - Bed frames to keep sheets off tender body parts
- Coping skills
  - Setting priorities
  - Getting out of the house
  - Seeking and accepting support
- Mayo Clinic Patient Education Tool

Follow-Up

- Physician
- Physical therapy
- Occupational therapy
- Laboratory data for underlying disease state
- Have the patient call the health care team immediately for tingling or weakness in hands or feet or for pain that is new.

Resources

- American Cancer Society: Managing Peripheral Neuropathy: https://www.cancer.org/treatment/treatments-and-side-effects/physical-side-effects/nervous-system/peripheral-neuropathy.html
- American Society of Clinical Oncology: Peripheral Neuropathy: http://www.cancer.net/navigating-cancer-care/side-effects/peripheral-neuropathy
- Center for Peripheral Neuropathy. (2022). About peripheral neuropathy. Available at http://peripheralneuropathycenter.uchicago.edu/learnaboutpn/aboutpn/whatispn/ (accessed March 6, 2022).
- ChemoCare: Peripheral Neuropathy: https://chemocare.com/chemotherapy/side-effects/numbness-tingling.aspx
- NCCN Guidelines for Patients: Survivorship Care for Cancer Related Late and Long Term Effects: https://www.nccn.org/patients/guidelines/content/PDF/survivorship-hl-patient.pdf

Bibliography

Grisdale, K. A., & Armstrong, T. S. (2014). Peripheral neuropathy. In D. Camp-Sorrell & R. A. Hawkins (Eds.), *Clinical manual for the oncology advanced practice nurse* (3rd ed.). Pittsburgh, PA: Oncology Nursing Press.

Mahon, S., & Carr, E. (2021). Peripheral neuropathy: Common side effect. *Clinical Journal of Oncology Nursing, 25*(6), 30.

Medline Plus Medical Encyclopedia. (2014). Peripheral neuropathy. Available at http://www.nlm.nih.gov/medlineplus/ency/article/000593.htm (accessed March 6, 2022).

Oncology Nursing Society. (2019). PEP topic: Peripheral neuropathy. Available at https://www.ons.org/practice-resources/pep/peripheral-neuropathy (accessed March 6, 2022).

Wilkes, G. M. (2014). Peripheral neuropathy. In C. H. Yarbro, M. H. Frogge, & M. Goodman (Eds.), *Cancer symptom management* (4th ed.). Sudbury, MA: Jones & Bartlett.

Pruritus/Xerosis

Nezar Ahmed Salim

Definition

- Pruritus (itch) is a common symptom that occurs in a varied range of skin diseases. It is a pathologic condition that triggers the sensory of discomfort, and itching is a symptom related to systemic and localized diseases.
- Xerosis is the medical name for dry skin. It comes from Greek: "xero" means "dry" and "osis" means "disease" or "medical disorder." A lack of moisture in the skin causes xerosis, which can be caused by aging (senile xerosis) or underlying diseases such as cancer.
- In older adults, xerosis is a prevalent cause of pruritus. The lower extremities are frequently affected. A pruritic, eczematous dermatitis may occur as a consequence of severe xerosis.
- Pruritus is a systemic issue with multiple causes. Stinging, pins and needles, tickling, crawling feeling, and pain are all terms that describe itching.
- It is estimated that pruritus is a manifestation of an underlying systemic disease in approximately 10% to 25% of affected patients with cancer.

Pathophysiology and Contributing Factors

- The risk of pruritus increases in immunocompromised patients.
- Patients receiving epidermal growth factor receptors (EGFRs) are more likely to develop pruritus.
- The incidence of pruritus in patients with cancer is higher in White patients than African American patients.
- A study of 85 patients treated with epidermal growth factor receptor inhibitor (EGFRI) found that xerosis affected (22.3%) of patients and pruritus (16.9%).

- The exact neurologic pathways that lead to itch are not fully understood.
- Histamine-sensitive nerve fibers play a role in the transmission of acute itch and itch in urticaria, whereas non-histamine nerve fibers play a role in the transmission of itch in most types of chronic itch, explaining why many types of chronic itch have a poor response to antihistamines.
- Histamines, proteases, cathepsins, gastrin-releasing peptides, opioids, substance P, nerve growth factor, interleukins, and prostaglandins, as well as their receptors, have all been identified as possible peripheral or central causes of pruritus.

A variety of systemic diseases, including malignancy, should be considered when a patient presents with generalized pruritus without any dermatologic manifestations.

Signs and Symptoms

- Pruritus may accompany other symptoms affecting the skin locally including:
  - Blisters
  - Bumps
  - Burning feeling
  - Cracking and/or scaling
  - Crusting
  - Discharge from sores, lesions, or pustules
  - Dryness
  - Pain
  - Peeling
  - Rash
  - Redness, warmth, or swelling

- Pruritus may accompany symptoms related to other body systems including:
  - Abdominal pain or cramping
  - Dry mouth
  - Nausea with or without vomiting
  - Rash or hives
  - Runny nose
  - Sneezing
  - Swelling

Assessment Tools

- Assessment should include dermatologic causes (local chemical reactions; skin disorders such as eczema, psoriasis, or infestation), systemic causes (opioid-induced pruritus, organ failure, endocrine dysfunction, connective tissue disorder), neuropathic causes, and psychological causes (psychiatric disorder) (see figure below).
- The intensity of the discomfort or distress can be assessed by using a 0 to 10 rating system.
- Check the area for signs of secondary infection.
- Check the family history for allergies, exposure to known infectious agents or insect bites, and other family members who may also be experiencing itching symptoms.
- Evaluate the patient's medication profile for potential causes, including chemotherapy and biologic medications.
- In patients who present without skin lesions or with only secondary skin lesions (e.g., excoriations, hyperpigmentation, or lichenification), consider the possibility of systemic, neurologic, or psychogenic causes.

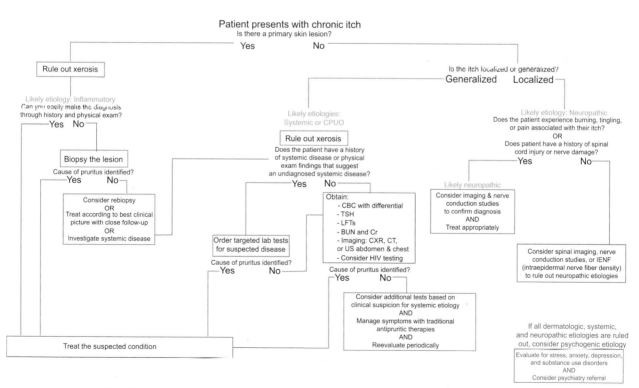

An Algorithm for Diagnosing and Managing the Patient With Chronic Pruritus. *BUN,* Blood urea nitrogen; *CBC,* complete blood count; *CPUO,* Chronic pruritus of unknown origin; *CT,* computed tomography; *CXR,* chest x-ray; *HIV,* human immunodeficiency virus; *LFTs,* liver function tests; *TSH,* thyroid-stimulating hormone; *US,* ultrasound. (From Lipman, Z. M., Ingrasci, G., & Yosipovitch G. [2021]. Approach to the patient with chronic pruritus. *Medical Clinics of North America, 105*[4], 699–721.)

- The following factors of the patient history, in addition to facts about the type of pruritus, may be important for diagnosis:
  - Thyroid problems, renal disease, human immunodeficiency virus (HIV) infection, or cancer in the past
  - Medication history
  - Travel history
  - Substance abuse and psychiatric history
- Check for signs of liver illness such as conjunctival pallor, thyromegaly, splenomegaly, or stigmata.
- Lymph nodes should be palpated for lymphadenopathy signs.

Laboratory and Diagnostic Tests

- Complete blood count (CBC) with differential to evaluate for myeloproliferative disease, malignancy, or iron deficiency.
- Serum bilirubin, alkaline phosphatase, transaminases to evaluate for liver diseases.
- Thyroid-stimulating hormone (TSH) to evaluate for thyroid gland disorders.
- Blood urea nitrogen (BUN) and creatinine to evaluate for renal disease.
- Chest radiograph to evaluate for adenopathy.

Differential Diagnoses

- Dry skin
- Hives
- Rash
- Eczema
- Psoriasis
- Chickenpox
- Insect bite
- Medications (opioid induced)
- Hormonal changes
- Infestations of the skin with a parasite, such as scabies or head lice
- Allergic reactions
- Shingles
- Blood disorders, such as anemia, polycythemia, multiple myeloma
- Kidney failure
- Liver disease, including hepatitis C, and cirrhosis
- Thyroid disease
- Diabetes
- AIDS

Interventions

- Depending on the severity and cause, use of topical, systemic, and behavioral interventions may be necessary.
  - Preventive treatment when possible; prevent dry skin or skin breakdown.
  - Topical treatments related to source of pruritus:

- Xerosis: Hydrate the skin by soaking in a warm/tepid bath and then patting dry and applying an occlusive moisturizer to trap in the moisture.
- Lotions should be alcohol and fragrance free; examples include Aquaphor, Vanicream, Moisturel, and Eucerin or Cetaphil.
- Soothing oatmeal baths and the use of cold packs can be helpful.
- Alcohol and spicy foods may worsen the itch.

Pharmacologic Interventions

- The triggering factors for pruritus and the severity of the pruritus have an impact on the treatment approach.
- Management consists of:
  - Treatment of the underlying cause (if applicable)
  - Elimination of aggravating factors
  - Pharmacologic, antipruritic therapies to reduce symptoms (see table below)

Topical Antipruritic Therapies

Topical Antipruritic Therapies	Example
Cooling lotions	• Calamine lotion • Lotion containing camphor • Menthol
Topical anesthetics	• Pramoxine • Lidocaine • Prilocaine (eutectic mixture of local anesthetics—EMLA) • Polidocanol • Ketamine • Amitriptyline
Topical antihistamines	• Doxepin • Diphenhydramine
Topical antiinflammatory agents	• Crisaborole
Topical capsaicin	• Capsaicin (8-methyl-N-vanillyl-6-nonenamide) is a substance derived from chili peppers that has been used for the treatment of chronic pain and pruritus

Systemic Therapies

- Oral antihistamines may give symptomatic relief in itching caused by histamine; however, they are not recommended for neuropathic pruritus.
- It is thought that antihistamines' sleepy effect enhances their antipruritic efficacy; however, a greater antihistamine dosage at bedtime may generate desired potentiation of the antipruritic effect by also giving this sedative effect.
- Successful treatment frequently necessitates a complex strategy that includes treating underlying conditions, removing aggravating factors, and receiving medical treatment (see table on next page).

Systemic Antipruritic Therapies

Topical Antipruritic Therapies	Example	Indications
Antihistamines	• Hydroxyzine • Diphenhydramine	Generalized pruritus. Because of their relative safety, wide availability, and cost, H₁ antihistamines are frequently the first systemic treatments used.
Antidepressants	• Mirtazapine • Fluvoxamine • Paroxetine • Sertraline • Doxepin	The evidence for antidepressant efficacy in persistent pruritus caused by malignancies, cholestasis, and chronic renal disease was reported in the literature. The effects of oral antidepressants on serotonin and histamine levels are thought to be the reason for their benefits.
Anticonvulsants	• Gabapentin • Pregabalin	Anticonvulsants are very effective in neuropathic pruritus caused by nerve compression, such as brachioradial pruritus and notalgia paresthetica.
Phototherapy	• Ultraviolet radiation	Although phototherapy is most commonly used to treat skin lesions in inflammatory dermatoses like psoriasis, it can also help patients with prurigo nodularis, uremia, polycythemia vera, psychogenic excoriations, and notalgia paresthetica who do not have a primary skin illness. The possibility to use phototherapy in patients with contraindications to systemic medicines, such as certain older adult patients on numerous drugs, is one of its benefits.
Opioid receptor antagonists	• Naltrexone • Nalmefene • Naloxone • Methylnaltrexone	In the treatment of uremic pruritus, opioid receptor agonists are used. These medications have also been used to treat other types of persistent pruritus.
Other agents	• Aprepitant • Thalidomide • Immunomodulating agents • Medical marijuana	Aprepitant's effectiveness may be related to its ability to prevent the binding of substance P (a pruritus mediator) to the neurokinin receptor. Thalidomide: thalidomide possesses central depressive, antiinflammatory, immunomodulatory, and neuromodulatory effects, and its efficacy can be achieved through a number of methods. Immunomodulating agents: reduce atopic itch immediately and have been linked to reduced pruritus in other disorders such as prurigo nodularis and hand eczema in case studies. In a patient with pruritus associated with lichen amyloidosis secondary to primary sclerosing cholangitis, medicinal marijuana medication was related with improvement and eventual remission of pruritus.

Nonpharmacologic Interventions

- Acupuncture or a transcutaneous electrical nerve stimulation (TENS) unit can be helpful in reducing pruritus.
- Behavioral techniques (e.g., distraction, relaxation techniques) may reduce the sensation of itching and break the cycle of itching and scratching.
- Psychotherapy is a broad and diverse area that can be used to change one's perception of itch or the actions connected with it.
- Textiles: clothing can either relieve or aggravate chronic pruritic skin conditions.
- When the origin of pruritus is known, pruritus can be divided into the categories as shown in the box below.

Categories of Pruritus

Dermatologic	Pruritus caused by skin problems. Xerosis, atopic dermatitis, psoriasis, urticaria, and cutaneous infections are examples.
Systemic	Diseases that impact other organ systems, such as chronic renal failure, liver illness, hematologic or lymphoproliferative disorders, and malignancy, are examples. This category also includes drug-induced pruritus.
Neurologic	Pruritus caused by diseases of the peripheral or central nervous system. Notalgia paresthetica, brachioradial pruritus, and multiple sclerosis are examples.
Psychogenic	Depression, anxiety, psychogenic excoriation, and delusional infestation fit in this category.
Mixed	Pruritus that can be related to several causes.

Patient Teaching

- Call the health care team if pruritus is not relieved.
- To reduce the risk of skin damage, gently bathe the affected area with warm water and mild soap to keep it clean and reduce the chance of bacterial infection.
- Minimize sun exposure and to use para-aminobenzoic acid (PABA)-free, ultraviolet A (UVA) and ultraviolet B (UVB) protection sunscreen containing zinc oxide or titanium dioxide with a sun protection factor of at least 30.
- When in the sun, wear a hat, sunglasses, and clothing that covers the skin.
- Stay away from chlorinated water, hot tubs, and lakes, as well as extreme hot and cold temperatures.
- Do not use topical antiacne drugs such retinoids, benzoyl peroxide, or salicylic acid since they can cause skin dryness, irritation, and burning.
- Use an alcohol-free, fragrance-free, and hypoallergenic moisturizer to avoid dry skin.
- Oatmeal baths, oral antihistamines, cold compresses, chilled creams, or pramoxine can help with itching (a local anesthetic).
- Drink enough water and eat nutritional meals because skin hydration and healing are dependent on appropriate water intake and good nutrition.
- Reassess after 2 weeks of treatment. If symptoms do not improve or worsen, contact the practitioner to discuss the next course of action.

Follow-Up

- Ascertain what the cause of the pruritus is and treat the underlying cause.
- Refer patient to a dermatology specialist for assistance in management.

Resources

- Mayo Clinic: http://www.mayoclinic.org/diseases-conditions/itchy-skin/basics/definition/CON-20028460?p=1

Bibliography

Almeida, T. C. D. C., Figueiredo, F. W. D. S., Barbosa Filho, V. C., de Abreu, L. C., Fonseca, F. L. A., & Adami, F. (2017). Effects of transcutaneous electrical nerve stimulation (TENS) on proinflammatory cytokines: Protocol for systematic review. *Systematic Reviews*, 6(1), 139.

Barbu, M. A., Niţipir, C., Voiosu, T., & Giurcăneanu, C. (2018). Impact of dermatologic adverse reactions on QOL in oncologic patients: Results from a single-center prospective study. *Romanian Journal of Internal Medicine = Revue Roumaine de. Medecine Interne*, 56(2), 96–101.

Bonchak, J. G., & Lio, P. A. (2020). Nonpharmacologic interventions for chronic pruritus. *Itch*, 5(1), e31.

Ceasovschih, A., Voloc, G., Şorodoc, V., Vâţă, D., Lupaşcu, C. D., Preda, C., & Şorodoc, L. (2022). From chronic pruritus to neuroendocrine tumor: A case report. *Experimental and Therapeutic Medicine*, 23(3), 189.

Chen, S. C., & Jhaveri, M. (2015). The efficacy of meditation for treatment of chronic pruritus: A pilot trial. *Journal of Investigative Dermatology*, 135, S41.

Chen, X. J., & Sun, Y. G. (2020). Central circuit mechanisms of itch. *Nature Communications*, 11(1), 3052.

Cho, S. I., Lee, J., Lim, J., Park, J. S., Kim, M., Kim, T. Y., … Jo, S. J. (2019). Pruritus in patients under targeted anticancer therapy: A multidimensional analysis using the 5-D itch scale. *Acta Dermato-Venereologica*, 99(4), 435–441.

Clabbers, J. M. K., Boers-Doets, C. B., Gelderblom, H., Stijnen, T., Lacouture, M. E., van der Hoeven, K. J. M., & Kaptein, A. A. (2016). Xerosis and pruritus as major EGFRI-associated adverse events. *Supportive Care in Cancer*, 24(2), 513–521.

Erickson, S., Nahmias, Z., Rosman, I. S., & Kim, B. S. (2018). Immunomodulating agents as antipruritics. *Dermatologic Clinics*, 36(3), 325–334.

Eucerin. (2022). *Xerosis—Symptoms, causes and solutions | Eucerin*. Available at https://int.eucerin.com/about-skin/indications/xerosis.

Fazio, S., & Yosipovitch, G. (2021). *Pruritus: Etiology and patient evaluation*.

Hu, X., Sang, Y., Yang, M., Chen, X., & Tang, W. (2018). Prevalence of chronic kidney disease-associated pruritus among adult dialysis patients: A meta-analysis of cross-sectional studies. *Medicine (Baltimore)*, 97(21), e10633. , May.

Kim, B. S., Berger, T. G., & Yosipovitch, G. (2019). Chronic pruritus of unknown origin (CPUO): Uniform nomenclature and diagnosis as a pathway to standardized understanding and treatment. *Journal of the American Academy of Dermatology*, 81(5), 1223–1224.

Kim, H. J., Zeidi, M., Bonciani, D., Pena, S. M., Tiao, J., Sahu, S., & Werth, V. P. (2018). Itch in dermatomyositis: The role of increased skin interleukin-31. *British Journal of Dermatology*, 179(3), 669–678.

Larson, V. A., Tang, O., Ständer, S., Kang, S., & Kwatra, S. G. (2019). Association between itch and cancer in 16,925 patients with pruritus: Experience at a tertiary care center. *Journal of the American Academy of Dermatology*, 80(4), 931–937.

Larson, V. A., Tang, O., Stander, S., Miller, L. S., Kang, S., & Kwatra, S. G. (2019). Association between prurigo nodularis and malignancy in middle-aged adults. *Journal of the American Academy of Dermatology*, 81(5), 1198–1201.

Lee, J., Lim, J., Park, J. S., Kim, M., Kim, T. Y., Kim, T. M., & Jo, S. J. (2018). The impact of skin problems on the quality of life in patients treated with anticancer agents: A cross-sectional study. *Cancer Research and Treatment*, 50(4), 1186–1193.

Lee, H. G., Stull, C., & Yosipovitch, G. (2017). Psychiatric disorders and pruritus. *Clinics in Dermatology*, 35(3), 273–280.

Lipman, Z. M., Ingrasci, G., & Yosipovitch, G. (2021). Approach to the patient with chronic pruritus. *Medical Clinics of North America*, 105(4), 699–721.

Mollanazar, N. K., Smith, P. K., & Yosipovitch, G. (2016). Mediators of chronic pruritus in atopic dermatitis: Getting the itch out? *Clinical Reviews in Allergy and Immunology*, 51(3), 263–292.

Olsen, M. M., LeFebvre, K. K., & Brassil, K. J. (Eds.). (2019). *Chemotherapy and immunotherapy guidelines and recommendations for practice*. Pittsburgh, PA: Oncology Nursing Society.

Oncology Nursing Society. (2017). *Skin reactions [Online] via the Web at.* Available at https://www.ons.org/pep/skin-reactions (Level VII).

Pepper, M. S., & May, M. (2018). Epidermal growth factor receptor inhibitor skin rash prophylaxis in a community oncology setting. *Journal of the Advanced Practitioner in Oncology*, 9(5), 489–495.

Pereira, M. P., Steinke, S., Bruland, P., Ständer, H. F., Dugas, M., Augustin, M., & Ständer, S. (2017). Management of chronic pruritus: From the dermatological office to the specialized itch center: A review. *Itch*, 2(2), e6.

Sanders, K. M., Nattkemper, L. A., & Yosipovitch, G. (2016). Advances in understanding itching and scratching: A new era of targeted treatments. *F1000Research*, 5, F1000 Faculty Rev-2042.

Ständer, S. (2016). Classification of itch. *Current Problems in Dermatology*, 50, 1–4.

Szepietowski, J. C., & Weisshaar, E. (Eds.). (2016). Itch—Management in clinical practice. *Current Problems in Dermatology (Basel)*. Bâle: Karger, 50, 86–93.

Szöllősi, A. G., Oláh, A., Lisztes, E., Griger, Z., & Tóth, B. I. (2022). Pruritus: A sensory symptom generated in cutaneous immuno-neuronal crosstalk. *Frontiers in Pharmacology*, 13, 745658.

United States Department of Health and Human Services, & National Institutes of Health—National Cancer Institute. (2017). Common terminology criteria for adverse events (CTCAE) (version 5.0) [Online]. Available at https://ctep.cancer.gov/protocoldevelopment/electronic_applications/docs/CTCAE_v5_Quick_Ref.

Pulmonary Symptom: Cough

Michele R. Gardom

Definition

- Cough is defined as a sudden, repetitive, spasmodic contraction of the thoracic cavity causing the release of air from the lungs accompanied by a distinctive sound.
- Coughing is a pulmonary protective reflex that clears the tracheobronchial tree.
- It is categorized as acute (<3 weeks) or chronic (>8 weeks).
- May become excessive and nonproductive, possibly harming the airway mucosa.

Pathophysiology and Contributing Factors

- Cough may occur voluntarily or reflexively (induced).
- Induced cough may be triggered by endogenous (mucus or inflammation) or exogenous (smoke, perfume, or cold air) sources.
- Vagal afferent nerves found in the airway mucosa and airway wall initiate the cough reflex, triggering a large inspiration followed by complete glottis closure (inspiratory phase). Closure of the glottis causes thorax compression and increased subglottic pressures (compression phase). This phase leads to the reopening of the glottis, causing peak expiratory airflow and ending with a decrease in expired volume (expiratory phase).
- Cough reacceleration occurs when multiple expulsive events happen during one inspiration. These additional

expulsive events help to move secretions or particles out of the airway.

- Excessive cough interferes with breathing and sleep and may cause headache, pain, nausea, vomiting, syncope, and urinary incontinence.
- Common causes of cough include asthma, chronic obstructive pulmonary disease (COPD), gastroesophageal reflux disease (GERD), and upper airway cough syndrome (formerly called postnasal drip syndrome).
- In oncology settings, cough is a common cause of distress in patients with lung cancer and may be due to underlying conditions such as infection or COPD, cancer, or side effects of cancer treatment.
  - Cough is a clinical symptom of immune checkpoint inhibitor (ICPi)-related pneumonitis, a serious complication occurring in 35% of cancer patients approximately 2 to 24 months after receiving ICPi therapy (see Dyspnea).
  - Radiation pneumonitis as another specific cause for cough. Seen in patients with radiation to the thorax and involves up to 14% of patients.
- Cough occurs in as many as 80% of cancer patients.

Signs and Symptoms

- Dyspnea
- Wheezing
- Fever
- Productive or nonproductive of sputum
- Hemoptysis
- Dry, tickling cough reported by lung cancer patients

Assessment Tools

- Comprehensive history:
  - Extent of cancer, past and current treatments, especially immunotherapy
  - Medication review of prescribed and over-the-counter medications with doses and frequencies being alert to use of angiotensin-converting enzyme (ACE) inhibitors
  - Presenting symptoms: Onset, location, duration, characteristics, relieving and aggravating factors
  - Changes in activities of daily living (ADLs)
  - Past medical history: COPD, asthma, GERD, allergies, tuberculosis (TB), human immunodeficiency virus (HIV)
  - Social history: Smoking history, exposure to environmental or occupational irritants
- Physical assessment
  - Oropharynx examination: assess for mucus or erythema
  - Pulmonary examination: assess respiratory muscles, lung sounds
  - Cardiovascular examination: jugular venous distention, wet lung sounds
- Common Terminology Criteria for Adverse Events (version 5.0)
  - Grade 1: Mild symptoms that may require nonprescription interventions
  - Grade 2: Moderate symptoms, medical intervention indicated; limiting instrumental ADLs
  - Grade 3: Severe symptoms; limiting self-care ADLs

Laboratory and Diagnostic Tests

- Sputum cytology, sputum culture to rule out infection
- Pulse oximetry to rule out hypoxia
- Chest radiographic film to rule out pneumonia and pneumonitis
- Computed tomography (CT) of chest and bronchoscopy if lung cancer or other tumor suspected
- Pulmonary function tests if asthma suspected
- Esophageal pH monitoring if GERD suspected

Differential Diagnoses

- Asthma
- Upper airway cough syndrome
- COPD
- Interstitial lung disease, pulmonary fibrosis
- Pulmonary emboli
- Infections such as pneumonia, bronchitis
- Superior vena cava (SVC) syndrome
- Pericardial or pleural effusion
- Tumors of the lung
- Lymphangitis carcinomatosis
- Paraneoplastic syndrome
- GERD
- Pneumonitis
- Transesophageal fistula

Interventions

- Treat the underlying cause
- According to the American College of Chest Physicians and the European Respiratory Society guidelines, a lack of credible evidence exists regarding effective interventions to manage acute and chronic cough and cough in patients with cancer.
- While the quality of evidence is low due to study methods and high risk of bias, some interventions demonstrated a positive effect for cough in cancer. Those pharmacologic and nonpharmacologic interventions are listed below.

Pharmacologic Interventions

In the oncology setting:
- Algorithmic approach:
  - Initial trial with demulcents
    - Simple linctus syrup, 5 mL three times daily (TID) or four times daily (QID) or,
    - Butamirate linctus (syrup) or glycerol-based linctus syrup
    - Many are available over-the-counter: Robitussin for dry coughs, Sinecod, Benylin Tickly Coughs are just a few
  - If no response to demulcents, try opiate derivatives titrated to acceptable side-effect profile

- Codeine, 30 to 60 mg qid (less preferred due to side effect profile)
- Dihydrocodeine, 10 mg tid
- Hydrocodone, 5 mg bid
- Methadone linctus, single-dose 2 mg (2 mL of 1 mg/mL solution)
- Morphine (Oramorph) 5 mg (single-dose trial; if effective, 5 to 10 mg slow-release morphine bid). For patients already taking morphine, consider adjusting their dose
- For opioid-resistant cough, try peripherally acting antitussives
  - Levodropropizine, 75 mg tid
- If no response to antitussives, local anesthetics may be helpful in certain cases, especially palliative care
  - Nebulized lidocaine, 5 mL of 0.2 tid

Nonpharmacologic Interventions

- Endobronchial brachytherapy at the lowest dose and fractionated schedule
- Brachytherapy and external beam radiation for select lung cancer patients
- Speech therapy and cough suppression exercises
  - Education
  - Strategies to control cough
  - Vocal hygiene training
  - Psychoeducation
  - Identifying cough triggers
  - Cough suppression techniques (pursed lip breathing, swallowing, sipping water)
  - Breathing exercises

Patient Teaching

- Dependent on interventions
- Encourage patient to take medications as prescribed.
- Encourage reduction in exposure to irritants.
- Provide smoking cessation resources and encourage maintenance of a smoke-free environment.

Follow-Up

- Dependent on etiology and treatment plan
- Refer patients to speech therapy if indicated

Resources

- Cancer.Net: Coping with cancer: Cough. Available at https://www.cancer.net/coping-with-cancer/physical-emotional-and-social-effects-cancer/managing-physical-side-effects/cough.
- National Institutes of Health; National Heart, Lung, and Blood Institute. Health topics: Cough. Available at https://www.nhlbi.nih.gov/health-topics/cough.

Bibliography

Conoscenti, C. S. (2017). Cough. In K. Kuebler (Ed.), *Integration of palliative care in chronic conditions: An interdisciplinary approach* (pp. 247–258) Pittsburgh: Oncology Nursing Society.

Harle, A., Molassiotis, A., Buffin, O., Burnham, J., Smith, J., Yorke, J., & Blackhall, F. H. (2020). A cross-sectional study to determine the prevalence of cough and its impact in patients with lung cancer: A patient unmet need. *BMC Cancer, 20*(1), 9.

Irwin, R. S., Dudiki, N., & French, C. L. (2020). Life-threatening and non-life-threatening complications associated with coughing: A scoping review. *Chest, 158*(5), 2058–2073.

Irwin, R. S., French, C. L., Chang, A. B., Altman, K. W., & CHEST Expert Cough Panel. (2018). Classification of cough as a symptom in adults and management algorithms: CHEST guideline and expert panel report. *Chest, 153*(1), 196–209.

Lee, K. K., Davenport, P. W., Smith, J. A., Irwin, R. S., McGarvey, L., Mazzone, S. B., … CHEST Expert Cough Panel. (2021). Global physiology and pathophysiology of cough: Part 1: Cough phenomenology CHEST guideline and expert panel report. *Chest, 159*(1), 282–293.

Molassiotis, A., Bailey, C., Caress, A., & Tan, J. Y. (2015). Interventions for cough in cancer. *Cochrane Database of Systematic Reviews, 5*, CD007881.

Molassiotis, A., Smith, J. A., Mazzone, P., Blackhall, F., Irwin, R. S., & CHEST Expert Cough Panel. (2017). Symptomatic treatment of cough among adult patients with lung cancer: CHEST guideline and expert panel report. *Chest, 151*(4), 861–874.

Morice, A. H., Millqvist, E., Bieksiene, K., Birring, S. S., Dicpinigaitis, P., Domingo Ribas, C., … Zacharasiewicz, A. (2020). ERS guidelines on the diagnosis and treatment of chronic cough in adults and children. *European Respiratory Journal, 55*(1), 1901136.

Pulmonary Symptom: Dyspnea

Michele R. Gardom

Definition

- A subjective experience of breathing discomfort involving distinct sensations of varying intensity
- Derived from interactions among multiple physiologic, psychological, social, and environmental factors and may induce secondary physiologic and behavioral responses
- An uncomfortable sensation or awareness of breathing
- May have a feeling of doom
- Subjective sensation of breathlessness
- Shortness of breath
- Described by patients as the:
  - Inability to get air or air hunger
  - Feeling of suffocation
- Severity may be related to the perception of dyspnea.
- Occurs in up to 70% of persons with advanced cancer
- Most common clinical symptom in lung cancer
- Most common clinical symptom of ICPi-induced pneumonitis

Pathophysiology and Contributing Factors

- Dyspnea is multifactorial and not entirely understood.
- Dyspnea may be caused by cancer, anemia, pulmonary and cardiac disease
- Although the respiratory center controls breathing, dyspnea results from cortical stimulation.
- The cortex overrides the respiratory center, stimulating chemoreceptors in the lung and respiratory muscles and mechanoreceptors.
- Respiratory effort increases along with increased use of respiratory muscles.

- Amplification of ventilatory requirements occurs.
- It can be acute or chronic and may occur with exertion or rest.
- Contributing factors include the following:
  - Hypoxia
  - Hypercapnia
  - Interstitial lung disease
  - Pleural or cardiac effusion
  - Malignancy: direct tumor effects, indirect tumor effects, or treatment-related causes
    - Prior treatment with ICPis, anthracycline-based chemotherapy, trastuzumab, or radiation therapy to the chest
  - COPD
  - Neuromuscular weakness
  - Bronchoconstriction or spasm
  - Airflow obstruction
  - Myocardial dysfunction
  - Anemia
  - Pain
  - Deconditioning
  - Thyroid disorders
  - Cardiovascular disease
  - Aspiration
  - Pneumonia
  - Anxiety
  - Radiation pneumonitis

Signs and Symptoms

- Air hunger
- Feeling of suffocation
- Cyanosis, pallor
- Anxiety
- Tachypnea
- Tachycardia
- Use of accessory muscles when breathing

Assessment Tools

- Comprehensive history:
  - Extent of cancer, past, and current treatments, especially immunotherapies, and date of last treatment
  - Medication review
  - Presenting symptoms: Onset, triggers, alleviating factors
  - Functional impact: Changes in ADLs
  - Past medical history: Cardiac disease, pneumonitis or other interstitial lung diseases, COPD, asthma, pneumonia, anxiety, diabetes
  - Social history
  - Psychological assessment
- Physical assessment and review of systems with emphasis on cardiopulmonary
  - Visual or verbal analog scale for dyspnea
  - Subjective descriptors/self-report
  - Respiratory rate and quality, use of accessory muscles
  - Oxygen saturation
  - Structured exercise test: 6-minute walk test

- Common Terminology Criteria for Adverse Events (version 5.0)
  - Grade 1: Shortness of breath with moderate exertion
  - Grade 2: Shortness of breath with minimal exertion; limiting instrumental ADL
  - Grade 3: Shortness of breath at rest; limiting self-care ADLs
  - Grade 4: Life-threatening; urgent care indicated
  - Grade 5: Death

Laboratory and Diagnostic Tests

- Pulse oximetry (may be within normal limits despite dyspnea)
- Complete blood count, blood chemistry, plasma brain natriuretic peptide (BNP) level
- Pulmonary function tests
- Maximal inspiratory pressure (MIP)
- Chest radiographic films to note the presence of pneumonia or cardiomyopathy
- Echocardiogram to determine left ventricular ejection fraction
- Arterial blood gas measurement (if clinically appropriate)

Differential Diagnoses

- Lung cancer
- COPD
- Pulmonary embolism
- Myocardial infarction
- Congestive heart failure
- Cardiomyopathy
- Anxiety/panic attack
- Pain
- Asthma
- Obesity

Interventions

- Treat the underlying cause

Pharmacologic Interventions

- Moderate evidence exists to support systemic opioids if no relief from nonpharmacologic interventions
  - Specific opioid of choice, route, and formulation should be guided by the patient's concurrent medications, comorbidities, clinical setting, and risk profile.
  - Oral opioids: typical choice for chronic dyspnea in cancer patients
  - Parenteral opioids: typical choice for acute severe dyspnea
- Evidence is weak for the following interventions, especially in patients with advanced cancer; clinicians should use their judgment when deciding benefit versus risk
  - Short-acting bronchodilators for bronchospasms
  - Systemic corticosteroids for obstructed or inflamed airway
  - Short-acting benzodiazepines for severe anxiety
- Insufficient evidence to support the use of diuretics, antidepressants, or neuroleptics
- Avoid β-blockers and nonsteroidal antiinflammatory drugs as they may cause dyspnea

Nonpharmacologic Interventions

- Moderate evidence exists to support the following, especially in patients with advanced cancer:
  - Using a handheld fan to blow cool air on the face: permits airflow to the trigeminal nerve
  - Oxygen for hypoxia only when SpO_2 ≤90% room air

Patient Teaching

- Take medications as directed
- Keep a dyspnea diary
- Report changes in sputum production
- Monitor temperature and report if greater than 100.5°F (38°C)
- Positioning for comfort; keep head tilted
- Exercise
- Nutrition
- Get rid of smoking and pet dander in the home.

Follow-Up

- Reinforce need for prompt communication with health care providers if future episodes of dyspnea occur or if interventions are not effective.

Resources

- Cancer.Net: Coping with cancer: Shortness of breath or dyspnea. Available at https://www.cancer.net/coping-with-cancer/physical-emotional-and-social-effects-cancer/managing-physical-side-effects/shortness-breath-or-dyspnea.

Bibliography

Brahmer, J. R., Lacchetti, C., Schneider, B. J., Atkins, M. B., Brassil, K. J., Caterino, J. M., … National Comprehensive Cancer Network. (2018). Management of immune-related adverse events in patients treated with immune checkpoint inhibitor therapy: American Society of Clinical Oncology clinical practice guideline. *Journal of Clinical Oncology, 36*(17), 1714–1768.

Fadol, A. (2021). Dyspnea: Common side effect. *Clinical Journal of Oncology Nursing, 25*(Suppl. 6), 341–352.

Hui, D., Bohlke, K., Bao, T., Campbell, T. C., Coyne, P. J., Currow, D. C., … Campbell, M. L. (2021). Management of dyspnea in advanced cancer: ASCO Guideline. *Journal of Clinical Oncology, 39*(12), 1389–1411.

Kocatepe, V., Can, G., & Oruç, Ö. (2021). Lung cancer-related dyspnea: The effects of a handheld fan on management of symptoms. *Clinical Journal of Oncology Nursing, 25*(6), 655–661.

Oncology Nursing Society. (2019, August 26). *Dyspnea*. Available at https://www.ons.org/pep/dyspnea?display=pepnavigator&sort_by=created&items_per_page=50 (accessed January 31, 2022).

Parshall, M. B., Schwartzstein, R. M., Adams, L., Banzett, R. B., Manning, H. L., Bourbeau, J., … American Thoracic Society Committee on Dyspnea. (2012). An official American Thoracic Society statement: Update on the mechanisms, assessment, and management of dyspnea. *American Journal of Respiratory Critical Care Medicine, 185*(4), 435–457.

Pulmonary Symptom: Pleural Effusion

Michele R. Gardom

Definition

- Accumulation of excess fluid in the pleural space

- Classified as *transudative* (from a systemic problem such as heart failure) or *exudative* (from a localized inflammatory or malignant dysfunction)
- Can be attributed to certain chemotherapy and immunotherapy agents
- Associated most commonly with lung, breast, or ovarian cancer; lymphoma; and cancer of unknown primary
- Approximately 45% of all pleural effusions are malignant; over 150,000 people are diagnosed with malignant pleural effusions (MPEs) in the United States each year

Pathophysiology and Contributing Factors

- Normally there is only 10 to 20 mL of pleural fluid, spread thinly over the visceral and parietal pleurae, which facilitates chest wall movement.
- Excess fluid is formed in, or fluid is removed from, the pleural space, resulting in imbalance between the osmotic and hydrostatic pressures controlling the secretion and reabsorption of pleural fluid.
- May be benign or malignant
- May result from direct tumor involvement or from indirect sequelae of disease progression due to pleural involvement or mediastinal cancer with blockage of lymphatics
- SVC syndrome
- Pericardial constriction
- Obstruction of mediastinal lymphatics by tumor
- Obstruction of pulmonary vessels by tumor or a pulmonary infarction
- Shedding of malignant cells into the pleural space
- Intraabdominal cancer draining through the right diaphragm

Signs and Symptoms

- Dependent on the amount and rate of fluid accumulation and comorbid illnesses (e.g., COPD, heart failure)
- MPEs usually develop slowly, are the most common cause of breathlessness, and reaccumulate more than 50% of the time
- Presenting symptoms:
  - Resting or exertional dyspnea
  - Cough: predominantly a dry cough
  - Pleuritic pain and chest discomfort
  - Weight loss from advancing cancer
  - Malaise

Assessment Tools

- Comprehensive history
  - Extent of cancer, past and current treatments, and date of last treatment
  - Patient history (both medical and oncologic). The temporal pattern of symptoms is important when assessing the cluster of symptoms experienced with the effusion.
- Physical examination
  - Vital signs: evaluate for pulsus paradoxus with SVC, respiratory rate, pulse rate

- Jugular venous pressure: increased, changes with respiration
- Distended chest veins and elevated jugular pulse with SVC
- Lung auscultation and percussion
  - Dullness to percussion measured on both sides of the chest, decreased breath sounds, egophony above the effusion
  - Absence of fremitus on affected side
  - Cardiac sounds: distant, gallop and murmur
- Common Terminology Criteria for Adverse Events (version 5.0):
  - Grade 1: Asymptomatic; clinical or diagnostic observations as no intervention needed
  - Grade 2: Symptomatic and interventions needed (diuretics, thoracentesis)
  - Grade 3: Symptomatic with respiratory distress and hypoxia; chest tube or pleurodesis required
  - Grade 4: Life-threatening respiratory compromise; intubation
  - Grade 5: Death

Laboratory and Diagnostic Tests

- Resting and ambulatory pulse oximetry
- Chest radiographic film
- Chest ultrasonography
  - Can detect small volumes (5 mL) of fluid
  - Useful in guiding thoracentesis as well as chest tube insertion
  - No radiation exposure
  - Can be repeated frequently at the bedside
- Chest CT scan with contrast: high-resolution scanning for pulmonary embolism depending on history
- Thoracentesis procedure with cytologic analysis of pleural fluid and assessment for symptom relief
- Video-assisted thoracoscopic surgery (VATS)
  - Used when thoracoscopy fails to confirm malignancy or tissue type remains in question

Differential Diagnoses

- Congestive heart failure
- Nephrotic syndrome
- Cirrhosis
- Infection
- Malignancy
- Hemothorax
- Pulmonary embolism
- Pancreatitis

Interventions

- Oxygen therapy if clinically appropriate
- Ultrasound-guided thoracentesis to reduce rates of pneumothorax; refrain from draining MPE in asymptomatic patients unless sampling is needed for diagnostic purposes

- Chest tube placement for drainage
- Indwelling pleural catheters (IPCs) or chemical pleurodesis as first line intervention for dyspnea due to MPE; associated with decreased length of stay
- Talc pleurodesis using talc slurry or talc poudrage for patients with symptomatic MPE and expandable lung
- External beam radiation therapy
- Pleuroperitoneal shunt
- Treatment of underlying malignancy in breast cancer or lymphoma
- PleurX catheter

Patient Teaching

- The patient and family should be educated that a malignant pleural effusion is a sign of advanced disease.
- The treatment plan should be based on patient goals, performance status, and general prognosis.
- If the patient is asymptomatic, observation alone is reasonable until symptoms occur.
- Provide information about specific procedures.

Follow-Up

- Provide routine follow-up to assess the effects of treatment.
- Plan for early diagnosis and intervention for recurrent pleural effusions.
- Assess patient goals to ensure that treatments are in keeping with the patient's wishes.
- An interdisciplinary approach should be used to provide continued education and support to the patient and family.
- Educate the patient or family when to contact the provider (e.g., if the patient becomes symptomatic or experiences a sudden change in respiratory status).

Resources

Cancer.Net: Coping with cancer: Fluid around the lungs or malignant pleural effusion. Available at https://www.cancer.net/coping-with-cancer/physical-emotional-and-social-effects-cancer/managing-physical-side-effects/fluid-around-lungs-or-malignant-pleural-effusion.

Bibliography

Dipper, A., Jones, H. E., Bhatnagar, R., Preston, N. J., Maskell, N., & Clive, A. O. (2020). Interventions for the management of malignant pleural effusions: A network meta-analysis. *Cochrane Database of Systematic Reviews*, 4(4), CD010529.

Feller-Kopman, D. J., Reddy, C. B., DeCamp, M. M., Diekemper, R. L., Gould, M. K., Henry, T., … Balekian, A. A. (2018). Management of malignant pleural effusions: An official ATS/STS/STR clinical practice guideline. *American Journal of Respiratory and Critical Care Medicine*, 198(7), 839–849.

Olsen, M. M., LeFebvre, K. B., & Brassil, K. J. (Eds.). (2019). *Chemotherapy and immunotherapy guidelines and recommendations for practice*. Pittsburgh: Oncology Nursing Society.

Shafiq, M., & Feller-Kopman, D. (2020). Management of malignant pleural effusions. *Clinics in Chest Medicine*, 41(2), 259–267.

Thomas, R., Roy, B., Maldonado, F., & Lee, Y. C. G. (2019). Management of malignant pleural effusions: What is new. *Seminars in Respiratory Critical Care Medicine*, 40(3), 323–339.

Principles of Symptom Management

4

Rash

Laura S. Wood

Definition

- A rash is a dermatologic reaction that can be treatment related or associated with a malignancy.
- Rashes are more commonly associated with targeted therapies but also occur with chemotherapy and other cancer therapies.
- With targeted therapies, the precise etiology of most rashes remains unclear but is thought to be related to pathway inhibition.
- Rashes may be associated with xerosis, pruritus, and/or pain.
- The incidence, severity, and timing of onset of rash associated with several targeted therapies may correlate with outcome.
- Rashes should be described by using phenotypic terms for appearance and location (see box below).

Phenotypic Terms Used to Describe Rashes

- Acneiform
- Acral erythema
- Bullous dermatitis or bullous pemphigoid
- Desquamation
- Erythema
- Erythema multiforme
- Erythroderma
- Folliculitis
- Lichenoid dermatitis, lichenoid drug eruption, or lichenoid planus
- Macule
- Morbilliform
- Nodule
- Papule
- Papulopustular
- Plaque
- Psoriasiform dermatitis
- Pustule
- Urticaria
- Vitiligo

From Balagula, Y., Rosen, A., Tan, B. H., Busam, K. J., Pulitzer, M. P., Motzer, R. J., … Lacouture, M. E. (2012). Clinical and histopathologic characteristics of rash in cancer patients treated with mammalian target of rapamycin inhibitors. *Cancer, 118*, 5078–5083; Sun, W., & Li, J. (2019). Skin toxicities with epidermal growth factor receptor tyrosine kinase inhibitors in cancer patients: A meta-analysis of randomized controlled trials. *Cancer Investigation, 37*, 253–264; Westphalen, C. B., Kukiolka, T., Garlipp, B., Hahn, L., Fuchs, M., Malfertheiner, P., … Waldschmidt, D. T. (2020). Correlation of skin rash and overall survival in patients with pancreatic cancer treated with gemcitabine and erlotinib-results from a non-interventional multi-center study. *BMC Cancer, 20*, 1–8; Uozumi, S., Enokida, T., Suzuki, S., Nishizawa, A., Kamata, H., Okano, T., … Yamaguchi, M. (2018). Predictive value of cetuximab-induced skin toxicity in recurrent or metastatic squamous cell carcinoma of the head and neck. *Frontiers in Oncology, 8*:616. Common terminology criteria for adverse events, (CTCAE) version 5.0: Available at https://ctep.cancer.gov/protocoldevelopment/electronic_applications/docs/ctcae_v5_quick_reference_5x7.pdf and https://ctep.cancer.gov/protocoldevelopment/electronic_applications/ctc.htm (accessed January 15, 2022).

Pathophysiology and Contributing Factors

- Many cancer drugs are associated with dermatologic toxicities due to pathway inhibition by cancer therapies.
- Receptors are expressed in the epidermal and follicular keratinocytes, sebaceous epithelium, and hair follicles.
- Inhibition of epidermal growth factor receptor (EGFR) may result in follicular occlusion due to lack of differentiation in the epithelium; this may cause sebaceous glands to produce a rosacea-like reaction that results in increased production of inflammatory mediators.
- Additional therapies associated with rash include mammalian target of rapamycin (mTOR) inhibitors, vascular endothelial growth factor (VEGF), mitogen-activated protein kinase (MEK), extracellular regulated kinase (ERK) inhibitors, checkpoint inhibitor therapies, and others.

Signs and Symptoms

- Rash associated with targeted therapies typically occurs within the first few weeks of treatment.
- Erythema, dry skin, pruritus, and pain may accompany the rash at any point in time.
- Areas of involvement, severity, and duration vary greatly.
- Eruptions associated with EGFR inhibitors commonly involve the seborrheic areas, the face, neck, retroauricular area, shoulders, upper trunk, and scalp.
- Erythematous papules may evolve into pustules with pus that dry out with the formation of yellow crusts.

Assessment Tools

- Patient history (both medical and oncologic)
  - Review of prior dermatologic reactions
  - Review of allergies and sensitivities to medications and environmental factors
- Physical examination including assessment of
  - Area of involvement
  - Appearance of the dermatologic reaction
  - Date of onset
    - Any change in type, extent, or severity of rash since its onset
  - Associated symptoms
    - Erythema, swelling, pruritus, blisters, desquamation
    - Determination of which side effects are affecting the patient. Treatment for mild or moderate side effects should be initiated before they become dose limiting.
- Common toxicity criteria for adverse events (CTCAE, version 5.0); https://ctep.cancer.gov/protocoldevelopment/electronic_applications/docs/ctcae_v5_quick_reference_5x7.pdf (see table on next page).

Dermatologic Terminology Criteria (CTCAE, Version 5.0)

	Grade 1	Grade 2	Grade 3	Grade 4
Dry skin	Covering <10% BSA and no associated erythema or pruritus	Covering 10%–30% BSA and associated with erythema or pruritus; limiting instrumental ADLs	Covering >30% BSA and associated with pruritus; limiting ADLs	—
Palmar-plantar erythrodysesthesia syndrome	Minimal skin changes or dermatitis (e.g., erythema, edema, hyperkeratosis) without pain	Skin changes (e.g., peeling, blisters, bleeding, fissures, edema, or hyperkeratosis) with pain; limiting instrumental ADL	Severe skin changes (e.g., peeling, blisters, bleeding, fissures, edema, or hyperkeratosis) with pain; limiting self-care ADL	—
Rash: acneiform	Papules and/or pustules covering <10% BSA, which may or may not be associated with symptoms of pruritus or tenderness	Papules and/or pustules covering 10%–30% BSA, which may or may not be associated with symptoms of pruritus or tenderness; associated with psychosocial impact; limiting instrumental ADL; papules and/or pustules cover >30% BSA with or without mild symptoms	Papules and/or pustules covering >30% BSA, with moderate or severe symptoms; limiting self-care ADL; associated with local superinfection with oral antibiotics indicated	Life-threatening consequences; papules and/or pustules covering any % BSA, which may or may not be associated with symptoms of pruritus or tenderness; and are associated with extensive superinfection with IV antibiotics indicated
Rash: maculopapular	Macules/papules covering <10% BSA with or without symptoms (e.g., pruritus, burning, tightness)	Macules/papules covering 10%–30% BSA, with or without symptoms (e.g., pruritus, burning, tightness); limiting instrumental ADL; rash covering >30% BSA with or without mild symptoms	Macules/papules covering >30% BSA, with moderate or severe symptoms; limiting self-care ADL	—

ADL, Activities of daily living; BSA, body surface area; IV, intravenous.
Adapted from National Cancer Institute. (2010). Common terminology criteria for adverse events (CTCAE), version 5.0. Available at https://ctep.cancer.gov/protocoldevelopment/electronic_applications/docs/ctcae_v5_quick_reference_5x7.pdf (accessed January 15, 2022).

Considerations for Diagnosing Cancer Therapy-Associated Rash

- Rash presentation: Appearance, area of involvement
- Associated symptoms: Pruritus, pain or burning, paresthesias
- Characteristics of secondary infection: Fluid or drainage from lesions, crusting, fever, or chills.
- Refer to dermatologist when:
  - Abrupt change in appearance of rash or its associated symptoms
  - Worsening of rash or associated symptoms in spite of several over-the-counter (OTC) or prescription topical interventions
  - Minimal or no response to oral corticosteroids, is grade ≥3, or is intolerable.
  - Atypical dermatologic manifestations unrelated to the rash

Laboratory and Diagnostic Tests

- Swab culture (to evaluate possible secondary infection)
- Biopsy (typically a punch biopsy)

Differential Diagnosis

- Folliculitis, often referred to as an acneiform eruption or acne-like rash, consists of inflammatory follicular papules and pustules.
- Bacterial culture may be appropriate but is often negative.

Interventions

- Treatment is based on the clinical phenotype and associated symptoms and focuses on maintaining quality of life while maximizing clinical outcomes.
- Evidence-based recommendations continue to evolve.
- Prophylactic strategies continue to evolve, and evolving data should be incorporated into clinical practice.

Pharmacologic Interventions

- Prophylactic approaches may decrease severity of the rash and improve quality of life.
- Use of topical or systemic steroids or antibiotics may be indicated (see box on next page).

Pharmacologic Interventions		
Topical Products	**Systemic Steroids**	**Systemic Antibiotics**
Diphenhydramine lotion	Dexamethasone	Clindamycin
Lac-Hydrin lotion	Methylprednisolone (Medrol dose pack)	Doxycycline
Clindamycin lotion or gel		Minocycline hydrochloride
Metrogel (topical Flagyl)		Trimethoprim/ sulfamethoxazole
Temovate (clobetasol propionate)		

Nonpharmacologic Interventions

- Initiation of cleansing and moisturizing skin care regimen with initiation of treatment
- Use mild soap and water for routine bathing
- Avoid topical products with fragrance or alcohol, which can dry the skin
- Nondeodorant, nonfragrance-containing soaps
- Frequent applications of lotion
- Use of lotions with higher dimethicone content to provide a higher degree of moisture barrier
- Water-based makeup (may also be used to camouflage rashes involving the face)
- Gentle makeup remover
- Avoidance of sun exposure and use of sunscreen with a strong sun protection factor (SPF) rating
- Multidisciplinary management including referral to dermatology

Patient Teaching

- Educate patient and family on adherence to the recommended skin care regimen.
- Emphasize prevention, early intervention, and ongoing management to maximize clinical benefit of therapy and quality of life.
- Follow good hygiene practices to avoid introduction of bacteria to potential open areas.
- Treatment interruptions and dose reduction may be needed for intolerable symptoms.
- Educate patient and family on early and ongoing communication with the health care team regarding interventions and management of rash.

Follow-Up

- Frequent follow-up to assess for clinical changes in rash, symptomatic changes, improvement, worsening, or development of new symptoms related to rash.
- Make referrals as appropriate, especially to a dermatologist and for psychosocial support if necessary.

Resources

- Cancer.Net: https://www.cancer.net
- Chemo Care (Cleveland Clinic): http://www.chemocare.com
- Multinational Association of Supportive Care in Cancer (MASCC): http://www.mascc.org
- National Comprehensive Cancer Network: http://www.nccn.org
- National Cancer Center Network Guidelines for patients. Immunotherapy side effects: Immune checkpoint Inhibitors: https://www.nccn.org/patients/guidelines/content/PDF/immunotherapy-se-ici-patient.pdf
- National Cancer Institute: Common terminology criteria for adverse events, version 5.0: https://ctep.cancer.gov/protocoldevelopment/electronic_applications/docs/ctcae_v5_quick_reference_5x7.pdf

Bibliography

Balagula, Y., Rosen, A., Tan, B. H., Busam, K. J., Pulitzer, M. P., Motzer, R. J., … Lacouture, M. E. (2012). Clinical and histopathologic characteristics of rash in cancer patients treated with mammalian target of rapamycin inhibitors. *Cancer, 118,* 5078–5083.

Barcenas, C. H., Hurvitz, S. A., Di Palma, J. A., Bose, R., Chien, A. J., Iannotti, N., … CONTROL Study Investigators. (2020). Improved tolerability of neratinib in patients with HER2-positive early-stage breast cancer: The CONTROL trial. *Annals of Oncology, 31,* 1223–1230.

Beech, J., Germetaki, T., Judge, M., Paton, N., Collins, J., Garbutt, A., … Saunders, M. P. (2018). Management and grading of EGFR inhibitor-induced cutaneous toxicity. *Future Oncology, 14,* 2531–2541.

Brahmer, J. R., Abu-Sbeih, H., Ascierto, P. A., Brufsky, J., Cappelli, L. C., Cortazar, F. B., … Ernstoff, M. S. (2021). Society for Immunotherapy of Cancer (SITC) clinical practice guideline on immune checkpoint inhibitor-related adverse events. *Journal for Immunotherapy of Cancer, 9*(6), e002435.

Chen, A. P., Setser, A., Anadkat, M. J., Cotliar, J., Olsen, E. A., Garden, B. C., & Lacouture, M. E. (2012). Grading dermatologic adverse events of cancer treatments: The common terminology criteria for adverse events, version 4.0. *Journal of the American Academy of Dermatology, 67,* 1025–1039.

Ding, J., Farah, M. H., Nayfeh, T., Malandris, K., Manolopoulos, A., Ginex, P. K., … Murad, M. H. (2020). Targeted therapy-and chemotherapy-associated skin toxicities: Systematic review and meta-analysis. *Oncology Nursing Forum, 47,* E149–E160.

Eaby-Sandy, B., & Lynch, K. (2014). Side effects of targeted therapies: Rash. *Seminars Oncology Nursing, 30,* 147–154.

Friedman, M. D., Lacouture, M., & Dang, C. (2016). Dermatologic adverse events associated with use of adjuvant lapatinib in combination with paclitaxel and trastuzumab for HER2-positive breast cancer: A case series analysis. *Clinical Breast Cancer, 16*(3), e69–e74.

Hofheinz, R. D., Deplanque, G., Komatsu, Y., Kobayashi, Y., Ocvirk, J., Racca, P., … Jatoi, A. (2016). Recommendations for the prophylactic management of skin reactions induced by epidermal growth factor receptor inhibitors in patients with solid tumors. *The Oncologist, 21,* 1483–1491.

Lacouture, M. E., Anadkat, M. J., Bensadoun, R. J., Bryce, J., Chan, A., Epstein, J. B., … MASCC Skin Toxicity Study Group. (2011). Clinical practice guidelines for prevention and treatment of EGFR inhibitor-associated dermatologic toxicities. *Supportive Care Cancer, 19,* 1079–1095.

Mahon, S. M., & Carr, E. (2021). Skin toxicities; common side effect. *Clinical Journal of Oncology Nursing, 25*(6), 32.

National Cancer Institute. (2010). Common terminology criteria for adverse events (CTCAE), version 5.0. Available at https://ctep.cancer.gov/protocoldevelopment/electronic_applications/docs/ctcae_v5_quick_reference_5x7.pdf (accessed February 2, 2022).

National Cancer Institute. (2020). National Comprehensive Cancer Network Guidelines for patients. Immunotherapy side effects: Immune checkpoint inhibitors. Available at https://www.nccn.org/patients/guidelines/content/PDF/immunotherapy-se-ici-patient.pdf (accessed February 2, 2022).

National Cancer Institute. (2021). National Comprehensive Cancer Network guidelines version 4.2021: Management of immunotherapy-related adverse toxicities. Available at NCCN.org (accessed February 2, 2022).

Ng, C. Y., Chen, C. B., Wu, M. Y., Wu, J., Yang, C. H., Hui, R. C., … Lu, C. W. (2018). Anticancer drugs induced severe adverse cutaneous drug reactions: An updated review on the risks associated with anticancer targeted therapy or immunotherapies. *Journal of Immunology Research, 2018,* 5376476.

Pepper, M. S., & May, M. (2018). Epidermal growth factor receptor inhibitor skin rash prophylaxis in a community setting. *Journal of the Advanced Practitioner in Oncology, 9,* 485–495.

Rossi, A. M., Hibler, B. P., Navarrete-Dechent, C., & Lacouture, M. E. (2020). Restorative oncodermatology: Diagnosis and management of dermatologic sequelae from cancer therapies. *Journal of the American Academy of Dermatology, 85*, 693–707.

Schneider, B. J., Naidoo, J., Santomasso, B. D., Lacchetti, C., Adkins, S., Anadkat, M., … Bollin, K. (2021). Management of immune-related adverse events in patients treated with immune checkpoint inhibitor therapy: ASCO Guideline update. *Journal of Clinical Oncology, 39*, 4073–4126.

Tsui, A., Edmondson, L., & Julius, J. (2021). An evaluation of the use of corticosteroids for the management of immune-mediated adverse events in cancer patients treated with immune checkpoint inhibitors. *Journal of the Advanced Practitioner in Oncology, 12*, 137–145.

Uozumi, S., Enokida, T., Suzuki, S., Nishizawa, A., Kamata, H., Okano, T., … Yamaguchi, M. (2018). Predictive value of cetuximab-induced skin toxicity in recurrent or metastatic squamous cell carcinoma of the head and heck. *Frontiers in Oncology, 8*, 616.

Wang, E., Kraehenbuehl, L., Ketosugbo, K., Kern, J. A., Lacouture, M. E., & Leung, D. Y. M. (2021). Immune-related cutaneous adverse events due to checkpoint inhibitors. *Annals of Allergy, Asthma & Immunology, 126*, 613–622.

Westphalen, C. B., Kukiolka, T., Garlipp, B., Hahn, L., Fuchs, M., Malfertheiner, P., … Waldschmidt, D. T. (2020). Correlation of skin rash and overall survival in patients with pancreatic cancer treated with gemcitabine and erlotinib-results from a non-interventional multi-center study. *BMC Cancer, 20*, 1–8.

Wiley, K., Ebanks, G. L., Jr., Shelton, G., Strelo, J., & Ciccolini, K. (2020). Skin toxicity: Clinical summary of the ONS Guidelines for cancer treatment-related skin toxicity. *Clinical Journal of Oncology Nursing, 24*, 561–565.

Williams, L. A., Ginex, P. K., Ebanks, G. L., Jr., Ganstwig, K., Ciccolini, K., Kwong, B. K., et al. (2020). ONS Guidelines for cancer treatment-related skin toxicity. *Oncology Nursing Forum, 47*, 539–556.

Wu, J., Liu, D., Offin, M., Lezcano, C., Torrisi, J. M., Brownstein, S., … Lacouture, M. E. (2021). Characterization and management of ERK inhibitor associated dermatologic adverse events: Analysis from a non-randomized trial of ulixertinib for advanced cancers. *Investigational New Drugs, 39*, 785–795.

Seizures

Carol Stein Blecher

Definition

- A seizure may be defined as a sudden overactivation of cerebral neurons that may cause changes in sensory and motor function. There may also be changes in autonomic function, behavior, and level of consciousness.

Pathophysiology and Contributing Factors

- Seizures are a symptom of irritation of the central nervous system (CNS) that results in an abnormal discharge of neurons.
- Cerebral function is disturbed by electrical discharges that are synchronous, abnormal, and excessive.
- This abnormal discharge of neurons can cause an alteration of consciousness or any other cerebral cortical function.
- Classification is either focal or generalized, but all seizures are characterized by sudden involuntary contraction of groups of muscles.
- Causes
  - Neuronal loss or scarring from surgery or head trauma
  - Primary brain cancer or metastatic brain tumors
  - Acquired immunodeficiency syndrome (AIDS) or a history of seizures

- Metabolic disturbances such as syndrome of inappropriate antidiuretic hormone (SIADH) secretion, hypoglycemia, hyponatremia, hypercalcemia (a late sign), hypocalcemia, hypomagnesemia, renal or hepatic failure, alcohol or drug withdrawal
- Chemotherapeutic agents including bevacizumab, blinatumomab, busulfan, CAR-T (chimeric antigen receptor-T cell therapy), carmustine, cisplatin, cyclosporine, cytarabine, cyclophosphamide, etoposide, gemcitabine, ifosfamide, interferon-alfa, intrathecal methotrexate, oxaliplatin, rituximab, vincristine
- Types
  - Primary generalized seizures
    - *Absence*: Brief loss of consciousness
    - *Myoclonic*: Sporadic (isolated), jerking movements
    - *Atonic*: Loss of muscle tone
    - *Tonic*: Muscle stiffness, rigidity
    - *Clonic*: Repetitive, jerking movements
    - *Tonic-clonic*: Unconsciousness, convulsions, muscle rigidity
  - Partial seizures: preceded by an aura
    - *Simple partial*: Characterized by focal activity with no loss of consciousness
    - *Complex partial*: Characterized by loss of consciousness
    - *Secondarily generalized*
  - Absence (petit mal): Brief, characterized by no obvious motor symptoms
  - Unclassified epileptic seizures characterized by abrupt onset, unconsciousness, involuntary motor activity, involuntary sensory activity, and incontinence. There is also a postictal state after the seizure that is characterized by somnolence or headache.

Signs and Symptoms

- Change in level of consciousness
- Aura before the event: an unusual feeling, smell, or sensation
- Change in muscle tone and movement
- Activity that is involuntary and uncontrolled
- A postictal state after the seizure is characterized by somnolence or headache
- No memory regarding the event

Assessment Tools

- History, including diagnosis and cancer treatment, current medications, presenting symptoms, changes in activities of daily living (ADLs), social history, family history, and history of recent infections
- Signs and symptoms, including clinical symptoms regarding the episode. This information may need to be obtained from an individual who observed the event because the patient may have no memory of the seizure.
- Neurologic examination evaluating for automatism (repetitive movements), hyperreflexia, positive Babinski sign, localized neurologic deficits

- Vital signs: orthostatic changes
- Skin examination for signs of intravenous (IV) drug abuse or trauma, including lacerations, bruises, and oral trauma
- Precipitating factors such as stress, exercise, alcohol, barbiturates, recreational drugs, fatigue, heat, flashing lights, focusing on a computer screen, driving, antihistamines, nonadherence to therapy
- National Cancer Institute (NCI) common toxicity criteria
  - Grade 1: brief partial seizure; no loss of consciousness
  - Grade 2: brief generalized seizure
  - Grade 3: new-onset seizures (partial or generalized); multiple seizures despite medical intervention
  - Grade 4: life-threatening consequences; prolonged repetitive seizures
  - Grade 5: death
- Physical Examination
- Neurologic examination
- Cranial nerve examination
- Motor examination
- Reflex examination
- Sensory examination
- Coordination examination

Laboratory and Diagnostic Tests

- Complete blood cell count (CBC) to rule out thrombocytopenia, which can cause intracerebral bleeding
- Chemistry studies to assess for SIADH, hypoglycemia, hyponatremia, hypercalcemia, hypocalcemia, hypomagnesemia, renal or hepatic failure
- Pregnancy test for women of childbearing age; because anticonvulsives are pregnancy category D, they can cause harmful effects to the fetus
- Drug screening for cocaine, crack cocaine, and heroin because these medications or their withdrawal can cause seizures
- Drug levels of current anticonvulsive medications
- Alcohol blood level
- Computed tomographic (CT) scan of the head to identify tumor, metastases, or head trauma
- Electroencephalogram (EEG) to differentiate seizure activity from psychogenic symptoms and motor activity caused by neuromuscular conditions
- Lumbar puncture to assess for infection (meningitis, abscess, toxoplasmosis) or meningeal carcinomatosis

Differential Diagnoses

- Alcohol withdrawal
- Cerebrovascular event
- Drug toxicity: busulfan, carmustine, cisplatin, cyclosporine, high-dose 5-fluorouracil (5-FU), ifosfamide, intrathecal methotrexate, cocaine, crack cocaine, and heroin
- Infectious meningitis, abscess, toxoplasmosis
- Metabolic imbalance
- Migraine headache
- Psychiatric disorders
- Tumor: primary brain tumor or metastatic disease
- Trauma

Interventions

Pharmacologic Interventions

- Carbamazepine (Tegretol) 600 to 1200 mg PO
- Diazepam (Valium) 2 to 10 mg PO bid to qid
- Gabapentin (Neurontin) 900 to 3600 mg PO
- Lamotrigine (Lamictal) 50 to 200 mg PO bid
- Levetiracetam (Keppra) 1000 to 3000 mg PO
- Lorazepam (Ativan) 1 to 8 mg PO
- Phenytoin (Dilantin) 300 to 400 mg PO
- Phenobarbital 60 to 200 mg PO at night
- Valproic acid (Depakote) 250 to 750 mg PO

Nonpharmacologic Interventions

- During an active seizure
  - Secure airway
  - Obtain IV access
  - Protect from injury
  - Provide oxygen supplementation
  - Obtain blood work: blood glucose level for hypoglycemia
  - If patient has a history of seizures and is taking antiseizure medications, monitor serum levels of anticonvulsants.
- If the seizure is caused by underlying metabolic disturbances, these should be corrected and any medications contributing to the conditions should be discontinued.
- If appropriate, transfer patient to the nearest emergency department.

Patient Teaching

- Instructions should include the following:
  - Follow seizure precautions.
  - Do not drive or operate dangerous machinery.
  - Report blurred vision, ataxia, or drowsiness caused by anticonvulsive medications to health care provider immediately.
  - Avoid alcohol while taking anticonvulsants.
  - Contact health care provider if
    - This is a first-time seizure.
    - A seizure lasts more than 2 to 5 minutes.
    - The person does not awaken or have normal behavior after a seizure.
    - Another seizure starts soon after a seizure ends.
    - The person had a seizure in water.
    - The person is pregnant, injured, or has diabetes.
    - The person does not have a medical ID bracelet (instructions explaining what to do).
    - There is anything different about this seizure compared with the person's usual seizures.

Follow-Up

- Monitor the patient's clinical state, seizure frequency, and serum anticonvulsant levels.
- CBC, chemistries, liver enzymes; monitor renal and hepatic function
- Patients who have a 2-year seizure-free period and no risk factors may be taken off the antiseizure medications. Anticonvulsive medication must be tapered slowly. Patients

with risk factors should be maintained on medication for 5 years.
- If the patient's disease is terminal, the seizure activity should be controlled with lorazepam or a barbiturate.
- Referrals should be made to a neurologist, a radiation oncologist, and an epilepsy center.

Resources
- Common terminology criteria for adverse events, version 5: https://ctep.cancer.gov/protocoldevelopment/electronic_applications/docs/ctcae_v5_quick_reference_8.5x11.pdf.
- Epilepsy Foundation of America: http://www.epilepsy.com/.
- Healthline: What you should know about seizures: https://www.healthline.com/health/seizures.
- Medline Plus. (2022). *Seizures.* Available at http://www.nlm.nih.gov/medlineplus/ency/article/003200.htm (accessed March 6, 2022).
- Medline Plus. (2022). *Epilepsy or seizures—Discharge.* Available at http://www.nlm.nih.gov/medlineplus/ency/patientinstructions/000128.htm (accessed March 6, 2022).
- MedlinePlus Patient Education Tools: http://www.nlm.nih.gov/medlineplus/ency/patientinstructions/000128.htm.

Bibliography

Common terminology criteria for adverse events, version 5. (2017). Available at https://ctep.cancer.gov/protocoldevelopment/electronic_applications/docs/ctcae_v5_quick_reference_8.5x11.pdf (accessed March 6, 2022).
Epilepsy Foundation of America. Homepage. Available at http://www.epilepsy.com/ (accessed March 6, 2022).
Gonzalez Castro, L. N., & Milligan, T. A. (2020). Seizures in patients with cancer. *Cancer, 126*(7), 1379–1389.
Schwartz, M. A. (2015). Neurological disturbances. In B. R. Ferrell, & N. Coyle (Eds.), *Textbook of palliative nursing* (4th ed.). New York: Oxford University Press.
Walker, J. G., & Le, E. M. (2014). Seizures. In D. Camp-Sorrell & R. A. Hawkins (Eds.), *Clinical manual for the oncology advanced practice nurse.* Pittsburgh, PA: Oncology Nursing Press.
Wilkes, G. M. (2014). Increased intracranial pressure. In C. H. Yarbro, M. H. Frogge, & M. Goodman (Eds.), *Cancer symptom management* (4th ed.). Sudbury, MA: Jones & Bartlett.
Zielke, K. A. (2008). Seizures. In K. K. Kuebler & P. Esper (Eds.), *Palliative practices A-Z* (2nd ed., pp. 211–213). Pittsburgh, PA: Oncology Nursing Society.

Sexual Dysfunction

Wendy H. Vogel

Definition
- Sexuality is a multidimensional concept that encompasses sexual self-concept, sexual function, sexual roles, sexual relationships, and sexual orientation. It includes intimacy and is not limited to just sexual function, intercourse, and reproduction. Sexuality is ultimately defined by each person.
- Sexual health is a component of overall health.
- Sexual dysfunction is a group of disorders, both physiologic and psychological, that adversely affect sexuality. This can include (but is not limited to) dyspareunia, loss of libido, impotence, infertility, anorgasmia, and delayed ejaculation.

- Estimates of prevalence of alterations in sexuality range from 40% to 100%. Long-term dysfunction may occur (50% of breast cancer survivors).
- Alterations in sexuality are underdiagnosed often because of health care professionals' discomfort, lack of knowledge, or embarrassment of the subject.

Pathophysiology and Contributing Factors
- Gonadal function is regulated by the anterior pituitary and the hypothalamus.
  - Hypothalamic hormones induce glandular secretions that control the hypothalamus and pituitary.
    - Luteinizing hormone-releasing hormone (LHRH) or gonadotropin-releasing hormone (GnRH), secreted by the hypothalamus, stimulates the pituitary to produce luteinizing hormone (LH) and follicle-stimulating hormone (FSH)
    - LH and FSH stimulate the testis to produce testosterone or the ovary to produce estrogen and progesterone, hormones that control sexual function
- Disruption of the neurovasculature of the genitalia or changes in hormonal status can occur secondary to cancer or cancer treatments.
- Chemotherapy, radiation therapy, or surgery may cause direct injury to gonads.
- Ovarian failure may be induced by radiation therapy, chemotherapy, hormonal therapy, surgery, or infection.
  - Estrogen deficiency, resulting in amenorrhea and vaginal and urogenital atrophy
  - Depletion of primordial follicles and oocytes, resulting in loss of fertility
  - Disruption of the hypothalamic-pituitary-gonadal axis
- Testicular aplasia, azoospermia, and erectile dysfunction in males may occur because of direct organ damage from surgery or radiation therapy or because of changes in hormonal status secondary to systemic cancer treatment (chemotherapy or hormonal therapy).
  - Disruption of the hypothalamic-pituitary-gonadal axis
  - Loss of or damage to germ cells and developing sperm
  - Leydig cell dysfunction resulting in decreased testosterone
  - Mechanical dysfunction resulting from surgery
- Other causes of sexual dysfunction include the following:
  - Medications (e.g., antihypertensives, anticonvulsants, antiemetics, psychotropic agents, narcotics, hormonal agents, histamine H_2 receptor blockers)
  - Alcohol, nicotine, cocaine, and other illegal drugs
  - Depression, stress, relationship difficulties
  - Body image (e.g., related to colostomy, head and neck surgery, amputation, cachexia, radiation skin changes, surgery)

Signs and Symptoms
- Women: Vaginal atrophy, thinning of the vaginal wall, dryness, dyspareunia, postcoital bleeding, premature menopause, decreased libido, impaired fertility, hot flashes,

emotional lability, mood changes, irritability, body image changes, sexual identity issues (see Menopausal Symptoms section)
- Men: Decreased testosterone, decreased libido, decreased to no production of semen, erectile dysfunction, ejaculatory difficulties, impotence, impaired fertility, gynecomastia, body image changes, sexual identity issues

Assessment Tools

- PLISSIT model (Permission, Limited Information, Specific Suggestions, Intensive Therapy)
- BETTER model (Bring up the topic, Explain the issue, Tell about resources, Time the discussion, Explain the side effects, Record the discussion)
- Men
  - International Index of Erectile Function
  - Brief Male Sexual Function Inventory
  - Sexual Health Inventory for Men
- Women
  - Brief Index of Sexual Functioning for Women
  - Changes in Sexual Functioning Questionnaire
  - Female Sexual Function Index
- Risk factors for sexual dysfunction
  - Increasing age
  - Certain medications
  - Psychological issues such as alterations in body image, depression, low self-esteem, decreased sense of femininity/masculinity, poor coping mechanisms, poor communication skills
  - Comorbidities such as arthritis, chronic obstructive pulmonary disease (COPD), diabetes, myocardial infarction, spinal cord injury
- Review medication list for medications that could be affecting sexual function.
- Assess relationship status, reasons, and incentives to be sexually active.
- Assess sexual functioning before cancer diagnosis and current sexual functioning.

Laboratory and Diagnostic Tests

- Females: FSH, LH, serum estradiol, mean estrone, human chorionic gonadotropin (hCG); genital, pelvic, and breast examination
- Males: testosterone, RigiScan, penile ultrasound studies, genital examination
- Both sexes as indicated: urinalysis if urinary tract symptoms are present, prolactin levels, rectal examination; testing for sexually transmitted diseases; fertility studies
- Computed tomography (CT), magnetic resonance imaging (MRI), or ultrasound of the abdomen/pelvis if vascular or neurologic damage is suspected

Differential Diagnoses

- Females: ovarian abnormalities, polycystic ovarian syndrome, ovarian neoplasia
- Hypothyroidism
- Pituitary tumors
- Adrenal abnormalities

Interventions

Pharmacologic Interventions

- Hormone replacement therapy (HRT) in postmenopausal women is a controversial subject because of various health risks, including breast cancer (see Menopausal Symptoms section).
- Testosterone replacement in men or women
  - Contraindicated in prostate cancer
  - In female patients, the route is not established nor is safety in hormonally related cancers.
- In the oncology patient, careful consideration should be given to hormone-related cancer, and the risks of cancer stimulation should be evaluated.
- Treatment of comorbidities affecting sexuality
- In females, menopausal symptoms should be treated as noted in Menopausal Symptoms on page 356.
- Medications for erectile dysfunction: sildenafil, vardenafil, tadalafil (contraindicated with concurrent use of nitrates or the α-blockers terazosin and doxazosin).

Nonpharmacologic Interventions

- Refer patients to a fertility preservation specialist before cancer treatment, as appropriate.
- Refer patients to a surgeon, urologist, or reconstructive surgeon as appropriate.
- Proactively approach patients about sexual dysfunction, giving them permission to ask questions or express concerns. Discuss common issues related to the type of treatment and some ways to work through it.
- Fatigue issues must be addressed.
- Advise smoking cessation, low to moderate alcohol intake, maintenance of a healthy weight, and exercise as tolerated.
- For dyspareunia (painful intercourse), recommend vaginal moisturizers or lubricants, position changes for comfort, relaxation exercises, stress reduction techniques, topical lidocaine, regular sexual activity, adequate foreplay, vaginal dilation; provide instruction in Kegel exercises, EROS clitoral therapy device.
- Vaginal lubricants, such as Replens (Auspharm, Australia), may be helpful for vaginal dryness (see Menopausal Symptoms section).
- For erectile dysfunction, penile suppositories, vacuum devices, penile injections, and penile implants may be used.
- For sexual issues related to colostomies or ileostomies
  - Refer to national organization resources.
  - Limit food intake before anticipated sexual activities.
  - Plan times for intimacy when bowel movement is less likely.
  - Empty pouch when intimacy is anticipated.
  - Roll up or tape down empty, flat ostomy bag.
  - Use decorative covers.
  - Review selection of ostomy products.
- Refer patients to a sex therapist or couples counseling as needed.
- Do not assume because a patient is elderly, terminally ill, or without a partner that sexual concerns are not an issue.

- Nurses must assume a nonjudgmental, open, caring attitude with all patients regardless of sexual orientation.

Patient Teaching

- Patients should understand the fertility risks and the potential for sexual dysfunction before undergoing cancer treatment.
- If hormonal therapy is considered, the risks and benefits must be fully explored with the patient.
- Reassure patients and significant others that there are many ways to express love and intimacy and that communication is key.
- Information regarding safe sex must be discussed with each oncology patient as part of chemotherapy teaching.
- Contraception discussion is needed for female patients of child-bearing age.
- Avoid sexual relations at times of low blood counts.
- Explore other means of sexual expression besides intercourse.

Follow-Up

- Provide follow-up as needed to assess symptom management.

Resources

- American Cancer Society: www.cancer.org
- Chemocare.org: www.chemocare.org
- National Cancer Institute: www.cancer.gov
- American Association of Sex Educators: www.aasect.org
- US Too International: www.ustoo.org/intimacy

Bibliography

Burns, K., Hoefgen, H., Strine, A., & Dasgupta, R. (2018). Fertility preservation options in pediatric and adolescent patients with cancer. *Cancer, 124*(9), 1867–1876.

Carter, J., Lacchetti, C., Andersen, B. L., Barton, D. L., Bolte, S., Damast, S., … Rowland, J. H. (2018). Interventions to address sexual problems in people with cancer: American Society of Clinical Oncology Clinical Practice Guideline Adaptation of Cancer Care Ontario Guideline. *Journal of Clinical Oncology, 36*(5), 492–511.

Del-Pozo-Lérida, S., Salvador, C., Martínez-Soler, F., Tortosa, A., Perucho, M., & Giménez-Bonafé, P. (2019). Preservation of fertility in patients with cancer (Review). *Oncology Reports, 41*(5), 2607–2614.

Del Pup, L., Villa, P., Amar, I., Bottoni, C., & Scambia, G. (2019). Approach to sexual dysfunction in women with cancer. *International Journal of Gynecological Cancer, 29*(3), 630–634.

Falk, S., & Dizon, D. (2020). Sexual health issues in cancer survivors. *Seminars in Oncology Nursing, 36*(1), 150981.

Faubion, S. S., Larkin, L. C., Stuenkel, C. A., Bachmann, G. A., Chism, L. A., Kagan, R., … Kingsberg, S. A. (2018). Management of genitourinary syndrome of menopause in women with or at high risk for breast cancer: Consensus recommendations from The North American Menopause Society and The International Society for the Study of Women's Sexual Health. *Menopause, 25*(6), 596–608.

Kamen, C. S., Alpert, A., Margolies, L., Griggs, J. J., Darbes, L., Smith-Stoner, M., … Norton, S. A. (2019). "Treat us with dignity": A qualitative study of the experiences and recommendations of lesbian, gay, bisexual, transgender, and queer (LGBTQ) patients with cancer. *Support Care Cancer, 27*(7), 2525–2532.

Kaplan, M. (2021). Sexual dysfunction: Common side effect. *Clinical Journal of Oncology Nursing, 25*(6), 16–20.

Krebs, L. (2014). Altered body image and sexual health. In C. Yarbro, D. Wujcik, & B. Gobel (Eds.), *Cancer symptom management* (4th ed.). Burlington, MA: Jones & Bartlett.

Krebs, L. (2018). Sexual and reproductive dysfunction. In C. Yarbro, D. Wujcik, & B. Gobel (Eds.), *Cancer nursing principles and practice* (8th ed.). Sudbury, MA: Jones & Bartlett.

Nashimoto, P., & Mark, D. (2015). Sexuality and reproductive issues. In C. Brown (Ed.), *A guide to oncology symptom management* (2nd ed.). Pittsburg, PA: Oncology Nursing Society.

National Comprehensive Cancer Network. (2021). NCCN1 Guidelines Version 3.2021 Survivorship: Sexual function. *The Journal of Clinical Oncology, 36*(19), 1994–2001.

Oktay, K., Harvey, B. E., Partridge, A. H., Quinn, G. P., Reinecke, J., Taylor, H. S., … Loren, A. W. (2018). Fertility preservation patients with cancer: ASCO Clinical Practice Guideline Update. *Journal of Clinical Oncology, 36*(19), 1994–2001.

Rees, M., Angioli, R., Coleman, R. L., Glasspool, R., Plotti, F., Simoncini, T., & Terranova, C. (2020). European Menopause and Andropause Society (EMAS) and International Gynecologic Cancer Society (IGCS) position statement on managing the menopause after gynecological cancer: Focus on menopausal symptoms and osteoporosis. *Maturitas, 134*, 56–61.

Schover, L. (2018). Sexual quality of life in men and women after cancer. *Climacteric, 22*(6), 553–557.

Stabile, C., Goldfarb, S., Baser, R. E., Goldfrank, D. J., Abu-Rustum, N. R., Barakat, R. R., … Carter, J. (2017). Sexual health needs and educational intervention preferences for women with cancer. *Breast Cancer Research and Treatment, 165*(1), 77–84.

Sleep Disturbances

Wendy H. Vogel

Definition

- Sleep disturbances include insomnia and hypersomnia.
  - Insomnia is the inability to sleep when needed; it may include difficulty falling asleep, difficulty maintaining sleep, or early-morning awakenings with difficulty resuming sleep.
  - Hypersomnia is the inability to maintain wakefulness when needed.
- Sleep disturbances are a common problem in oncology patients; they can be transient, chronic, or recurring and can affect quality of life.

Pathophysiology and Contributing Factors

- Sleep disturbances are common in oncology patients.
- Sleep impairment risk increases with age.
- The most common cause of insomnia is uncontrolled pain.
- Insomnia or hypersomnia can also occur because of use of certain medications, withdrawal from certain medications, anxiety, depression, hypoxia, sleep apnea, urinary frequency, pruritus, endocrine disorders, hot flashes, restless legs, sleeping during the day, caffeine intake, change in environment, or psychological stress.
- Insomnia could also be an independent disorder with no known etiology (primary insomnia).
- Cancer patients often complain of daytime sleepiness and nighttime insomnia.
- Sleep deprivation is linked to changes in mentation, such as a decline in cognitive function and behavioral changes.
- Studies have shown a decrease in certain immune functions associated with insomnia.
- Pathophysiology of sleep: an interrelated process involving the balance between being asleep and being awake, the circadian rhythm, and the cycles (stages) of sleep.
- There are two stages of sleep, non–rapid eye movement (NREM) sleep and rapid eye movement (REM) or dreaming

sleep. Circadian factors control the wake and sleep patterns over a 24-hour period. NREM sleep, REM sleep, and circadian rhythms may be disrupted in oncology patients.
- The normal amount of sleep needed to maintain healthy functioning varies from 6 to 10 hours per night.
- Types
  - Transient: lasting less than 2 weeks
  - Short-term: lasting between 2 and 4 weeks
  - Chronic: lasting longer than 4 weeks
- Incidence
  - The incidence of sleep disturbances ranges from 25% to 95% in oncology patients.
  - About 50% of these sleep disturbances are insomnias (in the general population, insomnia occurs in 30% to 35% of people).
  - Sleep disturbances are more likely during the initial diagnosis, during cancer treatments, and at the end of life.
  - Up to 44% of patients continue to report insomnia several years after diagnosis and treatment.

Signs and Symptoms

- Inability to fall asleep or sleeping too much
- Awakenings in the night, early-morning awakening, and inability to return to sleep, difficulty staying asleep
- Daytime sleepiness, daytime napping, fatigue, irritability, depression, anxiety, decreased concentration, irregular sleep schedules

Assessment Tools

- Routinely assess for sleep disturbances, including sleep quality, daytime sleepiness, and symptoms of insomnia. Include assessments of frequency, severity, and duration of symptoms
- Subjective Assessment Tools: Epworth Sleepiness Scale, Consensus Sleep Diary, Insomnia Severity Index, Pittsburgh Sleep Quality Index
- Knowing the patient's normal sleep habits enables the health care provider to establish a baseline normal pattern.
- Assess the amount and timing of daily physical exercise.
- Determine the bed partner or family member's perceptions of sleep disturbance.
- Bedtime/wake times
- Diet, caffeine, and alcohol intake
- Environmental conditions (e.g., lighting, noise, ventilation, bedding, temperature, positioning)
- Medication review
- Patient's belief about the cause of sleep disturbance
- Presence of daytime napping
- Pre-sleep routines (e.g., food and fluid intake, hygiene, stimulation)
- Total hours slept during a 24-hour period
- Assess for risk factors
  - Active chemotherapy treatment
  - Chronic medical illness (e.g., asthma, gastroesophageal reflux, and chronic obstructive pulmonary disease)
  - Depression/anxiety
  - Distress of symptoms such as pain, nausea, or diarrhea

- Fatigue
- Female sex
- Lower educational level
- Lower socioeconomic status
- Menstruation
- Older age
- Perimenopause
- Personal or family history of insomnia
- Recent life stressors
- Specific cancer type (e.g., breast, colorectal, prostate, ovarian, lung, hematologic, and malignant melanoma)
- Unpleasant environment
- Use of alcohol
- Shift work
- Polypharmacy
- Assess for medications known to cause insomnia
  - Amphetamines
  - Anticonvulsants
  - Biologicals (e.g., interferons, interleukins, tumor necrosis factor)
  - Bronchodilators
  - Caffeine
  - Chemotherapy
  - Corticosteroids
  - Decongestants
  - Dieting agents
  - Hormonal agents
  - Illicit drugs
  - Long-term use of analgesic medications
  - Monoamine oxidase inhibitors (MAOIs)
  - Selective serotonin reuptake inhibitors (SSRIs)
  - Theophyllines
- Physical examination
  - Neurologic assessment
  - Oropharyngeal examination, observing for anatomic obstruction

Laboratory and Diagnostic Tests

- No standard quantitative criteria exist to diagnose insomnia.
- A sleep study (polysomnography) may be useful in a primary sleep disorder such as narcolepsy, parasomnias, or sleep apnea (not indicated for evaluation of transient or chronic insomnia or insomnia associated with psychiatric disorders).
- It is useful to determine cause factors for sleep disturbances such as obstructive sleep apnea and periodic leg movements.
- A sleep journal (1- to 2-week log) may be helpful in obtaining the specific information related to the assessments described.
- Underlying physical and emotional causes should be ruled out and treated as necessary. This could include obtaining a urinalysis and a complete blood cell count.

Differential Diagnoses

- It is important to differentiate between a primary cause of sleep disturbance (e.g., narcolepsy, parasomnia) and secondary causes of sleep disturbance.
- Cancer-related fatigue

Interventions

- Rule out any physical or emotional causes of sleep disturbances. Management of these causes (e.g., uncontrolled pain, depression) may correct the sleep disturbance.

Pharmacologic Interventions

- For insomnia, benzodiazepines, benzodiazepine-receptor agonists, melatonin-receptor agonists, or sedative-hypnotics may be used.
- Medications should be closely monitored.
- Tolerance to short-acting benzodiazepines could occur in as little as 2 weeks, and these medications should be used intermittently and for as short a period as possible (ideally, no longer than 3 to 4 weeks).
- Tapering and then discontinuing the medication once a therapeutic point is reached should be considered.
- Pharmacotherapy is not recommended for chronic insomnia except for a short-term period and only as an adjunct to other treatment, such as cognitive behavioral treatment (see table below).
- Alternative treatments for insomnia (efficacy and safety not established):
  - Melatonin
  - Valerian root extract
  - THC (tetrahydrocannabinol)

Pharmacologic Treatment for Short-Term Insomnia

Class	Drugs	Benefits	Complications
Benzodiazepines	Clonazepam Lorazepam Oxazepam	Class of choice for short-term treatment Useful in insomnia caused by anxiety or restless legs Useful in insomnia that is refractory to other treatments	Long-acting agents may cause daytime drowsiness, dizziness, cognitive impairment Short-acting agents may have tolerance and dependence issues, rebound insomnia, daytime anxiety
Nonbenzodiazepines	Eszopiclone Zaleplon Zolpidem	More receptor selectivity Fewer residual side effects the next day Do not lead to tolerance and have less potential for abuse Quick onset of action	May cause amnesias, paresthesias, arthralgias, flu-like symptoms
Tricyclic antidepressants with sedative effects	Amitriptyline Doxepin Nortriptyline	Useful in depressed patients or insomnia from neuropathic pain High sedative effects	May cause dry mouth, somnolence, dizziness, constipation, palpitations
Second-generation antidepressants with sedative effects	Trazodone (low dose) Nefazodone Mirtazapine Silenor	Useful in depressed patients Mirtazapine can stimulate appetite and decrease nausea	May cause dry mouth, somnolence, dizziness, constipation
Antihistamines	Diphenhydramine Hydroxyzine	Useful for sedation, reducing nausea and vomiting	May cause daytime sedation and delirium, especially in elderly May cause constipation, urinary retention, and confusion
Melatonin-receptor agonists	Ramelteon	Useful with difficulty falling asleep; little to no hangover effect	Caution in mild-moderate hepatic impairment; poor bioavailability (need to avoid taking with meals with high fat content)
Dual orexin receptor antagonists	Suvorexant Lemborexant	May have fewer negative effects on cognitive performance, mood, and physical performance. Little hangover effect.	Somnolence. Potential for abuse. Could exacerbate depression

- Treatment for daytime hypersomnia
  - Psychostimulants such as methylphenidate or a cholinesterase inhibitor such as donepezil
  - Modafinil, a nonamphetamine stimulant, may be considered. Use in small doses, and give early in the day; this may help prevent daytime napping, thus improving insomnia

Nonpharmacologic Interventions

- Review medications; adjust timing so that patient does not have to awaken to take medications. Ensure that medications such as diuretics are taken no later than 3 PM.

- Instruct in good sleep hygiene. Sleep hygiene includes therapies for stimulus control, sleep restriction, and relaxation.
- Cognitive control techniques such as counting, refocusing, meditation, or guided imagery may assist in controlling racing thoughts or worries.
- Thought stopping is performed by repeating the word "the" or "stop" every 3 seconds.
- Relaxation training includes progressive muscle relaxation, biofeedback, yoga, hypnosis.
- Acupuncture
- Aromatherapy

Patient Teaching

- Educate the patient on sleep hygiene (specific behaviors that promote good sleep).
  - Stay in the bed only during the hours intended for sleep.
  - Establish a routine wake time and bedtime.
  - Avoid stimulants such as caffeine.
  - Refrain from exercising at least 6 hours before bedtime.
  - Decrease or eliminate nighttime use of tobacco products.
  - Determine the best sleep environment.
  - Do not nap during the day, or limit naps to 20 minutes, and avoid all naps after 3 PM.
  - Create a bedtime routine.
  - If not asleep within 15 to 20 minutes, get out of bed and do a nonstimulating activity until sleepy, then return to bed.
  - Avoid heavy foods at bedtime.
  - Keep a sleep log.
  - Remove bedroom clock.

Follow-Up

- Follow-up as indicated to assess pharmacologic success and as needed for cognitive-behavioral training.

Resources

- American Cancer Society: www.cancer.org
- American Academy of Sleep Medicine: http://www.aasmnet.org
- National Cancer Institute: http://www.cancer.gov/cancer topics/pdq/supportivecare/sleepdisorders/Health Professional/page1/AllPages
- National Institutes of Health, National Center on Sleep Disorder Research: http://www.nhlbi.nih.gov/about/org/ncsdr/
- OncoLink:https://www.oncolink.org/healthcare-professionals/nci/pqid-cdr00000627462

Bibliography

Chen, D., Yin, Z., & Fang, B. (2018). Measurements and status of sleep quality in patients with cancers. *Support Care Cancer*, 26(2), 405–414.

Garland, S., Mahon, K., & Irwin, M. (2019). Integrative approaches for sleep health in cancer survivors. *Cancer Journal*, 25(5), 337–342.

Garland, S. N., Xie, S. X., DuHamel, K., Bao, T., Li, Q., Barg, F. K., … Mao, J. J. (2019). Acupuncture versus cognitive behavioral therapy for insomnia in cancer survivors: A randomized clinical trial. *Journal of the National Cancer Institute*, 111(12), 1323–1331.

Matthews, E. (2018). Sleep disturbances. In C. Yarbro, D. Wujcik, & B. Gobel (Eds.), *Cancer symptom management* (8th ed.). Burlington, MA: Jones & Bartlett.

Matthews, E., Carter, P., Page, M., Dean, G., & Berger, A. (2018). Sleep-wake disturbance: A systematic review of evidence-based interventions for management in patients with cancer. *Clinical Journal of Oncology Nursing*, 22(1), 37–52.

Ozkaraman, A., Dügüm, Ö., Özen Yılmaz, H., & Usta Yesilbalkan, Ö. (2018). Aromatherapy: The effect of lavender on anxiety and sleep quality in patients treated with chemotherapy. *Clinical Journal of Oncology Nursing*, 22(2), 203–210.

Walker, W., & Borniger, J. (2019). Molecular mechanisms of cancer-induced sleep disruption. *International Journal of Molecular Sciences*, 20(11), 2780.

Xerostomia

Jennifer S. Webster

Definition

- Decrease in quantity of saliva, including complete absence, and changes in composition due to a lack of salivary secretion; referred to as dry mouth.
- May be acute or chronic.
- The most common acute and late side effect of radiation treatment for head and neck cancer is if the major salivary glands are affected by treatment.
- Often chronic, affecting taste, chewing, swallowing, speech, and oral comfort.
- Persistent xerostomia has a profound impact on a patient's quality of life.

Pathophysiology and Contributing Factors

- Saliva is critical to the protection and normal function of the oral cavity. Lack of saliva may impact nutritional status, diet quality, taste, dental integrity, and susceptibility to infectious oral microbes.
- Radiation therapy to the head and neck causes direct injury to salivary gland tissue and damages blood vessels. Damage depends on the total radiation dose and volume of tissue irradiated.
  - Major and minor salivary glands become atrophic and fibrotic.
  - Saliva consistency changes from thin and watery to thick, ropy, tenacious secretions.
  - Changes may be progressive for several months after radiation therapy and are irreversible.
- Surgical excision of head and neck tumors involving salivary glands may be causal.
- Chemotherapy is a contributing factor, although xerostomia related to standard-dose antineoplastics is typically mild and transient. High-dose chemotherapy used in hematopoietic stem cell transplant may cause long-lasting xerostomia in approximately 15% of patients.
- The advent of immuno-oncology agents such as nivolumab or pembrolizumab in the treatment of head and neck cancer suggests approximately 3% to 7% of these patients will experience xerostomia.
- Total body irradiation as a preparatory component of certain hematopoietic stem cell transplantation regimens may cause long-term salivary gland dysfunction.
- Chronic graft-versus-host disease in the setting of stem cell transplant may directly attack salivary tissue or cause inflammation, leading to xerostomia.
- Oral microbes, associated with poor oral health, are linked to adverse effects, such as xerostomia and dental caries, in patients receiving cancer treatment.

- Pharmacologic causes include anticholinergics, antidepressants, antihistamines, antihypertensives, diuretics, opiates, phenothiazines, and sedatives.
- Tobacco use, especially smoking cigarettes, reduces saliva flow.
- Gastroesophageal reflux may contribute.

Signs and Symptoms

- Dry mouth
- Thirst
- Poor mastication of food
- Dysphagia
- Gagging sensation
- Anorexia
- Gingival bleeding
- Halitosis
- Ulcerations in the oral cavity
- Dry and fissured lips and/or tongue
- Painful tongue (glossodynia)
- Sore throat
- Hoarseness and difficulty speaking
- Tenacious secretions
- Increase in dental caries
- Oral candidiasis
- Pain, mild to burning
- Difficulty wearing dentures
- Taste alterations
- Weight loss and malnutrition
- Infection
- Dehydration
- Sleep disturbances

Assessment Tools

- Common Terminology Criteria for Adverse Events (CTCAE), version 5.0, is a useful tool to measure the severity of xerostomia
- History and physical examination; clinical examination based on inspection of oral cavity:
  - Mucosa may appear dry, pale, atrophic, or hyperemic, with evidence of topical infections such as thrush.
  - The lips may be chapped or fissured, and the tongue may be dry and furrowed.
  - Ask the patient to describe the saliva (e.g., thin, watery, scant, thick, ropy).
  - Evaluate taste changes, increasing thirst, sensitivity/pain to spicy foods, and difficulty wearing dentures due to discomfort or poor fit.
  - Does patient have difficulty swallowing, chewing, or with speech?
  - Measure pain using a rating scale from 0 to 10 or a categorical scale (none, mild, moderate, and severe).
- Review of all prescription and over-the-counter medications.
- Review current oral hygiene and dental care.
- Assess nutritional status.

Laboratory and Diagnostic Tests

- Complete blood count (CBC) (to determine if patient is neutropenic)
- Blood, urine, and sputum cultures if systemic sepsis is suspected or patient has fever
- Culture of oral lesions or microbial overgrowth
- Sialometry—measurement of the rate of saliva production
- Biopsy taken from salivary glands in the lip, if ruling out Sjögren syndrome (an autoimmune disorder which attacks tear and salivary glands)

Differential Diagnoses

- Sjögren syndrome
- Oral cancer
- Malnutrition
- Dehydration
- Infection
- Dysphagia
- Anorexia
- Mucositis

Interventions

- If possible, treat the underlying cause to restore moisture and lubrication to the oral cavity.
- Most interventions are aimed at providing symptom relief.

Pharmacologic Interventions

- Amifostine (Ethyol), a radioprotective agent used as prophylaxis, has contradictory results, side effects, and cost that have prevented widespread routine adoption.
- Pilocarpine (Salagen): stimulates saliva production and may improve symptom relief, but results are not conclusive.
- Cevimeline (Evoxac): stimulates saliva production and may improve symptom relief, but results are not conclusive.
- Viscous lidocaine for pain

Nonpharmacologic Interventions

- Increased fluid intake during and between meals (e.g., water, nonacidic juices)
  - Frequent sips of water are the easiest and often the most effective technique to improve dry mouth.
  - Adding a slice of lemon or lime to drinking water may improve flavor and enhance output from the major salivary glands; however, highly acidic beverages should be avoided.
- Dental care using soft toothbrushes and fluoride toothpaste
- Fluoride gels and rinses: avoid those with alcohol, high sugar content, or strong flavors that can irritate
- Sugar-free candy or lozenges and sugar-free gum

- Avoidance of dry foods
- Nutritional status monitoring
- Avoidance of irritants such as tobacco, alcohol, carbonated beverages, caffeine, and spicy or acidic foods
- Saliva substitutes may be helpful in some situations, but are commonly not well accepted by patients.
- Acupuncture and transcutaneous nerve stimulation have been studied as both interventions and prophylaxis of xerostomia, with encouraging results, but further research is needed.
- Patient may benefit from a referral to a Speech or Swallowing specialist and a Nutritionist.

Patient Teaching

- Have a comprehensive dental evaluation before treatment is initiated.
- Report any pain, tenderness, or burning sensations in the oral cavity.
- Brush teeth three to four times daily, possibly with a high-fluoride toothpaste, using a soft toothbrush.
- Brush the tongue gently once a day with a soft toothbrush or tongue scraper.
- The use of topical fluoride is critical to control dental caries. Fluorides may be over the counter or highly concentrated prescription rinses or gels. Dental experts should guide fluoride choices.
  - Practice oral care daily using fluoride treatments during radiation therapy; wait 30 minutes afterward before rinsing, eating, or drinking.
  - Continue fluoride treatments with recommendations from dental professionals.
- Floss daily with unwaxed dental floss or alternative interproximal plaque-removing device.
- Rinse with nonalcoholic mouthwashes.
- Use moisturizer or lip balm regularly on the lips.
- After completion of therapy, irradiated patients with head and neck cancer require dental follow-up every 3 to 4 months to monitor for oral complications such as gingival deterioration or caries development.
- Report fever of 100.5°F (38°C) or greater.
- Follow dietary modifications.
- If approved by care team, use a cool mist humidifier in the bedroom to improve night sleep.

Follow-Up

- Assess the patient's current oral intake and ability to maintain adequate hydration and nutrition.
- Assess for pain unrelieved by pain medication.
- Reinforce the importance of communication with physician and nurse.

Resources

- McDonald, R. (2020). Cancer treatment-induced dry mouth is "much more consequential than it sounds." Available at https://www.curetoday.com/view/cancer-treatment-induced-dry-mouth-is-much-more-consequential-than-it-sounds- (accessed June 8, 2022).
- National Cancer Institute: Oral complications of chemotherapy and head/neck radiation (PDQ): Available at https://www.cancer.gov/about-cancer/treatment/side-effects/mouth-throat/oral-complications-hp-pdq#_592_toc (accessed June 2, 2022).
- Oncolink: Dry mouth (xerostomia): Available at https://www.oncolink.org/cancer-treatment/radiation/side-effects-of-radiation-therapy/dry-mouth-xerostomia (accessed June 8, 2022).

Bibliography

Aggarwal, P., Hutcheson, K. A., Garden, A. S., Mott, F. E., Lu, C., Goepfert, R. P., … Shete, S. (2021). Determinants of patient-reported xerostomia among long-term oropharyngeal cancer survivors. *Cancer, 127*(23), 4470–4480.

Barker, C. A., Wong, J. Y. C., & Yahalom, J. (2021). Total body irradiation. In L. L. Gunderson & J. E. Tepper (Eds.), *Clinical radiation oncology* (5th ed.). Philadelphia: Elsevier.

Cannon, G. M., Saba, N. F., & Harari, P. M. (2021). Oropharyngeal cancer. In L. L. Gunderson & J. E. Tepper (Eds.), *Clinical radiation oncology* (5th ed.). Philadelphia: Elsevier.

Dunnack, H. J., Judge, M. P., Cong, X., Salner, A., Duffy, V. B., & Xu, W. (2021). An integrative review of the role of the oral and gut microbiome in oral health symptomatology during cancer therapy. *Oncology Nursing Forum, 48*(3), 317–331.

Epstein, J. B., Smith, D. K., & Murphy, B. A. (2018). Oral health and survivorship: Late effects of cancer and cancer therapy. In I. Olver (Ed.), *The MASCC textbook of cancer supportive care and survivorship* (2nd ed.). Germany: Springer International Publishing.

Fazer, C. (2019). Checkpoint inhibitor immunotherapy for head and neck cancer: Incorporating care step pathways for effective side-effect management. *Journal of the Advanced Practitioner in Oncology, 10*(Suppl. 1), 37–46.

Jiang, N., Zhao, Y., Stensson, M., & Mårtensson, J. (2022). Effects of an integrated supportive program on xerostomia and saliva characteristics in patients with head and neck cancer radiated with a low dose to the major salivary glands: a randomized controlled trial. *BMC Oral Health, 22*(1), 199.

Levi, L. E., & Lalia, R. V. (2018). Dental treatment planning for the patient with oral cancer. *Dental Clinics of North America, 62*(1), 121–130.

Mercadante, V., Al Hamad, A., Lodi, G., Porter, S., & Fedele, S. (2017). Interventions for the management of radiotherapy-induced xerostomia and hyposalivation: A systematic review and meta-analysis. *Oral Oncology, 66*, 64–74.

Milano, M. T., Marks, L. B., & Constine, L. S. (2021). Late effects after radiation. In L. L. Gunderson & J. E. Tepper (Eds.), *Clinical radiation oncology* (5th ed.). Philadelphia: Elsevier.

Roesser, K. A. (2022). Stomatitis/xerostomia. In D. Camp-Sorrell, R. A. Hawkins, & D. G. Cope (Eds.), *Clinical manual for the advanced practice nurse* (4th ed.). Pittsburgh, PA: Oncology Nursing Society.

Vissink, A., Spijkervet, F. K. L., & Brennan, M. T. (2018). Xerostomia and dental problems in the head and neck radiation patient. In I. Olver (Ed.), *The MASCC textbook of cancer supportive care and survivorship* (2nd ed.). Germany: Springer International Publishing.

White, J. D. (2020). Complementary and alternative medicine. In J. O. Armitage, J. E. Tepper, M. B. Kastan, J. H. Doroshow, & J. E., Niederhuber (Eds.), *Ableoff's clinical oncology* (6th ed.). Netherlands: Elsevier.

Structural Emergencies

Jennifer S. Webster

Bowel Obstruction

Definition

- Bowel obstruction is interference with or cessation of the normal passage of intestinal contents through the gastrointestinal (GI) tract.
- The obstruction may be partial or complete.
- It may involve the small or large bowel.
- Paralytic ileus is a failure of normal motility in the absence of mechanical obstruction.
- Obstipation refers to intractable constipation refractory to normal interventions.

Epidemiology

- Patients with a history of cancer are at risk for obstruction. Colon cancer accounts for 25% to 40% of cases, followed by ovarian and gastric cancers.
- Obstructions can be caused by primary malignant neoplasms in any part of the bowel, abdomen, or pelvis or by metastases from many other sites.
- May be the presenting sign of an intraabdominal or pelvic malignancy.
- Patients with stage IV colon cancer and bowel obstruction upon presentation have a poorer prognosis than those without bowel obstruction, regardless of treatment.
- Treatment of malignancy can cause obstruction, such as fibrosis from radiation therapy or neurotoxic effects from chemotherapy.
- Nonmalignant obstructions include adhesions from previous operations, hernia, inflammatory bowel disease, fecal impaction, and bowel ischemia.
- Constipation occurs with palliative care and affects about 50% of patients admitted to hospice care; opioids are a primary contributor of constipation.

Pathophysiology

- Mechanical bowel obstruction, whether in the large or small bowel, is the result of a physical block to the passage of intestinal contents.
- The bowel normally secretes approximately 6 to 8 L daily.
- Functional bowel obstruction results from a loss of propulsive peristalsis (e.g., paralytic ileus, postoperative adhesions).
- Risk factors include the following:
  - History of abdominal or pelvic malignancies
  - Previous abdominal surgery (i.e., potential for adhesions)

- Inflammatory bowel disease
- Herniations of the abdominal wall
- Irradiation of the abdomen
- Opioid use
- Other supportive care medications such as ondansetron, anticholinergic agents
- Immobility
- Chemotherapy drugs, particularly vinca alkaloids and thalidomide or its derivatives
- Low fiber and fluid intake

Signs and Symptoms

- Presenting symptoms depend on the site of the obstruction.
- Symptoms of obstruction include anorexia, nausea, vomiting, abdominal distention, abdominal fullness, early satiety, dyspepsia, high-pitched bowel sounds, diminished or absent bowel sounds, abdominal or pelvic cramping, pain, constipation or conversely liquid stool, and obstipation.
- Patients with early bowel obstruction may have paradoxical diarrhea as the bowel attempts to push contents past the obstruction.
- Dyspnea may accompany abdominal distention.

Cancers Associated With Disorder

- Colon
- Ovarian
- Other abdominal cancers such as stomach, pancreatic, bladder, and endometrial
- All cancers have potential for bowel obstruction.

Diagnostic Tests

- Abdominal radiography is frequently the initial diagnostic modality.
- Computed tomography (CT) with contrast is the diagnostic test of choice.
- Contrast fluoroscopy is helpful if patient is clinically stable, and a partial small bowel obstruction is suspected.
- A complete blood cell count (CBC) guides clinical decision making. An elevated white blood cell (WBC) count suggests strangulation, and an elevated hematocrit may point to dehydration.
- Evaluation of electrolytes is important in cases of small bowel obstruction because acid-base disturbances are common due to vomiting and lack of fluid intake.

Differential Diagnosis

- Acute cholangitis
- Cholecystitis

5

- Cholelithiasis
- Constipation
- Diverticulitis
- Dysmenorrhea
- Endometriosis
- Inflammatory bowel disease

Treatment

Pharmacologic Management

- Octreotide inhibits the release of several GI hormones and reduces GI secretions and continues to be the agent of choice for malignant bowel obstruction.
- Antibiotics and antiemetics may be indicated.
- Correction of electrolyte imbalances.
- Role of corticosteroids in treating bowel obstruction is controversial, but they may be useful as adjuvant antiemetics.
- Evaluation and possible switching of prescribed opioids in patients undergoing treatment for chronic pain.

Nonpharmacologic Management

- Immediate treatment is bowel rest and intravenous fluid replacement.
- Nasogastric (NG) tubes are useful for decompression and drainage. A rectal tube may be needed to decompress the distal colon.
- Surgical intervention such as resection (i.e., removal of a portion of the bowel with or without the creation of an ostomy) may be necessary.
- Colorectal stents implanted with the use of endoscopy and fluoroscopy is an option for palliative treatment.

Nursing Interventions

- Symptom management: patient may experience a great deal of pain, nausea, vomiting, and dehydration until obstruction is relieved.
- Manage NG tubes
- Monitor fluid intake and output
- Care of surgical site and ostomy if needed. Referral to enterostomal therapist as appropriate.
- Emotional support and anxiety management
- Prevention of constipation can help prevent bowel obstruction; assess bowel function ongoing and provide early intervention if obstruction is not yet suspected.

Patient Teaching

- Identify early signs and symptoms, especially for patients at risk.
- Patient may need ostomy education and referral to ostomy support group for coping strategies
- Instruct patients to notify providers about constipation unrelieved with current modalities:
  - Note that common suggestions to prevent constipation with lifestyle modifications such as increasing fiber intake, fluid intake, and activity may be helpful in relatively healthy patients but show little efficacy in those with advanced cancer.

- Pharmacologic agents are frequently necessary to prevent constipation in patients with cancer and/or receiving opiates.

Follow-Up

- Provide a follow-up phone call following hospitalization to assess recovering bowel function.
- Continue a bowel regimen and encourage patient to track bowel movements with clear instructions about what to do if constipation occurs—that is, how many days without a bowel movement to wait before notifying the provider.

Bibliography

Alsharawneh, A., & Maddigan, J. (2021). The oncologic emergency of intestinal bowel obstruction: ED recognition and treatment outcomes. *Seminars in Oncology Nursing, 37*, 151207.

Biondo, S., Gálvez, A., Ramírez, E., Frago, R., & Kreisler, E. (2019). Emergency surgery for obstructing and perforated colon cancer: Patterns of recurrence and prognostic factors. *Techniques in Coloproctology, 23*(12), 1141–1161.

Davis, M., Hui, D., Davies, A., Ripamonti, C., Capela, A., DeFeo, G., … Bruera, E. (2021). Medical management of malignant bowel obstruction in patients with advanced cancer: 2021 MASCC guideline update. *Support Care Cancer, 29*, 8089–8096.

Hydzik, C., & Perialis, K. M. (2018). Gynecologic cancers. In L. Parks & M. Routt (Eds.), *Critical care nursing of the oncology patient* (pp. 117–156). Pittsburgh, PA: Oncology Nursing Society.

Jackson, P., & Cruz, M. V. (2018). Intestinal obstruction: Evaluation and management. *American Family Physician, 98*(6), 362–367.

Ledet, C. R., & Santos, D. (2020). Acute abdomen in cancer patients. In J. L. Nates & K. J. Price (Eds.), *Oncologic critical care* (pp. 847–856). Cham: Springer.

Wickham, R. J. (2017). Managing constipation in adults with cancer. *Journal of the Advanced Practitioner in Oncology, 8*(2), 149–161.

Young, S., & Justice, J. (2022). Large bowel obstruction. In F. F. Ferri (Ed.), *2022 Ferri's clinical advisor* (pp. 915–915.e2). Philadelphia: Elsevier.

Increased Intracranial Pressure

Definition

- Increased volume within the rigid cranium occupies space and increases pressure, disrupting normal brain activities and producing devastating effects.

Epidemiology

- Incidence is difficult to estimate in the oncology population. Primary brain tumors are associated with the highest risk of increased intracranial pressure (ICP) but make up less than 1.5% of new cancer diagnoses each year.
- The most common reason for increased ICP in the oncology population is metastatic disease. Approximately 20% to 40% of cancer patients develop metastatic disease to the brain. Melanoma, lung, breast, renal, and thyroid cancers have the highest incidence of brain metastases.
- Malignant cells from leukemias and lymphomas may invade the cerebrospinal fluid (CSF) and contribute to inflammation. The immunosuppressive therapies used for these hematologic malignancies may increase the risk of intracranial infection (e.g., meningitis, toxoplasmosis) or thrombocytopenia (intracranial hemorrhage) that can lead to ICP.

- Malignant tumor can obstruct outflow of CSF from the brain or cause local cerebral edema to develop, as can brain irradiation.
- Patients with an Ommaya reservoir, which is used to deliver chemotherapy medications directly into the CSF, may develop device-related obstruction, malposition, or infection that contributes to an increase in ICP.

Pathophysiology

- The adult skull is rigid, and its size is fixed.
- The three intracranial components are brain tissue, blood, and CSF.
- Increased volume inside the skull, whether from bleeding, injury, edema, primary or metastatic tumor, infection, or increased CSF production, increases pressure within the confined space of the skull.
- Initially, the body attempts to compensate by reducing blood or CSF volume in the skull, but response capabilities are limited. Pressure within the skull increases, and the patient experiences disruption of normal brain activities.
- Onset may be slow or rapid. Onset that occurs slowly allows the body to compensate more effectively, and symptoms may not be evident immediately.
- If unrecognized, ICP can progress to brain stem herniation and death.

Signs and Symptoms

- ICP may be initially difficult to detect in patients with slowly increasing intracranial volume.
- Signs and symptoms depend on the location of the pressure and the rate of increasing ICP.
- Altered mental status or level of consciousness is the most sensitive sign.
- Headache may worsen with bending over or Valsalva maneuvers.
- Patients may have nausea and vomiting.
- Focal changes depend on the location of pressure.
  - Changes in vision and pupil size
  - Speech changes such as slurring or inability to speak at a normal pace
  - Changes in handwriting and fine motor movements
  - Memory loss
  - Motor weakness
- Seizures may occur.
- The triad of hypertension, bradycardia, and respiratory depression is a late sign of brain stem compression and requires urgent intervention.
- Changes in vital signs should be monitored.
  - Widening pulse pressure in later stages
  - Decreased pulse with ongoing rise in ICP

Cancers Associated With Disorder

- Primary brain tumors
- Tumors that metastasize to the brain—see "Epidemiology" section
- Tumors with leptomeningeal (CSF) metastases, typically certain leukemias and lymphomas

Diagnostic Tests

- Contrast-enhanced magnetic resonance imaging (MRI) is preferred, but noncontrast CT is used in emergency situations when bleeding or hydrocephalus is suspected.
- Lumbar puncture to evaluate CSF if infection or malignant tumor cells are suspected.
- Positron emission tomography (PET) is used as a complement to MRI or CT to determine cerebral blood flow to the brain.
- Evaluation of CBC and chemistries assist in clinical decision making:
  - An elevated WBC indicate a potential infection such as meningitis or encephalitis.

  Altered electrolytes such as hyponatremia or diabetic keto-acidosis cause ICP.

Differential Diagnosis

- Acute nerve injury
- Blood dyscrasias
- Migraine headache
- Papilledema
- Stroke

Treatment

- Initial goal is to stabilize the patient and address emergent symptoms.
- If possible, implement definitive treatment of the underlying cause of ICP.

Pharmacologic Management

- Steroids reduce increased ICP related to edema due to brain tumors, cranial irradiation, or infection in the brain. However high doses of steroids should be a temporary measure due to side effects and conflicting data on clinical outcomes.
- Mannitol is an osmotic diuretic that decreases cerebral edema.
- Intravenous hypertonic saline pulls water into the intravascular space and away from the brain. Central venous access is required to avoid peripheral thrombophlebitis.
- Chemotherapy is primarily effective for chemotherapy-sensitive tumor types. May be administered by intrathecal route via lumbar puncture or Ommaya reservoir.
- Analgesics may be ordered to relieve pain and sedate the patient, which can help to minimize increases in ICP.
- Anticonvulsants for patients experiencing or at risk for seizures.

Nonpharmacologic Management

- Surgical interventions
  - Resection or debulking of a primary brain tumor
  - Evacuation of a blood clot
  - Shunt placement to divert CSF
- Radiation therapy
  - Used for unresectable brain tumors or diffuse metastases
  - May cause edema with inflammatory reaction or necrosis that can contribute to increased ICP

- Hyperventilation
  - Used only in emergencies or as a temporary therapy
  - Reduces carbon dioxide levels with subsequent cerebral vasoconstriction and drop in ICP
  - Short-term effect that can contribute to cerebral hypoxia
- Therapeutic hypothermia reduces brain metabolism and blood flow, therefore reducing ICP but is controversial and requires further study.
- Barbiturate coma decreases the cerebral metabolic rate and increases cerebral vasoconstriction, therefore lowering ICP, however can depress the myocardium, GI tract, and central nervous system.
- Maintain blood pressure, fluid and electrolyte balance, and temperature in normal range to prevent exacerbation of ICP.

Nursing Interventions

- Patient positioning: elevate head of the bed to at least 30 degrees (maximum 45 degrees) to facilitate venous drainage from the head.
- Maintain calm environment: avoid loud noises or bright lights.
- Perform serial neurologic assessments to monitor changes in neurologic status and to assess treatment efficacy.
- Maintain seizure precautions.
- Treat or prevent symptoms that can increase ICP, such as coughing, vomiting, straining at stool with constipation, or pain.

Patient Teaching

- Emphasize early identification of signs and symptoms.
- Teach strategies to maximize safety in activities of daily living (ADLs) and ambulation.
- Medication management includes anticonvulsants, steroids, and analgesics.
- Interventions to minimize increased ICP
  - Elevate head of bed.
  - Maintain calm environment.
  - Avoid coughing, vomiting, and the Valsalva maneuver, including straining with bowel movements; use cough suppressants, antiemetics, and stool softeners if needed.
  - Avoid lifting heavy objects or bending down at the waist.
- Use measures to enhance adaptation and rehabilitation if neurologic deficits continue.

Follow-Up

- Monitor signs and symptoms that suggest increased ICP during follow-up exams.
- Instruct patient and family to notify providers immediately with any signs or symptoms of increased ICP.

Bibliography

American Cancer Society. (2023). Facts and figures. Atlanta, GA: American Cancer Society. Available at https://www.cancer.org/content/dam/cancer-org/research/cancer-facts-and-statistics/annual-cancer-facts-and-figures/2023/2023-cancer-facts-and-figures.pdf

Brydges, N., & Brydges, G. J. (2021). Oncologic emergencies. AACN Advanced Critical Care, 32(3), 306–314.

Khorchid, Y. M., & Maldoff, M. (2020). Intracranial hemorrhage focused on cancer and hemato-oncologic patients. In J. L. Nates & K. J. Price (Eds.), Oncologic critical care (pp. 381–394). Cham: Springer.

Pandhi, A., Krishnan, R., Goyal, N., & Malkoff, M. (2020). Increased intracranial pressure in critically ill cancer patients. In J. L. Nates & K. J. Price (Eds.), Oncologic critical care (pp. 395–407). Cham: Springer.

Parks, L. (2018). Oncologic emergencies. In L. Parks & M. Routt (Eds.), Critical care nursing of the oncology patient (pp. 245–268). Pittsburgh, PA: Oncology Nursing Society.

Saria, M. G., & Kesari, S. (2021). Increased intracranial pressure: The use of an individualized ladder. Seminars in Oncology Nursing, 37(2), 151133.

Shelton, B. K., Skinner, J., & Baynes, M. (2018). Increased intracranial pressure. In M. Kaplan (Ed.), Understanding and managing oncologic emergencies: A resource for nurses (3rd ed., pp. 277–326). Pittsburgh, PA: Oncology Nursing Society.

Threlkeld, Z. D., & Scott, B. J. (2021). Neuro-oncologic emergencies. Neurologic Clinics, 39(2), 545–563.

Neoplastic Cardiac Tamponade

Definition

- Compression of the heart caused by accumulation of excessive fluid within the pericardial sac, resulting in decreased cardiac output. If untreated, cardiac tamponade leads to eventual cardiovascular collapse and death.

Epidemiology

- The incidence of neoplastic cardiac tamponade is unknown. It may go undetected until there is a significant decrease in cardiac output.
- It may be the presenting sign of an undetected malignancy.
- The most common primary malignant neoplasm causing tamponade is mesothelioma; the lymphomas and sarcomas are also implicated.
- Breast, lung and Hodgkin lymphoma are the cancers that most frequently metastasize to the pericardium resulting in effusion. Approximately 20% of patients have metastatic disease to the pericardium at autopsy.

Pathophysiology

- The pericardium is a two-layered sac that encloses the heart and great vessels.
- The pericardial space is created between the two membranes that protect the heart (i.e., parietal and visceral) and normally contains a very small amount of fluid (10 to 50 mL) that serves as a lubricant.
- When cancer cells invade the pericardial space, pericardial fluid osmotically accumulates (i.e., pericardial effusion), increasing pressure and compressing the heart. To maintain cardiac output, the body attempts to compensate by increasing the heart rate and peripheral vasoconstriction. Eventual failure of these compensatory mechanisms leads to decreased stroke volume and subsequent inadequate organ perfusion, resulting in cardiogenic shock and death.
- Onset may be slow or rapid:
  - A slow onset may be tolerated for weeks because the pericardium can stretch to accommodate up to 2 L of fluid.
  - An extremely rapid onset may cause death within a few minutes.

Signs and Symptoms

- Difficult to detect slowly accumulating effusions and may not be identified until fluid accumulation is significant. Patients may experience:

- gradually decreasing exercise capacity
- gradually increasing dyspnea upon exertion
- Hoarseness, cough or hiccups, difficulty swallowing (i.e., compression of trachea, esophagus, and nerves)
- Dyspnea, orthopnea
- Anxiety and restlessness
- Beck triad (indicates pericardial infusion and impending tamponade):
  - Muffled heart sounds
  - Arterial hypotension
  - Bilateral jugular venous distention
- Pericardial friction rub
- Decreased systolic blood pressure and increased diastolic pressure (i.e., narrowing of pulse pressure)
- Paradoxical pulse (i.e., decline in systolic blood pressure on inspiration)
- Other signs of decreased cardiac output: tachycardia, light-headedness, peripheral cyanosis, oliguria, and shock

Cancers Associated With Disorder

- Tumors most often associated with pericardial metastasis are lung cancer, breast cancer, leukemia, Hodgkin disease, and melanoma.
- Primary tumors are rare and are usually mesotheliomas or sarcomas.
- Lung and breast cancers can spread by direct extension or lymphatic metastasis.
- Lymphomas and leukemias typically spread by hematogenous routes.
- Radiation therapy of 4000 cGy or greater to the mediastinum can lead to immediate or long-term complications.

Diagnostic Tests

- Echocardiography is the imaging method of choice with a high degree of accuracy and allows for full assessment of the hemodynamic effects of the effusion.
- Routine chest radiographs initially reveal subtle changes and an enlarged pericardial silhouette.
- Electrocardiogram (ECG) findings may be nonspecific (e.g., sinus tachycardia).
- CT and MRI are noninvasive and reveal pleural effusion, masses, or pericardial thickening.
- Percutaneous pericardiocentesis is used only for large effusions or emergent cardiac tamponade to help relieve symptoms and obtain fluid for evaluation.
  - Fluid is aspirated and assessed for type of effusion: transudate (i.e., low protein level, usually from a nonmalignant cause) or exudate (i.e., high protein level, usually from a malignant cause).
  - Malignant cells are found in the pericardial fluid of approximately 60% of patients with cancer and effusions.

Differential Diagnosis

- Cardiogenic shock
- Pericarditis
- Pneumothorax
- Pulmonary embolism
- Tension pneumothorax

Treatment

- Primary goal is to remove the fluid and relieve or prevent impending cardiac collapse.
- Degree of intervention depends on the underlying disease status, comorbid conditions, and previous treatment.

Pharmacologic Management

- Mild tamponade may respond to diuretics and steroids (usually temporary).
- Chemotherapy is primarily effective for chemotherapy-sensitive tumor types.
- Pericardial sclerosis is instillation of agents (bleomycin, tetracycline, etc.) that cause irritation and subsequent fibrosis of the pericardial space; however, it is painful, and the success rate is approximately 50%.

Nonpharmacologic Management

- Surgical interventions
  - Pericardiocentesis and possible placement of a temporary catheter for further drainage or instillation of a sclerosing agent.
  - The pericardial window removes a section of the pericardium and inserts a small screen, which permits drainage of fluid into the pleural space. This procedure has a 90% response rate and is the preferred method of treatment.
  - A pericardectomy is the removal of all or part of the pericardium to relieve radiation-induced strictures or in those patients with recurring malignant effusions.
- Radiation therapy
  - Used successfully for radiosensitive tumors.
  - Cardiac tolerance is considered for radiation therapy (3500 to 4000 cGy).

Nursing Interventions

- Elevate head of bed and position patient to lean forward if needed to relieve dyspnea
- Monitor oxygenation and vital signs. Administer oxygen by face mask.
- Reduce patient energy expenditure, assist with ADLs
- Manage pain and anxiety
- Apply measures to enhance adaptation and rehabilitation.

Patient Teaching

- Emphasize early identification and reporting of signs and symptoms.
- Teach interventions to minimize severity of symptoms:
  - Elevate head of bed.
  - Arrange for oxygen at home if needed.
  - Review strategies to reduce energy expenditure if needed.
  - Discuss methods to manage pain and dyspnea.

Follow-Up

- Monitor for signs and symptoms of fluid reaccumulation and decreased cardiac output.
- Instruct patient and family to notify providers for signs or symptoms of returning cardiac effusion.

Oncologic Emergencies 5

Bibliography

Ghosh, A. K., Crake, T., Manisty, C., & Westwood, M. (2018). Pericardial disease in cancer patients. *Current Treatment Options in Cardiovascular Medicine, 20*(7), 60.

Kaplan, M. (2018). Cardiac tamponade. In M. Kaplan (Ed.), *Understanding and managing oncologic emergencies: A resource for nurses* (3rd ed., pp. 45–106). Pittsburgh, PA: Oncology Nursing Society.

Parks, L. (2018). Oncologic emergencies. In L. Parks & M. Routt (Eds.), *Critical care nursing of the oncology patient* (pp. 245–268). Pittsburgh, PA: Oncology Nursing Society.

Sargent, C., & Shelton, B. K. (2018). Cardiovascular complications. In L. Parks & M. Routt (Eds.), *Critical care nursing of the oncology patient* (pp. 195–244). Pittsburgh, PA: Oncology Nursing Society.

Spring, J., & Munshi, L. (2020). Oncologic emergencies: Traditional and contemporary. *Critical Care Clinics, 37*(1), 85–103.

Thandra, K., Salah, Z., & Chawla, S. (2020). Oncologic emergencies: The old, the new, and the deadly. *Journal of Intensive Care Medicine, 35*(1), 3–13.

Radiation Pneumonitis

Definition

- Radiation pneumonitis is a constellation of clinical, radiographic, and histologic findings reflecting acute toxicity due to inflammation of lung tissue exposed to radiation therapy.

Epidemiology

- Symptomatic injury may occur in up to 20% of cases and range from mild cough and dyspnea on exertion to respiratory failure.
- High-risk groups include the following:
  - Low pretreatment performance status
  - Comorbid lung disease such as chronic obstructive pulmonary disease (COPD)
  - Smoking history
  - Low pulmonary function tests
  - Elderly patients (disease tends to be more severe)
  - Lung cancer patients receiving an immune checkpoint inhibitor after concurrent chemoradiotherapy.
- Incidence and severity are related to the following:
  - Volume of lung irradiated
  - Dose, rate, and quality of radiation therapy
  - Concomitant chemotherapy (e.g., bleomycin, paclitaxel)
  - In lung cancer, tumor location in the lower lung
  - Lung cancer patients receiving an immune checkpoint inhibitor after concurrent chemoradiotherapy
  - History of previous radiation therapy
  - Baseline pulmonary function tests

Pathophysiology

- Radiation directly injures endothelial and epithelial cells, which results in alveolitis.
- Accumulation of inflammatory and immune cells takes place in the alveolar walls and spaces.
- Accumulation is thought to play a role in the development of pulmonary fibrosis or chronic inflammation and distorts the normal structures.
- Fibrosis is the repair process that follows; it thickens alveolar walls.
- Radiation pneumonitis usually occurs 2 to 9 months after radiation exposure but can evolve over months to years after initial damage.

Signs and Symptoms

- Dry cough is initially related to irritation of the main bronchus and decreased mucus production.
- One to 3 months after radiation therapy, symptoms may include dyspnea, productive cough, fever (usually low grade), and night sweats.
- More severe symptoms include acute respiratory distress with significant cough, dyspnea, hypoxia, fever, and tachycardia.

Cancers Associated With Disorder

- Radiation pneumonitis can be associated with any tumor type that is treated with radiation therapy alone to the chest and lung fields or in combination with chemotherapy.

Diagnostic Tests

- Chest radiographs may show diffuse haziness progressing to infiltrates within the irradiated area
- CT is an effective diagnostic tool in this setting
- Pulmonary function tests
- Arterial blood gases (ABGs)
- CBC with differential count: elevated WBC count and increased sedimentation rate

Differential Diagnosis

- Diagnosis is not difficult when clear demarcation visualized, and patient has a history of radiation therapy to the chest
- If the demarcation is unclear, differentials include ground-glass opacities or chronic airspace opacities

Treatment

- Prevention is the primary goal, including appropriate preassessment of underlying pulmonary impairment.
- Amifostine may be administered before radiation therapy to protect normal tissue and prevent damage; further studies are needed.

Pharmacologic Management

- Corticosteroids are the primary therapy.
- Antibiotics may be needed for a secondary infection.
- Bronchodilators and sedatives may be effective for symptom relief.

Nursing Interventions

- Monitor oxygenation and vital signs. Provide oxygen therapy as needed.
- Reduce patient activities to minimize energy expenditure, assist with ADLs.
- Assess adequate relief of symptoms such as pain and dyspnea.

Patient Teaching

- Identify critical symptoms or changes in status and report accordingly:
  - Chronic dry cough
  - Increased difficulty breathing

- Skin changes
- Use of accessory muscles
- Emphasize measures to minimize energy expenditure:
  - Frequent rest periods
  - Use of ready-made meals
  - Items used frequently within easy reach
- Ensure the patient understands and uses supportive therapies (e.g., morphine, oxygen, sedation).

Follow-Up

- Ongoing palliative care visits to optimize supportive therapies and quality of life
- Assess efficacy and tolerance of steroid therapy that is commonly employed to reduce the severity of the disease
- Patients and families should be offered counseling or support group therapy due to the potential for disease chronicity and worsening

Bibliography

Jang, J. Y., Kim, S. S., Song, S. Y., Kim, Y. J., Kim, S. W., & Choi, E. K. (2021). Radiation pneumonitis in patients with non-small cell lung cancer receiving chemoradiotherapy and an immune checkpoint inhibitor: A retrospective study. *Radiation Oncologist, 15*(1), 231.

Machtay, M., & Teba, C. V. (2020). Pulmonary complications of anticancer treatment. In J. E. Niederhuber, J. O. Armitage, M. B. Kastan, J. H. Doroshow, & J. E. Tepper (Eds.), *Ableoff's clinical oncology* (6th ed., pp. 715–724). Philadelphia: Elsevier.

Milano, M. T., Marks, L. B., & Constine, L. S. (2021). Late effects after radiation. In L. L. Gunderson & J. E. Tepper (Eds.), *Clinical radiation oncology* (5th ed., pp. 290–312). Philadelphia: Elsevier.

Slate, J. L. (2022). Radiation induced lung injury. In F. F. Ferri (Ed.), *2022 Ferri's clinical advisor* (pp. 915–915.e2). Philadelphia: Elsevier.

Spinal Cord Compression

Definition

- Spinal cord compression is caused by direct injury to the spinal cord that leads to progressive and permanent motor and sensory deficits if untreated; motor weakness usually occurs before sensory loss.

Epidemiology

- Occurs in 5% of oncology patient population
- Occurs in 20% of patient with metastases to the vertebral column
- Second most frequent neurologic complication of cancer
- Malignant spinal cord compression is a result of direct tumor compression of the spinal cord or tumor invasion of the vertebrae, with subsequent collapse onto the spinal cord.
- May be caused by metastases to the spinal column, leading to pain and potential collapse.
- May be the presenting manifestation of disease (e.g., multiple myeloma) although it more typically occurs in patients who are undergoing treatment for cancer.
- A significant association exists with the ability to walk at diagnosis and recovery from compression.

Pathophysiology

- The spinal cord is located within the epidural space in the spinal canal. Tumor may invade the epidural space and impinge on the cord or destroy vertebral bone, which collapses into the epidural space and compresses the cord.
- Compression of the cord produces edema and inflammation, leading to direct neural injury, vascular damage, and oxygen impairment.
- Level of cord involvement (e.g., cervical, thoracic, lumbar, sacral, cauda equina) determines the loss of function.
- Although not life-threatening, it represents a medical emergency. If untreated, it may progress to permanent paralysis.
- Rarely, primary tumors may arise in the spinal cord and cause compression.

Signs and Symptoms

- Depends on level of cord involvement
- Back pain: often the first symptom but significance may be unrecognized, can occur up to 6 months before diagnosis, and may be progressive. The pain is typically exacerbated by coughing, sneezing, or bending over.
- Leg (one or both) weakness, with or without sensory loss
- Muscle atrophy in lower extremities
- Autonomic dysfunction (late effect): loss of bowel and bladder function, urinary hesitancy or urgency, impotence

Cancers Associated With Disorder

- Highest risk from metastases of solid tumors (e.g., lung, breast, prostate, kidney)
- Cancers of the lung, breast, and prostate account for 50% of cases
- Occurs with some hematologic malignancies (e.g., lymphomas, multiple myeloma)

Diagnostic Tests

- Neurologic exam
- Imaging studies: MRI preferred; however, plain radiographs and CT are options. Plain films often used for vertebral blastic or lytic lesions, but contrast-enhanced MRI provides best definition of spinal lesions
- CBC with differential count and sedimentation rate to differentiate spinal cord compression from infection
- Chemistry profile, including calcium and liver function tests
- Lumbar punctures contraindicated because CSF removal may worsen spinal cord compression

Treatment

- Prompt diagnosis and treatment are crucial.
- Treatment is primarily palliation of symptoms and prevention of permanent disabilities.

Pharmacologic Management

- Corticosteroids
  - Reduce edema
  - Dose and duration based on patient response
- Pain management

- Chemotherapy
  - Indicated for chemotherapy-sensitive tumors (i.e., lymphoma or Hodgkin disease)
  - Adjuvant therapy in combination with radiation therapy or surgery
  - Bisphosphonates or denosumab to reduce pain and skeletal complications from vertebral metastases

Nonpharmacologic Management

- Radiation therapy
  - Reduces symptoms. May take up to 2 weeks for initial pain relief.
  - Initiated immediately after diagnosis.
  - Usual course of 2 to 4 weeks.
- Surgery
  - Surgical decompression is treatment of choice for patients whose tumors are not radiosensitive or for previously radiated sites.
  - Surgery is indicated with evidence of spinal instability or rapidly progressing loss of function.

Nursing Interventions

- Early recognition of signs and symptoms and ongoing assessment
- Monitor bowel and bladder output; patient may need catheterization and/or bowel program if autonomic nervous system is affected
- Initiate safety measures to prevent further injury
- Assist patient in adapting to neurologic or motor deficits
- Pain management

Patient Teaching

- Teach at-risk patients early recognition of signs and symptoms
- Mobility, safety
  - Maximize environmental safety such as eliminating throw rugs, installing grip bars in showers or use of shower chair
  - Side rails, low bed, items in easy reach
  - Promote use of walker to safely increase mobility
- Skin integrity
- Pain management
- Bowel elimination regimen
- Coping strategies for potential motor and sensory limitations including loss of sexual function

Follow-Up

- Monitor ongoing recovery in patients without deficits
- For patients with functional deficits and paraplegia
  - Referral to a rehabilitation center may be necessary to optimize functioning, depending on the patient's prognosis and ability to engage in therapy.
  - Assess family's ability to provide care for the disabled patient as needed.
  - Provide ongoing skin assessment, examining pressure points carefully.
  - Assess bowel and bladder care.
  - Assess comfort.

Bibliography

Antonarakis, E. S., & Carducci, M. A. (2020). Treatment of castration-resistant prostate cancer. In A. W. Partin, R. R. Dmochowski, L. R. Kavoussi, & A. Craig (Eds.), *Campbell-Walsh-Wein urology* (12th ed., pp. 3687–3706). Philadelphia: Elsevier.

Corn, B. W., Hahn, E., & Cherny, N. I. (2021). Palliative radiation medicine. In L. L. Gunderson & J. E. Tepper (Eds.), *Clinical radiation oncology* (5th ed., pp. 290–312). Philadelphia: Elsevier.

Crommett, J. W. (2020). Metastatic spinal cord compression. In J. L. Nates & K. J. Price (Eds.), *Oncologic critical care* (pp. 429–434). Cham: Springer.

Kaplan, M. (2018). Spinal cord compression. In M. Kaplan (Ed.), *Understanding and managing oncologic emergencies: A resource for nurses* (3rd ed., pp. 45–106). Pittsburgh, PA: Oncology Nursing Society.

Massel, D. H., & Maaieh, M. A. (2021). Surgical management update in metastatic diseases of the spine. *Operative Techniques in Orthopaedics, 31*(3), 100898.

Niglas, M., Tseng, S. L., Dea, N., Chang, E., Lo, S., & Sahgal, A. (2020). Spinal cord compression. In J. E. Niederhuber, J. O. Armitage, M. B. Kastan, J. H. Doroshow, & J. E. Tepper (Eds.), *Ableoff's clinical oncology* (6th ed., pp. 715–724). Philadelphia: Elsevier.

Parks, L. (2018). Oncologic emergencies. In L. Parks & M. Routt (Eds.), *Critical care nursing of the oncology patient* (pp. 245–268). Pittsburgh, PA: Oncology Nursing Society.

Spring, J., & Munshi, L. (2020). Oncologic emergencies: Traditional and contemporary. *Critical Care Clinics, 37*(1), 85–103.

Superior Vena Cava Syndrome

Definition

- Superior vena cava (SVC) syndrome is a complex of symptoms and physical findings associated with compression or obstruction of the SVC.
  - Caused by extrinsic tumor or internal thrombus
  - Results in compromised venous drainage of the head, neck, and upper extremities

Epidemiology

- Between 75% and 85% of SVC syndrome cases have a malignant cause:
  - About 80% of cases of neoplastic origin are related to lung cancer, most frequently small cell lung cancer, followed by non-Hodgkin lymphoma (NHL) and metastatic tumors
  - May be the presenting condition in lung cancer and NHL
- Nonmalignant causes include central venous catheter thrombus and cardiac surgery.
- Risk factors include presence of central venous catheters and pacemakers and previous radiation therapy to the mediastinum.

Pathophysiology

- The SVC is a thin-walled, low-pressure, major blood vessel.
  - Its primary function is to carry venous drainage from the head, upper extremities, and upper thorax to the heart.
  - The SVC is surrounded by rigid structures in the mediastinum and multiple lymph node chains.
  - It is easily compressed by direct tumor invasion, enlarged lymph nodes, or a thrombus within the vessel.
- Compression results in the following:
  - Increase in venous pressure in areas drained by the SVC

- Decrease in cardiac output as return of blood to the heart is impeded
- Life-threatening complications of respiratory failure and hemodynamic instability if the obstruction is severe

Signs and Symptoms

- Progression of physical findings can be gradual and insidious, or rapid and acute. Slower progression allows some collateral venous circulation to develop:
  - Facial swelling
  - Headache
  - Swelling of neck, arms, and hands. Rings and shirt collars may feel tight. Fine motor movements affected by swelling of fingers.
  - Neck and thoracic vein distention
  - Dyspnea (most common). Patient may begin to sleep more upright than usual to reduce discomfort from dyspnea.
  - Nonproductive cough
  - Cyanosis of the face and upper torso
  - Horner syndrome (i.e., ptosis, meiosis, and anhidrosis on one side of the face) due to pressure on cervical sympathetic nerves
- One of the hallmarks of SVC syndrome is the edema and venous distension of the upper torso and extremities does not extend to the lower extremities
- Symptoms may be aggravated by lowering the head (e.g., bending forward, coughing)
- Symptoms may gradually subside over the day as fluid drains from upper torso
- Late signs and symptoms due to cerebral edema and airway compromise include the following:
  - Severe headache
  - Irritability
  - Visual disturbances
  - Change in level of consciousness
  - Stridor, orthopnea, tachypnea

Cancers Associated With Disorder

- Lung cancer
- Lymphoma involving the mediastinum
- Breast cancer metastasis
- Other solid tumors that metastasize to the mediastinal lymph nodes

Diagnostic Tests

- Radiographs are the initial test (approximately 10% to 15% of patients have normal findings)
  - Superior mediastinal widening in approximately 66%
  - Pleural effusions in about 25%
  - Hilar mass in 12%
- CT of chest with contrast preferred
- MRI (patient may not be able to tolerate lying flat for extended period)
- Endobronchial ultrasound bronchoscopy for tissue diagnosis
- Laboratory data

- ABGs
- Coagulation studies if venous thrombus is suspected
- Serum tumor markers if tumor growth is suspected

Differential Diagnosis

- Cardiac tamponade
- Pneumonia, acute respiratory distress syndrome
- Chronic obstructive pulmonary disease
- Mediastinitis
- Thoracic aortic aneurysm

Treatment

- Early identification of patients at risk is essential.
- Treatment depends on etiology of SVC syndrome and severity of symptoms. Goals are to provide rapid palliation or relief of symptoms and attempt to resolve the underlying condition.

Pharmacologic Management

- Corticosteroids may reduce the inflammatory component and cerebral edema and improve venous blood flow.
- Chemotherapy for chemotherapy-sensitive tumors
- Fibrinolytic or anticoagulation therapy for obstructing venous thrombus
- Diuretics (limited effect)

Nonpharmacologic Management

- Radiation therapy
  - Gold standard for SVC syndrome in lung cancer and frequently used in other tumor types
  - Emergency therapy in cases of acute respiratory distress
  - Many radiation fractionation protocols are effective
- Removal of the central venous catheter combined with anticoagulation
- Percutaneous implantation of endovascular stents is associated with a high success rate and low morbidity.

Nursing Interventions

- Monitor oxygenation and vital signs
- Elevate head of bed
- Oxygen therapy to relieve dyspnea
- Remove rings and restrictive clothing
- Avoid venipunctures or blood pressure measurement on upper extremities
- Elevate upper arms to promote venous return
- Monitor skin integrity
- Elevate upper arms to promote venous return
- Monitor for bleeding if anticoagulation methods were needed
- Manage patient nausea, constipation, or cough to avoid Valsalva maneuver

Patient Teaching

- Emphasize early recognition and reporting of signs and symptoms:
  - Tight rings or watch
  - Swollen arms or fingers

Oncologic Emergencies ⑤

- Diminished fine motor movements such as buttoning a shirt
- Headache, visual changes, or altered mental status due to cerebral edema
- Family members may notice face, neck, and arm swelling before the patient does

Follow-Up

- When SVCS is secondary to an internal thrombus, anticoagulation therapy and subsequent monitoring are indicated.
- If SVCS has a malignant cause, palliative or supportive care may be needed.

Bibliography

Brydges, N., & Brydges, G. J. (2021). Oncologic emergencies. *AACN Advanced Critical Care*, 32(3), 306–314.

Gupta, A., Kim, N. D., Kalva, S., Reznik, S., & Johnson, D. H. (2020). Superior vena cava syndrome. In J. E. Niederhuber, J. O. Armitage, M. B. Kastan, J. H. Doroshow, & J. E. Tepper (Eds.), *Ableoff's clinical oncology* (6th ed., pp. 775–785). Philadelphia: Elsevier.

Matos, V. J. (2020). Superior vena cava syndrome in critically ill cancer patients. In J. L. Nates & K. J. Price (Eds.), *Oncologic critical care* (pp. 1253–1263). Cham: Springer.

Michaud, G. (2022). Superior vena cava syndrome. In F. F. Ferri (Ed.), *2022 Ferri's clinical advisor* (pp. 1440–1441). Philadelphia: Elsevier.

Parks, L. (2018). Oncologic emergencies. In L. Parks & M. Routt (Eds.), *Critical care nursing of the oncology patient* (pp. 245–268). Pittsburgh: Oncology Nursing Society.

Shelton, B. K. (2018). Superior vena cava syndrome. In M. Kaplan (Ed.), *Understanding and managing oncologic emergencies: A resource for nurses* (3rd ed., pp. 561–587). Pittsburgh, PA: Oncology Nursing Society.

Spring, J., & Munshi, L. (2020). Oncologic emergencies: Traditional and contemporary. *Critical Care Clinics*, 37(1), 85–103.

Trudeau, A., Bean, D., Fleming, D., Boado, G., Samuels, N., & Kurup, R. (2018). Diagnostic snapshot: Acute edema in the oncology patient. *Journal of the Advanced Practitioner in Oncology*, 9(6), 677–679.

Urologic Emergencies

Jennifer S. Webster

Cystitis

Definition

- Cystitis is a painful bladder disorder caused by diffuse inflammation of the bladder epithelium.
- The inflammatory lesion or process compromises the ability to store urine in the lower urinary tract.
- It is associated with cancer symptoms, treatment side effects, and disease sequelae.
- Hemorrhagic cystitis often arises from anticancer chemotherapy or radiation therapy for pelvic malignancies and is characterized by diffuse inflammation and bleeding from the bladder mucosa. Sudden onset of dysuria and hematuria most frequently results from use of the cytotoxic alkylating agents ifosfamide and cyclophosphamide.

Epidemiology

- In the individual with cancer, cystitis is most frequently related to the following:
  - Carcinoma of the bladder in 75% to 85% of patients with gross or microscopic hematuria
  - Irritable bladder symptoms in about 20% of cases
  - Drug-induced cystitis
  - BK virus is the most common viral cause
- Patients undergoing hematopoietic stem cell transplantation are at highest risk.
- Radiation-induced cystitis occurs after external beam radiation therapy and pelvic irradiation.
- With the advent of immune checkpoint inhibitors for treatment of certain cancers there are case reports of immunotherapy related cystitis, but it is uncommon.

Pathophysiology

- The mucosal lining of the bladder is made of many layers of epithelial cells susceptible to irritation or damage.
- Symptoms have several causes:
  - Tumor invasion
  - Infection
  - Chemotherapy
  - Radiation therapy
- Symptoms may be similar for different causes, but tumor invasion is usually more insidious and produces gross hematuria.
- Chemotherapy-induced cystitis is a result of:
  - Unchanged drug that is excreted in the urine and damaged tissues
  - Metabolites of cytotoxic drugs, which are excreted into the renal system and reside in the bladder for extended periods. The most common example is acrolein, a metabolite of ifosfamide and cyclophosphamide, which contributes to uric acid crystal formation that damages the bladder epithelium.
- Some symptoms are expected consequences of immune system stimulation and inflammatory reactions (e.g., bacillus Calmette-Guérin [BCG] used to treat superficial bladder cancer).
- Radiation-induced cystitis is caused by external beam or interstitial irradiation to the pelvis and can damage the urethra, impair blood flow, and induce fibrosis, stricture, or atrophy.

Signs and Symptoms

- Urinary frequency
- Mild burning to excruciating pain in the bladder, lower abdomen, perineum, or vagina
- Low back pain
- Urinary urgency
- Incontinence
- May or may not have white blood cells (WBCs) or red blood cells (RBCs) in the urine

Cancers Associated With Disorder

- Bladder cancer or invasion of bladder by tumors in the pelvis
- Ovarian, cervical, uterine, rectal, prostate, or colon cancers
- Any cancer that requires radiation to the pelvic area
- Any tumor type treated with systemic cytotoxic drugs
  - Cyclophosphamide
  - Ifosfamide
  - Busulfan
  - Thiotepa (rare)
- Intravesicular treatment with BCG, thiotepa (rare) or mitomycin (rare)

Diagnostic Tests

- Detailed urinalysis
  - Urine dipstick
  - pH
  - Microscopic analysis
- Urine culture (midstream or sterile specimen)
- Urine cytologic examination
- Intravenous pyelogram (IVP)
- Cystoscopy
- Renal and bladder ultrasonography

Differential Diagnosis

- Infectious: recurrent urinary tract infection (UTI), vaginitis
- Gynecologic: pelvic inflammatory disease, pelvic mass, endometriosis

- Urologic: overflow incontinence or bladder outlet obstruction, bladder cancer, chronic pelvic pain, interstitial cystitis/bladder pain syndrome
- Neurologic: Parkinson disease, multiple sclerosis, spinal stenosis or tumor, cerebral vascular accident
- Other: Hernia, inflammatory bowel disease, diverticulitis, gastrointestinal malignancy, adhesions, trauma

Treatment

- Type of treatment is determined by the cause and severity of cystitis.
- Preventive strategies, particularly in immunocompromised patients, are essential.

Pharmacologic Management

- Antimicrobial therapy as indicated
- IV hydration
- Management of viral hemorrhagic cystitis is primarily supportive with hydration, diuresis, and bladder irrigation.
- Systemic administration of thiols can prevent or ameliorate the bladder damage related to acrolein production; the most widely used is mercaptoethane sulfonate (MESNA); however, there is continuing debate about its efficacy.
- Symptomatic management of BCG-induced cystitis includes urinary system–specific analgesics or opioids and antispasmodics.
- Hyperbaric oxygen is a rare treatment modality but appears to be safe and effective in case reports.
- For continued bleeding despite other measures, a sclerosing agent such as formalin may be inserted directly into the bladder.

Nonpharmacologic Management

- Maintain oral hydration of at least 1500 mL/day unless contraindicated. Avoid fluids with caffeine, alcohol, or high acidity.
- Bladder irrigation for patients at highest risk of hemorrhagic cystitis (i.e., those receiving high doses of ifosfamide or cyclophosphamide). Irrigation dilutes acrolein and decreases contact time of uric acid crystals with the bladder lining. However, there is some question about its effectiveness.
- Warm moist heat to lower back
- Warm baths

Patient Teaching

- Maintain hydration (at least 1500 mL daily). Ask patient to notify health care team if 1500 mL cannot be maintained due to nausea, vomiting, pain, or other factors.
- Encourage frequent bladder emptying.
- Create a voiding diary: for one 24-hour period patient tracks time and volume of urine to create baseline information. Further time periods can be used to follow patient progress.
- Teach and encourage patient to perform pelvic floor exercises (i.e., Kegel exercises) for urinary incontinence.
- Minimize foods or fluids known to promote acidic, concentrated urine. Avoid caffeine, alcohol, and carbonated beverages. Although avoidance of acidic beverages such as citrus juice is often advised, cranberry juice is frequently suggested, which is also acidic. The use of cranberry juice in this setting remains inconclusive.
- Avoid bladder catheterization.

Follow-Up

- Continue to monitor for signs and symptoms of infection.
- Monitor for ongoing complications of cystitis as indicated.
- Inform the patient to notify providers if symptoms arise.

Bibliography

Almalag, H. M., Alasmari, S. S., Alrayes, M. H., Binhameed, M. A., Alsudairi, R. A., Alosaimi, M. M., … Alarfaj, A. S. (2021). Incidence of hemorrhagic cystitis after cyclophosphamide therapy with or without mesna: A cohort study and comprehensive literature review. *Journal of Oncology Pharmacy Practice, 27*(2), 340–349.

Boorjian, S. A., Raman, J. D., & Baracoas, D. A. (2021). Evaluation and management of hematuria. In A. W. Partin, R. R. Dmochowski, L. R. Kavoussi, C. A. Peters, & R. R. Dmochowski (Eds.), *Campbell-Walsh-Wein urology* (12th ed., pp. 247–259.e3). Philadelphia: Elsevier.

Botta, L. M., & Botta, G. P. (2018). Hemorrhagic cystitis: Treatment with hyperbaric oxygen therapy in patients with acute lymphoblastic leukemia. *Clinical Journal of Oncology Nursing, 22*(6), E146–E151 (Online exclusive).

Cooper, K. L., Badalato, G. M., & Rutman, M. P. (2021). Infections of the urinary tract. In A. W. Partin, R. R. Dmochowski, L. R. Kavoussi, C. A. Peters, & R. R. Dmochowski (Eds.), *Campbell-Walsh-Wein urology* (12th ed., pp. 1129–1201.e14). Philadelphia: Elsevier.

Kennedy, L. B., & Salama, A. (2020). A review of cancer immunotherapy toxicity. *CA: A Cancer Journal for Clinicians, 70*(2), 86–104.

Martin, S. E., Begun, E. M., Samir, E., Azaiza, M. T., Allegro, S., & Abdelhady, M. (2019). Incidence and morbidity of radiation-induced hemorrhagic cystitis in prostate cancer. *Urology, 131*, 190–195.

Matz, E. L., & Hsieh, M. H. (2017). Review of advances in uroprotective agents for cyclophosphamide- and ifosfamide-induced hemorrhagic cystitis. *Urology, 100*, 16–19.

Moldwin, R. M., & Hanno, P. M. (2021). Interstitial cystitis/bladder pain syndrome and related disorders. In A. W. Partin, R. R. Dmochowski, L. R. Kavoussi, C. A. Peters, & R. R. Dmochowski (Eds.), *Campbell-Walsh-Wein urology* (12th ed., pp. 1224–1250.e16). Philadelphia: Elsevier.

Visintini, C., Venturini, M., Botti, S., Gargiulo, G., & Palese, A. (2019). Nursing management of haemorrhagic cystitis in patients undergoing haematopoietic stem cell transplantation: A multicentre Italian survey. *Mediterranean Journal of Hematology and Infectious Diseases, 11*(1), e2019051.

Urinary Tract Infection

Definition

- In a lower UTI, the bladder epithelium undergoes inflammatory changes when colonized with an infectious agent.
- Bacteria are present in the urine (i.e., bacteriuria).
- UTIs can be symptomatic or asymptomatic.
- WBCs may be found in the urine (i.e., pyuria).

Epidemiology

- One of the most common conditions treated by physicians
- Females have a much higher rate of infection than males throughout their lifespan. Up to 60% of US women will have at least one UTI during their lifetime compared to 5% of US men. Ten percent of adult women have at least one UTI per year.
- Highest rates are among the elderly, also the age group most likely to have cancer
  - 20% for women older than 65 years
  - 10% for men older than 65 years

- Most common bacteria: *Escherichia coli*, *Enterobacter*, and *Staphylococcus* species
- Most common infection acquired in the health care setting
- One of the most common causes of acute confusion or delirium in older adults
- Men have increased protective factors:
  - Longer urethral length
  - Scrotum that provides a physical barrier
- Common causes of male dysuria:
  - Foreskin in early life
  - Enlarged prostate in middle and later life
- Women are at higher risk:
  - Shorter urethral length than men
  - Urethra exits close to vagina and rectum
- Common causes of female dysuria:
  - Use of spermicide vaginally or with condoms
  - Sexual intercourse
  - Pregnancy
  - Estrogen deficiency in postmenopausal women
- Other contributing factors:
  - Inefficient bladder emptying
  - Catheterization of the urinary tract
  - History of previous infections
  - Immune deficiency disorders such as human immunodeficiency virus (HIV) infection, cancer, or diabetes mellitus
  - Children and elders with constipation

Pathophysiology

- The urinary tract, adjacent to the bacteria-rich lower gastrointestinal tract, produces and stores urine. The periurethral area is typically colonized with gut and other flora, some capable of causing a UTI.
- Urination flushes bacteria from the urethral orifice. Periurethral pathogens occasionally enter the urethra and ascend, reaching the bladder and resulting in a UTI.
- UTIs can involve mucosal tissue (e.g., cystitis) or soft tissue (e.g., pyelonephritis, prostatitis).
- They may result in the spread of infection from the urinary tract to the bloodstream (i.e., urosepsis), with subsequent increased risk of death.
- In urethritis, inflammation and infection are limited to the urethra only or to the urethra and vagina in women; infection is usually caused by a sexually transmitted pathogen.
- Acute pyelonephritis is an infection of the renal parenchyma and renal pelvis caused by ascending cystitis.

Signs and Symptoms

- Asymptomatic bacteriuria: Urine culture reveals significant growth of a pathogen, but the patient has no symptoms of a UTI.
- Symptomatic UTI
  - Bladder irritability
  - Suprapubic pain
  - Dysuria
  - Urgency
  - Frequency

- Fever
- Strong or foul odor in urine
- Cloudy urine
- Hematuria

Cancers Associated With Disorder

- Not associated with specific malignancies
- Women with cancer have the highest risk

Diagnostic Tests

- Urine dipstick
  - Leukocyte esterase: finding indicates neutrophils in urine; results not valid in neutropenic patients
  - Protein
  - pH
  - Urinalysis
  - Urine culture
  - Microscopic analysis

Differential Diagnosis

- Differentiation between UTI and bacteriuria
  - Pyuria alone versus inflammation
  - Bacteriuria without pyuria versus colonization
  - Pyuria versus bacteriuria versus nitrites versus infection

Treatment

Pharmacologic Management

- Antimicrobial therapy

Nonpharmacologic Management

- Maintain hydration
- Avoid unnecessary catheterizations; minimize length of catheterization if catheterized
- Indwelling urinary catheter care:
  - Use sterile technique when inserting catheter
  - Use evidence-based guidelines for care
  - Remove catheter at the earliest opportunity
- The use of cranberry (*Vaccinium microcarpum*) for prevention and treatment of UTIs is the subject of numerous research studies; however, the evidence is not conclusive. The expected benefit of long-term adherence to cranberry products may be overestimated but can be suggested as an option for women with recurrent UTIs.

Patient Teaching

- Emphasize identification and reporting of signs and symptoms.
- Ensure fluid intake of at least 1 to 2 L/day. Hydration is probably adequate if voided urine is clear to light yellow.
- Teach proper toileting techniques.
- Avoid bladder irritants (spicy foods, carbonated and caffeinated drinks). Although avoidance of acidic beverages such as citrus juice is often advised, cranberry juice is frequently suggested, which is also acidic. The use of cranberry juice in this setting remains inconclusive but can be suggested as an option for women with recurrent UTIs.
- Avoid catheterizations.

Follow-Up

- Monitor for recurrence of signs and symptoms.
- Repeat urinalysis as needed during ambulatory visits.

Bibliography

Cooper, K. L., Badalato, G. M., & Rutman, M. P. (2021). Infections of the urinary tract. In A. W. Partin, R. R. Dmochowski, L. R. Kavoussi, C. A. Peters, & R. R. Dmochowski (Eds.), *Campbell-Walsh-Wein urology* (12th ed., pp. 1129–1201.e14). Philadelphia: Elsevier.

Dest, V. M. (2016). Radiation therapy: Toxicities and management. In C. H. Yarbro, D. Wujcik, & B. H. Gobel (Eds.), *Cancer nursing* (8th ed., pp. 375–416). Burlington, MA: Jones & Bartlett.

Gersch, C. (2021). Concepts of care for patients with urinary problems. In D. D. Ignatavicius, M. L. Workman, C. R. Rebar, & N. M. Heimgartner (Eds.), *Medical-surgical nursing: Concepts for interprofessional collaborative care* (10th ed., pp. 1325–1353). St. Louis: Elsevier.

Mantzorou, M., & Giaginis, C. (2018). Cranberry consumption against urinary tract infections: Clinical state of- the-art and future perspectives. *Current Pharmaceutical Biotechnology, 19*(13), 1049–1063.

Moldwin, R. M., & Hanno, P. M. (2021). Interstitial cystitis/bladder pain syndrome and related disorders. In A. W. Partin, R. R. Dmochowski, L. R. Kavoussi, C. A. Peters, & R. R. Dmochowski (Eds.), *Campbell-Walsh-Wein urology* (12th ed., pp. 1224–1250.e16). Philadelphia: Elsevier.

McCoy, C., Paredes, M., Allen, S., Blackey, J., Nielsen, C., Paluzzi, A., … Radovich, P. (2017). Catheter-associated urinary tract infections: Implementing a protocol to decrease incidence in oncology populations. *Clinical Journal of Oncology Nursing, 21*(4), 460–465.

Urinary Tract Obstruction

Definition

- A drop in urine outflow may indicate failure of the kidneys to filter blood and produce urine (i.e., oliguria or anuria).
- Urinary stasis or blockage of urine transport from upper to lower urinary tracts indicates an obstruction.
- Obstruction of the urinary tract may occur at multiple levels:
  - Ureter
  - Bladder
  - Urethra
  - Obstruction blocks the urine flow, causing it to back up and damage one or both kidneys.
  - Cancer can involve the urinary tract by direct extension, encasement, or invasion. Obstruction can also occur from metastases.

Epidemiology

- Many cases go undetected until there is a significant decrease in urinary output.
- Bladder outlet obstruction in men is most commonly caused by benign prostatic hypertrophy (BPH).
- Cervical cancers cause most ureteral obstructions in women.
- Risk factors include the following:
  - Ureteral stones
  - Bladder stones
- Urinary tract tumors
- Retroperitoneal fibrosis and/or urethral strictures may result from radiation therapy to the pelvic area.
- BPH (i.e., enlarged prostate)
- Inflammatory response to infection

Pathophysiology

- Urine is transported from the renal papilla to the bladder through the upper urinary tract to the lower urinary tract (i.e., bladder and urethra). Active transport depends on smooth muscle contractibility.
- Blockage causes an accumulation of urine and subsequent distention.
- Pressure builds directly on the tissue and causes structural damage.
- Tubular filtrate pressure may increase within the nephron because drainage in the urinary collecting system is impaired.
- Acute or chronic renal failure results.
- Renal failure with uremia and elevated serum potassium levels compromises cardiac function.

Signs and Symptoms

- Symptoms depend on whether the obstruction is acute or chronic, unilateral or bilateral, complete or partial, with or without infection.
- Flank pain
  - Bilateral or unilateral
  - Intermittent or chronic
  - Moderate or severe:
    - Pain in an acute obstruction is typically unrelenting, excruciating, and may radiate to lower abdomen
    - Chronic obstruction may be relatively painless
- Urinary tract infection
  - Fever
  - Difficulty or pain while urinating
  - Nausea or vomiting
- Hypertension
- Renal failure
- Edema
- Decreased urine output
- Hematuria (i.e., microscopic or gross)

Cancers Associated With Disorder

- Tumors of nearby organs
- Colon cancer
- Cervical cancer
- Uterine cancer

Diagnostic Tests

- Radiographic studies
  - Kidney, ureter, and bladder (KUB) study
  - IVP
  - Abdominal ultrasonography
  - Renal ultrasonography
  - Abdominal CT
  - Magnetic resonance urography
- Laboratory studies
  - Complete blood cell count (CBC)
  - Blood urea nitrogen (BUN) and creatinine levels
  - Urinalysis

Differential Diagnosis

- Nephrolithiasis
- Prostatitis
- Diabetes mellitus
- Sickle cell anemia
- Priapism

Treatment

Pharmacologic Management

- Pain management
- Urine alkalinization to prevent stone formation
- Steroids
- Antibiotics to manage infections
- Chemotherapy to reduce invasive cancer or tumor obstruction

Nonpharmacologic Management

- Radiation therapy for management of invasive disease
- Extracorporeal shock wave lithotripsy (ESWL) for noninvasive stone management
- Catheterization and balloon dilation of ureteral strictures
- Surgery
  - Although temporary relief from the obstruction can be achieved without surgery, the cause of the obstruction must be removed and the urinary system repaired.
  - Stents in the ureter or in renal pelvis may provide short-term relief of symptoms. Nephrostomy tubes, which drain urine from the kidneys through the back, may be used to bypass the obstruction.
- Foley catheter to manage urethral obstruction

Patient Teaching

- Recognize and report early signs of urinary problems.
- Manage hypertension, and monitor blood pressure frequently.
- Maintain hydration of 1 to 2 L of fluid per day. Ask patient to contact care team if unable to meet this goal due to nausea, vomiting or pain.
- Citrus juices and fruits may assist in the prevention of certain types of ureter or bladder stones.
- Manage pain.
- Appropriately manage drainage tubes.

Follow-Up

- Monitor urinary output, urinalysis as appropriate.
- Monitor renal function tests as appropriate.

Bibliography

Gersch, C. (2021). Concepts of care for patients with urinary problems. In D. D. Ignatavicius, M. L. Workman, C. R. Rebar, & N. M. Heimgartner (Eds.), *Medical-surgical nursing: Concepts for interprofessional collaborative care* (10th ed., pp. 1325–1353). St. Louis: Elsevier.

Hofer, M. D., Liu, J. S., & Morey, A. F. (2017). Treatment of radiation-induced urethral strictures. *Urologic Clinics of North America, 44*(1), 87–92.

Nakada, S. Y., & Best, S. L. (2021). Management of upper urinary tract obstruction. In A. W. Partin, R. R. Dmochowski, L. R. Kavoussi, C. A. Peters, & R. R. Dmochowski (Eds.), *Campbell-Walsh-Wein urology* (12th ed., pp. 1942–1981.e7). Philadelphia: Elsevier.

Peters, C. A., & Meldrum, K. K. (2021). Pathophysiology of urinary tract obstruction. In A. W. Partin, R. R. Dmochowski, L. R. Kavoussi, C. A. Peters, & R. R. Dmochowski (Eds.), *Campbell-Walsh-Wein urology* (12th ed., pp. 776–797.e8). Philadelphia: Elsevier.

Oncologic Emergencies

5

Metabolic Emergencies

Kristen Maloney

Adrenal Failure

Definition

- In adrenal failure, the adrenal gland is unable to produce adequate amounts of cortical hormones in response to physiologic demands.
- Glucocorticoids, which are required for the normal function of all cells, are normally secreted from the adrenal cortex in large quantities during times of physiologic stress to maintain homeostasis.
- Adrenal failure can be primary (i.e., Addison disease) or secondary and caused by a lack of adrenocorticotropic hormone (ACTH), also called *corticotropin* or *cosyntropin.*

Epidemiology

- Overall prevalence of adrenal insufficiency varies based on geographic location.
- Primary adrenal insufficiency is rare, most often associated with congenital adrenal hyperplasia, which occurs in 1 in 12,000 to 15,000 people.
- Secondary adrenal insufficiency is seen more often and is most commonly seen in patients with pituitary tumors.

Pathophysiology

- The adrenal cortex produces cortisol that helps to regulate metabolism and the stress response and aldosterone that helps to control blood pressure.
- Adrenal failure results from destruction or dysfunction of the hypothalamic-pituitary-adrenal axis that regulates the hypothalamus, pituitary gland, and adrenal glands.
- Primary adrenal insufficiency or adrenal failure is caused by damage to the adrenal glands.
  - Most common causes: autoimmune adrenalitis and *Mycobacterium tuberculosis* infection
  - Less common causes: bilateral hemorrhage of the glands, malignancies, acquired immunodeficiency syndrome (AIDS), and fungal infections
  - Medication-related causes: anticoagulants, tyrosine kinase inhibitors, ketoconazole, fluconazole, etomidate, phenobarbital, phenytoin, and rifampin
- Secondary adrenal insufficiency or adrenal failure results from reduced secretion of corticotropin-releasing hormone (CRH) by the hypothalamus or ACTH by the pituitary gland.
  - Causes include: abrupt discontinuation of long-term administration of glucocorticoids, metastatic cancers to the brain or adrenals, pituitary infarction, surgery or radiation, and central nervous system disturbances (e.g., basilar skull fracture, infection).

- Medication-related causes: glucocorticoid therapy, fluticasone, megestrol acetate, medroxyprogesterone, ketorolac tromethamine, tyrosine kinase inhibitors, checkpoint inhibitors, and opiates.

Signs and Symptoms

- Ninety percent of both adrenal glands must be nonfunctioning before clinical symptoms are seen.
- Generalized symptoms
  - Fatigue and weakness
  - Hypotension
  - Nausea, vomiting, diarrhea, and abdominal pain
  - Tachycardia
  - Failure to thrive
  - Anorexia
  - Hyperpigmentation
  - Headache
- Electrolyte abnormalities associated with aldosterone deficiency
  - Hyperkalemia
  - Hyponatremia
- Electrolyte abnormalities associated with cortisol deficiency
  - Hypoglycemia
  - Hypercalcemia

Cancers Associated With Disorder

- Metastases to the adrenals or pituitary
  - Including craniopharyngiomas, meningiomas, intrasellar, and suprasellar metastases
- Solid cancers with a risk for adrenal gland metastasis
  - Breast cancer
  - Malignant melanoma
  - Lung cancer
  - Colon cancer
  - Esophageal cancer
  - Rectal cancer
- Hematologic cancers (non-Hodgkin lymphoma)
  - Primary involvement of the adrenal gland in hematologic cancers is rare
  - Secondary involvement of the adrenal gland in hematologic cancers occurs in up to 20% of cases
  - Primary adrenal lymphoma (rare)

Diagnostic Tests

- Low cortisol production is necessary for a diagnosis of adrenal insufficiency.
  - Cortisol level greater than 18 µg/dL indicates normal adrenal function.

- Cortisol level less than 3 µg/dL indicates adrenal insufficiency.
- Cortisol levels are evaluated in the morning, when serum cortisol levels are at their peak.
- Cortisol circulates bound to albumin, and the level may be falsely low in patients with an albumin level less than 2.5 g/dL.
- ACTH stimulates production and release of cortisol from the adrenal gland cortex.
  - The ACTH level is elevated in primary adrenal insufficiency.
  - The ACTH level is low or normal in secondary adrenal insufficiency.
  - The ACTH stimulation test assesses adrenal insufficiency.
    - Draw a blood sample to determine the baseline cortisol level.
    - Administer 0.25 mg (250 µg) of cosyntropin intravenously.
    - Draw samples for cortisol levels at 30 and 60 minutes after dosing.
    - Normal function is between 500 and 550 nmol/L, but the result depends on the assay used.
  - In primary adrenal insufficiency, no rise is seen in cortisol levels because the adrenal gland is dysfunctional.
  - In secondary adrenal insufficiency, a normal response is seen; a serum cortisol level of more than 18 µg/dL at either time point is normal.
- Serum potassium level
  - Elevated in primary adrenal insufficiency
  - Normal in secondary adrenal insufficiency
- Serum sodium level is decreased.
- Serum glucose level is decreased.

Differential Diagnosis

- Primary adrenal failure
  - Autoimmune adrenalitis
  - Tuberculosis, histoplasmosis, or HIV infection
- Secondary adrenal failure
  - Pituitary adenomas

Treatment

- Treatment is prompt replacement of corticosteroids.
- Glucocorticoids are the main form of therapy for all forms of adrenal failure.
  - Hydrocortisone (10 to 25 mg/day)
    - Given in divided doses two to three times per day
    - Most of the dose taken in the morning hours to reflect normal body cortisol secretion
    - Last dose is taken 4 to 6 hours prior to bed to avoid sleep disturbances
  - May require lower dose, particularly for secondary adrenal insufficiency.
  - Smallest dose that improves symptoms is recommended.
  - Short half-life mimics normal cortisol circadian rhythm.
- Stress-dose steroids

- For minor stress (e.g., fever, cold, surgery with local anesthesia), two to three times the usual daily dose.
- For major stress (e.g., major surgery with anesthesia, trauma or disease requiring intensive care) dosing is controversial, but a significant increase in the dose is recommended, for example, 150 mg/day intravenously over the first 24 hours and reduce to 100 mg/day intravenously.
- Follow patient and then switch to oral form and taper.
- Consider this treatment for patients experiencing septic shock not resolved with fluid resuscitation and vasopressor agents.
- Mineralocorticoids are needed in addition to glucocorticoids for patients with primary adrenal insufficiency.
  - Required for patients with concomitant aldosterone deficiency resulting in persistent hyperkalemia.
  - Fludrocortisone (0.05 to 0.2 mg/day) is given as a single dose in the morning, and the dose is adjusted according to symptoms.
  - Monitoring includes orthostatic blood pressure, serum sodium level, serum potassium level, and plasma renin concentration (PRC).
- Treatment for adrenal crisis includes the following considerations:
  - Hydrocortisone 100 mg bolus intravenously, followed by 200 mg daily via continuous infusion or 50 mg bolus every 6 hours intravenously or intramuscularly.
  - Intravenous fluids either normal saline or 5% dextrose in isotonic saline.

Patient Teaching

- The patient and caregiver should understand stress factors and recognize and report signs of an adrenal crisis.
- The patient should wear a medical alert bracelet or necklace stating the need for glucocorticoids in the event of an emergency.
- The patient and caregiver should recognize signs and symptoms of illness that may require dose adjustments of glucocorticoid.

Follow-Up

- Consider an endocrinology consultation.
- Hydrocortisone may be needed during periods of stress.
- Monitor symptoms for signs of crisis.
- Provide emotional support to the patient during a crisis as needed.

Bibliography

Husebye, E. S., Pearce, S. H., Krone, N. P., & Kämpe, O. (2021). Adrenal insufficiency. *Lancet*, 397(10274), 613–629.

Moini, J., Badolato, C., & Ahangari, R. (2020). Adrenal cortex tumors. In *Epidemiology of endocrine tumors* (pp. 295–318). Philadelphia: Elsevier.

Pazderska, A., & Pearce, S. H. (2017). Adrenal insufficiency—Recognition and management. *Clinical Medicine (London, England)*, 17(3), 258–262.

Richard, R. P., Grishaw, J. A., & Enfield, K. B. (2019). Adrenal emergencies in critically ill cancer patients. In J. Nates & K. Price (Eds.), *Oncologic critical care*. Cham: Springer.

Rushworth, R. L., Torpy, D. J., & Falhammar, H. (2019). Adrenal crisis. *The New England Journal of Medicine*, 381(9), 852–861.

Oncologic Emergencies

5

Hypercalcemia of Malignancy

Definition

- Hypercalcemia of malignancy is an abnormally high level of calcium (i.e., serum calcium >11 mg/dL or ionized calcium >1.35 mmol/L).
- Rate of calcium mobilization from bone exceeds the renal threshold for calcium excretion.
- Two mechanisms can cause hypercalcemia: humoral hypercalcemia of malignancy (HHM) and local osteolytic hypercalcemia (LOH).

Epidemiology

- Hypercalcemia of malignancy occurs in up to 30% of all cancer patients.
- It is the most common oncologic emergency.

Pathophysiology

- Parathyroid hormone (PTH), 1,25-dihydroxyvitamin D (vitamin D), and calcitonin assist in regulation of calcium and bone metabolism.
- Stimulation of calcium resorption from bones and kidneys is supported by PTH.
- Vitamin D, which is released in response to low calcium levels, promotes absorption of calcium from dietary intake.
- Calcitonin decreases calcium levels in the body.
- Osteoblasts are cells that secrete an extracellular matrix for bone formation.
- Osteoclasts are large, multinucleate cells that absorb bone tissue during growth and healing. They breakdown tissue by releasing a proteolytic enzyme that dissolves the bone matrix and releases calcium into the extracellular space.
- LOH accounts for 20% of hypercalcemia of malignancy cases.
- Tumor cells infiltrating bone (i.e., bone metastasis) locally secrete cytokines that directly stimulate osteoclasts to resorb bone and inhibit osteoblasts, resulting in increased release of calcium into the extracellular fluid and the systemic circulation.
- HHM accounts for 80% of hypercalcemia of malignancy cases.
- Systemic cytokines secreted by tumor cells promote the release of calcium and phosphate from bone, increasing calcium resorption in the kidney.
- Parathyroid hormone–related protein (PTHrP) is the principal mediator of cancer-related hypercalcemia in patients with solid tumors. It acts similar to PTH and increases renal and bone resorption of calcium.
- Vitamin D–mediated hypercalcemia
  - Vitamin D may be activated by certain lymphomas, increasing calcium absorption in the gut.
  - Dehydration develops due to the effects of hypercalcemia and impairs renal excretion of calcium.

Signs and Symptoms

- Based on serum calcium levels, hypercalcemia of malignancy is categorized as mild, moderate, or severe.

- Most symptoms are seen in the gastrointestinal, neurologic, musculoskeletal, renal, and cardiovascular systems.
- Patients with mild hypercalcemia (10.5 to 11.9 mg/dL) may report the following symptoms:
  - Nausea, vomiting, abdominal cramping, and loss of appetite
  - Restlessness, difficulty concentrating, and confusion
  - Fatigue and generalized weakness
  - Excessive thirst (i.e., polydipsia), frequent urination (i.e., polyuria), and nocturia
- Patients with moderate hypercalcemia (12 to 13.9 mg/dL) may report the following as their calcium levels increase in addition to symptoms of mild hypercalcemia:
  - Constipation, increased bloating, and abdominal pain
  - Psychosis and increased drowsiness
  - Increased weakness and bone pain
  - Feelings of dehydration
  - Palpitations and increasing anxiety (reflecting electrocardiographic [ECG] changes)
- Patients with severe hypercalcemia (>14 mg/dL) may experience the following symptoms in addition to those listed for mild and moderate hypercalcemia:
  - Ileus
  - Seizures and possible coma
  - Ataxia and pathologic fractures
  - Oliguria, renal insufficiency, and possible renal failure
  - Continued ECG changes and cardiac arrest

Cancers Associated With Disorder

- Greatest risk factors for hypercalcemia
  - Solid tumor diagnoses: breast, squamous cell lung, and prostate cancer
  - Hematologic cancer diagnoses: multiple myeloma and lymphoma
- Primary breast, lung, and multiple myeloma cancers account for 50% of all cases of hypercalcemia in the United States and Europe

Diagnostic Tests

- Serum calcium level greater than 11 mg/dL
- Ionized serum calcium level greater than 1.35 mmol/L
- Serum albumin level is measured with calcium because calcium circulates bound to albumin.
  - Decreased albumin level may give a false-normal calcium value.
  - Corrected calcium level is the total serum calcium (mg/dL) + (4.0 − serum albumin [g/dL]) × 0.8.
- The PTH level is typically low, except in rare cases of a PTH-secreting tumor.
- A PTHrP level greater than 1 pmol/L is a specific indicator of malignancy.

Differential Diagnosis

- Primary or secondary hyperparathyroidism
- Renal failure
- Paget disease of bone
- Medications and supplements (e.g., thiazides, lithium, large doses of vitamins A or D)

Treatment
Pharmacologic Management

- Effective long-term management is treatment of the underlying disease.
- Continuing management requires pharmacologic measures to inhibit bone resorption and promote renal calcium excretion.
- Immediate goal is to restore fluid and electrolyte balance.
- Hydration is achieved with isotonic (0.9%) saline solution.
  - Rate of infusion depends on the severity of dehydration, level of serum calcium, and patient's ability to tolerate a high rate of infusion and large volume of fluid.
    - Typically 1 to 2 L fluid bolus is given, followed by maintenance of fluids at a rate of 100 to 150 mL/h, ensuring urine output of 100 mL/h.
  - Hydration results in an approximately 2-mg/dL decrease in the serum calcium level.
  - Clinical improvement usually is seen within 24 hours, but the effect is temporary.
- Diuresis
  - A loop diuretic, such as 20 to 40 mg of furosemide, is given intravenously every 12 hours.
  - Diuresis enhances calcium excretion.
  - Thiazide diuretics are contraindicated due to inhibition of urinary excretion of calcium.
- Bisphosphonates and bone-modifying agents
  - They are used to prevent pathologic fracture, spinal cord compression, and hypercalcemia.
  - They inhibit normal and pathologic bone resorption by affecting osteoclasts and may inhibit adhesion of tumor cells to bone matrix.
  - All agents may cause osteonecrosis of the jaw.
  - They are administered intravenously because of poor oral absorption.
  - Zoledronic acid (4 mg given intravenously over 15 minutes every 3 to 4 weeks) has proved to be more effective than pamidronate.
- Use of corticosteroids
  - Used mostly in patients with hematologic malignancies, specifically multiple myeloma
  - Use of a combination of hydrocortisone 200 to 400 mg/day for 3 to 4 days, followed by prednisone 10 to 20 mg/day for 7 days or prednisone 40 to 60 mg/day for 10 days
  - Steroids should be used with caution, given side effects such as hyperglycemia, hypertension, muscle weakness, and further immunosuppression
  - Calcitonin is given intramuscularly or subcutaneously in a dose of 4 to 8 IU/kg every 6 to 12 hours.
    - It inhibits osteoclast-mediated bone resorption.
    - Calcitonin promotes urinary calcium and sodium excretion.
    - It decreases the serum calcium level in 2 to 6 hours.
    - Resistance to effects develops within a few days of instituting therapy.
  - Denosumab is a monoclonal antibody approved for hypercalcemia in malignancy.
    - It is used after a failed response to bisphosphonate therapy.
    - Given as a subcutaneous injection of 120 mg weekly for 1 month, followed by monthly with monitoring of calcium levels for continued dosing.
    - Side effects include arthralgias, nausea, diarrhea, dyspnea, hypocalcemia, and osteonecrosis of the jaw.
- Dialysis rapidly reduces the serum calcium level in patients who cannot tolerate aggressive hydration.

Patient Teaching

- Teach the patient and caregiver to recognize and report signs and symptoms of hypercalcemia.
- Discuss with the patient and caregiver how to maintain safety if the patient becomes confused.
- Educate the patient and caregiver about appropriate ways to maintain safe activity levels.
- The patient and caregiver are taught to take the patient's weight daily and monitor oral intake.

Follow-Up

- Continue to monitor serum calcium levels and laboratory values related to renal function.
- Monitor fluid intake and output.
- Monitor for early signs and symptoms of hypercalcemia such as confusion and for fatigue and nausea, which can indicate recurrence.

Bibliography

Asonitis, N., Angelousi, A., Zafeiris, C., Lambrou, G. I., Dontas, I., & Kassi, E. (2019). Diagnosis, pathophysiology and management of hypercalcemia in malignancy: A review of the literature. *Hormone and Metabolic Research*, 51(12), 770–778.

Kaplan, M. (2018). Hypercalcemia of malignancy. In C. H. Yarbro, D. Wujcik, & B. H. Gobel (Eds.), *Cancer nursing: Principles and practice* (8th ed., pp. 1107–1134). Burlington: Jones & Bartlett.

Klemencic, S., & Perkins, J. (2019). Diagnosis and management of oncologic emergencies. *The Western Journal of Emergency Medicine*, 20(2), 316–322.

Parks, L. (2018). Oncologic emergencies. In M. M. Findlay & L. Parks (Eds.), *Critical care nursing of the oncology patient*. Pittsburgh: Oncology Nursing Society.

Quintero, A., Racedo, J., & Fernández, M. G. (2019). Electrolytic abnormalities related to calcium in critically ill cancer patients. In J. Nates & K. Price (Eds.), *Oncologic critical care*. Cham: Springer.

Zagzag, J., Hu, M. I., Fisher, S. B., & Perrier, N. D. (2018). Hypercalcemia and cancer: Differential diagnosis and treatment. *CA: A Cancer Journal for Clinicians*, 68(5), 377–386.

Hypoglycemia

Definition

- Hypoglycemia is an abnormal decrease in serum glucose levels.
- Insulin-like growth factor, secreted by tumor cells, binds with insulin receptors, decreasing the blood glucose level.
- The diagnosis depends on three criteria (Whipple triad):
  - Signs and symptoms of hypoglycemia
  - Low plasma glucose concentration when the signs and symptoms occur
  - Resolution of signs and symptoms with treatment
- Glucose level of less than 40 mg/dL requires immediate treatment.
- Hypoglycemia can be mild to severe with various complications.

Epidemiology

- Up to 18% of patients with cancer have diabetes.
- As the number of cancer cases increases, especially among older adults, diabetes will become a significant comorbid condition.
- Of the patients with diabetes, 90% to 95% have type 2 diabetes.
- Higher risk of complications exists, resulting in higher mortality rates and hospitalizations in cancer patients with diabetes.

Pathophysiology

- Normal brain function relies on a continuous supply of glucose in the circulation.
- The body maintains normal glucose levels through the following mechanisms:
  - Decreased insulin secretion when glucose levels decrease
  - Increased glucagon secretion
  - Increased epinephrine secretion
  - If those mechanisms fail, glucose levels continue to decline.
- Type 1 diabetes is an autoimmune disease in which pancreatic β-cells are destroyed, resulting in insufficient production or no production of insulin.
- Type 2 diabetes occurs when the body becomes resistant to insulin and the pancreas can no longer produce the amount of insulin needed to support the body's needs.
- Paraneoplastic syndrome, in which tumor cells secrete insulin-like growth factor 2 (IGF-2), may occur.
  - IGF-2 interacts with insulin receptors and IGF receptors, stimulating glucose uptake by muscle and fat and potentially by tumor cells while hepatic glucose output is suppressed.
  - IGF-2 may provide a survival signal for oncogene-induced abnormal cancer cell growth by increasing glucose consumption and use by the tumor and by inhibiting apoptosis.

Signs and Symptoms

- Symptoms of hypoglycemia are categorized as neuroglycopenic or neurogenic.
- Neuroglycopenic symptoms
  - Behavioral changes (e.g., fatigue, confusion)
  - Seizures
  - Loss of consciousness
  - Diaphoresis
  - Pallor
- Neurogenic symptoms
  - Palpitations
  - Tremor
  - Sweating
  - Hunger
  - Anxiety
  - Paresthesias

Cancers Associated With Disorder

- Insulin-like growth factors are involved in the following cancers:
  - Breast
  - Prostate
  - Colon
  - Lung
  - Head and neck squamous cell
- Non–islet cell tumors
- Mesenchymal tumors
- Hepatocellular carcinoma
- Fibrous pleural tumor

Diagnostic Tests

- Blood glucose levels are classified according to the National Cancer Institute (NCI) Common Terminology Criteria for Adverse Events (CTCAE):
  - Grade 1: less than 55 mg/dL (lower limit of normal [LLN])
  - Grade 2: less than 55 to 40 mg/dL
  - Grade 3: less than 40 to 30 mg/dL
  - Grade 4: less than 30 mg/dL
  - Grade 5: death
  - Level less than 40 mg/dL establishes severe hypoglycemia.
- Serum insulin level
  - Increased with an insulinoma (i.e., insulin-producing tumor of the pancreas)
  - Increased with exogenous insulin administration
  - Decreased with tumor-associated hypoglycemia
- Serum C peptide level
  - Increased with insulinoma
  - Decreased with tumor-associated hypoglycemia
  - Decreased with hypoglycemia from exogenous insulin administration

Differential Diagnosis

- Drug-induced hypoglycemia
- Surreptitious or therapeutic insulin administration
- Oral hypoglycemic agents
- Critical illness (e.g., infection, sepsis)
- Hormone deficiency
- Non–islet cell tumor
- Insufficient food intake or starvation
- Chronic liver disease
- Adrenal or pituitary failure

Treatment

- Treatment is based on the underlying cause.
  - If related to a malignancy, treating the cancer is the only effective method to correcting hypoglycemia long term.
  - Approximately 15 to 20 g of glucose can reverse hypoglycemia.
- If the patient can tolerate oral intake, supply approximately 15 g of carbohydrate (i.e., 4 to 6 oz. of fruit juice, 1 tablespoon of sugar, honey, or corn syrup or 3 to 5 glucose tablets).
- If the patient cannot tolerate oral intake, glucagon (1 mg given subcutaneously or intramuscularly) is administered; may repeat one to two times as needed.
- The glucose level should be checked 15 minutes after giving carbohydrate or glucagon.
  - If glucose remains below 70 mg/dL, repeat the carbohydrate serving
  - Recheck blood sugar after 15 minutes

- Severe hypoglycemia requires immediate treatment.
  - Rapid intravenous push of 25 g of a 50% dextrose solution
  - Continuous intravenous infusion of glucose may be needed.

Patient Teaching

- Education is key for the patient and caregiver.
  - Understanding early signs and symptoms of hypoglycemia is critical for patient and caregiver.
- The patient should always carry the following for emergency use:
  - Glucose tablets, fruit juice, and a carbohydrate snack
  - A glucagon kit should be available and kept with the patient.
- The patient should report episodes of hypoglycemia to his or her provider.
- The patient should keep a diary of blood sugar trends.
- Support of an oncology pharmacist in the outpatient setting is recommended, as available.

Follow-Up

- The glucose level should be monitored regularly.
- The underlying cause should be corrected if possible.

Bibliography

Al-Taie, A., Izzettin, F. V., Sancar, M., & Köseoğlu, A. (2020). Impact of clinical pharmacy recommendations and patient counselling program among patients with diabetes and cancer in outpatient oncology setting. *European Journal of Cancer Care, 29*(5), e13261.

American Diabetes Association. (2019). 6. Glycemic targets: Standards of Medical Care in Diabetes—2019. *Diabetes Care, 42*(Suppl. 1), S61–S70.

Carlson, J. N., Schunder-Tatzber, S., Neilson, C. J., & Hood, N. (2017). Dietary sugars versus glucose tablets for first-aid treatment of symptomatic hypoglycaemia in awake patients with diabetes: A systematic review and meta-analysis. *Emergency Medicine Journal: EMJ, 34*(2), 100–106.

Kittah, N. E., & Vella, A. (2017). Management of endocrine disease: Pathogenesis and management of hypoglycemia. *European Journal of Endocrinology, 177*(1), R37–R47.

National Cancer Institute. (2017). *Common terminology criteria for adverse events (CTCAE)*. Available at https://ctep.cancer.gov/protocolDevelopment/electronic_applications/docs/CTCAE_v5_Quick_Reference_5x7.pdf.

Oguz, S. H., Unluturk, U., Lacin, S., Gurlek, A., & Yalcin, S. (2019). Hypoglycemia and hyperglycemia in critically ill cancer patients. In J. Nates & K. Price (Eds.), *Oncologic critical care*. Cham: Springer.

Parks, L. (2018). Oncologic emergencies. In M. M. Findlay & L. Parks (Eds.), *Critical care nursing of the oncology patient*. Oncology Nursing Society.

Seaquist, E. R., Anderson, J., Childs, B., Cryer, P., Dagogo-Jack, S., Fish, L., … Vigersky, R. (2013). Hypoglycemia and diabetes: A report of a workgroup of the American Diabetes Association and the Endocrine Society. *The Journal of Clinical Endocrinology and Metabolism, 98*(5), 1845–1859.

Syndrome of Inappropriate Antidiuretic Hormone

Definition

- Syndrome of inappropriate antidiuretic hormone (SIADH) secretion is an endocrine paraneoplastic syndrome in which inappropriate secretion of antidiuretic hormone (ADH) is produced by malignant cells or the posterior pituitary gland, resulting in water excess and dilutional hyponatremia.
- Malignant cells can synthesize, store, and release ADH independent of normal physiologic controls.
- Hyponatremia is classified as follows:
  - Mild: 125 to 135 mEq/L
  - Moderate: 115 to 125 mEq/L
  - Severe: less than 115 mEq/L (i.e., medical emergency)

Epidemiology

- SIADH occurs in up to 30% of cancer patients.
- SIADH occurs in 4% to 15% of hospitalized patients and is a common electrolyte disorder.
- Associated with increased mortality and length of stay in hospitalized patients with cancer.
- It is often seen in patients with lung cancer:
  - In 15% to 44% of patients with small cell lung cancer, dependent on hyponatremia definitions
  - In 2% to 4% of patients with non–small cell lung cancer, dependent on hyponatremia definitions

Pathophysiology

- ADH is normally produced by the hypothalamus, stored in the posterior pituitary gland, and released in response to changes in plasma osmolality.
- The activated form of ADH is arginine vasopressin (AVP).
- Release of AVP causes renal tubules to resorb increased amounts of sodium and water. AVP is released in response to the following:
  - Plasma osmolality differences
  - Plasma volume changes
- SIADH is characterized by unregulated production of ADH.
  - Cancer cells can inappropriately synthesize and release ADH that is unregulated by negative feedback mechanisms.
  - Kidneys are stimulated to conserve water, leading to increased free water in the extracellular fluid and dilutional serum hyponatremia.
  - Kidneys excrete small amounts of concentrated urine with increased sodium osmolality.
- Increased free water is distributed through intracellular pathways, which can cause cerebral edema (i.e., water intoxication).
- Cerebral edema leads to disruption of neural function and may lead to death.

Signs and Symptoms

- Symptoms are primarily neurologic and gastrointestinal.
  - Neurologic examination and volume status must be assessed.
- The severity of symptoms is related to the degree of hyponatremia and rapidity of onset.
- Early manifestations:
  - Thirst
  - Anorexia
  - Nausea and vomiting
  - Weight gain without edema
  - Muscle cramps

- Headache
- Weakness
- Lethargy and irritability
- More symptoms develop as the sodium level falls below 120 mg/dL (resulting from cerebral edema):
  - Hyporeflexia
  - Confusion and combativeness
  - Oliguria
- Symptoms of severe hyponatremia (<110 to 115 mg/dL):
  - Seizures
  - Coma
  - Death if hyponatremia is severe or rapid in onset

Cancers Associated With Disorder

- Solid cancers
  - Small cell and non–small cell lung cancers
  - Head and neck cancers
  - Gastrointestinal cancers
  - Brain cancer
  - Pituitary tumors
- Hematologic cancers, specifically leukemia and lymphoma
- Chemotherapeutic agents associated with SIADH:
  - Vinca alkaloids (e.g., vincristine)
  - Platinum-based agents (e.g., cisplatin)
  - Alkylating agents (e.g., cyclophosphamide)
  - Methotrexate

Diagnostic Tests

- Diagnostic tests are key to treatment of SIADH
- Serum osmolality (<280 mOsm/kg)
- Serum sodium level (<135 mmol/L)
- Urine sodium (>20 mEq/L)
- Urine osmolality greater than serum osmolality
- Decreased blood urea nitrogen level
- Decreased creatinine level
- Elevated serum ADH level
- Decreased uric acid level
- Decreased albumin level
- Assessment of volume status of patient remains important

Differential Diagnosis

- Central nervous system
  - Infection
  - Trauma
  - Guillain-Barré syndrome
- Pulmonary system
  - Tuberculosis
  - Pneumonia
- Effects of chemotherapeutic agents and other drugs
  - Antidepressants (e.g., tricyclic, selective serotonin reuptake inhibitors [SSRIs])
  - Opioids
  - Barbiturates
  - Nonsteroidal antiinflammatory drugs (NSAIDs)
- Renal failure
- HIV and AIDS

Treatment

- Goals include treatment of the underlying malignancy and management of hyponatremia.
- Strict monitoring of intake and output to assess volume status.
- Monitoring serum sodium is essential because treatment is based on severity.
- Management of mild hyponatremia
  - Patient should be placed on fluid restriction (1000 mL/day).
  - Serial neurologic assessments should be performed.
  - Medication reconciliation should be performed.
- Management of moderate hyponatremia
  - Patient should be placed on fluid restriction (1000 mL/day).
  - Serial neurologic assessments should be performed.
  - Medication reconciliation should be performed.
  - Consider use of demeclocycline in patients with chronic hyponatremia (900 to 1200 mg/day)
    - Impairs effect of ADH on renal tubules
    - Facilitates free water excretion
    - Not used frequently due to potential side effects of hematologic changes, nephrotoxicity, photosensitivity, and nephrogenic diabetes insipidus
- Management of severe hyponatremia
  - Patient should be placed on fluid restriction (1000 mL/day).
  - Serial neurologic assessments should be performed.
  - Medication reconciliation should be performed.
  - Use of 3% saline solution
  - Severe symptoms: 100 mL of 3% NaCl infused intravenously over 10 minutes, repeat twice as needed
  - Mild to moderate symptoms: 3% NaCl infused at 0.5 to 2 mL/kg/h
    - Slow infusion prevents a rapid increase of sodium and pulmonary edema.
  - Use of a loop diuretic (e.g., furosemide, bumetanide, ethacrynic acid)
    - Dose is 20 mg twice daily with hypertonic saline solution infusion.
    - It induces loss of free water.
- Untreated SIADH or too-rapid correction may result in severe neurologic impairment or death.
  - Osmotic demyelination syndrome can occur within 2 to 6 days of too-rapid correction.
  - Endothelial cells in the brain can be damaged from dehydration.
  - The blood-brain barrier can break down.
- If seizures result with too-rapid correction of sodium, dexamethasone (10 to 20 mg) and mannitol (50 g given intravenously) should be given immediately.
- Mild hypovolemic hyponatremia may be treated with isotonic (0.9%) saline solution given intravenously or, if tolerated, oral salt tablets, which may result in little or no net change in the sodium level.
- Recommended rate of correction is no more than 12 mEq/L/day over 2 to 3 days.

Patient Teaching

- The patient should monitor daily weights and report changes to the health care provider.
- Instruct the patient about the importance of fluid restriction. Explain the use of a chart to monitor fluid intake and output.
- Teach the patient and caregiver about the signs and symptoms of hyponatremia, including gastrointestinal and neurologic symptoms.

Follow-Up

- Monitor the patient's weight.
- Record fluid intake and output.
- Monitor laboratory values, including levels of serum sodium, urine sodium, and urine osmolality.
- Monitor use of medications that may contribute to SIADH.
- Complete neurologic checks according to the severity of hyponatremia.

Bibliography

Berardi, R., Antonuzzo, A., Blasi, L., Buosi, R., Lorusso, V., Migliorino, M. R., … Peri, A. (2018). Practical issues for the management of hyponatremia in oncology. *Endocrine, 61*(1), 158–164.

Burst, V., Grundmann, F., Kubacki, T., Greenberg, A., Rudolf, D., Salahudeen, A., … Grohé, C. (2017). Euvolemic hyponatremia in cancer patients. Report of the Hyponatremia Registry: An observational multicenter international study. *Supportive Care in Cancer, 25*(7), 2275–2283.

Filippatos, T., Elisaf, M., & Liamis, G. (2018). Pharmacological management of hyponatremia. *Expert Opinion on Pharmacotherapy, 19*(12), 1337–1344.

Higdon, M. L., Atkinson, C. J., & Lawrence, K. V. (2018). Oncologic emergencies: Recognition and initial management. *American Family Physician, 97*(11), 741–748.

Hoorn, E. J., & Zietse, R. (2017). Diagnosis and treatment of hyponatremia: Compilation of the guidelines. *Journal of the American Society of Nephrology: JASN, 28*(5), 1340–1349.

Keenan, A. (2018). Syndrome of inappropriate antidiuretic hormone. In C. H. Yarbro, D. Wujcik, & B. H. Gobel (Eds.), *Cancer nursing: Principles and practice* (8th ed., pp. 1197–1206). Burlington: Jones & Bartlett.

Parks, L. (2018). Oncologic emergencies. In M. M. Findlay & L. Parks (Eds.), *Critical care nursing of the oncology patient.* Oncology Nursing Society.

Peri, A., Grohé, C., Berardi, R., & Runkle, I. (2017). SIADH: Differential diagnosis and clinical management. *Endocrine, 55*(1), 311–319.

Tasler, T., & Bruce, S. D. (2018). Hyponatremia and SIADH: A case study for nursing consideration. *Clinical Journal of Oncology Nursing, 22*(1), 17–19.

Workeneh, B. T., Jhaveri, K. D., & Rondon-Berrios, H. (2020). Hyponatremia in the cancer patient. *Kidney International, 98*(4), 870–882.

Tumor Lysis Syndrome

Definition

- Tumor lysis syndrome (TLS) is a spectrum of electrolyte abnormalities that can occur after the initiation of cytotoxic therapy that causes the breakdown of large numbers of malignant cells.
- Most often noted to occur in patients with highly proliferative hematologic malignancies.
- Different grading systems exist for TLS:
  - Cairo-Bishop defines TLS through laboratory criteria at presentation and within 7 days of treatment, using a grading system of five levels for severity
  - NCI CTCAE defines TLS using a grading system of only three levels for severity

Epidemiology

- TLS risk of severity depends on the following:
  - Tumors larger than 8 to 10 cm (e.g., abdominal mass, mediastinal mass)
  - Tumor cells with a high proliferation rate
  - Extensive lymph node involvement
  - Bulky tumors associated with lymphadenopathy or hepatosplenomegaly
- Elevated pretreatment lactate dehydrogenase (LDH) level
- Preexisting conditions
  - Chronic renal insufficiency
  - Oliguria
  - Dehydration
  - Hypotension
  - Ascites
  - Exposure to nephrotoxins (e.g., vancomycin, aminoglycosides)

Pathophysiology

- Antineoplastic agents kill cells rapidly, increasing the cellular contents (i.e., potassium, phosphorus, and uric acid) released into the bloodstream.
- TLS results from inadequate excretion of the contents from the body and causes the following:
  - Hyperkalemia
  - Hyperuricemia
  - Hyperphosphatemia
  - Hypocalcemia
- The inability of the kidneys to clear the intracellular byproducts from the bloodstream can lead to life-threatening hemodynamic and renal complications:
  - Cardiac arrhythmias
  - Renal failure
  - Acute respiratory distress syndrome (ARDS)

Signs and Symptoms

- Caused by electrolyte abnormalities
- Most likely to occur 24 to 48 hours after starting chemotherapy treatment
  - Can occur as early as 12 hours and as late as 72 hours after starting chemotherapy treatment
- May last up to 7 days after therapy is completed
- Early signs
  - Weakness
  - Muscle cramps
  - Nausea, vomiting
  - Diarrhea
  - Lethargy
  - Paresthesias
- Late signs
  - Multiorgan failure, renal and cardiac most commonly noted
  - Paralysis
  - Bradycardia
  - Hypotension
  - Oliguria
  - Edema

- Cardiac irritability
- Laryngospasm
- Flank pain
- Hematuria
- Crystalluria
- Tetany
- Renal failure
- Seizures
- Cardiac arrest

Cancers Associated With Disorder

- TLS most commonly occurs in hematologic cancers.
  - High-grade lymphomas
  - Acute leukemia
- It is less common in solid cancers.
  - Breast cancer
  - Small cell lung cancer
  - Medulloblastoma
- Specific treatments associated with an increased risk of TLS include:
  - Chemotherapy
  - Radiation therapy
  - Hormonal therapy
  - Corticosteroids
  - Monoclonal antibodies
  - Immunotherapies
  - Biologic agents

Diagnostic Tests

- Basic metabolic panel (e.g., electrolytes, renal function)
- Liver function test
- Urinalysis

Differential Diagnosis

- Acute nephrocalcinosis
- Acute renal failure

Treatment

- Identify persons at increased risk for TLS.
  - Factors to consider should include:
    - Patients with preexisting renal disease
    - Patients experiencing hyperphosphatemia or hyperuricemia pre-treatment
    - Patients with acidic urine
    - Patients with hypovolemia or hypotension
- Monitor laboratory data.
  - Depending on the risk of TLS, samples may be drawn every 4 to 8 hours for analysis.
- Initiate preventative measures such as intravenous hydration:
  - Administer 24 to 48 hours before therapy begins and continue for up to 72 hours after therapy is completed.
  - Amount of hydration depends on the patient's age and comorbidities
  - Normal saline solution or 5% dextrose in water (D_5W) is used as the hydration fluid before, during, and after treatment.

- Goal to maintain urine output at 2 mL/kg/h or 100 mL/h during treatment
- Excessive hydration is contraindicated for persons with poor cardiac status because it may lead to fluid overload.
- Loop diuretics (e.g., furosemide) can be used to help decrease fluid retention and overload.
- Allopurinol, a xanthine oxidase inhibitor, is used to reduce the serum uric acid level.
  - It can be given orally or intravenously.
  - Parenteral dosing 200 to 400 mg/m^2/day in a single infusion or in divided infusions
  - Oral dose of 600 to 800 mg should be given 24 to 48 hours before treatment.
  - It blocks the enzyme xanthine oxidase and decreases the production of uric acid.
  - Deposits of uric acid in the kidney are decreased.
- Rasburicase, a recombinant urate oxidase, can be used instead of allopurinol or as prevention or initial therapy for TLS.
  - Dose is 0.2 mg/kg given intravenously over 30 minutes for up to 5 days.
  - May be recommended for patients with preexisting renal or cardiac dysfunction
  - It is contraindicated for patients with a glucose-6-phosphate dehydrogenase (G6PD) deficiency.
- Hemodialysis is used when the level of potassium is greater than 6 mEq/L, uric acid is greater than 10 mEq/L, phosphorus is greater than 10 mEq/L, or calcium phosphate is greater than 70 mg^2/dL.
- Treat electrolyte abnormalities.
  - Manage mild hyperkalemia (i.e., potassium level <6.5 mEq/L).
    - Sodium polystyrene sulfonate (i.e., Kayexalate), given orally or by retention enema, can lower potassium levels.
    - Monitor dietary intake of potassium.
  - Manage severe hyperkalemia (i.e., potassium level >6.5 mEq/L or ECG changes).
    - Calcium gluconate if ECG changes are apparent
    - Hypertonic glucose (e.g., 50% dextrose) given intravenously
    - Regular insulin
    - Sodium bicarbonate
    - Loop diuretics
  - Manage hyperphosphatemia.
    - Decreased phosphorus levels help to normalize calcium levels.
    - Give phosphate-binding, aluminum-containing antacids.
    - Consider hypertonic glucose and an insulin infusion.
    - Monitor dietary intake of phosphorus.
  - Manage hypocalcemia.
    - Treat only if symptomatic.
    - Calcium level is not corrected unless the patient is symptomatic or has a positive Chvostek or Trousseau sign.
    - Administer calcium gluconate.

- Manage hyperuricemia.
  - Continue aggressive intravenous hydration.
  - Increase dose of allopurinol.
  - If maximum dose is reached, start rasburicase.

Patient Teaching

- The patient and caregiver should be able to describe the signs and symptoms of TLS and report them to the provider.
- The patient and caregiver should understand the purpose of frequent laboratory draws that can indicate electrolyte abnormalities.
- Encourage the patient to increase fluid intake before and after chemotherapy and monitor daily weight.
- Provide dietary education about the intake of potassium-, calcium-, and phosphorus-rich foods.
- The patient and caregiver should understand current medications and the impact on TLS.

Follow-Up

- Continue to monitor for signs and symptoms of TLS.
- Monitor laboratory findings and treat electrolyte imbalances as needed.

- Maintain monitoring of fluid intake and output.
- Assess daily weight.
- Continue to monitor cardiac function and assess ECG changes.

Bibliography

Brydges, N., & Brydges, G. J. (2021). Oncologic emergencies. *AACN Advanced Critical Care, 32*(3), 306–314.

Goodrich, A. (2021). Advanced practice perspectives on preventing and managing tumor lysis syndrome and neutropenia in chronic lymphocytic leukemia. *Journal of the Advanced Practitioner in Oncology, 12*(1), 59–70.

Gupta, A., & Moore, J. A. (2018). Tumor lysis syndrome. *JAMA Oncology, 4*(6), 895.

National Cancer Institute. (2017). *Common terminology criteria for adverse events (CTCAE)*. Available at https://ctep.cancer.gov/protocolDevelopment/electronic_applications/docs/CTCAE_v5_Quick_Reference_5x7.pdf.

Rahmani, B., Patel, S., Seyam, O., Gandhi, J., Reid, I., Smith, N., & Khan, S. A. (2019). Current understanding of tumor lysis syndrome. *Hematological Oncology, 37*(5), 537–547.

Vioral, A. (2018). Tumor lysis syndrome. In C. H. Yarbro, D. Wujcik, & B. H. Gobel (Eds.), *Cancer nursing: Principles and practice* (8th ed., pp. 1207–1224). Burlington: Jones & Bartlett.

Wagner, J., & Arora, S. (2017). Oncologic metabolic emergencies. *Hematology/Oncology Clinics of North America, 31*(6), 941–957.

Williams, S. M., & Killeen, A. A. (2019). Tumor lysis syndrome. *Archives of Pathology & Laboratory Medicine, 143*(3), 386–393.

Oncologic Emergencies

5

Hematologic Emergencies

Jeanene (Gigi) G. Robison

Deep Vein Thrombosis

Definition

- Deep vein thrombosis (DVT) is a condition in which a blood clot forms in a vein, mostly in the deep veins of legs or pelvis. The thrombus (clot) formation may cause either a partial or complete occlusion of blood flow in the deep veins.
- Distal DVT (also known as isolated distal DVT, calf DVT, or below-the-knee DVT) occur when the blood clot develops inside the leg veins below the knee. The extension of the clot in proximal (above the knee) veins and the migration of a clot to the lungs (pulmonary embolism [PE]) are the most common complications.
- PE is when the blood clot dislodges and travels in the blood, particularly to the pulmonary arteries.
- Venous thromboembolism (VTE) is a term that includes both DVT and PE.

Epidemiology

- VTE, comprised of DVT and PE, is a common complication in cancer patients and is associated with significant morbidity and mortality.
- VTE is third most common cardiovascular pathology by its prevalence after myocardial infarction and stroke, with about 900,000 cases and 300,000 deaths in the U.S. annually.
- VTE has an annual incidence of 1 to 2 per 1000 population.
  - Mortality is high; death occurs within 30 days in about 6% of patients with DVT, primarily through PE, and in 13% of patients with PE.
- After 3 to 6 months of anticoagulation, VTE recurs in up to 40% of patients within 10 years.
- VTE is second overall leading cause of death for patients with cancer, and there is an approximately two-fold increase in fatal PE in patients with cancer.
- VTE occurs two to four times more frequently in patients with cancer than in those without cancer
  - VTE may be a marker of advanced stage cancer or of a more biologically aggressive tumor.
- COVID-19 infection is associated with profound coagulopathy, including DVT and PE. Incidence of VTE is up to 35% in patients with severe cases of COVID-19.
- DVT is the most preventable cause of death among hospitalized or recently hospitalized patients.
  - Two million Americans are affected with DVT yearly.
  - Approximately 200,000 hospital visits are due to DVT.
  - About 50% of persons with DVT have symptoms; the other 50% are asymptomatic and do not receive treatment, which increases the risk of a significant complication.
- Routine use of tools for prognostic scoring of DVT and PE is not recommended.
  - American Society of Hematology guidelines reviewed prognostic performance of multiple tools and found that their discrimination ability and validation was limited.
  - In certain circumstances, such as when patients are undecided or the balance between risks and benefits is uncertain, prognostic scoring tools for DVT may be useful.
- Increased risk for DVT:
  - Cancer-related risk factors
    - Cancer, which can cause a hypercoagulable state: Stomach and pancreas cancer are very high risk; lung, lymphoma, gynecologic, bladder, and testicular cancer are high risk
    - Hematologic malignancies, especially multiple myeloma, due to hyperviscosity state, and acute promyelocytic leukemia (APL)
  - Patient-related risk factors
    - Prechemotherapy platelet count (350×10^9/L or higher)
    - Hemoglobin level less than 10 g/dL
    - Prechemotherapy leukocyte count higher than 11×10^9/L
    - Obesity (body mass index [BMI] ≥ 35 kg/m^2 or higher)
    - Associated diseases (e.g., cardiac disease, peripheral vascular disease, chronic renal disease, chronic obstructive pulmonary disease [COPD], diabetes, acute, and chronic infections)
    - Chronic inflammation (e.g., inflammatory bowel disease), chronic autoimmune disease, chronic infections—are permanent/persistent VTE risk factors
    - Hypercoagulable state (prior VTE [DVT or PE], blood clotting disorders, disseminated intravascular coagulation [DIC])
    - More than half of patients who have a PE have an accompanying clot in their lower limb
    - COVID-19 infection, which may result in hypercoagulable state
    - Conditions that promote venous stasis, such as prolonged bed rest or prolonged immobility resulting from pain, trauma, surgery, or paralysis
    - Confined to bed in hospital for ≥ 3 days with an acute illness ("bathroom privileges")—is a major transient VTE risk factor

- Admission to hospital less than 3 days with an acute illness, confined to bed out of hospital ≥3 days with an acute illness, leg injury with reduced mobility—is a minor transient VTE risk factor
- Conditions that cause vessel damage, such as burns or fractures
- Treatment-related risk factors
  - Use of red blood cell (RBC) growth factors
  - Recent general surgery with any anesthesia (>30 minutes) or trauma—is a major transient VTE risk factor.
  - Recent general surgery with any anesthesia (<30 minutes) or trauma—is a minor transient VTE risk factor.
  - Chemotherapy, with correlation between development of PE and patient receiving cisplatin, carboplatin, gemcitabine, and paclitaxel
  - Bevacizumab in lung cancer patients, especially small cell lung cancer (SCLC)
  - Therapy for multiple myeloma patients with thalidomide or lenalidomide in combination with doxorubicin, multiagent chemotherapy, or high-dose dexamethasone (≥480 mg/month)
  - Medications such as antiestrogens (tamoxifen, raloxifene) and estrogens
  - Medications that induce endothelial damage, such as some vasopressor agents (e.g., dopamine), contrast medium, high-dose antibiotics, and antiphospholipid antibodies (associated with systemic lupus erythematosus [SLE])
  - Use of a central venous catheter
  - Radiation therapy

Pathophysiology

- Patients with cancer have a higher incidence of DVT because clot formation is a common complication of malignancy.
  - Thrombus formation occurs in the cardiovascular system.
  - Embolus (i.e., thromboembolism), which is a traveling clot, may be formed when part of the thrombus is dislodged.
- Pathogenesis of VTE in cancer patients likely includes the release of procoagulants and cytokines from cancer cells, direct endothelial damage, and down-regulation of endogenous anti-coagulants.
  - Prothrombotic activity of tumor cells plays an important role in occurrence of PE
- Pathogenesis of VTE in COVID-19 patients is a combination of classic VTE (macrothrombosis) and diffuse microthrombosis with endothelial damage in the lungs, directly caused by the coronavirus.
- Three mechanisms (i.e., Virchow triad) are integral to thrombus formation:
  - Abnormal blood flow because venous stasis predisposes to blood clot formation
    - A venous thrombus is primarily comprised of erythrocytes, platelets, and leukocytes, bound together by fibrin. It is formed in sites of vessel damage and

areas of stagnant blood flow, such as valve pockets of deep veins of lower extremities (calf) or extends proximately.
    - Pooling allows coagulation factors to accumulate and increases the chance of platelet aggregation and clot formation.
    - Hyperviscosity occurs due to high levels of plasma proteins, fibrinogen, white blood cells (WBCs), or platelets in bloodstream.
    - May also be caused by external compression of blood vessels, which is caused by the tumor and impedes blood flow (e.g., superior vena cava syndrome).
  - Endothelial vessel injury
    - Tumor invasion of the blood vessels
    - Proinflammatory cytokines (e.g., interleukin-1, interleukin-6, tumor necrosis factor-β), which are secreted by tumor, downregulate anticoagulation factors and create an environment for thrombus formation.
  - Enhanced activation of clotting factors
    - Procoagulant is secreted by tumor cells and induces a hypercoagulable state.
    - Tissue factor and cancer procoagulant can directly activate factor X, which initiates the clotting pathway.
    - Elevated levels of plasma activator inhibitor 1 (PAI-1) have been linked to an increased risk of DVT in persons with or without cancer.

Signs and Symptoms

- Clinical manifestations of DVT
  - Unilateral swelling in an extremity
  - Pain or heaviness in extremity
  - Unexplained persistent calf cramping
  - Swelling in face, neck, or supraclavicular space
  - Catheter dysfunction, if catheter is present
  - A dull ache, tight feeling, or frank pain in the calf, which is made worse with standing or walking and is made better with elevation
  - Localized tenderness or pain over the involved vein
  - Tender, palpable venous cord of the involved vein
  - Swollen calf or thigh of affected extremity; measurement of calf swelling of more than 3 cm in circumference in the symptomatic leg
  - Warmth and erythema of affected extremity
  - Dilated superficial venous collateral vessels (non-varicose)
  - Possible low-grade fever
  - Post-thrombotic syndrome (PTS): occurs later after person develops DVT, with signs/symptoms including leg pain, tenderness, leg fatigue, persistent swelling, erythema, pigmentation, or ulceration.
- Assessment for Homans sign:
  - Calf pain is a positive sign and is produced by dorsiflexion of foot with knee bent in 30 degrees of flexion.
  - Positive results found for less than 50% of patients.
  - High incidence of false-positive results
  - Test for Homans sign may cause an embolism; therefore, it should not be performed if DVT is suspected.

- Signs/symptoms of PE may be first indication of DVT.
  - PE signs/symptoms may include dyspnea, chest pain, tachypnea, tachycardia, apprehension, and syncope

Cancers Associated With Disorder

- Stomach and pancreas cancer (very high risk for PE)
- Lung (SCLC and non–small cell lung cancer [NSCLC]), lymphoma, gynecologic (e.g., ovarian, endometrial), bladder and testicular cancer (high risk for PE)
- Colorectal cancer and mucin-secreting gastrointestinal tumors
- Breast, prostate, and intracranial carcinomas—low risk for PE
- APL, multiple myeloma, and myeloproliferative disorders

Diagnostic Tests

- Laboratory tests
  - Complete blood count (CBC) with a platelet count
  - Prothrombin time (PT) and activated partial thromboplastin time (aPTT) ± fibrinogen
  - Liver and kidney function tests
  - D-dimer—testing is recommended by some experts, stating that D-dimer levels are raised in most patients with DVT (sensitivity 94% to 96%); however, national guidelines do not support the use of D-dimer testing.
- Radiologic imaging tests (initial):
  - Venous ultrasonography (VUS) of lower extremity
    - Initial test of choice for diagnosis of DVT
    - Low cost, noninvasive, highly sensitive, and specific for symptomatic DVT
    - Less accurate than venography
    - Less sensitive and specific for detecting proximal and calf DVT for the high-risk postoperative patient who does not have symptoms
    - If test results are positive, combined with results of labs and physical assessment, then treat patient for DVT
    - If test results are negative or inconclusive, then perform additional imaging tests.
- Radiologic imaging tests (subsequent): may be appropriate to use if initial venous ultrasound results were negative or inconclusive
  - Repeat VUS of lower extremity
  - CT scan with contrast
    - Spiral CT and CT angiography have been used to diagnose DVT
  - Magnetic resonance venogram (MRV) with contrast
    - May be alternative to venography
    - Very useful for detecting thrombi in the pelvic vein
  - Consider venography with possible clot extraction or thrombolysis
    - Identifies DVT by infusing contrast material into the venous system by a catheter in foot
    - Positive result: obstruction of flow of dye within the vein, indicating a thrombus
    - Gold standard for diagnosing DVT
    - Used when diagnosis of DVT remains unclear after evaluation and initial testing

- Not the first choice of diagnostic tests because it is expensive, invasive, and carries significant side effects resulting from hypersensitivity reactions to the contrast medium

Differential Diagnosis

- Calf muscle strain or tear
- Intramuscular hematoma
- Cellulitis, superficial phlebitis
- COVID-19 infection
- Obstruction of lymphatics by tumor, from irradiation or lymph node dissection
- Acute arterial occlusion
- Ruptured Baker cyst
- Chronic venous insufficiency
- Lymphangitis or fibrositis
- Kidney, liver, or heart disease (usually has bilateral edema)
- Hypoalbuminemia

Treatment

- Surgical placement of inferior vena cava (IVC) filter.
  - An endoluminal filter is used to interrupt blood flow through the IVC. Retrievable filter is preferred.
  - Indicated in cancer patients who have a contraindication to anticoagulants and have a DVT located in proximal lower extremity (pelvic/iliac/IVC or femoral/popliteal)
  - Filters may not be beneficial and may increase the risk of recurrent DVT
  - Not recommended for persons with proximal DVT, significant preexisting cardiovascular disease, or PE with hemodynamic compromise.
- Consider catheter removal in patients with catheter-related DVT.

Pharmacologic Management

- Prevention
  - Goal: Prevent DVT
  - VTE prophylaxis options for hospitalized medical oncology patients:
    - Dalteparin (Fragmin) 5000 units subcutaneous daily (category 1)
    - Enoxaparin (Lovenox) 40 mg subcutaneous daily (category 1)
    - Fondaparinux (Arixtra) 2.5 mg subcutaneous daily (category 1)—should be avoided in patients weighing less than 50 kg
    - Unfractionated heparin (UFH) 5000 units subcutaneous every 8 to 12 hours (category 1)
  - VTE prophylaxis options for ambulatory medical oncology patients:
    - Apixaban (Eliquis) 2.5 mg PO twice daily
    - Rivaroxaban (Xarelto) 10 mg PO once daily
    - Dalteparin (Fragmin) 200 units/kg subcutaneous daily × 1 month, then 150 units/kg subcutaneous daily × 2 months
    - Enoxaparin (Lovenox) 1 mg/kg subcutaneous daily × 3 months, then 40 mg subcutaneous daily

- VTE prophylaxis options for surgical oncology patients:
  - Apixaban (Eliquis) 2.5 mg PO every 12 hours × 28 days
  - Dalteparin (Fragmin) 5000 units subcutaneous daily × 28 days
  - Enoxaparin (Lovenox) 40 mg subcutaneous daily × 28 days
- VTE prophylaxis for patients with multiple myeloma and ≤3 points by IMPEDE score or less than 2 points by SAVED score
  - Aspirin 81 to 325 mg once daily
- VTE prophylaxis for patients with multiple myeloma and ≥4 points by IMPEDE score or ≥2 points by SAVED score
  - Low-molecular-weight heparin (LMWH) (equivalent to 40 mg of enoxaparin once daily), or
  - Rivaroxaban (Xarelto) 10 mg daily or
  - Apixaban (Eliquis) 2.5 mg twice daily or
  - Fondaparinux (Arixtra) 2.5 mg daily or
  - Warfarin (target international normalized ratio [INR] of 2.0 to 3.0)
- Management of DVT
  - Anticoagulant therapy
    - Anticoagulation therapy is the mainstay treatment for VTE (DVT and PE). It aims to reduce mortality, thrombus extension, recurrence, and risk of PTS
    - Anticoagulant therapy interrupts thrombosis and allows the lytic system to dissolve the clot that is in the blood vessel
    - Vitamin K antagonists (VKAs), such as warfarin, are oral agents that are used for long-term anticoagulation after thromboembolism occurs and for secondary prophylaxis. Agents may be initiated concurrently with heparin
    - For patients with DVT and/or PE, who have completed primary treatment and will continue to receive secondary prevention, national guidelines recommend using anticoagulation over aspirin
  - Home treatment is recommended over hospital treatment:
    - Treating persons with DVT at home, rather than in the hospital setting, decreased the risk of PE
    - Home treatment is appropriate for persons with low risk of complications. This is not the recommendation for patients who have conditions that would require hospitalization, have limited or no support at home, cannot afford medications, or have a history of poor compliance
  - Therapeutic anticoagulation treatment for VTE (DVT or PE) constitutes acute management in hemodynamically stable patients:
    - Direct oral anticoagulants (DOACs), also known as oral factor Xa inhibitors, are preferred for patients without gastric or gastroesophageal lesions: Apixaban (Eloquis; category 1), edoxaban (Savaysa; category 1), and rivaroxaban (Xarelto)

- LMWH—preferred for patients with gastric or gastroesophageal lesions): Dalteparin (Fragmin; category 1) and enoxaparin (Lovenox).
- If above regimens are not appropriate or available: Dabigatran
- Fondaparinux
- UFH (category 2B)
- Warfarin
- Monitoring INR in patients who are on VKA therapy (e.g., warfarin)
  - For patients with DVT and/or PE, who have completed primary treatment and will continue VKA therapy as secondary prevention, it is recommended that the INR range is 2.0 to 3.0.
  - For patients with breakthrough DVT and/or PE during therapeutic VKA treatment, it is suggested to use LMWH over DOAC therapy.
- Duration of anticoagulation
  - Recommended duration of anticoagulation therapy is minimum time of 3 months, or as long as active cancer or cancer therapy.
  - Recommendation is for a shorter course (3 to 6 months), versus a longer course (6 to 12 months), for primary treatment of DVT or PE, whether provoked by a transient risk factor, chronic risk factor, or unprovoked.
- Consider catheter-directed therapy (pharmacomechanical thrombolysis or mechanical thrombectomy) in appropriate persons with DVT.

Nonpharmacologic Management

- Maintain patient on bed rest for the first 5 to 7 days, with leg elevation for acute DVT and PE.
- Perform frequent leg exercises (i.e., range of motion [ROM] or isometric), if bedridden
  - Every 1 to 2 hours while awake to improve venous flow
  - Includes heel pumping and ankle circles for 10 to 12 repetitions
- Use mild analgesics and warm compresses for comfort of persons with acute DVT and acute PE
- Use compression stockings
  - Apply compression (anti-embolic) stockings or hose before surgery
  - Apply pneumatic compression stockings or devices postoperatively to stimulate circulation and prevent DVT and PE
  - Remove compression stockings or devices for 15 to 20 minutes, every 8 hours, or per facility policy
  - Assess skin color and peripheral perfusion in extremities with compression stockings or devices daily
- Encourage frequent ambulation, if tolerated, after 5 to 7 days of bed rest
- Elevate foot of bed by 15 to 20 inches with slight knee flexion.
  - Do not exceed 45 degrees with leg elevation
- Do not perform the Homans test after DVT is diagnosed or Homans test result is positive, since this could lead to development of PE

- Place pillows behind knees and elevate legs
  - Avoid popliteal pressure, which is produced by crossing the legs
- Do not massage the legs of persons with DVT or PE
- Encourage regular position changes to prevent hypoventilation
- Avoid smoking and caffeine to prevent vasoconstriction
- Maintain adequate hydration
- Administer supplemental oxygen by nasal cannula to maintain a PaO_2 higher than 80 mm Hg in persons with acute DVT and acute PE

Patient Teaching

- Goals
  - Define DVT
  - Identify signs/symptoms of DVT to report to health care provider
  - Understand lab and diagnostic testing, nursing care and treatments related to managing DVT
  - Stimulate patient's circulation
  - Prevent recurrent DVTs
  - Maintain patient safety by identifying signs/symptoms of bleeding and avoiding injury and bleeding while on anticoagulant therapy
  - Prevent respiratory complications
  - Understand how to administer the anticoagulant and identify med side effects
- Teach patient the purpose of laboratory and diagnostic tests, nursing care, and treatments for VTE
- Teach patient ways to stimulate the circulation to prevent DVT.
  - Change position regularly
  - Move the toes, feet, and legs often (e.g., wiggle the toes, flex/rotate the foot and ankles, tighten the calves)
  - Avoid sitting or standing for long periods
  - Make frequent stops on long trips in order to move around
  - Avoid constrictive clothing or devices
  - Perform ROM or isometric exercises
  - Wear the pneumatic compression stockings or devices as ordered
- Teach patient other strategies to prevent recurrent DVT/PE.
  - Ambulate soon after surgery
  - Drink 8 to 10 glasses of fluid per day
  - Quit smoking
  - Avoid caffeine intake
  - Take actions to lose weight, if obese
  - Increase vitamin E in diet, which is important for health of heart and blood vessels
  - Keep legs elevated to promote venous return
  - Keep legs straight and do not cross one leg over another leg
  - Avoid pressure on back of knees (i.e., popliteal area) to prevent clot from forming
- Teach patient to maintain safety while on anticoagulation therapy by identifying any bleeding signs/symptoms and following precautions to avoid injury and bleeding

- Identify and report any excessive bleeding, abnormal wounds, unusual pain or swelling; cyanosis or toe/foot pain
- Avoid any contact sports that could lead to serious injury
- Use soft toothbrush for oral care
- Avoid substances that can irritate the tissues of the mouth and gums, such as hot or spicy foods, alcoholic beverages, and mouthwashes that contain alcohol
- Use an electric razor if there is a need to shave
- Avoid blowing nose vigorously, clean nares with a cotton swab or tissue
- Use saline nose drops and sprays and a small amount of moisturizing ointment (e.g., petroleum jelly) inside the nostrils to prevent nosebleeds
- Check home for environmental hazards, and identify and remove bump and fall risks (e.g., throw rugs, clutter from rooms and pathways)
- Wear rubber gloves or garden gloves to protect hands when doing household or yard work
- Do not walk barefoot; wear shoes or slippers to protect the feet
- Teach patient ways to prevent complications, including respiratory compromise.
  - Ambulate frequently
  - Use incentive spirometry
- Teach patient how to administer medications and to understand their side effects
  - Teach patients to take their anticoagulant medication (e.g., warfarin) at the same time every day, and to not double up on the dose if they forget to take a dose
  - Teach patients, who are taking subcutaneously administered medications (e.g., LMWH), how to take these meds at home
  - Teach patients how blood counts (e.g., CBC with platelet count, PT/INR, etc.) will be monitored, as part of requirement for monitoring effectiveness of medications
- Teach patient, who is taking warfarin, to maintain diet consistent in amount of vitamin K.
  - Foods that are high in vitamin K: green leafy vegetables (e.g., spinach, kale) and liver
  - Foods that contain small amounts of vitamin K: milk, meats, eggs, cereal, fruits, and vegetables
  - Recommended daily allowances of vitamin K are 80 μg/day for men and 65 μg/day for women.
  - Patients should not take supplemental vitamin K because it increases blood clotting.

Follow-Up

- Continue to closely monitor cancer patients, who have been diagnosed with venous thrombosis, since they may have a more aggressive tumor biology and poor prognosis
- Monitor for signs and symptoms of subsequent or recurrent DVT or PE.
- Monitor laboratory findings to determine the continuation or resolution of DVT or PE.
- Reconcile medications at both hospital discharge and during provider follow-up visits.

- Screen for economic and social support (including housing, nutritional, financial, and spiritual support).
  - Make referrals, where available, to meet these needs
  - Provide additional resources, such as home equipment or assistance, as needed, to address the severe complications of DVT (e.g., PE)
- Refer patient for nutritional counseling about vitamin K in their diet, if needed.

Bibliography

Ahmed, M. H., Ghanem, H. M., & Khalil, S. S. (2020). Assessment of nurses' knowledge and practice about venous thrombo embolism for cancer surgery patients. *Assiut Scientific Nursing Journal*, 8(20), 13–20.

Asakura, H., & Ogawa, H. (2021). COVID-19-associated coagulopathy and disseminated intravascular coagulation. *International Journal of Hematology*, 113(1), 45–57.

Balabhadra, S., Kuban, J. D., Lee, S., Yevich, S., Metwalli, Z., McCarthy, C. J., … Sheth, R. A. (2020). Association of inferior vena cava filter placement with rates of pulmonary embolism in patients with cancer and acute lower extremity deep venous thrombosis. *JAMA Network Open*, 3(7), e2011079.

Barp, M., Carneiro, V. S., Amaral, K. V., Pagotto, V., & Malaquias, S. G. (2018). Nursing care in the prevention of venous thromboembolism: An integrative review. *Revista Eletrônica Enfermagem*, 20, v20a14.

Budnik, I., & Brill, A. (2018). Immune factors in deep vein thrombosis initiation. *Trends in Immunology*, 39(8), 610–623.

Cha, S. I., Shin, K. M., Lim, J. K., Yoo, S. S., Lee, S. Y., Lee, J., … Jung, C. Y. (2018). Pulmonary embolism concurrent with lung cancer and central emboli predict mortality in patients with lung cancer and pulmonary embolism. *Journal of Thoracic Disease*, 10(1), 262–272.

El-Said, A., & El-sol, H. (2018). Nursing discharge plan: Prevent further pulmonary embolism. *Mansoura Nursing Journal*, 5(1), 183–189.

Giustozzi, M., Agnelli, G., Del Toro-Cervera, J., Klok, F. A., Rosovsky, R. P., Martin, A. C., … Huisman, M. V. (2020). Direct oral anticoagulants for the treatment of acute venous thromboembolism associated with cancer: A systematic review and meta-analysis. *Thrombosis and Haemostasis*, 120(07), 1128–1136.

Kirkilesis, G., Kakkos, S. K., Bicknell, C., Salim, S., & Kakavia, K. (2020). Treatment of distal deep vein thrombosis. *Cochrane Database of Systematic Reviews*, 4.

Kraaijpoel, N., Bleker, S. M., Meyer, G., Mahé, I., Muñoz, A., Bertoletti, L., … UPE Investigators. (2019). Treatment and long-term clinical outcomes of incidental pulmonary embolism in patients with cancer: An international prospective cohort study. *Journal of Clinical Oncology*, 37(20), 1713–1720.

Kruger, P. C., Eikelboom, J. W., Douketis, J. D., & Hankey, G. J. (2019). Deep vein thrombosis: Update on diagnosis and management. *Medical Journal of Australia*, 210(11), 516–524.

Levi, M., & Iba, T. (2021). COVID-19 coagulopathy: Is it disseminated intravascular coagulation? *Internal and Emergency Medicine*, 16(2), 309–312.

Li, Y., Shang, Y., Wang, W., Ning, S., & Chen, H. (2018). Lung cancer and pulmonary embolism: What is the relationship? A review. *Journal of Cancer*, 9(17), 3046–3057.

Lin, H. F., Liao, K. F., Chang, C. M., Lin, C. L., Lai, S. W., & Hsu, C. Y. (2018). Correlation of the tamoxifen use with the increased risk of deep vein thrombosis and pulmonary embolism in elderly women with breast cancer: A case–control study. *Medicine*, 97(51), e12842.

Najm, M. A., Jassim, A. H., & Mohammed, T. R. (2020). Critical care nurses' knowledge about pulmonary embolism in respiratory care unit in Baghdad teaching hospitals. *Indian Journal of Forensic Medicine & Toxicology*, 14(3), 895.

National Comprehensive Cancer Network. (2021). *NCCN clinical practice guidelines in oncology (NCCN guidelines): Cancer-associated venous thromboembolic disease. Version 3.2021—November 15, 2021.* Available at www.nccn.org (accessed February 17, 2021).

National Comprehensive Cancer Network. (2022). *NCCN clinical practice guidelines in oncology (NCCN guidelines): Multiple myeloma. Version 4.2022—December 14, 2021.* Available at www.nccn.org (accessed February 19, 2021).

Ortel, T. L., Neumann, I., Ageno, W., Beyth, R., Clark, N. P., Cuker, A., … Zhang, Y. (2020). American Society of Hematology 2020 guidelines for management of venous thromboembolism: Treatment of deep vein thrombosis and pulmonary embolism. *Blood Advances*, 4(19), 4693–4738.

Qdaisat, A., Kamal, M., Al-Breiki, A., Goswami, B., Wu, C. C., Zhou, S., … Yeung, S. J. (2020). Clinical characteristics, management, and outcome of incidental pulmonary embolism in cancer patients. *Blood Advances*, 4(8), 1606–1614.

Rodriguez, A. L. (2014). Bleeding and thrombotic complications. In C. Yarbro, D. Wujcik, & B. H. Gobel (Eds.), *Cancer symptom management* (4th ed., pp. 287–316). Jones & Bartlett.

Soumagne, T., Lascarrou, J. B., Hraiech, S., Horlait, G., Higny, J., d'Hondt, A., … Piton, G. (2020). Factors associated with pulmonary embolism among coronavirus disease 2019 acute respiratory distress syndrome: A multicenter study among 375 patients. *Critical Care Explorations*, 2(7), e0166.

Suh, Y. J., Hong, H., Ohana, M., Bompard, F., Revel, M. P., Valle, C., … Yoon, S. H. (2021). Pulmonary embolism and deep vein thrombosis in COVID-19: A systematic review and meta-analysis. *Radiology*, 298(2), E70–E80.

Thachil, J., Khorana, A., & Carrier, M. (2021). Similarities and perspectives on the two C's—Cancer and COVID-19. *Journal of Thrombosis and Haemostasis*, 19(5), 1161–1167.

Turner Story, K. (2014). Deep vein thrombosis. In D. Camp-Sorrell, & R. A. Hawkins (Eds.), *Clinical manual for the oncology advanced practice nurse* (3rd ed., pp. 349–361). Oncology Nursing Society.

Voicu, S., Bonnin, P., Stépanian, A., Chousterman, B. G., Le Gall, A., Malissin, I., … Mégarbane, B. (2020). High prevalence of deep vein thrombosis in mechanically ventilated COVID-19 patients. *Journal of the American College of Cardiology*, 76(4), 480–482.

Zambakari, C., & Zambakari, N. (2021). *Pulmonary embolism: Everything you should know.* Phoenix, AZ: Desert Haven Home Care. Available at https://papers.ssrn.com (accessed February 20, 2022).

Zhou, X., Cheng, Z., Luo, L., Zhu, Y., Lin, W., Ming, Z., … Hu, Y. (2021). Incidence and impact of disseminated intravascular coagulation in COVID-19 a systematic review and meta-analysis. *Thrombosis Research*, 201, 23–29.

Disseminated Intravascular Coagulation

Definition

- DIC is a life-threatening, systemic clotting disorder.
- DIC is characterized by both hypercoagulation and bleeding. Multiorgan dysfunction, which is a final complication, is caused by widespread intravascular thrombosis (comprised of fibrin-platelet clots deposited in the microcirculation). Simultaneously, bleeding complications are caused by excessive consumption of platelets and coagulation factors.
- Two types of DIC
  - Acute (hemorrhagic) DIC develops quickly. It can lead to excessive blood clotting in the small vessels, which may cause organ dysfunction and failure (e.g., hepatic, kidney, or respiratory failure). It can also lead to serious bleeding, and a common presenting symptom is bleeding into organs.
  - Chronic (thrombotic) DIC occurs with exposure of a smaller amount of thrombin over a longer time period (weeks to months). Platelets and clotting factors are consumed more slowly than in acute DIC, and the person may be able to compensate. There are more blood clotting complications and symptoms in persons with chronic DIC. Cancer is a common cause of chronic DIC

Epidemiology

- One percent of inpatients, and 30% to 50% of patients with sepsis, are believed to suffer from DIC.
- Patients with APL are at increased risk of DIC due to release of procoagulant activity from the leukemic cells.
- Incidence of DIC is increased in cancer patients with advanced disease (stages III to IV), liver metastasis, presence of necrosis in tumor specimen, advanced age, and males.

- COVID-19 infections are associated with profound coagulopathy
  - Incidence of DIC is higher in more severe cases of COVID-19
  - Incidence of DIC has been reported in COVID-19 non-survivors, ranging from 5% to 71.4%, and COVID-19 survivors, ranging from 0% to 0.6%
- Chronic (thrombotic) DIC is the most common coagulation disorder that occurs in cancer patients.
- DIC is associated with a high mortality rate; however, this is typically due to the underlying disease
  - It is difficult to estimate frequency of DIC in oncology patients, since this is often diagnosed on autopsy

Pathophysiology

- Normal coagulation system: hemostasis is maintained by a balance between the processes of clot formation (i.e., thrombosis) and clot breakdown (i.e., fibrinolysis).
- DIC: A clotting disorder resulting from excessive pathologic production of thrombin and fibrin in blood
  - This gives rise to a hypercoagulation state, which is characterized by formation of small and large thrombi, tissue lesions, and organ failure
  - Due to impact of thrombin on coagulation cascade, platelets and clotting factors are consumed
  - Secondary fibrinolysis occurs, and this ultimately leads to excessive bleeding
- DIC always occurs secondary to an underlying pathologic condition:
  - Neoplastic conditions (e.g., leukemia, especially APL; lymphoma; adenocarcinomas of lung, breast, prostate, colorectal, gastric, and pancreatic origin; malignancies of epithelial tumors [e.g., head and neck, pharyngeal, laryngeal])
  - Sepsis or severe infections
    - Gram-negative or gram-positive bacterial infection
    - Viral infection (e.g., COVID-19, varicella, hepatitis, cytomegalovirus [CMV])
    - Parasitic infection, malaria
  - Severe toxic or immunologic reactions: hemolytic transfusion reaction, transplant rejection, severe anaphylaxis
  - Severe trauma or tissue injury:
    - Organ destruction (acute pancreatitis, glomerulonephritis)
    - Acute liver disease: obstructive jaundice, acute hepatic failure, intrahepatic or extrahepatic cholestasis
    - Organ shock of any kind (e.g., septic or cardiogenic shock, heat stroke, malignant hyperthermia)
  - Pregnancy and obstetric complications: amniotic fluid embolism, intrauterine fetal death, pre-eclampsia, abruptio placentae, therapeutic abortion
  - Placement of prosthetic devices (e.g., intraperitoneal shunt, LeVeen or Denver shunts, and aortic balloon assist devices)
  - Vascular abnormalities or stasis:
    - Abdominal aortic aneurysm, vasculitis, malignant hypertension, grafts

- Microangiopathic hemolytic anemia (MHA): thrombotic thrombocytopenic purpura (TTP), hemolytic uremic syndrome (HUS)
- Hematologic diseases: polycythemia vera, paroxysmal nocturnal hemoglobinuria
- In thrombus development, four pathologic mechanisms can occur simultaneously and stimulate a procoagulant state in DIC:
  - Thrombin production is enhanced
    - Overwhelming thrombogenic stimulus occurs (i.e., infection, malignancy, or trauma)
    - Triggers intrinsic or extrinsic pathway of clotting cascade that leads to excessive circulating thrombin in blood
    - Thrombin converts fibrinogen to fibrin
    - Clotting factors are consumed (e.g., platelets, fibrinogen, factor V, factor VIII, C protein, and antithrombin)
    - Results in multiple fibrin clots circulating in bloodstream
    - Platelets are trapped by excess fibrin clots
    - Leads to formation of microvascular and macrovascular fibrin thrombi (i.e., stationary blood clots)
  - Anticoagulant pathways, which tightly regulate thrombin, are suppressed
  - Fibrinolytic system, which breaks down clots, is suppressed by high plasma levels of PAI-1
  - Proinflammatory cytokines (primarily interleukin-6 and tumor necrosis factor-α) are activated.
- When part of the thrombus is dislodged, an embolus (i.e., thromboembolus) is formed. The traveling clot can lead to diffuse microvascular obstruction and can cause ischemia, impaired organ perfusion, and end-organ damage.
- Fibrinolysis
  - Normally, the fibrinolytic system is activated after clot formation. This controls how large the clot becomes and reopens the healed blood vessel over time.
  - Tissue plasminogen activator (tPA) converts plasminogen to plasmin.
  - Plasmin release causes enzymatic lysis of the fibrin clot.
  - Fibrin clots break down, which causes release of fibrin-split products, also called fibrin-degradation products (FDPs).
  - Fibrinolysis process may become uncontrolled in patients with DIC.
    - FDPs are not effectively removed from circulation and accumulate in the bloodstream.
    - Accumulation of FDPs contributes to bleeding and hemorrhaging, that is observed in patients with DIC.
  - Platelets and clotting factors are consumed at rate greater than body's ability to replace them during thrombosis, which leads to increased bleeding.

Signs and Symptoms

- Signs and symptoms in subclinical DIC
  - Changes in laboratory results (e.g., coagulation studies, renal function tests [RFTs], liver function tests [LFTs]) may be present
  - Signs and symptoms may be absent

- Signs and symptoms of bleeding, which is often the first obvious sign with acute (hemorrhagic) DIC:
  - Overall
    - Fever
  - Skin and oral cavity symptoms
    - Bleeding ranging from oozing to frank, life-threatening hemorrhaging
    - Bleeding from any invasive site, including a wound, incision, injection site, and intravenous or central line
    - Gingival or mucosal bleeding from oral cavity
    - Ecchymosis, hematomas and epistaxis
    - Pallor, sluggish capillary refill, and cool, clammy skin
    - Petechiae, purpura, ecchymosis, hemorrhagic bullae
    - Purpura fulminans, which is a rare and serious condition that includes widespread hemorrhagic skin necrosis and tissue thrombosis
    - Acral cyanosis (i.e., generalized sweating with cold, mottled fingers and toes)
    - Jaundice
  - Respiratory symptoms
    - Respiratory distress, including shortness of breath, dyspnea, air hunger, hypoxia, cyanosis
    - Hemoptysis
    - Tachypnea
    - Abnormal lung sounds (e.g., crackles, rubs, wheezing), stridor, and accessory muscle use
    - Hemothorax
  - Cardiovascular symptoms
    - Changes in vital signs: hypotension or tachycardia
    - Weak and thready pulse or narrow pulse pressure
    - Decreased peripheral pulses
    - Changes in color and temperature of extremities
    - Venous distention
    - Cardiac tamponade (e.g., muted heart sounds, hypotension, pulsus paradoxus, angina, palpitations)
    - Shock
  - Gastrointestinal symptoms
    - Hematemesis or coffee-ground emesis
    - Nausea, vomiting, anorexia, and weakness
    - Dysphagia
    - Abdominal tenderness, cramping, pain, or distention
    - Hyperactive or hypoactive bowel sounds
    - Diarrhea
    - Positive results for the guaiac stool test, frank blood in stool, or tarry stool
    - Hemorrhoids
  - Genitourinary and gynecologic symptoms
    - Hematuria (sometimes with a burning sensation), dysuria, frequency, and pain on urination
    - Decreased urinary output
    - Renal dysfunction/failure
    - Menorrhagia (e.g., heavily prolonged vaginal bleeding, suprapubic pain, cramping)
  - Neurologic symptoms
    - Symptoms may be caused by intracerebral bleeding and may include:
      - Headache and vertigo
      - Mental status changes (e.g., lack of orientation, restlessness, confusion, lethargy, obtundation, coma)
      - Changes in level of consciousness or pupil size and reactivity
      - Sensory or motor strength changes
      - Speech changes
      - Seizures
  - Ocular and ears/nose/throat symptoms
    - Scleral or subconjunctival hemorrhage; periorbital edema
    - Visual disturbances (e.g., blurring, diplopia, absent or altered fields of vision, nystagmus)
    - Eye or ear pain
    - Petechiae on nasal or oral mucosa; epistaxis; tenderness or bleeding from gums
  - Musculoskeletal symptoms
    - Warm, swollen, sore, or painful joints
    - Decreased mobility of joints (usually unilateral); stiffness in joints
- Signs and symptoms of clotting, which are seen with both acute and chronic (thrombotic) DIC
  - Cardiac and or respiratory dysfunction or failure (e.g., shortness of breath, stroke, myocardial infarction, pulmonary embolus, shock, death)
  - Changes in color and temperature of extremities (e.g., pain, warmth, swelling of extremity with DVT in upper or lower extremity), which could progress to gangrene
  - Central nervous system dysfunction (e.g., headache, speech changes, paralysis with stroke)
  - Renal dysfunction or acute kidney failure related to renal system clotting
  - Liver dysfunction or failure

Cancers Associated With Disorder

- APL, which is commonly associated with acute DIC
- Myeloproliferative diseases, including acute myelogenous leukemia (AML) and chronic myelogenous leukemia (CML)
- Lymphoproliferative diseases, including acute lymphoblastic leukemia (ALL) and lymphomas (especially immunoblastic lymphoma and Hodgkin disease)
- Solid cancers, such as mucin-secreting adenocarcinomas and prostate, lung, breast, gastric, biliary, colon, melanoma, and ovarian cancers

Diagnostic Tests

- Primary laboratory tests for diagnosing DIC
  - Platelet count is usually decreased
    - Normal platelet count: 150,000 to 400,000/mm^3
    - Moderate decrease in platelet count: 50,000 to 100,000/mm^3
    - Severe decrease in platelet count: less than 50,000/mm^3 (see the table on the next page)
  - Fibrinogen level is usually decreased
    - Normal fibrinogen level: 1.8 to 4.0 g/L or 180 to 400 mg/dL

- Moderate decrease in fibrinogen level: 1.1 to 1.5 g/L or 110 to 150 mg/dL
- Severe decrease in fibrinogen level: ≤1.0 g/L, or less than 100 mg/dL
- Acute (hemorrhagic) DIC: extreme and rapid decrease in fibrinogen
- Chronic (thrombotic) DIC: fibrinogen is rarely decreased and may increase due to a hypercoagulable state
- FDPs titer is increased
  - Normal FDP: less than 10 µg/mL
  - Mild increase in FDP: 10 to 20 µg/mL
  - Moderate increase in FDP: greater than 20 to less than 40 µg/mL
  - Severe increase in FDP: ≥40 µg/mL
- D-dimer assay (often combined with the FDP titer) value is increased (see table on this page)
  - Normal value in SI units is less than 0.5 µg/mL—fibrinogen equivalent units (FEU), or in conventional units is less than 250 ng/mL—D-dimer units.
  - D-dimer levels are excessively elevated in COVID-19 patients.
  - Patients with COVID-19, who had elevated D-dimer levels (>2.0 µg/mL) and FDP levels demonstrated greater in-hospital mortality and poor prognosis
- Coagulation tests
  - Results of coagulation tests may be nonspecific in DIC, since changes in PT, aPTT, and INR may be related to liver impairment, vitamin K deficiency, or other causes
  - PT: normally is 11 to 14 seconds; is usually prolonged in DIC (see table on this page)
  - INR: normally is 1 to 1.2 times normal; is usually prolonged or higher in DIC
  - aPTT: normally is 30 to 40 seconds; may be prolonged in DIC
  - PT/APTT ratio is usually increased
  - Thrombin time (TT): normally is 7 to 12 seconds; is usually prolonged in DIC
  - TAT, a coagulation marker, and PIC, a fibrinolytic activation marker, may be helpful to evaluate coagulopathy in patients with COVID-19
- Laboratory tests to determine accelerated coagulation
  - Antithrombin III level is decreased.
  - Fibrinopeptide A level is increased.
  - Prothrombin activation peptide level is increased.
  - Thrombin-antithrombin complex concentration is increased.
- Laboratory tests to determine accelerated fibrinolysis
  - Plasminogen level is decreased.
  - α_2-Antiplasmin levels: decreased
- Laboratory tests to identify thrombotic microangiopathy (TMA)
  - von Willebrand factor (VWF)/ADAMTS-13 ratio
  - VWF antigen and activity
- Laboratory tests to identify microvascular hemolysis
  - RBC morphology: presence of schistocytes (i.e., RBC fragments) on a peripheral blood smear are increased in 25% to 50% of patients with DIC.

- Other tests to assist in diagnosis of DIC:
  - Vitamin K deficiency (PT is screening test; diagnosis confirmed by PIVKA-II)
  - Bilirubin level and blood urea nitrogen (BUN): may be elevated
  - CBC: Hemoglobin level may be decreased (anemia)
  - Protein C and Protein S levels: may be decreased
  - Hemoccult testing of stool, emesis, and nasogastric tube secretions
  - Urine dipstick testing for blood
  - Imaging studies: usually not indicated for DIC, except to identify underlying cause.
    - Radiologic studies: used to assess internal bleeding or thrombosis.
    - Posteroanterior and lateral radiographs: used to rule out acute respiratory distress syndrome (ARDS).
    - Administer platelets and clotting factors before performing invasive studies. Perform studies with caution due to risk of bleeding.

International Society on Thrombosis and Haemostasis Diagnostic Criteria for Disseminated Intravascular Coagulation

Lab Test	Parameter	Score
Platelet count	>100 × 10⁹/L	0
	50–100 × 10⁹/L	1
	<50 × 10⁹/L	2
D–dimer (often combined with FDP levels)	No increase	0
	Moderate increase (1–10 times upper limit of normal)	2
	Strong increase (>10 times upper limit of normal)	3
Fibrinogen	>1.0 g/L, or >100 mg/ dL	0
	≤.0 g/L, or ≤100 mg/ dL	1
Prothrombin time prolongation	>3 sec	0
	3–6 sec	1
	>6 sec	2
	Overt DIC is score ≥5	

DIC, Disseminated intravascular coagulation; *FDP*, fibrin-degradation product. Modified from Arachchillage, D. R. J., & Laffan, M. (2020). Abnormal coagulation parameters are associated with poor prognosis in patients with novel coronavirus pneumonia. *Journal of Thrombosis and Haemostasis*, 18(5), 1233–1234; McCracken, C., & Martin, R. (2018). Disseminated intravascular coagulation: A case-based approach. In *ONS Congress Presentation* (May 17, 2018). Washington, DC. https://ons.confex.com/ons/2018/meetingapp.cgi/Session/1506; Nitipir, C., Neagu, A. M., Iaciu, C., Alexandra, M., Constantinescu, C. P., Pituru, S., . . . Stanciu, A. E. (2019). New biomolecules for the treatment of disseminated intravascular coagulation. *Romanian Biotechnological Letters*, 24(4), 580–585; Wada, H., Matsumoto, T., Suzuki, K., Imai, H., Katayama, N., Iba, T., & Matsumoto, M. (2018). Differences and similarities between disseminated intravascular coagulation and thrombotic microangiopathy. *Thrombosis Journal*, 16(1), 14.

Differential Diagnosis (May Be Concurrent With DIC)

- COVID-19 coagulopathy or pneumonia
- Malignancy or hematologic diseases
- Sepsis, severe infection, or shock
- Severe toxic or immunologic reaction; cytokine release syndrome
- Massive blood loss
- Heparin-induced thrombocytopenia (HIT)
- Vitamin K deficiency
- Vascular disorders or stasis

- TMA: TTP or HUS
- Organ destruction or failure: Lungs (ARDS), liver, kidneys
- Pregnancy and obstetric complications

Treatment

- Use multidisciplinary team to manage DIC in patients with thrombotic and/or hemorrhagic complications, including intensive care unit (ICU) doctors, hematologic specialists, biomedical researchers, surgeons, and availability of a Blood Transfusion Center
- Treat underlying or predisposing conditions causing DIC
- Support of the patient's hemodynamic status
- Manage signs and symptoms related to bleeding or thrombosis
  - Acute (hemorrhagic) DIC: Focus on transfusion support and oxygen for bleeding
  - Chronic (thrombotic) DIC: Focus on anticoagulation

Pharmacologic Management

- Prevent progression of DIC in patients with subclinical DIC (e.g., lab changes without bleeding or clotting signs/symptoms)
  - Consider prophylactic anticoagulation
- Eliminate or treat the underlying condition to remove the trigger for DIC. This is the main principle of DIC management
  - Administer appropriate chemotherapy if malignancy is the cause. Examples:
    - Patient with NSCLC and genetic driver mutation (ROSI-1): treated with entrectinib, and DIC resolved
    - Patient with adenocarcinoma of lung, who harbored both epidermal growth factor receptor (EGFR) mutation and *EML4-ALK* fusion gene and developed DIC: treated with Osimertinib, which is a third-generation EGFR tyrosine kinase inhibitor, and DIC resolved
    - Patient with BRAF-mutated melanoma, developed DIC: treated with dabrafenib and trametinib and DIC resolved
    - Patients with APL, who were treated with oral arsenic and all-trans-retinoic acid: Group 1 (DIC score of 4) consumed less platelets as compared to group receiving IV arsenic trioxide; and Group 2 (DIC score <4) had a prompt recovery of fibrinogen levels
  - Administer antibiotics if infection is the cause
  - Avoid medications that interfere with platelet function (e.g., nonsteroidal antiinflammatory drugs [NSAIDs], aspirin)
- Provide hemodynamic supportive care
  - Indication: usually for acute (hemorrhagic) DIC
  - Administer fluid replacement to treat hypotension
  - Use oxygen therapy to treat hypoxia
  - Administer intravenous vasopressors (e.g., dopamine) to maintain blood pressure
  - Administer diuretics or intravenous fluids to maintain central venous pressure
- Use platelet transfusions
  - Indication: Acute (hemorrhagic) DIC

- Platelet transfusion may be indicated for patients with DIC and with platelet count of 50,000/mm^3, if patients are actively bleeding or have a high risk of bleeding
  - Platelet transfusions may be indicated for patients with DIC and with platelet count of 20,000/mm^3, with or without symptoms
- Target goal for correcting platelet count after platelet transfusion:
  - 20,000 to 30,000/mm^3 for most patients with DIC
  - More than 50,000/mm^3 for patients with DIC, who have intracranial or life-threatening hemorrhage
- Dose: 1 to 2 units of platelets per 10 kg, or 1 platelet unit per day
- Use washed, packed red blood cells (PRBCs)
  - Indication:
    - Acute (hemorrhagic) DIC and anemia secondary to bleeding related to DIC
    - Patient has signs/symptoms of active bleeding and hemoglobin level less than 8 g/dL
  - Target goal: Maintain hemoglobin in range of 6 to 10 g/dL
  - Washed, packed RBCs are preferred to whole blood because of fewer complications related to fluid overload and immune response
- Use fresh frozen plasma (FFP)
  - Indication: Acute (hemorrhagic) DIC
  - Contains all the necessary clotting factors and inhibitors
  - Corrects deficiency of clotting factors and replaces clotting factors that were depleted during active bleeding
  - Give only to patients who are experiencing substantial bleeding and have abnormal coagulation values
    - INR greater than 2.0
    - aPTT greater than 2 × normal
    - Fibrinogen less than 100 mg/dL
  - Monitor for worsening of congestive heart failure after FFP administration
  - Dose: Initial doses start at 15 mg/kg, or 1 to 2 units FFP
  - No evidence supports that FFP infusion stimulates ongoing activation of coagulation.
- Use cryoprecipitate
  - Indication: Acute (hemorrhagic) DIC
    - Corrects deficiency of clotting factors
    - Since it contains higher concentrations of fibrinogen than in FFP, it is indicated for patients with substantial active bleeding and severe hypofibrinogenemia (e.g., fibrinogen level that is consistently <1 g/L, or 100 mg/dL)
    - It may correct severe fibrinogen deficiency that persists after FFP replacement
  - Contains fibrinogen, factor VIII, VWF, factor XIII, and fibronectin
  - Ensure ABO compatibility, whenever possible
  - Dose: 8 to 10 units of cryoprecipitate if fibrinogen is less than 1 g/L or less than 100 mg/dL
- Use fibrinogen concentrate
  - Indication: Acute (hemorrhagic) DIC
  - Dose: 3 g
  - Goal: may raise the plasma fibrinogen level by 1 g/L
  - Consider if volume is an issue for the patient

- Use prothrombin complex concentrate (PCC)
  - PCC is a medication is a Factor IX complex, made up of clotting factors II, IX, and X (e.g., Beriplex [Kcentra], Octaplex)
  - Consider PCC in actively bleeding patients if FFP transfusion is not possible
  - Consider PCC if volume is an issue for the patient
  - Black box warning: could stimulate DIC by activating the clotting cascade
- Use intravenous or subcutaneous heparin or LMWH
  - Indication:
    - Patients with chronic (thrombotic) DIC, in which thrombosis predominates (e.g., solid tumors)
    - Patients with acute DIC who are bleeding despite ongoing appropriate treatment (e.g., blood transfusion)
  - MOA: Heparin is an anticoagulant that activates antithrombin, which inactivates clotting factors, primarily thrombin and factor 10A. This action suppresses formation of fibrin and inhibits further thrombus formation
  - Consider heparin only if a platelet count of 50,000/mm^3 or higher can be supported
  - If using UFH: Use low-dose infusion (6 to 10 units/kg/hr) with no bolus dose
  - Heparin is expected to have anticoagulant, antiviral, and anti-inflammatory effects and is effective in treating thrombosis in COVID-19 patients
  - Contraindications: history of APL, central nervous system disorders, diffuse gastrointestinal bleeding, open wounds, recent surgery (due to increased risk of hemorrhage), and obstetric complications that require surgical intervention
- Use fibrinolytic inhibitor medications
  - Indication: Treat patients with acute (hemorrhagic) DIC, who are experiencing significant bleeding, have failed to respond to other treatments for DIC, and FDPs are thought to be inhibiting patient's platelets
    - Rarely used to treat patients with DIC
    - Not indicated for patients with subclinical (asymptomatic) DIC or patients with severe DIC, who are suffering from organ failure
  - Use ε-aminocaproic acid (Amicar) or tranexamic acid (Lysteda)
    - Indication: Can be used in severe cases in which bleeding does not respond to other therapies
    - MOA: Antifibrinolytic agents inhibit the plasmin-plasminogen system
    - Administration: Always give in combination with heparin to mitigate the prothrombic effect
    - Primary side effect: Clotting, which can lead to organ failure from large vessel thrombosis
    - Consider for patients who have significant hemorrhage after transfusion of blood component therapy or for patients with strong fibrinolysis, such as those with prostate cancer
    - Not shown to be effective in APL
- Use of antithrombin III concentrates (AT III)
  - May be used to supplement low levels of AT III in patients with DIC
  - May be given IV or subcutaneous
  - Use is controversial

Nonpharmacologic Management

- Recognize relevant lab changes and signs/symptoms of DIC early.
- Monitor laboratory results and trends (e.g., platelets, fibrinogen, D-dimer, FDP, PT, aPTT) every 6 hours for patients who are in acute (hemorrhagic) phase of DIC.
  - Acute (hemorrhagic) phase of DIC: assess lab results every 6 hours
  - Chronic (thrombotic) or subclinical (asymptomatic) phase of DIC: assess labs results less often
- Monitor hemodynamic signs/symptoms, vital signs, neurologic signs, and all sites of active bleeding every 2 to 4 hours during the acute (hemorrhagic) phase of DIC, or as indicated.
- Monitor amount of bleeding to determine efficacy of therapeutic measures:
  - Count Peri-Pads
  - Weigh affected dressings
  - Measure bloody drainage
- Monitor weights daily and assess intake/output every 1 to 2 hours during acute phase of DIC to assess for dehydration or fluid overload.
- Measure abdominal girth every 4 hours if abdominal bleeding is suspected.
- Apply direct pressure or apply pressure dressings or sandbags to sites of active bleeding.
- Elevate sites of active bleeding, if possible.
- Assess role of spirituality in patient's life, and impact of receiving blood products.
- Assist with activities of daily living and ambulation to avoid skin bumps or scrapes, and to minimize heavy lifting or straining.
- Use thrombocytopenic precautions to minimize bleeding: Use an electric razor, not a straight-edged razor; use a soft toothbrush; avoid flossing if this causes bleeding or if patient did not normally floss; wear protection on feet when ambulating
- Promote safety:
  - Supervise closely during ambulation
  - Ensure clear pathways for walking
  - If hospitalized, place bed in low locked position, two side rails up, call bell within reach
- Assess available resources for patient and caregivers
- Provide emotional support and resources for patient and caregivers

Patient Teaching

- Goals for patient with DIC:
  - Reverse the hypercoagulable state
  - Maintain normal coagulation levels
- Define DIC and the condition of simultaneous bleeding and clotting

- Differentiate between acute (hemorrhagic) and chronic (thrombotic) phases of DIC
- Describe signs and symptoms of acute and chronic DIC
- Teach patient about critical signs/symptoms of bleeding to report, such as bruising, red rash, headache, black stools, blood in the urine or stools, and bleeding from the gums, nose, eyes, vagina, rectum, wound, or central venous catheter site
- Teach patient about critical signs/symptoms related to thrombosis to report, such as shortness of breath; chest pain; changes in color/temperature/swelling of extremities; changes in mental status (e.g., headaches, speech changes, paralysis)
- Teach patient/family to save urine, stool, and emesis for the nurse to check for blood, when indicated
- Explain purpose of the laboratory tests, nursing care, and treatments for DIC
- Teach patients self-care measures to maximize their safety:
  - Use an electric razor, not a straight-edged razor
  - Maintain the bed in a low position with the side rails up
  - Minimize activities that could trigger bleeding; avoid contact sports and heavy lifting
  - Take precautions against accidental bleeding because even minor scrapes or bumps can result in bleeding
- Teach possible risks related to injury/falls: bleeding, head injury, fractured bones
- Teach fall precautions if the patient is at risk for falls:
  - Clear pathways in room and hallway to maintain safety during ambulation
  - Remove throw rugs and items that can obstruct the pathway in their home
  - Walk carefully and change positions gradually
- Teach patients to avoid over-the-counter medications that may interfere with normal platelet function, such as aspirin and NSAIDs (e.g., ibuprofen, naproxen sodium)
- Teach patients to minimize activities that contribute to development of additional clots and increase circulation in the lower extremities:
  - Avoid tight or restrictive clothing
  - Use compression stockings to promote venous return
  - Elevate legs when possible; do not sit with legs crossed or dangle feet on side of bed
  - Do not use pillows under the knees or a knee gatch
  - Instruct patient to wiggle toes and feet and to rotate ankles, especially when in bed

Follow-Up

- Patients in acute (hemorrhagic) phase of DIC often require hospitalization for close monitoring of signs/symptoms and laboratory results, and for continuing treatment.
- Patients who are in chronic (thrombotic) phase of DIC, or patients who have survived the acute phase of DIC, may be carefully monitored in the outpatient setting.
  - Continue to monitor for signs/symptoms of DIC
  - Support and manage new and long-term sequela related to DIC
  - Monitor laboratory findings (especially CBC with diff, D-dimer, FDP, and coagulation studies) to determine whether DIC is continuing or resolving

- Monitor D-dimer, especially in COVID-19-positive patients
- Reconcile medications at ICU discharge, hospital discharge, and follow-up visits
- Screen for economic and social support (including housing, nutritional, financial, and spiritual support).
  - Make referrals, where available, to meet these needs
  - Provide additional resources, such as home equipment or assistance, for severe complications of DIC (e.g., organ dysfunction) and activity limitations
  - Schedule a home assessment with home nursing care and physical therapy, if needed
- Consult a hematologist if DIC is diagnosed during the initial evaluation or if bleeding continues despite therapy interventions.

Bibliography

Adelborg, K., Larsen, J. B., & Hvas, A. M. (2021). Disseminated intravascular coagulation: Epidemiology, biomarkers, and management. *British Journal of Haematology*, 192(5), 803–818.

Arachchillage, D. R. J., & Laffan, M. (2020). Abnormal coagulation parameters are associated with poor prognosis in patients with novel coronavirus pneumonia. *Journal of Thrombosis and Haemostasis*, 18(5), 1233–1234.

Asakura, H., & Ogawa, H. (2021). COVID-19-associated coagulopathy and disseminated intravascular coagulation. *International Journal of Hematology*, 113(1), 45–57.

Boral, B. M., Williams, D. J., & Boral, L. I. (2016). Disseminated intravascular coagulation. *American Journal of Clinical Pathology*, 146(6), 670–680.

Chandrashekar, V. (2012). DIC score: Statistical relationship with PT, APTT, and simplified scoring systems with combinations of PT and APTT. *ISRN Hematology*, 2012, 579420.

Chuang, J., Uche, A., Gupta, R., Margolin, K., & Kim, P. (2019). Fulminant disseminated intravascular coagulation as initial presentation of BRAF-mutated melanoma. *Case Reports in Oncological Medicine*, 2019, 9246596.

Delaney, E., Nikolai, C., & Coe, K. (2020). Metabolic emergencies. In J. M. Brandt (Ed.), *ONS core curriculum for oncology nursing* (6th ed.). Elsevier.

Ding, R., Wang, Z., Lin, Y., Liu, B., Zhang, Z., & Ma, X. (2018). Comparison of a new criteria for sepsis-induced coagulopathy and International Society on Thrombosis and Haemostasis disseminated intravascular coagulation score in critically ill patients with sepsis 3.0: A retrospective study. *Blood Coagulation and Fibrinolysis*, 29(6), 551–558.

Dumache, R., Daescu, E., Ciocan, V., Mureşan, C., Talida, C., Gavrilita, D., & Enache, A. (2021). Molecular testing of SARS-CoV-2 infection from blood samples in disseminated intravascular coagulation (DIC) and elevated D-dimer levels. *Clinical Laboratory*, 67(1). https://doi.org/10.7754/Clin.Lab.2020.200704.

Fujita, K., Naka, M., Ito, T., Kanai, O., Maekawa, K., Nakatani, K., & Mio, T. (2021). Successful management of a lung cancer patient harbouring both EGFR mutation and EML4-ALK fusion gene with disseminated intravascular coagulation. *Respiratory Medicine Case Reports*, 33, 101393.

Iba, T., Di Nisio, M., Thachil, J., Wada, H., Asakura, H., Sato, K., & Saitoh, D. (2018). A proposal of the modification of Japanese Society on Thrombosis and Hemostasis (JSTH) disseminated intravascular coagulation (DIC) diagnostic criteria for sepsis-associated DIC. *Clinical and Applied Thrombosis/Hemostasis*, 24(3), 439–445.

Iba, T., & Levy, J. H. (2020). Sepsis-induced coagulopathy and disseminated intravascular coagulation. *Anesthesiology*, 132(5), 1238–1245.

Iba, T., Levy, J. H., Warkentin, T. E., Thachil, J., van der Poll, T., Levi, M., … The Scientific and Standardization Committee on Perioperative and Critical Care of the International Society on Thrombosis and Haemostasis. (2019). Diagnosis and management of sepsis-induced coagulopathy and disseminated intravascular coagulation. *Journal of Thrombosis and Haemostasis*, 17(11), 1989–1994.

Levi, M. (2019). Disseminated intravascular coagulation in cancer: An update. *Seminars in Thrombosis and Hemostasis*, 45(4), 342–347.

Levi, M., & Iba, T. (2021). COVID-19 coagulopathy: Is it disseminated intravascular coagulation? *Internal and Emergency Medicine*, 16(2), 309–312.

Lillicrap, D. (2020). Disseminated intravascular coagulation in patients with 2019-nCoV pneumonia. *Journal of Thrombosis and Haemostasis*, 18(4), 786–787.

McCracken, C., & Martin, R. (2018). Disseminated intravascular coagulation: A case-based approach. In *ONS Congress Presentation* (May 17, 2018). Washington, DC. https://ons.confex.com/ons/2018/meetingapp.cgi/Session/1506

Nitipir, C., Neagu, A. M., Iaciu, C., Alexandra, M., Constantinescu, C. P., Pituru, S., … Stanciu, A. E. (2019). New biomolecules for the treatment of disseminated intravascular coagulation. *Romanian Biotechnological Letters, 24*(4), 580–585.

Oben, P., & Fein, V. (2019). Comprehensive review of oncological emergencies seen in clinical practice. *Medical Studies/Studia Medyczne, 35*(1), 69–81.

Squizzato, A., Hunt, B. J., Kinasewitz, G. T., Wada, H., Ten Cate, H., Thachil, J., … Di Nisio, M. (2016). Supportive management strategies for disseminated intravascular coagulation. An international consensus. *Thrombosis and Haemostasis, 115*(5), 896–904.

Tang, N., Li, D., Wang, X., & Sun, Z. (2020). Abnormal coagulation parameters are associated with poor prognosis in patients with novel coronavirus pneumonia. *Journal of Thrombosis and Haemostasis, 18*(4), 844–847.

Wada, H., Matsumoto, T., Suzuki, K., Imai, H., Katayama, N., Iba, T., & Matsumoto, M. (2018). Differences and similarities between disseminated intravascular coagulation and thrombotic microangiopathy. *Thrombosis Journal, 16*(1), 14.

Woodford, R., Lu, M., Beydoun, N., Cooper, W., Liu, Q., Lynch, J., & Kasherman, L. (2021). Disseminated intravascular coagulation complicating diagnosis of ROS1-mutant non-small cell lung cancer: A case report and literature review. *Thoracic Cancer, 12*(17), 2400–2403.

Xiao, J., Li, S., Zhai, X., Liu, X., Chen, Y., & Huang, M. (2020). The genomic profile and potential predictive circulating cytokines of gastric cancer combine disseminated intravascular coagulation. *Journal of Clinical Oncology, 38*(15), e16543.

Zhang, L., Yan, X., Fan, Q., Liu, H., Liu, X., Liu, Z., & Zhang, Z. (2020). D-dimer levels on admission to predict in-hospital mortality in patients with Covid-19. *Journal of Thrombosis and Haemostasis, 18*(6), 1324–1329.

Zhou, X., Cheng, Z., Luo, L., Zhu, Y., Lin, W., Ming, Z., … Hu, Y. (2021). Incidence and impact of disseminated intravascular coagulation in COVID-19 a systematic review and meta-analysis. *Thrombosis Research, 201*, 23–29.

Zhu, H. H., Guo, Z. P., Jia, J. S., Jiang, Q., Jiang, H., & Huang, X. J. (2018). The impact of oral arsenic and all-trans-retinoic acid on coagulopathy in acute promyelocytic leukemia. *Leukemia Research, 65*, 14–19.

Hemolytic Uremic Syndrome

Definition

- HUS is a rare blood clotting disorder involving TMA. This complex, multisystemic disease is characterized by the clinical trial of MHA, thrombocytopenia, and acute kidney injury.
- Shiga toxin-associated hemolytic uremic syndrome (STEC-HUS) is also referred to as typical HUS, diarrhea-associated HUS, or infection-associated HUS. It is classically a disease of children. It is caused by infection with *Escherichia coli*, which produces the Shiga toxin. This toxin produces bacteria that act on endothelial lining of intestine and cause hemorrhagic enterocolitis.
- *Streptococcus pneumoniae* hemolytic uremic syndrome (SP-HUS) is also a disease of children. Children affected by SP-HUS are younger with more severe hematologic and renal disease and require longer hospital stays. DIC often occurs concurrently with SP-HUS.
- Atypical HUS (aHUS) is also termed "complement-mediated TMA." It usually results from defective regulation of complement pathway. It is a syndrome of MHA, thrombocytopenia, and acute renal failure without a diarrhea prodrome.

Epidemiology

- Overall incidence of HUS is 1 to 2 cases per 100,000 per year, with the most cases attributed to STEC-HUS.

- Typical HUS, or STEC-HUS, accounts for 85% to 95% of cases of HUS.
  - Most cases in previously healthy children, with peak incidence of 3 to 5 years old; some adult cases
  - STEC-HUS is the leading cause of acute renal failure in children aged less than 3 to 5 years old
  - Can occur in sporadic form, such as microepidemics, or as community-wide food-borne outbreaks
  - Prognosis is good overall and renal function usually returns when triggering factor is removed and/or when anti-complement therapy is administered
    - Mortality associated with STEC-HUS is reported to be approximately 3%.
    - Patients presenting with the highest leukocyte counts, especially greater than 25,000 cells/mL, are at greatest risk of dying
- SP-HUS:
  - About 5% of cases of HUS are associated with invasive infections by *S. pneumoniae*
  - Incidence has decreased since introduction of polyvalent vaccine (in some countries)
- aHUS (complement-mediated HUS, or diarrhea-negative HUS); occurs in 5% to 10% of cases of HUS
  - Rare disease; affects one to two persons out of every 1 million Americans.
  - Manifests in early childhood; some cases in older adults
  - May be sporadic or familial
  - Children and adults often have recurrent episodes
  - Can be triggered by infection (and diarrhea may be present at presentation), vaccinations, or pregnancy
  - Prognosis is poor in patients with recurrent aHUS, and acute renal failure and death occur in 54% of cases
- Therapy-related HUS
  - May occur after recent (<200 days) hematopoietic stem cell transplantation (HSCT) or use of TMA-associated drugs (e.g., cyclosporine)
  - Incidence in cancer patients is about 5%
  - Delayed and potentially fatal complication after HSCT
- Cobalamin C deficiency-HUS
  - Rare cause of HUS—seen within the first year of life
- Factors increasing risk of HUS
  - Infections, particularly:
    - Infections with Shiga toxin–producing *E. coli* (STEC)
    - Infections with *S. pneumoniae*
  - Immune-related:
    - Disorders of complement system
    - Immune disorders, such as SLE and acquired immunodeficiency syndrome (AIDS)
  - HSCT-related
    - High-dose chemotherapy conditioning regimens (e.g., HSCT)
    - Graft-rejection after HSCT
  - Medication-related
    - Chemotherapy regimens, especially with mitomycin C
    - Immunosuppressant drugs (e.g., cyclosporin, tacrolimus)
  - Disorders interfering with degradation of VWF

- Pregnancy, hemolysis, or hemolysis, elevated liver enzymes, low platelets (HELLP) syndrome (i.e., HELLP)
- Elevated levels of liver enzymes
- Factors increasing the risk of patients with typical HUS needing dialysis
  - Most significant factors were: Peak leukocyte count greater than 20,000; anuria; hemoglobin level over 9.5 g/dL at time of admission
  - Other risk factors included: plasma creatinine, lactate dehydrogenase (LDH), peak urea value

Pathophysiology

- Trigger for HUS is endothelial damage.
  - In STEC-HUS, the Shiga toxin causes damage to endothelial lining of intestine.
  - In aHUS, endothelial damage can be caused by defects in complement system, which acts as a central defense of innate immunity
  - Endothelial damage leads to platelet aggregation, thrombocytopenia, and subsequent renal, neurologic, and pulmonary dysfunction
  - Renal vasculature is primarily affected in patients with all forms of HUS and often results in irreversible renal damage in patients with aHUS
- STEC-HUS (Typical HUS or diarrhea-positive HUS)
  - Caused by infections with STEC (with the predominant serotype is O157:H7)
  - Shiga toxin–producing bacteria cause hemorrhagic enterocolitis. The toxin induces epithelial cell injury in colon, which results in abdominal pain and bloody diarrhea.
  - Frequently associated with diarrhea and acute renal failure
  - When Shiga toxin enters the bloodstream, neutrophils and monocytes transport it to the kidneys
    - Shiga toxin binds to and activates platelets
    - It promotes platelet aggregation by directly damaging renal endothelial cells or by other mechanisms
    - Tissue factor is released, which renders the vessel wall prothrombotic
- SP-HUS
  - Thompsen-Friedenreich cryoantigen is present on RBCs, platelets, glomeruli, and hepatocytes.
    - The cryoantigen is exposed to neuraminidase, which is produced by all subtypes of *S. pneumoniae*.
    - The cryoantigen interacts with IgM antibodies, resulting in agglutination.
- aHUS (complement-mediated HUS, or diarrhea-negative HUS)
  - Body loses its ability to control activation of the complement system, which is sometimes the result of a genetic mutation
    - Complement system is a group of proteins that is part of innate immune system. It enhances, or complements, the ability of the antibodies and phagocytes (including granulocytes, monocytes, and macrophages) to rid the body of pathogens and damaged or dead cells.
    - Complement protein 5 (C5), one member of the complement system, plays an important role in destroying foreign or damaged cells.

- Normally, control mechanisms keep C5 and other complement proteins from attacking healthy cells.
- In aHUS, these control mechanisms fail and uncontrolled C5 begins to damage healthy cells.
- Eculizumab can effectively inhibit immune system, by blocking activation of C5. This drug has been proven to be very effective in reversing clinical presentation in aHUS patients.
- Chronic, often progressive disease; Not associated with the Shiga toxin or diarrhea
- Sporadic form of aHUS is triggered that may accelerate activation of complement system:
  - Autoimmune disease (SLE, AIDS, complement disorders)
  - Disorders interfering with degradation of VWF
  - Infections (e.g., Glomerulonephritis, *S. pneumoniae*)
  - Surgery, trauma, transplantation
  - Cancer
  - Malignant hypertension
  - Medications (e.g., cyclosporin)
  - Postpartum
- Familial form of aHUS is rare but associated with a significant risk of morbidity and mortality
- Prognosis is poor in subgroup of patients with recurrent aHUS, since they have a strong association with diseases of complement system
  - Patients in this subgroup often have end-stage renal disease and require kidney transplant
  - Patients in this subgroup commonly have severe arterial hypertension and require multidrug therapy.
- Cobalamin C deficiency-HUS
  - A rare cause of HUS that is caused by recessive mutations of the methylmalonic aciduria (cobalamin deficiency) CblC type with *MMACHC* gene.
  - Presentation is typically within the first year of life.

Signs and Symptoms

- Signs/symptoms that may occur in all forms of HUS:
  - Fever
  - Shortness of breath, pallor, extreme fatigue: may correlate with degree of anemia
  - Petechiae, easy bruising, unexplained bruises due to thrombocytopenia; occurs in 70% of patients
  - Unusual bleeding, such as bleeding from nose and mouth, or blood in urine due to thrombocytopenia
  - Swelling of legs, feet or ankles, and less often in face, hands, feet due to renal dysfunction
- STEC-HUS (typical HUS, or infection-associated HUS) signs and symptoms
  - Gastrointestinal symptoms:
    - Diarrhea (often watery and progresses to overtly bloody) due to hemorrhagic colitis (toxin is acting on endothelial lining of intestine)
    - Nausea, vomiting
    - Intense abdominal pain, cramping, bloating
    - Can progress to bowel necrosis and perforation
  - Renal symptoms: Anuria (51%), oliguria (29%)

- Major CNS symptoms (33%): seizures, impaired consciousness, hemiparesis (occurs due to microvascular thrombosis in CNS, resulting in focal areas of infarction and necrosis; parenchymal hemorrhage; cerebral edema; and leukoencephalopathy)
- Minor CNS symptoms (14%): Lethargy, irritability
- Hypertension (34%)
- Cardiovascular symptoms: myocardial infarction, congestive heart failure, dilated cardiomyopathy
- TMA presents 5 to 7 days after the intestinal Shiga toxin infection
- Extrarenal manifestations:
  - Transaminase level: elevated (49%)
  - Amylase level: elevated (15%)
  - Pulmonary hemorrhage, pleural effusion
  - Pancreatitis and resulting pancreatic enzyme elevation, diabetes mellitus, and cholecystitis
- *S. pneumoniae* HUS signs and symptoms
  - Typically presents with pneumonia
  - Direct Coombs test (DAT) is positive for hemolytic anemia
- aHUS signs and symptoms
  - Renal impairment or failure (e.g., oliguria, anuria): abnormally low urine output occurs in all patients.
  - Other renal symptoms may include listlessness, confusion, weight loss, nausea/vomiting, weight gain, edema, severe hypertension, proteinuria, encephalopathy (due to toxins not being cleared by kidneys)
  - Thrombocytopenia, petechiae, easy bruising, or bleeding may or may not be present
  - Shortness of breath, tachycardia, pale skin, or weakness that may correlate with the degree of anemia, which occurs in most patients
  - Neurologic symptoms, such as seizures, loss of vision, loss of balance, confusion, and nystagmus
  - Gastrointestinal symptoms: colitis, abdominal pain, pancreatitis, nausea/vomiting, gastroenteritis, diarrhea (not overtly bloody)
  - Jaundice, due to liver not metabolizing all of the damaged RBCs
  - Cardiovascular symptoms: severe hypertension, arterial thrombosis, vascular stenosis, DVT, stroke, heart attack
- Among bone marrow transplant (BMT) recipients, onset of HUS typically occurs 30 to 875 days after the procedure and manifests with a triad of symptoms:
  - MHA: hematuria and fatigue
  - Thrombocytopenia with increased bleeding or hemorrhaging
  - Renal insufficiency with increased creatinine, reduced creatinine clearance, and fluid retention

Cancers Associated With Disorder

- Adenocarcinomas, including gastric cancer, lung cancer, and breast cancer
- Lymphoma

Diagnostic Tests

- Diagnostic criteria for HUS
  - MHA

- Thrombocytopenia
- Acute renal failure
- Possible diarrhea
- Laboratory tests
  - CBC with a platelet count
    - Anemia, with an average hemoglobin decreased to 7 to 9 g/dL
    - Thrombocytopenia, with platelet count less than 50,000 cells/mm^3 or 50% decrease from previous count
  - Diagnostic criteria for MHA
    - Schistocytes in peripheral blood smear (>1%, or >3 schistocytes per high-power microscopic field). These are split RBCs that indicate MHA, and their presence is hallmark for diagnosing TTP and HUS
    - Reticulocyte count: increased
    - Bilirubin level (mainly indirect reacting): increased
    - Serum haptoglobin levels: decreased
    - Free plasma hemoglobin: increased in severe cases.
    - Elevated reticulocyte counts
  - Serum ADAMTS13 activity
    - Important to promptly quantify ADAMTS13 antigen, activity, and autoantibodies, in order to differentiate from other thrombotic microangiopathies (TMAs), such as TTP
    - Is usually normal in person with HUS
  - Infection/diarrhea assessment
    - Blood, stool, and/or urine cultures to identify infection as an underlying cause of HUS
    - Positive stool culture for *E. coli* (serotype O157:H7); Positive for antibody to Shiga toxin
    - Rapid test for malaria, dengue; IgM antibodies for dengue, leptospirosis (if suspected)
  - Renal function test results:
    - BUN: elevated
    - Serum creatinine: elevated
    - Estimated glomerular filtration rate: decreased
  - Comprehensive metabolic panel (CMP)
    - LDH: elevated due to hemolysis
    - Electrolyte levels: elevated due to renal impairment
    - Serum bilirubin level: elevated due to significant RBC hemolysis
  - Direct Coombs test (also known as direct antiglobulin test [DAT])
    - Determines whether RBCs have been coated in vivo with immunoglobulin, complement, or both.
    - Negative result: nonautoimmune, nondrug-induced hemolytic anemia
    - Positive result: autoimmune, drug-induced hemolytic anemia
  - Coagulation tests
    - PT, aPTT, factor V, factor VIII, fibrinogen: usually normal levels
    - FDP level: may be elevated.
    - TT: may be prolonged.
  - Blood levels of complement C3
  - Troponin T or troponin I levels to rule out cardiac involvement

- Liver function tests to rule out liver involvement (usually normal)
- Blood type and screen tests to prepare for provision of blood products
- Hepatitis A, B, or C and human immunodeficiency virus (HIV) testing of blood products to exclude an underlying viral precipitant
- Urinalysis, with proteinuria, microscopic hematuria, and granular or red cell casts as the most consistent findings
- Renal biopsy may be considered in patients with:
  - Unclear diagnosis of HUS
  - Unsatisfactory clinical response, to determine extent of renal damage and help in prognosis; and
  - Distinguish between causes of allograft dysfunction, including recurrent aHUS
- Radiologic evaluation
  - Renal sonogram or renal angiogram
  - Intravenous pyelogram
  - CT of the abdomen to determine kidney involvement
  - CT of the chest, abdomen, and pelvis with or without tumor markers to assess for underlying malignancy
  - Electrocardiogram (ECG) or echocardiogram to document or monitor cardiac damage

Differential Diagnosis

- Diagnosis of HUS can be difficult, since there can be overlap with TTP, autoimmune disease, and a spectrum of pregnancy-related problems.
  - Some patients may concurrently have an autoimmune disorder (e.g., SLE, antiphospholipid antibody syndrome) and TTP
- Hematuria related to:
  - Other diseases (e.g., infection, intrinsic kidney disease, benign prostatic hypertrophy)
  - Medications (e.g., ifosfamide, high-dose cyclophosphamide, intravesical chemotherapy)
  - Radiation therapy (e.g., pelvic irradiation, prostate seed implants)
- Systemic malignancy can cause thrombocytopenia and MHA without signs of DIC.
- Malignant hypertension can cause thrombocytopenia, MHA, renal failure, and severe neurologic abnormalities.
- Systemic infection or sepsis, typically viral (e.g., CMV, adenovirus, herpes simplex virus) or severe bacterial (e.g., meningococcus, pneumococcus), but may be fungal
- DIC
- HUS (diarrhea positive or negative)
- HIT
- Vasculitis
- Drugs: quinine, simvastatin, interferon, calcineurin inhibitors
- Complications for persons undergoing HSCT:
  - Graft-versus-host disease
  - Hepatic sinusoidal obstruction syndrome
  - CMV

- Pregnancy—associated conditions can cause MHA, thrombocytopenia, renal failure, and minor neurologic abnormalities:
  - HELLP
  - Eclampsia
- Differential diagnosis of TTP and HUS
  - TTP and HUS are distinct diseases with different causes and demographics.
    - Many patients are inaccurately diagnosed with "TTP-HUS disorder" on basis of clinical and laboratory findings only.
  - Similar clinical and laboratory features, which occur in both patients with TTP and patients with HUS, include:
    - Thrombocytopenia: platelet count less than 150,000/mm^3 or $\geq$25% decrease in platelets from baseline
    - MHA: schistocytes present on peripheral smear, elevated LDH, decreased haptoglobin, decreased hemoglobin and hematocrit
    - Plus or minus one of the following clinical symptoms due to localized microvascular thrombosis: (1) Neurologic symptoms (confusion, seizures, or other cerebral abnormalities); (2) Renal impairment (elevated creatinine, decreased estimates GFR, elevated blood pressure, abnormal urinalysis); (3) Gastrointestinal symptoms (diarrhea $\pm$ blood, nausea/vomiting, abdominal pain, gastroenteritis)
  - Clinical and laboratory features that differentiate patients with TTP from patients with HUS include:
    - ADAMTS13 deficiencies are the cause of both acquired and congenital TTP; ADAMTS13 does not play a role in pathogenesis of HUS
    - Platelets are less than 30,000/mm^3 in TTP, and thrombocytopenia is less severe in HUS
    - Etiology of STEC-HUS: associated with Shiga toxin–associated hemorrhagic colitis
    - Clinical presentation of TTP patients: dominated by hemorrhages and neurologic symptoms. Renal involvement (e.g., proteinuria, microscopic hematuria) is common, but oliguric acute renal failure is unusual.
    - Clinical presentation of HUS patients: significant renal impairment or failure is the dominant clinical feature
    - Treatment of TTP patients: Therapeutic plasma exchange (TPE), corticosteroids, and drugs (e.g., rituximab, caplacizumab)
    - Treatment of HUS patients: Insulting factors are removed, supportive care is given (IV fluids, PRBC transfusion, dialysis) and anti-complement therapy (e.g., eculizumab or ravulizumab) is administered. Patients with HUS have a lack of a complete response to plasma exchange

Treatment

- Typical HUS (diarrhea-positive HUS)
  - Supportive care
    - Fluid and electrolyte management after oliguric renal failure develops. Although persons with HUS may be dehydrated, fluids are given judiciously due to risk of kidney impairment.
    - PRBC transfusions to treat anemia
    - Blood pressure control medications
    - Hemodialysis
  - Use of systemic antibiotics is controversial
    - Early studies suggested a risk of progression to HUS with systemic antibiotics, which were administered to patients with STEC-HUS and enterocolitis, and later studies have presented conflicting data
    - Menne and colleagues (2012) reported that macrolide antibiotic administration for patients with STEC-HUS resulted in no worsened disease activity, reduction of long-term *E. coli* carriage, and ultimately decreased incidence of seizure activity
  - Avoid antimotility agents, and opioids, which are associated worsening of disease
  - Avoid NSAIDs, which can decrease renal blood flow
- aHUS (diarrhea-negative HUS)
  - Plasma exchanges, which benefit about one-third of children, except for the subgroup with membrane cofactor protein mutations
  - Terminal complement inhibitor eculizumab

Pharmacologic Management

- Prevention
  - Early and cautious fluid resuscitation, in the setting of enterocolitis before development of STEC-HUS, may improve renal and neurologic outcomes
  - Vigorous pre-transplantation parenteral or oral hydration
  - Continuous bladder irrigation with normal saline solution
- Management
  - Anti-complement therapy (eculizumab and ravulizumab)
    - Eculizumab (Soliris) and ravulizumab (Ultomiris) are complement C5-inhibitors and are indicated for patients with aHUS
    - Kim and colleagues (2018) reported that eculizumab blocks the terminal complement pathway and has been successfully used in the treatment of aHUS. Several guidelines for aHUS recommend eculizumab as first-line therapy in children with aHUS, and life-long eculizumab therapy is generally recommended
    - Barbour and colleagues (2021) reported that ravulizumab administered every 8 weeks was efficacious with an acceptable safety profile for the long-term treatment of adults with aHUS and provided additional clinical benefit beyond 6 months of treatment
    - Eculizumab therapy has very effectively reversed TMA and reduced mortality and morbidity
    - For aHUS, treatment with eculizumab has been successful

- For typical HUS, eculizumab may be effective in treating patients with diarrhea-positive HUS
- Both drugs have a black box warning for increased susceptibility to life-threatening meningococcal infection. Patients should be immunized with meningococcal vaccine at least 2 weeks before starting either drug.
- FFP infusion
  - Pathogen-reduced FFP is preferred
  - Repetitive plasma infusions increase risk of infection
  - Initial dose: recommended volume is 60 to 65 mL/kg/week
  - Maintenance dose: recommended volume is 20 mL/kg/week
- TPE is less effective in HUS, with response rates of 20% to 30%, compared with response rates of 80% in classic TTP
- Provide Cobalamin supplementation
  - This is indicated for rare cases of Cobalamin C deficiency HUS that is caused by recessive mutations
- Provide immunizations, including hepatitis A and B

Nonpharmacologic Management

- Remove factors that are triggering the HUS and causing injury to endothelium
  - If chemotherapy drugs (e.g., mitomycin, gemcitabine) are suspected to be the cause of the TMA/HUS, then the first intervention should be to stop administration of the drug
  - Immunosuppressants (e.g., cyclosporin, ticlopidine, clopidogrel) have been associated with TMA and therefore need to be discontinued
  - Avoid platelet transfusions
    - Platelet transfusions are contraindicated because they can worsen microvascular thrombi
- Nephrology consultation to determine the most appropriate renal therapy
- Intravenous fluids
- Renal replacement therapy (e.g., peritoneal dialysis, hemodialysis)
  - May be successful for patients with recurrent aHUS
  - Kidney transplantation not recommended for patients with soluble complement disorders (e.g., aHUS)
    - Failure rate is about 70% for renal transplantation complicated by recurrence of disease
- Liver transplantation
  - Combined renal and liver transplantation is a logical form of treatment for typical HUS, because factors H and I are synthesized in the liver
  - Transplantation is not recommended for persons with complement disorders (aHUS)

Patient Teaching

- Goals
  - Define HUS
  - Identify signs/symptoms of HUS to report to health care provider

- Understand lab and diagnostic testing, nursing care and treatments related to managing HUS
- Prevent relapse of HUS
- Maintain patient safety by identifying signs/symptoms of bleeding and avoiding injury and bleeding while experiencing thrombocytopenia
- Describe goals of therapy for HUS:
  - Blood cell counts (especially platelets and hemoglobin) return to normal levels
  - Symptoms (e.g., bleeding, renal, and neurologic abnormalities) subside
- Provide patients with verbal and written educational materials on HUS
- Define HUS
- Describe signs/symptoms, and report symptoms, such as increased bleeding, blood in urine, decreased urine output, swelling in extremities, and mental status changes
- Teach patient purpose of laboratory tests, nursing care, and treatments for HUS
- Teach patient/family to save urine, stool, and emesis for nurse to check for blood
- Encourage patient to drink 8 to 10 glasses of fluid daily, if kidney function is adequate
- Teach patients self-care measures to maximize their safety:
  - Use electric razor, not straight-edged razor
  - Maintain bed in low position with side rails up
  - Clear pathways in room and hallway
  - Minimize activities that can trigger bleeding
  - Avoid contact sports and lifting
  - Take precautions against accidental bleeding because even minor scrapes or bumps can cause bleeding
- Teach fall precautions if the patient remains at risk for falls
  - In the home, remove throw rugs and items that can obstruct pathways
  - Wear shoes that fit appropriately
  - Walk carefully, and change positions gradually
- Teach patients to avoid over-the-counter medications that may interfere with normal platelet function such as aspirin and NSAIDs (e.g., ibuprofen, naproxen sodium)
- Teach patients to minimize activities that contribute to development of additional clots and to increase circulation in the lower extremities:
  - Avoid tight or restrictive clothing
  - Use compression stockings to promote venous return
  - Elevate legs when possible
  - Wiggle toes and feet, and rotate ankles, especially when in bed
  - Do not sit with legs crossed
  - Do not dangle feet on the side of the bed
  - Do not use pillows under the knees or a knee gatch
- Teach patient about critical signs/symptoms and to report bruising, red rash, headache, black stools, blood in the urine or stools, and bleeding from the gums, nose, eyes, vagina, rectum, wound, or central venous catheter site

Follow-Up

- Continue to monitor for signs and symptoms of HUS.
- Monitor appropriate laboratory findings (especially platelet count and hemoglobin or hematocrit) to determine the continuation or resolution of HUS.
- Reconcile medications at ICU discharge, hospital discharge, and follow-up visits.
- Screen for economic and social support (including housing, nutritional, financial, and spiritual support).
  - Make referrals, where available, to meet these needs
  - Provide additional resources, such as home equipment or assistance, as needed
- Monitor BMT recipients treated with high-dose chemotherapy for potential long-term sequelae, including HUS.

Bibliography

Bagga, A., Khandelwal, P., Mishra, K., Thergaonkar, R., Vasudevan, A., Sharma, J., … Indian Society of Pediatric Nephrology. (2019). Hemolytic uremic syndrome in a developing country: Consensus guidelines. *Pediatric Nephrology*, 34(8), 1465–1482.

Barbour, T., Scully, M., Ariceta, G., Cataland, S., Garlo, K., Heyne, N., … 311 Study Group Members. (2021). Long-term efficacy and safety of the long-acting complement C5 inhibitor ravulizumab for the treatment of atypical hemolytic uremic syndrome in adults. *Kidney International Reports*, 6(6), 1603–1613.

Cody, E. M., & Dixon, B. P. (2019). Hemolytic uremic syndrome. *Pediatric Clinics of North America*, 66(1), 235–246.

Del Cogliano, M. E., Pinto, A., Goldstein, J., Zotta, E., Ochoa, F., Fernández-Brando, R. J., … Bentancor, L. V. (2018). Relevance of bacteriophage 933W in the development of hemolytic uremic syndrome (HUS). *Frontiers in Microbiology*, 9, 3104.

Exeni, R. A., Fernandez-Brando, R. J., Santiago, A. P., Fiorentino, G. A., Exeni, A. M., Ramos, M. V., & Palermo, M. S. (2018). Pathogenic role of inflammatory response during Shiga toxin-associated hemolytic uremic syndrome (HUS). *Pediatric Nephrology*, 33(11), 2057–2071.

Gulleroglu, K., Fidan, K., Hançer, V. S., Bayrakci, U., Baskin, E., & Soylemezoglu, O. (2013). Neurological involvement in atypical hemolytic uremic syndrome and successful treatment with eculizumab. *Pediatric Nephrology*, 28, 827–830.

Khalid, M., & Andreoli, S. (2019). Extrarenal manifestations of the hemolytic uremic syndrome associated with Shiga toxin-producing *Escherichia coli* (STEC HUS). *Pediatric Nephrology*, 34(12), 2495–2507.

Kim, S. H., Kim, H. Y., & Kim, S. Y. (2018). Atypical hemolytic uremic syndrome and eculizumab therapy in children. *Korean Journal of Pediatrics*, 61(2), 37–42.

Kremer Hovinga, J. A., Heeb, S. R., Skowronska, M., & Schaller, M. (2018). Pathophysiology of thrombotic thrombocytopenic purpura and hemolytic uremic syndrome. *Journal of Thrombosis and Haemostasis*, 16(4), 618–629.

Legendre, C. M., Licht, C., Muus, P., Greenbaum, L. A., Babu, S., Bedrosian, C., … Loirat, C. (2013). Terminal complement inhibitor eculizumab in atypical hemolytic-uremic syndrome. *New England Journal of Medicine*, 368, 2169–2181.

Mele, C., Remuzzi, G., & Noris, M. (2014). Hemolytic uremic syndrome. *Seminars in Immunopathology*, 36(4), 399–420. https://doi.org/10.1007/s00281-014-0416-x

Menne, J., Nitschke, M., Stingele, R., Abu-Tair, M., Beneke, J., Bramstedt, J., … EHEC-HUS Consortium. (2012). Validation of treatment strategies for enterohaemorrhagic *Escherichia coli* O104:H4 induced haemolytic uraemic syndrome: Case-control study. *BMJ*, 345, e4565.

Percheron, L., Gramada, R., Tellier, S., Salomon, R., Harambat, J., Llanas, B., … Garnier, A. (2018). Eculizumab treatment in severe pediatric STEC-HUS: A multicenter retrospective study. *Pediatric Nephrology*, 33(8), 1385–1394.

Scully, M., Cataland, S., Coppo, P., de la Rubia, J., Friedman, K. D., Kremer Hovinga, J., … International Working Group for Thrombotic Thrombocytopenic Purpura. (2017). Consensus on the standardization of terminology in thrombotic thrombocytopenic purpura and related thrombotic microangiopathies. *Journal of Thrombosis and Haemostasis*, 15(2), 312–322.

Scully, M., Hunt, B. J., Benjamin, S., Liesner, R., Rose, P., Peyvandi, F., ... British Committee for Standards in Haematology. (2012). Guidelines on the diagnosis and management of thrombotic thrombocytopenic purpura and other thrombotic microangiopathies. *British Journal of Haematology*, *158*, 323–335.

Wijnsma, K. L., Duineveld, C., Wetzels, J. F. M., & van de Kar, N. C. A. J. (2019). Eculizumab in atypical hemolytic uremic syndrome: Strategies toward restrictive use. *Pediatric Nephrology*, *34*(11), 2261–2277.

Ylinen, E., Salmenlinna, S., Halkilahti, J., Jahnukainen, T., Korhonen, L., Virkkala, T., ... Saxén, H. (2020). Hemolytic uremic syndrome caused by Shiga toxin-producing *Escherichia coli* in children: Incidence, risk factors, and clinical outcome. *Pediatric Nephrology*, *35*(9), 1749–1759.

Zuber, J., Frimat, M., Caillard, S., Kamar, N., Gatault, P., Petitprez, F., ... Frémeaux-Bacchi, V. (2019). Use of highly individualized complement blockade has revolutionized clinical outcomes after kidney transplantation and renal epidemiology of atypical hemolytic uremic syndrome. *Journal of the American Society of Nephrology*, *30*(12), 2449–2463.

Pulmonary Embolism

Definition

- PE is invasion of thrombus (blood clot), which has been detached from its original source, and travels with blood flow into pulmonary arteries or one of its branches. A very large embolus may lodge in main pulmonary artery, and smaller emboli pass to more distal branches of the pulmonary artery, causing partial or total occlusion of blood vessels.
- PE is a life-threatening complication of DVT.
- Incidental PE (IPE), or unsuspected PE (UPE), is when cancer-associated PE events are found incidentally on radiographic testing performed for diagnostic or staging purposes, and for treatment response evaluation in cancer patients.

Epidemiology

- VTE, comprised of DVT and PE, is a common complication in cancer patients and is associated with significant morbidity and mortality.
- VTE incidence and prevalence:
  - VTE is the third most common cardiovascular pathology by its prevalence after myocardial infarction and stroke, with about 900,000 cases and 300,000 deaths in U.S. annually
  - VTE has an annual incidence of 1 to 2 per 1000 population. Mortality is high; Death occurs within 30 days in about 6% of patients with DVT, primarily through PE, and in 13% of patients with PE
  - After 3 to 6 months of anticoagulation, VTE recurs in up to 40% of patients within 10 years
  - VTE is the second overall leading cause of death for patients with cancer, and there is an approximately two-fold increase in fatal PE in patients with cancer
  - VTE occurs two to four times more frequently in patients with cancer than in those without cancer. VTE may be a marker of advanced stage cancer or of a more biologically aggressive tumor
- Incidence and prevalence of PE:
  - PE is gradually considered to be the third most common disease in the vascular disease category

- In one study with cancer patients ($n = 4492$), 5.1% of patients developed a new PE after their initial DVT diagnosis
- PE is common in lung cancer patients, with a pooled incidence of 3.7%
- PE is incidentally diagnosed in up to 5% of cancer patients on routine imaging scans
- COVID-19 infection is associated with a profound coagulopathy, including PE. Incidence of VTE is up to 35% in patients with severe cases of COVID-19
- Up to 80% of emboli are small and clinically undetectable because the pulmonary circulation has several sources of collateral flow
- Pulmonary infarction occurs in 10% to 15% of cases, usually in persons with cardiopulmonary disease, and a high mortality rate is associated with large or multiple emboli
- Increased risk for DVT/PE:
  - *Cancer-related risk factors*
    - Cancer is a permanent/persistent risk factor for VTE
    - Cancer, which can cause a hypercoagulable state: Stomach and pancreas cancer are very high risk; lung, lymphoma, gynecologic, bladder, and testicular cancer are high risk
    - Hematologic malignancies, especially multiple myeloma, due to hyperviscosity state, and APL
  - *Patient-related risk factors*
    - Prechemotherapy platelet count (350×10^9/L or higher)
    - Hemoglobin level less than 10 g/dL
    - Prechemotherapy leukocyte count higher than 11×10^9/L
    - Obesity (BMI $\geq$35 kg/m^2 or higher)
    - Associated diseases (e.g., cardiac disease, peripheral vascular disease, chronic renal disease, COPD, diabetes, acute and chronic infections)
    - Chronic inflammation (e.g., inflammatory bowel disease), chronic autoimmune disease, chronic infections—are permanent/persistent VTE risk factors
    - Hypercoagulable state (prior VTE [DVT or PE], blood clotting disorders, DIC)
    - More than half of patients who have a PE have an accompanying clot in their lower limb
    - COVID-19 infection, which may result in hypercoagulable state
    - Conditions that promote venous stasis, such as prolonged bed rest or prolonged immobility resulting from pain, trauma, surgery, or paralysis
    - Confined to bed in hospital for $\geq$3 days with an acute illness ("bathroom privileges")—is a major transient VTE risk factor
    - Admission to hospital less than 3 days with an acute illness, confined to bed out of hospital $\geq$3 days with an acute illness, leg injury with reduced mobility—is a minor transient VTE risk factor
    - Conditions that cause vessel damage, such as burns or fractures

- *Treatment-related risk factors*
  - Use of RBC growth factors
  - Recent general surgery with any anesthesia (>30 minutes) or trauma—is a major transient VTE risk factor.
  - Recent general surgery with any anesthesia (<30 minutes) or trauma—is a minor transient VTE risk factor.
  - Chemotherapy, with correlation between development of PE and patient receiving cisplatin, carboplatin, gemcitabine, and paclitaxel
  - Bevacizumab in lung cancer patients, especially SCLC
  - Therapy for multiple myeloma patients with thalidomide or lenalidomide in combination with doxorubicin, multiagent chemotherapy, or high-dose dexamethasone (≥480 mg/month)
  - Medications such as antiestrogens (tamoxifen, raloxifene) and estrogens
  - Medications that induce endothelial damage, such as some vasopressor agents (e.g., dopamine), contrast medium, high-dose antibiotics, and antiphospholipid antibodies (associated with SLE)
  - Use of a central venous catheter
  - Radiation therapy

Pathophysiology

- See "Pathophysiology of DVT" regarding clot formation (Virchow triad).
  - When blood clot is detached from the original source, the embolus travels with the blood flow.
  - Embolus may also be a fat globule, air, tumor, amniotic fluid, other tissue fragment, clumped bacteria, or a foreign body.
  - Embolism may migrate from a distal vein to the IVC, right atrium and right ventricle and enter the pulmonary artery.
  - A very large embolus may lodge in the main pulmonary artery, and smaller emboli pass to more distal branches of the pulmonary artery.
  - When embolus lodges in the pulmonary artery or one of its branches, it can cause partial or total occlusion of the vessel.
- Pathogenesis of VTE in cancer patients likely includes the release of procoagulants and cytokines from cancer cells, direct endothelial damage, and down-regulation of endogenous anti-coagulants. Prothrombotic activity of tumor cells plays an important role in occurrence of PE.
- Pathogenesis of VTE in COVID-19 patients is a combination of classic VTE (macrothrombosis) and diffuse microthrombosis with endothelial damage in the lungs, directly caused by the coronavirus.
- PE may result from mechanical occlusion of a regional pulmonary artery.
  - Perfusion and ventilation changes occur in the section of lung supplied by the artery.
- Lung volumes and compliance are usually reduced.
- Pulmonary shunting may cause hypoxia.
- Pulmonary artery pressure may become elevated.
- If the PE is massive, the right ventricle may be unable to generate enough pressure to maintain adequate cardiac output.
- Right ventricular failure can increase right arterial pressure, and cardiogenic shock can ensue.

Signs and Symptoms

- Severity of clinical manifestations of PE depends on: (1) size of embolus (e.g., patients with small emboli may exhibit few or no symptoms), and (2) patient's pre-existing cardiopulmonary status.
- Up to 75% of PE cases have no initial observable symptoms.
- Clinical presentation is important in guiding management since PE can be difficult to diagnose with tests.
- Most frequent signs/symptoms of PE:
  - Shortness of breath, or dyspnea (usually with a sudden onset). Severity can vary from mild to severe, and from intermittent to progressive
  - Chest pain (often anginal type at onset) that worsens with deep breathing and later becomes pleuritic
  - Tachycardia
  - Tachypnea (respiratory rate >24 breaths/min)
  - Apprehension
  - Syncope
- Less frequent signs/symptom of PE
  - Anxiety and restlessness
  - Thrombophlebitis symptoms: warmth, erythema, and palpable, cordlike veins
  - Respiratory crackles or rales, diminished breath sounds, and wheezing
  - Cough, hemoptysis (usually a later symptom), and bloody sputum
  - Low-grade fever
  - Diaphoresis
  - Non-pleuritic chest pain
  - Hypotension, cyanosis, and pleural rub
  - Back or abdominal pain, lower extremity pain, tenderness, or swelling
- Signs/symptoms of massive PE:
  - Acute right ventricular failure
  - Systemic hypotension
  - Sudden death

Cancers Associated With Disorder

- Stomach and pancreas cancer (very high risk for PE)
- Lung (SCLC and NSCLC), lymphoma, gynecologic (e.g., ovarian, endometrial), bladder, and testicular cancer (high risk for PE)
- Colorectal cancer and mucin-secreting gastrointestinal tumors
- Breast, prostate, and intracranial carcinomas—low risk for PE
- APL, multiple myeloma, and myeloproliferative disorders

Diagnostic Tests

- Laboratory tests
  - CBC with a platelet count
  - PT and aPTT
  - Liver and kidney function tests
  - D-dimer—testing is recommended by some authors, stating D-dimer levels are raised in most patients with DVT (sensitivity 94% to 96%); however, national guidelines do not support the use of D-dimer testing.
- Radiologic workup—Initial Evaluation
  - Chest radiograph
    - Elevation of a hemidiaphragm and pulmonary infiltrates are most identified in patients with PE.
    - Findings are often determined to be abnormal, but they are frequently related to a history of COPD or cardiac disease, rather than PE.
  - ECG
    - Tachycardia and nonspecific ST-T wave changes are most often observed but are not diagnostic for PE.
- Radiologic workup—Subsequent Imaging
  - Computed tomography angiography (CTA), with contrast
    - CTA is used to assess for right ventricular enlargement or dysfunction.
    - Improved resolution has led to enhanced visualization of pulmonary arteries to subsegmental level, which has resulted in higher sensitivity for PE and increased incidence of IPE findings
    - If results are negative, evaluate for other causes.
    - If results are positive, initiate treatment for PE.
  - X-Ray pulmonary angiography with contrast
    - Angiography is rarely used unless coupled with clot extraction or thrombolytic therapy.
    - If results are negative, evaluate for other causes.
    - If results are positive, initiate treatment for PE.
  - Ventilation-perfusion (VQ) scan (lung scan)
    - Used if CTA is contraindicated (e.g., renal insufficiency, allergy to contrast is refractory to anaphylaxis prophylaxis).
    - A negative result (normal scan) rules out clinical PE; evaluate for other causes.
    - A low or intermediate result indicates a possible PE; use clinical judgment.
    - A positive result, in conjunction with clinical signs, definitively indicates the need for immediate treatment of PE.

Differential Diagnosis

- Myocardial infarction, congestive heart failure, pericardial tamponade, or dissecting aortic aneurysm
- Infection (e.g., pneumonia, pneumonitis, pleuritis, pericarditis, endocarditis)
- COVID-19 infection
- Pneumothorax, pleural effusions (PE can lead to pleural effusions), pulmonary fibrosis, or COPD
- Superior vena cava syndrome

- Gastrointestinal abnormalities (e.g., esophageal rupture, ulcers, gastritis)
- Anxiety disorder with hyperventilation

Treatment

- Surgical placement of an IVC filter to prevent PE in recurrent DVT is advocated for cancer patients who have a contraindication to anticoagulants.
  - Procedure uses an endoluminal filter to interrupt blood flow through the IVC.
  - A retrievable filter is preferred.
  - In a large study ($n = 88,585$), results indicate that IVC filter placement reduced development of PE in patients with very-high-risk, high-risk, and low-risk malignant neoplasms. Also, study results demonstrate significant improvement in PE-free survival in high-risk patients with coagulopathy, intracranial hemorrhaging, and upper GI bleeding.
  - IVC filter is not recommended for persons with proximal DVT, significant preexisting cardiovascular disease, or PE with hemodynamic compromise.
- Rescue thrombolysis/thrombectomy or embolectomy (rare) is performed as a surgical procedure or as a catheter technique under radiographic guidance.
  - Considered in hemodynamically stable patients with PE, who deteriorate despite anticoagulation.
- Thrombolytic therapy (e.g., streptokinase, recombinant tPA), which may be administered either catheter-directed or systemic, and is followed by anticoagulation, is recommended for patients with PE with hemodynamic compromise. This reduces mortality and may reduce the risk of subsequent PE.
- Consider catheter removal in patients with catheter-related DVT.

Pharmacologic Management

- Prevention
  - Goal: Prevent DVT so that PE does not occur.
  - VTE prophylaxis options for hospitalized medical oncology patients:
    - Dalteparin (Fragmin) 5000 units subcutaneous daily (category 1)
    - Enoxaparin (Lovenox) 40 mg subcutaneous daily (category 1)
    - Fondaparinux (Arixtra) 2.5 mg subcutaneous daily (category 1)—should be avoided in patients weighing less than 50 kg
    - UFH 5000 units subcutaneous every 8 to 12 hours (category 1)
  - VTE prophylaxis options for ambulatory medical oncology patients:
    - Apixaban (Eliquis) 2.5 mg PO twice daily
    - Rivaroxaban (Xarelto) 10 mg PO once daily
    - Dalteparin (Fragmin) 200 units/kg subcutaneous daily × 1 month, the 150 units/kg subcutaneous daily × 2 months

- Enoxaparin (Lovenox) 1 mg/kg subcutaneous daily × 3 months, then 40 mg subcutaneous daily
- Extended VTE prophylaxis options for surgical oncology patients:
  - Apixaban (Eliquis) 2.5 mg PO every 12 hours × 28 days
  - Dalteparin (Fragmin) 5000 units subcutaneous daily × 28 days
  - Enoxaparin (Lovenox) 40 mg subcutaneous daily × 28 days
- VTE prophylaxis for patients with multiple myeloma and ≤3 points by IMPEDE score or less than 2 points by SAVED score
  - Aspirin 81 to 325 mg once daily
- VTE prophylaxis for patients with multiple myeloma and ≥4 points by IMPEDE score or ≥2 points by SAVED score
  - LMWH (equivalent to 40 mg of enoxaparin once daily), or
  - Rivaroxaban (Xarelto) 10 mg daily or
  - Apixaban (Eliquis) 2.5 mg twice daily or
  - Fondaparinux (Arixtra) 2.5 mg daily or
  - Warfarin (target INR of 2.0 to 3.0)
- Management of PE
  - Anticoagulant therapy
    - Anticoagulation therapy is the mainstay treatment for VTE. It aims to reduce mortality, thrombus extension, recurrence, and risk of PTS.
    - Anticoagulant therapy interrupts thrombosis and allows the lytic system to dissolve the clot that is in the pulmonary vessel.
    - International guidelines suggest the same anticoagulant treatment for cancer patients with incidentally detected PE as those with symptomatic PE.
    - UFH is the traditional standard for initial treatment of PE because of its rapid onset of action. PE usually responds to treatment.
    - VKAs, such as warfarin, are oral agents that are used for long-term anticoagulation after thromboembolism occurs and for secondary prophylaxis. Agents may be initiated concurrently with heparin.
    - For patients with DVT and/or PE, who have completed primary treatment and will continue to receive secondary prevention, national guidelines recommend using anticoagulation over aspirin.
  - Home treatment is recommended over hospital treatment:
    - Treating persons with DVT at home, rather than in the hospital setting, decreased the risk of PE.
    - Home treatment is appropriate for persons with low risk of complications. This is not the recommendation for patients who have conditions that would require hospitalization, have limited or no support at home, cannot afford medications, or have a history of poor compliance.
  - Therapeutic anticoagulation treatment for VTE (DVT or PE) constitutes acute management in hemodynamically stable patients:

- DOACs—also known as oral factor Xa inhibitors—are preferred for patients without gastric or gastroesophageal lesions: Apixaban (Eloquis; category 1), Edoxaban (Savaysa; category 1), and rivaroxaban (Xarelto)
- LMWH—preferred for patients with gastric or gastroesophageal lesions): Dalteparin (Fragmin; category 1) and enoxaparin (Lovenox).
- If above regimens are not appropriate or available: Dabigatran
- Fondaparinux
- UFH (category 2B)
- Warfarin
- Monitoring INR in patients who are on VKA therapy (e.g., warfarin)
  - For patients with DVT and/or PE, who have completed primary treatment and will continue VKA therapy as secondary prevention, it is recommended that the INR range is 2.0 to 3.0.
  - For patients with breakthrough DVT and/or PE during therapeutic VKA treatment, it is suggested to use LMWH over DOAC therapy.
- Duration of anticoagulation
  - Recommended duration of therapy is minimum time of 3 months, or as long as active cancer or cancer therapy.
  - Recommendation is for a shorter course (3 to 6 months), versus a longer course (6 to 12 months), for primary treatment of DVT or PE, whether provoked by a transient risk factor, chronic risk factor, or unprovoked.
  - For PE, recommend indefinite anticoagulation while cancer is active, under treatment, if risk factors for recurrence persist, or if patient has recurrent, unprovoked VTE.

Nonpharmacologic Management

- Maintain patient on bed rest for the first 5 to 7 days, with leg elevation for acute DVT and PE.
- Perform frequent leg exercises (i.e., ROM or isometric), if bedridden
  - Every 1 to 2 hours while awake to improve venous flow
  - Includes heel pumping and ankle circles for 10 to 12 repetitions
- Use mild analgesics and warm compresses for comfort of persons with acute DVT and acute PE.
- Administer supplemental oxygen by nasal cannula to maintain a PaO_2 higher than 80 mm Hg in persons with acute DVT and acute PE.
- Encourage frequent ambulation, if tolerated, after 5 to 7 days of bed rest.
- Apply compression (anti-embolic) stockings or hose before surgery.
- Use pneumatic compression stockings or devices postoperatively to stimulate circulation and prevent DVT and PE.
- Remove compression stockings or devices for 15 to 20 minutes, every 8 hours, or per facility policy.

- Assess skin color and peripheral perfusion in extremities with the compression stockings or devices daily.
- Elevate foot of bed by 15 to 20 inches with slight knee flexion. Do not exceed 45 degrees with leg elevation.
- Avoid popliteal pressure, which is produced by crossing the legs. Place pillows behind knees and elevate legs.
- Do not massage the legs of persons with DVT or PE.
- Encourage regular position changes to prevent hypoventilation.
- Avoid smoking and caffeine to prevent vasoconstriction.
- Maintain adequate hydration.
- Do not perform the Homans test after DVT is diagnosed or the test result is positive, since this could lead to development of PE.

Patient Teaching

- Goals
  - Define DVT and PE
  - Identify signs/symptoms of DVT and PE to report to health care provider.
  - Understand lab and diagnostic testing, nursing care and treatments related to managing PE.
  - Stimulate patient's circulation.
  - Prevent recurrent DVTs and PEs.
  - Maintain patient safety by identifying signs/symptoms of bleeding and avoiding injury and bleeding while on anticoagulant therapy.
  - Prevent respiratory complications.
  - Understand how to administer the anticoagulant and identify med side effects.
- Teach patient to identify and report signs/symptoms of VTE.
  - Define DVT and PE
  - Identify and report signs/symptom of DVT and PE
    - DVT: Leg pain or swelling; other signs of subsequent or/recurrent DVT; signs of thrombophlebitis
    - PE: Shortness of breath; chest pain that worsens with deep breathing; fast heart rate; fast breathing rate; uneasiness; feeling faint
- Teach patient purpose of laboratory and diagnostic tests, nursing care, and treatments for VTE.
- Teach patient ways to stimulate the circulation to prevent DVT.
  - Change position regularly
  - Move the toes, feet, and legs often (e.g., wiggle the toes, flex/rotate the foot and ankles, tighten the calves)
  - Avoid sitting or standing for long periods
  - Make frequent stops on long trips in order to move around
  - Avoid constrictive clothing or devices
  - Perform ROM or isometric exercises
  - Wear the pneumatic compression stockings or devices as ordered
- Teach patient other strategies to prevent recurrent DVT/PE.
  - Ambulate soon after surgery
  - Drink 8 to 10 glasses of fluid per day

- Quit smoking
- Avoid caffeine intake
- Take actions to lose weight, if obese
- Increase vitamin E in diet, which is important for health of heart and blood vessels
- Keep legs elevated to promote venous return
- Keep legs straight and do not cross one leg over another leg
- Avoid pressure on back of knees (i.e., popliteal area) to prevent clot from forming
- Teach patient to maintain safety while on anticoagulation therapy by identifying any bleeding signs/symptoms and following precautions to avoid injury and bleeding.
  - Identify and report any excessive bleeding, abnormal wounds, unusual pain or swelling; cyanosis or toe/foot pain
  - Avoid any contact sports that could lead to serious injury
  - Use soft toothbrush for oral care
  - Avoid substances that can irritate the tissues of the mouth and gums, such as hot or spicy foods, alcoholic beverages, and mouthwashes that contain alcohol
  - Use an electric razor, if there is a need to shave
  - Avoid blowing nose vigorously and clean nares with cotton swab or tissue
  - Use saline nose drops and sprays and small amount of moisturizing ointment (e.g., petroleum jelly) inside nostrils to prevent nosebleeds
  - Check home for environmental hazards and identify and remove bump and fall risks (e.g., throw rugs, clutter from rooms and pathways).
  - Wear rubber gloves or garden gloves to protect hands when doing household or yard work.
  - Do not walk barefoot and wear shoes or slippers to protect the feet
- Teach patient ways to prevent complications, including respiratory compromise.
  - Ambulate frequently
  - Use incentive spirometry
- Teach patient how to administer medications and to understand the side effects.
  - Teach patients to take their anticoagulant medication (e.g., warfarin) at the same time every day, and to not double up on the dose if they forget to take a dose
  - Teach patients, who are taking subcutaneously administered medications (e.g., LMWH), how to do so at home
  - Teach patient about side effects of their anticoagulant medication
  - Teach patients how the blood counts (e.g., CBC with platelet count, PT/INR, etc.) will be monitored, as part of the requirement for monitoring the medications
- Teach patient, who is taking warfarin, to maintain a diet consistent in the amount of vitamin K.
  - Foods that are high in vitamin K: green leafy vegetables (e.g., spinach, kale) and liver.
  - Foods that contain small amounts of vitamin K: milk, meats, eggs, cereal, fruits, and vegetables.

- Recommended daily allowances of vitamin K are 80 μg/day for men and 65 μg/day for women.
- Patients should not take supplemental vitamin K because it increases blood clotting.

Follow-Up

- Continue to closely monitor cancer patients, who have been diagnosed with venous thrombosis, since they may have a more aggressive tumor biology and poor prognosis
- Monitor for signs and symptoms of subsequent or recurrent DVT or PE.
- Monitor laboratory findings to determine the continuation or resolution of DVT or PE.
- Reconcile medications at hospital discharge and follow-up visits
- Screen for economic and social support (including housing, nutritional, financial, and spiritual support).
  - Make referrals, where available, to meet these needs
  - Provide additional resources, such as home equipment or assistance, to address the severe complications of DVT (e.g., PE)
- Refer patient for nutritional counseling about vitamin K in their diet, if needed.

Bibliography

Ahmed, M. H., Ghanem, H. M., & Khalil, S. S. (2020). Assessment of nurses' knowledge and practice about venous thrombo embolism for cancer surgery patients. *Assiut Scientific Nursing Journal, 8*(20), 13–20.

Asakura, H., & Ogawa, H. (2021). COVID-19-associated coagulopathy and disseminated intravascular coagulation. *International Journal of Hematology, 113*(1), 45–57.

Balabhadra, S., Kuban, J. D., Lee, S., Yevich, S., Metwalli, Z., McCarthy, C. J., … Sheth, R. A. (2020). Association of inferior vena cava filter placement with rates of pulmonary embolism in patients with cancer and acute lower extremity deep venous thrombosis. *JAMA Network Open, 3*(7), e2011079.

Barp, M., Carneiro, V. S., Amaral, K. V., Pagotto, V., & Malaquias, S. G. (2018). Nursing care in the prevention of venous thromboembolism: An integrative review. *Revista Eletrônica Enfermagem, 20*, v20a14.

Budnik, I., & Brill, A. (2018). Immune factors in deep vein thrombosis initiation. *Trends in Immunology, 39*(8), 610–623.

Cha, S. I., Shin, K. M., Lim, J. K., Yoo, S. S., Lee, S. Y., Lee, J., … Jung, C. Y. (2018). Pulmonary embolism concurrent with lung cancer and central emboli predict mortality in patients with lung cancer and pulmonary embolism. *Journal of Thoracic Disease, 10*(1), 262–272.

Davies, M. (2014). Pulmonary embolism. In D. Camp-Sorrell, & R. A. Hawkins (Eds.), *Clinical manual for the oncology advanced practice nurse* (3rd ed., pp. 273–280). Oncology Nursing Society.

El-Said, A., & El-sol, H. (2018). Nursing discharge plan: Prevent further pulmonary embolism. *Mansoura Nursing Journal, 5*(1), 183–189.

Giustozzi, M., Agnelli, G., Del Toro-Cervera, J., Klok, F. A., Rosovsky, R. P., Martin, A. C., … Huisman, M. V. (2020). Direct oral anticoagulants for the treatment of acute venous thromboembolism associated with cancer: A systematic review and meta-analysis. *Thrombosis and Haemostasis, 120*(7), 1128–1136.

Kraaijpoel, N., Bleker, S. M., Meyer, G., Mahé, I., Muñoz, A., Bertoletti, L., … UPE Investigators. (2019). Treatment and long-term clinical outcomes of incidental pulmonary embolism in patients with cancer: An international prospective cohort study. *Journal of Clinical Oncology, 37*(20), 1713–1720.

Levi, M., & Iba, T. (2021). COVID-19 coagulopathy: Is it disseminated intravascular coagulation? *Internal and Emergency Medicine, 16*(2), 309–312.

Levy, J. H., Iba, T., & Gardiner, E. E. (2021). Endothelial injury in COVID-19 and acute infections: Putting the pieces of the puzzle together. *Arteriosclerosis, Thrombosis, and Vascular Biology, 41*(5), 1774–1776.

Li, Y., Shang, Y., Wang, W., Ning, S., & Chen, H. (2018). Lung cancer and pulmonary embolism: What is the relationship? A review. *Journal of Cancer, 9*(17), 3046–3057.

Lin, H. F., Liao, K. F., Chang, C. M., Lin, C. L., Lai, S. W., & Hsu, C. Y. (2018). Correlation of the tamoxifen use with the increased risk of deep vein thrombosis and pulmonary embolism in elderly women with breast cancer: A case-control study. *Medicine, 97*(51), e12842.

Najm, M. A., Jassim, A. H., & Mohammed, T. R. (2020). Critical care nurses' knowledge about pulmonary embolism in respiratory care unit in Baghdad teaching hospitals. *Indian Journal of Forensic Medicine & Toxicology, 14*(3), 895.

National Comprehensive Cancer Network. (2021). *NCCN clinical practice guidelines in oncology (NCCN guidelines): Cancer-associated venous thromboembolic disease. Version 3.2021—November 15, 2021.* Available at www.nccn.org (accessed February 17, 2021).

National Comprehensive Cancer Network. (2022). *NCCN clinical practice guidelines in oncology (NCCN guidelines): Multiple myeloma. Version 4.2022—December 14, 2021.* Available at www.nccn.org (accessed February 19, 2021).

Nguyen, E., Caranfa, J. T., Lyman, G. H., Kuderer, N. M., Stirbis, C., Wysocki, M., … Kohn, C. G. (2018). Clinical prediction rules for mortality in patients with pulmonary embolism and cancer to guide outpatient management: A meta-analysis. *Journal of Thrombosis and Haemostasis, 16*(2), 279–292.

Ortel, T. L., Neumann, I., Ageno, W., Beyth, R., Clark, N. P., Cuker, A., … Zhang, Y. (2020). American Society of Hematology 2020 guidelines for management of venous thromboembolism: Treatment of deep vein thrombosis and pulmonary embolism. *Blood Advances, 4*(19), 4693–4738.

Qdaisat, A., Kamal, M., Al-Breiki, A., Goswami, B., Wu, C. C., Zhou, S., … Yeung, S. J. (2020). Clinical characteristics, management, and outcome of incidental pulmonary embolism in cancer patients. *Blood Advances, 4*(8), 1606–1614.

Qiu, M., Meng, Y., Wang, H., Sun, L., Liu, Z., Kan, S., … Zhang, S. (2021). Concurrence of gastric cancer and incidental pulmonary embolism may be a prognostic factor for advanced gastric cancer patients with incidental pulmonary embolism. *Cancer Management and Research, 13*, 7637–7644.

Rodriguez, A. L. (2014). Bleeding and thrombotic complications. In C. Yarbro, D. Wujcik, & B. H. Gobel (Eds.), *Cancer symptom management* (4th ed.). Jones & Bartlett.

Soumagne, T., Lascarrou, J. B., Hraiech, S., Horlait, G., Higny, J., d'Hondt, A., … Piton, G. (2020). Factors associated with pulmonary embolism among coronavirus disease 2019 acute respiratory distress syndrome: A multicenter study among 375 patients. *Critical Care Explorations, 2*(7), e0166.

Suh, Y. J., Hong, H., Ohana, M., Bompard, F., Revel, M. P., Valle, C., … Yoon, S. H. (2021). Pulmonary embolism and deep vein thrombosis in COVID-19: A systematic review and meta-analysis. *Radiology, 298*(2), E70–E80.

Thachil, J., Khorana, A., & Carrier, M. (2021). Similarities and perspectives on the two C's—Cancer and COVID-19. *Journal of Thrombosis and Haemostasis, 19*(5), 1161–1167.

Zambakari, C., & Zambakari, N. (2021). *Pulmonary embolism: Everything you should know.* Desert Haven Home Care. Available at https://papers.ssrn.com (accessed February 20, 2022).

Sepsis and Septic Shock

Definition

- *Early sepsis:* Persons with infection and bacteremia are at risk for developing sepsis. Although no formal definition for early sepsis exists, early identification of those persons who are at risk is critical to prevent sepsis and to decrease mortality related to sepsis and septic shock
- *Sepsis:* A life-threatening organ dysfunction caused by a dysregulated host response to infection
  - This overwhelming systemic infection can lead to septic shock and multiple organ dysfunction syndrome (MODS)
- *Septic shock:* subset of sepsis causing particularly profound circulatory, cellular, and metabolic abnormalities
  - It is an infection-related circulatory dysfunction

- Hypotension results, which requires vasopressors to maintain mean arterial pressure (MAP) of 65 mm Hg or greater, and with a serum lactate level greater than 2 mmol/L (or 18 mg/dL), in the absence of hypovolemia

Epidemiology

- Sepsis and septic shock are major healthcare problems. Annually, sepsis and septic shock impacts millions of people around the world each year and causes death in one in three and one in six of those it affects
- Bloodstream infections (BSI) are associated with significant morbidity, mortality, and cost
  - An estimated 575,000 to 677,000 episodes and 79,000 to 94,000 deaths per year are attributable to nosocomial BSI in North America
  - These infections are the sixth-leading cause of death in Canada, and seventh-leading cause of death in the United States
  - Mortality rate for septic shock is 40% greater than mortality rate for sepsis
- Centers for Disease Control and Prevention (2022) reports the following annual statistics related to sepsis:
  - At least 1.7 million adults in America develop sepsis
  - Nearly 270,000 Americans die as a result of sepsis
  - One in three patients who dies in a hospital has sepsis
  - Sepsis, or the infection causing sepsis, starts outside of the hospital in nearly 87% of cases
- Despite new advances in critical care support techniques, 30% to 45% of patients die following hospitalization with severe sepsis and septic shock
- Among cancer patients, the incidence of sepsis is:
  - Approximately 25%, and the associated mortality rate is 28%
  - Approximately 10% to 20% among patients who have had a febrile neutropenic event
  - Greater among patients with hematologic malignancies than in those with solid tumors
- Risk factors for sepsis or septic shock
  - Compromised immune system, which may be due to:
    - Neutropenia (severe risk when absolute neutrophil count [ANC] <500 cells/mm^3; moderate risk when ANC is 500 to 1000 cells/mm^3), especially febrile neutropenia
    - Hematologic malignancies
    - High-dose chemotherapy, especially for patients undergoing BMT/HSCT
    - Radiation therapy, especially total body irradiation
    - Protein-calorie malnutrition
    - Significant antibiotic use
  - Invasive medical devices: central venous catheters, urinary catheter, drain
  - Adults with advanced age, who are 65 years old or older; or children younger than 1 year old
  - Bacteremia, community acquired pneumonia
  - ICU admission, previous hospitalization, sepsis survivors
  - Chronic medical conditions, such as diabetes, cancer, lung disease, and kidney disease

- Genetic factors
- Infections most often associated with sepsis: lung (pneumonia), urinary tract infections (UTI), skin infections (often due to breakdown of skin and mucous membranes), endovascular infections, and intra-abdominal infections

Pathophysiology

- Phases of Septic Shock Cascade
  - Infection or bacteremia
    - Bacteria, viruses, or fungi circulate in the bloodstream, and release their toxins
    - Host tissue has inflammatory response to invasion by microorganisms and releases cell components (e.g., neutrophils, macrophages, monocytes, plasma cells) into bloodstream
    - Mature neutrophils are first line of defense against bacterial infection. Production of neutrophils and other WBCs can be impaired by chemotherapy and radiation
  - Early sepsis
    - Clinical evidence of systemic inflammatory response to invasion by microorganisms
    - Systemic inflammatory response syndrome (SIRS) criteria include two or more of the following: (1) temperature greater than 38° C (100.4° F) or less than 36° C (96.8° F), (2) heart rate greater than 90 beats/min, (3) respiratory rate greater than 20 breaths/min or PaCO$_2$ less than 32 mm Hg, (4) WBC count greater than 12,000 cells/mm^3, WBC count less than 4000 cells/mm^3, or more than 10% immature (band) cells in peripheral blood.
  - *Sepsis* is a documented infection with presence of two or more of SIRS criteria.
    - Blood lactate levels are measured, since elevated blood lactate levels are associated with increased mortality in patients with sepsis
    - Coagulation studies are performed, since sepsis or severe infections can activate the coagulation system and lead to a hypercoagulable state
    - An estimated 30% to 50% of patients with sepsis are believed to suffer from DIC
    - COVID-19 infections are associated with coagulopathy and DIC
  - *Severe sepsis* is dysfunction of one or more organ systems.
  - *Septic shock* is acute circulatory failure characterized by hypotension that does not respond to fluid hydration.
    - MAP is measured, since this is a key determinant of mean systemic filling pressure, which in turn is the major driver of venous return and cardiac output
  - MODS
    - Dysfunction or failure of two or more organs
    - Immediate treatment required to maintain homeostasis
    - MODS can lead to death

- Pathogens that can cause sepsis
  - Bacterial infections are the most common source of sepsis (45% to 50% of septic shock cases).
    - Gram-positive organisms are most common cause of BSIs in the United States. Incidence in prevalence related to increased use of vascular access devices. Most common include *Staphylococcus aureus*; *Enterococcus* spp.; and *S. pneumoniae*.
    - Gram-negative organisms remain a substantial contributor to incidence of BSI. Most common include *E. coli; Klebsiella pneumoniae,* and *Pseudomonas aeruginosa.*
  - Viruses
    - Viruses may cause significant infectious complications in patients who are immunocompromised
    - Potent cytokine release mechanisms in response to COVID-19 infections appear to be leading to acute lung injury, ARDS, marked coagulopathy, and multiple organ failure, which frequently require intensive-care support
  - Fungal infections can result in severe morbidity and mortality for oncology patients.
    - Most common organism causing fungal infection: Candida
  - Anaerobes and protozoa: can also cause septic shock.

Signs and Symptoms

- Signs and symptoms of infection may be subtle or absent, especially in neutropenic patients.
- Single screening tools for sepsis or septic shock: recommendations per international guidelines for "Surviving Sepsis Campaign":
  - Guidelines recommend: SIRS, NEWS (National Early Warning Score), or MEWS (Modified Early Warning Score)
  - Guidelines do not recommend qSOFA (quick Sequential Organ Failure Score) or SOFA
- One screening tool is SIRS. SIRS criteria identify persons at risk for sepsis or septic shock, who manifest with two or more of the following:
  - Fever, elevated temperature (≥38° C or 100.4° F) or low temperature (<36° C, or 96.8° F)
  - Elevated heart rate (>90/min)
  - Elevated respiratory rate (>20/min or $PaCO_2$ <32)
  - Abnormal WBC count (WBC >12,000/mL, WBC <4000/mL, or WBC >10% immature forms or blasts)
- Sepsis signs and symptoms
  - Vital sign changes:
    - Temperature: usually elevated (≥38° C or 100.4° F)
    - Heart rate less than 90 bpm
    - Respiratory rate greater than 20 respirations/min or respiratory distress
    - Hypotension: systolic BP ≤90 mm Hg, or a reduction of 40 mm Hg from baseline
    - MAP less than 70
  - WBC count elevated
  - Documented infection (positive cultures; imaging results)
  - General symptoms:

- Fever, shivering, feeling very cold
- Extreme pain or discomfort
- Skin:
  - Breaks in skin integrity, redness, tenderness, lesions
  - Clammy or sweaty skin
  - Warm and flushed in early sepsis; skin feels cool as sepsis progresses, allowing blood to be diverted to vital organs
- Catheter sites or wounds: erythema, inflammation, tenderness, purulent drainage
  - Purulent drainage may not be seen in neutropenic patients, who are unable to exhibit signs of infection
- Oral mucosa: erythema, ulceration, tenderness
- Respiratory symptoms: Shortness of breath, dyspnea, cough
- Cardiovascular: edema
- GI: abdominal pain, distention, firmness, guarding
- GU: lesions or abscess, decreased urine output
- Neurologic: Confusion, disorientation
- Signs and symptoms of septic shock:
  - Patient requires vasopressors to maintain an initial target MAP of 65 mm Hg or greater, and
  - Lactic acidosis (serum lactate level >2 mmol/L, or >18 mg/dL), in absence of hypovolemia (e.g., despite adequate fluid status)
- Organ dysfunction in sepsis/septic shock may manifest as:
  - Cardiovascular: hypotension, tachycardia, arrythmias, decreased capillary refill time
  - Respiratory: tachypnea, shortness of breath, decreased breath sounds, crackles or wheezes, hypoxia, pulmonary edema, ARDS
  - Skin: may progress to cold, pale, clammy skin; decreased perfusion, resulting in acrocyanosis; mottling
  - Renal: oliguria, anuria, or azotemia
    - Urine output less than 0.5 mL/kg/hr for at least 2 hours without hypovolemia
  - Central nervous system: mental status changes, confusion, agitation, obtundation, coma
  - GI: nausea, vomiting, decreased GI motility, ileus, stress ulcers, GI blood loss
  - Hepatic: elevated liver enzymes, jaundice
  - Hematologic: neutropenia or neutrophilia, thrombocytopenia, DIC

Cancers Associated With Disorder

- Leukemia, especially acute leukemia and chronic lymphocytic leukemia
- Lymphoma (e.g., Hodgkin disease, non-Hodgkin lymphoma)
- Multiple myeloma
- Disease with bone marrow metastasis
- Solid tumors

Diagnostic Tests

- Assessments to diagnose sepsis/septic shock and monitor clinical response:
  - Temperature, heart rate, respiratory rate, blood pressure
  - Pulse oximetry

- Skin color
- Mental status
- Intake and output
- MAP: invasive monitoring
- Laboratory tests
  - CBC and differential
    - Assess for neutropenia, leukocytosis, thrombocytopenia, anemia
  - CMP: Assesses electrolytes (increased glucose) and uric acid
    - Electrolytes: increased glucose
    - Creatinine: greater than 0.5 mg/dL
  - Liver function test: Results are elevated
  - Renal function test: Results show increased BUN and creatinine levels
  - Coagulation studies: Results show prolonged PT or aPTT, decreased fibrinogen level, increased D-dimer, and increased FDP level
  - Arterial blood gas (ABG) determinations show an increased lactic acid level.
- Cultures: Obtain the following cultures at the first suspicion of sepsis:
  - Immediate blood cultures from two peripheral sites or from a peripheral site and a central venous access site, if central venous access is in place
  - Urine culture & sensitivity and cultures of sputum, drainage, stool, wound, and central line site, as appropriate
- Imaging studies
  - Posteroanterior and lateral chest radiographs to rule out infection (e.g., pneumonia)
  - Chest tomography (CT if chest radiographic results are suspicious)
  - Venogram or spiral chest CT to diagnose PE as source of fever
  - ECG or echocardiograms when cardiac source of infection is suspected
  - Doppler ultrasound for diagnosing venous thrombosis as a source of fever
  - Lumbar puncture when neurologic infection is suspected
- Ongoing evaluation
  - Vital signs: temperature, heart rate, respiratory rate, blood pressure
  - Strict intake and output measurements
  - Daily weights
  - Pulse oximetry and ABG determinations
  - Antibiotic levels, as indicated
  - CBC, chemistry panel, electrolytes, liver and renal function tests, and serum lactate level
  - Serologies and cultures for viral diseases

Differential Diagnosis

- Specific infection (e.g., pneumonia, UTI, etc.) and specific pathogen (e.g., bacterial, fungal, viral)
- Tumor-associated fever, especially in lymphoma, acute leukemia, chronic leukemia, multiple myeloma, solid tumors, and metastases to liver or central nervous system

- Febrile response related to drug administration (e.g., amphotericin B, ganciclovir, interferons, interleukins) may occur at start of therapy or 1 to 2 weeks later.
- Allergic reaction to drugs or blood products
- Nosocomial fever
- DIC

Treatment

- Sepsis and septic shock are medical emergencies.
  - Early identification and appropriate, immediate treatment and resuscitation in initial hours after development of sepsis improves patient outcomes
- In a study of sepsis admissions to 509 hospitals in the U.S. (n = 1,012,410), mortality was lower in hospitals with higher compliance with achieving the sepsis bundles successfully.
  - Sepsis bundles include standard approaches, such as:
    - Early identification of sepsis
    - Monitoring serum lactate levels
    - Obtaining cultures to identify the causative agent
    - Starting antibiotics in a timely manner to treat the infection
    - Administering fluids and medications to support the patient's hemodynamic status
- In a study related to preventability of sepsis-associated mortality (n = 568), researchers found that suboptimal care, most commonly delays in antibiotics, was identified in 68 of 300 sepsis-associated deaths
- International guidelines recommend that patients, who have sepsis or septic shock and require ICU admission, are admitted to the ICU within 6 hours.
- For adults with suspected sepsis or septic shock, but unconfirmed infection:
  - Continuously re-evaluate and search for alternative diagnoses
  - Discontinue empiric antimicrobials if an alternative cause of illness is demonstrated or strongly suspected
- For adults with possible sepsis without shock:
  - Rapidly assess likelihood of infectious versus non-infectious causes of acute illness.
  - Promptly remove intravascular access devices that are a possible source of sepsis or septic shock, after other vascular access has been established.
  - Manage clinical manifestations of infection or sepsis.

Pharmacologic Management

- Prevention
  - Prophylactic antibiotics may be administered to neutropenic patients.
  - WBC growth factors (e.g., granulocyte colony-stimulating factor, granulocyte-macrophage colony-stimulating factor) may be administered to decrease length of neutropenia and decrease incidence of infection after chemotherapy administration.
  - Antifungal agents, including nystatin, clotrimazole, fluconazole, and amphotericin B, may be administered prophylactically.

- VTE prophylaxis
  - Pharmacologic VTE prophylaxis: Use LMWH
  - May consider combining LMWH treatment with mechanical VTE prophylaxis (e.g., IVC filter placement surgically)
- Management
  - Establish vascular access and initiate aggressive fluid resuscitation.
  - Obtain blood cultures at first suspicion of sepsis.
  - Administer empiric, broad-spectrum antibiotics, which cover common gram-negative and gram-positive organisms, immediately after obtaining blood cultures for adults with possible septic shock or a high likelihood of sepsis.
    - Administer empiric antibiotics ideally within 1 hour of recognition of signs/symptoms of sepsis.
    - For adults with sepsis or septic shock, who are at high risk of methicillin-resistant *Staphylococcus aureus* (MRSA), use empiric antimicrobials with MRSA coverage.
  - Empiric antifungal therapy
    - Initiated when patient remains febrile for 5 to 7 days after empiric antibiotic therapy is started.
    - Amphotericin B is drug of choice.
  - Antiviral agents (e.g., acyclovir, ganciclovir) and various formulations of immunoglobulin are used to prevent and treat viral infections.
  - Antipyretic therapy (primarily acetaminophen) is administered to:
    - Decrease patient's temperature, and
    - Minimize discomforts of fever (e.g., chills, seizures, delirium)
  - Fluid resuscitation for adults with sepsis or septic shock
    - May be administered to manage sepsis-induced hypoperfusion or septic shock (including hypotension or oliguria)
    - Recommendation: Give at least 30 mL/kg of IV crystalloid fluid (e.g., normal saline solution, lactated Ringer solution) within the first 3 hours of resuscitation.
    - Crystalloids are first-line fluids for resuscitation. Lactated Ringer solution is recommended over normal saline.
    - Colloid solutions (e.g., albumin, dextran, plasma protein fraction) are also used. Albumin may be used in patients who have received large volumes of crystalloids
    - Not recommended: using starches or gelatin for resuscitation
  - Vasopressors for adults with sepsis or septic shock
    - Norepinephrine is recommended as first-line agent over other vasopressors.
    - Use other vasopressor options, including dopamine (high-quality evidence to support use) and vasopressin (moderate-quality evidence to support use).
    - Add vasopressin, instead of increasing norepinephrine dose, for patients on norepinephrine with inadequate MAP levels.
    - Add epinephrine if patient's MAP levels do not increase while on norepinephrine and vasopressin
    - Start vasopressors peripherally to restore MAP; do not delay initiation of vasopressors if a central venous access is not secured.
- Insulin therapy for adults with sepsis or septic shock
  - Initiate insulin therapy at a glucose level of ≥180 mg/dL
- Sodium bicarbonate therapy
  - Indicated for persons with severe metabolic acidemia (pH ≤7.2) and acute kidney injury (acute kidney injury classification score [AKIN] score 2 or 3)
  - Sodium bicarbonate therapy is not recommended to improve hemodynamics or reduce vasopressor requirements
- High-dose vitamin C therapy
  - Subnormal plasma vitamin C concentrations are common in critically ill patients, including those with sepsis.
  - Lower plasma vitamin C levels (especially levels averaging around 18 μM) correlate with higher incidence of organ failure and worse outcomes in septic patients.
  - Multiple studies have demonstrated decreased mortality in patients who have received moderate doses of vitamin C (25 mg/kg every 6 hours × 3 days) or high doses of vitamin C (1500 mg every 6 hours × 4 days or until ICU discharge).

Nonpharmacologic Management

- Wear personal protective equipment (PPE) when caring for persons with COVID-19 infection
  - Use standard PPE, including gloves, gown, and eye protection (such as face shield or safety goggles)
  - Use fitted respirator masks (N95 respirators, FFP2, or equivalent), as opposed to surgical/medical masks, when performing aerosol-generating procedures on patients with COVID-19, in addition to standard PPE
    - Aerosol-generating procedures include open suctioning, tracheostomy insertion/care; administering nebulized treatment; endotracheal intubation, manual ventilation, CPR
- Manage sepsis urgently, by obtaining cultures immediately and starting antibiotics within 1 hour of presentation of signs/symptoms.
- Monitor patient with suspected or confirmed infection/sepsis/septic shock:
  - Vital signs every 4 hours, or as clinically indicated
  - Changes in laboratory values
    - Report significant changes, including increased WBC count and organism growth in cultures
  - Signs and symptoms of infection
    - Obtain order for culture of suspicious sites of infection
  - Signs and symptoms of fluid overload
    - Including rales, edema, and weight gain
  - Intake and output every 4 to 8 hours, or as clinically indicated
    - Goal is for urine output to be 0.5 mL/kg/hr

- Pulse oximetry results and patient's response to oxygen therapy
- Use physical methods to control elevated body temperature (fever):
  - Includes: tepid baths, sponging, cool washcloths, ice packs, cooling blankets, air conditioning, fans, and blankets during periods of chilling
- Implement strategies to prevent infection:
  - Good hand hygiene
  - Neutropenic precautions, per institutional procedure
- Implement strategies to provide supportive care
  - Administer oxygen as ordered
    - Begin oxygen therapy to maintain SpO_2 at 94% (e.g., nasal canula, non-rebreather mask, or mechanical ventilation, if needed)
    - Start supplemental oxygen if SpO_2 is less than 90% in adult patients with COVID-19
  - Provide patient with high-calorie, high-protein diet to ensure proper nutrition
  - Encourage hydration (e.g., drinking 8 to 10 glasses of fluid/day)

Patient Teaching

- Discuss goals of care and prognosis with patients and families:
  - Prevent septic shock with prompt recognition of signs/symptoms of infection and sepsis and with prompt management of infection
  - Assist patient to progress toward hemodynamical stability when sepsis is managed according to current evidence
  - Prognosis: This is a life-threatening, medical emergency
    - Despite new advances in critical care support techniques, 30% to 45% of patients die following hospitalization with severe sepsis and septic shock
- Define sepsis and septic shock
- Describe signs/symptoms of sepsis and septic shock.
- Explain purpose of laboratory tests (especially WBC/ANC), diagnostic tests, nursing care, and treatments for sepsis/septic shock.
- Teach patient self-care activities to prevent or minimize risk of infection:
  - Wash hands frequently
  - Keep body clean by bathing daily
  - Wash hands after using bathroom
  - Brush teeth at least twice daily and floss once daily
  - Drink 8 to 10 glasses of fluid per day
  - Turn, cough, and deep-breathe to maintain optimal respiratory functioning
  - Avoid large crowds, people who are sick, and infants, children, and adults who have been vaccinated within past 3 weeks
  - Do not clean up cat litter or clean up excreta from animals
- Verify that patient and family understand how to take patient's temperature and provide additional teaching as needed.
- Teach patient:
  - Rationale and schedule for oral prophylactic antibiotics or WBC growth factors, if indicated
  - Rationale and schedule for having blood drawn for a CBC
  - Importance of reporting temperature ≥100.4° F and symptoms of infection, such as redness, swelling, warmth, pain, or drainage

Follow-Up

- Reconcile medications at ICU discharge, hospital discharge, and follow-up visits
- Include information about the hospital/ICU stay, sepsis and related diagnoses, treatments, and common impairments after sepsis in written and verbal hospital discharge summary
- Screen for economic and social support (including housing, nutritional, financial, and spiritual support)
  - Make referrals, where available, to meet these needs
  - Provide additional resources, such as home equipment or assistance, as needed
- Follow-up with clinicians to continue to:
  - Assess and follow-up for physical, cognitive, and emotional problems after hospital discharge
  - Support and manage new and long-term sequela related to sepsis/septic shock
  - Monitor laboratory findings, especially CBC with diff, to determine continuation or resolution of sepsis

Bibliography

Alhazzani, W., Møller, M. H., Arabi, Y. M., Loeb, M., Gong, M. N., Fan, E., … Rhodes, A. (2020). Surviving sepsis campaign: Guidelines on the management of critically ill adults with Coronavirus Disease 2019 (COVID-19). *Intensive Care Medicine, 46*(5), 854–887.

Angus, D. C., & van der Poll, T. (2013). Severe sepsis and septic shock. *New England Journal of Medicine, 369,* 840–851.

Asakura, H., & Ogawa, H. (2021). COVID-19-associated coagulopathy and disseminated intravascular coagulation. *International Journal of Hematology, 113*(1), 45–57.

Centers for Disease Control and Prevention. (2022). *Get ahead of sepsis—Know the risks. Spot the signs. Act fast.* Available at: https://www.cdc.gov/patient-safety/features/get-ahead-of-sepsis.html (accessed March 17, 2022).

Delaney, E., Nikolai, C., & Coe, K. (2020). Metabolic emergencies. In J. M. Brandt (Ed.), *ONS core curriculum for oncology nursing* (6th ed.). St. Louis, MO: Elsevier.

Ding, R., Wang, Z., Lin, Y., Liu, B., Zhang, Z., & Ma, X. (2018). Comparison of a new criteria for sepsis-induced coagulopathy and International Society on Thrombosis and Haemostasis disseminated intravascular coagulation score in critically ill patients with sepsis 3.0: A retrospective study. *Blood Coagulation and Fibrinolysis, 29*(6), 551–558.

Evans, L., Rhodes, A., Alhazzani, W., Antonelli, M., Coopersmith, C. M., French, C., … Levy, M. (2021). Surviving sepsis campaign: International guidelines for management of sepsis and septic shock 2021. *Intensive Care Medicine, 47*(11), 1181–1247.

Goulden, R., Hoyle, M. C., Monis, J., Railton, D., Riley, V., Martin, P., … Nsutebu, E. (2018). qSOFA, SIRS and NEWS for predicting inhospital mortality and ICU admission in emergency admissions treated as sepsis. *Emergency Medicine Journal, 35*(6), 345–349.

Holford, P., Carr, A. C., Jovic, T. H., Ali, S. R., Whitaker, I. S., Marik, P. E., & Smith, A. D. (2020). Vitamin C—An adjunctive therapy for respiratory infection, sepsis and COVID-19. *Nutrients, 12*(12), 3760.

Kahn, J. M., Davis, B. S., Yabes, J. G., Chang, C. H., Chong, D. H., Hershey, … Angus, D. C. (2019). Association between state-mandated protocolized sepsis care and in-hospital mortality among adults with sepsis. *JAMA, 322*(3), 240–250.

Kashiouris, M. G., L'Heureux, M., Cable, C. A., Fisher, B. J., Leichtle, S. W., & Fowler, A. A. (2020). The emerging role of vitamin C as a treatment for sepsis. *Nutrients, 12*(2), 292.

Levi, M. (2018). Pathogenesis and diagnosis of disseminated intravascular coagulation. *International Journal of Laboratory Hematology, 40*(Suppl 1), 15–20.

Levi, M., & Iba, T. (2021). COVID-19 coagulopathy: Is it disseminated intravascular coagulation? *Internal and Emergency Medicine, 16*(2), 309–312.

Nitipir, C., Neagu, A. M., Iaciu, C., Alexandra, M., Constantinescu, C. P., … Stanciu, A. E. (2019). New biomolecules for the treatment of disseminated intravascular coagulation. *Romanian Biotechnological Letters, 24*(4), 580–585.

Rhodes, A., Evans, L. E., Alhazzani, W., Levy, M. M., Antonelli, M., Ferrer, R., … Dellinger, R. P. (2017). Surviving sepsis campaign: International guidelines for management of sepsis and septic shock: 2016. *Intensive Care Medicine, 43*(3), 304–377.

Savage, R. D., Fowler, R. A., Rishu, A. H., Bagshaw, S. M., Cook, D., Dodek, P., … Daneman, N. (2016). Pathogens and antimicrobial susceptibility profiles in critically ill patients with bloodstream infections: A descriptive study. *Canadian Medical Association Open Access Journal, 4*(4), E569–E577.

Singer, M., Deutschman, C. S., Seymour, C. W., Shankar-Hari, M., Annane, D., Bauer, M., … Angus, D. C. (2016). The third international consensus definitions for sepsis and septic shock (Sepsis-3). *JAMA, 315*(8), 801–810.

Tallon, J., Browning, B., Couenne, F., Bordes, C., Venet, F., Nony, P., … Tayakout-Fayolle, M. (2020). Dynamical modeling of pro- and anti-inflammatory cytokines in the early stage of septic shock. *In Silico Biology, 14*(1–2), 101–121.

Viviano, D. L. (2014). Shock. In D. Camp-Sorrell, & R. A. Hawkins (Eds.), *Clinical manual for the oncology advanced practice nurse* (3rd ed.). Oncology Nursing Society.

Zafer, M. M., El-Mahallawy, H. A., & Ashour, H. M. (2021). Severe COVID-19 and sepsis: Immune pathogenesis and laboratory markers. *Microorganisms, 9*(1), 159.

Zitella, L. (2014). Infection. In C. Yarbro, D. Wujcik, & B. Gobel (Eds.), *Cancer symptom management* (4th ed., p. 131). Jones and Bartlett.

Thrombotic Thrombocytopenic Purpura

Definition

- TTP is a rare and life-threatening TMA. Microthrombi, which are rich in platelets and VWF, form in smaller blood vessels and cause organ ischemia, hemolysis of RBCs, and consumption of platelets.
- TTP is characterized by three criteria:
  - Laboratory criteria (MHA and severe thrombocytopenia), which occur in absence of other causes
  - Severe deficiency of ADAMTS13 (activity <10%), which is the only biologic marker for TTP
  - Clinical criteria (multi-visceral ischemic symptoms, including neurologic, renal, cardiac, and gastrointestinal symptoms, and fever)

Epidemiology

- Annual incidence of TTP in patients with severe ADAMTS13 deficiency (<5% activity) is approximately 1.74 cases per 100,000 adults.
- Age: TTP has been described in patients 1 to 90 years old, and incidence peaks during the third decade.
- TTP is idiopathic in about one-third of cases, and thus occurs abruptly and independent of any other associated condition.
- Without treatment, most persons with TTP rapidly deteriorate and die.
  - Mortality rate is 90% if left untreated
  - Current mortality rate remains between 10% and 20%, despite using plasma exchange.
- Risk factors and causes of TTP
  - Predisposing Risk Factors
    - Female gender: occurs 1.5 to 2 times more often in females
    - Black ethnicity
    - HLA-DRB1*11

- Obesity
- Primary factors causing ADAMTS13 severe deficiency
  - Immune-mediated (i.e., autoantibodies due to autoimmune diseases): SLE, antiphospholipid antibody syndrome, scleroderma, Wegener granulomatosis, Sjögren syndrome
  - Gene mutations: Hereditary TTP is an autosomal-recessive disorder; is very rare
- Secondary factors causing increase in VWF levels
  - Inflammatory diseases/infection: rheumatoid arthritis, polyarthritis, endocarditis, pancreatitis, sepsis
  - Systemic disease: Malignant hypertension, systemic vasculitis
  - Medications: Chemotherapy drugs (e.g., gemcitabine, carmustine, mitomycin C, pentostatin), cyclosporine, iodine, oral contraceptives, statins, quinine, ticlopidine, clopidogrel, trimethoprim-sulfamethoxazole, vancomycin, zoledronic acid
  - COVID-19 infection and vaccine are associated with coagulopathies and autoimmune TTP; low ADAMTS13 plasma levels are associated with increased mortality in seriously ill COVID-19 patients
  - During pregnancy or postpartum period
- Cancer-related causes of TTP/MHA:
  - Malignancies: lymphoma, HSCT, advanced cancer with MHA

Pathophysiology

- Two categories of TTP
  - Hereditary (congenital) TTP: due to inherited deficiency of ADAMTS13
    - Results from deficiency of the ADAMTS13 enzyme caused by inherited frameshift and point mutations in the *ADAMTS13* gene.
    - This rare disease is an autosomal recessive disorder, which is associated with the formation of platelet microthrombi in small blood vessels.
  - Acquired (classic) TTP:
    - Due to deficiency of ADAMTS13 caused by autoantibodies directed against ADAMTS13.
    - Main clinical features of classic TTP are fever, hemolytic anemia, thrombocytopenia, and neurologic and renal abnormalities.
- Cancer-related TTP/TMA
  - Related to differential diagnoses and cancer, some literature refers to malignancy-related TMA, and not TTP, and other references refer to cancer-associated TTP
    - Cause of secondary (cancer-associated) TTP/TMA is less well understood because ADAMTS13 activity is usually not as depressed as in classic TTP, and ADAMTS13 inhibitors cannot be detected.
    - In some cases, cause appears to be endothelial cell damage, although formation of thrombi resulting in vessel occlusion may not be essential in pathogenesis.
    - Manifestations of cancer-associated TTP are less pronounced, hemany patients do not exhibit the full syndrome of TTP at diagnosis.
- Normal function of VWF

- VWF (factor VIII-related antigen) is a large glycoprotein that is:
  - Present in plasma and endothelium
  - Synthesized exclusively by endothelial cells and megakaryocytes
- Functions of VWF:
  - Involved in blood clotting and is essential in promoting homeostasis
  - Binds to other proteins and forms circulating complexes, especially with factor VIII, a coagulant protein that activates factor X in intrinsic coagulation pathway
  - Prevents the rapid degradation of factor VII
  - Plays a crucial role in platelet aggregation
- In normal physiologic conditions, endothelial cell injury activates release of ultra-large von Willebrand factor (ULVWF) multimers from endothelial cells into blood.
  - In healthy persons, ULVWF multimers usually do not circulate because they are rapidly broken down into smaller units by normal proteolysis, specifically through action of plasma enzyme called ADAMTS13
  - ADAMTS13 action occurs after ULVWF multimers are released into blood
  - Smaller VWF multimers are less adhesive to platelets

- Normal function of ADAMTS13
  - It is an enzyme (disintegrin-like and metalloproteinase with a thrombospondin type 1 motif, member 13) that cleaves VWF
  - Plays a fundamental role in regulation of hemostasis and thrombosis
- TTP: Deficiency of ADAMTS13, either absent by congenital defect or inhibited by specific autoantibodies
  - Deficiency of ADAMTS13 leads to accumulation of ULVWF multimers, which are prothrombogenic.
  - ULVWF multimers are released into blood and are hyper-adhesive to platelets, causing spontaneous platelet aggregates.
  - Microthrombi form where there is high shear stress (e.g., arterioles, capillaries) and are comprised of large amounts of ULVWF, platelet aggregates, and little or no fibrin.
  - The VWF-platelet aggregates induce:
    - Thrombosis in microvasculature: tissue ischemia in various organs results (e.g., brain, heart, kidneys)
    - Spontaneous platelet aggregation: platelets are consumed, and thrombocytopenia results
    - MHA: RBCs encounter thrombotic obstruction and fibrin strands in microvasculature, and they are sheared. Result is anemia and schistocytes present on peripheral blood smear (see figure below).

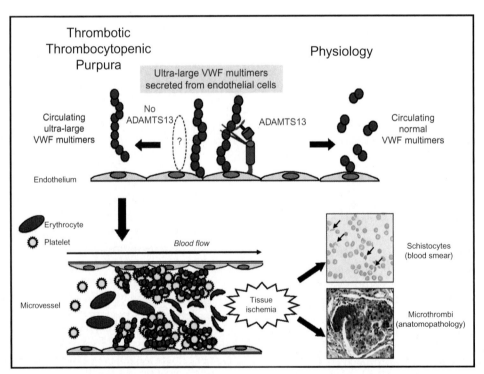

Pathophysiology for Thrombotic Thrombocytopenic Purpura (TTP). In physiologic conditions, ULVWF multimers released from endothelial cells are cleaved by ADAMTS13 in smaller VWF multimers, less adhesive to platelets. In thrombotic thrombocytopenic purpura, because of the absence of functional ADAMTS13 (either absent by congenital defect or inhibited by specific autoantibodies), ULVWF multimers are released into the blood and bind spontaneously to platelets to form aggregates within the arterial and capillary microvessels. The VWF–platelet aggregates are large enough to form microthrombi inducing tissue ischemia, platelet consumption, and microangiopathic hemolytic anemia (schistocytes on blood smear). (From Joly, B. S., Coppo, P., Veyradier, A. [2017]. Thrombotic thrombocytopenic purpura. *Blood, 129,* 2836–2846.)

Signs and Symptoms

- Fever (37.5° C/99.5° F): occurs in 75% of patients
- Neurologic: occur in 70% to 80% of patients; often intermittent and variable
  - Confusion or dizziness
  - Headache
  - Change in mental status (e.g., forgetfulness, trouble concentrating)
  - Paresis
  - Aphasia, dysarthria, and visual problems
- Major neurologic abnormalities: occur in 10% to 35% of patients.
  - Coma
  - Seizure
  - Stroke and focal abnormalities
  - Encephalopathy
- Thrombocytopenia/Anemia:
  - Petechiae, easy bruising, or bleeding due to thrombocytopenia occurs in most patients, and symptoms are typically moderate to severe
  - Shortness of breath, tachycardia, pallor, fatigue, and weakness may correlate with the degree of anemia, which occurs in most patients
  - Other: epistaxis, gingival bleeding, hematuria, menorrhagia, hemoptysis, gastrointestinal bleeding, retinal/choroidal hemorrhaging
  - Purpura occurs in more than 90% of cases
- Renal impairment: proteinuria, microscopic hematuria, decreased renal function
- Cardiac symptoms: chest pain, heart failure, hypotension
- Gastrointestinal symptoms: abdominal pain
- Jaundice: may result from microangiopathic hemolytic anemia (i.e., MHA), hyperbilirubinemia
- Cancer patients diagnosed with TTP will have many of the signs and symptoms of classic TTP, but they are less pronounced. Specifically:
  - Fever is usually not seen at the onset but almost always occurs during the illness
  - Renal involvement (e.g., proteinuria and microhematuria) is common
    - Decreased renal function occurs in 40% to 80% of patients
  - Abdominal pain occurs in 10% to 30% of patients
  - Heart involvement occurs infrequently
  - Lung involvement occurs rarely and may include alveolar and interstitial infiltrates

Cancers Associated With Disorder

- Lymphoma
- Cancers being treated by BMT or HSCT
- Advanced cancers with MHA

Diagnostic Tests

- Five primary diagnostic criteria for acquired (classical) TTP
  - MHA (schistocytes present on peripheral smear and low hemoglobin)
- Severe thrombocytopenia (<30,000/mL)
- ADAMTS13 activity less than 10%
- Fever, neurologic abnormalities, renal insufficiency: may or may not be present (60% have neurologic symptoms at presentation)
- With or without cause for TMA
  - Some experts state that deficiency in ADAMTS13 activity is required for diagnosis of TTP; other experts state that a diagnosis of TTP must be considered in the event of thrombocytopenia and MHA alone
- Diagnostic criteria for congenital TTP:
  - ADAMTS13 activity less than 5%
  - Absence of antibody and confirmation of homozygous or compound heterozygous defects of *ADAMTS13* gene.
  - Severe jaundice in neonates: red flag
  - Unexplained thrombocytopenia in children or adults: red flag
- Laboratory tests
  - CBC with a platelet count
    - Anemia, with an average hemoglobin decreased to 7 to 9 g/dL
    - Thrombocytopenia, with platelet count less than 50,000 cells/mm^3 or 50% decrease from previous count
  - Diagnostic criteria for MHA
    - Schistocytes in peripheral blood smear (>1%, or >3 schistocytes per high-power microscopic field). These are split RBCs that indicate MHA, and their presence is hallmark for diagnosing TTP and HUS.
    - Reticulocyte count: increased
    - Bilirubin level (mainly indirect reacting): increased
    - Serum haptoglobin levels: decreased
    - Free plasma hemoglobin: increased in severe cases.
    - Elevated reticulocyte counts
  - Serum ADAMTS13 activity
    - Promptly quantifying ADAMTS13 antigen, activity, and autoantibody has a crucial role in the diagnosis and management of TTP and can help differentiate from other TMAs
    - Normal plasma ADAMTS13 activity levels range from 0.65 to 1.79 international unit/mL
    - In persons with TTP, the serum ADAMTS13 activity level may be less than 5% to 10%, distinguishing TTP from HUS
    - Multiple versions of ADAMTS13 assays exist, and testing takes time
    - It is appropriate to treat a person, who may have all of the clinical and laboratory symptoms of TTP, with a normal serum ADAMTS13 activity level
  - LDH level
    - Increased due to hemolysis
  - CMP
    - Electrolyte levels: increased due to renal impairment
    - Serum BUN and creatinine: increased in 40% to 80% of patients with TTP
    - Serum bilirubin level: increased
    - Liver function tests: rule out liver involvement

- Direct Coombs test (also known as DAT)
  - Determines whether RBCs have been coated in vivo with immunoglobulin, complement, or both.
  - Negative result: indicates nonautoimmune, nondrug-induced hemolytic anemia
  - Positive result: indicates autoimmune, drug-induced hemolytic anemia
- Coagulation tests
  - PT, aPTT, factor V, factor VIII, and fibrinogen: Usually normal values
  - FDP level: may be normal to slightly elevated.
  - TT: may be prolonged.
- Urinalysis
  - Proteinuria, microscopic hematuria, and granular or red cell casts as the most consistent findings
- Blood or urine cultures
  - To identify infection as an underlying cause of TTP
- Troponin T or troponin I levels to rule out cardiac involvement
- Blood type and screen tests to prepare for provision of blood products
- Hepatitis A, B, or C and HIV testing of blood products to exclude an underlying viral precipitant
- Pregnancy test for women of child-bearing age
- Stool culture, to assess for *E. coli* if having diarrhea
- Radiologic evaluation
  - Renal sonogram, renal angiogram, intravenous pyelogram to assess renal function
  - CT or MRI of brain to determine neurologic involvement
  - CT of chest, abdomen, and pelvis, with or without tumor markers, to assess for underlying malignancy
  - ECG or echocardiogram to document or monitor cardiac damage

Differential Diagnosis

- Diagnosis of TTP can be difficult, since there can be overlap with HUS, autoimmune disease, and a spectrum of pregnancy-related problems.
  - Some patients may concurrently have an autoimmune disorder (e.g., SLE, antiphospholipid antibody syndrome) and TTP
- Hematuria related to:
  - Other diseases (e.g., infection, intrinsic kidney disease, benign prostatic hypertrophy)
  - Medications (e.g., ifosfamide, high-dose cyclophosphamide, intravesical chemotherapy)
  - Radiation therapy (e.g., pelvic irradiation, prostate seed implants)
- Systemic malignancy can cause thrombocytopenia and MHA without signs of DIC.
- Malignant hypertension can cause thrombocytopenia, MHA, renal failure, and severe neurologic abnormalities.
- Systemic infection or sepsis, typically viral (e.g., CMV, adenovirus, herpes simplex virus) or severe bacterial (e.g., meningococcus, pneumococcus), but may be fungal.
- DIC
- HUS (diarrhea positive or negative)

- HIT
- Vasculitis
- Drugs: quinine, simvastatin, interferon, calcineurin inhibitors
- Complications for persons undergoing HSCT:
  - Graft-versus-host disease
  - Hepatic sinusoidal obstruction syndrome
  - CMV
- Pregnancy-associated conditions can cause MHA, thrombocytopenia, renal failure, and minor neurologic abnormalities:
  - HELLP
  - Eclampsia
- Differential diagnosis of TTP and HUS
  - TTP and HUS are distinct diseases with different causes and demographics.
    - Many patients are inaccurately diagnosed with "TTP-HUS disorder" on basis of clinical and laboratory findings only.
  - Similar clinical and laboratory features, which occur in both patients with TTP and patients with HUS, include:
    - Thrombocytopenia: platelet count less than 150,000/mm^3 or $\geq$25% decrease in platelets from baseline
    - MHA: schistocytes present on peripheral smear, elevated LDH, decreased haptoglobin, decreased hemoglobin and hematocrit
    - Plus or minus one of the following clinical symptoms due to localized microvascular thrombosis: (1) Neurologic symptoms (confusion, seizures, or other cerebral abnormalities; (2) Renal impairment (elevated creatinine, decreased estimates GFR, elevated blood pressure, abnormal urinalysis); (3) Gastrointestinal symptoms (diarrhea $\pm$ blood, nausea/vomiting, abdominal pain, gastroenteritis)
  - Clinical and laboratory features that differentiate patients with TTP from patients with HUS include:
    - ADAMTS13 deficiencies are the cause of both acquired and congenital TTP; ADAMTS13 does not play a role in pathogenesis of HUS
    - Platelets are less than 30,000/mm^3 in TTP, and thrombocytopenia is less severe in HUS
    - Etiology of STEC-HUS: associated with Shiga toxin–associated hemorrhagic colitis
    - Clinical presentation of TTP patients: dominated by hemorrhages and neurologic symptoms. Renal involvement (e.g., proteinuria, microscopic hematuria) is common, but oliguric acute renal failure is unusual.
    - Clinical presentation of HUS patients: significant renal impairment or failure is the dominant clinical feature
  - Treatment responses that differentiate patients with TTP from patients with HUS include:
    - Treatment of TTP patients: TPE, corticosteroids, and drugs (e.g., rituximab, caplacizumab)
    - Treatment of HUS patients: Insulting factors are removed and anti-complement therapy (e.g., eculizumab) is administered. Patients with HUS have a lack of a complete response to plasma exchange

Treatment

- An early diagnosis of TTP is crucial, but it may be difficult due to the lack of explicit diagnostic criteria.
- When diagnosis of TTP is made, begin TPE as soon as possible.

Pharmacologic Management

- Prevention
  - Hydration
    - Vigorous, parenteral, or oral pre-transplantation hydration before BMT or HSCT
  - Thromboprophylaxis
    - When platelet count is greater than 50,000/mm^3, administer thromboprophylaxis with LMWH and aspirin.
  - Rituximab
    - Use rituximab for patients with TTP who are in remission but still have low plasma ADAMTS13 activity with no clinical signs/symptoms.
    - Per ISTH guidelines, this is a conditional recommendation in the context of very low certainty of evidence.
  - Plasma infusion or watch and wait
    - For patients with congenital TTP, who are in remission, ISTH panel recommends either plasma infusion or watch and wait strategy.
    - Per ISTH guidelines, this is a conditional recommendation in the context of very low certainty of evidence.
- Management
  - TPE
    - TPE, also known as "plasmapheresis" and "apheresis," is a procedure in which plasma in blood is removed and replaced with another fluid (e.g., FFP or cryoprecipitate-poor plasma). This is first-line therapy for TTP.
    - FFP or cryoprecipitate-poor plasma more effective than albumin.
    - Removes or reduces circulating antibodies against ADAMTS13 and replenishes blood levels of enzyme ADAMTS13.
    - Reverses platelet consumption, which is responsible for thrombus formation and the symptoms associated with TTP.
    - Treatment with plasma exchange should be started as soon as possible, preferably within 4 to 8 hours of diagnosis, due to high risk of preventable, early deaths in persons who present with MHA and thrombocytopenia, in the absence of any other identifiable cause.
    - Most patients with an early diagnosis of TTP enter remission with this procedure.
    - Recommendation to administer solvent/detergent plasma, which is preferred over FFP, in treating patients with TTP undergoing plasma-exchange procedures.

- Corticosteroids
  - Add corticosteroids to TPE for treatment of acute TTP in patients experiencing a first acute event and experiencing a relapse of TTP. This recommendation is part of ISTH guidelines for treatment of TTP.
  - ISTH panel did not recommend preferred dose and type of corticosteroid (methylprednisolone or prednisone), since special attention needs to be given to adverse events of corticosteroids and susceptible populations (e.g., cancer, diabetes mellitus, hypertension, psychiatric comorbidities, advanced age).
  - Mechanism of action: Corticosteroids may suppress autoantibodies, inhibiting ADAMTS13 activity.
- Rituximab
  - Add Rituximab to standard treatment (e.g., TPE and corticosteroids) in patients with acute TTP
  - This recommendation is for patients with acute TTP, who are experiencing their first acute event or experiencing a relapse.
  - According to ISTH panel, this is a conditional recommendation in context of very low certainty evidence.
  - In one study ($n = 50$), 100% of new-onset cases of TTP and 84.61% of refractory cases of TTP achieved remission, when started on Rituximab
- Caplacizumab
  - Add caplacizumab to standard treatment (e.g., TPE and corticosteroids) in patients experiencing a first event or relapse of TTP
  - This is a conditional recommendation by ISTH, in the context of moderate certainty evidence.
  - Capacizumab, approved in 2018 for treatment of adults experiencing an acute episode of TTP. It is an anti-VWF humanized bivalent variable-domain-only immunoglobulin fragment.
  - Mechanism of action: inhibits interaction between VWF multimers and platelets.
  - Scully and colleagues (2019) conducted a study in 145 patients and compared treatment efficacy of caplacizumab and standard TTP treatment (plasma exchange and glucocorticoids) versus placebo and standard TTP treatment. Results demonstrated faster normalization of platelet count; lower incidence of composite of TTP-related deaths, recurrence of TTP, or thromboembolic event during the treatment period; and a lower rate of recurrence of TTP during the trial than placebo.
  - Völker and colleagues (2020) conducted a study in 60 patients, who were treated with caplacizumab, plasma exchange, and corticosteroids at 29 different medical centers (standard clinical care settings). They reported that caplacizumab was effective in the treatment of acute TTP and led to a rapid normalization of platelet count (e.g., > 150K). Their data also suggest that plasma exchange can be stopped when platelet values rise above 100,000 to 150,000/mm^3.

Oncologic Emergencies

⑤

- Bortezomib
  - Add Bortezomib to standard treatment (e.g., TPE, corticosteroids, and rituximab) in patients experiencing severe, refractory TTP
- Discontinue drugs that induce TTP.
  - For a patient undergoing allogeneic HSCT in whom TTP develops while on cyclosporine, recommendation is to discontinue cyclosporine and initiate tacrolimus.
  - However, removing the drug may not reverse the TTP, and GVHD may worsen.
- Packed RBCs may be transfused, based on severity of anemia and amount of bleeding.
- Platelet transfusions are usually not indicated to treat TTP, due to potential for generating platelet-rich microthrombi
  - Severe thrombocytopenia alone is not an appropriate indication for platelet transfusion in patients with classic TTP.
  - Platelet transfusion may be indicated for intracranial bleeding, which is documented by CT or MRI, or for life-threatening bleeding. Platelets may be transfused slowly.
  - Complications associated with platelet transfusions in persons with TTP include development or progression of neurologic symptoms and acute renal failure.
- Measuring outcomes for treatment of TTP
  - Clinical Response (pre-remission): defined as:
    - Platelet counts $\geq$150,000/mm^3
    - LDH less than 1.5 upper limit of normal
    - No clinical evidence of new or progressive ischemic organ injury
  - Exacerbation (post-clinical response and pre-remission): defined as:
    - Platelet counts decrease to less than 150,000/mm^3 (with other causes of thrombocytopenia excluded)
    - With or without clinical evidence of new or progressive ischemic organ injury
  - Occurs within 30 days of stopping TPE or anti-VWF therapy
  - Clinical Remission: Sustained clinical response with either:
  - No TPE or no anti-VWF therapy for $\geq$30 days or
    - With attainment of ADAMTS13 remission (partial or complete), whichever occurs first
  - ADAMTS13 remission
    - Partial: ADAMTS13 activity $\geq$20% to less than LLN
    - Complete: ADAMTS13 activity $\geq$LLN
  - Clinical Relapse: defined as:
    - After a clinical remission, platelet counts decrease to less than 150,000/mm^3 (with other causes of thrombocytopenia ruled out), with or without clinical evidence of new ischemic organ injury
    - Clinical relapse must be confirmed by documentation of severe ADAMTS13 deficiency

- ADAMTS13 Relapse: defined as:
  - After an ADAMTS13 remission (partial or complete), the ADAMTS13 level decreases to less than 20%

Nonpharmacologic Management

- Determine if religious beliefs affect willingness to receive blood products
- Nephrology consultation: needed to determine most appropriate renal therapy.
- Splenectomy has a 50% success rate at best.
- Renal replacement therapy
  - May include peritoneal dialysis and hemodialysis (minority of patients with TTP)
  - May be successful treatment for patients with recurrent cancer-associated TTP
- Assist patient/family with coping
  - Assess available resources for patient and caregiver support
  - Provide positive feedback to patients/caregivers through coaching and listening
  - Suggest resources, such as psychological counseling and pastoral care services for emotional and spiritual support

Patient Teaching

- Goals
  - Define TTP
  - Describe signs/symptoms of TTP and identify signs/symptoms of TTP to report to health care provider.
  - Understand lab and diagnostic testing, nursing care and treatments related to managing TTP
  - Prevent relapse of TTP
  - Maintain patient safety by identifying signs/symptoms of bleeding and avoiding injury and bleeding while on anticoagulant therapy
- Describe goals of therapy for TTP:
  - Blood cell counts (especially platelets and hemoglobin) return to normal levels.
  - Symptoms (e.g., bleeding, neurologic abnormalities) subside.
- Provide patients with verbal and written educational materials on TTP.
- Define TTP, and describe signs/symptoms.
- Teach patient the purpose of laboratory tests, nursing care, and treatments for TTP.
- Ask the patient to report symptoms such as bleeding and mental status changes.
- Teach patients self-care measures to minimize bleeding and maximize their safety:
  - Use an electric razor, not a straight-edged razor
  - Maintain the bed in a low position with side rails up
  - Clear pathways in the room and hallway
  - Minimize activities that could trigger bleeding
  - Avoid contact sports and heavy lifting
  - Take precautions against accidental bleeding because even minor scrapes or bumps could result in bleeding

- Teach fall precautions if the patient is at risk for falls
  - In the home, remove throw rugs and items that can obstruct pathways
  - Wear shoes that fit appropriately
  - Walk carefully and change positions gradually
- Teach patients to avoid over-the-counter medications that may interfere with normal platelet function such as aspirin and NSAIDs (e.g., ibuprofen, naproxen sodium).
- Teach patient ways to stimulate the circulation in lower extremities and minimize activities that could lead to development of clots:
  - Change position regularly
  - Move toes, feet, and legs often (e.g., wiggle the toes, flex/rotate the foot and ankles, tighten the calves)
  - Avoid sitting or standing for long periods
  - Make frequent stops on long trips to move around
  - Avoid constrictive clothing or devices
  - Perform ROM or isometric exercises
  - Wear the pneumatic compression stockings or devices as ordered
- Teach patient and family to observe and save urine, stool, and emesis for nurse to check for blood.
- Teach patient to report critical signs and symptoms such as bruising, red rash, headache, black stools, blood in the urine or stools, and bleeding from gums, nose, eyes, vagina, rectum, wound, or central venous catheter site.

Follow-Up

- Short-term follow-up
  - Monitor CBC and other labs as appropriate daily during the acute phase to determine the continuation or resolution of TTP.
  - Monitor patient one to two times per week until hemoglobin, hematocrit, and platelet levels become stable.
    - After remission occurs, patients gradually need fewer routine blood counts
  - Monitor for signs/symptoms of recurrent TTP
  - Platelet count is necessary when symptoms of any illness occur to diagnose a possible recurrence of TTP in a timely manner.
- Long-term follow-up
  - Monitor platelet counts frequently during the first year of initial treatment because patients often relapse during this time.
  - Provide additional resources such as home equipment or assistance as needed.

Bibliography

Albiol, N., Awol, R., & Martino, R. (2020). Autoimmune thrombotic thrombocytopenic purpura (TTP) associated with COVID-19. *Annals of Hematology, 99*(7), 1673–1674.

Asakura, H., & Ogawa, H. (2021). COVID-19-associated coagulopathy and disseminated intravascular coagulation. *International Journal of Hematology, 113*(1), 45–57.

Bazzan, M., Montaruli, B., Sciascia, S., Cosseddu, D., Norbiato, C., & Roccatello, D. (2020). Low ADAMTS 13 plasma levels are predictors of mortality in COVID 19 patients. *Internal and Emergency Medicine, 15*(5), 861–863.

Cuker, A., Cataland, S. R., Coppo, P., de la Rubia, J., Friedman, K. D., George, J. N., … Scully, M. (2021). Redefining outcomes in immune TTP: An international working group consensus report. *Blood, 137*(14), 1855–1861.

Delaney, E., Nikolai, C., & Coe, K. (2020). Metabolic emergencies. In J. M. Brant (Ed.), *Core curriculum for oncology nursing* (6th ed.). Elsevier.

Joly, B. S., Coppo, P., & Veyradier, A. (2017). Thrombotic thrombocytopenic purpura. *Blood, 129*(21), 2836–2846.

Kim, W. H., Park, J. B., Jung, C. W., & Kim, G. S. (2015). Rebalanced hemostasis in patients with idiopathic thrombocytopenic purpura. *Platelets, 26*(1), 38–42.

Kremer Hovinga, J. A., Heeb, S. R., Skowronska, M., & Schaller, M. (2018). Pathophysiology of thrombotic thrombocytopenic purpura and hemolytic uremic syndrome. *Journal of Thrombosis and Haemostasis, 16*(4), 618–629.

Levi, M. (2019). Disseminated intravascular coagulation in cancer: An update. *Seminars in Thrombosis and Hemostasis, 45*(4), 342–347.

Levi, M., & Iba, T. (2021). COVID-19 coagulopathy: Is it disseminated intravascular coagulation? *Internal and Emergency Medicine, 16*(2), 309–312.

Marietta, M., Franchini, M., Bindi, M. L., Picardi, F., Ruggeri, M., & De Silvestro, G. (2016). Is solvent/detergent plasma better than standard fresh-frozen plasma? A systematic review and an expert consensus document. *Blood Transfusion, 14*(4), 277–286.

Patriquin, C. J., Thomas, M. R., Dutt, T., McGuckin, S., Blombery, P. A., Cranfield, T., … Scully, M. (2016). Bortezomib in the treatment of refractory thrombotic thrombocytopenic purpura. *British Journal of Haematology, 173*(5), 779–785.

Rathnayaka, R. N., Ranathunga, P. A. N., & Kularatne, S. A. (2019). Thrombotic microangiopathy, hemolytic uremic syndrome, and thrombotic thrombocytopenic purpura following hump-nosed pit viper (Genus: *Hypnale*) envenoming in Sri Lanka. *Wilderness and Environmental Medicine, 30*(1), 66–78.

Raval, J. S., Mazepa, M. A., Brecher, M. E., & Park, Y. A. (2014). How we approach an acquired thrombotic thrombocytopenic purpura patient. *Transfusion, 54*(10), 2375–2382.

Saha, M., McDaniel, J. K., & Zheng, X. L. (2017). Thrombotic thrombocytopenic purpura: pathogenesis, diagnosis and potential novel therapeutics. *Journal of Thrombosis and Haemostasis, 15*(10), 1889–1900.

Scully, M., Cataland, S., Coppo, P., de la Rubia, J., Friedman, K. D., Kremer Hovinga, J., … International Working Group for Thrombotic Thrombocytopenic Purpura. (2017). Consensus on the standardization of terminology in thrombotic thrombocytopenic purpura and related thrombotic microangiopathies. *Journal of Thrombosis and Haemostasis, 15*(2), 312–322.

Scully, M., Cataland, S. R., Peyvandi, F., Coppo, P., Knöbl, P., Kremer Hovinga, J. A., … HERCULES Investigators. (2019). Caplacizumab treatment for acquired thrombotic thrombocytopenic purpura. *New England Journal of Medicine, 380*(4), 335–346.

Shah, N., & Sarode, R. (2013). Thrombotic thrombocytopenic purpura—What is new? *Journal of Clinical Apheresis, 28*(1), 30–35.

Starke, R., Machin, S., Scully, M., Purdy, G., & Mackie, I. (2007). The clinical utility of ADAMTS13 activity, antigen and autoantibody assays in thrombotic thrombocytopenic purpura. *British Journal of Haematology, 136*(4), 649–655.

Terrell, D. R., Williams, L. A., Vesely, S. K., Lämmle, B., Hovinga, J. A., & George, J. N. (2005). The incidence of thrombotic thrombocytopenic purpura-hemolytic uremic syndrome: All patients, idiopathic patients, and patients with severe ADAMTS-13 deficiency. *Journal of Thrombosis and Haemostasis, 3*(7), 1432–1436.

Tso, A. C. Y., Sum, C. L. L., & Ong, K. H. (2020). Reference range for ADAMTS13 antigen, activity and anti-ADAMTS13 antibody in the healthy adult Singapore population. *Singapore Medical Journal, 63*(4), 214–218.

Völker, L. A., Kaufeld, J., Miesbach, W., Brähler, S., Reinhardt, M., Kühne, L., … Menne, J. (2020). Real-world data confirm the effectiveness of caplacizumab in acquired thrombotic thrombocytopenic purpura. *Blood Advances, 4*(13), 3085–3092.

Yocum, A., & Simon, E. L. (2021). Thrombotic thrombocytopenic purpura after Ad26.COV2-S vaccination. *The American Journal of Emergency Medicine, 49*, 441.e3–441.e4.

Zheng, X. L., Vesely, S. K., Cataland, S. R., Coppo, P., Geldziler, B., Iorio, A., … Peyvandi, F. (2020). ISTH guidelines for treatment of thrombotic thrombocytopenic purpura. *Journal of Thrombosis and Haemostasis, 18*(10), 2496–2502.

Survivorship

Carrie Tompkins Stricker and Rupa Ghosh-Berkebile

Introduction and Epidemiology

A cancer survivor is defined as a person diagnosed with cancer, from the time of diagnosis through the balance of their life (National Cancer Institute [NCI], 2022). Cancer survivors are thus very diverse and include those living with cancer and those free of cancer. Using this broadest of definitions, cancer survivorship encompasses a continuum that spans from initial diagnosis and treatment with curative intent through to cancer-free survival, as well as living with cancer through and beyond intermittent periods of active disease, and/or continuous treatment for metastatic disease, and ultimately end-of-life (Hewitt et al., 2006). While the term *survivor* is intended to capture a group of people with a history of cancer; some survivors are uncomfortable referring to themselves with this label (National Comprehensive Cancer Institute [NCCN], 2022). However, the National Coalition for Cancer Survivorship (NCCS, 2021) State of Survivorship Survey did discover that 85% of participants considered themselves to be "survivors," and the likelihood of identifying with this label increased over time following diagnosis and movement through, and in some cases, beyond, the treatment (NCCS, 2021).

Advances in cancer screening, treatment, and care have contributed to the exponential growth of cancer survivors, including an estimated 18 million cancer survivors living in the United States as of January 1, 2022, representing 5.4% of the total U.S. population (NCI, 2022). This number is expected to approach 22.5 million by 2032 (American Cancer Society [ACS], 2022). The lifetime probability of developing cancer is 39.5% (NCI, 2022). In the United States, one of two men and one of three women are expected to develop cancer (ACS, 2022). Among people diagnosed with cancer, 69% are expected to be alive after 5 years and nearly half (47%) are now living 10 or more years (ACS, 2022). Furthermore, survival rates continue to grow, thanks to both the aging population and the improvements in screening and early detection previously discussed (Siegel et al., 2021). Detailed statistics describing the cancer survivor population, including breakdown by gender, age, cancer diagnosis, and time since treatment, are available on the NCI website (NCI, 2022), including accompanying graphs and charts. Of note, 67% of cancer survivors in the United States are estimated to be age 65 or older, and nearly half are living 10 or more years beyond their cancer diagnosis (ACS, 2022). As such, a majority of cancer survivors simultaneously are either at risk for and/or are currently experiencing other age-related diseases, which may be exacerbated by the long-term toxic effects of the cancer treatments themselves. Chronologic age may not match physical age due to these synergistic effects. Furthermore, this "silver tsunami" will persist; such older adults, often with complex health needs, will continue to dominate the survivor population over the next quarter century (Bluethmann et al., 2016).

With this growing number of cancer survivors comes health care delivery challenges. The terms "cancer survivors" and "cancer survivorship care" are related but distinct, with the first term describing the population and the second defining the care organized around and delivered to that population and the individuals within it. Keeping in mind the broad definition of a cancer survivor above, the cancer survivorship care continuum can be seen as starting with risk assessment and intervention at the time of cancer diagnosis and persisting throughout the entire cancer care trajectory (see the figure on next page) (National Academies of Sciences, Engineering, and Medicine [NASEM], 2018). Cancer survivors require specialized care both during and after acute treatment period(s), as they may continue to cope with the long-term and late effects of cancer treatment, including risk for secondary conditions, long after some acute treatment effects may have resolved. This chapter will focus on evolving trends in the delivery of quality survivorship care, including a significant emphasis on incorporation of survivorship care plans (SCPs) as one mechanism for the delivery of quality survivorship care.

History of Cancer Survivorship and Standards for Survivorship Care

Cancer survivorship as a field has a rich history, and attention to and understanding of related concepts have evolved tremendously over the past several decades. Seminal cancer survivorship events over time have shaped our understanding of both what a cancer survivor is and what the field of cancer survivorship addresses (Stricker, 2021).

In addition to the understanding of the term cancer survivor evolving from "victim" to "survivor," to now a term used by some, "thriver" (NCCS, 2021), there has more recently been increasing attention to specific subpopulations and trajectories of care. These include "long-term survivorship" and postacute treatment (NASEM, 2018), as well as the term "meta-vivor," which was recently proposed to describe the subpopulation of cancer survivors living with metastatic disease as a population with unique needs that deserves special emphasis (Mollica et al., 2022a). It is important, however, to note that "previvors," a term defining a population of individuals who have not had cancer yet are at increased risk for developing cancer due to inheritance of genetic predispositions (e.g., *BRCA*-1, *BRCA*-2), are considered a distinct population from cancer survivors, although many experience similar (and also unique) needs.

From a historical perspective, the seminal Institute of Medicine (IOM) report *From Cancer Patient to Cancer Survivor: Lost in Transition* (Hewitt et al., 2006) and a 2014 American Society of Clinical Oncology (ASCO) report were pivotal in driving efforts to focus care of cancer survivors after treatment. The 2006 IOM report outlined essential elements of quality survivorship care as the following, and both the IOM (2006) and ASCO (2014) reports included a recommendation to provide a personalized SCP to each individual completing active treatment. In 2015, this growing momentum led to two major accreditation organizations (i.e., American College of Surgeons' Commission on Cancer [CoC] and the National Accreditation Program for Breast Centers [NAPBC]) adding survivorship care standards to their requirements, including mandating the delivery of SCPs to individuals completing initial cancer treatment with curative intent (CoC, 2014; NAPBC, 2018). To incentivize centers to provide quality and cancer care, the Centers for Medicare and Medicaid Innovation (CMMI) launched the oncology-focused model (OCM) of payment in 2015 (CMS.gov, 2022). A mandated component of care transformation activities in the OCM was also the delivery of SCPs. As such, the period of time from 2006 to 2018 was characterized by the growth of programs and initiatives focused on SCP delivery at cancer centers and oncology practices, particularly those participating in OCM and/or the CoC and NAPBC accreditation programs (NASEM, 2018). Unfortunately, implementation of other recommendations central to enhancing the quality of cancer survivorship care remained largely absent from comprehensive cancer control plans at centers around the country, including crucial components such as the development and implementation of evidence-based guidelines for cancer survivorship care and quality survivorship care measures (Mollica et al., 2020). National policy and organizational recommendations evolved to encompass a more comprehensive and longitudinal view of survivorship care in 2018 (NASEM, 2018; Blaes et al., 2020), given the lack of consistent evidence supporting the benefit of SCPs (Blaes et al., 2020), the challenges inherent in their delivery (Mayer et al., 2014), and the emerging evidence that too great a focus on mandating their delivery distracted from the development and implementation of more all-encompassing and holistic programs of survivorship care (Stricker, 2021). The 2018 NASEM workshop extended and refined the recommendations from the earlier IOM workshop and report, *From Cancer Patient to Cancer Survivor: Lost in Transition*, which identified prevalent gaps in comprehensive and coordinated care for posttreatment survivorship and served as an urgent call to all those involved with cancer treatment to focus on improving the care delivered to patients *after treatment* (Hewitt et al., 2006). Taken together, these two IOM/NASEM reports on cancer survivorship communicate that survivorship care should focus on palliation of symptoms, prevention of late effects, and health promotion across the entire cancer care trajectory, including *but not limited to* the posttreatment period (Hewitt et al., 2006; NASEM, 2018).

In September 2019, the CoC made substantial revisions to the survivorship standard, replacing standard 3.3, "Survivorship Care Plan," with standard 4.8, "Survivorship Program." The date for implementation was January 1, 2021 (CoC, 2019). The new standard reflects a shift in emphasis from isolated delivery of a document to a specific population to development of a comprehensive program directed at delivering cancer survivorship care to meet the specific needs of all cancer survivors. The SCP is included as a part of the program but is no longer a required element for maintaining accreditation. The program is run by a team of interdisciplinary providers, managed by a survivorship program coordinator. The new standard allows for flexibility using specific strategies to meet the goal. The survivorship team determines a list of services and programs to be offered on site or by referral to meet the needs of cancer survivors. These may include but are not limited to: treatment summaries and SCPs; screening programs for new cancers; surveillance programs for cancer recurrence, rehabilitation, nutritional, psychological, and psychiatric services; referrals to cardio-oncology, sexual health, and fertility preservation specialists; financial support services; physical activity programs; and support groups and educational seminars for survivors. The survivorship program coordinator submits annual documentation of a minimum of three services that will be offered and developed to meet the needs of cancer survivors, as well as the resources needed to improve those services if barriers were encountered (CoC, 2019). The NAPBC standard 2.20 continues to require accredited breast centers to provide care plans to 50% of patients who have completed active treatment for cancer within 6 months of completing treatment (NAPBC, 2017).

What Is Survivorship Care?

Consistent with the broader definition of cancer survivors as individuals from the time of diagnosis through the balance of life, *survivorship services*—at some centers—are seen as an umbrella term for a range of comprehensive care services provided throughout the course of diagnosis, treatment, and after treatment, and are sometimes also called *supportive care services*. Encompassed within this definition of survivorship care, however, remains the postacute treatment period, which includes follow-up care that is essential for cancer survivors and includes a focus on the numerous long-term and late side effects and the potential risks that are unique to each survivor. Survivorship care is comprehensive, coordinated care that addresses the physical, emotional, spiritual, financial, psychosocial, and practical issues of each patient. Consistent with the IOM (2006) and NASEM (2018) reports, the NCCN defined standards for quality survivorship care in their survivorship guidelines as follows (NCCN, 2022):

1. Prevention of new and recurrent cancers and other late effects
2. Surveillance for cancer spread, recurrence, or second cancers
3. Assessment of late psychosocial and physical effects
4. Intervention for consequences or cancer and treatment (e.g., medical, symptoms, psychological distress, financial and social concerns)
5. Coordination of care between primary care providers (PCPs) and specialists to ensure that all of the survivor's health needs are met, and
6. Planning for ongoing survivorship care

What Do Cancer Survivors Prioritize and Desire for Cancer Survivorship Care?

Input from cancer survivors themselves can help us define what might best represent quality cancer survivorship care. Mead et al. (2020) asked cancer survivors to identify their top priorities for survivorship care. The box below illustrates survivors' needs for better understanding of and expectation setting for dealing with the chronic and long-term nature of survivorship, and clear desire for better care coordination and teamwork that is directed at achieving comprehensive, holistic, "whole-person" care. Their perspectives support the recommendations and focus of NCCN, NASEM, and other organizations and professional bodies, as well as the CoC's shift in September 2019 to broadening its accreditation requirement from a singular focus on delivery of SCPs to the now more comprehensive standard 4.8, "Survivorship Program" (American College of Surgeons Commission on Cancer [CoC], 2019). Unfortunately, as illustrated by the results of the NCCS (2021) survey, there remain both great gaps in the degree to which these needs are being met, as well as substantial heterogeneity in individual survivor experiences. In particular, racial, ethnic, and socioeconomic disparities exist in both the care received and the outcomes experienced by cancer survivors (Alfano et al., 2019b).

Survivors' Priorities and Wishes for Cancer Survivorship Care

Survivors' Principles
- Principle 1. Underscoring the chronic nature of survivorship to prepare survivors
- Principle 2. Creating an integrated, holistic system to better manage ongoing issues in survivorship

Practice Priorities at the *Individual* Survivor Level
- Priority 1. Understanding expectations of survivorship care and how to "live with cancer"
- Priority 2. Having peer networks for emotional and social support
- Priority 3. Getting information and resources to help manage care
- Priority 4. Getting mental health support

Practice Priorities at the *Interpersonal* Level
- Priority 5. Having supportive and responsive providers
- Priority 6. Being an empowered and engaged patient
- Priority 7. Engaging in meaningful communication and shared decision-making between providers and survivors

Practice Priorities at the *Organizational* Level
- Priority 8. Seamless care coordination and transitions across providers
- Priority 9. Offering practical support to help manage life after cancer
- Priority 10. Creating infrastructure/processes to increase access and facilitate continuous care
- Priority 11. Providing a full spectrum of care without access barriers

From Mead, K. H., Raskin, S., Willis, A., Arem, H., Murtaza, S., Charney, L., & Pratt-Chapman, M. (2020). Identifying patients' priorities for quality survivorship: conceptualizing a patient-centered approach to survivorship care. *Journal of Cancer Surviv*orship, 14, 939–958.

Scope of a Treatment Summary and Survivorship Care Plan

A treatment summary and survivorship care plan (TS/SCP) is a personalized document containing a summary of the patient's treatment, implications of the diagnosis and treatment for follow-up care, and recommended health behaviors. The care plan is intended to serve as a roadmap for cancer survivors. It shows them which providers they should see and when. It also allows providers to share detailed information about the patient's treatment, potential long-term risks associated with it, and the appropriate screening recommendations (Mayer et al., 2014; NCCN, 2022).

The key components of the TS are:
1. Contact information for the treating institutions and providers
2. Specific diagnosis, histologic subtype, clinical and pathologic stage of disease
3. Surgery: year and month, name of procedure and location
4. Systemic therapy: start and end dates of therapy, names of systemic therapy agents
5. Radiation therapy: start and end dates of therapy, anatomic location of treatment, total dose and fractions delivered
6. If applicable, genetic or hereditary risk factors, predisposing conditions, and genetic testing results, if performed

The key components of the SCP are:
1. Potential schedule of follow-up clinical visits: location, frequency, and providers responsible
2. Disease-specific cancer surveillance tests for recurrence: location, frequency, anticipated imaging or laboratory testing, and providers responsible for ordering, testing, and follow-up on results
3. Cancer screening for early detection of new primary cancers: location, frequency of testing, who is responsible for ordering testing and follow-up on results
4. Other periodic testing and examinations and provider responsible (usually the PCP)
5. Possible symptoms of cancer recurrence; can be a general statement such as "any new, unusual, and/or persistent symptoms should be brought to the attention of your cancer care team."
6. Potential long-term and/or late effects associated with treatment, ongoing toxicities or adverse effects from treatments received, as well as symptoms that may indicate the presence of late-effect conditions
7. List of practical concerns (e.g., work/employment, parenting and childcare, financial stress/insurance, emotional or mental health) and resources for the survivors, including referrals to appropriate specialists such as cancer rehabilitation and psychosocial care providers.
8. General information emphasizing the importance of healthy weight, nutrition, adequate physical activity, sunscreen use, smoking cessation, reduction in alcohol use and their effects on cancer prevention

Models of and Approaches to Survivorship Care

In an effort to address care gaps and improve upon the quality of cancer survivorship care, a number of models of survivorship care delivery have been developed and implemented. There is no consensus, however, as to which models are most effective, for which particular populations, and for the achievement of specific outcomes. Models and systems for survivorship care have been previously well described (Chan et al., 2021), and a detailed description is beyond the scope of this chapter. However, the most common models described in the literature are the oncologist- or specialist-led, nurse- or advanced practice provider (APP)-led, consultative, integrated, multidisciplinary, general survivorship, shared oncology/PCP, and primary care-led (Chan et al., 2021). There is also the pediatric long-term follow-up model (McCabe & Jacobs, 2012). One predominant model has been oncologist- (or specialist-) led survivorship care. However, due to the growing oncology physician shortage and growing demands on physicians' time, it is not sustainable for oncologists alone to be accountable for all aspects of cancer survivors' care indefinitely, nor is it often feasible for oncologists to conduct a lengthy visit to address all aspects of a cancer survivor's needs (Chan et al., 2021). Hence, other models must be considered. PCP-led or shared oncologist/PCP-led models have been of great interest for this and other reasons, but they also have their own challenges to implementation and sustainability, including the PCP shortage and the need for additional education and training in survivorship care (Potosky & Han, 2011). There are growing numbers of PCP educational resources available, but little evidence showing their clinical effectiveness (Chan et al., 2022). Such models of care have been evaluated, and there is at least one ongoing randomized trial (NIH, 2022) investigating the efficacy of PCP versus shared models of care that incorporates tailored education and training of PCPs as part of the intervention. Finally, nurse- and/or APP-led models of survivorship care have been widely implemented, and evaluations of these models have shown some benefit with respect to cost, psychosocial issues, health promotion, and healthy lifestyle activities, as well as patient and caregiver experiences (Chan et al., 2021). Overall, there has been no evidence to date of any significant difference in effectiveness across survivorship care models, and more research and evaluation are thus needed (Chan et al., 2021). One approach to delivering on these objectives that has emerged across many cancer centers and practices has been to conduct a comprehensive survivorship assessment at the first posttreatment visit (a "transition visit") to identify potential issues that may affect quality of life and create a plan to mitigate them; these visits are often conducted by nurses and/or APPs (Mayer et al., 2016). Using such a one-time transition visit as a platform for the delivery of SCPs was shown to be equivalent to two other approaches in one randomized trial of three different approaches (Snyder et al., 2022).

When patients were surveyed about preference for which provider(s) deliver their survivorship care, the results were dependent on the type of care that was needed. The survey showed that 25% of survivors were comfortable with the PCP-led model of care, and 50% were comfortable with follow-up care in a multidisciplinary survivorship clinic. Survivors preferred their oncologist or their team to provide survivorship care for long-term and late effects, recurrence, and cancer-related screenings, but were comfortable with their PCP handling preventive care and other comorbidities (Attai et al., 2022). This and other evidence show there is no "one size fits all" approach; the best model of care will vary between care facilities and patient populations based on need, feasibility, and many other factors.

Regardless of model, cancer programs and the oncology nurses involved in their administration should be aware that—to be compliant with the CoC *Survivorship Program* standards updated in 2019—any model of survivorship care delivery must be overseen by a survivorship program that is run by a team of interdisciplinary providers and managed by a survivorship program coordinator, the latter who is often a nurse (CoC, 2019).

Personalized Survivorship and Risk-Stratified Care Pathways: The Path Forward?

Given both the individualized needs of cancer survivors, a widely heterogeneous population, and the workforce challenges previously discussed, risk-stratified models of survivorship care may advance more personalized and sustainable survivorship care (Alfano et al., 2019a; Biddell et al., 2021; Kline et al., 2018; Stricker, 2021). Decades of research and practice in implementing risk-stratified pathways in the U.K. have demonstrated that such approaches are both cost-effective and care-efficient and achieve high-quality outcomes such as reducing unmet patient/survivor needs (National Health Service [NHS], n.d.). Personalized survivorship care in the U.K. and also Australia has involved triaging survivors to care pathways after the completion of acute cancer treatment, based on their current care needs as well as the risk for issues and needs later in survivorship (Biddle et al., 2021; NHS, n.d.). The U.K. pathways are divided into three tiers, with pathways tailored to survivors with *low*, *intermediate*, and *high* risks and/or needs, based on standardized assessment and disease-/treatment-specific criteria (Kline et al., 2018; NHS, n.d.). Each pathway includes direction on both the focus and the provision of primary care, comorbidity management, and disease prevention, plus cancer-specific follow-up care. *Low*-risk/need survivor pathways emphasize supporting patients in self managing their cancer-specific needs outside of cancer surveillance. The *intermediate* pathway employs a shared care model, wherein a limited number of clinicians see patients for cancer-related needs, but self-management and primary care are emphasized. Finally, *high-risk/need* survivors receive complex case management delivered by a multidisciplinary clinical team.

Stakeholders participating in the NASEM (2018) workshop on *Long-Term Cancer Survivorship* proposed a vision for risk-stratified survivorship care pathways for the U.S. context. This proposal focuses on the organization of care for survivors between oncology and primary care at a time point beginning 5 years following the completion of initial cancer treatment. Similar to the U.K. approach, pathways are divided into low-, intermediate-, and high-risk tiers (Kline et al., 2021). A more detailed proposal for risk-stratified pathways for personalized survivorship care has been proposed as well, including more prescriptive and detailed guidance for implementation (Biddell et al., 2021).

While these pathways have not yet been widely implemented and/or evaluated in the United States, there is a great need for oncology nurses to help drive forward innovative approaches aligned with this proposal, especially given the ever-growing workforce shortages in the United States combined with the growing numbers of survivors (U.S. Department of Health and Human Services, Health Resources and Services Administration, National Center for Health Workforce Analysis, 2022). Systematic processes and infrastructure, including appropriate use of technology, will be crucial to the success and sustainability of these and other models of survivorship care delivery (Alfano et al., 2019b; Biddell et al., 2021; Stricker, 2021).

Personalized Survivorship Care Delivery Beginning at Diagnosis

Although risk-stratified pathways for survivorship care in the United States certainly hold great potential, substantial opportunity to prevent and/or mitigate harm will be lost if only implemented postacute treatment. Implementing such pathways proximal to diagnosis not only aligns conceptually with expanded definitions of cancer survivorship as beginning at the time of cancer diagnosis, but also optimizes the ability to mitigate toxicity, prevent disability, optimize long-term health, and maximize participation in cutting-edge research across the cancer continuum. Alfano et al. (2022) propose that achieving such survivorship care—re-defined as being from diagnosis forward—must be grounded in a team medicine approach plus seven additional core components. Furthermore, they posit that four key innovations will be needed to build this "evolved model of care" (p. 922); specifically,

> *(1) A team medicine approach that connects oncology, primary care, subspecialists and programs, researchers, and patients and their caregivers; (2) a prospective surveillance model that proactively assesses symptoms, function, and social determinants of health addressed through timely referrals; (3) a comprehensive approach that begins at diagnosis and continues throughout oncology care and into post-treatment follow-up for patients who transition; and (4) planning for and pilot testing new care models that ensure the right people, processes, and technology are in place, and leadership is supportive (Alfano et al., 2022, p. 922).*

This refined model of care holds potential for optimizing outcomes and preventing and mitigating toxicities not only for cancer survivors who eventually transition to postacute follow-up care, but also for subpopulations of cancer survivors, more broadly defined, who receive prolonged antineoplastic therapy (either continuous and/or intermittent treatment), including those who have metastatic disease, that is, "meta-vivors" (Mollica et al., 2022a). NCCN guidelines also reinforce the principle that comprehensive assessment and care planning are best undertaken before treatment begins, so that potential problems can be prevented or minimized to avoid significant adverse effects on the quality of life of cancer survivors and their families (NCCN, 2022). NCCN proposes a detailed survivorship assessment to facilitate this process (NCCN, 2022) and recommends periodic follow-up on identified issues.

Nursing Role in Survivorship Care Delivery

There is an enormous opportunity for oncology nurses and APPs who are already working as part of the treatment team to deliver survivorship care, including the creation and delivery of care plans (Klemp, 2015), should this be a focus of the cancer care system's survivorship efforts. Understanding the diagnoses, having an active role in treatment, being able to identify the end of treatment, regularly assessing patient needs (e.g., rehabilitation, counseling, nutrition, practical issues, financial burden), and practicing care coordination as part of their everyday jobs position oncology nurses and APPs to create and deliver SCPs and provide comprehensive survivorship care, more broadly defined (Mayer, 2022; Stricker, 2021). Furthermore, the escalating oncology workforce crisis is such that a shortage of over 1500 oncologists is anticipated in the United States by 2025, given a projected 40% rise in demand for services concurrent with only a projected rise of 25% in supply of oncologists (ASCO, 2021). The opportunity for nurse practitioners (NPs) to help fill this provider gap is especially important, given a current national workforce of approximately 325,000, of which between 5350 and 7000 are estimated to specialize in oncology (American Association of Colleges of Nursing [AACN], 2021). In 2018, a survey of oncology APPs showed that 81% of NPs and 86.2% of physician assistants reported involvement with follow-up care of cancer survivors (Bruinooge, 2018). Given the broader definition of cancer survivorship that extends beyond just the postacute care of individuals following completion of acute treatment means that *all* oncology nurses, including advanced practice nurses, will play pivotal roles in survivorship care delivery (Washko et al., 2022). As such, oncology nurses are perfectly positioned to be leaders of the transformative change needed to improve cancer survivorship care and outcomes by applying many of the principles and evolving methodologies detailed in this chapter.

References

Alfano, C. M., Jefford, M., Maher, J., Birken, S. A., & Mayer, D. K. (2019a). Building personalized cancer follow-up care pathways in the United States: Lessons learned from implementation in England, Northern Ireland, and Australia. *American Society of Clinical Oncology educational book. American Society of Clinical Oncology. Annual Meeting, 39*, 625–639.

Alfano, C. M., Leach, C. R., Smith, T. G., Miller, K. D., Alcaraz, K. I., Cannady, R. S., … Brawley, O. W. (2019b). Equitably improving outcomes for cancer survivors and supporting caregivers: A blueprint for care delivery, research, education, and policy. *CA: A Cancer Journal for Clinicians, 69*(1), 35–49.

Alfano, C. M., Oeffinger, K., Sanft, T., & Tortorella, B. (2022). Engaging TEAM medicine in patient care: Redefining cancer survivorship from diagnosis. American Society of Clinical Oncology educational book. *American Society of Clinical Oncology. Annual Meeting, 42*, 1–11.

American Association of Colleges of Nursing (AACN). (2021). *2020–2021 Enrollment and graduations in baccalaureate and graduate programs in nursing.* AACN.

American Cancer Society (ACS). (2022). *Cancer treatment & survivorship facts & figures 2022–2024.* Atlanta: American Cancer Society.

American Cancer Society of Clinical Oncology (ASCO). (2021). 2021 Snapshot state of the oncology workforce in America. *JCO Oncology Practice, 17*(5), 249.

American College of Surgeons' Commission on Cancer (CoC). (2019). *Optimal resources for cancer care 2020 standards (updated April 2022).* Available at https://www.facs.org/media/whmfnpppx/2020_coc_standards.pdf (accessed August 4, 2022).

Attai, D. J., Katz, M. S., Streja, E., Hsiung, J. T., Marroquin, M. V., Zavaleta, B. A., & Nekhlyudov, L. (2022). Patient preferences and comfort for cancer survivorship models of care: Results of an online survey. *Journal of Cancer Survivorship*. https://doi.org/10.1007/s11764-022-01177-0

Biddell, C. B., Spees, L. P., Mayer, D. K., Wheeler, S. B., Trogdon, J. G., Rotter, J., & Birken, S. A. (2021). Developing personalized survivorship care pathways in the United States: Existing resources and remaining challenges. *Cancer, 127*(7), 997–1004.

Blaes, A. H., Adamson, P. C., Foxhall, L., & Bhatia, S. (2020). Survivorship care plans and the Commission on Cancer standards: The increasing need for better strategies to improve the outcome for survivors of cancer. *Journal of Oncology Practice, 16*(8), 447–450.

Bluethmann, S., Mariotto, A., & Rowland, J. (2016). Anticipating the "silver tsunami" prevalence trajectories and comorbidity burden among older cancer survivors int the United States. *Cancer Epidemiology Biomarkers Prevention, 25*, 1029–1036.

Bruinooge, S. S., Pickard, T. A., Vogel, W., Hanley, A., Schenkel, C., Garrett-Mayer, E., … Williams, S. F. (2018). Understanding the role of advanced practice providers in oncology in the United States. *Journal of the Advanced Practitioner in Oncology, 9*(6), 585–598.

Center for Medicare & Medicaid Services (CMS). (2022). *The oncology care model*. Available at https://innovation.cms.gov/innovation-models/oncology-care. Last updated August 4, 2022.

Chan, R. J., Agbejule, O. A., Yates, P. M., Emery, J., Jefford, M., Koczwara, B., … Nekhlyudov, L. (2022). Outcomes of cancer survivorship education and training for primary care providers: A systematic review. *Journal of Cancer Survivorship, 16*, 279–302.

Chan, R. J., Crawford-Williams, F., Crichton, M., Joseph, R., Hart, N. H., Milley, K., … Nekhlyudov, L. (2021). Effectiveness and implementation of models of cancer survivorship care: An overview of systematic reviews. *Journal of Cancer Survivorship: Research and Practice, 17*(1), 197–221.

Commission on Cancer (CoC). (2014). *Accreditation committee clarifications for standard 3.3 survivorship care plan*. Available at https://www.facs.org/publications/newsletters/coc-source/special-source/standard33 (accessed March 4, 2016).

Hewitt, M., Greenfield, S., & Stovall, E. (2006). *From cancer patient to cancer survivor: Lost in transition*. Institute of Medicine. The National Academies Press.

Klemp, J. R. (2015). Survivorship care planning: One size does not fit all. *Seminars in Oncology Nursing, 13*(1), 67–72.

Kline, R. M., Arora, N. K., Bradley, C. J., Brauer, E. R., Graves, D. L., Lunsford, N. B., … Ganz, P. A. (2018). Long-term survivorship care after cancer treatment—summary of a 2017 National cancer policy forum workshop. *Journal of the National Cancer Institute, 110*(12), 1300–1310.

Kline, R. M., Temple, L. K. F., & Nekhlyudov, L. (2021). Implementing quality colon cancer survivorship care: A practical proposal for a path forward. *JCO Oncology Practice, 17*(2), 77–84.

Mayer, D. K. (2022). *Future directions in cancer survivorship research*. https://cancercontrol.cancer.gov/sites/default/files/2022-02/mayer-webinar-abbreviated.pdf.

Mayer, D. K., Deal, A. M., Crane, J. M., Chen, R. C., Asher, G. N., Hanson, L. C., … Rosenstein, D. L. (2016). Using survivorship care plans to enhance communication and cancer care coordination: results of a pilot study. *Oncology Nursing Forum, 43*(5), 636–645.

Mayer, D. K., Nekhlyudov, L., Snyder, C. F., Merrill, J. K., Wollins, D. S., & Shulman, L. N. (2014). American Society of Clinical Oncology clinical expert statement on cancer survivorship care planning. *Journal of Oncology Practice, 10*(6), 345–351.

McCabe, M. S., & Jacobs, L. A. (2012). Clinical update: Survivorship care—Models and programs. *Seminars in Oncology Nursing, 28*(3), e1–e8. https://doi.org/10.1016/j.soncn.2012.05.001. PMID: 22846488.

Mead, K. H., Raskin, S., Willis, A., Arem, H., Murtaza, S., Charney, L., & Pratt-Chapman, M. (2020). Identifying patients' priorities for quality survivorship: conceptualizing a patient-centered approach to survivorship care. *Journal of Cancer Survivorship, 14*, 939–958.

Mollica, M. A., Falisi, A. L., Geiger, A. M., Jacobsen, P. B., Lunsford, N. B., Pratt-Chapman, M. L., … Nekhlyudov, L. (2020). Survivorship objectives in comprehensive cancer control plans: A systematic review. *Journal of Cancer Survivorship, 14*(2), 235–243. https://doi.org/10.1007/s11764-019-00832-3. Epub 2020 Jan 17. PMID: 31953645.

Mollica, M. A., Smith, A. W., Tonorezos, E., Castro, K., Filipski, K. K., Guida, J., … Gallicchio, L. (2022a). Survivorship for individuals living with advanced and metastatic cancers: National Cancer Institute meeting report. *Journal of the National Cancer Institute, 114*(4), 489–495.

Mollica, M. A., Falisi, A. L., Geiger, A. M., Jacobsen, P. B., Lunsford, N. B., Pratt-Chapman, M. L., … Nekhlyudov, L. (2022b). Survivorship objectives in comprehensive cancer control plans: a systematic review. *Journal of Cancer Survivorship, 14*(2), 235–243.

NAPBC Standards and Resources. (2018). Available at https://www.facs.org/quality-programs/cancer-programs/national-accreditation-program-for-breast-centers/standards-and-resources/.

National Academies of Sciences, Engineering, and Medicine (NASEM). (2018). *Long-term survivorship care after cancer treatment: Proceedings of a workshop*. The National Academies Press.

National Accreditation Program for Breast Centers (NAPBC). (2017). *NAPBC standards manual, 2018 edition: standard 2.20, Breast cancer survivorship care*. Available at https://www.facs.org/media/pofgxojm/napbc_standards_manual_2018.pdf (accessed August 4, 2022).

National Cancer Institute (NCI) (2022). *Statistics: Office of Cancer Survivorship: Statistics and Graphs*. Available at https://cancercontrol.cancer.gov/ocs/statistics/statistics.html; last updated August 11, 2022 (accessed August 15, 2022).

National Coalition for Cancer Survivorship (NCCS). (2021). *State of survivorship survey: 2021*. Available at https://canceradvocacy.org/wp-content/uploads/NCCS-2021-Survivorship-Survey-Full-Report-Final.pdf (accessed August 4, 2022).

National Comprehensive Cancer Institute. (2022). *NCCN Clinical practice guidelines in oncology: Survivorship, version 1.2022*. Available at https://www.nccn.org/professionals/physician_gls/pdf/survivorship.pdf (accessed July 31, 2022).

National Institutes of Health (NIH). (2022). *Erin Hahn (PI): The EPICS (Engaging Primary care in Cancer Survivorship) study: A trial of novel models of care for cancer survivors*. Available at https://reporter.nih.gov/search/VngQzqZeF0WDK0a6iN1sqA/project-details/10418631.

NHS. (n.d.). *Innovation to implementation: Stratified pathways of care for people living with or beyond cancer—A 'how to guide'*. Available at https://www.england.nhs.uk/wp-content/uploads/2016/04/stratified-pathways-update.pdf.

Potosky, A., & Han, P. K. (2011). Differences between primary care physicians' and oncologists' knowledge, attitudes and practices regarding the care of cancer survivors. *Journal of General Internal Medicine, 26*(12), 1403–1410.

Siegel, R. L., Miller, K. D., Fuchs, H. E., & Jemal, A. (2021). Cancer statistics, 2021. *CA: A Cancer Journal for Clinicians, 71*(1), 7–33.

Snyder, C., Choi, Y., Blackford, A. L., DeSanto, J., Mayonado, N., Rall, S., … SSCP Stakeholder Advisory Board. (2022). Simplifying survivorship care planning: A randomized controlled trial comparing 3 care plan delivery approaches. *Journal of the National Cancer Institute, 114*(1), 139–148. https://doi.org/10.1093/jnci/djab148. PMID: 34302474; PMCID: PMC8755486.

Stricker, C. T. (2021). *Survivorship care challenges: Navigating changing concerns*. Plenary session at JADPRO LIVE, the Annual Meeting of the Advanced Practitioners' Society of Hematology Oncology (APSHO); October 2021 (virtual).

U.S. Department of Health and Human Services, Health Resources and Services Administration, National Center for Health Workforce Analysis. (2022). *Health workforce shortage areas*. U.S. Department of Health and Human Services. Available at https://data.hrsa.gov/topics/health-workforce/shortage-areas (accessed October 30, 2022).

Washko, M., Holt, M., Deal, A., Heiling, H., Hoover, R., & Mayer, D. K. (2022). Unmet needs in survivors on and off cancer treatment: A comparative survey. *Clinical Journal of Oncology Nursing, 26*(4), 335–342.

Palliative Care

Anna Weber

Introduction

Health care professionals usually are not as comfortable dealing with issues related to death and dying as they are with supporting the patient through curative treatment. Knowledge and skill in providing physical and emotional comfort to dying patients and their families are essential in providing optimal care to persons with advanced, progressive diseases. Palliative care is growing specialty that focuses on promoting the best possible quality of life (QOL) for patients facing life-threatening illness through optimal management of physical, psychosocial, emotional, and spiritual symptoms. This specialty grew out of the hospice movement and is continuing to evolve as more palliative care teams are integrated into health care systems, more palliative care content is taught in schools of medicine and nursing, and more research is conducted to support an evidence base for palliative interventions.

Definition

Palliative care is a philosophy of care and a highly organized system for delivering care. Palliative care focuses on expert assessment and management of pain and other symptoms, assessment and support of caregiver needs, and coordination of care. This specialized care attends to the physical, functional, psychological, practical, and spiritual consequences of a serious illness. It is a person- and family-centered approach to care, providing people living with serious illness relief from the symptoms and stress of an illness. Palliative care is inclusive of all people with serious illness, regardless of setting, diagnosis, prognosis, or age (National Consensus Project for Quality Palliative Care [NCP], 2018). Palliative care expands the traditional disease model of medical treatment to include the goals of enhancing QOL for the patient and family, optimizing function, assisting with decision-making, and providing opportunities for personal growth. It can be delivered concurrently with life-prolonging care or as the main focus of care. Palliative care is distinguished from routine symptom management by the following:

- The interdisciplinary approach
- Focus on physical, psychological, social, and spiritual needs
- Inclusion of the family in the unit of care

The box below summarizes the practice guidelines outlined by the NCP (2018).

Clinical Practice Guidelines for Quality Palliative Care

1. Structure and processes of care
   a. Since palliative care is holistic in nature, it is provided by a team of physicians, advanced practice registered nurses, physician assistants, nurses, social workers, chaplains, and others based on need. The palliative care team works with other clinicians and community service providers supporting continuity of care throughout the illness trajectory and across all settings, especially during transitions of care. Depending on care setting and patient population, interdisciplinary team (IDT) members may be certified palliative care specialists in their discipline and/or have additional training in palliative care. Primary care and other clinicians work with interdisciplinary colleagues to integrate palliative care into routine practice.
   b. An interdisciplinary comprehensive assessment of the patient and family forms the basis for the development of an individualized patient and family palliative care plan.
   c. In collaboration with the patient and family, the IDT develops, implements, and updates the care plan to anticipate, prevent, and treat physical, psychological, social, and spiritual needs.
   d. The IDT has defined processes to ensure access, quality, and continuity of care, especially during transitions of care.
   e. Palliative care is provided in any care setting, including private residences, assisted living facilities, rehabilitation, skilled and intermediate care facilities, acute and long-term care hospitals, clinics, hospice residences, correctional facilities, and homeless shelters.
   f. Education, training, and professional development are available to the IDT.
   g. Care is coordinated and characterized as the right care at the right time throughout the course of an individual's disease(s) or condition. The IDT recognizes that transitions of care occur within care settings, between care settings, and between care providers. Care transitions are anticipated, planned, and coordinated to ensure patient goals are achieved.
   h. Providing palliative care to patients with a serious illness and their families has an emotional impact, therefore the IDT creates an environment of resilience, self-care, and mutual support.
   i. In its commitment to continuous quality improvement, the IDT develops, implements, and maintains a data-driven process focused on patient- and family-centered outcomes using established quality improvement methodologies.
   j. Recognizing limitations in reimbursement for interdisciplinary palliative care, the IDT endeavors to secure funding for long-term sustainability and growth.
2. Physical aspects of care
   a. The palliative care IDT endeavors to relieve suffering and improve QOL, as defined by the patient and family, through the safe and timely reduction of the physical symptoms and functional impairment associated with serious illness.
   b. The IDT assesses physical symptoms and their impact on well-being, QOL, and functional status.
   c. Interdisciplinary care plans to address physical symptoms, maximize functional status, and enhance QOL are developed in the context of the patient's goals of care, disease, prognosis, functional limitations, culture, and care setting. An essential component of palliative care is ongoing management of physical symptoms, anticipating changes in health status, and monitoring of potential risk factors associated with the disease and side effects due to treatment regimens.

Clinical Practice Guidelines for Quality Palliative Care—cont'd

d. The palliative care team provides written and verbal recommendations for monitoring and managing physical symptoms.

3. Psychological and psychiatric aspects of care
   a. The IDT assesses and addresses psychological and psychiatric aspects of care based on the best available evidence to maximize patient and family coping and QOL.
   b. A core component of the palliative care program is a grief and bereavement program available to patients and families based on assessment of needs.

4. Social aspects of care
   a. The IDT includes a social worker with the knowledge and skills to assess and support mental health issues, provide emotional support, and address emotional distress and QOL for patients and families experiencing the expected responses to serious illness. The IDT has the training to assess and support those with mental health disorders, either directly, in consultation, or through referral to specialist level psychological and/or psychiatric care.
   b. The IDT screens for, assesses, and documents psychological and psychiatric aspects of care based upon the best available evidence to maximize patient and family coping and QOL.
   c. The IDT manages and/or supports psychological and psychiatric aspects of patient and family care including emotional, psychosocial, or existential distress related to the experience of serious illness, as well as identified mental health disorders. Psychological and psychiatric services are provided either directly, in consultation, or through referral to other providers.
   d. The IDT provides recommendations for monitoring and managing long-term and emerging psychological and psychiatric responses and mental health concerns.

5. Spiritual, religious, and existential aspects of care
   a. Patient and family spiritual beliefs and practices are assessed and respected. Palliative care professionals acknowledge their own spirituality as part of their professional role and are provided with education and support to address each patient's and family's spirituality.
   b. The spiritual assessment process has three distinct components—spiritual screening, spiritual history, and a full spiritual assessment. The spiritual screening is conducted with every patient and family to identify spiritual needs and/or distress. The history and assessment identify the spiritual background, preferences, and related beliefs, values, rituals, and practices of the patient and family. Symptoms, such as spiritual distress and spiritual strengths and resources, are identified and documented.
   c. The IDT addresses the spiritual needs of the patient and family.
   d. Patient and family spiritual care needs can change as the goals of care change or patients move across settings of care.

6. Cultural aspects of care
   a. The IDT delivers care that respects patient and family cultural beliefs, values, traditional practices, language, and communication preferences and builds upon the unique strengths of the patient and family. Members of the IDT works to increase awareness of their own biases and seeks opportunities to learn about the provision of culturally sensitive care. The care team ensures that its environment, policies, procedures, and practices are culturally respectful.
   b. The IDT ensures that patient and family preferred language and style of communication are supported and facilitated in all interactions.

c. The IDT uses evidence-based practices when screening and assessing patient and family cultural preferences regarding health care practices, customs, beliefs and values, level of health literacy, and preferred language.

d. A culturally sensitive plan of care is developed and discussed with the patient and/or family. This plan reflects the degree to which patients and families wish to be included as partners in decision-making regarding their care. When hosting meetings to discuss and develop the plan, the IDT ensures that patient and family linguistic needs are met.

7. Care of the patient at the end of life
   a. The IDT includes professionals with training in end-of-life care, including assessment and management of symptoms, communicating with patients and families about signs and symptoms of approaching death, transitions of care, and grief and bereavement. The IDT has established structures and processes to ensure appropriate care for patients and families when the end of life is imminent.
   b. The IDT assesses physical, psychological, social, and spiritual needs, as well as patient and family preferences for setting of care, treatment decisions, and wishes during and immediately following death. Discussions with the family focus on honoring patient wishes and attending to family fears and concerns about the end of life. The IDT prepares and supports family caregivers throughout the dying process, taking into account the spiritual and cultural background and preferences of the patient and family.
   c. In collaboration with the patient and family and other clinicians, the IDT develops, implements, and updates (as needed) a care plan to anticipate, prevent, and treat physical, psychological, social, and spiritual symptoms. The care plan addresses the focus on end-of-life care and treatments to meet the physical, emotional, social, and spiritual needs of patients and families. All treatment is provided in a culturally and developmentally appropriate manner.
   d. During the dying process, patient and family needs are respected and supported. Post-death care is delivered in a manner that honors patient and family cultural and spiritual beliefs, values, and practices.
   e. Bereavement support is available to the family and care team, either directly or through referral. The IDT identifies or provides resources, including grief counseling, spiritual support, or peer support, specific to the assessed needs. Prepared in advance of the patient's death, the bereavement care plan is activated after the death of the patient and addresses immediate and longer-term needs.

8. Ethical and legal aspects of care
   a. The core ethical principles of autonomy, substituted judgment, beneficence, justice, and nonmaleficence underpin the provision of palliative care.
   b. The provision of palliative care occurs in accordance with federal, state, and local regulations and laws, as well as current accepted standards of care and professional practice.
   c. The patient's preferences and goals for medical care are elicited using core ethical principles and documented.
   d. Within the limits of applicable state and federal laws, current accepted standards of medical care, and professional standards of practice, person-centered goals form the basis for the plan of care and decisions related to providing, forgoing, and discontinuing treatments.

Data from National Consensus Project for Quality Palliative Care. (2018). *Clinical practice guidelines for quality palliative care* (4th ed.). Richmond, PA: National Coalition for Hospice and Palliative Care. Available at https://www.nationalcoalitionhpc.org/ncp.

Palliative care should be initiated at the diagnosis of a life-threatening or chronic, progressive illness and continued throughout the course of the illness across all care settings. As illustrated in the figure on the next page, palliative care is started along with life-prolonging therapies at the initial diagnosis of a life-threatening illness. As the disease progresses, there is greater emphasis on palliative interventions than life-prolonging interventions. Hospice care is part of the palliative care continuum when the emphasis is no longer on life prolongation but primarily on comfort. In the United States, this is often defined as the last 6 months of life and is based on the eligibility requirements for hospice benefits under Medicare.

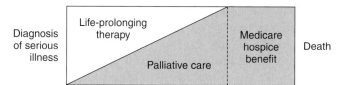

Palliative Care's Place in the Course of Illness. (From National Consensus Project for Quality Palliative Care. [2018]. *Clinical practice guidelines for quality palliative care* [4th ed.]. Pittsburgh, PA: National Coalition for Hospice and Palliative Care.)

Palliative Care in Persons With Cancer

Palliative care and its many components are beneficial to patient and family health and well-being. Integrating palliative care into a patient's usual cancer care soon after a diagnosis of advanced cancer can improve their QOL and mood, and may even prolong survival (National Cancer Institute, 2021). The expertise of the palliative care IDT can be especially helpful in four key areas (Ramchandran & von Roenn, 2013):

- Advanced disease with a prognosis of less than 1 year
- Significant symptom burden from the disease or from treatment
- Significant social or psychological distress
- Poor functional status

Models of Palliative Care Delivery

Palliative care services are most effective when integrated into the care setting. Various models are used to facilitate access to the expertise of the palliative care team and include one or some combination of the following:

- Internal consultation team in an acute or rehabilitation hospital, nursing home, or free-standing inpatient hospice
- External consultation team in an acute or rehabilitation hospital, nursing home, or free-standing inpatient hospice
- Dedicated inpatient unit in an acute or rehabilitation hospital, nursing home, or free-standing inpatient hospice
- Hospital- or private practice–based outpatient palliative care practice or clinic
- Hospice- or private practice–based palliative care in the home care setting

Hospice and Palliative Care

The figure above illustrates that hospice care is part of the palliative care continuum when life-prolonging therapies are no longer providing benefit. The focus of care is on comfort and quality of living by affirming life and viewing dying as a normal process. Services provided by the hospice IDT include pain and symptom management, psychosocial and spiritual support, assistance and support with direct caregiving, and bereavement care for the patient and family. The practice guidelines outlined by the NCP (2018) (see box in the next column) also apply to the organized, comprehensive services available through hospice programs.

The Hospice Medicare Benefit

Eligibility Criteria (Required of the Patient)

- Have Medicare Part A
- Be certified as having a terminal diagnosis with a prognosis of 6 months or less by a physician
- Accept palliative care (for comfort) instead of care to cure the illness
- Choose hospice care instead of other Medicare-covered treatments for the terminal illness and related conditions
- Enroll in a Medicare-approved hospice program

Services Covered (All Services for the Terminal Illness)

- Physician services
- Nursing care
- Medical equipment
- Medical supplies
- Prescription drugs
- Hospice aide and homemaker services
- Physical and occupational therapy
- Speech-language pathology services
- Social work services
- Dietary counseling
- Grief and loss counseling for the patient and family
- Short-term inpatient care (for pain and symptom management)
- Short-term respite care
- Any other Medicare-covered services needed to manage the terminal illness and related conditions, as recommended by the hospice team

Services Not Covered

- Treatment intended to cure the terminal illness and/or related conditions
- Prescription drugs (except for symptom control or pain relief)
- Care from any provider that is not arranged by the hospice medical team
- Room and board
- Care in an emergency room, inpatient facility care, or ambulance transportation that is not arranged by the hospice team or is unrelated to the terminal illness and related conditions

Benefit Period

- There are two 90-day periods followed by an unlimited number of 60-day periods.
- At the start of each period of care, the hospice medical director or other hospice doctor must recertify that the patient is terminally ill.

Payment for Service

- Hospice programs are paid a per diem rate to provide all the services, and there is no deductible.
- The patient may be required to pay a copayment of up to $5 per prescription for outpatient prescription drugs for pain and symptom management.
- The patient may be required to pay 5% of the Medicare-approved amount for inpatient respite care.

From Centers for Medicare and Medicaid Services. (2021). *Medicare and hospice benefits*. CMS Product No. 11361. Baltimore, MD: U.S. Department of Health and Human Services. Available at https://www.medicare.gov/Pubs/pdf/11361-Medicare-Hospice-Getting-Started.pdf (accessed December 17, 2021).

Medicare, some state Medicaid programs, and some private insurance companies require that patients have a prognosis of 6 months or less to be eligible for hospice services. However, the median length of stay in hospice programs in 2019 was only 18 days (National Hospice and Palliative Care Organization, 2021). Barriers that interfere with initial and timely referrals to hospice programs include the following (Friedman et al., 2002):

- Discomfort in discussing end-of-life care issues by patients, family members, and health care professionals
- Difficulty in determining a prognosis of 6 months or less
- Lack of information or misinformation about hospice care by patients, family members, and health care providers

- Real or perceived requirement to discontinue life-prolonging therapies to receive hospice services

Eligibility requirements and an outline of the services provided under the Medicare hospice benefit are listed in the box on the previous page. Hospices receive a per diem rate from Medicare to pay for all services related to the terminal illness. Traditional Medicare coverage remains in place for services related to problems other than the identified terminal illness. Many private insurance companies have hospice benefits that are similar to those provided under Medicare.

The services from hospice programs are much more comprehensive than can be provided under a traditional home care insurance benefit, giving the patient and family more physical, clinical, psychosocial, emotional, and spiritual support over a longer period of time than is available under other benefits. Patients whose residence is a long-term care facility receive these same benefits in addition to the services provided by the facility.

Services not paid for under the Medicare hospice benefit include the following:

- Treatment or medications intended to cure the terminal illness rather than for symptom control
- Care from any provider or in any facility that is not arranged by the hospice team
- Room and board

Because Medicare does not pay for room and board at nursing homes, patients who qualify for skilled care in a long-term care facility may have less out-of-pocket expense by using their "skilled days" before enrolling in a hospice program. This is unfortunate because many of these patients and families could benefit from the expertise and support of the hospice team during this difficult time. Palliative care teams in long-term care facilities, when available, can address the symptom management and support needs of this population of patients.

References

Friedman, B., Harwood, K., & Shields, M. (2002). Barriers and enablers to hospice referrals: An expert overview. *Journal of Palliative Medicine, 5,* 73–81.

National Cancer Institute. (2021). *Palliative care in cancer.* Available at https://www.cancer.gov/about-cancer/advanced-cancer/care-choices/palliative-care-fact-sheet (accessed December 1, 2021).

National Consensus Project for Quality Palliative Care (NCP). (2018). *Clinical practice guidelines for quality palliative care* (4th ed.). Pittsburgh, PA: National Coalition for Hospice and Palliative Care. Available at https://www.nationalcoalitionhpc.org/wp-content/uploads/2020/07/NCHPC-NCPGuidelines_4thED_web_FINAL.pdf (accessed December 1, 2021).

National Hospice and Palliative Care Organization. (2021). *NHPCO's facts and figures.* Available at https://www.nhpco.org/hospice-care-overview/hospice-facts-figures/ (accessed December 2, 2021).

Ramchandran, K. J., & von Roenn, J. H. (2013). What is the role for palliative care in patients with advanced cancer? In N. E. Goldstein & R. S. Morrison (Eds.), *Evidence-based practice of palliative medicine* (pp. 276–280). Philadelphia: Elsevier.

Bibliography

Ferrell, B., Coyle, N., & Paice, J. A. (2015). *Oxford textbook of palliative nursing* (4th ed.). New York: Oxford University Press.

Goldstein, N. E., & Morrison, R. S. (2013). *Evidence-based practice of palliative medicine.* Philadelphia: Elsevier Saunders.

Final Hours

Mary E. Murphy and Terri Gross

Introduction

Patients in the final hours and days before death may experience a variety of emotional, psychosocial, spiritual, and physical symptoms. Patients, families, health care workers, and physicians may misdiagnose or refuse to identify the signs and symptoms of imminent death. Barriers include the diagnosis, age, religion, and moral beliefs, along with denial and apprehension about discussing the dying process or ongoing treatment options.

Failure to identify a patient's terminal state may lead to inappropriate diagnostic testing, futile treatment, and mismanagement of end-of-life symptoms that would be better managed with palliative or hospice care. Estimation of a short-term prognosis may be complex because of the diagnosis, disease trajectory, and patient and care provider's emotional value system. An honest conversation about functional decline and prognosis is needed to allow the patient and family to identify their goals of care.

Similar physical and psychosocial characteristics are seen during the final weeks, days, and hours of a patient's life. The period is often divided into two major categories: the preactive phase and the active phase of dying. The following symptoms are seen during the preactive phase, which is 7 to 14 days before death.

- Increased weakness
- Need for assistance with activities of daily living increasing to total care needs
- Bed-to-chair or bed-bound status
- Increased sleeping
- Disorientation, confusion, or episodes of near-death awareness
- Decreasing food and fluid intake
- Fever
- Incontinence of bowel and bladder/constipation or urinary retention
- Swallowing difficulty, including a need to discontinue or alter the route of medication
- Restlessness, agitation, withdrawal, loss of bowel and bladder control, withdrawal from family and friends, fear of the dying process, or asking when it will happen
- Increased spiritual needs, visions of deceased friends and family members
- Family and caregiver fatigue

The following symptoms are seen during the active phase, which is 2 to 3 days before death:
- Altered vital signs
  - Lowered blood pressure
  - Lowered or elevated temperature
  - Abnormal respiratory pattern (e.g., apnea, Cheyne-Stokes breathing)
  - Heart rate (i.e., faded, muffled, or rapid)
- Decreased level of consciousness
- Terminal respiratory congestion
- Cool, dusky, or mottled skin
- Decreased responsiveness to external stimuli
- Limited oral intake
- Restlessness, agitation, staring, disconnectedness, viewing of environment from a distance (symptoms vary according to the person and time of the event, but some patients experience last-minute surges of energy)
- Crying out, moaning, whimpering when touched
- Pain
- Urinary or bowel incontinence

Nursing Considerations Before Death

Discuss the following issues with the patient or family members:
- Review advance directives and durable power of attorney for health care (DPOA-HC) status and code status.
- Review with the patient and family the DPOA for financial issues.
- Review wishes about the desire for an autopsy and cremation or burial. Offer resources for funeral plans and phone numbers.
- Explore the family's need to be present at the time of death and obtain list of family members to call. Obtain information on how far from the patient the family is located to determine if the request can be achieved.
- Review goals of care such as palliation or active treatment.
- Address hydration and feeding concerns.
- Review signs and symptoms of the terminal phase.
- Review treatment and medication modalities to relieve symptoms. Avoid the use of medical jargon. Offer open, honest, and supportive concern.
- Provide a supportive environment in which to deliver bad news.
- Be aware of rituals, traditions, and rites that may be important to care or related to religious or cultural beliefs.
- Support storytelling and journaling.
- Identify what support is available at the time of death and in the days following.
- Address unfinished business, goals, or family concerns.
- Check for potential posttraumatic stress disorder (PTSD) concerns.
- Coach families in distress to accomplish four tasks:
  - Ask for forgiveness

- Say thank you
- Say I love you
- Say good-bye

Palliative Therapy Options for End-of-Life Patients

Pain Management

- Use observation scales (e.g., Universal Pain Assessment tool, Pain Assessment in Advanced Dementia [PAINAD]) that are appropriate to the level of alertness and current situation and are approved at the facility where the staff members are working.
- Never discontinue opioids or benzodiazepines if unable to swallow them. Seek alternative routes to provide patient comfort.

Dyspnea

- Use oxygen for support.
- Elevate the head of the bed.
- Suction mildly as needed.
- Use benzodiazepines and low-dose opioids.

Dehydration

- Provide mouth and lip care.
- Offer sips of fluids as appropriate.
- Discuss food and fluid issues.

Incontinence

- Provide skin care.
- Use a Foley catheter (assess for bladder distention).
- Use incontinence barriers.
- Provide manual impaction removal with the use of a suppository only if the patient has distention and discomfort.

Confusion and Agitation

- Use benzodiazepines and phenothiazines.

Respiratory Congestion or Death Rattle

- Suction only if necessary.
- Elevate the head of the bed.
- Manage medications:
  - Hyoscyamine (Levsin)
  - Atropine
  - Scopolamine

Physical Care

- Provide mouth care.
- Continue turning and positioning for comfort.
- Provide skin care.
- Provide safety.
- Provide emotional care.
- Provide a quiet environment or sounds that are comforting (e.g., tapes, voices).
- Engage in storytelling (i.e., past pleasant events).
- Call the patient by name.
- Explain who is in the room, and state who you are and what you will be doing.

Special Considerations

- Increased preparation is needed for some diagnoses and expected symptoms:
  - Hemorrhage
  - Seizures
  - Severe and uncontrolled terminal agitation
  - Children or younger patients
  - PTSD
  - Management of severe symptoms, for example, pain, nausea, vomiting, dyspnea, obstructed airway

Nursing Care After Death

- Clarify who needs to be present or notified before the body is removed.
- Determine whether any ritual (e.g., poem, prayer) should take place.
- Remove personal items (e.g., rings, hair) and document who they were given to or where they were secured.
- Offer support services based on individual or family religious values and support systems.
- Identify ongoing support needs as well as high-risk needs and resources.
- Prepare the body.
- Say final good-byes.

Last-Minute Concerns

- No one can predict the time of death, which may be associated with symptoms, significant events in the patient's life (e.g., birthdays, holidays, anniversaries), or other events that are outside of everyone's control.

Bibliography

American Association of Colleges of Nursing. (2020). End of Life Nursing Education Consortium (ELNEC). Available at www.aacnnursing.org/ELNEC (accessed December 19, 2021).

Bobb, B. T. (2015). Urgent syndromes at the end of life. In B. Ferrell, et al. (Eds.), *Care of the imminently dying*, HPNA palliative nursing manuals (online ed.). New York: Oxford Academic. Available at https://doi.org/10.1093/med/9780190244286.003.0003 (accessed March 15, 2023).

Byock, I. (1997). *Dying well: The prospects for growth at end-of-life*. Riverhead Press.

Campbell, M., Donesky, D., Sarkosy, A., & Reinke, L. F. (2021). Treatment of dyspnea in advanced disease and at the end of life. *Journal of Hospice and Palliative Care*, 23(5), 406–420.

Dudgeon, D. (2015). Dyspnea, death rattle, and cough. In B. Ferrell, et al. (Eds.), *Care of the imminently dying*, HPNA palliative nursing manuals (online ed.). New York: Oxford Academic. Available at https://doi.org/10.1093/med/9780190244286.003.0002 (accessed March 15, 2023).

Heidrich, D. E., & English, N. K. (2015). Delirium. In B. Ferrell, et al. (Eds.), *Care of the imminently dying*, HPNA palliative nursing manuals (online ed.). New York: Oxford Academic. Available at https://doi.org/10.1093/med/9780190244286.003.0001 (accessed March 15, 2023).

Huang, L., Tai, C., Longcoy, J., & McMillan, S. C. (2021). The mutual effects of perceived spiritual needs on quality of life in patients with advanced cancer and family caregivers. *Journal of Hospice and Palliative Care*, 23(4), 323–330.

National Coalition for Hospice and Palliative Care, Clinical Practice Guidelines for Quality Palliative Care. (2018). *Care of the patient nearing end of life* (4th ed.). Available at Nchr_NCPGGUIDLINES_4th ED WEB_final.pdf. Domain 7 (accessed December 19, 2021).

National Institute on Aging. (2017). Providing care and comfort at end of life. Available at www.nia.nih.gov (accessed December 19, 2021).

Loss, Grief, and Bereavement

Anna Weber

Introduction

People with cancer and their family members experience multiple losses throughout the cancer experience, including body image changes, loss of control over time and schedules, loss of the ability to fulfill usual roles at work or home, and the ultimate loss of life. Grief is a normal and expected reaction to these losses. Oncology nurses play an important role in supporting individuals through the normal grieving process and in identifying individuals who may require additional support for complicated grief.

Definition

Several terms are used when discussing grief and bereavement (Corless & Meisenhelder, 2019; Rando, 1984; Shear, 2015).
- *Loss:* The absence of an object, position, ability, or attribute
- *Grief:* The psychological, social, and somatic responses to loss
- *Anticipatory grief:* The psychological, social, and somatic responses to an anticipated loss
- *Mourning:* The outward and active expression of grief through participation in various death and bereavement rituals that vary by culture.
- *Bereavement:* The state of having suffered a loss or the period of time during which grief and mourning occur; the first year after a loss is usually the most difficult.
- *Complicated grief:* Intense grief after the death of a loved one that lasts longer than expected according to social norms and causes functional impairment.
  Many factors affect grief and bereavement:
- Support systems (e.g., children, organizations, family)
- Previous experiences
- Suddenness of the event
- Coping mechanisms
- Relation to and significance of the person or event
- Knowledge and understanding
- Timing of the event
- Life sequence of the event
- Concurrent stresses
- Rituals and expectations
- Religion, spirituality, and culture
- Boundaries
- Financial burden or support
- Events from diagnosis to death
- Role in the family and community
- Personal value system (e.g., body image, self-concept)
- Role in the family (i.e., internal or external)
- Perception of the loss, esteem, or identity
- Future goals (i.e., what will not be)

Normal Manifestations of Grief

Manifestations of grief include social, physical, and cognitive-emotional reactions, which can vary widely from one individual to another. There is no right way to grieve.

Social Manifestations
- Restlessness and inability to sit still
- Feeling uncomfortable around other people or social withdrawal
- Feeling of not wanting to be alone
- Lack of ability to initiate and maintain organized patterns of activity

Physical Manifestations
- Anorexia and weight loss or overeating and weight gain
- Heart palpitations, nervousness, tension, or panic
- Shortness of breath
- Tightness in the throat
- Inability to sleep
- Lack of energy and feelings of physical exhaustion
- Headaches, muscular aches, and gastrointestinal distress

Cognitive-Emotional Manifestations
- Sadness and crying
- Forgetfulness or difficulty concentrating
- Feelings of anger or guilt
- Mood swings
- Sense of helplessness
- Yearning for the deceased
- Dreams of the deceased

Grief Theories

Grief theories provide a framework to help explain an individual's response to grief and the process of adjusting to a loss. The following three theories show the evolution of our understanding of the grief process.
1. *Stages of grief:* Denial, anger, bargaining, depression, and acceptance (Kübler-Ross, 1969).
2. *Tasks of grief work:* Accept reality of loss, experience the pain of the loss, adjust to the environment without the deceased person, and withdraw emotionally from the deceased by forming an ongoing relationship with the memories of the deceased in a way that allows the individual to continue with life (Worden, 2018).
3. *Dual-process model of coping with bereavement:* Understanding the dynamic nature of grief as involving oscillation between loss-oriented coping (i.e., working through the loss) and restoration-oriented coping (i.e., mastering new tasks, reorganizing life, and developing a new identity) (Stroebe & Schut, 2010).

Complicated Grief

- *Prolonged grief:* Persistent and severe yearning for the deceased beyond 6 months after the loss (Killikelly & Maercker, 2018). Prolonged grief disorder is recognized as a mental disorder causing significant distress and disability, and it is included in the *Diagnostic and Statistical Manual of Mental Disorders*, 5th ed. (DSM-V). Given disagreement about the definitions of complicated grief and prolonged grief, the DSM-V created another disorder called persistent complex bereavement disorder, listed in the appendix as a disorder requiring further study (American Psychiatric Association, 2013).
- *Disenfranchised grief:* Grief that occurs when the loss cannot be openly acknowledged. Examples of disenfranchised grief include the death of a person in a nonsanctioned relationship (e.g., extramarital affair, homosexual partner), loss from miscarriage or abortion, or the loss of the essence of the individual before the actual death, such as with severe dementia (Doka, 2002).

Support and Counseling

Facilitating uncomplicated grief for persons after loss can be provided using 10 principles described by Worden (2018).
- Help the survivor actualize the loss
- Help the survivor identify and experience feelings
- Assist living without the deceased
- Help find meaning in the loss
- Help find ways to remember the deceased
- Provide time to grieve
- Interpret normal behavior
- Allow for individual differences
- Examine defenses and coping styles
- Identify pathology and refer

References

American Psychiatric Association. (2013). *Diagnostic and statistical manual of mental disorders* (5th ed.). Washington, DC: American Psychiatric Association.

Corless, I. B., & Meisenhelder, J. B. (2019). Bereavement. In B. R. Ferrell, N. Coyle, & J. A. Paice (Eds.), *Oxford textbook of palliative nursing* (5th ed.). New York: Oxford University Press.

Doka, K. J. (2002). *Disenfranchised grief: New directions, challenges, and strategies for practice.* Research Press.

Killikelly, C., & Maercker, A. (2018). Prolonged grief disorder for ICD-11: The primacy of clinical utility and international applicability. *European Journal of Psychotraumatology, 8*(Suppl 6), 1476441.

Kübler-Ross, E. (1969). *On death and dying.* New York: Macmillan.

Rando, T. (1984). *Grief, dying, and death: Clinical interventions for caregivers.* Champaign, IL: Research Press Company.

Shear, M. K. (2015). Complicated grief. *New England Journal of Medicine, 372*(2), 153–160.

Stroebe, M., & Schut, H. (2010). The dual process model of coping with bereavement: A decade on. *Omega, 61,* 273–389.

Worden, J. W. (2018). *Grief counseling and grief therapy* (5th edition): *A handbook for the mental health practitioner.* New York, NY: Springer Publishing Company.

Communication

Lisa Kennedy Sheldon

Communication and Patient-Centered Care

Communication between health care providers and patients is the foundation of high-quality cancer care. Whether verbal, written, or virtual, these skills are especially important for oncology clinicians, who must regularly adjust their approach to meet the changing physiologic and psychosocial needs of patients after a cancer diagnosis. To promote comprehensive care, timely communication is needed among the members of interprofessional oncology team as well as with primary care providers and specialists in palliative and end-of-life care.

Effective communication in cancer care links specific provider behaviors with patient outcomes (de Haes & Bensing, 2009; Street et al., 2009). For example, when providers share information with patients, the desired outcome is increased patient autonomy and decision making; however, too much information may increase patient uncertainty and anxiety. Communication by clinicians requires a balance between delivering factual information about managing the disease and compassionately talking with patients about their concerns (Eggly et al., 2009). Patient-provider communication should be tailored to the needs—physical, emotional, spiritual, decisional—of patients and caregivers (Li et al., 2020).

According to the sentinel Institute of Medicine (IOM) publication, patient-clinician communication in cancer care has six main functions (Epstein & Street, 2007):
1. Fostering healing relationships
2. Exchanging information
3. Responding to emotions
4. Managing uncertainty
5. Making decisions
6. Enabling patient self-management

Oncology clinicians use verbal and nonverbal skills to promote trust with patients and provide an atmosphere in which patients are comfortable asking questions and sharing concerns. It is well known that communication between people occurs both verbally with written and spoken words, and nonverbally (e.g., body posture, facial expressions). It is important that providers tailor their verbal and nonverbal communication to the individual patient incorporating values, beliefs, culture, ethnicity, and preferred method of communicating. In addition, communication should address health and technological literacy, especially if communication occurs via virtual means such as telehealth. Finally, including the patients' caregivers in important discussions provides additional support for patients and information about the needs outside of the hospital setting.

Nonverbal cues from patients often contain essential information about their condition and concerns that enhance what is communicated verbally. It is interesting that nonverbal behaviors such as body posture or eye glances may indicate patient concerns. Sometimes nonverbal cues such as guarding or bracing may indicate symptoms such as pain or dyspnea. For example, a subdued demeanor with lack of eye contact may indicate deeper emotions and concerns. Information from verbal and nonverbal cues provides a more comprehensive picture of the patient that can help to direct assessment and interventions. Interpreting nonverbal cues may be more challenging with telehealth strategies as only the head and shoulders may be in the frame. On the other hand, family members or caregivers may also be present and contribute information that enhances clinician understanding of the patient's issues.

Telehealth and Communication

Providers can promote effective communication in a variety of modalities during face-to-face and telehealth encounters, and electronic health records (see the table on the next page). Nurses have used forms of telehealth such as telephone triage for decades. The coronavirus pandemic of 2020 rapidly increased the use of telehealth modalities to reach patients during the public health emergency. Most nurses have not been specifically trained in what has been called "webside manner" (Warshaw, 2018) as the abilities needed to deliver care remotely through monitors or other mobile devices. This skill set is being studied and incorporated into the education of health care providers including nurses. Key elements include how to position a video camera, maintain eye contact, and effectively engage patients and family members. In addition, assessment may include the use of digital monitoring to provide additional information.

7

Behaviors by Oncology Clinicians That Promote or Inhibit Communication

Promote Communication	Inhibit Communication
Body posture and camera angle, such as facing the patient, closer distance (as culturally appropriate), leaning forward, sitting centered in the screen	Greater distance, blocking with the computer, crossed arms
Direct eye gaze to patient or camera (as culturally appropriate)	Looking away or at a chart or computer screen, not staying in the screen
Pauses and listens	Interrupting the patient, speaking faster, dominating the conversation content
More expression in voice and face, nodding	Greater distance, less expression, loud voice
Smiling	Less or no smiling
Open-ended questions	Dominating conversation, limiting questions
Soliciting the patient's expectations, goals of care and preferences, determining advanced care directives	Telling the patient options without asking about preferences
Use of questions about emotions or concerns	Providing factual information and directing the focus of the conversation
Promoting partnership, building with the patient	Providing information and prescribing treatment

In oncology care, communicating with patients and families occurs primarily around four areas:

1. Information about diagnosis, treatment, and symptom management
2. Education about treatment plan
3. Assessment of psychosocial and emotional responses to the disease, treatment, symptoms, and prognosis
4. Discussions about patient preferences and values, goals of care, and advanced care planning

Information Sharing

Oncology providers provide information with patients that promotes shared decision making. Cancer care can be complex making tailored communication essential for patient understanding for informed treatment decision making. As specialists in cancer care, providers must interpret and clearly share information in words that are appropriate for patients' language and literacy levels. For example, for clinicians, a *positive biopsy result* means that evidence of disease has been found, but the term may be misinterpreted as a good finding or indicating absence of disease by people not in health care professions. In addition, survivorship care involves sharing follow-up plans for monitoring, primary care and selfcare, requiring engaged patients and written communication such as treatment summaries and survivorship care plans. Both visits and documentation improve the delivery of coordinated and comprehensive care.

It is important to understand the patient's knowledge about cancer and treatment and preferences for care delivery. For example, the clinician should ask for permission from patients to discuss their condition. For example, the clinician may inquire, "Tell me what you know about your illness." When patients are not receptive to having a discussion about their illness, the next question becomes, "With whom would you like me to talk?" It is important to explore the patient's usual decision-making practices, such as consulting with family or clergy. Questions might include:

- How do you make decisions?
- Whom do you include in making decisions?
- If you cannot make decisions, who will make them for you?

Education About Treatment Plan

Patient education about treatment is essential to promote adherence, set realistic expectations, and improve patient outcomes. This is increasingly important due to numerous treatment options including oral therapies and home infusions. Information can be shared verbally in a conversation and then reinforced with written material, videos, telehealth visits, or internet resources. Confirmation is an important step to ensure patients have the information they need to make decisions about their care and improve self-management of treatment regimen and communicate symptoms and adverse events. To check that the patient has understood the message, the provider may say, "Talk with me about your understanding of the diagnosis" or "Tell me what you understand about what we have discussed so far." These open-ended statements allow patients to describe their level of understanding in their own words and provide a foundation for the next steps in the conversation such as clarification or additional information to fill gaps.

Psychosocial and Emotional Responses

Oncology providers care for people adjusting to changes in health, adapting to a cancer diagnosis and treatment and new expectations for the future. By virtue of the time spent with patients, nurses often hear patients' psychosocial concerns. This is especially true at vulnerable points in the cancer trajectory such as new diagnosis, cancer recurrence, changes in treatment or withdrawal of treatment, when patients and families are prone to more anxiety and fear. Oncology nurses have an obligation to assess patient concerns at these vulnerable points and during routine care (see box below).

Vulnerable Points

1. Waiting for diagnostic and genetic test results
2. Giving the diagnosis
3. Discussing prognosis, survival, and treatment plan
4. Sharing "bad news" when the disease recurs or progresses, the treatment no longer is effective, or there is new metastatic disease
5. Assessing new symptoms or severe adverse effects of treatment
6. Stopping active treatment and transitioning to end-of-life and hospice care

Oncology nurses have a critical role in communication with patients and caregivers. They spend the most time in direct contact with patients during care delivery. Some of these conversations may be around difficult topics such as advancing disease, ineffective treatment, or uncontrolled symptoms. Wittenberg et al. (2018) describe the COMFORT curriculum as one method to train nurses in key communication skills around difficult topics. This curriculum focuses on whole patient assessment and includes eliciting the patient's story, addressing health literacy needs, being mindful of clinician burnout, and communicating with both the patient and caregivers.

Discussions occurring at vulnerable points along the care trajectory are sometimes called *bad news conversations*. The SPIKES protocol can provide structure for the delivery of difficult information during these conversations (Baile et al., 2000).

S (setting): Use privacy and quietness, include all parties who need to be there, and prevent distractions.

P (perception): Assess what the patient and family know and their perceptions of the situation first. Ask open-ended questions such as the following:

"What is your understanding of why your family member is in the hospital?"

"What have you been told about your illness?"

"How do you feel the treatment has been working?"

I (invitation or information): Ask directly how much and what kind of information the patient and family wish to know.

K (knowledge): Communicate the bad news honestly while being direct and caring, provide information in small segments, and check for comprehension.

E (empathy): Acknowledge and validate the emotions and reactions; use active listening.

S (summarize and strategize): Review what was said; ensure and verify comprehension; and present plan for further intervention, treatment, palliation, or hospice.

Assessment of Psychosocial Concerns

People often have emotional and psychological responses to a diagnosis of cancer. The IOM emphasized psychosocial care for patients in its landmark 2007 report: *Cancer Care for the Whole Patient: Meeting Psychosocial Health Needs* (IOM, 2007). In addition, accreditation standards for cancer centers have been developed by the American College of Surgeons Commission on Cancer (2020a, 2020b) and include assessment of psychosocial concerns of people with a diagnosis of cancer and a referral pathway for those with significant distress.

Psychosocial assessment requires tools that measure concerns and detect significant distress. For example, the National Comprehensive Cancer Network (NCCN) has been advocating for screening of distress since 1999 and created a tool, the distress thermometer, for use in clinical practice (NCCN, 2021). It contains a visual scale of 0 (no distress) to 10 (extreme distress) displayed on a thermometer. If a patient scores 4 or higher on the scale, referrals and interventions are warranted to address specific concerns. The tool also has 38 items for practical, family, emotional, spiritual or religious, or physical problems. Because of the simplicity of the tool, oncology nurses can administer it and refer to the primary oncology team for distress levels of 4 or higher or unrelieved physical symptoms.

More specific tools are available for assessing specific conditions such as the Patient Health Questionnaire (PHQ-9) for depression (Spitzer et al., 1999) (see box below).

Measures of Distress, Anxiety, Depression, Fear, and Worry

- National Comprehensive Cancer Network (NCCN) Distress Thermometer (DT)
- Hospital Anxiety and Depression Scale (HADS)
- State Trait Anxiety Inventory (STAI)
- Center for Epidemiologic Studies Depression (CES-D)
- Beck Depression Inventory
- Structured Clinical Interview
- Functional Assessment of Cancer Treatment (FACT)
- Worry Scale
- Fear Questionnaire
- Padua Inventory

Assessment of concerns requires evidence-based approaches to assessment, treatment, and referral of significant psychosocial issues. The NCCN (2021) and the American Society of Clinical Oncology (ASCO, 2014) have developed evidence-based guidelines to assess and manage distress including anxiety and depression associated with cancer.

The NCCN Distress Thermometer (NCCN, 2021) (0 = no distress to 10 = extreme distress) is commonly used in clinical settings. It enables discussion and treatment of distress as part of routine care. The thermometer includes a corresponding list of problems to determine if a patient's distress arises from practical problems, family problems, emotional problems, spiritual/religious concerns, and/or physical problems or symptoms. This free resource is translated into 46 languages for global accessibility.

In 2014, ASCO released a new evidence-based clinical practice guideline on managing depression and anxiety in adult patients with cancer. This guideline was adapted from the Pan-Canadian Practice Guideline: Screening, Assessment and Care of Psychosocial Distress (Depression, Anxiety) in Adults With Cancer (NCCN, 2021).

Specific aspects of communication between patients and clinicians may improve assessment and detection of psychosocial concerns. For example, patients are more descriptive about their concerns if a clinician initiates the conversation (Heyn et al., 2013). In another study, patients who expressed their concerns more often and those expressing more explicit emotion were more likely to have their concerns assessed and treated (Sheldon et al., 2015). Nurses can play an active role in initiating discussions about psychosocial concerns including self-report tools and encourage their patients to speak about their concerns, allowing the oncology team to further assess patient needs.

Responding to Concerns

Deciding on the appropriate interventions to respond to patient concerns is based on evidence-based strategies and clinician experience. Promoting patient-centered communication in cancer care should give emphasis to responding and managing patients' emotions. Providers should assess, recognize, and elicit patients' emotional concerns and develop emotional regulation skills among patients and improve their ability to cope with emotional distress (Sardessai-Nadkarni & Street, 2022).

One common concern of oncology providers is how to react to negative emotions such as anger or profound sadness. Some of the most effective strategies for providers include nonverbal skills such as psychological availability, presence, respect, listening, eye contact, and touch as appropriate. However, strong emotions from patients may also prompt emotional responses in providers that may impede therapeutic communication. Specific communication skills may be useful in addressing emotion during conversations with patients. The NURSE mnemonic may be applied in these situations (Kaplan, 2010) (see box below).

NURSE Mnemonic for Responding to Emotions

N: Name the emotion or feeling expressed by the patient.
"What I said made you … [emotion]."
"You seem ….[emotion] today."

U: Understand or acknowledge the emotional reaction as reasonable.
"Given what you have been through, it is understandable that you would be …..[emotion]."

R: Respect the patient's abilities and challenges.
"You have been through a lot and were able to care for yourself and your family."
"It's probably frustrating not to be able to work like you always have."

S: Supportive statements demonstrate that the provider is prepared to support the patient.
"I am here to help you."
"Let me know what you need."

E: Ask the patient to elaborate the emotion.
"Tell me more about how being sad affects you."
"What do you do when you feel this way?"

The NURSE mnemonic is a guide to provide structure during emotionally laden conversations, making it easier for providers to continue the conversation. Providers may not always agree with patients' responses, but they can continue to demonstrate understanding, and respect, and provide support. The NURSE therapeutic responses express respect and appreciation for the patient's abilities to cope with difficult situations.

Uncertainty

Living after a cancer diagnosis means learning strategies to live with uncertainty. Patients may fear recurrence, uncontrolled symptoms such as pain, or a potentially shortened life. An unpredictable future may create a pervasive sense of unease that results in chronic anxiety and decreased pleasure in the present. The intensity, duration, and extent of these feelings differentiate normal from abnormal responses to the stress of cancer. Assessment of general distress using self-report tools such as the NCCN Distress Thermometer is a first step in understanding the extent and type of concerns. Patients often offer hints rather than directly expressing their fears, especially at points of vulnerability (see Communication Skills When Discussing Transitions in Care box in the next column).

Palliative Care

Palliative care is a component of all cancer care including active treatment and end-of-life care. Conversations at the time of transition from curative treatment to palliative treatment when cure is no longer possible may be difficult for patients and families (see box below). Although palliative care discussions often include goals of care and advanced care planning, symptom management is a vital component of all cancer care. Some patients may see palliative care as a less aggressive approach to cancer treatment or the oncology providers "giving up" on them. They may ask about the meaning of palliative care and how it differs from hospice care. Providers can approach these concerns by discussing that palliative care is a part of all good cancer care. End-of-life care occurs when cancer treatment is stopped and hospice and/or comfort care is the principal approach. These decisions are made with patients and families and are framed in ways that patients do not feel abandoned.

Communication Skills When Discussing Transitions in Care

- Recognize patient responses to the situation.
- Establish the patients and family or caregivers' understanding of current condition.
- Discuss patient values, priorities, preferences, and goals of care.
- Respond to emotions (e.g., NURSE pneumonic).
- Discuss changes in care goals if treatment or disease trajectory changes.
- Update Advance Care Planning documents as needed.
- Promote understanding of transitions.
- Address the family or caregivers' concerns.
- Plan for next steps and refer the patient as needed for additional services including home care and hospice.

When the focus of care changes from curative cancer treatment to hospice and end-of-life care, patients and a family is useful in planning the next steps. Oncology providers may focus on goals of care, symptom management, and maintenance of quality of life (Tulsky, 2005). A family meeting may help to honor patient requests and facilitate informed choices. If the family is unable to visit due to hospital policies or isolation, remote modalities such as conference calls and virtual meetings may allow family members to join the meeting. Communication during a family meeting is structured to establish both patient and family goals (see box below).

Family Meetings

- Clearly state the agenda.
- Make partnership statements.
- Check the patient and family or caregiver's understanding of the situation.
- Reinforce the patient's level of decision making and give permission to ask questions.
- Clarify, empathize, and normalize.
- Validate, respect, summarize, and offer help.
- Make partnership statements.
- Ask open questions.
- Summarize, check understanding, and plan the next steps.

Special communication strategies are needed to address complex issues. Providers may need to frame messages when discussing sensitive issues such as withdrawal of interventions and do-not-resuscitate orders. The table on the next page provides some communication that may not be helpful as well as suggestions for sensitive approaches to discussions with the patients and families.

Transition to Hospice Care: Communication Mistakes and Solutions

Communication to Avoid	Helpful Communication
There is nothing more to be done.	Although we cannot shrink the cancer, we can improve quality of life.
If your heart stops, would you want us to do everything? They would pound on your chest and put in a breathing tube.	What do you know about cardiopulmonary resuscitation? It will not prolong your life and may increase your suffering.
He has failed third-line chemotherapy.	The treatment did not work. The cancer is very aggressive (i.e., the patient is not a failure).
If we discuss hospice and end-of-life care, he will give up hope.	This discussion may allow him to feel prepared and supported.
The cancer has advanced or progressed. He is in denial.	Where do you see things going? What is your understanding of your condition?

Caring for Providers

Many situations in cancer care may provoke strong reactions in patients and providers. These human responses require acknowledgment and reflection so that they do not stifle other professional and personal interactions. For oncology providers, job stress can lead to burnout and lack of satisfaction with clinical care. On the other hand, positive emotional communication (PEC) has been seen across the care trajectory including the end-of-life (Terrill et al., 2018). In fact, positive emotions are common in nurses, caregivers, and patients at end-of-life and do not decline closer to death. Specific training in communication skills, self-awareness, and self-care strategies can reduce burnout especially during stressful times challenging circumstances such as a pandemic. Self-care strategies for handling stress include the following:

- Journaling
- Support groups for debriefing and grieving
- Self-reflection exercises
- Training in self-awareness of emotional responses including savoring, taking joy, and using humor to patient care
- Mindfulness training and meditation

Conclusion

Communication among patients, families, and oncology providers is essential for creating healing environments that improve the treatment of the disease, management of symptoms, and improved well-being and quality of life. Effective communication includes sharing information, addressing psychosocial needs, and creating meaning. Verbal and nonverbal forms of communication provide information about the patient's needs and responses to care. This information enlightens treatment of the disease, palliation of symptoms, and care at the end of life. Compassionate communication requires an understanding of the patient's preferences, beliefs, and psychosocial and emotional needs.

Providers may also experience stress and emotional situations arising during cancer care. They can benefit from training in self-care to improve their well-being and communication

with patients and families. Ultimately, combining the art and science of communication improves the delivery of cancer care and enhances the well-being of all people.

References

American College of Surgeons Commission on Cancer. (2020a). *Cancer program standards: Ensuring patient-centered care.* Available at http://www.facs.org/cancer/coc/programstandards2012.html (accessed January 10, 2022).

American College of Surgeons Commission on Cancer. (2020b). *Optimal resources for cancer care.* Available at https://www.facs.org/-/media/files/quality-programs/cancer/coc/optimal_resources_for_cancer_care_2020_standards.ashx.

American Society of Clinical Oncology (ASCO). (2014). *Practice guideline: Screening, assessment and care of psychosocial distress (depression, anxiety) in adults with cancer.* Alexandria, VA: ASCO.

Baile, W. F., Buckman, R., Lenzi, R., Glober, G., Beale, E. A., & Kudelka, A. P. (2000). SPIKES—A six-step protocol for delivering bad news: Application to the patient with cancer. *The Oncologist, 5*(4), 302–311. Available at http://theoncologist.alphamedpress.org/content/5/4/302 (accessed March 12, 2016).

de Haes, H., & Bensing, J. (2009). Endpoints in medical communication research, proposing a framework of functions and outcomes. *Patient Education and Counseling, 74,* 287–294.

Eggly, S. S., Albrecht, T. L., Kelly, K., Prigerson, H. G., Sheldon, L. K., & Studts, J. (2009). The role of the clinician in cancer clinical communication. *Journal of Health Communication, 14*(Suppl 1), 66–75.

Epstein, R. M., & Street, R. L. (2007). *Patient-centered communication in cancer care: Promoting healing and reducing suffering.* Bethesda: National Cancer Institute.

Heyn, L., Finset, A., & Ruland, C. M. (2013). Talking about feelings and worries in cancer consultations: The effects of an interactive tailored symptom assessment on source, explicitness, and timing of emotional cues and concerns. *Cancer Nursing, 36*(2), E20–E30.

Institute of Medicine (IOM). (2007). *Cancer care for the whole patient: Meeting psychosocial health needs.* National Academies Press. Available at https://www.ncbi.nlm.nih.gov/books/NBK52822/.

Kaplan, M. (2010). SPIKES: A framework for breaking bad news to patients with cancer. *Clinical Journal of Oncology Nursing, 14*(4), 514–516.

Li, J., Luo, X., Cao, Q., Lin, Y., Xu, Y., & Li, Q. (2020). Communication needs of cancer patients and/or caregivers: A critical literature review. *Journal of Oncology, 2020,* 7432849.

National Comprehensive Care Network (NCCN). (2021). NCCN clinical practice guidelines in oncology: Distress management. Version 1.2022. Includes NCCN distress thermometer. Available at https://www.nccn.org/professionals/physician_gls/pdf/distress.pdf (accessed January 10, 2022).

Sardessai-Nadkarni, A. A., & Street, R. L., Jr. (2022). Understanding the pathways linking patient-centered communication to cancer survivors' emotional health: Examining the mediating roles of self efficacy and cognitive reappraisal. *Journal of Cancer Survivorship.*

Sheldon, L. K., Blonquist, T. M., Hilaire, D. M., Hong, F., & Berry, D. L. (2015). Patient cues and symptoms of psychosocial distress: What predicts assessment and treatment of distress by oncology clinicians? *Psycho-Oncology, 24*(9), 1020–1027.

Spitzer, R. L., Kroenke, K., Williams, J. B. (1999). Validation and utility of a self-report version of PRIME-MD: The PHQ primary care study. Primary Care Evaluation of Mental Disorders. Patient Health Questionnaire. JAMA, 282(18), 1737–1744.

Street, R. L., Jr., Makoul, G., Arora, N. K., & Epstein, R. M. (2009). How does communication heal? Pathways linking clinician-patient communication to health outcomes. *Patient Education and Counseling, 74*(3), 295–301. https://doi.org/10.1016/j.pec.2008.11.015.

Terrill, A. L., Ellington, L., John, K. K., Latimer, S., Xu, J., Reblin, M., & Clayton, M. F. (2018). Positive emotion communication: Fostering well-being at end of life. *Patient Education and Counseling, 101*(4), 631–638.

Tulsky, J. A. (2005). Beyond advance directives: Importance of communication skills at the end of life. *Journal of the American Medical Association, 294,* 359–365.

Warshaw, R. (2018, April 24). *From bedside to webside: Future doctors learn how to practice remotely.* Special to AAMCNews. Available at https://www.aamc.org/news-insights/bedside-webside-future-doctors-learn-how-practice-remotely.

Wittenberg, E., Reb, E., & Kanter, E. (2018). Communicating with patients and families around difficult topics in cancer care using the COMFORT Communication curriculum. *Seminars in Oncology Nursing, 34*(3), 264–273.

Socio-Cultural Considerations

Nimian Bauder

Definition of Culture

Culture comprises the values, beliefs, norms, and practices of a particular group that are learned and shared. It guides thinking, decisions, and actions in a patterned way (Leininger, 1991) and includes the following:

- Country of origin, length or location of current residence, and reasons for migration
- Communication, including native language, willingness to share personal thoughts or feelings, use of touch and by whom, meaning of eye contact, time orientation, and format of names
- Family roles, including who is the decision maker, caregiver, or spokesperson; gender-related roles; and role of the extended family
- Workforce issues, including current employment, economic impact of illness, and educational preparation
- Biologic differences, including skin color, physical attributes, differences in incidence of illnesses, and variations in drug metabolism
- Therapy-compromising behaviors such as use of alcohol, tobacco, and recreational drugs and participation in health promotion and safety practices
- Nutrition, including the meaning of food, types of foods eaten, food rituals, and dietary practices
- Pregnancy and childbearing practices
- Death rituals
- Spirituality, including identifying with a formal religion or cult, meaning of life, use of prayer or meditation, and relationship between spiritual beliefs and health practices
- Health care practices, including practices that impact health promotion and prevention practices, who is responsible for health care, beliefs about the meaning of illness and health, barriers to health care, and beliefs about acceptance of treatments, drugs, blood transfusions, and loss of organs
- Health care practitioners, including the role of traditional and folk practitioners; age, gender, and race of the health care provider; and acceptance of care by the patient and family (see the figure on this page).

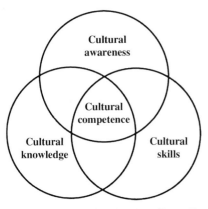

The three domains of cultural competence. (From Shay, A. [2019]. *Assistive technology service delivery: A practical guide for disability and employment professionals.* London: Elsevier.)

Providing Culturally Competent Care

Culturally competent care is a process, not an end point, in which the nurse works to provide care within the cultural context of the patient, family, or community Abualhaija (2021). The registered nurse practices with cultural humility and inclusiveness. It includes the following:

- Demonstrates respect, equity, and empathy in actions and interactions with all health care consumers
- Respects consumer decisions without bias
- Participates in lifelong learning to understand cultural preferences, worldviews, choices, and decision-making processes of diverse consumers
- Reflects upon personal and cultural values, beliefs, biases, and heritage
- Applies knowledge of differences in health beliefs, practices, and communication patterns without assigning value to the differences
- Addresses the effects and impact of discrimination and oppression on practice within and among diverse groups

- Uses appropriate skills and tools for the culture, literacy, and language of the individuals and population served
- Communicates with appropriate language and behaviors, including the use of qualified health care interpreters and translators in accordance with consumer needs and preferences
- Serves as a role model and educator for cultural humility and the recognition and appreciation of diversity and inclusivity
- Identifies the cultural-specific meaning of interactions, terms, and content
- Advocates for policies that promote health and prevent harm among diverse health care consumers and groups
- Promotes equity in all aspects of health and health care
- Advances organizational policies, programs, services, and practices that reflect respect, equity, and values for diversity and inclusion (American Nurses Association [ANA], 2021).

Assessment Model

The assessment model is delineated by the acronym CONFHER:

- **C** (communication): What language does the patient speak? What words does the patient use for common health terms (e.g., pain, fever)?
- **O** (orientation): What cultural group does the patient identify with? What are the values that influence the patient? How long has the patient been in the United States?
- **N** (nutrition): What are the patient's food preferences? Are there food taboos? Are there concerns about artificial nutrition and hydration?
- **F** (family relationships): How is the family defined, and who is in the family? Who is the decision maker in the family? What are the roles of the men, women, and children?
- **H** (health beliefs): What are the beliefs about health and illness? Are there conflicts with Western medicine? Who is consulted about health concerns? What does illness mean to the culture? What beliefs may interfere with delivery of care?
- **E** (education): What is the patient's learning style and education level? What is the patient's occupation?
- **R** (religion): What are the patient's religious beliefs? Do the beliefs have an impact on health care and illness? (Fong, 1985)

ADDRESSING Framework

The ADDRESSING framework facilitates remembering some of the key social identities to consider when getting to know someone's cultural identity (see figure below).

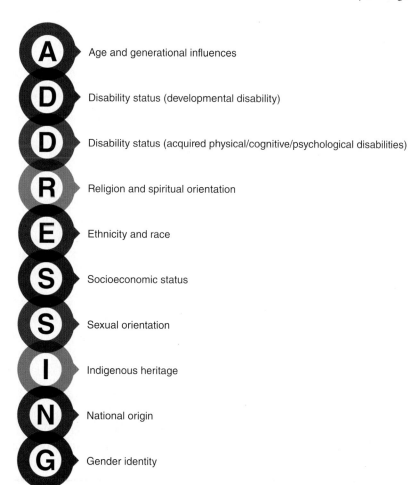

ADDRESSING Framework. (Hays, P. A. (2022). Addressing Cultural Complexities in Counseling and Clinical Practice: An Intersectional Approach (4th edition). Washington DC: American Psychological Association.)

Barriers to Cultural Competence

- Ethnocentrism: using one's customs or values to judge others. Can manifest as feelings of superiority or discrimination with respect to one's own group or culture over another group or culture.
  - The nurse's cultural background
  - The culture of Western health care
- Stereotyping: making assumptions that an individual reflects all characteristics associated with a group. Can lead to erroneous misrepresentations of diverse cultural groups, age groups, and gender identity.
  - Assuming, for instance, a Latino patient has limited English proficiency and arranging for an interpreter before confirming this
  - Assuming an Asian male patient is stoic about pain and will not ask for pain medication (see table below) (Andrews et al., 2020).

Overview of the Primary Barriers and How They Influenced Various Aspects of Health Care Delivery/Reception

Primary Barriers to Culturally Competent Care	Areas of Health Care Service Delivery/Reception Affected
Language barriers	<ul><li>Practitioner-patient/caregiver communication</li><li>Establishment of rapport</li><li>Information provision and instruction</li><li>Engagement in intervention/therapy</li></ul>
Cultural barriers	<ul><li>Practitioner-patient/caregiver communication</li><li>Establishment of rapport</li><li>Diagnosis</li><li>Decision-making on treatment</li><li>Establishment in intervention/therapy</li></ul>
Limited resources	<ul><li>Practitioner-patient/caregiver communication</li><li>Establishment of rapport</li><li>Diagnosis</li><li>Assessments</li><li>Engagement in intervention/therapy</li></ul>

From Grandpierre, V., Milloy, V., Sikora, L., Fitzpatrick, E., Thomas, R., & Potter, B. (2018). Barriers and facilitators to cultural competence in rehabilitation services: A scoping review. *BMC Health Services Research, 18*(1), 23.

Combating Implicit Bias and Stereotypes

Implicit bias refers to the attitudes or stereotypes that affect our understanding, actions, and decisions in an unconscious manner. An implicit bias can make us susceptible to unintentionally acting in ways that are inconsistent with our values. Although you do not choose to have an implicit bias, you can choose to be aware of it and combat its effects.

Two important first steps are to:
- Recognize that we all have implicit biases and that implicit bias can negatively affect clinical interactions and outcomes
- Accept the responsibility to identify and understand your implicit biases

- The box below presents the next steps you can take to confront your implicit biases and reduce stereotypic thinking. Consistent and conscious use of these strategies can help you create a habit of nonbiased thinking.

Overcoming Implicit Bias and Stereotypes or Ways to Overcome

Stereotype replacement	Become aware of the stereotypes you should hold and create nonstereotypical alternatives to them
Counter-stereotypic imaging	Remember or imagine someone from a stereotyped group who does not fit the stereotype
Individuating	See each person as an individual, not a group member; pay attention to things about them besides the stereotypes of their group
Perspective-taking	Imagine the perspective of someone from a group different than your own ("Put yourself in the other person's shoes.")
Contact	Seek ways to get to know people from different social groups. Build your confidence by interacting with people who are different from you. Seek opportunities to engage in discussions in safe environments, spend time with people outside your usual social groups, or volunteer in a community different from your own.
Emotional regulation	Reflect on your "gut feelings" and negative reactions to people from different social groups. Be aware that positive emotions during a clinical encounter make stereotyping less likely.
Mindfulness	Keep your attention on the present moment so you can recognize a stereotypic thought before you act on it.

From Office of Minority Health. (n.d.). *Combating implicit bias and stereotypes*. US Department of Health and Human Services. Available at https://thinkculturalhealth.hhs.gov/assets/pdfs/resource-library/combating-implicit-bias-stereotypes.pdf (accessed January 19, 2022).

National Standards for Culturally and Linguistically Appropriate Services

The National Standards for Culturally and Linguistically Appropriate Services (CLAS) aim to improve health care quality and advance health equity by establishing a framework for organizations to serve the nation's increasingly diverse communities. The CLAS standards are inclusive of all cultures and are designed to address the needs of racial, ethnic, and linguistic populations that experience unequal access to health services (Andrews et al., 2020). There are a total of 15 standards (Office of Minority Health. n.d.).

Principal Standard

1. Provide effective, equitable, understandable, and respectful quality care and services that are responsive to diverse cultural health beliefs and practices, preferred languages, health literacy, and other communication needs.

Governance, Leadership, and Workforce

2. Advance and sustain organizational governance and leadership that promotes CLAS and health equity through policy, practices, and allocated resources.

3. Recruit, promote, and support a culturally and linguistically diverse governance, leadership, and workforce that are responsive to the population in the service area.

4. Educate and train governance, leadership, and the workforce in culturally and linguistically appropriate policies and practices on an ongoing basis.

Communication and Language Assistance

5. Offer language assistance to individuals who have limited English proficiency or other communication needs at no cost to them to facilitate timely access to all health care and services.

6. Inform all individuals of the availability of language assistance services clearly and in their preferred language, both verbally and in writing.

7. Ensure the competence of individuals providing language assistance, recognizing that the use of untrained individuals or minors as interpreters should be avoided.

8. Provide easy-to-understand print and multimedia materials and signage in the languages commonly used by the populations in the service area.

Engagement, Continuous Improvement, and Accountability

9. Establish culturally and linguistically appropriate goals, policies, and management accountability, and infuse them throughout the organization's planning and operations.

10. Conduct ongoing assessments of the organization's CLAS-related activities and integrate CLAS-related measures into assessment measurement and continuous quality improvement activities.

11. Collect and maintain accurate and reliable demographic data to monitor and evaluate the impact of CLAS on health equity and outcomes and to inform service delivery.

12. Conduct regular assessments of community health assets and needs, and use the results to plan and implement services that respond to the cultural and linguistic diversity of populations in the service area.

13. Partner with the community to design, implement, and evaluate policies, practices, and services to ensure cultural and linguistic appropriateness.

14. Create conflict- and grievance-resolution processes that are culturally and linguistically appropriate to identify, prevent, and resolve conflicts or complaints.

15. Communicate the organization's progress in implementing and sustaining CLAS to all stakeholders, constituents, and the general public.

Strategies for Promoting Cultural Competence in the Organization

In 2013, the Office of Minority Health released the enhanced National CLAS Standards, which are a comprehensive set of 15 guidelines that inform, guide, and facilitate practices related to culturally and linguistically appropriate health services. An accompanying implementation initiative resulted in development of the Blueprint for Advancing and Sustaining CLAS Policy and Practice and provided specific and systematic guidance for implementing each standard.

Social Determinants of Health

Social determinants of health (SDOH) are the conditions in the environments where people are born, live, learn, work, play, worship, and age that affect a wide range of health, functioning, and quality-of-life outcomes and risks (see box below).

SDOH can be grouped into five domains:

1. *Economic stability:* Earning a steady income allows people to meet their health needs. People with economic instability cannot afford healthy foods, health care, and housing.

2. *Education access and quality:* People with higher levels of education are more likely to be healthier and live longer.

3. *Health care access and quality:* People without insurance are less likely to have a primary care provider, and they may not be able to afford the health care services and medications they need.

4. *Neighborhood and built environment:* People's well-being and health are affected by their neighborhoods and environments. Racial/ethnic minorities and people with low incomes are more likely to live in places with high rates of violence, unsafe air or water, and other health and safety risks.

5. *Social and community context:* People's relationships and interactions with family, friends, co-workers, and community members can have a major impact on their health and well-being. (Office of Disease Prevention & Health Promotion, 2021).

Social Determinants of Health

Economic Stability
- Employment
- Food Insecurity
- Housing Instability
- Poverty

Education
- Early Childhood Education & Development
- Enrollment in Higher Education
- High School Graduation
- Language and Literacy

Social and Community Context
- Civic Participation
- Discrimination
- Incarceration
- Social Cohesion

Health and Health Care
- Access to Health Care
- Access to Primary Care
- Health Literacy

Neighborhood and Built Environment
- Access to Foods That Support Healthy Eating Patterns
- Crime and Violence
- Environmental Conditions
- Quality of Housing

From Office of Disease Prevention & Health Promotion. (2021). *Social Determinants of Health.* Available at https://health.gov/healthypeople/objectives-and-data/social-determinants-health (accessed January 19, 2022).

Nursing Practice Considerations

7

The *Future of Nursing 2020–2030* provides several examples of SDOH in which nurses should address, and include education, employment, health systems and services, housing, income and wealth, the physical environment, public safety, the social environment (including structures, institutions, and policies), and transportation. Everyone is affected by SDOH. Some people with more education or higher income will have better health because they may be able to make more informed choices, have better access to health care, and have the ability to pay for health care (Wakefield et al., 2021).

The immediate living environment of the patient also has a direct impact on the risk of cancer. The environment plays an important role in access to medical care and early diagnosis. Social factors are a strong determinant of morbidity and mortality (Rogers et al., 2020). Individuals living in poverty have higher cancer mortality rates, mainly due to reduced access to care and out-of-pocket expenses. Individuals living in poverty may not have health insurance and avoid being examined or seeking health care for fear of cost (Alcaraz et al., 2020).

Consideration of Social Determinants of Health

SDOH also contribute to wide health disparities and inequities. In order to improve health disparities, SDOH must be addressed. A patient's health is dependent on what occurs outside of the medical and health care environments. It is important for nurses to consider what occurs outside of the health care facility; therefore, nurses have an ethical obligation to consider patients' SDOH and address any gaps. Nurses are uniquely positioned to assist in addressing SDOH. They are often the first and most frequent contact with patients. They can assist by:

- Identifying risk through screening
- Conducting a community health needs assessment
- Creating individual and community-targeted solutions
- Leading interprofessional teams to increase community referrals
- Creating community partnerships
- Serving as advocates for patients and communities
- Addressing inequalities and social needs within communities
- Advocating for policy change (Wakefield et al., 2021).

Assessing Patients Social Risks and Needs

Identifying the social needs and social risks of patients is an important first step. A multisite survey conducted in a large integrated health system found that most patients support clinical social needs screening and intervention (Rogers et al., 2020). The Agency for Healthcare Research and Quality (AHRQ) offers several tools online to help identify a patient's current social needs and their risks for developing social needs. It is also important to share this information with the team to ensure proper care coordination and resource allocation.

- *HealthBegins Upstream Risks Screening Tool* includes questions about 14 SDOH.
- *WellRx* is a validated 11-item clinical screener for nonmedical social needs.

- *Kaiser Permanente's Your Current Life Situation (YCLS) survey* captures a range of social and economic needs, including living situation, housing, food, utilities, childcare, debts, medical needs, transportation, stress, and social isolation.
- *Protocol for Responding to and Assessing Patients' Assets, Risks, and Experiences (PRAPARE)* includes 17 core questions and four optional questions about SDOH. Its implementation guide includes the four electronic health record (EHR) tools, technical resources, best practices, multiple tested workflows, and other resources (AHRQ, 2021).

Cancer Health Disparities

Cancer health disparities, also known as cancer disparities, are adverse differences between certain population groups in cancer measures, such as incidence (new cases), prevalence (all existing cases), morbidity (cancer-related health complications), mortality (deaths), survivorship and quality of life after cancer treatment, burden of cancer or related health conditions, screening rates, and stage at diagnosis (National Cancer Institute [NCI], 2015). Cancer incidence and mortality rates are markedly different among the four major minority groups in the United States. Although cancer incidence and death rates in the United States are generally declining, the risk of certain cancers or deaths among minority groups is still increasing. Cancers in minorities are detected at a later stage compared with non-Hispanic Whites.

- Blacks
  - Collectively, Black men and Black women have the highest death rate and shortest survival of any racial/ethnic group in the United States for most cancers.
  - Death rate for cancer among Blacks is 29% higher for men and 14% higher for women compared with non-Hispanic Whites.
  - Prostate cancer is the most commonly diagnosed cancer in Black men, and breast cancer is the most common in Black women.
  - Esophageal cancer is the number two cause of death for Black men aged 35 to 54 years.
  - Colorectal cancer incidence is 40% higher in Blacks than Whites in the United States.
  - Inequalities among Blacks are complex and reflect social and economic differences.
- Hispanic/Latinx
  - Hispanic men and women are generally less likely to be diagnosed at an early stage.
  - They have the lowest rates of tobacco-related cancers because of their low rates of smoking.
  - They have the highest rate for cancers associated with infection, including cancers of the liver (i.e., hepatitis B infection), stomach (i.e., *Helicobacter pylori*), cervix (i.e., human papillomavirus), and gall bladder, depending on countries of origin.
  - Hispanic men and women have a higher risk of stomach cancer before 50 years of age.
- Asian and Pacific Islanders
  - They have the lowest overall cancer incidence and mortality rates.

- They have the highest rates for cancers of the liver and stomach, similar to Hispanics.
- They are 70% more likely to have stomach cancer.
- Asian and Pacific Islander men are twice as likely to die from stomach cancer as compared to non-Hispanic White men.
- American Indians and Alaska Natives
  - They have the highest kidney cancer incidence and mortality rates, likely due to the prevalence of smoking, obesity, and hypertension.
  - They have the highest liver cancer incidence and mortality rates.
  - Most prevalent cancers: biliary, nasopharyngeal, testicular, cervical, and renal.

(American Cancer Society, 2019, 2021; Office of Minority Health, 2021).

Nurses need to consider socio-cultural factors to better meet patient needs, in lieu of the SDOH that influence cancer outcomes. A starting point is for nurses to assess social and cultural identities and identify disparities that could interfere with access to quality cancer care. Better awareness and identification of cultural differences and social challenges can help nurses provide referrals to resources and provide effective, high-quality cancer care.

References

Abualhaija, N. (2021). Clarifying cultural competence in nursing: A concept analysis approach. *Journal of Cultural Diversity*, 28(1), 3–14. Available at https://core.ac.uk/download/pdf/287028169.pdf.

Agency for Healthcare Research and Quality (AHRQ). (2021). *SDOH & practice improvement*. https://www.ahrq.gov/sdoh/practice-improvement.html (accessed January 19, 2022).

Alcaraz, K. I., Wiedt, T. L., Daniels, E. C., Yabroff, K. R., Guerra, C. E., & Wender, R. C. (2020). Understanding and addressing social determinants to advance cancer health equity in the United States: A blueprint for practice, research, and policy. *CA: A Cancer Journal for Clinicians*, 70(1), 31–46.

American Cancer Society. (2019). *Cancer facts and figures for African Americans 2019–2021*. Available at https://www.cancer.org/content/dam/cancer-org/research/cancer-facts-and-statistics/cancer-facts-and-figures-for-african-americans/cancer-facts-and-figures-for-african-americans-2019-2021.pdf (accessed January 19, 2022).

American Cancer Society. (2021). *Cancer facts and figures for Hispanic/Latino People 2021–2023*. https://cancercontroltap.smhs.gwu.edu/news/cancer-facts-figures-hispanicslatinos-2021-2023 (accessed January 19, 2022).

American Nurses Association. (2021). *Nursing: Scope and standards of practice* (4th ed.). ANA.

Andrews, M. M., Boyle, J. S., & Collins, J. (2020). *Transcultural concepts in nursing care* (8th ed.). Wolters Kluwer.

Fong, C. M. (1985). Ethnicity and nursing practice. *Topics in Clinical Nursing*, 7(3), 1–10.

Grandpierre, V., Milloy, V., Sikora, L., Fitzpatrick, E., Thomas, R., & Potter, B. (2018). Barriers and facilitators to cultural competence in rehabilitation services: A scoping review. *BMC Health Services Research*, 18(1), 23.

Leininger, M. (1991). Transcultural nursing: The study and practice. *Imprint*, 38, 55–66.

National Cancer Institute (NCI). (2015, February 17). *Cancer health disparities definitions and examples*. Available at https://www.cancer.gov/about-nci/organization/crchd/about-health-disparities/definitions (accessed January 19, 2022).

Office of Disease Prevention & Health Promotion. (2021). *Social determinants of health*. Available at https://health.gov/healthypeople/objectives-and-data/social-determinants-health (accessed January 19, 2022).

Office of Minority Health. (n.d.). *ADDRESSING framework*. US Department of Health and Human Services. Available at https://thinkculturalhealth.hhs.gov/assets/pdfs/resource-library/addressing-framework.pdf (accessed January 19, 2022).

Office of Minority Health. (2021). *Cancer and Asian Americans*. US Department of Health and Human Services. https://minorityhealth.hhs.gov/omh/browse.aspx?lvl=4&lvlid=46 (accessed January 19, 2022).

Office of Minority Health. (n.d.). *Combating implicit bias and stereotypes*. US Department of Health and Human Services. Available at https://thinkculturalhealth.hhs.gov/assets/pdfs/resource-library/combating-implicit-bias-stereotypes.pdf (accessed January 19, 2022).

Office of Minority Health. (n.d.). *CLAS standards*. US Department of Health and Human Services. Available at https://thinkculturalhealth.hhs.gov/clas/standards (accessed January 19, 2022).

Rogers, A. J., Hamity, C., Sharp, A. L., Jackson, A. H., & Schickedanz, A. B. (2020). Patients' attitudes and perceptions regarding social needs screening and navigation: Multi-site survey in a large integrated health system. *Journal of General Internal Medicine*, 35(5), 1389–1395. https://doi.org/10.1007/s11606-019-05588-1.

Wakefield, M. K., Williams, D. R., Menestrel, S. L., & Flaubert, J. L. (2021). *The future of nursing 2020-2030: Charting a path to achieve health equity*. The National Academies Press. Available at https://nap.nationalacademies.org/catalog/25982/the-future-of-nursing-2020-2030-charting-a-path-to (accessed May 18, 2023).

Ethical Considerations

Jesee Jay Castro

Introduction

Ethical considerations play a major role in oncology nursing practice and excellent patient and family care. The American Nurses Association (ANA) established a framework for nursing practice, which includes the following:

1. Practice with unconditional compassion and respect.
2. Have a commitment to the patient, whether an individual, family, or group.
3. Promote and advocate for health and safety.
4. Take responsibility for providing optimal care (and recognizing what is beyond the scope of practice).
5. Respect self and others, preserving integrity, safety, and professional growth.
6. Take responsibility for a healthy work environment.
7. Contribute to professional practice, education, and administration.
8. Collaborate in community efforts to meet health care needs.
9. Take responsibility for articulating nursing values to shape policy and practice.

Ethics is derived from the Greek term *ethos*, meaning "customs, conduct, or character." It involves the study of how a person determines right and wrong. Analytical thinking and reasoning must be employed when faced with complex choices, and the benefits and risks of each choice should be thoroughly articulated and communicated.

Ethical dilemmas arise when conflicting values are associated with decision options, and it is essential to carefully weigh each option before a decision is made. In the event of an ethical dilemma, an organizational ethics committee can be consulted to weigh risks and benefits according to ethical principles.

Key Ethical Theories

- *Ethical relativism:* Morality is understood in the context of culture.
- *Feminist theory:* Feminist ethics attempt to revise traditional ethics to the extent that the system depreciates or devalues women's moral experience. The philosophy is also concerned with decisions in the context of how the patient, family, others who depend on one another, and the community may be affected.
- *Deontology:* Ethical decisions are those for which the intentions are good; the good intention is the primary value rather than the outcome.
- *Utilitarianism:* The philosophy supports what is best for the majority. The value of the decision is based on its usefulness; the outcome is the primary value rather than the intention.

Key Ethical Principles

- *Fidelity:* Duty to alleviate suffering and commitment to caring for others.
- *Respect for persons:* Unconditional positive regard for others (includes truth telling, also known as veracity).
- *Autonomy:* Self-determination, which is based on effective informed consent.
- *Nonmaleficence:* Avoiding harm; the core of the medical oath and nursing ethics
- *Beneficence:* Doing good (i.e., implies that nurses are competent to provide good care); core principle of patient advocacy.
- *Human rights:* Basic rights and freedom from arbitrary interference or restriction that are based on moral principles and thought to belong to all persons; this includes maintaining confidentiality and respecting diversity.
- *Justice:* Fairness related to equal distribution of resources in the context of a benefit-burden analysis.
- *Paternalism:* Health care professionals in positions of authority make decisions about diagnosis, prognosis, and treatment based partly on their own beliefs and restrict the freedom and responsibilities of those subordinate to them.

Framework for Ethical Decision-Making

- Gather and document relevant data.
- Assess the social and interpersonal dynamics of the issue at hand.
- Determine the ethical issue apart from other dimensions (e.g., legal, institutional, medical).
- Identify relevant assumptions, beliefs, and values of all stakeholders.
- Determine core values of the issue at hand.
- Determine whether conflicts exist related to these values (i.e., ethical dilemmas).
- Identify ethically acceptable options and their consequences.
- Provide options and make choices.
- Support choices.
- Evaluate the outcome, and assess for process improvements.
- Consider patients' social determinants in health.

Effective Informed Consent

- Informed consent depends on an ethical and legal commitment to explain the risks, benefits, and alternatives needed to make a decision.
- Patient understanding must be ensured.
- Patient participation is important and is verified by asking questions and clarifying meanings (e.g., surgical consent, blood transfusion consent, research participation).

Requirements for Effective Informed Consent

- Adequate decision-making capacity (i.e., decision-maker able to weigh benefits and risks)
- Adequate time for a thorough discussion of the benefits and risks of each option
- Inclusion of the family and others in the discussion at the patient's request
- Lack of coercion
- Elicitation of patient's preference
- Provision of a surrogate decision-maker, including the following:
  - Health care power of attorney (HCPOA) (i.e., substituted judgment)
  - Next-of-kin (i.e., substituted judgment)
  - Guardianship
  - The physician acting in the best interest of the patient (if the patient lacks capacity and has no other surrogate)
- Accurate documentation of the discussion
- Agreement of the patient or decision-maker to the treatment plan

Elements of Decision-Making Capacity

- Ability to understand information regarding medical treatment options and consequences of choices
- Ability to evaluate the information, comparing benefits and risks of each option
- Ability to communicate a choice that remains consistent over time (i.e., new information may cause a different choice to be made)
- Lack of any of the previous criteria constitutes a lack of decision-making capacity

Barriers to Ethical Decision-Making and Effective Informed Consent

- Language and other communication barriers (i.e., lack of proper interpreters)
- Culture and religious beliefs (if the discussion is refused because of these influences)
- Lack of adequate time to discuss all options (i.e., benefits vs. risks)
- Altered capacity (i.e., physical, mental, or emotional)
- Confirmation bias (i.e., staff tendency to easily go along with a decision if it aligns with their own values regardless of established informed consent)
- Coercion
- Literacy
- Legal disputes
- Pandemic restrictions for family visitations
- Staff negligence to provide or establish all criteria in the "Requirements for an Effective Informed Consent" section

Factors That May Impair Decisional Capacity

Patients with cancer may have impaired decision-making capacity, either temporarily or permanently. The following situations require frequent monitoring to find a time when the patient has optimal decisional capacity:

- Cognitive impairment
- Delirium
- Weakness
- Depression or anxiety
- Uncontrolled pain and symptoms
- Grief
- Sleep deprivation
- Medications, for example, opioids and benzodiazepines

Common Ethical Issues in Oncology

- Life-sustaining treatments, especially at the end of life
- Treatment choices in the context of quality-of-life goals
- Artificial nutrition or hydration
- Medical futility
- Sedation for refractory symptoms at the end of life
- Family requests to withhold information from the patient
- Assisted suicide and euthanasia
- Ethical decisions for children (When do they have decisional capacity?)
- Moral distress of professional staff and others (i.e., moral distress can exist when the right course of action is known but people are unable to take it for any reason)
- Impact of moral distress of others on the patient
- Clinical trials and research
- Hospital visitation and number of visitors in the midst of infection concerns (e.g., pandemics) and health care setting logistics

Role of the Nurse in Ethical Decision-Making

- Provide education and support the health care team in explaining options, benefits, and risks
- Offer support to the patient and family as they consider options
- Facilitate communication between all involved parties
- Serve as an advocate for the patient
- Serve as a witness according to the guidelines of the organization
- Provide thorough and accurate documentation of discussions, questions, responses, and choices
- Evaluate complex cases
- Utilization of appropriate gender-affirming care
- Attend and facilitate family meetings
- Recognize their own implicit bias

Ethical Support for Nursing

- Administrative policies and leadership staff
- Ethics committee
- Nurse Practice Act
- ANA code of ethics with interpretive guidelines
- Peer support
- Bioethics networks (state or local community)

Bibliography

Berlinger, N., Wynia, M., Powell, T., Hester, D. M., Milliken, A., Fabi, R., … Jenks, N. P. (2020). *Ethical framework for health care institutions responding to novel Coronavirus SARS-CoV-2 (COVID-19): Guidelines for institutional ethics services responding to COVID-19.* Garrison, NY: The Hastings Center.

Crico, C., Sanchini, V., Casali, P. G., & Pravettoni, G. (2020). Evaluating the effectiveness of clinical ethics committees: A systematic review. *Medicine, Health Care and Philosophy, 24*(1), 135–151.

Dellasega, C., & Kanaskie, M. L. (2021). Nursing ethics in an era of pandemic. *Applied Nursing Research, 62*, 151508.

FitzGerald, C., & Hurst, S. (2017). Implicit bias in healthcare professionals: A systematic review. *BMC Medical Ethics, 18*(1), 19.

Ghose, S., Radhakrishnan, V., & Bhattacharya, S. (2019). *Ethics of cancer care: Beyond biology and medicine. ecancer.* Available at https://ecancer.org/en/journal/article/911-ethics-of-cancer-care-beyond-biology-and-medicine.

Hugelius, K., Harada, N., & Marutani, M. (2021). Consequences of visiting restrictions during the COVID-19 pandemic: An integrative review. *International Journal of Nursing Studies, 121*, 1–10.

Kimberly, L. L., Folkers, K. M., Friesen, P., Sultan, D., Quinn, G. P., Bateman-House, A., ... Salas-Humara, C. (2018). Ethical issues in gender-affirming care for youth. *Pediatrics, 142*(6), 1–9.

Long, K. L., Ingraham, A. M., Wendt, E. M., Saucke, M. C., Balentine, C., Orne, J., & Pitt, S. C. (2021). Informed consent and informed decision-making in high-risk surgery: A quantitative analysis. *Journal of the American College of Surgeons, 233*(3), 337–345.

McDermott-Levy, R., Leffers, J., & Mayaka, J. (2018). Ethical principles and guidelines of global health nursing practice. *Nursing Outlook, 66*(5), 473–481.

Schwan, B. (2021). Responsibility amid the social determinants of health. *Bioethics, 35*(1), 6–14.

Silva, M. D., Genoff, M., Zaballa, A., Jewell, S., Stabler, S., Gany, F. M., & Diamond, L. C. (2016). Interpreting at the end of life: A systematic review of the impact of interpreters on the delivery of palliative care services to cancer patients with limited English proficiency. *Journal of Pain and Symptom Management, 51*(3), 569–580.

Varkey, B. (2021). Principles of clinical ethics and their application to practice. *Medical Principles and Practice, 30*(1), 17–28.

Quality and Safety

Julie Ponto

Quality and Safety in Oncology

Quality programs and initiatives in oncology help to ensure that individuals with cancer and their families receive care that is based on evidence and aligns with national and, in some cases, international standards. Quality and safety are closely related concepts in oncology because of the unique treatment modalities that can pose safety concerns. For example, hazardous drugs and radiation therapies are key elements in oncology practice that require unique safety standards. Safety systems and procedures are designed to ensure that patients, their families, and health care workers are not harmed. This chapter outlines several programs, initiatives, and standards that promote quality and safety in settings where cancer care is delivered.

Chemotherapy Quality and Safety

American Society of Clinical Oncology (ASCO) and Oncology Nursing Society (ONS) Chemotherapy Administration Safety Standards (https://www.ons.org/ascoons-chemotherapy-administration-safety-standards)

- Originally published in 2009, the protocol outlined 31 chemotherapy safety standards related to staffing, preparation, and administration of chemotherapy, monitoring, and other principles of safe practice in outpatient settings.
- Revised in 2012 to incorporate inpatient settings and in 2013 to include oral chemotherapy.
- Revised in 2016 to include pediatric oncology, double check during preparation, use of minibag for vinca alkaloids, and medication labeling.
- Standards reorganized into four domains:
  - Creating a safe environment—staffing and general
  - Treatment planning, patient consent, and education
  - Ordering, preparing, dispensing, and administering chemotherapy
  - Monitoring after chemotherapy is administered, including adherence, toxicity, and complications (Neuss et al., 2017)

Radiation Therapy Quality and Safety

The American Society for Radiation Oncology (ASTRO) (https://www.astro.org/) offers several guidelines and safety programs for radiation oncology clinicians.

- Target Safely (https://www.astro.org/Patient-Care-and-Research/Patient-Safety/Target-Safely)
  - multipronged initiative addressing practice, regulatory, patient and professional safety, and quality issues related to the safe administration of radiation therapy

- Radiation Oncology Incident Learning System (RO-ILS) (https://www.astro.org/Patient-Care-and-Research/Patient-Safety/RO-ILS)
  - secure and nonpunitive system of tracking radiation-related incidents for the purpose of shared learning, safety, and quality improvement (QI) within the field of radiation oncology
- Safety is no Accident (https://www.astro.org/Patient-Care-and-Research/Patient-Safety/Safety-is-no-Accident)
  - Consensus reference guide containing practice standards, guidelines, tools, and resources
- ASTRO Accreditation Program for Excellence (APEx) (https://www.astro.org/Daily-Practice/Accreditation)
  - Voluntary certification program for radiation oncology practices
  - Standards of practice for certification based on:
    - The process of care
    - The radiation oncology team
    - Safety
    - Quality management
    - Patient-centered care
  - On-site survey conducted by medical physicist and radiation oncologist or other radiation oncology personnel
  - Successful practices receive APEx certification for 3 or 4 years
- ASTRO practice guidelines and consensus statements (https://www.astro.org/Patient-Care-and-Research/Clinical-Practice-Statements)
  - topical, evidence-based guidelines and statements related to the use of radiotherapy for specific cancer diagnoses
  - relate to screening, prevention, and treatment
  - include consensus guidelines, white papers, and model policies

Surgery Quality and Safety

The American College of Surgeons (ACOS) offers programs on quality and safety to optimize the standards of surgical care and ethical practice.

- ACOS Commission on Cancer (CoC) (https://www.facs.org/quality-programs/cancer/coc)
  - Develops cancer care standards, provides quality and safety programs and resources, and offers an oncology accreditation program
    - Accreditation based on *Optimal Resources for Cancer Care* (2020) (https://www.facs.org/quality-programs/cancer/coc/standards/2020)

- Applicants submit evidence of meeting nine accreditation standards and receive an on-site survey demonstrating compliance with all standards
- Accreditation is awarded in 3-year accreditation cycles
- ACOS National Accreditation Program for Breast Centers (https://www.facs.org/quality-programs/napbc)
  - Consortium program focused on improving quality care for individuals with diseases of the breast
  - Accreditation based on *National Accreditation Program for Breast Centers Standards Manual* (2018) six categories:
    - Center leadership
    - Clinical services
    - Research
    - Community outreach
    - Profession education
    - Quality improvement
  - Accreditation evaluation includes initial site visit and re-accreditation visit every 3 years
- ACOS National Accreditation Program for Rectal Centers (https://www.facs.org/quality-programs/cancer/naprc)
  - Collaborative program focused on ensuring quality, multidisciplinary care for individuals with rectal cancer
  - Accreditation based on *Optimal Resource for Rectal Cancer Care* (2020) in eight categories:
    - Institutional administrative commitment
    - Program scope and governance
    - Facilities and equipment resources
    - Personnel and services resources
    - Patient care: expectations and protocols
    - Data surveillance and systems
    - Quality improvement
    - Education: professional and community outreach
- National Cancer Database (NCDB) (https://www.facs.org/quality-programs/cancer/ncdb)
  - Joint effort with the American Cancer Society (ACS) to analyze cancer data from CoC-accredited cancer programs
  - Data are used to analyze cancer trends, create benchmarks, and inform QI efforts
  - Data reflect hospital (e.g., type of accredited program), patient (e.g., age, diagnosis, gender, race or ethnicity, income, insurance status), and treatment (e.g., surgery, chemotherapy, radiation therapy) quality indicators

Oncology Professional Organizations' Initiatives on Quality and Safety

Oncology Nursing Society Quality and Safety Resources

- ONS Quality Improvement Registry (https://www.ons.org/make-difference/quality-improvement/quality-improvement-registry)
  - Provides QI and evidence-based practice (EBP) information and resources in key topics in oncology nursing practice (e.g., cancer-related fatigue, skin toxicity, anxiety/depression)
  - Identifies key metrics for each topic

- Role-Specific Core Competencies (https://www.ons.org/acq-search?search=role+competencies&source=Competencies)
  - ONS publications on role-specific competencies describe the required skills and responsibilities of nurses in many oncology nursing roles:
    - Oncology nurse generalist
    - Oncology nurse navigator
    - Oncology clinical trials nurse
    - Oncology nurse practitioner
    - Oncology clinical nurse specialist
    - Leadership
    - Undergrad-pre-licensure
  - Competency articles can be used to determine expected behaviors of oncology nurses, establish consistent role responsibilities, and develop job descriptions for newly created oncology roles
- ONS Standard for Educating Nurses who Administer Chemotherapy and Biotherapy (https://www.ons.org/sites/default/files/ONS_Standard_Educating_Nurses_Chemo_Pathway_Web_111016.pdf?ref=CO)
  - Algorithm for ONS/Oncology Nursing Certification Corporation (ONCC) educational programs tailored to frequency of administration
  - ONS Fundamentals of Chemotherapy Immunotherapy Administration
  - ONS/ONCC Chemotherapy Immunotherapy Certificate Course
- Additional ONS Courses and Resources (www.ons.org)
  - ONS Developing a Culture of Quality course
  - ONS/ONCC Radiation Therapy Certificate Course
  - Searchable index of course offerings, articles, blogs, events, guidelines, web pages
  - Chemotherapy Biotherapy articles and texts (Coyne et al., 2019; Olsen et al., 2019; Von Ah et al., 2019)

American Society of Clinical Oncology Quality and Safety Initiatives

- Quality Oncology Practice Initiative (QOPI) (https://practice.asco.org/quality-improvement/quality-programs/quality-oncology-practice-initiative)
  - Provides an opportunity for oncology practices to participate tracking multiple quality measures (e.g., core, symptoms, breast, colorectal, end of life).
  - Participants receive quality reports and can benchmark quality measure results with other de-identified practices.
  - Multiple program tracks are available including certification track, international sites, and low-/middle-income country (LMIC) tracks.
- QOPI Certification Program (QCP) (https://practice.asco.org/quality-improvement/quality-programs/qopi-certification-program)
  - Performance-based certification program based on QOPI and standards adapted from the 2016 ASCO/ONS Chemotherapy Administration Safety Standards (Neuss et al., 2017)

- Practice must participate in QOPI quality measure chart abstraction
  - Practice applies for certification, submits evidence of meeting select ASCO/ONS Chemotherapy Administration Safety Standards, and receives an on-site survey.
  - Practices that successfully meet the standards, receive a 3-year QOPI certification.
- Cancer-LinQ (https://www.cancerlinq.org/)
  - Health information technology initiative that aggregates and analyzes data from patient records to promote rapid learning and improve patient outcomes
- ASCO Guidelines, Tools, and Resources (https://www.asco.org/practice-patients/guidelines)
  - Address many aspects of oncology practice, such as assays and predictive markers; prevention, screening, treatment, and follow-up of specific cancers; and supportive care (Woofter et al., 2021)

General Health Care Quality and Safety Initiatives

The Joint Commission (TJC)

TJC, formerly called the Joint Commission on Accreditation of Healthcare Organizations (JCAHO), accredits more than 22,000 health care organizations and certifies many quality and safety programs (https://www.jointcommission.org/)

- Disease-Specific Care Certification Program (https://www.jointcommission.org/accreditation-and-certification/certification/certifications-by-setting/hospital-certifications/disease-specific-care-certification/)
  - TJC does not offer a general certification program in oncology, an oncology practice can apply for certification in specific areas of cancer care (e.g., breast cancer, colorectal cancer, leukemia, lymphoma) in the Disease-Specific Care Certification Program.
  - Programs self-select a minimum of four performance measures related to clinical processes or outcomes and/or program activity.
- Advanced Certification Program for Palliative Care for hospital inpatient programs (https://www.jointcommission.org/accreditation-and-certification/certification/certifications-by-setting/hospital-certifications/palliative-care-certification/)
  - To be eligible for certification, a hospital must do the following:
    - Follow an organized approach supported by an interdisciplinary team of health professionals
    - Use standardized clinical practice guidelines, or EBP
    - Have the ability to direct the clinical management of patients and coordinate care
    - Provide a full range of palliative care services to hospitalized patients 24 hours a day, 7 days a week, with on-site or on-call staff
    - Use performance measurement to improve quality over time
    - Collect data for standardized performance measures

- Requires palliative care programs to collect and analyze data on at least four performance measures that are evidence-based, relevant, valid, and reliable
- National Patient Safety Goals (NPSGs) (https://www.jointcommission.org/standards/national-patient-safety-goals/)
  - Updated each year based on emerging patient safety concerns, TJC identifies key
  - Patient safety goals organized into programs or settings of care (e.g., ambulatory health care, critical access hospital, home care, hospital, long-term care)
  - NPSGs are developed and updated by a multidisciplinary team of experts, including nurses, physicians, pharmacists, risk managers, clinical engineers, and others who identify emerging safety issues in health care
  - Hospital, ambulatory health care, nursing care, and office-based surgery safety goals provide a basis on which to build oncology safety standards

National Academy of Medicine (Formerly Institute of Medicine)

National Academy of Medicine (NAM) periodically publishes consensus reports, meeting proceedings, and special monographs addressing topics relevant to cancer care safety and quality (https://www.nap.edu/). Recent examples include the following:

- Diagnosing and Treating Adult Cancers and Associated Impairments (2021)
- Childhood Cancer and Functional Impacts Across the Care Continuum (2021)
- Advancing Progress in the Development and Implementation of Effective, High-Quality Cancer Screening (2021)
- Addressing the Adverse Consequences of Cancer Treatment (2021)
- Opportunities and Challenges for Using Digital Health Applications in Oncology (2021)
- Delivering High Quality Cancer Care: Charting a New Course for a System in Crisis (2013)
  - Identified the significant patient care and workforce issues confronting the United States regarding the growing number of individuals with cancer, particularly older adults.
  - Recommendations address care coordination, cost, research, technology, competencies of the cancer workforce, end-of-life care, and reduction of disparities.
  - Specifically recommended development of a national quality reporting program for cancer care, establishment of a public reporting system, identification of meaningful quality measures, and development of a national reporting infrastructure.

Quality and Safety Education in Nursing

Begun in 2005 as a collaboration among the Robert Wood Johnson Foundation, the American Association of Colleges of Nursing (ACCN), and the University of North Carolina, it was created to improve quality and safety education in prelicensure through graduate nursing education (https://qsen.org/).

- Six competencies comprise the Quality and Safety Education in Nursing (QSEN) initiative: patient-centered care, teamwork and collaboration, EBP, QI, safety, and informatics.
- QI and safety competencies reflect knowledge, skills, and attitudes required of nurses and are categorized by level of education.
- Numerous resources are available for staff education and development, including literature reviews, learning modules, videos, and webinars.

Occupational Safety and Health Administration

The Occupational Safety and Health Administration (OSHA) develops and monitors workplace standards to ensure workplace safety (https://www.osha.gov/).

- Provides education and training, enforces rules and regulations related to workplace safety issues, including the administration of hazardous drugs and ionizing radiation.
- Maintains a large database of workplace safety issues with search and query functionality.

National Institute for Occupational Safety and Health

The National Institute for Occupational Safety and Health (NIOSH) (https://www.cdc.gov/niosh/index.htm) is the US agency organized within the Centers for Disease Control and Prevention responsible for conducting research and making recommendations for the prevention of work-related injury and illness.

- NIOSH List of Antineoplastic and Other Hazardous Drugs in Healthcare Settings, 2016 (https://www.cdc.gov/niosh/docs/2016-161/)
  - Reference for recommendations on antineoplastic and other hazardous drug preparations, including transport, administration, and disposal.
  - No recommended exposure limits are established for hazardous drugs.
  - Factors affecting workplace exposure include drug handling (i.e., preparation, administration, or disposal), amount of drug prepared, frequency and duration of drug handling, potential for absorption, use of ventilated cabinets, personal protective equipment (PPE), and work practices.
  - Detailed recommendations in the report include assessing hazards in the workplace, handling drugs safely, and using and maintaining equipment properly (see box on this page).
- Closed System Drug-Transfer Device (CSTD) (https://www.cdc.gov/niosh/topics/hazdrug/cstd.html)
  - NIOSH recommends health care workers use a CSTD throughout the hazardous drug-handling chain, from pharmaceutical compounding to patient dose administration.
  - CSTDs should be used as part of a hazardous drug safety program and used in conjunction with other engineering controls.

United States Pharmacopeial (USP) General Chapter 800

The USP General Chapter 800 provides national guidelines for handling hazardous drugs with the intent to reduce exposure for health care personnel and communities (https://www.usp.org/compounding/general-chapter-hazardous-drugs-handling-healthcare).

- The USP Compounding Expert Committee develops General Chapter 800
- Education courses and safety updates regarding USP 800 are offered (https://www.usp.org/compounding/general-chapter-hazardous-drugs-handling-healthcare)
- A resource of frequently asked questions (FAQ) regarding USP 800 is provided on the USP website (https://www.usp.org/frequently-asked-questions/hazardous-drugs-handling-healthcare-settings)

NIOSH Recommendations for Administering Hazardous Drugs

1. Administer drugs safely by using protective medical devices (e.g., needleless systems, closed systems) and techniques (e.g., priming of IV tubing by pharmacy personnel inside a ventilated cabinet, inline priming with nondrug solutions).
2. Wear PPE (including double gloves, goggles, and protective gowns) for all activities associated with drug administration, such as opening the outer bag, assembling the delivery system, delivering the drug to the patient, and disposing of all equipment used to administer drugs.
3. Attach drug administration sets to the IV bag and prime them before adding the drug to the bag.
4. Never remove tubing from an IV bag containing a hazardous drug.
5. Do not disconnect tubing at other points in the system until the tubing has been thoroughly flushed.
6. Remove the IV bag and tubing intact when possible.
7. Place disposable items directly into a yellow chemotherapy waste container and close the lid.
8. Remove outer gloves and gowns, and bag them for disposal in the yellow chemotherapy waste container at the site of drug administration.
9. Double bag the chemotherapy waste before removing inner gloves.
10. Consider double bagging all contaminated equipment.
11. Wash hands with soap and water before leaving the drug administration site.

IV, Intravenous; *NIOSH*, National Institute for Occupational Safety and Health; *PPE*, personal protective equipment.

From Department of Health and Human Services, Centers for Disease Control and Prevention. (2004). *NIOSH alert: Preventing occupational exposure to antineoplastic and other hazardous drugs in health care settings.* Publication number 2004-165. Available at https://www.cdc.gov/niosh/docs/2004-165/pdfs/2004-165.pdf?id=10.26616/NIOSHPUB2004165 (accessed February 3, 2022).

References

Coyne, E., Northfield, S., Ash, K., & Brown-West, L. (2019). Current evidence of education and safety requirements for the nursing administration of chemotherapy: An integrative review. *European Journal of Oncology Nursing, 41,* 24–32.

Neuss, M. N., Gilmore, T. R., Belderson, K. M., Billett, A. L., Conti-Kalchik, T., Harvey, B. E., … Olsen, M. (2017). 2016 Updated American Society of Clinical Oncology/Oncology Nursing Society Chemotherapy administration safety standards, including standards for pediatric oncology. *Oncology Nursing Forum, 44*(1), 31–43.

NIOSH. (2016). *NIOSH list of antineoplastic and other hazardous drugs in healthcare settings, 2016.* By Connor, T. H., MacKenzie, B. A., DeBord, D. G., et al. U.S. Department of Health and Human Services, Centers for Disease Control and Prevention, National Institute for Occupational Safety and Health, DHHS (NIOSH) Publication Number 2016-161 (Supersedes 2014-138).

Olsen, M., LeFebvre, K., & Brassil, K. (2019). *Chemotherapy and immunotherapy guidelines and recommendations for practice.* Pittsburgh: Oncology Nursing Society.

Von Ah, D., Brown, C. G., Brown, S. J., Bryant, A. L., Davies, M., Dodd, M., ... Cooley, M. E. (2019). Research agenda of the oncology nursing society: 2019-2022. *Oncology Nursing Forum, 46*(6), 654–669.

Woofter, K., Kennedy, E. B., Adelson, K., Bowman, R., Brodie, R., Dickson, N., ... Paschall, M. (2021). Oncology medical home: ASCO and COA standards. *JCO Oncology Practice, 17*(8), 475–492.

Evidence-Based Practice

Diane Cope

Definition

- Evidence-based practice (EBP) is the purposeful use of current evidence for making decisions about the care of a patient.
- EBP integrates the best evidence with clinical expertise and the patient's desires, values, and needs to facilitate clinical decision-making.

Goals of Evidence-Based Practice

- EBP provides the highest quality of care to patients and their families.
- EBP provides practicing nurses with the best and most current evidence.
- EBP resolves problems in the clinical setting.
- EBP reduces variations in nursing care.
- EBP promotes effective nursing interventions.
- EBP assists with efficient and effective decision-making.

Five Steps of Evidence-Based Practice

- Step 1: Ask a searchable clinical question.
- Step 2: Find the best evidence to answer the question.
- Step 3: Critically appraise the evidence.
- Step 4: Apply the evidence with clinical expertise, taking the patient's wants and needs into consideration.
- Step 5: Evaluate the effectiveness and efficiency of the process.

Step 1: Ask a Searchable Clinical Question

- Use the PICOT format.
- The PICOT variables provide a framework for searching electronic databases for the most relevant articles to address the clinical question:
  P: patient population of interest
  I: intervention or area of interest
  C: comparison intervention or group
  O: outcome
  T: time

Step 2: Find the Best Evidence to Answer the Question

- Consider scheduling a meeting with a science librarian.
- Identify key searchable words or phrases from the clinical question.
- Combine searches using the Boolean connector *AND* to limit and refine the search; *OR* to expand the search.
- Select relevant databases to search for the evidence:
  - Cochrane Database of Systematic Reviews (www.cochrane.org)
  - Database of Abstracts of Reviews of Effects
  - PubMed/Medline (www.ncbi.nlm.nih.gov/pubmed)
  - Cumulative Index to Nursing and Allied Health Literature (CINAHL) (https://www.ebsco.com/products/research-databases/cinahl-database)
  - National Guideline Clearinghouse (www.guideline.gov)

Step 3: Critically Appraise the Evidence

- Research literature is systematically examined to appraise its trustworthiness, value, and relevance in a particular context.
- Strong evidence fulfills the requirements of three criteria:
  - *Quality*: randomized, controlled trials (RCTs) to avoid selection bias
  - *Validity*: outcomes that are large and statistically significant
  - *Size*: trials with large numbers of patients
- Levels of evidence (i.e., hierarchy of evidence) (see table below) are assigned to studies based on the methodologic quality of their design, validity, and applicability to patient care, factors that determine the grade (i.e., strength) of the recommendation.
  - Many scales for levels of evidence exist and use three to seven levels.
  - Although standardized definitions of the levels of evidence are lacking, systematic reviews or meta-analyses of RCTs and EBP guidelines are considered the strongest level of evidence, and expert opinions are considered the weakest level of evidence to guide practice decisions.
  - High levels of evidence may not exist for all clinical questions.

Hierarchy of Evidence

Evidence Level	Type of Evidence*	Type of Evidence†
I	Randomized, controlled trial (RCT) Meta-analysis of RCTs	Systematic review or meta-analysis
II	Quasi-experimental study	RCT
III	Nonexperimental study Qualitative study Meta-synthesis	Controlled trial without randomization
IV		Case-control or cohort study
V		Descriptive study Systematic review of qualitative or descriptive studies
VI		Descriptive study Qualitative study
VII		Opinion or consensus

*Using the system of Dang, D., Dearholt, S. L., Bissett, K., Ascenzi, J., & Whalen, M. (2021). *Johns Hopkins evidence-based practice for nurses and healthcare professionals: Model and guidelines* (4th ed.). Indianapolis, IN: Sigma Theta Tau International.
†Using the system of Melnyk, B. M., & Fineout-Overholt, E. (Eds.). (2018). *Evidence-based practice in nursing and healthcare: A guide to best practice* (4th ed.). Philadelphia: Lippincott Williams & Wilkins.

- Types of studies
  - *Systematic review:* An article in which the authors have systematically searched for, appraised, and summarized all of the medical literature for a specific topic.
  - *Meta-analysis:* A systematic review that uses quantitative methods to combine and reanalyze results from the combined studies to summarize results based on the pool of studies.
  - *RCT:* Study that includes patients randomized to an experimental group or a control group of those not receiving the intervention. The groups are evaluated over time for the variables or outcomes of interest.
  - *Quasi-experimental study:* An interventional study in which subjects are not randomly assigned to treatment groups or a control group.
  - *Nonexperimental study:* A study in which data are collected without introducing an intervention, usually descriptive in nature.
  - *Cohort study:* Research that identifies two groups (i.e., cohorts) of patients (i.e., one group that received the exposure or intervention and one that did not), with the cohorts followed to examine the outcomes.
  - *Case-control study:* Research that identifies patients who have the outcome of interest (i.e., cases) and persons without the same outcome (i.e., controls) to determine the exposure of interest.
  - *Descriptive study:* Research that examines individual characteristics or circumstances and the frequency in which they occur in a population.
  - *Qualitative study:* A study of phenomena that are difficult or impossible to quantify mathematically that is performed by collection of narrative data that is analyzed for cross-cutting themes.
  - *Expert opinion:* Handbooks, encyclopedias, textbooks, and clinical experience of respected authorities

Step 4: Apply the Evidence With Clinical Expertise, Taking the Patient's Wants and Needs Into Consideration

- Applies the evidence to the patient or their family, or both.
- Incorporates clinical knowledge gained over time.
- Incorporates the patient's unique situation, desires, and values.

Step 5: Evaluate the Effectiveness and Efficiency of the Process

- After implementation, evaluation is performed to determine whether the practice resulted in positive outcomes.

- Outcome measurement
  - How are outcomes measured?
  - Who performs the measurement?
  - Do instruments exist for measurement of the outcomes?

Oncology Nursing Society Putting Evidence Into Practice

The Oncology Nursing Society (ONS) coordinates Putting Evidence into Practice (PEP) projects that summarize evidence-based interventions for the care of patients.

- Systematic reviews that are conducted by oncology nurses cover a wide array of topics.
- Categories of assessment
  - *Recommended for practice:* interventions for which effectiveness has been established
  - *Likely to be effective:* interventions for which evidence is less well established
  - *Benefits balanced with harms:* clinicians advised to consider the risk–benefit ratio
  - *Effectiveness not established:* insufficient data are available, or data may not be of adequate quality to determine the effectiveness of an intervention
  - *Effectiveness unlikely:* effectiveness of an intervention is less well established
  - *Not recommended for practice:* ineffectiveness or harm demonstrated

Relevance of Evidence-Based Practice to Nursing Practice

- Nursing practice should be based on science rather than tradition.
- EBP improves patient outcomes.
- EBP decreases unnecessary procedures.
- EBP empowers nursing through sound knowledge.

Bibliography

Dang, D., Dearholt, S. L., Bissett, K., Ascenzi, J., & Whalen, M. (2021). *Johns Hopkins evidence-based practice for nurses and healthcare professionals: Model and guidelines* (4th ed.). Indianapolis, IN: Sigma Theta Tau International.

Melnyk, B. M., & Fineout-Overholt, E. (Eds.). (2018). *Evidence-based practice in nursing and healthcare: A guide to best practice* (4th ed.). Philadelphia: Lippincott Williams & Wilkins.

Mitchell, S. A., & Friese, C. R. (2022). *Decision rules for summative evaluation of a body of evidence.* Available at https://www.ons.org/explore-resources/pep/decision-rules-summative-evaluation-body-evidence (accessed January 10, 2022).

Oncology Nursing Society. (2022). *Evidence-based practice learning library.* Available at https://www.ons.org/learning-libraries/evidence-based-practice (accessed January 10, 2022).

Polit, D. F., & Beck, C. T. (2019). *Nursing research: Generating and assessing evidence for nursing practice* (11th ed.). Philadelphia: Lippincott Williams & Wilkins.

Nurse Navigation*

Darcy Burbage

Introduction

The role of patient navigation is typically credited to the foundational work led by Dr. Harold P. Freeman in the 1990s with low-income women diagnosed with breast cancer in Harlem, New York. Dr. Freeman created the nation's first navigation program in response to concerns identified regarding health care disparities among vulnerable populations, including low-income and racial/ethnic minority groups (Freeman & Rodriguez, 2011). The program provided a framework to ensure available access to timely care and support systems to help eliminate financial, social, and cultural barriers to care. As a result of navigation interventions delivered, significant shifts were noted in terms of earlier stage at diagnosis and improved survival. These demonstrated successes in Harlem, New York, led to widespread national attention regarding the important role patient navigation can play in improving cancer outcomes and reducing health care disparities. Fast forward 30 years, and the role of navigation has evolved into a valued part of cancer programs and an essential component of quality care. Funds from multiple sources, including private foundations, community organizations, and local, state, and federal governments, along with health systems, have been allocated to advance the efforts of navigation and further expand adoption of the service with the overall intent of reducing health care disparities (Freeman & Rodriguez, 2011).

Definitions of Navigation

C-Change, a collaborative organization involving cancer leaders from public, private, and not-for-profit groups, is frequently cited as first defining navigation in 2005 as "individualized assistance offered to patients, families, and caregivers to help overcome health care system barriers and facilitate timely access to quality medical and psychosocial care" (C-Change, 2005). In 2010, President Obama signed the Patient Protection and Affordable Care Act, which required navigation programs to become part of health care. Currently, they are required components of the Oncology Care Model, a novel episode-based payment system developed by the Center for Medicare and Medicaid Services (Karam, 2020). Other organizations have adopted and embraced this definition of navigation, including the American College of Surgeons Commission on Cancer (2020), which revised their cancer program standards to include a component related to patient navigation services. "Patient navigation," also be referred to as "lay navigation," takes into account that non–health care providers are serving in navigation roles as well as nurses. Social workers may also function in navigation positions.

Models of Navigation

The first navigation program created by Dr. Freeman consisted predominantly of two interventions: access to free and low-cost mammography services paired with individualized assistance in obtaining timely diagnosis and initiation of treatment. His program engaged community members in cancer outreach efforts who were deemed to be successful because of their inherent knowledge of and sensitivity to the community's cultural and language barriers.

Since the inception of the initial navigation program, Dr. Freeman has identified and vetted nine core principles of patient navigation that remain foundational today (Freeman & Rodriguez, 2011):

1. Patient navigation is a patient-centric health care service delivery model.
2. Patient navigation serves to virtually integrate a fragmented health care system for the individual patient.
3. The core function of patient navigation is the elimination of barriers to timely care across all segments of the health care continuum.
4. Patient navigation should be defined with a clear scope of practice that distinguishes the roles and responsibilities of the navigator from those of all other providers.
5. Delivery of patient navigation services should be cost-effective and commensurate with the training and skills necessary to navigate an individual through a particular phase of the care continuum.
6. The determination of who should navigate should be determined by the level of skills required at a given phase of navigation.
7. In a given system of care, there is the need to define the point at which navigation begins and the point at which navigation ends.
8. There is a need to navigate patients across disconnected systems of care, such as primary care sites and tertiary care sites.
9. Patient navigation systems require coordination.

As additional navigation programs have been implemented, various models and adaptations have evolved. Various navigation models, along with key characteristics and potential program advantages, are outlined in the table on the next page.

Models of navigation deemed to be most effective have been specifically designed to meet the needs of a defined population and an individual cancer program. A common notion among experienced navigators and program administrators is that "one size does *not* fit all" when it comes to navigation programs and interventions. Rather, thoughtful assessment and program planning are essential to create a program that best meets the needs of one's community.

---

* The author would like to acknowledge Karyl Blaseg, RN, MN, OCN for her contributions to the previous edition of this book.

Examples of Navigation Models

	Community	Professional
Community/Lay Navigation Versus Professional Navigation		
Characteristics	Non–health care professional • Typically, a member of the community served • May or may not be a cancer survivor	Health care professional • Registered nurse • Social worker • Others (e.g., advanced practice registered nurse, mammography technologist)
	Volunteer or paid employee, full- or part-time May or may not be embedded within a health care system	Paid employee, full- or part-time Typically embedded within a health care system
Advantages	Lower program costs	Professional scope of practice allowing for greater patient education and supportive care Good working knowledge of complex health care systems
	Keen awareness of financial, social, and cultural barriers Great potential for cultural diversity	
Site-Specific Navigation Versus Setting-Specific Navigation		
	Site-Specific	**Setting-Specific**
Characteristics	Professional or community/lay navigator Dedicated to single or multiple types of cancers	Professional or community/lay navigator Focused on a single aspect of care, such as • Outreach/prevention/screening • Genetics/high-risk surveillance • Diagnostic Mammography Center • Financial • Inpatient unit • Integrative health • Oral therapy • Survivorship • Palliative/supportive care
Advantages	Commonly embedded within health care system Focused on timely coordination of multidisciplinary care Professional scope of practice allowing for greater patient education and supportive care Clinical expertise regarding specific types of cancers and national care guidelines Good working knowledge of complex health care systems	Narrow scope of responsibilities, which may facilitate hard-wiring of specific processes
Mixed Model Navigation		
Characteristics	Combination of one or more of the above models	
Advantages	Potential for more cost-effective utilization of resources Potential for greater diversity Recognition for the positive attributes of both professional and community/lay navigators	

Roles, Responsibilities, and Core Competencies

Specific roles and responsibilities of navigators vary according to the navigation model created, defined start and end points for navigation, and extent of services provided. Despite this variability, core fundamental roles can be identified among navigators. These include identification and resolution of barriers to care, coordination of timely access to care, facilitation of open communication and collaboration, and provision of emotional support. Competence has largely been associated with the knowledge, skills, and attitudes required to fulfill a specific navigation role. A clearly defined competency framework is essential to establishing the role expectations and responsibilities for a navigator.

Cantril et al. (2019) evaluated the role, scope of work, and educational preparation of the oncology nurse navigator (ONN) between two health systems. Results of their work demonstrated striking inconsistencies between academic preparation, responsibilities, scope of work, and even job titles, lending support to the importance of consistency in the standardization of the ONNs' role, ongoing validation and evaluation of competencies, and integration and tracking of metrics to measure success (Cantril et al., 2019).

The National Coalition of Oncology Nurse Navigators (NCONNs), which later disbanded, developed the first set of core competencies for ONNs in 2009. Similar efforts were undertaken by the Academy of Oncology Nurse and Patient Navigators (AONN+) which was founded with the goal of providing a network for professionals involved in and interested in navigation to better manage the complexities of cancer treatment throughout the care continuum. Since their inception, the AONN+ has collaborated on developing metrics, establishing certification, and providing education for both professional and lay navigators (AONN+, 2020).

Building upon the initial role delineation study conducted by the Oncology Nursing Society (ONS) in 2010, a second study was conducted in 2016 to better understand the core responsibilities and job functions and potential changes of this specialty area. Data obtained from participants further helped to define the knowledge, tasks, and skills specific to the ONN role and led to revisions to the ONS Position Statement and Core Competencies for ONNs, which also included development of the Oncology Nurse Navigation Care Model (ONNCM) to reflect how the ONN affects each phase of the cancer care continuum (Oncology Nursing Society, 2017, 2018).

In 2017, the ONS revised their ONN core competencies to address four key areas along with defining the role of the novice and expert ONN in achieving these competencies (Oncology Nursing Society, 2017). To align with these competencies, ONS released its own position statement specifically addressing the role of the ONN throughout the cancer continuum (Oncology Nursing Society, 2018). The position statement supports that nurses in ONN roles should practice in accordance with the ONS ONN core competencies as applicable to their practice setting recognizing that the role of the ONN should be tailored to meet the needs of the patient in their practice setting (Oncology Nursing Society, 2018).

The second ONS-conducted role delineation study noted that the role of the ONN has quickly evolved since 2010 (Lubejko et al., 2017). While similar to results obtained from the first role delineation study, several additional key areas emerged that set apart the ONN role from that of the clinic or staff nurse. Most important is that the ONN serves as the essential point of contact for patients and caregivers throughout the cancer continuum. Roles delineated in the study include the following:

Tasks

- Ensure timely *access* to appropriate care throughout the cancer continuum
- Identify and assist patients with individual *barriers* to care
- *Coordinate care* to ensure timely and smooth transitions throughout the cancer continuum
- Facilitate *communication* among patients, providers, and other agencies
- Facilitate distress screening
- Survivorship care planning

Knowledge Areas

- Pathophysiology of cancer
- Multimodality treatment planning
- Goals of care
- Symptom management
- Quality of life
- Evidence-based practice guidelines

Skills

- Communication
- Collaboration
- Critical thinking
- Problem solving
- Advocacy
- Multitasking
- Time management
- Patient and family education

Considerations for Building a Successful Navigation Program

Program Preparations

Those with the vision to create a successful navigation program must engage the support of administrative leadership and key stakeholders including providers, patients, other staff, and local community organizations. The desire to develop a navigation program may be prompted by an accreditation standard or funding requirement of an external agency. However, even if that is the impetus, it is important to take time to conduct a thorough community and cancer-program needs assessment to clearly identify and understand existing needs for which navigation services can effectively address and positively impact patient care. A robust needs assessment might include information from local community health reports, local and state cancer registries, the Centers for Disease Control and Prevention and National Cancer Institute databases, and the American Cancer Society Cancer Facts and Figures data to identify concerning trends in access to care, stage at diagnosis, and increasing rates of incidence or mortality. Also, key pieces of information can be gleaned through community focus groups with patients, families, and caregivers affected by cancer to learn firsthand the barriers and challenges experienced when seeking cancer care and any gaps in the health care delivery system (Cantril et al., 2019; American College of Surgeons, 2020).

Once the needs assessment has been completed and analyzed, the structure of the navigation program can be developed along with identified goals and objectives. Key considerations when establishing the program framework include clearly identifying the start and end points for navigation interventions, aligning the program with organizational priorities, and setting realistic program goals and objectives. Objectives direct the focus of a program and should be used to break down large, long-term goals into manageable and achievable pieces. Once goals and objectives have been determined, measures should be identified to assess program performance, processes, and the achievement of defined objectives. Most sustainable and successful navigation programs have been established over time by starting small and building incrementally through continuous process improvements and program expansion as objectives are achieved and positive outcomes are demonstrated (AONN+, 2020).

Job descriptions should be established and should clearly define position requirements reflective of program needs, along with key roles and responsibilities. Along with the creation of job descriptions, high-level process maps should be outlined to clearly identify the scope of responsibilities, system bottlenecks, and where patient navigation attention might initially be focused. Standard operating procedures (SOPs) should be documented. SOPs set role expectations by outlining the specific steps associated with various responsibilities and tasks required of the patient navigator. These documents should be reviewed on an established schedule (i.e., annually or biennially) and updated to reflect process and role changes (Kline et al., 2019).

Successful Onboarding

The importance of hiring the right person and providing meaningful orientation and training for a navigation program cannot be overemphasized. Consideration must first be given to the specific navigation model to be implemented and to determine whether this program would best be served with a professional or a community/lay navigator. Further thought should then be given to specific qualities and characteristics of the desired candidate, including cultural competence, superb communication skills, thorough familiarity with disease processes, sound knowledge of resources, and demonstrated leadership skills. An orientation checklist provides a structured "roadmap" for the orientation process and helps to direct the patient navigator in obtaining a broad understanding and solid knowledge base of the organization's systems, processes, and overall culture.

Aside from orientation to the specific organization and role expectations, a number of navigation training programs as well as online program resources and toolkits are available for those just getting started in the role. Some examples include:

- Training Programs
  - Equipping the Novice Oncology Nurse Navigator An Oncology Nursing Society (ONS) Collaboration with the AONN+: https://www.ons.org/courses/equipping-novice-oncology-nurse-navigator-ons-collaboration-aonn
  - Patient Navigator Training Collaborative: http://www.patientnavigatortraining.org
  - EduCare: http://www.educareinc.com
  - The George Washington Cancer Institute https://smhs.gwu.edu/gwci/survivorship/center-advancement-cancer-survivorship-navigation-and-policy-casnp/patient-navigator
  - Harold P. Freeman Patient Navigation Institute: http://www.hpfreemanpni.org
  - Smith Center for Healing and the Arts: http://www.smithcenter.org
- Program Development Resources
  - Association of Community Cancer Centers (ACCC): https://www.accc-cancer.org/projects/patient-navigation-project/patient-navigation-tools
  - The Boston Medical Center Patient Navigation Toolkit: https://sites.bu.edu/coeinwomenshealth/resources/avontoolkits/
  - Oncology Nurse Navigator Toolkit: https://www.ons.org/clinical-practice-resources/ons-oncology-nurse-navigator-toolkit
  - National Academies of Science, Engineering, and Medicine: Establishing Effective Patient Navigation Programs in Oncology. https://www.nap.edu/catalog/25073/establishing-effective-patient-navigation-programs-in-oncology-proceedings-of-a-workshop
  - Patient Navigation in Cancer Care (Pfizer, Inc.): http://www.patientnavigation.com

Program Evaluation

The Navigation Assessment Tool can assess the growth potential of both new and existing patient navigation programs (Swanson et al., 2012). This document was developed by consensus and structured in a matrix format with 16 identified core measures that represent important elements in building a strong navigation program, each with up to five levels

of maturity. The intent of this tool was to provide an institutional self-assessment of the maturity of individual programs and to offer a structure to systematically expand the depth and breadth of patient navigation services provided. This tool outlined 16 core measures of the Navigation Assessment Tool as follows:

1. Key stakeholders
2. Community partnerships
3. Acuity system/patient risk factors
4. Quality improvement measures
5. Marketing of the navigation program
6. Percentage of patients offered patient navigation
7. Continuum of navigation
8. Support services available and used by the navigation team
9. Tools for reporting navigator statistics
10. Financial assessment
11. Focus on disparities
12. Navigator responsibilities
13. Patient identification process
14. Navigator training
15. Engagement with clinical trials
16. Multidisciplinary care/conference involvement

Flucke and Sullivan-Moore (2021) developed another standardized assessment tool specific to the needs of patients in rural areas, recognizing rural patients that experience greater challenges accessing oncology services, leading to a higher risk of dying as compared to individuals living in urban areas. This unique tool is another resource to assist navigators in providing individualized patient care and allow for tracking of barriers over time, as well as aligning with program goals and accreditation standards (Flucke & Sullivan-Moore, 2021).

Outcomes and Performance Measures

The literature on navigation is rapidly expanding, with evidence showing the positive impact navigation has on improving clinical outcomes and the overall patient experience. Despite positive outcome themes that have emerged (e.g., screening access, time to diagnostic resolution and treatment, satisfaction levels, health care costs and resource utilization, access to community-based resources), concern exists regarding inconsistencies in reporting outcomes as well as program variations, making it challenging to compare outcomes and advance the scientific evidence related to navigation.

Until recently, recommendations for standardizing navigation-sensitive metrics were not available. In response to these concerns, the American Cancer Society organized the National Patient Navigation Leadership Summit in 2010 with the intent of establishing a national consensus on core program metrics and outcome measures related to patient navigation across the cancer continuum (Esparza & Calhoun, 2011). As a result of this Summit, the National Cancer Policy Forum convened a two-day conference on establishing effective patient navigation programs in oncology, which led to a task force to standardize program metrics to determine benchmarks for navigation programs in order to improve patient care delivery and quality cancer care outcomes. In 2020, the AONN+ published its navigation metrics toolkit, a comprehensive guide for navigation programs to measure the impact and reach of the role of navigation. Core navigation metrics identified by the study team include five overarching areas: navigator competencies, navigator caseload, barriers to care, psychosocial distress screening, and interventions (AONN+, 2020).

Future of Navigation

The navigation role has demonstrated significant strides over the past 30 years and has documented the positive impact navigation can have on reducing the financial, social, and cultural burdens of cancer while improving clinical outcomes. Initiatives related to navigation continue to build momentum through focused efforts and widespread adoption as organizations increasingly recognize these benefits. The role of navigation continues to be a consistent and core element of accreditation standards, Accountable Care Organizations and Medical Home initiatives across the country. The future holds endless possibilities for navigation and the need to ensure continuity of care across the health care continuum.

References

Academy of Oncology Nurse and Patient Navigators. (2020). *Navigation metrics toolkit*. Available at https://www.aonnonline.org/navigation-metrics.

American College of Surgeons. (2020). *Commission on Cancer. Ensuring patient-centered care*: Cancer program standards. Available at https://www.facs.org/quality-programs/cancer/coc/standards/2020.

Cantril, C., Christensen, D., & Moore, E. (2019). Standardizing roles: Evaluating oncology nurse navigator clarity, educational preparation, and scope of work within two healthcare systems. *Clinical Journal of Oncology Nursing, 23*(1), 52–59.

C-Change. (2005). *Cancer patient navigation*. C-Change.

Esparza, A., & Calhoun, E. (2011). Measuring the impact and potential of patient navigation. *Cancer, 117*(suppl. 15), 3535–3536.

Flucke, N., & Sullivan-Moore, C. P. (2021). Patient assessment: Using the Oncology Nurse Navigator Patient Assessment for rural and other resource poor settings. *Clinical Journal of Oncology Nursing, 25*(6), 729–734.

Freeman, H. P., & Rodriguez, R. I. (2011). History and principles of patient navigation. *Cancer, 117*(suppl. 15), 3539–3542.

Karam, S. (2020). New roles in oncology nurse navigation. *ONS Voice*, 1–4.

Kline, R. M., Rocque, G. B., Rohan, E. A., Blackley, K. A., Cantril, C. A., Pratt-Chapman, M. L., & Shulman, L. N. (2019). Patient navigation in cancer: The business case to support clinical needs. *Journal of Oncology Practice, 15*(11), 585–590.

Lubejko, B. G., Bellfield, S., Kahn, E., Lee, C., Peterson, N., Rose, T., & McCorkle, M. (2017). Oncology Nurse Navigation: Results of the 2016 role delineation study. *Clinical Journal of Oncology Nursing, 21*(1), 43–50.

Oncology Nursing Society. (2017). *Oncology nurse navigator core competencies*. Oncology Nursing Society.

Oncology Nursing Society. (2018). *Role of the oncology nurse navigator throughout the cancer trajectory*. Oncology Nursing Society.

Swanson, J. R., Strusowski, P., Mack, N., & DeGroot, J. (2012). Growing a navigation program: Using the NCCCP Navigation Assessment Tool. *Oncology Issues, 27*(4), 36–45.

Patient Education

Leah A. Scaramuzzo

Patient education is a critical component of almost every nursing intervention. It involves more than just telling patients to take their medications or manage their symptoms. Rather, it encompasses skill building and helping patients learn when, how, and even why to make changes. Patient education requires a baseline needs assessment of the patient and caregiver in order to comprehensively address needs adequately (see the table on next page). Understanding and overcoming educational, ethnic, sociocultural, and spiritual barriers should be incorporated into every education plan. Ultimately, the process should build patient knowledge and skills and enable patients and their caretakers to participate actively in their care and contribute to positive outcomes. Education that patients can understand will contribute greatly to their satisfaction with care, promote adherence to plans of care, and increase the quality of their lives.

What Are the Challenges of Providing Patient Education?

- Shorter hospitalizations and therefore less time to teach
- Ambulatory clinic visits with limited time allocated for patient education
- Increased complexity of care at home and need for more comprehensive education
- Patients' seeking information from at least one other source besides the physician
- Information on the Internet that may be misleading, subject to interpretation, or is clearly incorrect
- Literacy level or difficulty interpreting and retaining information
- Anxiety, physical symptoms, or medications that may affect concentration and recollection

Need for Varied Teaching Methods

Although many clinicians believe they have given adequate instruction or information during a patient visit, they may fail to realize that patients do not retain everything they are told while in the examination room, clinic, or hospital. Patients retain:

- 20% of what they hear
- 30% of what they see
- 50% of what they see and hear
- 70% of what they see, hear, and say
- 90% of what they see, hear, say, and do

Content needs to be reinforced by various learning methods. Combining different methods—written materials, verbal instruction, demonstration, and patient participation—during the learning process makes it more likely that patients will retain the information provided.

Outcomes of Patient Education

- Promote communication between patient and health care provider
- Reduce uncertainty
- Encourage participation in decision making
- Increase adherence to the plan of care
- Maximize self-care skills
- Increase ability to cope with health status
- Promote healthy lifestyles and behaviors
- Increase empowerment and autonomy
- Reduce health care expenditures

Mandates and Standards for Patient Education

- American Hospital Association (AHA)—*A Patient's Bill of Rights*
- The Federal Plain Language Guidelines—*The Plain Language Action and Information Network (PLAIN)*: a community of federal employees dedicated to the idea that citizens deserve clear communications from government
- National Health Education Standards—*The Joint Committee on National Health Education Standards*: written expectations for what students should know and be able to do by grades 2, 5, 8, and 12 to promote personal, caregiver, and community health. These standards provide a framework for curriculum development, selection, instruction, and student assessment in health education.
- National Culturally and Linguistically Appropriate Services (CLAS) Standards—*Department of Health and Human Services, Office of Minority Health*: helps organizations address cultural and language differences between people who provide information and services and the people they serve. The principal standard is to provide effective, equitable, understandable, and respectful quality care and services that are responsive to diverse cultural health beliefs, practices, preferred languages, health literacy, and other communication needs.
- American Society of Clinical Oncology/Oncology Nursing Society Chemotherapy Administration Safety Standards Including Standards for Pediatric Oncology

Role of the Nurse in Patient Education

Definition	Roles
To determine the patient's knowledge base and his or her need to know: • Assess learning barriers and best means to learn • Assess preference for brief or plentiful information	Identify the potential learner: • Patient, caregiver, spouse, significant other Identify barriers that may influence learning outcomes: • Physical • Sensory (vision/hearing) • Emotional, e.g., anxiety • Readiness to learn • Denial of need to learn • Cultural, religious • Cognitive • Literacy level, educational level • Social determinants • Special learning needs • Speech • Financial concerns • Language (non–English speaking) Identify preferred learning method: • Reading • Pictures • Video • Listening • Demonstration
To develop and strategize the best means to educate the patient/caregiver	Identify expressed educational needs/concerns: • Diagnosis–disease process, plan of care and treatment options • Procedures, preoperative and postoperative teaching • Medical equipment and skills • Pain and symptom management • Cancer treatments and side effect management • Medications • Nutrition, drug/food interactions • Community resources, coping strategies, advance directives • Activity • Personal hygiene • Prevention of infection • Speech and hearing evaluations • Discharge planning • Other areas as identified by the patient/caregiver
To prioritize and execute teaching content to ensure that the learner's needs are met and self-care activities vital to ongoing physical and psychological well-being are taught	Establish an environment that encourages patients and families to ask questions, learn, and participate: • Provide respect • Offer privacy • Establish eye contact • Listen attentively • If possible, sit with patient/caregiver Mutually determine goals and time frame Methods of teaching: • Explanation • Demonstration • Written • Audio/visual Settings: • In-person • Telephone • Telehealth
To determine whether the content has been learned	Verbalize understanding via the teach-back method: • Ask patient to explain in his or her own words the information shared. • Example: "Share with me what you will explain to your wife about your medicines for nausea and vomiting and how you will take them." Identify need for further information or reinforcement

Education Theories

- *Behavioral Learning Theory:* Learning is based on observable behaviors (e.g., relaxation)
- *Cognitive Learning Theory:* Internal processes lead to learning (e.g., creation of mnemonic for symptoms to call the physician)
- *Social Learning Theory:* Learning takes place based on watching and imitating others
- *Motivational Learning Theory:* Learning results from personal cues (e.g., "I want to be here for my children, so I have to quit smoking")
- *Adult Learning Theory:* Uses approaches that are problem-based, collaborative, and less didactic; the six principles of adult learners are:
  1. They are internally motivated and self-directed
  2. They bring life experiences and knowledge to learning experiences
  3. They are goal oriented
  4. They are relevancy oriented
  5. They are practical
  6. They like to be respected

Learner Barriers to Education

- Lack of emotional readiness
  - Anxiety, lack of support system, motivation
  - Risk-taking behaviors
  - Frame of mind in accordance with Maslow's hierarchy of needs (e.g., if basic needs are not met, learning cannot occur)
- Lack of experiential readiness
  - Level of aspiration
  - Past coping mechanisms
  - Cultural background
  - Social determinants (food, shelter, etc.)
  - Locus of control, assertiveness
- Limited cognitive ability
  - Extent to which information can be processed
  - Behavioral objectives + cognitive ability = learning
  - Knowledge versus competence
  - Competency validation
  - Health literacy + activation = health outcomes

Barriers to Providing Effective Patient Education

- Lack of awareness regarding the patient's level of health literacy
- Lack of time to talk with the patient and answer questions
- Inaccurate simplification of complex scientific information
- A view that simplifying information means "dumbing it down"
- Concerns about offending skilled readers
- Staff turnover and need for periodic training
- Lack of staff buy-in or interest

Health Education Goals

- Inform and instruct
- Empower and motivate
- Prevent problems and complications

- Enhance quality of life
- Supplement information given verbally

Health Literacy

Definition

Health literacy is the ability to obtain, process, understand, and act on health care information. Examples include:

- Reading consent forms and medicine labels
- Understanding written and oral information
- Acting on procedures and instructions

Health Literacy in the United States

- The health of 90 million people may be at risk because of difficulty understanding and acting on health information.
- Only 12% of adults have proficient health literacy.
- Literacy skills are a stronger predictor of an individual's health status than age, income, employment status, education level, or racial/ethnic group.
- One out of five American adults reads at the fifth grade level or below.
- The average American reads at the eighth to ninth grade level, yet most health care materials are written above the 10th grade level.
- More than 66% of adults in America age 60 and older have inadequate or marginal literacy skills.
- According to the Center for Health Care Strategies, a disproportionate number of minority group members and immigrants have limited literacy.

High-Risk Groups

- Elderly individuals
- Minority group members
- Immigrants
- Poor people
- Homeless people
- Prisoners
- People with limited education

Possible Results of Low Health Literacy

- Poor health outcomes such as higher rates of hospitalization, less frequent use of preventive services, higher health care costs
- Poor patient adherence to treatment protocols and medications including oral therapy
- Medication or treatment errors
- Poor self-care management strategies
- Lack of participation in informed decision making, healthy lifestyle choices, cancer prevention and screening
- Difficulty navigating the health care system
- Higher rates of missed appointments

Indirect Indicators of Reading Problems

- Mouthing words
- Pointing to text as it is read
- Complaints of poor eyesight or wrong glasses (see the box on this page)

Attributes of a Health Literate Health Care Organization

1. Has leadership that makes health literacy integral to its mission, structure, and operations.
2. Integrates health literacy into planning, evaluation measures, patient safety, and quality improvement.
3. Prepares the workforce to be health literate and monitors progress.
4. Includes populations served in the design, implementation, and evaluation of health information and services.
5. Meets the needs of populations with a range of health literacy skills while avoiding stigmatization.
6. Uses health literacy strategies in interpersonal communications and confirms understanding at all points of contact.
7. Provides easy access to health information and services and navigation assistance.
8. Designs and distributes print, audiovisual, and social media content that is easy to understand and act on.
9. Addresses health literacy in high-risk situations, including care transitions and communications about medicines.
10. Communicates clearly what health plans cover and what individuals will have to pay for services.

From Brach, C., Keller, D., Hernandez, L. M., Baur, C., Parker, R., Dreyer, B., … Schillinger, D. (2012). Ten attributes of health literate health care organizations. NAM Perspectives, Discussion Paper. Washington, DC: National Academy of Medicine. https://doi.org/10.31478/201206a.

Health Education Materials

Advantages of Printed Educational Materials

- Consistency of message content
- Flexibility of delivery
- Portability and reusability
- Low cost to produce and update
- Permanence of information
- Reinforcement of verbal instructions

Goals of Patient Education Materials

Patient education materials should ensure patient and caregiver ability to do the following:

- Read prescription bottles and appointment slips
- Understand informed consents and discharge instructions
- Follow diagnostic test instructions
- Read health education materials
- Complete health insurance applications

Outcomes of Providing Understandable Health Care Instructions

- Improved treatment adherence
- Decreased hospitalization and return visits to the hospital or emergency room
- Improved health outcomes

Developing Written Materials

- Define target audience: involve audience in planning and writing. Ensure material is relevant and appropriate for the patient's literacy level, age, sex, and culture.
- Identify key points of the material to impart.
- Determine the tone: aim for a friendly and conversational tone.
- Ascertain readability: ensure material is easy to read and understand; have more than one person review it.
- Use common words; give examples to explain uncommon words.
- Use short sentences.
- Include interaction, if possible.
- Place key information first.

- Use headers.
- Use serif type and lowercase lettering, for example, Times New Roman.
- Use 12- to 14-point fonts.
- Avoid using capital letters.

Content and Organization

- Content should be verified by subject matter experts.
- The purpose of the material should be clear to the audience.
- Present only the most important information.
- New information should be related to what the audience already knows.
- Retention of information is lower when the content is unfamiliar.
- Organize content to convey the meaning of the material and to motivate the learner.
- Examples should be limited to those that the audience can understand and relate to.
- Summarize points throughout the text.

Organizing Principles

- Use short titles that convey meaning clearly.
- Include a table of contents.
- Repeat important information in bulleted lists.
- Keep related ideas together; present only one idea per paragraph.
- State the main idea in the first sentence of the paragraph.
- Keep sentences short and simple.

Appropriate Language and Format

- Language should not exceed sixth grade reading level.
- Limit sentences to one idea.
- Avoid complicated medical terms, acronyms, and words of three or more syllables.
- If a medical term must be used, define it clearly and provide a glossary of terms.
- Consider linguistic capabilities and possible limitations of the target audience.
- Use large print for those with visual problems.
- Keep the tone reader-friendly.
- Address patients' needs and questions in terms that reassure rather than frighten.
- Use positive phrases such as "Avoid smoking" instead of "Do not smoke."
- Use a clear, concise, and friendly format if patients are anxious or nervous.

Motivational Principles

- Focus on what audience should know or do.
- Use the active voice.
- Use questions as headings.

Linguistic Principles

- Use one and two-syllable words.
- Use words that are easily understood by the target audience.
- Avoid multiple clauses and double negatives.
- Define unfamiliar terms.
- Use contractions.

Plain Language

Plain language is a strategy for making written and oral information easier to understand. Keep information conversational. For example:

- Original sentence: "It is now well established that the substance currently under investigation is effective for the duration of a minimum of 4 hours."
- Revised to: "The tablet being tested works for at least 4 hours."

Strategies for Developing Culturally Appropriate Materials

- Be familiar with beliefs and values if addressing a specific group of patients.
- If language barriers exist, provide information in patients' native language.
- Include the audience's beliefs and values.
- Collaborate with community organizations.
- Choose words that show respect.
- Use graphics, pictures, and examples.
- Field-test materials and involve the target audience in development.

Tone

- Be reader-friendly.
- Address patients' needs.
- Capture and hold readers' attention.
- Be realistic but reassuring.
- Tell the truth.
- Avoid negatives.

Formatting Educational Materials

- Write simple, catchy titles.
- Keep the page layout simple.
- Use an unjustified right-hand margin.
- Use Times New Roman font for easier reading.
- Use bulleted lists; number bullets and lists if there is an order.
- Title each list or table.
- Use black ink on light-colored paper that is heavy, dull-coated, and matte.
- Make liberal use of white space to help rest the eyes.
- Present some material in tables, diagrams, drawings, and photographs.

Readability Statistics

- Assesses the reading difficulty of printed material.
- Reading statistics formulas should not be the sole basis for evaluating reading materials; context and other factors must also be considered.
- Most common instruments are the following:
  - Flesch-Kincaid grade level scale
  - Fry graph
  - FOG scale (Gunning FOG formula)
  - Simple Measure of Gobbledygook (SMOG) index
    - Readability assessment tools are available at http://www.readabilityformulas.com/free-readability-formula-tests.php

Tools for Assessing Health Literacy

- Reading Recognition Tests
- Suitability Assessment of Materials (SAM)
- Wide Range Achievement Test (WRAT)
- Slosson Oral Reading Test
- Rapid Estimate of Adult Literacy in Medicine (REALM)

- Medical Achievement Reading Test
- Peabody Individual Achievement Test
- Test of Functional Health Literacy in Adults (TOFHLA)

Using Technology in Patient Education

- The World Wide Web
  - More than 50% of Americans use it to obtain health information
  - Viewers can watch videos of procedures, ask questions, or receive information
  - Online health seekers use the Web to
    - Search for health information
    - Research a diagnosis or prescription
    - Prepare for surgery or how to best recover
    - Get online tips from other patients and caregivers about symptom management
    - Keep caregivers and friends informed of a loved one's condition
  - Nurses play an important role in teaching patients how to evaluate information (see table below)

How to Evaluate Health Information on the Internet

Question	Criteria
Who	
Who sponsors the site? Who funds the site?	• Should be easily found on every major page of the site. • Does it sell advertising or is it sponsored by a pharmaceutical company? (".org" and ".gov" sites are unbiased and reliable; ".com" sites are businesses that may promote their sales) • Is there an editorial board? (if so, may be more reliable)
Who chooses and reviews the information?	• Do the reviewers have professional or scientific qualifications? (will increase reliability)
What	
What is the purpose of the site? What information is provided or claimed?	• Look at the "About This Site" link
Is it unbiased?	• Is it too good to be true? • Are sources or references listed? • Can the information be verified on another site? • What amount of information is given? • What personal information does the site collect, and why? • Are topics covered completely, or are links given for more information?
Where	
Where was the site developed?	• Government agencies ".gov" • Colleges and universities ".edu" • Institutions and organizations ".org" or ".net" • Commercial sites ".com"
When	
When was the site published, reviewed, and updated?	• Medical information must be current • Even if the information has not changed, date of review should be noted on site
How	
How does the site look?	• Is it easy to use? • Is the spelling and grammar correct? • Do the links work?
How does the site interact with visitors?	• Can you contact someone with questions or feedback?

- Social Media
  - Communication format for people with similar interests to share information
  - Five core sites for benchmarking and research:
    - Facebook, Instagram, Pinterest, LinkedIn, and Twitter
  - Used to educate, empower, send messages, and gather information on public perceptions about health
  - Potential risks: may market/show unhealthy behaviors such as smoking, breech in confidentiality/protection of personal health information
- Webcasts and Webinars
  - Mechanisms to deliver presentations with audio and/or video
  - Webcasts allow for participant interaction
  - Useful when trying to reach learners in broad geographic locations
  - Risk: can be frustrating for learner and instructor if not able to communicate
- E-Mail
  - Inexpensive and quick way to communicate with patients
  - Allows patients time to gather thoughts and retain written information from clinician's response
  - Risk: need to ensure privacy for patient's computer and health care organization (Health Insurance Portability and Accountability Act [HIPAA])
- Online chats
  - Online conversation in real time
  - Useful for ongoing education or information exchange
  - Benefits patients who are homebound or isolated
  - Risk: fast pace; may be difficult to keep up with conversation, potential for inaccurate information shared among nonprofessionals
- Telehealth
  - Delivering education content via telehealth technology (videoconferencing)
  - Virtual platforms can be cellular or Internet based
  - Ability for patients to learn from home environment
  - Others can join educational session including family located across the county
  - Avoids additional trip to health care facility for education
  - Requires computer or smart phone and experience with technology
- Patient Portal
  - Secure web-based servers that provide patient access, communicate with their health care team, and share education
  - Promotes the interoperability of information, creating the ability to view, transmit, and download information online
  - Access to patient education materials
  - Increase transparency to health information
- Patient Decision Aids
- Tools created for patients to share in decision making about health care options
  - Examples include leaflets, videos, DVDs, websites
- Provides information on options including the potential pros and cons

- Reduces feeling uninformed
- Assists patients with clarifying and communicating their own values about the different options available
- Do not advise patients to choose one option over another
- Does not replace health care providers' consultation
- Helps patients to make informed, values-based decisions with their health care provider

Professional Resources: Patient Education

- Association of Community Cancer Centers (ACCC) online health literacy gap assessment tool: accc-cancer.org/health-literacy.
- Agency for Healthcare Research and Quality (AHRQ)—Health Literacy: https://www.ahrq.gov/health-literacy/index.html.
- AHRQ—Health Literacy Universal Precautions Toolkit: http://www.ahrq.gov/professionals/quality-patient-safety/quality-resources/tools/literacy-toolkit/.
- The Cancer Patient Education Network: http://www.cancerpatienteducation.org/.
- Centers for Disease Control and Prevention—Health Literacy: https://www.cdc.gov/healthliteracy/index.html.
- Centers for Disease Control and Prevention—tips for creating easy-to-read print materials your audience will want to read and use: http://www.cdc.gov/healthliteracy/pdf/Simply_Put.pdf.
- Health Literacy Online: A Guide for Simplifying the User Experience—from the Office of Disease Prevention and Health Promotion, guides administrators, providers, and educators in presenting information to low literacy individuals using the web: https://health.gov/healthliteracyonline/.
- Health Literacy Studies—this site is designed for professionals in health and education who are interested in health literacy: http://www.hsph.harvard.edu/healthliteracy/.
- Institute for Healthcare Advancement: Health Literacy Solutions Center—Health Care Education Association: https://www.hcea-info.org/.
- The Joint Commission "Speak Up" initiatives: http://www.jointcommission.org/speakup.aspx.
- MedinePlus: https://medlineplus.gov/healthliteracy.html.
- National Institutes of Health Clear Communication—defines health literacy, states health literacy objectives in, and links to more information: http://www.nih.gov/clearcommunication/healthliteracy.htm.
- National Academies of Sciences Engineering Medicine—Roundtable on Health Literacy: https://www.nationalacademies.org/our-work/roundtable-on-health-literacy.
- PLAIN—a community of federal employees from many different agencies and specialties: PlainLanguage.gov.
- Project to Review and Improve Study Materials (PRISM) at the Group Health Center for Health Studies—a resource that shows research teams how to create consent forms and other patient materials in plain language: https://www.grouphealthresearch.org/about-us/capabilities/research-communications/prism/.

Patient Resources: Cancer Patient Education

- American Cancer Society: http://www.cancer.org.
- Cancer Care: http://www.cancercare.org.
- Cancer.com: https://www.cancer.com.
- Cancer Support Community: https://www.cancersupportcommunity.org/.
- Cancer.Net: http://www.cancer.net.
- Livestrong: https://www.livestrong.org/.
- Medical Library Association—Recommended Websites for Cancer Information: https://www.mlanet.org/page/recommended-websites-for-cancer-information.
- National Cancer Institute: http://www.cancer.gov.
- National Comprehensive Cancer Network (NCCN): https://www.nccn.org/patientresources/patient-resources/guidelines-for-patients.
- National Library of Medicine's Medline Plus: https://medlineplus.gov/cancers.html.
- Oncolink: http://www.oncolink.org.

Bibliography

Bastable, S. B. (2019). *Nurse as educator: Principles of teaching and learning for nursing practice* (5th ed.). Burlington, MA: Jones & Barlett.
Blevins, S. (2018). The art of patient education. *Medsurg Nursing, 27*(6), 401.
Bremer, D., Klockmann, I., Jaß, L., Härter, M., von dem Knesebeck, O., & Lüdecke, D. (2021). Which criteria characterize a health literate health care organization?—A scoping review on organizational health literacy. *BMC Health Services Research, 21*(1), 664.
Cartwright, L. A., Dumenci, L., Cassel, J. B., Thomson, M. D., & Matsuyama, R. K. (2017). Health literacy is an independent predictor of cancer patients' hospitalizations. *Health Literacy Research and Practice, 1*(4), e153–e162.
Centers for Disease Control and Prevention (CDC). Office of the Associate Director for Communication. (2019). *Clear communication index: A tool for developing and assessing CDC public communication products user guide.* Available at https://www.cdc.gov/ccindex/pdf/ClearCommUserGuide.pdf.
Cutilli, C. C. (2020). Excellence in patient education: Evidence-based education that "sticks" and improves patient outcomes. *Nursing Clinics, 55*(2), 267–282.
Doak, C. C., Doak, L. G., & Root, J. H. (1996). The literacy problem. In C. C. Doak, L. G. Doak, & J. H. Root (Eds.), *Teaching patients with low literacy skills* (2nd ed.). Philadelphia: J.B. Lippincott.
Dunn, P. (2017). Enhancing informal patient education in nursing practice: A review of the literature. *Journal of Nursing Education and Practice, 7*(2), 18–24.
Finkelman, A., & Kenner, C. (2009). *Teaching IOM: Implications of the Institute of Medicine reports for nursing education* (2nd ed.). Silver Spring, MD: American Nurses Association.
Fleary, S. A., Paasche-Orlow, M. K., Joseph, P., & Freund, K. M. (2019). The relationship between health literacy, cancer prevention beliefs, and cancer prevention behaviors. *Journal of Cancer Education, 34*(5), 958–965.
Nass, S., Alper, J., Balogh, E., et al. (Eds.). (2020). National Academies of Sciences, Engineering, and Medicine; Health and Medicine Division; Board on Health Care Services; Roundtable on Health Literacy; National Cancer Policy Forum. In *Health literacy and communication strategies in oncology: Proceedings of a workshop.* Washington, DC: National Academies Press (US).
National Academies of Sciences, Engineering, and Medicine, Health and Medicine Division, Board on Population Health and Public Health Practice, & Roundtable on Health Literacy. (2018). *A proposed framework for integration of quality performance measures for health literacy, cultural competence, and language access services: Proceedings of a workshop.* Washington, DC: National Academies Press (US).
Papadakos, J. K., Hasan, S. M., Barnsley, J., Berta, W., Fazelzad, R., Papadakos, C. J., … Howell, D. (2018). Health literacy and cancer self-management behaviors: A scoping review. *Cancer, 124*(21), 4202–4210.
Rodriguez, E. S. (2018). Using patient portals to increase engagement in patients with cancer. *Seminars in Oncology Nursing, 34*(2), 177–183.
Watson, J. (2018). Social media use in cancer care. *Seminars in Oncology Nursing, 34*(2), 126–131.
Yen, P. H., & Leasure, A. R. (2019). Use and effectiveness of the teach-back method in patient education and health outcomes. *Federal Practitioner: For the Health Care Professionals of the VA, DoD, and PHS, 36*(6), 284–289.

Note: Page numbers followed by f indicate figures, t indicate tables, and b indicate boxes.